Basic Science of PET Imaging

Magdy M. Khalil
Editor

Basic Science of PET Imaging

Springer

Editor
Magdy M. Khalil
Medical Biophysics
Department of Physics
Faculty of Science
Helwan University
Cairo
Egypt

ISBN 978-3-319-40068-6 ISBN 978-3-319-40070-9 (eBook)
DOI 10.1007/978-3-319-40070-9

Library of Congress Control Number: 2016957323

Printed on acid-free paper

This Springer imprint is published by Springer Nature
The registered company is Springer International Publishing AG Switzerland
The registered company address is Gewerbestrasse 11, 6330 Cham, Switzerland

أهدي هذ الكتاب إلي أمي
غفر الله لها و تغمدها بر حمته
I dedicate this book to my Mother.
God Bless her at all times.

Preface

This book *Basic Science of PET Imaging* was designed to be a daughter element of the parent book *Basic Sciences of Nuclear Medicine* (Springer, Khalil MM (Ed), 2011) with special focus on positron emission tomography (PET) imaging with its rather extended scientific disciplines and clinical applications. The rapid growth and advances in medical imaging in general and in PET imaging in particular have motivated and required a dedicated volume recording this historical moment in the lifetime of nuclear medicine and molecular imaging. I think the release of the book is timely as it captures a snapshot of one of the most important and dynamically changing fields of medicine.

PET imaging technologies and their clinical and biomedical applications have become an integral part and indispensable tool in daily practice of modern medicine. It was a very exciting mission to collect most if not all of scientific bases and underlying fundamental concepts about PET imaging in a single volume. This has been made with careful attention to describe the basic scientific principles, highlighting new advances and shedding light on recent developments in most of the covered topics. The power of PET imaging is currently not residing only in diagnostic workup of oncology, cardiology, and neurology and other diseases but also stem from its ability to work with other modalities in an integrated fashion in the new era of personalized or precision medicine.

In the last few decades, there were several exciting developments in most aspects of PET imaging technology that have made it an attractive, invaluable, and clinically rich imaging modality. I believe that the future of PET is bright with promising findings that will help our patients, the core of the work, get diagnosed in their early disease development and supporting physicians in taking the most accurate decision in treatment and management. The multidisciplinary collaboration that is taking place among physics, chemistry, biology, mathematics, engineering, and biomedical as well as medical professions in shaping nuclear medicine and molecular imaging has changed the way how new educational courses of molecular imaging and therapeutics would be designed and presented. I wish this textbook would be a good source for those educational programs.

Here I am presenting all chapters individually highlighting the most notable points and angles that characterize each chapter.

Chapter 1 has initiated the marathon of PET imaging by explaining some fundamental concepts and principles in radiation physics starting from the electromagnetic radiation and atomic models going through production of radiopharmaceuticals, radioactivity and modes of decay, interactions of radiation with matter, and positron-emitting radionuclides and finally describing some practically useful radiation detection and measurement devices.

Chapter 2 was written with special focus on radiation protection and safety parameters including shielding calculations and PET facility design, staff exposure, and optimization. X-ray computed tomography (CT) was the second important part of the chapter concentrating on technology developments, factors controlling dose in clinical examinations, as well as dose metrics such as CT dose index (CTDI) and its variants, dose length product, size-specific dose estimate, and effective dose. Other measures of CT dosimetry like diagnostic reference levels and optimization of CT image, attenuation correction, and whole body imaging were also described with some emphases placed on quality control of CT scanners.

Chapter 3 was dedicated to PET internal dosimetry with some details on radiation dose calculation scheme, biokinetic analysis and study design, animal data collection that includes tissue extraction and small animal imaging, small animal dosimetry, human imaging procedures, as well as dealing with kinetic analyses. Calculations of organ dose and standardized dose tables, patient-individualized dosimetry, and radiation dose concerns for pregnant/lactating mothers were also provided.

Chapter 4 covered labeling strategies used in the synthesis of PET radiopharmaceuticals. The authors discussed the commonly used positron-emitting radionuclides and electrophilic as well as nucleophilic substitution-based F18 labeling. Aliphatic and aromatic nucleophilic fluorination was also incorporated as well as F18 labeling of biomolecules. Labeling strategies of carbon-11 tracers were also mentioned with some details on methylation reactions, carbonylation reactions, and reactions with organometallic Grignard reagents. Other important labeling approaches for oxygen-15 and nitrogen-13 were mentioned. The emerging and the current G68-labeling methods were also outlined along with a discussion of the Ga3+ ions' physicochemical and labeling properties and associated chelation chemistry including conventional and new bifunctional chelators.

Chapter 5 was placed subsequent to Chap. 4 to describe the quality control procedures required for the release of PET radioactive drugs into the clinic. Most of the quality parameters including visual inspection, pH control, radiochemical and radionuclidic identity, half-life determination, radiochemical and radionuclidic purity, chemical purity, residual solvent determination, enantiomeric purity, sterility, and bacterial endotoxin test were explained. Analytical techniques of high-performance liquid chromatography (HPLC), thin layer chromatography (TLC), gas chromatography, and gamma spectrometry were described. Validation of analytical procedures and characteristics required, namely, specificity, precision, accuracy, linearity and range, detection limit, quantitation limit, and robustness, was discussed. Quality control of C11 tracers taking C11-methionine as an example as well as Ga68 radiopharmaceuticals taking ^{68}Ga-edotreotide as an example was also presented.

Chapters 6 and 7 were written to circumvent the regulatory aspects of PET tracer production in European countries and the United States, respectively. The former chapter has emphasized the development of pharmaceutical regulations and regulatory agencies as well as some attributes of a qualified person.

Regulatory framework and manufacturing authorization, clinical trials, magistral approach, and documentation were described. Drug development and approval steps were also explained along with data needed for submission and scientific writing. Good manufacturing practice (GMP) was presented with its required elements and components. Other topics such as new European clinical trial regulations, recognition of special status of radiopharmaceuticals, risk assessment approaches, and quality by design were also discussed.

Chapter 7 has made real focus on the framework of US regulations surrounding radiopharmaceutical production as well as the Food and Drug Administration (FDA) Modernization Act (the Modernization Act) of 1997. Discussion is extended to cover compounded and non-compounded PET drugs; current good manufacturing practice (cGMP); unique aspects of PET drug production; Part 210, 211, and 212 of 21 Code of Federal Regulations (CFR) and significant differences; quality assurance; quality control; personnel and resources; facilities and equipment; production and process controls; laboratory controls; finished drug product controls and acceptance criteria; packaging and labeling; distribution and complaint handling; and records. Other topics delineated were the *United States Pharmacopeia* (USP) < 823 > and revised USP < 823>, inspection of the PET drug production facility including types of FDA inspections, selection of inspection coverage, major issues identified in 2013/2014 PET drug inspections, and other related topics.

Chapter 8 provided details of PET instrumentation and physical principles underlying the detection theory of annihilation radiation, coincidence logic, and electronic collimation. Types of events, scintillation detectors, photosensors, detector design and geometry, data acquisition, and signal processing were described. System characteristics such as sensitivity, spatial resolution, energy resolution, coincidence timing resolution, count rate performance, multimodality PET/CT highlighting motivation, and review of fusion imaging of software and hardware approaches were also described. Attenuation correction, scatter correction, random correction, and issues related to PET/CT imaging protocols including low-dose and contrast injection were discussed. TOF technology was prominently outlined. Advances in PET imaging that include new photosensors, organ-specific imaging, and multimodality PET/MR were also briefly discussed.

Chapter 9 focused on PET/MR with some details of many technical and physical aspects of this relatively new hybrid imaging technology. Topics covered were system design of PET/MR scanners, technical challenges, as well as solutions implemented. PET imaging system and MR scanner hardware design and requirements were discussed. Different approaches devised for attenuation correction, data acquisition, imaging workflow, and motion correction were also explained, with the chapter closing with opportunities, challenges, and future directions of PET/MR imaging systems.

Chapter 10 has dealt with PET/CT scanner performance, acceptance testing, and quality control checks that should be performed for optimal operation. A comprehensive coverage of the topic and its various elements was made such as instrumental detection and data flow, detection and system calibration, acceptance testing considering NEMA performance parameters and other tests, and routine quality assurance that covers daily, monthly/quarterly, and annual tests in addition to the use of PET scanners in clinical trials.

Chapter 11 was designed to discuss image reconstruction algorithms used in PET imaging classifying them into analytical versus iterative-based reconstruction methods. Advantage of iterative reconstruction was discussed along with requirements posed to yield significant improvements in image quality and quantitative accuracy. This has been discussed together with analysis of image properties and PET data corrections, such as normalization, attenuation, and scatter correction. Recent updates were also highlighted covering time-of-flight image reconstruction as well as parametric image reconstruction.

Chapter 12 has special focus on image processing tools and new measures introduced to support risk stratification, treatment response assessment, and prognosis. Morphological versus conventional image features of PET data were discussed together with static and dynamic data set. Extension to PET/CT and PET/MR was also made to utilize the unique features provided by combining morphological and molecular-based scanning procedures. Application of PET in radiotherapy treatment planning was also pointed out in the chapter with emphases on using PET in tumor delineation or biological target definition. PET image characteristics such as robustness and stability of extracted image features and improved PET-based outcome models as well as an outlook at improved PET-based outcome models were explained.

Chapter 13 discussed quantitative PET imaging highlighting the differences between static and dynamic data acquisition, describing the different types of information that can be extracted from each approach. Standardized uptake value (SUV) and its pros and cons, SUV variants, total disease burden, factors affecting quantitative results, response to treatment and evaluation criteria, and finally tumor texture analysis were covered.

Chapter 14 covered kinetic modeling and tracer kinetic analysis. The chapter outlined important definitions, assumptions, and solutions of 1-tissue compartment model (1TC), 2TC model, and 3TC model, general solution, as well as parameter estimation of PET data. Linearization of the kinetic model and use of graphical techniques such as Logan plot and Patlak plot were described, in addition to a discussion on spectral derivation and analysis. Physiological and biological basis of compartmental model was integrated within the chapter contents to provide more insight on underlying concepts behind derivation of quantitative parameters. Arterial input function and time activity curve, continuous infusion, and reference region model were also described and demonstrated.

Chapter 15 talked about partial volume effect and correction techniques with some details of historical background and varieties of methods/algorithms used in research and practice. Topics covered were point spread function, tissue fraction effect, deconvolution, motion, and partial volume. The correction techniques were also detailed including region-based, voxel-based, and combined methods. Practical consideration of partial volume correction was also described such as accuracy, resolution, co-registration, segmentation, and sampling. Alternative methods/approaches were outlined with clinical applications in cardiology, neurology, and oncology.

Chapter 16 covered motion artifact problems in PET/CT image acquisition. Illustrative description of artifacts caused by respiratory motion, mis-registration, and frequency of occurrence was explained. Average CT of less than 1 mSv to reduce mis-registration, benefits of average CT for radiation therapy, and 4D-PET as well as 4D-PET/CT data acquisition were demonstrated.

Chapter 17 stated the molecular basis and physiologic fundamentals of different PET tracers besides their utility in disease detection and patient diagnosis. F18-Fluorodeoxyglucose (F18-FDG) and tracers beyond were comprehensively described in many areas of cancer metabolism, angiogenesis, hypoxia, apoptosis, proliferation, growth factor receptors, somatostatin receptors, bone metabolism, chemokine receptor, as well as tracers used in multidrug resistance of cancer therapy.

Chapter 18 described the application of F18-FDG PET imaging in a number of oncologic disorders including lung, lymphoma, breast, malignant melanoma, head and neck, thyroid, esophageal, and colorectal cancers in addition to gynecological such as cervical and ovarian malignancies. Other topics of response monitoring, pitfalls, PET in clinical trials, and future outlook were also presented.

Chapter 19 dealt with cardiac PET imaging covering technical background and clinical applications. Major headings of the chapter were instrumentation, cardiac PET tracers, myocardial perfusion imaging, stress protocols, data interpretation, quantification of myocardial blood flow and flow reserve, ECG gating, and cardiac PET tracers. Moreover, the discussion is extended to highlight metabolic cardiac imaging including carbohydrate metabolism, fatty acid metabolism, oxidative metabolism, viability imaging, metabolic alteration studies, and quantification of metabolism, myocardial and vascular inflammation, and cell signaling. The latter has been classified into neurocrine, endocrine, paracrine, autocrine, juxtacrine, and matricrine pathways. The chapter is closed with discussions on cardiac PET in clinical trials and future directions.

Chapter 20 talked about PET in neurological and psychiatric disorders emphasizing technical advances and clinical applications. Many topics have been covered and included such as new aspects of long-standing diagnostic applications, role of F18-FDG in neurodegenerative disease, role of FDG in various conditions, contributions of FDG and other PET tracers to epilepsy characterization, important physiologic measures such as regional and global cerebral blood flow, oxygen extraction fraction, and tissue viability and amyloid imaging. The use of PET inclusion/progression parameter in clinical trials, drug development and dose finding by occupation/displacement, and biodistribution of new candidate compounds were also described. Additional points such as studying indirect neurochemical effects of acute pharmaceuticals and interventions onto radioligand targets, pressing diagnostic questions acceded by early investigatory tracers, pathophysiological studies of neurotransmission, targets of radioligands/radiosubstrates, ion channel-coupled receptors, enzymes, and enzyme transporters have been mentioned as well.

Chapter 21 was placed to discuss the role of PET/CT in pediatric malignancies. Technical and clinical considerations of PET imaging in pediatric population were discussed. Tumors of the sympathetic nervous system and lymphoma including Hodgkin and non-Hodgkin with evaluation of response, relapse, or recurrence were demonstrated. Other pediatric disorders such as leukemia, tumors of the brain and central nervous system, osseous and soft tissue malignancy, nephroblastoma, hepatoblastoma, and thyroid malignancy were also described and outlined.

Chapter 22 focused on the role of PET/CT in radiotherapy treatment planning with an introduction that sheds light on the importance of integrating PET data into the planning strategy. Applications of PET in treatment planning for a number of critical malignancies were also discussed such as lung, head and neck, esophageal, breast, lymphoma, myeloma, brain, gynecological, colorectal, and prostate malignancies. The last section of the chapter discusses the important role of imaging hypoxia in radiotherapy and treatment outcome.

PET imaging technologies have become ever-fast-moving disciplines, and every effort was made to produce this volume covering basic principles along with recent advances in most aspects. It was aimed to be easy to read, illustrative, and scientifically rich without compromising other necessary requirements of different readers who are coming from various backgrounds. I would therefore appreciate comments, remarks, or any observation that the reader may find necessary for corrections or useful points for future update.

In this respect, I am so grateful to all the authors for their time and efforts to contribute and place their broad area of expertise in their writing. I am again thankful to all of them as without their participation this volume would not have been possible. I hope this book would be a valuable reference for practitioners and newcomers in the field as well for those involved in different educational programs. Researchers are also important targets since new developments and advances have been incorporated in many areas throughout the book chapters.

Thank you.

Magdy M. Khalil
Giza, Egypt
10th Feb, 2016

Acknowledgments

Thanks go to my God, for without him nothing can come into existence. I am so grateful and indebted to my parents who always are the driving and motivating force to my success and progress. I wish them all the best herein and thereafter. Special thanks go to my wife and my children who sacrificed a lot of their time for the sake of completion of this book. I am grateful to Springer Publishing and the editorial team for their efforts in bringing this volume out to the reader. I am thankful to all colleagues, friends, mentors, and professors who are too many to mention over the years for their time, collaborations, and advices. I would like also to take this opportunity to acknowledge and send my thanks and appreciation to all authors who were really professional and eminent at all stages of writing this textbook. I give thanks again for their time, efforts, and high expertise that have been shown very clearly in their respective chapters. Last but not least, I would like to express my deepest gratitude to my colleagues in the Department of Physics, Faculty of Science, Helwan University, Cairo, Egypt, for their support and encouragement.

رَبِّ أَوْزِعْنِي أَنْ أَشْكُرَ نِعْمَتَكَ الَّتِي
أَنْعَمْتَ عَلَيَّ وَعَلَى وَالِدَيَّ وَأَنْ أَعْمَلَ
صَالِحًا تَرْضَاهُ وَأَدْخِلْنِي بِرَحْمَتِكَ فِي
عِبَادِكَ الصَّالِحِينَ

"My Lord!

Grant me the power and ability that I may be grateful for Your favors which You have bestowed on me and on my parents, and that I may do righteous good deeds that will please You, and admit me by Your mercy among Your righteous servants.

Contents

Part I Physics, Radiation Safety and Dosimetry of PET

1 **Basic Radiation Physics** 3
Taher Hosny, Eman Al-Anezi, and Magdy M. Khalil

2 **Radiation Safety and CT Dosimetry in PET/CT Imaging** 37
Debbie Peet and Sue Edyvean

3 **Radiation Dosimetry of PET Imaging** 65
Michael G. Stabin

Part II PET Chemistry and Regulation of PET Radiopharmaceuticals

4 **Chemistry of PET Radiopharmaceuticals: Labelling Strategies** 79
Stefano Boschi and Filippo Lodi

5 **Quality Control of PET Radiopharmaceuticals** 105
Filippo Lodi and Stefano Boschi

6 **Regulation of PET Radiopharmaceuticals Production in Europe** 127
James R. Ballinger and Jacek Koziorowski

7 **Regulatory Aspects of PET Radiopharmaceutical Production in the United States** 145
Joseph C. Hung

Part III PET Physics and Instrumentation

8 **PET Physics and Instrumentation** 173
Srilalan Krishnamoorthy, Jeffrey P. Schmall, and Suleman Surti

9 **PET/MR: Basics and New Developments** 199
Magdy M. Khalil

10 **PET Calibration, Acceptance Testing, and Quality Control** 229
Magnus Dahlbom

Part IV PET Image Reconstruction, Processing and Quantitation

11 PET Image Reconstruction: Methodology and Quantitative Accuracy 259
Bing Bai and Evren Asma

12 Image Processing and Analysis of PET and Hybrid PET Imaging 285
Issam El Naqa

13 Basics and Advances of Quantitative PET Imaging 303
Magdy M. Khalil

14 Compartmental Modeling in PET Kinetics 323
Hiroshi Watabe

Part V PET Imaging Artifacts and Correction Techniques

15 Partial Volume Correction in PET Imaging 355
Kjell Erlandsson

16 Motion Artifacts and Correction Techniques in PET/CT 379
Tinsu Pan

Part VI Scientific and Clinical Basis of PET Applications

17 Physiologic and Molecular Basis of PET in Cancer Imaging .. 399
Abhishek Mahajan and Gary Cook

18 Clinical Applications of PET/CT in Oncology 429
Abhishek Mahajan and Gary Cook

19 Cardiac PET Imaging: Principles and New Developments ... 451
Ran Klein and Robert A. deKemp

20 PET in Neurological and Psychiatric Disorders: Technologic Advances and Clinical Applications 485
Andreas Matusch and Tina Kroll

21 Role of PET/CT in Pediatric Malignancy 537
Joe Barfett, Reza Vali, and Amer Shammas

22 Role of PET/CT in Radiotherapy Treatment Planning 577
Maria Picchio, Elena Incerti, and Nadia Di Muzio

Index 609

Contributors

Eman Al-Anezi Nuclear Medicine and Cyclotron Department, King Hamad Univrsity Hospital, Busaiteen, Bahrain

Evren Asma, PhD Toshiba Medical Research Institute USA, Inc, Vernon Hills, IL, USA

Bing Bai, PhD Toshiba America Medical Systems, Inc, Tustin, CA, USA

James R. Ballinger, PhD Division of Imaging Sciences and Biomedical Engineering, King's College London, London, UK

Joe Barfett, MD Saint Michael Hospital, University of Toronto, Toronto, ON, Canada

Stefano Boschi, PhD Department of Nuclear Medicine, PET Radiopharmacy, S.Orsola-Malpighi University Hospital, Bologna, Italy

Gary Cook, MB BS, MSc, MD, FRCR, FRCP Division of Imaging Sciences and Biomedical Engineering, King's College London and Guy's & St. Thomas' PET Centre, St Thomas' Hospital, London, UK

Magnus Dahlbom, PhD, DABR Department of Molecular and Medical Pharmacology, David Geffen School of Medicine at UCLA, Nuclear Medicine Clinic, Los Angeles, CA, USA

Robert deKemp, PhD, PEng, PPhys National Cardiac PET Centre, Cardiac Imaging, The University of Ottawa Heart Institute, Ottawa, ON, Canada

N. Di Muzio, MD Department of Radiation Oncology, IRCCS San Raffaele Scientific Institute, Milan, Italy

Sue Edyvean, MSc Public Health England, Chilton, UK

Issam El Naqa, PhD, DABR Physics Division, Department of Radiation Oncology, University of Michigan, Ann Arbor, MI, USA

Kjell Erlandsson, PhD Institute of Nuclear Medicine, University College London, London, UK

Taher Hosny Nuclear Medicine and Cyclotron Department, King Hamad University Hospital, Busaiteen, Bahrain

Department of Biophysics, Faculty of Science, Cairo University, Cairo, Egypt

Joseph C. Hung, PhD., BCNP, FASHP, FAPhA Mayo Clinic, Rochester, NY, USA

E. Incerti, MSc Department of Nuclear Medicine, IRCCS San Raffaele Scientific Institute, Milan, Italy

Magdy M. Khalil, PhD Medical Biophysics, Department of Physics, Faculty of Science, Helwan University, Cairo, Egypt

Ran Klein, PhD Department of Nuclear Medicine, The Ottawa Hospital, Ottawa, ON, Canada

Jacek Koziorowski, PhD Department of Radiology and Department of Medical and Health Sciences, Linköping University, Linköping, Sweden

Srilalan Krishnamoorthy, PhD Department of Radiology, Perelman School of Medicine, University of Pennsylvania, Philadelphia, PA, USA

Tina Kroll, MD Institute of Neuroscience and Medicine (INM-2), Research Centre Juelich, Juelich, Germany

Filippo Lodi, PhD Nuclear Medicine Unit, PET Radiopharmacy, Azienda Ospedaliero Universitaria di Bologna, Policlinico St.Orsola-Malpighi, Bologna, Italy

Abhishek Mahajan, MBBS, MD Department of Radiodiagnosis, Tata Memorial Hospital, Mumbai, India

Andreas Matusch, MD Institute of Neuroscience and Medicine (INM-2), Research Centre Juelich, Juelich, Germany

Tinsu Pan, PhD Department of Imaging Physics, M.D. Anderson Cancer Center, The University of Texas, Houston, TX, USA

Debbie Peet, MSc University Hospitals of Leicester, Leicester, UK

M. Picchio, MD Department of Nuclear Medicine, IRCCS San Raffaele Scientific Institute, Milan, Italy

Jeffrey P. Schmall, PhD Department of Radiology, Perelman School of Medicine, University of Pennsylvania, Philadelphia, PA, USA

Amer Shammas, MD University of Toronto, The Hospital for Sick Children, University of Toronto, Toronto, ON, Canada

Division Head of Nuclear Medicine, Department of Diagnostic Imaging, The Hospital for Sick Children, Toronto, ON, Canada

Michael G. Stabin, PhD, CHP Department of Radiology and Radiological Sciences, Vanderbilt University, Nashville, TN, USA

Suleman Surti, PhD Department of Radiology, Perelman School of Medicine, University of Pennsylvania, Philadelphia, PA, USA

Reza Vali, MD Medical Imaging Department, Department of Diagnostic Imaging, University of Toronto, The Hospital for Sick Children, Toronto, ON, Canada

Hiroshi Watabe, PhD Division of Radiation Protection & Safety Control, Cyclotron and Radioisotope Center, Tohoku University, Sendai, Japan

Part I

Physics, Radiation Safety and Dosimetry of PET

1 Basic Radiation Physics

Taher Hosny, Eman Al-Anezi, and Magdy M. Khalil

Contents

1.1 **Introduction** 4

1.2 **Electromagnetic Radiation** 4
1.2.1 Wave/Particulate Nature of Radiation 5
1.2.2 Duality Principle 5

1.3 **Atomic Models** 6
1.3.1 History of Atomic Models 7
1.3.2 Bohr Model 8
1.3.3 Quantum Mechanics Model 8

1.4 **Structure of the Atom** 9
1.4.1 Mass and Energy 9
1.4.2 Atomic Mass Unit 9
1.4.3 Binding Energy and Mass Defect 10
1.4.4 Nuclear Stability 12

1.5 **Production of Radiopharmaceuticals** 13
1.5.1 Reactor Production Using Neutrons 13
1.5.2 Accelerator Production Using Charged Particles 14
1.5.3 Specific Activity 17
1.5.4 Saturation Yield 17

1.6 **Radioactivity** 18
1.6.1 Modes of Decay 18
1.6.2 Radioactive Decay Equations 22

1.7 **Interaction of Radiation with Matter** 23
1.7.1 Photoelectric Effect 23
1.7.2 Compton Effect 24
1.7.3 Pair Production 25
1.7.4 Linear and Mass Attenuation Coefficient 25

1.8 **Positron Emitter Radionuclides** 26
1.8.1 Exposure Rate Constant 27

1.9 **Radiation Detection and Measurements** 28
1.9.1 Gas-Filled Detector 28
1.9.2 Well Counter 30
1.9.3 Scintillation Detectors 31
1.9.4 Neutron Detectors 33
1.9.5 Solid State Detectors 34

References and Further Reading 35

T. Hosny
Nuclear Medicine and Cyclotron Department, King Hamad University Hospital, Busaiteen, Bahrain

Biophysics Department, Faculty of Science, Cairo University, Giza, Egypt
e-mail: Taher_Hosny@outlook.com

E. Al-Anezi
Nuclear Medicine and Cyclotron Department, King Hamad University Hospital, Busaiteen, Bahrain
e-mail: Eman-al-anzy@hotmail.com

M.M. Khalil, PhD (✉)
Medical Biophysics, Department of Physics, Faculty of Science, Helwan University, Cairo, Egypt
e-mail: Magdy_khalil@hotmail.com

Abstract

This chapter provides a comprehensive overview of essential radiation physics required to understand many fundamental concepts of nuclear medicine in general and positron emission tomography (PET) imaging in particular. We aimed to introduce the most important elements of radiation physics as tightly related to daily practice and routine activities performed in clinical environment. Topics covered in this chapter have discussed definition of electromagnetic radiation, atomic models, atomic structure, radio-

M.M. Khalil (ed.), *Basic Science of PET Imaging*, DOI 10.1007/978-3-319-40070-9_1

activity and radioactive modes of decay; production of radiopharmaceuticals including medical cyclotrons, saturation yield and reactor-produced radionuclides; and interaction of radiation with matter, linear and mass attenuation coefficients as well as mostly commonly used radiation detection and measurement devices. As this is the first chapter in the book, we made every effort to cover as many aspects that might come across the reader throughout or facilitate the understanding of other chapters.

1.1 Introduction

Radiation physics does broaden our understanding of many facts and theories that underlie clinical application of radioisotopes in medicine and other areas of biomedical research. More specifically, nuclear medicine practitioners are among those that must always keep an eye not only on fundamental radiation and nuclear physics but also on how this can be utilized and applied in practice. Many of the achievements in nuclear medicine were in large part related to those concepts with particular benefits to diagnostic imaging and radionuclide therapy. Therefore, it is an important course for those who attempt to learn the underlying bases such as the structure of the atom, electron as well as nuclear binding energy, radioactivity and its associated formulae, units and conversions in addition to production of radiopharmaceuticals, interaction of radiation with matter and other safety and radiation protection devices and measurements. Electromagnetic radiation and its associated wide spectrum, duality principle, structure of the atom, atomic models proposed over the years, mass defect and nuclear binding energy and other important issues are among the first topics that we will start with.

1.2 Electromagnetic Radiation

Electromagnetic radiation (EM) consists of self-sustaining oscillating electric and magnetic fields at right angles but in phase and perpendicular to each other and to the direction of propagation as shown in Fig. 1.1. It does not require a supporting medium and travels through empty space at the speed of light. EM radiation exhibits wave properties as well as particulate properties (duality principle). All different kinds of electromagnetic radiation (microwaves, radio waves, infrared, x-ray, gamma ray, etc.) differ in one important property which is its specific wavelength. When electromagnetic radiation is spread out according to its wavelength, the result is electromagnetic spectrum as explained in Fig. 1.2. The electromagnetic spectrum is divided into five major types of radiation. These include radio waves (including microwaves), light (including ultraviolet, visible and infrared), heat radiation and ionizing radiation such as x-rays and gamma rays.

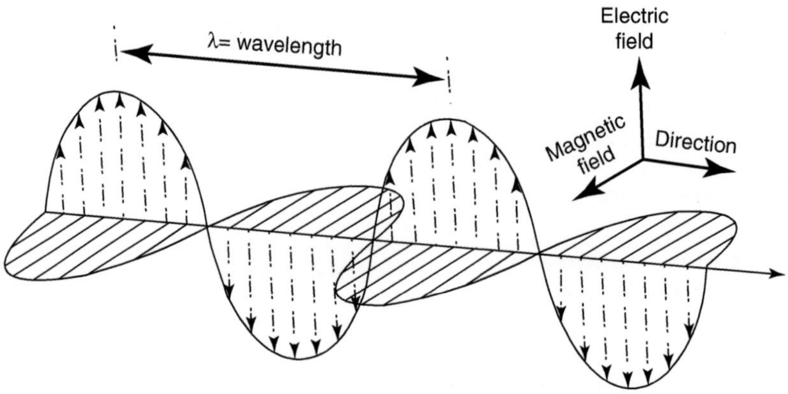

Fig. 1.1 Electric and magnetic field propagated as a transverse wave perpendicular to each other and perpendicular to the direction of propagation

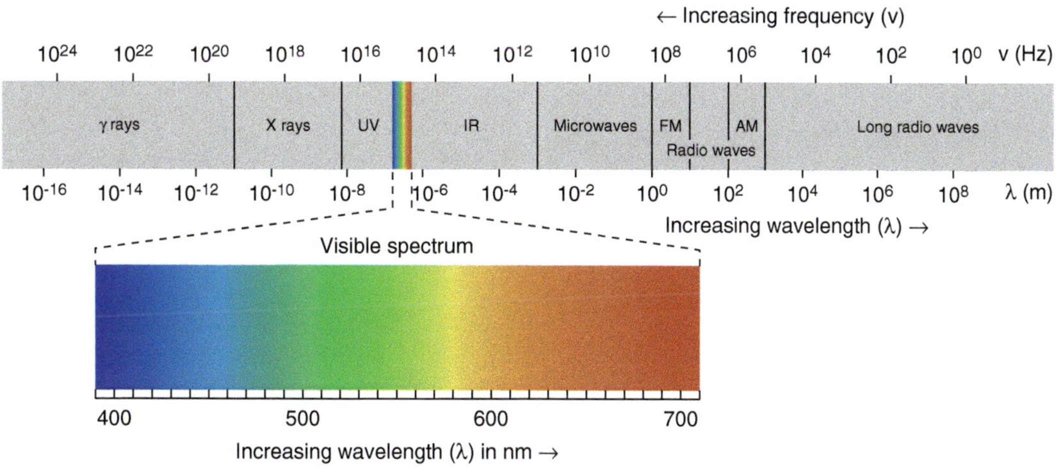

Fig. 1.2 Electromagnetic spectrum: Waves with shorter wavelength will have high frequency and vice versa. Ionizing radiation with high frequency is more energetic and can induce biological effects

1.2.1 Wave/Particulate Nature of Radiation

Although wave and particle having different physical characteristics, electromagnetic radiation can behave as both at once (wave-like and particle-like). Many experiments showed that radiation is sometimes behaves as wave and sometimes behaves as particle concluding that wave and particle cannot be separated, only together the phenomena can be explained. This has been proposed by a number of scientists leading to the theory of wave – particle duality.

1.2.2 Duality Principle

The duality principle describes the elementary particles and electromagnetic radiation in terms of wave and particle-like characteristics. It was not originated from a single scientist or revealed from only one experiment. Max Plank has stated that energy is transferred in a form of packets or quanta, while Albert Einstein thought of light as particle-like or localized in packets of discrete energy in contrast to its original definition as wave-like properties. Another contribution came from the phenomenon of photoelectric effect proposed also by Einstein. He stated that the emission of photoelectrons from metal plates does occur if and only if the incident photons on photoemissive plate have a threshold wavelength of energy that is able to liberate electrons from the metal. Then, Louis de Broglie proposed that electrons and other particles can behave as waves and has wavelength and frequencies. While this proposal was in 1927, the announcement of the understanding of the wave and particle aspects of matter was carried out in 1928. See Fig. 1.3.

Radiation can be described in terms of packet of energy, called photons. The energy of a photon is given by

$$E\ (\text{photon}) = h\nu = hc/\lambda \qquad (1.1)$$

where h is plank's constant ($h = 6.625\ 6 \times 10^{-34}$ J s); ν and λ are characteristics frequency and wavelength, respectively; and c is the speed of light in vacuum (Table 1.2).

Waves are characterized by frequency, wavelength and phase. Electromagnetic radiation is massless with no charge, while wavelength and frequency of oscillating fields are related to each other by the following equation:

$$c = \lambda \nu \qquad (1.2)$$

However, they are still affected by gravity.

It is of relevance to mention here that many diagnostic imaging modalities rely heavily on physical properties of different electromagnetic radiations. For example, in x-ray computed tomography (CT), a uniform x-ray beam interacts with

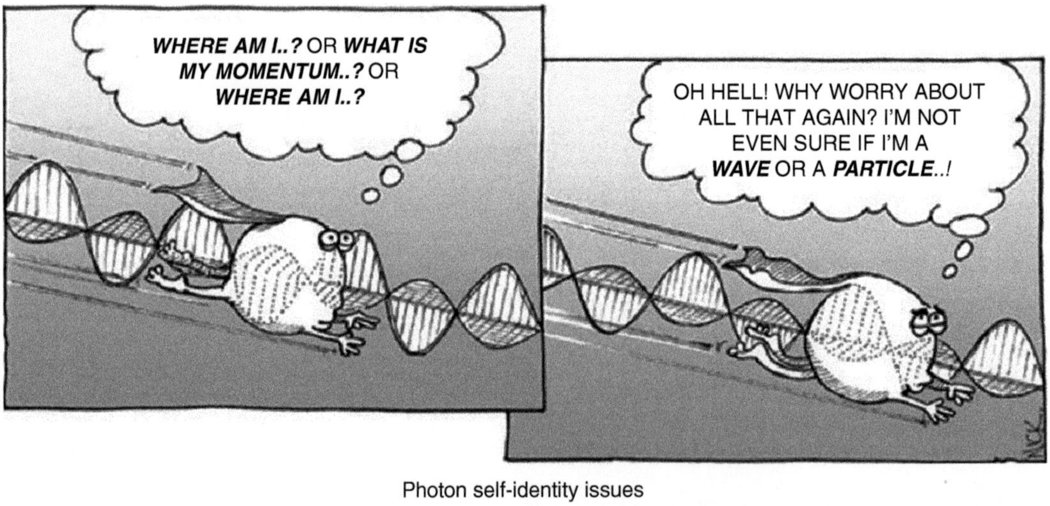

Fig. 1.3 Duality principle: Particles and electromagnetic radiation possess waves and particle characteristics (From http://www.lab-initio.com/quantum.html)

the human tissues, and the transmitted amount is measured by the CT detector to reveal an image that reflects the attenuation properties of the tissue covered in the scanning beam. Radiologic techniques such as fluoroscopy, angiography and x-ray radiography are also dependent on x-ray radiations in eliciting important diagnostic information for a wide range of human diseases and abnormalities.

Electromagnetic radiation is also associated with nuclear medicine in the sense that gamma emission is used in many diagnostic purposes utilizing the powerful penetrating capabilities of the radiation beam. This essentially takes place when patient is injected with pharmaceutical compound labelled to gamma-emitting radionuclide. After radiopharmaceutical administration, the body tissue will be the source of gamma ray emission that is used in the imaging process.

Another application of electromagnetic radiation in clinical practice is magnetic resonance (MR) imaging which is different from other imaging techniques such as CT and nuclear medicine, as it uses radio frequency (i.e. radio wave) as energy source rather than ionizing radiation. The procedure requires the usage of a strong magnetic field for spin alignment of hydrogen nuclei in the body. The spin synchronizes as the radio-frequency pulse matches the nuclear resonance frequency of the protons.

While radio wave energy is consistent with energy of nuclear spin in magnetic field, microwave matches rotational energy of the molecule. The infrared (IR) region in the spectrum lies beyond the region that the human eye perceives as red light. The absorption of infrared light causes increases in the frequencies at which the bonds between atoms stretch and bend. This is the idea behind infrared spectroscopy where there is a sort of matching between the IR radiation energy and the frequency of a specific molecular motion usually bond bending or stretching. However, the higher-frequency ultraviolet radiation that lies above the visible limit of the light spectrum is matching to different electronic transition states. In summary:

- Radio → nuclear spin in magnetic field
- Microwave → rotation
- Infrared → vibration
- Ultraviolet → electronic

1.3 Atomic Models

Atom is considered as the basic building unit of an element. An atom is the smallest unit of element that retains its physical and chemical properties. Each known element has atoms differ from the atoms of other elements; this gives each element a unique atomic structure. Many atomic models were proposed, and some have been adopted as ways to describe the atom. Neither of them is perfect, but they have relative contribu-

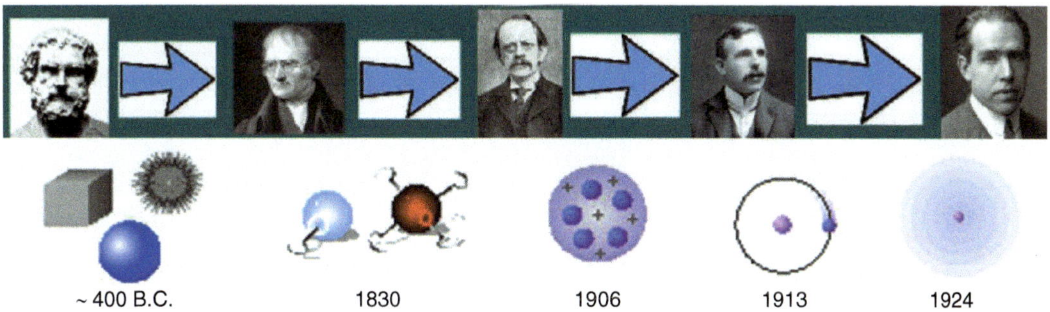

Fig. 1.4 Serial time line of atomic models proposed over the years and described by the following scientists (*left to right*): Democritus, Dalton, Thomson, Rutherford and Bohr. Taken from http://www.K12tlc.net/content/atomhist.htm

tions towards understanding these building blocks. See Figure 1.4 serial time line of atomic models.

1.3.1 History of Atomic Models

The first atomic model described in the literature is dated back to the Greek philosopher Democritus. He postulated the existence of invisible atoms, which are characterized only by quantitative properties such as size, shape and motion. His model described the atom as indivisible spheres representing the smallest piece of an element that still behave like the entire chunk of matter. There were no significant advances in definition and characterization of the atom until the English chemist John Dalton started to look at this in the 1800s. Dalton shared the same thoughts and impression as Democritus about atom in the sense that it is tiny and indivisible particles, but he introduced new assumptions about atom. The main assumptions of Dalton model were:

- All matter was composed of atoms, indivisible and indestructible. While all atoms of an element are identical and have the same properties, different elements have atoms of different size and mass.
- All compounds are composed of combinations of these atoms in defined ratios.
- Atoms can combine to form different compounds (e.g. carbon and oxygen combine to form carbon monoxide CO and carbon dioxide CO_2).
- Chemical reactions resulted in rearrangement of the reacting atoms.

In 1897, J.J. Thomson discovered the electron in series of experiments designed to study the nature of electric discharge in a high-vacuum cathode ray tube. In 1904, Thomson introduced a new atom model that differs from pervious atom models suggesting that the atom is uniform sphere of positively charged matter in which electrons are positioned by electrostatic forces.

A monumental breakthrough came in 1911 based on experimental results when Ernest Rutherford and his colleagues Hans Geiger and Ernest Marsden conducted the famous gold foil experiment intended to determine angles through which a beam of alpha particles (helium nuclei) would scatter after passing through a thin foil of gold. It was a new but exciting moment when they found few alpha particles recoiled almost directly backwards. It was Rutherford's interpretation that this happen when a positively charged and relatively heavy target particle, such as the proposed nucleus, could account for such strong repulsion. The negative electrons that balanced electrically the positive nuclear charge were regarded as travelling in circular orbits around the nucleus (Fig. 1.5) like planets that move around the stars, and therefore this model was called planetary model.

The planetary model was greatly inconsistent with Thomson's hypothesis in which the atom is a mixture of positive and negative particles that uniformly mixed throughout the atom. Based on the classical electromagnetic theory, however, the model failed to solve stability problem of the atom as the electrons lose energy and falling into the nucleus under the influence of attraction forces. The model proposed by Rutherford relied heavily on classical physics and was superseded in a few years by the Bohr atomic model, which

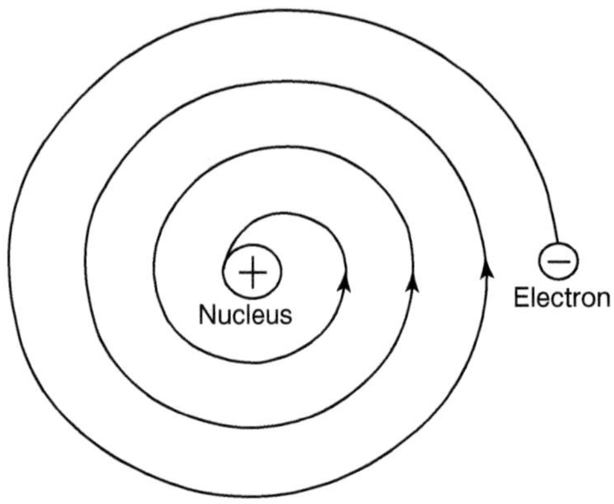

Fig. 1.5 Planetary model: In this model Rutherford proposed that electrons move in circular path around a central positive mass. This was contradicted by the fact that revolution makes electron lose energy while moving in spiral path and fall into the positively charged nucleus under influence of attraction force

incorporated some early quantum theory in combination with some classical concepts.

1.3.2 Bohr Model

In 1913, Bohr introduced a new model to explain atom stability. Bohr model of the atom was the first model that incorporated quantum theory and was the predecessor of wholly quantum-mechanical models. The model focused on electron description and based on spectroscopic observations. Bohr built up his model with the following postulates:

- The electron exists in certain energy levels (stationary states) with circular movement around the nucleus.
- Transition between these stationary states is accompanied with emission or absorption of electromagnetic radiation. The energy difference between these two energy levels is given by

$$\Delta E = \hbar v \tag{1.3}$$

  where ħ (i.e. *h* bar) or sometimes reduced plank's constant is commonly associated with angular momentum and given by

$$\hbar = h / 2\pi \tag{1.4}$$

- Quantization of orbit. The only allowed orbits (stationary states) are those for which the angular momentum L is

$$L = n\hbar$$

  where n is principal quantum number and takes values of 1,2,3,….., n and cannot be less than one.

Bohr's postulates were experimentally confirmed in experiments of Franck and Hertz (German scientists) in 1913 who studied the inelastic scattering of electrons of mercury atoms. This experiment showed that the energy levels of mercury atom were discrete. However, Bohr's model had no way of approaching non-periodic quantum-mechanical phenomena, like scattering. Furthermore, although Bohr' model served to predict energy levels, it was not able to explain transition rates between levels. Finally, the model was successful only for one-electron atoms like hydrogen and fails even for helium. To correct these drawbacks, one needs to apply a more completely quantum-mechanical treatment of atomic structure, and such an approach is used in Schrödinger theory.

1.3.3 Quantum Mechanics Model

The quantum mechanics model is derived from the quantum theory in which electron location and momentum are governed by the wave function. This hypothesis is denoted as uncertainty principle (Heisenberg principle) and states that the position and momentum of the electron can't be determined simultaneously with the same high precision. Stated another way, the more the precision in determining the electron location, the low the probability of determining the momentum and vice versa. The theory used the term orbitals to describe the location of the electrons, which are volumes in space used to define the probability distribution function. Four quantum numbers were introduced to define the electrons and their orbitals around the nucleus:

1. Principle quantum number (n): it is an integer number that indicates electron energy and orbital size, and it is the same number intro-

duced by Bohr. It takes values $n=0,1,2,\ldots\ldots$, while the maximum number of electrons in certain energy level is equal to $2n^2$.
2. Angular quantum number (l) describes the orbital shape of a particular principal quantum number. It divides energy shells or levels into subshells (sublevels). These sublevels represented by letters like *s*, *p*, *d* and *f*. Angular quantum number takes values $l=0,1,2\ldots,n-1$.
3. Magnetic quantum number, m_l ($m_l = -l,\ldots, 0,\ldots, +l$) specifies the orientation in space of an orbital of a given energy (n) and shape (l). This number divides the subshell into individual orbitals which hold the electrons; there are $2l+1$ orbitals in each subshell.
4. Spin quantum number, m_s ($m_s = +½$ or $-½$) defines the orientation of the spin axis of an electron. An electron can spin in only one of two directions.

1.4 Structure of the Atom

As mentioned earlier, an atom is the main building block of matter. The atomic mass is concentrated in the nucleus which considered the heaviest portion of the atom. The positively charged nucleus contains particles of nearly equal mass, protons and neutrons, electrically balanced with negatively charged electrons moving in certain orbitals around it. Any element can be represented as

$$ {}^{A}_{Z}X $$

where *A* atomic mass number is the sum of protons number *Z* and neutrons number *N*. The atomic number *Z* equals also the number of electrons in stable nuclei. It is not applicable to have two different elements having the same atomic number. The periodic table is arranged by order of increasing atomic number, which is always an integer. On the other hand, different forms of the same element can have different masses (i.e. have same atomic number) which are called isotopes, while those that have the same number of neutrons are called isotones. Isobars are nuclide with different numbers of protons and neutrons but with the same mass number. Examples of the three different nomenclatures are described in Table 1.1.

1.4.1 Mass and Energy

Mass and energy were considered two different quantities. Early 1900s, Einstein proved by his equation that neither mass nor energy was conserved separately. Thus, the mass can be converted to energy and vice versa while total mass- energy was conserved. In the following section the conversion of mass and energy will be demonstrated.

1.4.2 Atomic Mass Unit

The first atomic weight was initially proposed by *John Dalton* in 1803 as the mass of the hydrogen atom, H-1. Then it was suggested by *Wilhelm Ostwald* that it can best expressed in terms in units of 1/16 of the weight of the oxygen atom. Atomic mass can be measured by approximating the weight of a proton or neutron which indicates the masses of atom nucleons. The atom mass is expressed by a unified unit called the atomic mass unit denoted by the symbol *u*. In 1961, the international union of pure and applied chemistry had adopted and defined the modern applications of atomic mass unit and related it to the mass of carbon-12.

The definition of the atomic masses has been based on the unified mass scale considering one mole of carbon-12 which by conversion equals 12 g as the best reference nuclide. Determination of ^{12}C atom mass in grams using Avogadro's number divided on the total number of the individual atom nucleons indicates the masses of these nucleons which used to convert one atomic mass unit (1 u) to grams. Therefore, the atomic mass unit is one-twelfth ^{12}C atom in its electronic and nuclear ground state:

Table 1.1 Some examples of isotopes, isobars and isotones

Isotopes	Same *Z*	${}^{16}_{8}O$	${}^{17}_{8}O$	${}^{18}_{8}O$
		$Z=8$		
Isobars	Same *A*	${}^{18}_{9}F$		${}^{18}_{8}O$
		$A=18$		
Isotones	Same *N*	${}^{19}_{9}O$		${}^{18}_{8}O$
		$N=10$		

$$1\ \text{u} = \frac{1}{12} m\left({}^{12}_{6}\text{C}\right)$$

$$\text{Thus, mass of one atom of } {}^{12}\text{C} = \frac{12\text{g/mol}}{6.022\ 141\ 29 \times 10^{23}\ \text{atoms/mol}}$$
$$= 1.992\ 646\ 705 \times 10^{-23}\ \text{g/atom}$$

$$\text{The mass per nucleon} = \frac{1.992\ 646\ 705 \times 10^{-23}\ \text{g/atom}}{12}$$
$$= 1.660\ 538\ 921 \times 10^{-24}\ \text{g}$$

Then, 1 u = $1.660\ 538\ 921 \times 10^{-27}$ kg.

Now the mass of proton and neutron in terms of atomic mass unit can be determined by using its actual mass in grams:

$$\text{Proton mass}\left(m_{\text{p}}\right) = \frac{1.672\ 621\ 777 \times 10^{-27}}{1.660\ 538\ 921 \times 10^{-27}} = 1.007\ 276\ 467\ \text{u}$$

$$\text{Neutron mass}\left(m_{\text{n}}\right) = \frac{1.674\ 927\ 351 \times 10^{-27}}{1.660\ 538\ 921 \times 10^{-27}} = 1.008\ 664\ 916\ \text{u}$$

Conversion of the energy unit from the SI scale to the unified atomic mass unit is being done by using Einstein's mass-energy relationship ($E = mc^2$ where c is the speed of light in vacuum) taking into account that 1 eV = $1.602\ 176\ 565 \times 10^{-19}$ kg.m^2/s. Inserting this quantity of mass 1 u = $1.660\ 538\ 921 \times 10^{-27}$ into Einstein's equation and applying conversion factors, the nucleons mass equivalent energy can be determined.

$$E = mc^2 \tag{1.4}$$

$$= 1\ \text{u}\left(\frac{1.660\ 538\ 921 \times 10^{-27}\ \text{kg}}{\text{u}}\right) \times \left(299\ 792\ 458\ \text{m/s}\right)^2 \left(\frac{1\ \text{N}}{1\ \text{kg}.\frac{\text{m}}{\text{s}^2}}\right)\left(\frac{1\ \text{J}}{N.m}\right)$$

$$= 1.492\ 417\ 955 \times 10^{-10}\ \text{J}\left(\frac{1\ \text{MeV}}{1.602\ 176\ 565 \times 10^{-13}\ \text{J}}\right)$$

$$= 931.494\ 060\ 9\ \text{MeV}$$

Some of the constants and conversion factors used in the above derivations can be found in Table 1.2 which provides a number of useful physical quantities and constants used in converting mass into energy and vice versa.

1.4.3 Binding Energy and Mass Defect

For all nuclei, the mass of the nucleus that have been formed is always less than the total composed

Table 1.2 Summary of several physical quantities and constants in atomic and nuclear scale used in mass-energy conversion

Quantity	Symbol	Numerical value	Unit
Avogadro's number	N_A	6.022 141 29 × 10^{23}	mol^{-1}
Speed of light in vacuum	C	299 792 458	m/s
Electron volt	eV	1.602 176 565 × 10^{-19}	J
Atomic mass unit-kilogram relationship	1 u	1.660 538 921 × 10^{-27}	kg
Atomic mass unit-electron volt relationship	1 u (C^2)	931.494 061 × 10^6	eV
Atomic mass unit-joule relationship	1 u (C^2)	1.492 417 954 × 10^{-10}	J
electron Volt-atomic mass unit relationship	1 eV/C^2	1.073 544 150 × 10^{-9}	u
Electron mass Energy equivalent	m_e	9.109 382 91 × 10^{-31}	kg
	m_e	5.485 799 094 6 × 10^{-4}	u
	$m_e C^2$	8.187 105 06 × 10^{-14}	J
	$m_e C^2$	0.510 998 928	MeV
Proton mass Energy equivalent	m_p	1.672 621 777 × 10^{-27}	kg
	m_p	1.007 276 466 812	u
	$m_p C^2$	1.503 277 484 × 10^{-10}	J
	$m_p C^2$	938.272 046	MeV
Neutron mass Energy equivalent	m_n	1.674 927 351 × 10^{-27}	kg
	m_n	1.008 664 916 00	u
	$m_n C^2$	1.505 349 631 × 10^{-10}	J
	$m_n C^2$	939.565 379	MeV

Source: NIST (2010 CODATA recommended values)

masses of the contributing nucleons. This is due to conversion of that mass difference to the required energy for holding these nucleons together (i.e. the conversion of mass to binding energy). This mass difference is known as the mass defect and represents the binding energy which is defined as the amount of energy that need to be supplied to a nucleus to completely separate its constituent nucleons. The mass defect can be calculated by adding up the masses of the constituent particles and then subtracting the known mass of that atom:

$$\Delta m = \left[Z\left(m_{\text{proton}} + m_{\text{electron}}\right) + (A - Z)m_{\text{neutron}}\right] - m_{\text{atom}} \tag{1.5}$$

where:

Δm = mass defect (u)

m_{proton} = mass of a proton

m_{electron} = mass of electron

m_{neutron} = mass of neutron

m_{atom} = mass of the nuclide

Z is the atomic number and A is the mass number.

Since 1 u is equivalent to 931.5 MeV of energy as calculated in Sect. 1.4.2, the binding energy can be calculated by

$$\text{B.E.} = \Delta m\left(\frac{931.5\ \text{MeV}}{1\ \text{u}}\right)$$

Example

Calculate the mass defect of ^{235}U provided that the mass of the atom is 235.043 9 u?

Solution:

The atomic number of the ^{235}U is 92. The mass defect can be calculated by using Eq. 1.5.

$$\Delta m = \left[Z\left(m_{\text{proton}} + m_{\text{electron}}\right) + (A - Z)m_{\text{neutron}}\right] - m_{\text{atom}}$$

$$\Delta m = \left[92\left(1.007\ 28 + 5.485\ 79 \times 10^{-4}\right) + (235 - 92)1.008\ 66\right] - 235.043\ 9$$

$$= 1.914\ 71\text{u}$$

1.4.4 Nuclear Stability

Since Earth formation, there were about 275 stable nuclides found in nature, and more than 2000 nuclides are known to be unstable (i.e. radioactive). The constituents of the unstable nuclei are not arrayed in the lowest potential energy states; therefore, the nucleus undergoes spontaneous decay with time in such a way that this excess energy is emitted forming new nuclide. A study of the characteristics of the naturally stable nuclides provides clues of instability factors of the radioactive nuclides. An *N*/*Z* diagram of the 'line of stability' relates the naturally stable nuclides extending from $Z=1$ for hydrogen up to $Z=83$ for ^{209}Bi to those radioactive according to their neutron and proton numbers. Very long-lived nuclides are shown at the end of the line of stability although of their instability.

A major measure of nuclear stability is the neutron-proton ratio, as a result of the coulomb repulsion and exchange forces between them. Referring to Fig. 1.6 and closer look into light nuclei, the line of stability shows that neutron and proton numbers are equal ($N \approx Z$). For heavy nuclei, the coulomb repulsion between the protons is substantial, and extra neutrons are needed to supply additional binding energy to hold the nucleons together. Thus, the line of stability shows $N \approx 1.5\ Z$, that is heavy stable nuclides have nearly 50 % more neutrons than protons. From $Z > 83$ all heavier nuclides are unstable. Radioactive nuclides surround the line of stability; nuclides lying above the line are said to be

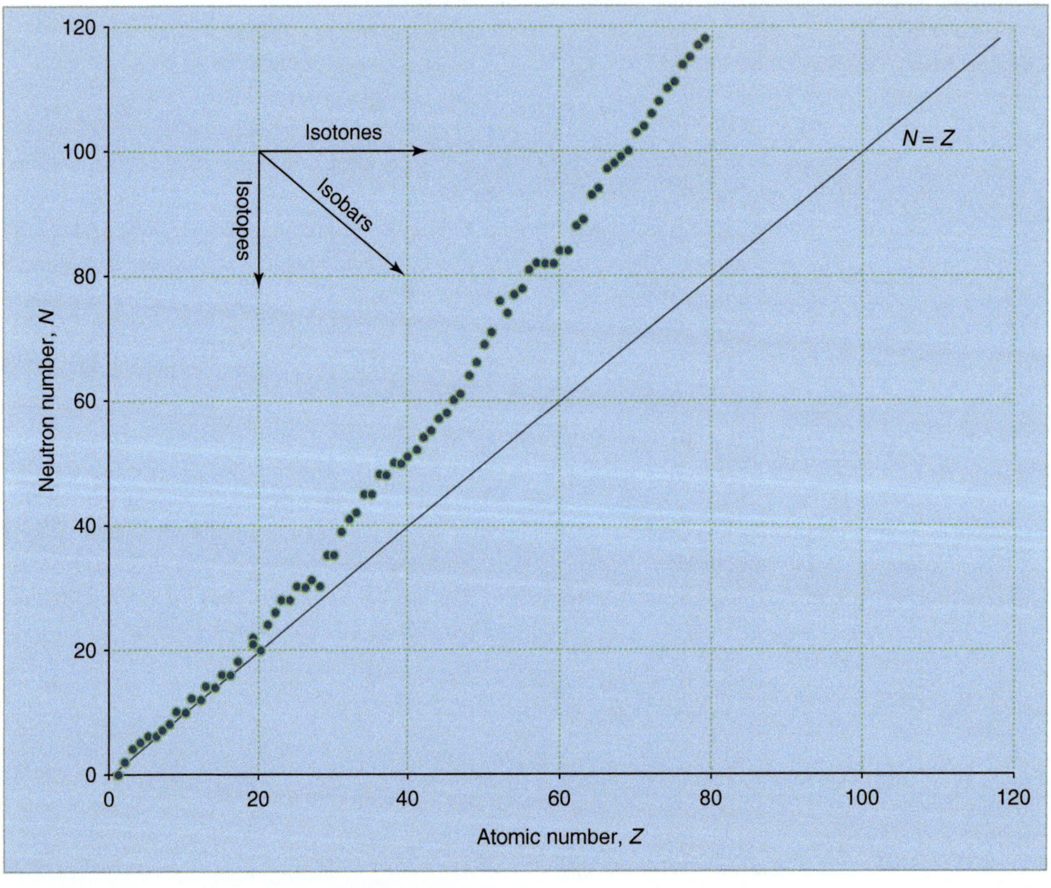

Fig. 1.6 Neutron number (*N*) versus atomic number (*Z*) for nuclides found in nature. The deviation of the stable nuclei from the line of identity (i.e. $Z=N$) is obvious and has been attributed to an increase in neutron number to moderate proton repulsion

'proton deficient', whereas nuclides lying below the line are 'neutron deficient'. Radioactive nuclei attempt to reach the stability by different modes of radioactive decay which is going to be discussed later. In the *N/Z* diagram (Fig. 1.6), the excess-neutron number is seen as the vertical distance between the stable nuclides and the diagonal $N=Z$ line. From the frequency distribution of stable isobars, isotopes and isotones, it has been concluded that even numbers of identical nucleons are more stable than odd numbers of the same nucleons (oddness of both *Z* and *N* tends to lower the nuclear binding energy).

1.5 Production of Radiopharmaceuticals

Nuclear medicine is a unique medical specialty that uses radiopharmaceuticals for diagnostic or therapeutic purposes. The diagnostic role is to interrogate valuable functional information about disease biochemistry not only on the cellular or subcellular level but also extend to extract molecular and genetic information. The other good facet of nuclear medicine is its ability to target but treat critical diseases using therapeutic radionuclides. Diagnostic radiopharmaceutical is a radioactive drug that is administered in a tracer quantity with no pharmacological effect on human body. Radiopharmaceuticals can be broadly classified into two different categories, single photon emitters that are commonly used in conventional gamma camera imaging examinations and positron emitter-based radiopharmaceuticals. The former class of compounds are commonly labelled with ^{99m}Tc solution eluted from molybdenum-99 generators. Radionuclides such as ^{201}Tl, ^{67}Ga, ^{111}In-, ^{123}I and ^{131}I belong also to the same class and have several diagnostic or therapeutic applications.

The other class of radiopharmaceuticals are based on labelling with positron emitters (such as ^{18}F, ^{11}C, ^{13}N, ^{15}O, etc.) and used in PET imaging applications such as oncology, cardiology and neurology. These kinds of radiotracers require medical cyclotrons and other essential infrastructures that include radiochemistry production facility, analytical and quality control equipments and other radiation detection and measurements devices. More details about medical cyclotron will be discussed later.

Since naturally occurring radioisotopes are relatively long half-lived and not handled well with human body, an artificially produced radioisotope which is cyclotron or reactor produced is being used. However, on-site radionuclide production is often required for positron emitter radionuclides with short half-lives such as ^{15}O (2.04 min), ^{13}N (10 min) and ^{11}C (20.38 min) which requires a local production to avoid loss of the material due to continuous decay. Since the radioisotopes need to be incorporated into some form of pharmaceutical, it should also be capable of being produced in a form which is amenable to chemical, pharmaceutical and sterile processing.

In March 2000, the fluorine-18-labelled glucose or F-18 fluoro-2-deoxyglucose (F-18 FDG) received Food and Drug Administration FDA approval for usage to evaluate and diagnose oncology patients although the first production was in 1978 for neurological applications. It is worth mentioning that first applications of FDG were focused on neurology and cardiac imaging, but its importance in oncology was realized on a later stage. F18-FDG limitations such as low specific targeting in PET imaging were an incentive for development of new PET tracers with special targeting capabilities. Newly developed PET traces are more specific and allow for imaging biological processes, such as angiogenesis, hypoxia, proliferation, apoptosis and many others. The expression of different receptors can be visualized like the somatization receptor 2, gene expression and dopamine and serotonin receptors in addition to large spectrum of potential cellular and molecular targets. Some of these approaches have found their way forward to the clinic, while others are still under extensive research and clinical evaluation.

1.5.1 Reactor Production Using Neutrons

Artificially produced radionuclide takes place in nuclear reactor by means of fission reaction or by using neutron flux to activate special target

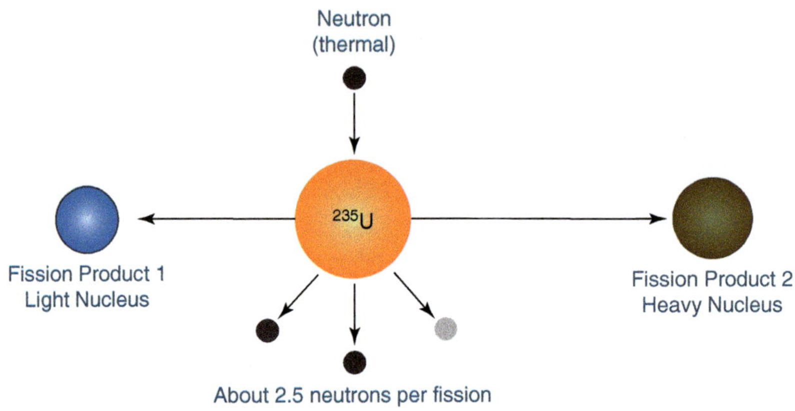

Fig. 1.7 Spontaneous fission reaction; ^{235}U splits into two fission nuclei accompanied with neutrons release which in turn induce another fission reaction (chain reaction initiation)

material located in reactor core. Naturally occurring radioactive material especially heavy nuclei (^{235}U) undergoes spontaneous fission reaction; see Fig. 1.7. The result of such a reaction is two lighter fission fragments and few fission neutrons in addition to large amount of energy released. The fission neutrons will in turn initiate further fission reaction or what is called chain reaction. As the reactor uses the newly generated neutrons to keep fission reaction going on, on average one fission neutrons induce one more fission, so the process is self-sustaining chain reaction.

Since N/Z ratio is high for fission fragments, it will undergo β^- decay until either stable nuclei are reached or relatively long half-life nuclide is reached and extracted from the reaction. The most important isotope produced in this way is ^{99}Mo which decays into ^{99m}Tc through β^-decay with half-life 2.75 days. The daughter nuclide (^{99m}Tc) has very important clinical value in nuclear medicine and in wide variety of diagnostic examinations. The production of ^{99}Mo by a fission reaction is represented as $^{235}U\ (n, f)\ ^{99}Mo$.

In this reaction, uranium/aluminium alloy (containing uranium enriched to 45 % ^{235}U) is used as target material. The typical yield of ^{99}Mo is in the order of (4–10 Ci) per g of ^{235}U irradiated for 50–200 h in a neutron flux of 1.5×10^{14} n cm^2 s^{-1}.

Molybdenum-99 production can also take place through neutron activation in which target material (MoO_3) is irradiated by neutron flux (n, γ) reaction for 1 week.

$$^{98}\mathrm{Mo}(n,\ \gamma)^{99}\ \mathrm{Mo}$$
$$^{98}_{42}\mathrm{Mo} + {}^{1}_{0}n \rightarrow {}^{99}_{42}\mathrm{Mo} + \gamma$$

In this method of production, yield depends on neutron flux, neutron energy, target material and reaction activation cross section. Radionuclides production by (n, γ) reaction having poor specific activity as the produced nuclide and target material are isotopes and cannot be chemically separated. Other radionuclides used for diagnostic and therapeutic application in nuclear medicine such as^{131}I, ^{153}Sm, ^{90}Y, ^{89}Sr, etc., are reactor produced.

1.5.2 Accelerator Production Using Charged Particles

Charged particle (protons, deuterons and alpha particles) accelerated by means of particle accelerator should possess sufficient kinetic energy to penetrate coulomb repulsion forces surrounding the nucleus. In this kind of radionuclide production, electrically charged particles are being accelerated to very high energy in range of MeV and then extracted towards target material initiating nuclear reaction for certain period of time in order to obtain sufficient amount of radionuclide. Radionuclide production takes place in charged particle accelerator by different nuclear reactions. The (p, n) reaction is one of the most reactions used for this purpose where irradiated atoms gain one proton accompanied by emission of neutron. The most common example is the production of F-18 from heavy water as shown here:

$$^{18}_{8}\text{O}(p,n)^{18}_{9}\text{F}$$

Another common nuclear reaction used is (*d*, *n*) in which the target nucleus will catch the accelerated particle (deuteron), subsequently the produced radionuclide atomic number and mass number each increases by one. The (*d*, *n*) reaction is given by:

$$^{A}_{Z}X(d,n)^{A+1}_{Z+1}X$$

An example of a radionuclide that is produced by deuteron irradiation is oxygen-15, and this reaction is written as

$$^{14}\text{N}(d,n)^{15}\text{O}$$

There are many different types of particle accelerator including the Van de Graaff accelerator, cyclotron, synchrocyclotron, synchrotron and linear accelerator although they are different types, but the main concept is still the same. Charged particles are accelerated in the presence of electric or magnetic field or both to reach the desired energy for extraction towards its target. Charged particle accelerators can produce radionuclides with high specific activity than reactor did.

1.5.2.1 Medical Cyclotrons

The first medical applications of cyclotron start at the University of California, Berkeley, when Lawrence and his brother John quickly demonstrated the clinical importance of cyclotron-produced radioisotopes in disease research. In 1936, they started to produce radioactive phosphorus for leukaemia and polycythaemia treatment. These were the first therapeutic applications of artificially produced radioisotopes on human patients.

By 1938, the Berkeley 27 in. (later upgraded to 37 in.) cyclotron had produced ^{14}C, ^{24}Na, ^{32}P, ^{59}Fe and ^{131}I radioisotopes, among many others that were used for medical research. Nowadays medical cyclotrons widely use medium energy 10–20 MeV for routine production of positron emitters (^{18}F, ^{11}C, ^{13}N, ^{15}O,...) for synthesis of radiopharmaceuticals used in diagnostic purposes. Other commercially available medical cyclotrons (Fig. 1.8a) are in energy range 18–24 MeV for traditional positron emitters production as well as for single photon emitters production (^{123}I, ^{111}In, ^{67}Ga, ^{57}Co, ^{99m}Tc) as diagnostic biomarkers and other applications in SPECT imaging.

Cyclotron first designed to accelerate the positive ions H^+ and $^2H^+$, but after that cyclotron design changed to accelerate negative ions hydrogen or deuteron. Positive ion cyclotron acceleration does not need as much vacuum as negative ion cyclotron acceleration, but it results in cyclotron metal part activation, and it has complicated extraction beam system which became more simple in negative ion cyclotrons giving the flexibility to use dual beam production with similar or different beam currents.

The cyclotron consists of a large cylindrical chamber placed between the poles of a huge electromagnet. The magnet system consists of magnet itself, magnet poles made of low-carbon steel and magnet coils made of hollow copper conductors. Inside the chamber, two big hollow D-shaped copper electrodes (Dees) are connected to a very high voltage oscillating with high radio frequency in range of 20–30 MHz and an ion source located at the centre of chamber where the ionization process of hydrogen or deuteron gas takes place. The radio-frequency (RF) system (particle acceleration) includes RF generator, RF cable and RF cavity. The chamber is kept under very high vacuum (e.g. 10^{-07} mbar) by means of vacuum system (e.g. diffusion and mechanical pump).

The cyclotron operation takes place through a master PC station which allows an operator to set up irradiation parameters (beam current and irradiation time) and have a control over many of the cyclotron operations and functions overseeing the production process step by step in a diagrammatic manner. Some of these parameters to be followed are ion source, target, foil and probe currents, Dee voltage, gas flow and other critical RF settings as well as helium cooling pressure. Ionization starts as high purity gas (H_2, D_2) that pass through the ion source with predefined flow rate. Ionization

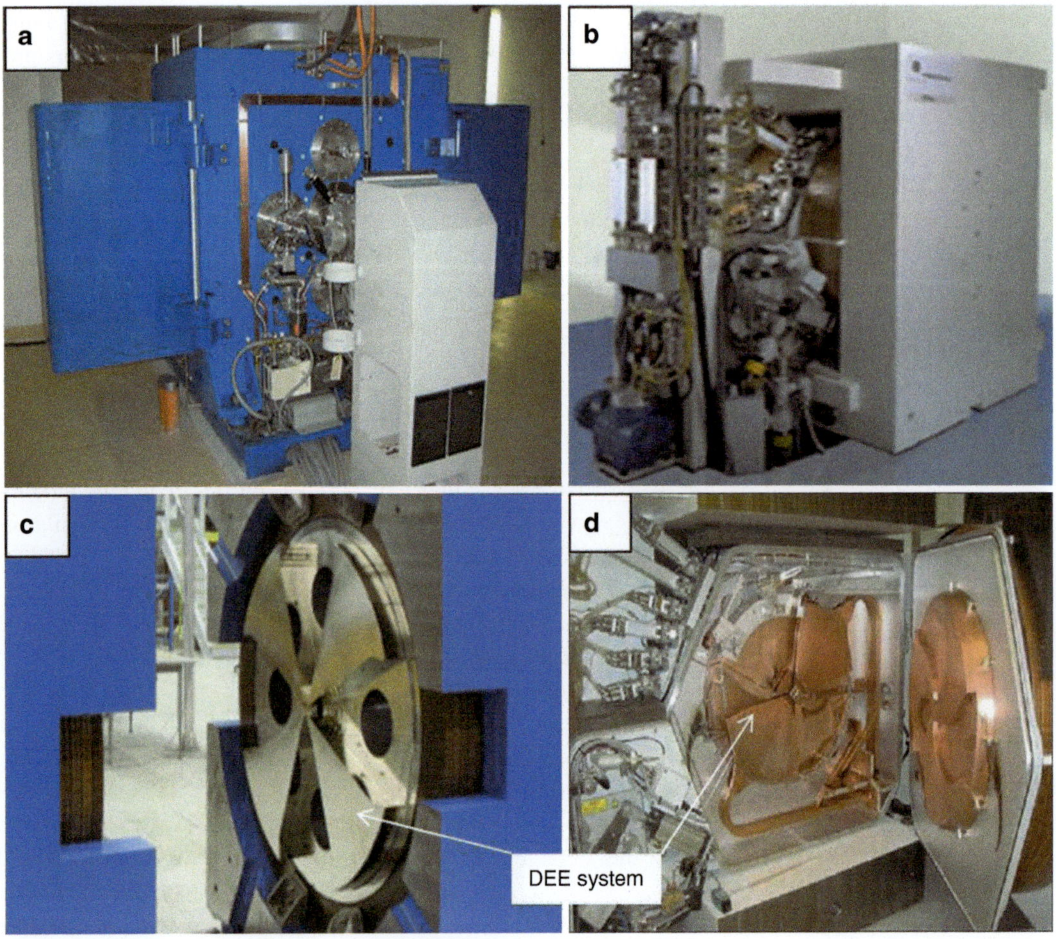

Fig. 1.8 Medical cyclotron for radiopharmaceuticals productions. (**a**) ACS cyclotron TR-24 (24 MeV) high current cyclotron for production of PET and SPECT radionuclides (Courtesy of ACS, Inc.). (**b**) GE PETtrace 800 series medical cyclotron (16.5/8.4 MeV) (Courtesy of GE Health Care). (**c**, **d**) are their respective Dee's system

of such gas is then followed by injection of ionized particles into the chamber centre between the Dees where constant magnetic field is applied along ionized particle path. The role of applied magnetic field during particle acceleration is to focus on and maintain accelerated particle in spiral path (for explanation, see Fig. 1.9). The force of applied magnetic field is given by

$$F = qvB \tag{1.6}$$

And the centripetal force can be described as

$$F = \frac{mv^2}{r} \tag{1.7}$$

where B magnetic field strength is in Tesla, r particle's radius in metre, q particle's charge in coulomb and m particle's mass in kg. From Eqs. 1.6 and 1.7,

$$qvB = \frac{mv^2}{r} \tag{1.8}$$

Hence, particle velocity v is represented by

$$v = \frac{qBr}{m} \tag{1.9}$$

And particle frequency in spiral path is

$f = \dfrac{v}{2\pi r}$, substitute for v so

$$f = \frac{qBr}{2\pi rm} \tag{1.10}$$

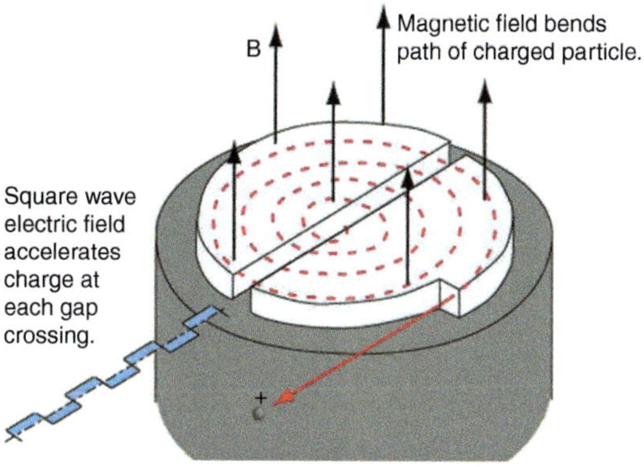

Fig. 1.9 Schematic diagram showing particle path in a cyclotron as well as the applied magnetic and electric field. Ion source located at the centre of high-vacuum chamber, negative ions being maintained by magnetic field accelerated by RF until reach extraction radius then directed to the target body by thin carbon foil (From http://hyperphysics.phy-astr.gsu.edu/hbase/hph.html)

Hence,

$$f = \frac{qB}{2\pi m} \tag{1.11}$$

At resonance condition between the high-frequency electric field (RF) and the circular motion frequency

$$f = f_{\text{oscillator}} \text{ or } qB = 2\pi \, \mathrm{mf}_{\text{oscillator}}$$

Under resonance condition, as the particle completes half revolution, the polarity of the field will change. The particle will again be accelerated across the gap; its velocity will increase so that now it will move in a circular path of greater radius, but its frequency will not be affected and the process of acceleration continues. Hence, the maximum kinetic energy achievable by the accelerated particle is given by

$$E = \frac{1}{2}mv^2 \tag{1.12}$$

Using Eq. 1.9 to substitute for v in Eq. 1.12.

$$E = \frac{B^2 r^2}{2}\left(\frac{q^2}{m}\right) \tag{1.13}$$

Once the required kinetic energy is gained by the accelerating particles, the positively charged ions (H^+ and $2H^+$) are extracted by means of a stripping foil technique in which thin carbon foil is placed at the extraction radius to strip electrons as the negatively charged accelerated ions passing through it (Fig. 1.10). Subsequently, the direction and curvature of the positively charged beam path change (opposite direction) towards the selected target, and bombardment starts for radionuclide production.

The target system where the bombardment and nuclear reactions takes place can be liquid, gas or solid target. Heat dissipation on the target should be removed by means of cooling applied by water cooling system and high purity helium gas. At the end of bombardment, the activity will transfer to specific synthesis modules where the chemical reaction and labelling under preset conditions of temperature and pressure take place to have the final radiopharmaceuticals.

1.5.3 Specific Activity

Specific activity is defined as activity per unit mass of the radioisotope (mCi/g, Bq/mol) including radioactive and nonradioactive molecules. Since one mole of any element contains Avogadro's number of atoms, so for calculation standardization, it is good to represent specific activity in unit activity/mol. Specific activity has an important role in PET radiopharmaceuticals because of possible competition between cold and radioactive molecules with noticed uptake reduction in different tissue.

1.5.4 Saturation Yield

Saturation yield of radionuclide production is represented as the maximum activity produced per unit microampere (mCi/μA), and it is given by:

$$(\text{mCi}/\mu\text{A}) = \frac{A_0}{I\left(1 - e^{\lambda t}\right)} \tag{1.14}$$

where A_0 is activity (mCi) at the end of bombardment (EOB), $\left(1 - e^{\lambda t}\right)$ is saturation factor, t is irradiation time in minutes, λ is decay constant of

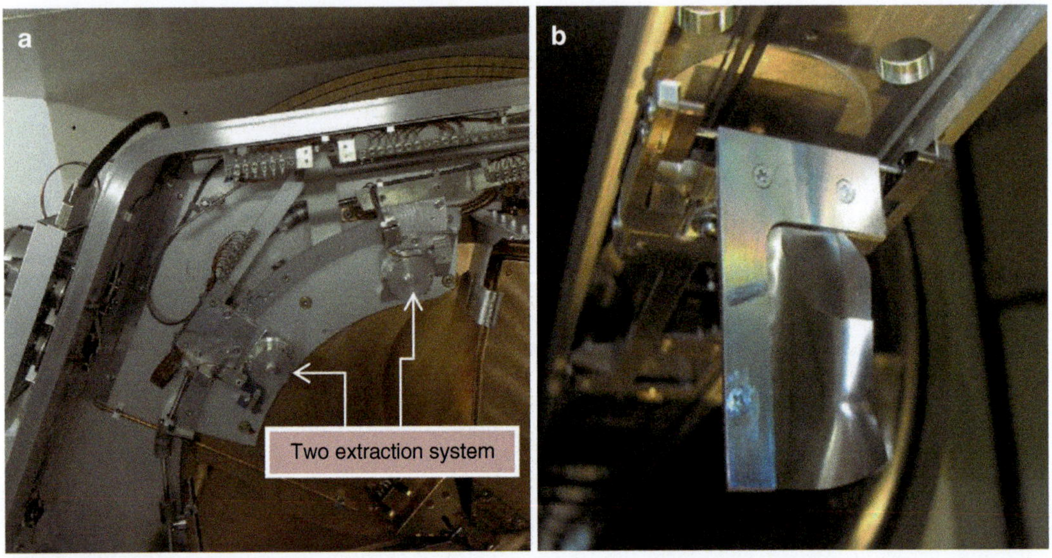

Fig. 1.10 Cyclotron extraction system. (**a**) GE PETtrace 800 extraction system. One extraction system for each target set allowing dual beam production (Courtesy of GE Health Care) and (**b**) used and cracked extraction foil (From www.triumf.ca)

isotope of interest and I is the beam current in (μA).

Saturation factor is defined as the production rate of isotope during irradiation time of the target for a time t. Saturation factor approaches unity within 5–7 half-lives of irradiation time of radionuclide produced. At that point, equilibrium between production rate and decay occurs.

The above equation is valid for thin target while there is no beam attenuation. For thick target (beam is completely absorbed in the target) where there is variations in beam energy because of gradual energy loss due to interactions of charged particles with electrons, target yield depends on other factors such as energy and stopping power, and it is given by:

$$Y = \frac{1.03 \times 10^5}{Z \times A} \int_{E_{in}}^{E_{out}} \frac{\sigma(E)}{dE/dX} dE \quad \text{for } t >> T_{1/2}$$

where Y is the thick target yield (μCi/μA), Z atomic number of charged particle, A mass number of target nuclei, dE/dX stopping power of charged particle in MeV/g, $\sigma(E)$ cross section in mbarn, t irradiation time, $T_{1/2}$ half-life of isotope, E_{in} incident energy of the particle and E_{out} exiting energy of the particle.

1.6 Radioactivity

As mentioned previously, all heavy (large) nuclei (i.e. $Z>83$) are structurally unstable (unstable nucleus) and therefore radioactive. Sooner (nanosecond) or later (thousands of years), those unstable nuclei change to more stable nuclear configurations through various processes of spontaneous radioactive decay that involve emission of energetic particles such as alpha, beta and gamma. Thus, unstable radionuclide (parent) transforms to more stable nuclide (daughter) throughout various radioactive decay modes that will be discussed in the following sections.

1.6.1 Modes of Decay

1.6.1.1 Alpha Decay

Alpha particle (^4_2He) is the nucleus of the helium atom and consists of two protons and two neutrons. From the stability standpoint, the alpha particle has very stable configurations and plays an important role in reducing the heavy weight of some radioactive nuclei transforming them into less excited or ground state. The position of those radionuclides on the N/Z diagram determines its mode of

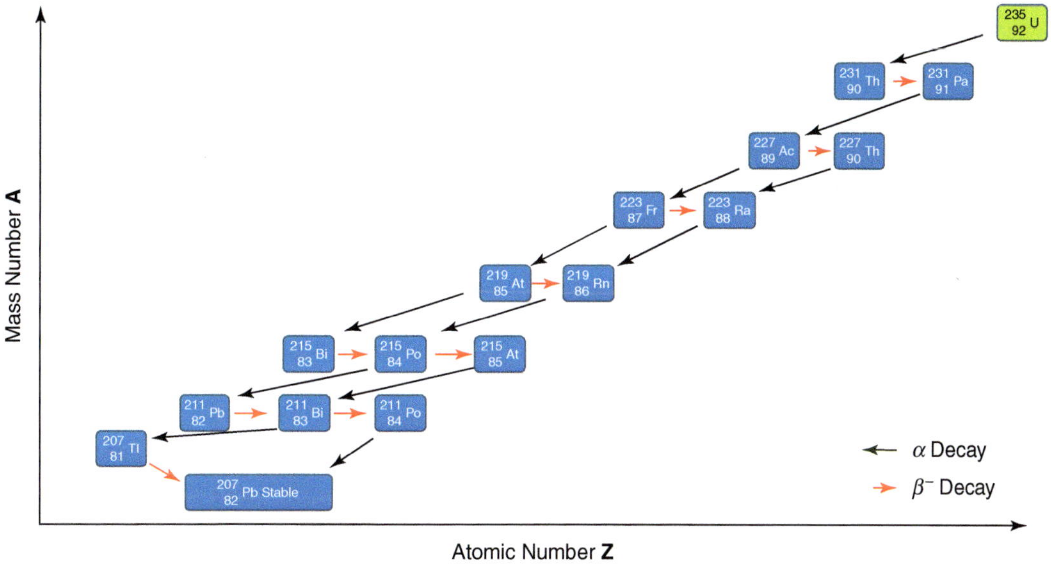

Fig. 1.11 ^{235}U decay series: unstable ^{235}U decays to stable ^{207}Pb nuclei through alpha and beta decay modes

radioactive decay; for heavy large nuclei (Z>83), they need to reduce their A, Z and N numbers to reduce large mass and charges to achieve the stability through the emission of several helium-4 nucleus (^4_2He nuclei – alpha particle). Each emission of alpha particle reduces the mass by 4; some heavy radionuclides (^{235}U) reach its stability through a chain of transformation that need several alpha particle emission (decay series) before a stable nuclide (^{207}Pb) is achieved. The decay series of such a transformation can be seen in Fig. 1.11; the decay modes include those leading to ejection of an alpha particle (α) or a beta particle (β^-).

Radium-226 is a typical example of alpha decay; see decay scheme in Fig. 1.12.

$$^{226}_{88}\text{Ra} \rightarrow {}^{222}_{86}\text{Rn} + {}^4_2\text{He} + 4.87\ \text{MeV}$$

Although the alpha particles are monoenergetic and their kinetic energy is below 10 MeV (in range 4–9 MeV), it can penetrate the parent nucleus coulomb barrier of 30 MeV due to quantum-mechanical effect of tunnelling (tunnelling through the barrier).

1.6.1.2 Beta Minus (β^-) Decay

Small radionuclide (Z<83) of unstably high N/Z ratio indicates an excess of neutrons (proton deficient), lie above the line of stability. Beta minus

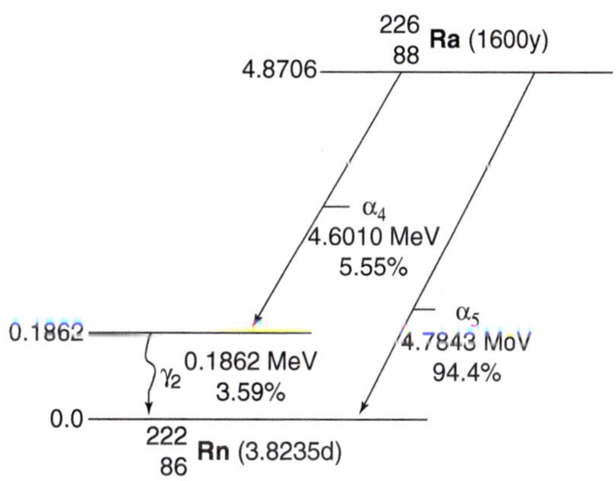

Fig. 1.12 ^{226}Ra decay scheme

decay transforms a neutron into a proton and eject one electron (beta particle) plus antineutrino, leading those nuclei closer to the line of stability by adding more positive charge (charges increase on the nucleus and a slight reduction of mass), thus, changing only the atomic number Z of the parent by one unit (+1) leaving the atomic mass A constant (isobar daughter).

$$n \rightarrow p + \overline{e} + \overline{v_e}$$

$$^A_Z P \rightarrow {}_{Z+1}^{\ \ A}D + \overline{e} + \overline{v_e}$$

Unlike the alpha particles (monoenergetic), the beta particles are being emitted with a range of energies (MeV) forming a continuous spectrum (not all the beta particles being emitted with the same energy value); some of them reaches a maximum energy denoted by $E_{\beta max}$, whereas others are emitted with smaller energy. Thus, the energy released from this transformation is distributed randomly between the electron (beta particle) which has most of it and the antineutrino.

There are some radionuclides of medical interest that undergo decay solely by β^- emission (^{3}H, ^{14}C, ^{32}P and ^{90}Y) or combination of (β^-, γ) emission (^{131}I, ^{133}Xe and ^{137}Cs). Radionuclide can be used either as diagnostic radiopharmaceuticals or as therapeutic products. Pure beta-emitting radionuclides (e.g. Yettrium-90, ^{90}Y) are mainly used with therapeutic purposes, to deliver high-dose rate on tumours due to their high linear energy transfer (LET) and range of deposition in tissue several mm to cm.

^{90}Y is one of the radionuclides that is most widely used in nuclear medicine therapeutic applications. Thanks to its long β particle range, ^{90}Y allows a uniform irradiation of large tumours commonly expressing heterogeneous perfusion and hypoxia. The average energy of β^- emissions from ^{90}Y is 0.9367 MeV and maximum of 2.27 Mev (see Fig. 1.13, ^{90}Y decay scheme), with a mean tissue penetration of 2.5 mm and a maximum of 11 mm. However, ^{90}Y-labelled SIR –microspheres (diameter ~30 μm) are used in selective internal radiation therapy for the treatment of hepatocellular carcinoma (HCC) and potentially other diseases metastatic to the liver. ^{131}I radionuclide is being used in both diagnostic and therapy (combination of emission); it is used for the treatment of variety of thyroid disorders, benign and malignant. The decay scheme for ^{131}I indicates emission of six beta minus particles of varying energies and emission of 14 gamma rays of different energies. Thus, 90 % of the tissue damage from ^{131}I is caused by beta particles due to the LET rate for beta minus particles, which is much higher than for gamma rays.

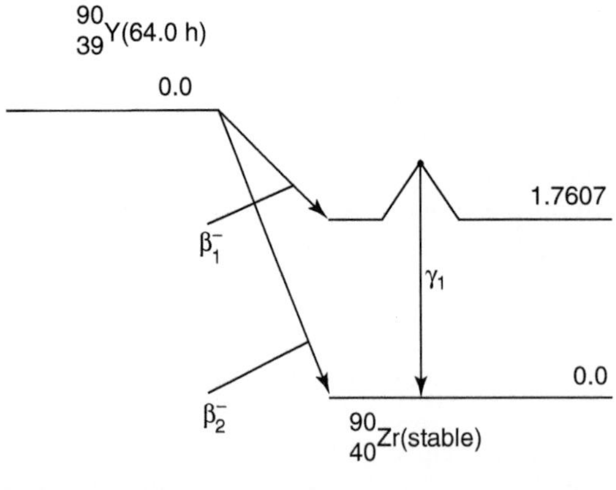

Fig. 1.13 ^{90}Y decay scheme

1.6.1.3 Positron (β+) Decay

Proton-rich radio nuclei (lie below the line of stability) achieve their stability by a nuclear change which requires either a positive charged electron emission (positron decay) or a capture of orbital electron (electron capture). Radioactive transformation by positron (β^+) emission is occurred by rearrangement of the protons and neutrons of the nucleus binding in a way they could supply the essential energy ($E = 1.022$ MeV) for this transformation which yield a neutron, create positive electron and eject a neutrino and reducing the atomic number by one. The energy 1.022 MeV is being consumed in producing two electron masses as a product of the decay (Fig. 1.14).

$$p \to +e^+ + \nu_e$$
$$^A_Z P \to {}_{Z-1}^{A} D + e^+ + \nu_e$$

An example of (β^+) decay:

$$^{18}_{9}\mathrm{F} \to {}^{18}_{8}\mathrm{O} + {}^{0}_{1}e + \nu + Q + \text{orbital electron}$$

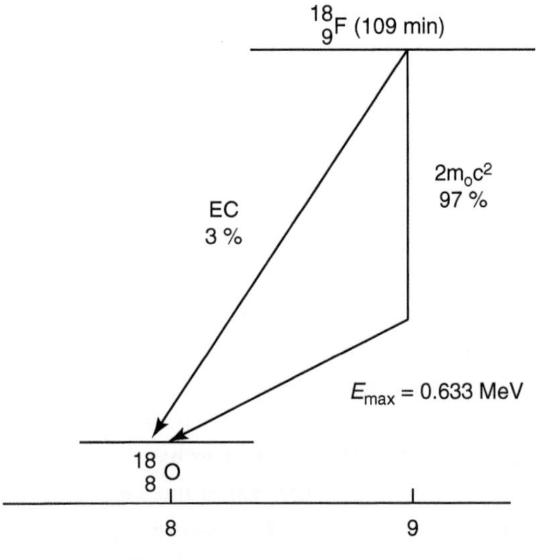

Fig. 1.14 ^{18}F decay scheme

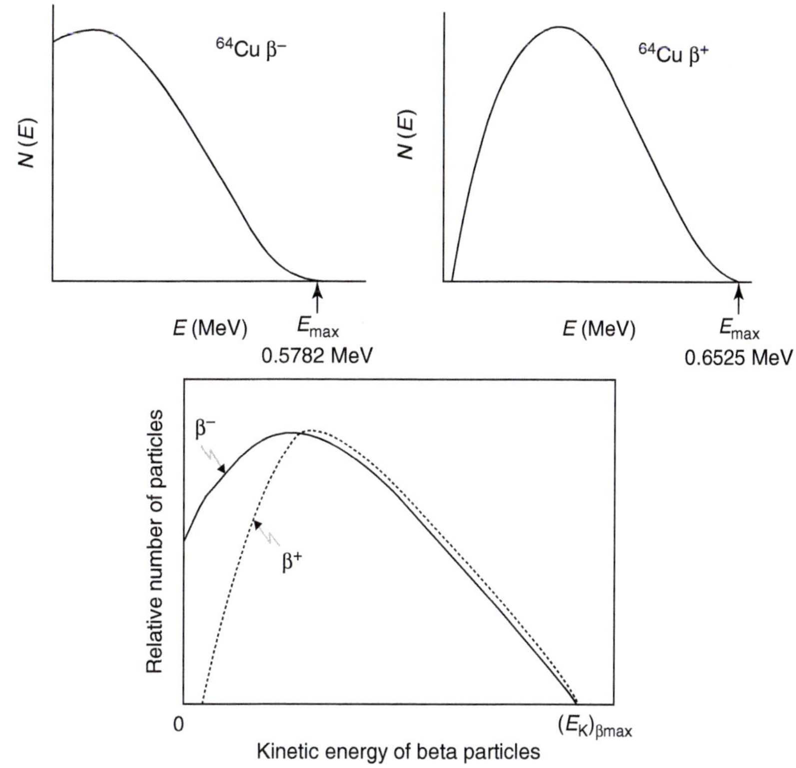

Fig. 1.15 Beta particles energy spectrum for $^{64}_{29}Cu$ undergoing β^- (*top left*) and β^+ (*top right*) emissions with maximum energy 0.579 and 0.653 MeV to reach stable nuclides $^{64}_{30}Zn$ and $^{64}_{28}Ni$, respectively (Adapted from Martin James [3]). Difference in energy spectrum of beta minus and beta plus is also shown in the bottom figure (Adapted from Podgorsak [23])

Similarly to beta minus, the beta plus is continuously distributed in an energy spectrum skewed to the right as shown in Fig. 1.15 (charge effects cause shift to higher energies).

The average energy $\overline{E_\beta}$ of the spectrum is approximately one-third of the end point energy (maximum energy $E_{\beta\ max}$); the general relationship for the average kinetic energy of the beta particles is:

$$\overline{E_{\beta^+}} = \frac{1}{3} E_{\beta^+\ max} \times \left(1 + \frac{\sqrt{E_{\beta^+\ max}}}{4}\right) \quad \text{for } \beta^+ \text{ decay} \tag{1.15}$$

$$\overline{E_{\beta^-}} = \frac{1}{3} E_{\beta^-\ max} \times \left(1 - \frac{\sqrt{Z}}{50}\right)\left(1 + \frac{\sqrt{E_{\beta^-\ max}}}{4}\right) \quad \text{for } \beta^- \text{ decay} \tag{1.16}$$

where $\overline{E_{\beta^-}}$ and $\overline{E_{\beta^+}}$ are in MeV.

1.6.1.4 Electron Capture (EC)

As mentioned earlier, the proton-rich nuclei undergo radioactive transformation indicated by capture of orbital electron. This happens when the sufficient energy is not available for positron emission ($E < 1.022$ MeV); the only way to reduce number of protons in proton-rich nuclei would be the capture of an orbital electron. Due to de Broglie wave pattern of the orbiting electrons, they could come close to or pass through the unstable nucleus allowing capture to occur yielding Z reduction by 1, N increase by 1, and the mass number A remains the same. The capture from the close atom shells (K with 90 % capture probability, L (10 %) and M (1 %)) leaves vacancy which then filled by a higher energy level electron, and characteristic radiation is emitted with probability of Auger process; for more details, refer to Sect. 1.7.1.

^{55}Fe is a radionuclide undergoes such a transformation to reach the nuclear stability.

$$p + \bar{e} \rightarrow n + v_e$$
$${}^{A}_{Z}P + \bar{e} \rightarrow {}_{Z-1}^{A}D + v_e$$

$${}^{55}_{26}\mathrm{Fe} + {}^{0}_{-1}e \rightarrow {}^{55}_{25}\mathrm{Mn} + v + Q$$

Although positron emission occurs more frequently among light elements and electron capture among heavier elements, unstable nucleus has energy of $E \geq 1.022$ MeV and reaches stability by positron emission accompanied with electron capture mode of decay. ^{11}C and ^{18}F are radionuclides of medical interest that undergo such competitive decay (β^+ and EC). See Fig. 1.16.

1.6.1.5 Isomeric Transition

Most of radioactive decay yields a daughter nucleus in an excited state relieved in less than 10^{-9} s by gamma emission. However, some daughter nuclei may be formed in excited states that could exist long enough to be measurable.

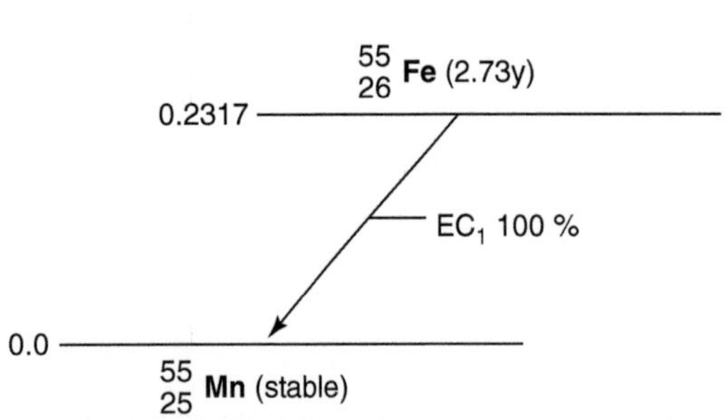

Fig. 1.16 ${}^{55}_{26}Fe$ decay scheme illustrates positron emission accompanied with electron capture

Such a "long-lived" excitation represents a metastable (or isomeric state). To relieve the excitation energy of that state, emission of gamma rays is carried out. An example of such decay is the production of ^{99m}Tc by radioactive transformation of ^{99}Mo; see Fig. 1.17 ^{99}Mo decay chain. ^{99m}Tc is decayed considerably with almost 6 h half-life, and it is relieved to the ground state of ^{99}Tc throughout the gamma ray emission.

1.6.2 Radioactive Decay Equations

The fundamental law of radioactive decay is based on the fact that the decay, i.e. the transition of a parent nucleus to a daughter nucleus is a purely statistical process. The disintegration (decay) probability is a fundamental property of an atomic nucleus and remains equal in time.

Mathematically this law is expressed as

$$dN = \lambda N.dt$$
$$\lambda = (-dN/dt)/N$$

where λ is the decay constant and it is unique value for each radioisotope.

($-dN/dt$) is the disintegration rate, and the negative sign signifies that N is decreasing with time. N is the number of radioactive nuclei. By integration and applying the boundary conditions in the beginning, $t=0$ and $N=N_0$, we obtain

$$\mathrm{In}\left(\frac{N}{N_o}\right) = -\lambda t$$

Subsequently the equation of exponential decay $N=N_o\, e^{-\lambda t}$

Or in terms of activity

$$A = A_o e^{-\lambda t} \quad (1.17)$$

Half-life time ($t_{1/2}$) is the time required for radioactivity to reach half of its original value and is related to the decay constant through the relation:

$$T_{1/2} = 0.693/\lambda \quad (1.18)$$

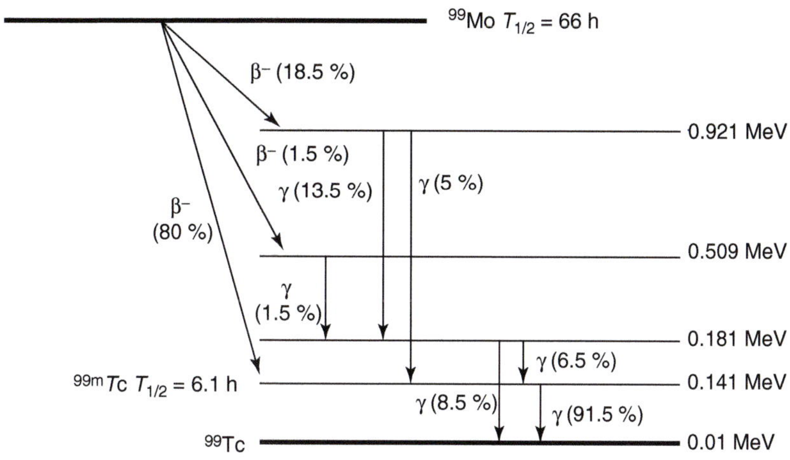

Fig. 1.17 ^{99}Mo decay scheme, 80 % of ^{99}Mo undergoes beta minus decay to reach metastable technetium-99 which disintegrates to stable technetium-99 through emission of 140 keV gamma rays

This can be easily derived if we substitute the activity *A* or number of atoms *N* by (½)*A* or (½)*N* receptively in the two equations above while denoting $t = T_{1/2}$.

1.7 Interaction of Radiation with Matter

Ionizing radiation either heavy or light charged particles or electromagnetic waves (such as gamma rays, x-rays, etc.) do interact in different modes with matter. Energetic charged particles interact with matter by losing kinetic energy via excitation and ionization. Excitation and ionization occur when charged particles lose energy by interacting with orbital electrons. Excitation is the transfer of some of the incident particle's energy to electrons in the absorbing material, rising electron to higher energy level. In excitation, the energy transferred to an electron does not exceed its binding energy. Following excitation, the electron loses energy going to its original energy level, with the emission of the lost excitation energy in the form of electromagnetic radiation or Auger electrons. If the transferred energy exceeds the binding energy of the electron, then ionization occurs in which the electron is ejected from the atom.

Sometimes the ejected electrons possess sufficient energy to produce secondary ionization. Light charged particles as positrons during passing through absorbing material lose their energy due to interaction with electrons of absorber atoms and come to almost rest; recombination of positron and electron will initiate annihilation process. Photon detection of the annihilation process is the basis upon which PET imaging has been conceptualized.

1.7.1 Photoelectric Effect

In the photoelectric effect, all of the incident photon energy is transferred to the inner most electron of the absorber, which is ejected from the atom. The kinetic energy of the ejected electron (E_e in Eq. 1.19) is equal to difference between incident photon energy (E_i) and binding energy of the orbital electron (E_b) (Fig. 1.18a). Therefore, for photoelectric interaction to occur, the energy of incident photon should be equal to or slightly above the binding energy of ejected electron. As a result of this interaction, the atom becomes unstable and ionized with vacancy in the inner most energy shell. Subsequently, electron from higher energy level will fill this gap with emission of characteristic x-ray (K, L, M, etc.). Alternatively, the emitted radiation due to electron transition may result in bombarding an orbital electron in the same atom producing what is called Auger electron, named after one of the discoverers Pierre Victor Auger (Fig. 1.18b).

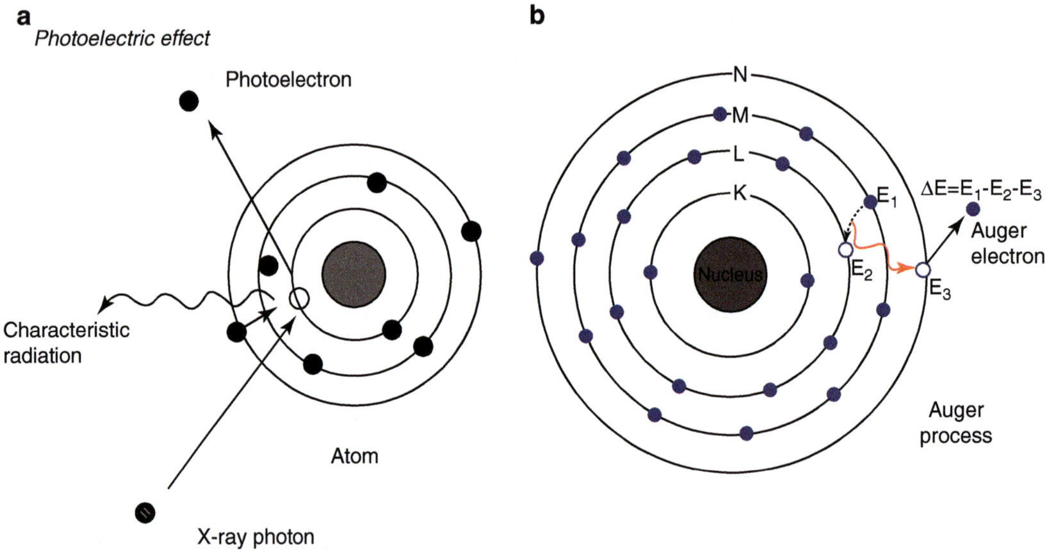

Fig. 1.18 Photoelectric effect and Auger electron process. (**a**) Photoelectric interaction; gamma rays interact with most inner shell; energetic electron is ejected with energy equal to difference between incident photon energy and K-shell binding energy and (**b**) Auger electron

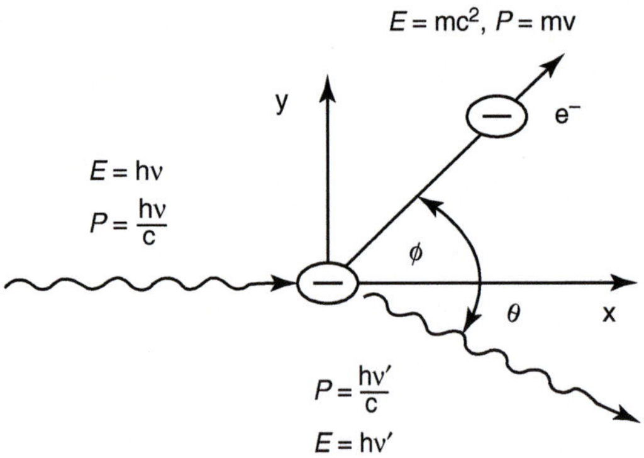

Fig. 1.19 In Compton scattering, incident photon interacts with free electron and deflected by angle θ with energy equal to the difference between incident photon energy and recoil electron

The probability of characteristic x-ray emission decreases as the atomic number of the absorber decreases and thus does not occur frequently for diagnostic energy photon interactions in soft tissue. The probability of this interaction decreases with increasing energy of the incident photon, but increases with increasing atomic number of the absorber.

$$E_e = E_i - E_b \tag{1.19}$$

1.7.2 Compton Effect

Compton scattering is an inelastic collision between gamma ray and valence electron of an atom whose binding energy is much less than gamma ray energy. It is the most prevailing interaction of gamma ray with soft tissue in energy range used for diagnostic purposes. In this mechanism incident gamma photon transfers some of its energy to an electron that assumed to be in rest and known as recoil electron resulting in scattered gamma photon by angle $\underline{\theta}$ with respect to its original path as shown in Fig. 1.19. The energy transferred to the electron is varying depending on the scattered photon angle and can be calculated by applying the laws of conservation of energy and momentum:

$$h\dot{\upsilon} = \frac{h\upsilon}{1+\left(\frac{h\upsilon}{m_e c^2}\right)(1+\cos\theta)} \tag{1.20}$$

where $m_e c^2$ is the rest mass energy of electron (0.511 MeV, refer to Table 1.2). The probability of Compton scattering increases linearly with atomic number of absorber material.

1.7.3 Pair Production

If the gamma ray energy exceeds 1.022 MeV (rest mass energy for two electrons) and passes near to the nucleus, pair production interaction will take place. Conversion of gamma ray energy into two particles (electron and anti-electron) each with mass m_ec^2 but opposite electrostatic charge and the total kinetic energy is approximately equal to $hv-2m_ec^2$; therefore, all energy in excess that required to create the pair will be shared by the positron-electron pair as a kinetic energy. After production of a pair, the positron and electron lose their kinetic energy by excitation, ionization and bremsstrahlung as any high-energy electron. When the positron expended all of its kinetic energy, it recombines with an electron, and annihilation phenomenon takes place with production of two photon quanta each of 0.511 MeV released at angle of $180° \pm 0.25°$ relative to each other.

1.7.4 Linear and Mass Attenuation Coefficient

Linear attenuation coefficient (μ_l) is a constant that determines the fraction of radiation beam loss per unit thickness of the absorber because of beam absorption or scatter; in other words, it is a measure of the probability of interaction of photons with matter per unit length. It can be expressed by the following formula:

$$\text{Linear attenuation coefficient } (\mu_l) = \frac{\%\,\text{Reduction in intensity}}{\text{Absorber thickness (cm)}}\,\text{cm}^{-1}$$

Linear attenuation coefficient is specific for each absorber material, but any change in absorber density will change linear attenuation coefficient value. Using mass attenuation coefficient eliminates density dependence of linear attenuation coefficient. Mass attenuation coefficient (μ_m) is given by

$$\mu_m = \frac{\mu_l}{\rho}\ \text{cm}^2/\text{gm} \qquad (1.21)$$

where ρ is absorber density in gm/cm^3 and μ linear attenuation coefficient in cm^{-1}

The total linear attenuation coefficients μ is defined as the sum of photoelectric, Compton and pair production attenuation coefficients:

$$\mu = \tau + \sigma + k \qquad (1.22)$$

where τ, σ and k are linear attenuation coefficients of photoelectric, Compton interaction and pair production, respectively.

For 511 keV photons produced by positron annihilation, the primary mechanism for photon interaction with matter (one or both annihilation photons) is by Compton interaction while photoelectric absorption is being negligible. From energy dependence point of view, the probability of photoelectric interactions is inversely proportional with cubic photon energy ($1/E^3$); as a result, extreme drop in the probability of photoelectric interaction occurs in a certain absorber material as energy increases, while in Compton interaction, the energy of incident photon must be greater than the electron's binding energy. Therefore, photoelectric interaction is the most preferable interaction for low-energy photons, but as the incident photon energy increases, Compton interaction becomes the most predominant one (Fig. 1.20).

Also, the probability of photoelectric interactions is directly proportional with cubic atomic number of the material (Z^3); thus, the photoelectric interaction is predominant for high Z material. On the other hand, Compton interaction probability depends on electron density (number of electrons/g), and therefore the probability of Compton scattering per unit mass is almost independent of atomic number, and the probability of Compton scattering per unit volume is approximately proportional to the density of the material. In comparison to other elements, the absence of neutrons in the hydrogen atom results in an approximate doubling of electron density. Thus, hydrogenous materials have a higher

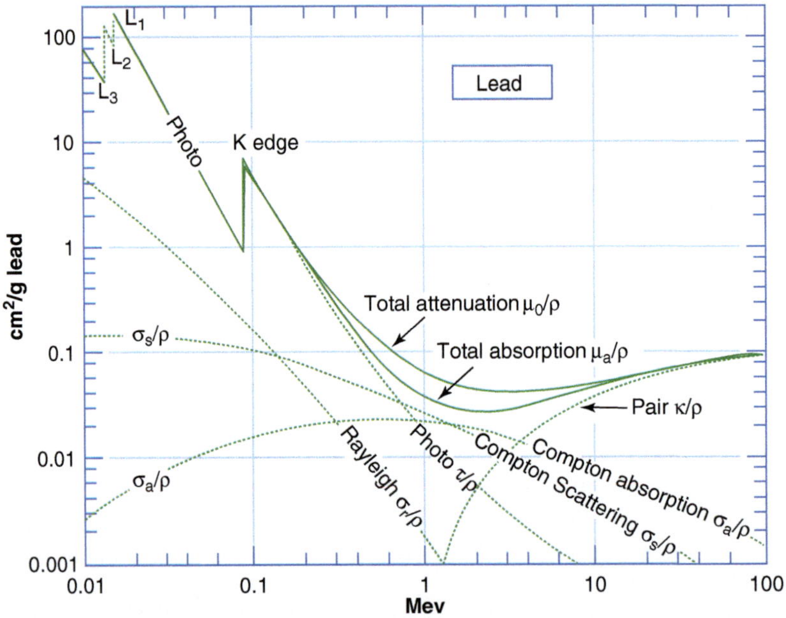

Fig. 1.20 The mass attenuation coefficient of lead (atomic number 82) for gamma rays, plotted versus gamma energy and the contributions by the three interaction effects. Photoelectric effect dominates at low energy. Above 5 MeV, pair production starts to dominate. Compton scattering is the most common interaction at intermediate energies

probability of Compton scattering than a non-hydrogenous material of equal mass.

The product of this form of interaction is that primary photon changes the direction (secondary scattered photon) and loses part of its energy. In addition, the atom where the interaction occurred is ionized. However, when a photon passes through a thickness of absorber material, the probability that it will experience an interaction (removal of photons) is a function of photon energy together with composition and thickness of the absorber. Under conditions of narrow-beam geometry, the transmission of a monoenergetic photon beam through an absorber is described by an exponential function:

$$I(x) = I(0)e^{-\mu_1 x} \tag{1.23}$$

where $I(0)$ is the intensity of the un-attenuated photon beam and $I(x)$ is the intensity of photon beam measured at a thickness x through an absorber of linear attenuation coefficient μ_l. The total linear attenuation coefficient of 511 keV gamma rays in tissue is 0.096 cm^{-1}; this corresponds to 7 cm half value layer (HVL = ln2/μ_l). In PET instrumentation, the two annihilation photons interact before escaping the object that is being imaged. The result is that the primary photons are being removed or attenuated from the line of response (LOR) and a potential detection of scattered photons in a different LOR.

1.8 Positron Emitter Radionuclides

As explained above, radionuclides undergoing (β^+) decay are called positron emitters. They differ in the energy of emitted positrons and thus differ in the positron range inside the tissues (the range that the positron travels in tissue depends on the emission energy and the electron density of the surrounding tissue). These radionuclides are used to label a wide variety of pharmaceutical compounds that interrogate disease biochemistry using PET imaging techniques. Briefly, the pharmaceutical interacts with the body through a metabolic process; the radionuclide allows that interaction to be followed, mapped and measured (two annihilation

Table 1.3 The commonly used positron emitters in PET imaging and their physical properties

Radionuclide	Half-life	E_β *max* MeV	$\overline{E_\beta}$ MeV	Percentage of β^+ decays (%)	β^+ max range (mm)	β^+ mean range (mm)	Production method
C-11	20.4 min	0.96	0.39	99	4.1	1.1	Cyclotron
N-13	9.96 min	1.19	0.49	100	5.1	1.5	Cyclotron
O-15	123 s	1.72	0.73	100	7.3	2.5	Cyclotron
F-18	110 min	0.635	0.24	97	2.4	0.6	Cyclotron
Ga-68	68.3 min	1.9	0.84	88	8.2	2.9	Generator (from Ge-68)
Rb-82	78 s	3.35	1.52	95	14.1	5.9	Generator (from Sr-82)

Source: Refs. [2, 6]

photons detected in coincidence). Table 1.3 lists some clinically useful positron emitter radionuclides.

Higher positron energy means a longer effective positron range (the average distance from the emitting nucleus to the end of the positron range) travelling through tissue. For example, in water ^{18}F has low-energy positrons (0.635 MeV) with a very short range (2.4 mm) compared to ^{82}Rb which has high-energy positrons (3.4 MeV) and a longer range (14.1 mm). However, the half-life of radionuclides plays an important role in the availability of the clinical application. Carbon-11, nitrogen-13 and oxygen-15 with very short half-lives can only be used to study processes that have rapid uptake. Fluorine-18 with an approximately 2 h half-life allows more time for synthesis, tracer uptake and for imaging particularly in diagnostic applications of oncology.

1.8.1 Exposure Rate Constant

Before discussing the emission rate and exposure levels of positron emitter radionuclides, it would be appropriate to understand some basic definitions in this context. In terms of energy levels, one can note that radiation of energy >20 keV (lower energy does not contribute to radiation exposure) interacts with an absorbing medium (air or patient) to deposit energy producing positive and negative ions or what is called ionization. The amount of ionization of air caused by a γ-ray or x-ray source is defined as exposure, whereas the sum of the kinetic energy of all charged particles produced by interactions from a source of x-rays or γ-rays (through Compton scatter, photoelectric absorption or pair production) per kg of air is known as air kerma. The relationship between exposure, *X*, and air kerma, *K*, can be calculated as:

$$K(\mathrm{Gy}) = X(R) \times 0.00869$$

The radiation exposure level from gamma and x-ray sources can be estimated from the exposure rate constant Γ which is defined as the exposure rate in μSv/h from 1 mCi (37 MBq) of a radionuclide at a distance of 1 m. Each radionuclide has a specific value of exposure rate constant (Table 1.4). Precisely, while calculating the exposure rate constant of radionuclide, all emitted radiations from that source must be considered, and adjustments should be made for any attenuating medium (air or patient) between the source and the point of interest. Therefore, each radionu-

Table 1.4 Summary of exposure rate constant for different radionuclides used in nuclear medicine procedures

Nuclide	Half-life (h)	Dose rate constant μSv.m^2/MBq.h	
		Point source	Patient
Ga-67	78.1 h	0.028	0.011
Tc-99m	6.02 h	0.0195	0.0075
In-111	2.8 days	0.086	0.03
I-123	13 h	0.041	0.015
I-131	8.06 days	0.0575	0.023
Xe-133	5.3 days	0.135	0.006
F-18	110 min	0.143	0.092

Source: Refs. [10, 13]

clide represents an exposure rate constant for a point source geometry different than being in vivo (patient body). Due to body attenuation (the body absorbs some of the annihilation radiation), the dose rate from the patient is reduced by a significant factor (self-absorption). For example, the exposure rate of ^{18}F as a point source is 0.143 μSv.m²/MBq.h, whereas the patient exposure rate is significantly lower (0.092 μSv.m²/MBq.h) accounting for 36 % photon reduction.

The exposure rate in air at a given distance:

$$\Gamma = \frac{1}{4\pi}\sum_i (\mu_{en}/\rho)_i Y_i E_i \qquad (1.24)$$

where (μ_{en}/ρ) is the mass-energy absorption coefficient in air for photons of energy E_i emitted by the nuclide with yield Y_i. To estimate the exposure rate (dose rate) from a source of (mCi) activity at a certain distance (m), the following relation may be used:

$$D(\mu Sv/h) = \frac{\Gamma A}{d^2} \qquad (1.25)$$

where Γ is the exposure rate constant also known as gamma constant (μSv m²/MBq h), A is the activity (MBq) and d is the distance (m). In radiation shielding, it is therefore of economic value to use the most appropriate exposure rate constant provided the different conditions including the type of radionuclide, exposure rate constant, uptake time, imaging time, occupancy factors and other variables that may exist in PET or SPECT imaging environments. See Chap. 2 for further details on facility design and other shielding calculations.

1.9 Radiation Detection and Measurements

Radiation detection and measurements are cornerstone activities in nuclear medicine daily practice. It includes many of the hot laboratory equipments, radio-pharmacy, radiation safety and protection, assay counting as well as scanning examinations. All of these require similar or different concepts of radiation detection and/or measurements. We will discuss here the most important radiation equipments involved in dose measurements and counting taking the most typical examples which are dose calibrator and well counter. Other detection devices such as gas-filled detectors, scintillator as well as semiconductor-based detection systems will also be outlined.

1.9.1 Gas-Filled Detector

Gas-filled detectors consist of a chamber filled with a volume of pressurized gas usually at a pressure of one atmosphere or less, to enhance interactions of radiation as it passes through the medium. Radiation that passes through the medium results in gas molecule ionization, followed by collection of the ion pairs with the application of a voltage between the two electrodes. Ions produced are collected as current and amplified to record the resultant signal. The collection of the ion pairs is a function of the applied voltage, radiation energy, intensity levels and type of the gas.

At very low voltage (<10 V), not all the ion pairs could drift towards the electrodes and be collected; some ion pairs recombine to form the original molecule (not enough acceleration). This region is called the region of *recombination.* As voltage increases (>10 V), recombination becomes negligible, and the entire ion pairs can be collected efficiently by the electrodes. The applied voltage changes do not affect the produced current, current remains the same as it called the saturation current, and it is proportional to the deposit ionization energy of the incoming radiation (alpha, beta, gamma). Hence, the region is called the *ionization region* (50–300 V).

Raising the applied voltage to a higher value provides the ion pairs (primary ionization) with a higher energy and velocities and enables them to collide with the medium forming a secondary ionization. Hence, increasing the voltage that provides each electron with the enough energy to produce a secondary ionization, a multiplication of charges and amplification of the produced ionization is proportional to the initial ionization. This region is called the *proportional region.* Beyond that voltage range, the proportionality

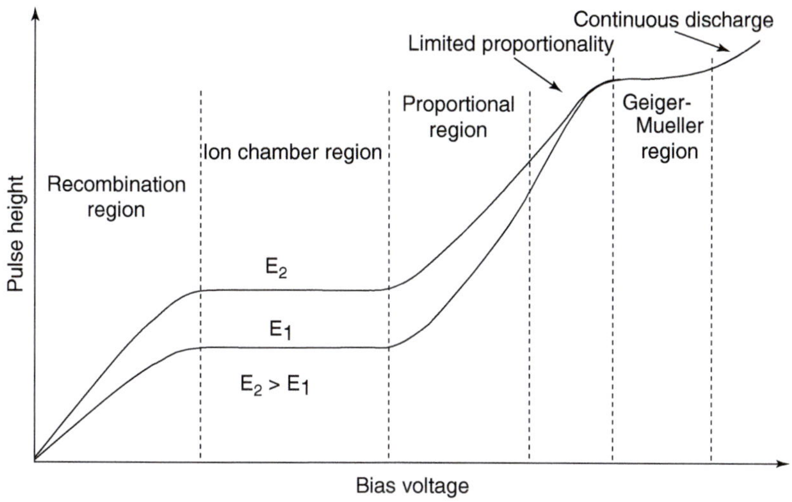

Fig. 1.21 Types of operational voltage regions of gas-filled detector as a result of two different energies of incident photons

becomes limited as the multiplication of charges increases rapidly (limited *proportionality* region). Further increased voltage, the yielded current is of identical behaviour for all types of radiations forming a plateau as voltage increases. This region is referred to *Geiger-Mueller* region. At very high voltage, *continuous discharge* region begins in which a spontaneous ionization is taking place inside the chamber; using a detector at such high voltage might destroy it. Figure 1.21 is showing the various operating voltage regions.

Different types of radiation lead to different ion pair production, since the interaction of the ionizing particle/photons with gas molecules is different. Alpha, beta and gamma radiation could be detected using the gas-filled detector types (i.e. ionization chamber, proportional counter and Geiger-Mueller counter).

An important application of ionization chamber principle is for CT dosimetry measurement purposes through the usage of CT ionization pencil chamber. The ionization pencil chamber is used for the evaluation of computed tomography dose index (CTDI) either in air or mounted in acrylic or polymethyl methacrylate (PMMA) phantoms (head, 16 cm, and body, 32 cm in diameter for adult). It is a pencil-shaped chamber with about 10 cm sensitive length specifically designed for x-ray beam measurements and can be connected to electrometer. It has an excellent energy and partial volume response along its entire length. Hence, it produces an accurate dose estimate by irradiating its entire volume. It also provides uniform response to incident radiations in every angle around its axis and therefore can fit the dosimetric conditions required for dose estimate in CT imaging procedures. Figure 1.22 is showing an ionization chamber and PMMA phantoms used in CT dosimetry. Further details on CT dosimetry can be found in Chap. 2.

1.9.1.1 Dose Calibrator

Dose calibrator contains an argon gas-filled ionization chamber coupled to a high voltage power supply and an electronic circuit that converts and displays chamber response in units of activity. The ionization chamber is under high pressure (increases detection sensitivity), sealed (eliminates the need for temperature and pressure correction) and contains two electrodes having an electric potential between them. A beam of ionizing radiation passes through the chamber and produces electrical charges that are collected by positive (anode) and negative (cathode) electrodes forming total amount of current (time-averaged ionization current). This amount of current is measured by using sensitive current-measuring devices called electrometers (quantify very small electric currents of fA to μA, corresponding to

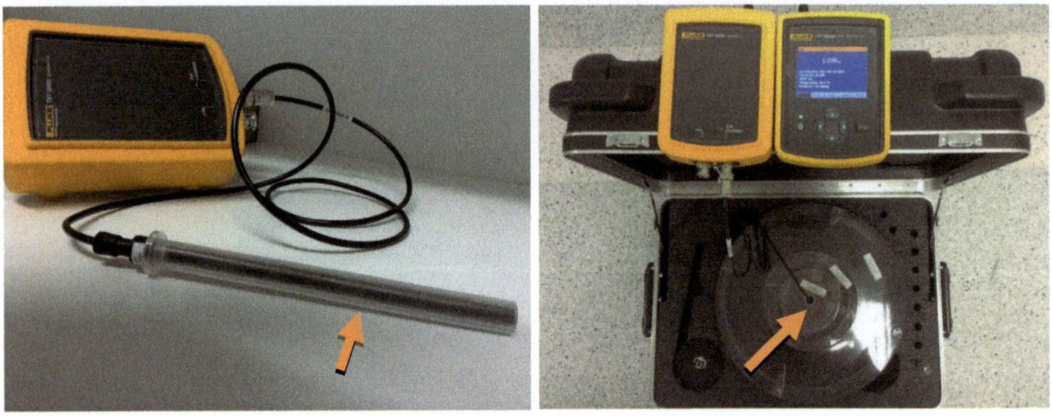

Fig. 1.22 Photographs showing one of the commercially available ionization chamber that is in operation in our laboratory (Courtesy of Fluke Biomedical). *Arrows* indicate ionization chamber (*left*) inserted into one of the phantom wells used in CT calibration (*right*)

10^{-15} and 10^{-6} Ampere, respectively). The current generated in the circuit is proportional to the activity of the measured quantity. Shielding is used around the chamber to reduce the effect of background radiation and to reduce unnecessary operator exposure.

A dose calibrator is used for assaying activities of radiopharmaceutical (γ-rays emitters) of relatively large quantities (i.e. MBq range) placed in vials and syringes. It is calibrated to read directly in units of activity (becquerels or curies) with the ability of choosing the radionuclide type and volume (specifying calibration factor). Dose calibrator's chamber response depends on the specified radionuclide source geometry, its type of decay, energy of emission and source position inserted. For example, the chamber response to pure gamma emitter radionuclide (^{99m}Tc) is different than for a combination of beta and gamma emission (e.g.^{131}I). However, calibration factors assure the accurate activity reading for a selected radionuclide source in the specific geometry being used.

Despite the high range of activity that the dose calibrator can measure, it is relatively insensitive and cannot accurately assay activities less than 1 μCi. Furthermore, the ionization chamber has no ability to distinguish photons of different energies as is possible with detectors having pulse-height analysis capabilities. However, dose calibrators are of great importance in nuclear medicine departments to check every radiopharmaceutical dose that is received or dispensed. Also, they are used to assay the activity of various types of radiopharmaceuticals prior to clinical usage. Therefore, dose calibrator's operation must be checked in a daily basis to assure the desired continued accuracy of the dosage assays (≤5 % accuracy), and several quality control tests need to be performed and repeated at specific intervals (see Table 1.5).

1.9.2 Well Counter

Well counter is a highly efficient radiation detector for counting low-level radioactive samples such as blood or urine collected from radioactive patients, wipes of contamination and any source of activity in the range of micro-curies. Well counters consist of a single solid cylindrical crystal of thallium-doped sodium iodide-NaI(Tl) detector with a hole in the centre for a sample to be placed. It is coupled to photomultiplier tube (PMT) and its associated electronics such as preamplifier, amplifier, pulse-height analyzer (PHA) and scalar-timer. Dimensions of such NaI(Tl) crystal detectors are in the range of:

- 4.5–12.7 cm diameter
- 5–12.7 cm long

Table 1.5 Recommended quality control programmes for a local dose calibrator

Test type	Frequency	Acceptance criteria
High voltage	Daily	Comparable with the manufacture's tolerances
Zero adjustment	Daily	Comparable with the manufacture's tolerances
Background	Daily	Within normal range comparable with the environmental facility
Constancy (check source)	Daily, annually	Within ±5 % of the decay corrected initial value
Accuracy	Annually	Within ±5 % of the decay corrected initial value
Reproducibility (precision)	Annually	Within ±1 % of the average measurements
System linearity	Annually	Within ±5 % of the expected values
	Quarterly	Within ±2 %
Supplier equivalence	Annually	Differences ≤ ±10
	Acceptance (initially established)	Differences ≤ ±5

Table taken from Ref. [9]
Daily means every 24 h starting at 12:00 a.m.

And the well dimension can have the following measures:

- 1.6–3.8 cm diameter
- 3.8–7 cm depth length

A thickness of 5 cm or greater of lead is commonly placed around the detector to reduce background counting levels. Small well counters are used for low-energy gamma rays detection (<200 keV), whereas larger well counters are used for high-energy gamma rays.

Since the inserted sample in the well counter is surrounded by the scintillation crystal, NaI(Tl) detectors have high intrinsic and geometric detection efficiencies of gamma rays; only small amounts of activity can be counted up to about 1 μCi (37 kBq). At higher activities, serious dead time problems do emerge leading to count rate underestimation. The detection efficiency of well counter device is a function of photon energy and detector thickness. For example, the detection efficiencies of a commercially available well counter installed in our laboratory for the radionuclides ^{99m}T, ^{131}I and ^{18}F are 81.66 %, 28.70 % and 28.25 %, respectively.

1.9.3 Scintillation Detectors

Although scintillation mechanism is one of the oldest technical methods for detection of ionizing radiation, it is still widely used as a radiation detector. As outlined above, there are a number of available technologies that can be used in photon detection with relative advantages and technical merits. Scintillator detectors can be used with cost-effective and feasible manner to be incorporated in many imaging systems. It has been used in the manufacturing of SPECT systems, survey metres for energy discrimination and high-efficient radiation detectors as well as in PET imaging scanner including clinical and preclinical systems. Scintillation detectors can be classified into:

I. Inorganic scintillation detectors, e.g. alkali halide scintillator (NaI, CsI, etc.) in the form of solid crystal
II. Organic scintillators which can be pure organic crystal, liquid organic solutions or polymers known as plastic scintillators

The basic difference between organic and inorganic scintillator is the light production mechanism. In case of inorganic scintillator, the light emitted by an inorganic crystal is primarily due to the crystal structure, whereas organic substances exhibit luminescence by virtue of molecular properties.

The ideal scintillation material should possess the following properties:

1. *High stopping efficiency.* Scintillator material should have high efficiency for converting incident radiation energy into emitted luminescence. Scintillator with high effective Z and high density is a better candidate as the former is proper for photoelectric interaction, while the later serves to dominate Compton interaction.
2. *High-energy resolution.* This feature plays an important role in removing scattered radiation. It can be improved by using crystals of high light output and efficient electronic circuitry.
3. *Transparency.* The medium should be transparent to wave length of its own emission for good light conversion and reduction of light loss. The light readout photosensor should also have optical properties that fit the wavelength range of the emitted photon quanta from the scintillator.
4. *Short decay constant.* Short decay constant is a desired property that helps improve coincidence timing resolution as well as an important factor in count rate performance and reduction of dead time. Random coincidences can also be reduced by using crystal of short decay time. Crystals of short decay time are also better candidates in time of flight applications.
5. *High light yield.* The material should be of good optical yield and has a size large enough to use as practical detector. As the crystal dimension decreases in size to improve spatial resolution, as in block detector design of PET scanners, it is necessary to have a scintillator of high light output. As outlined above, light yield also improves timing and energy resolution.

No material can fit all of these properties, and therefore it is usually a trade-off process favouring some properties over the others. For diagnostic purpose, the use of inorganic alkali halide crystal doped with thallium such as NaI(Tl) is widely applied in gamma camera and SPECT imaging systems. In PET imaging, BGO crystal and LSO-type detectors occupy the most important class of scintillator in the market with much interest given to the later due to its better physical properties that fit into state-of-the-art PET clinical applications. Table 1.6 summarizes the physical properties of some crystals used in PET imaging scanners.

The scintillation light is emitted isotropically and optically coupled to the photocathode of a PMT. Scintillation photons incident on the photocathode liberate electrons through the photoelectric effect, which are then accelerated by a strong electric field in the PMT. As these photoelectrons

Table 1.6 Physical properties of some useful inorganic scintillation crystals used in PET

	NaI(TI)	BGO	GSO:Ce	LSO:Ce	LYSO:Ce	$LaBr_3$	BaF_2
Density (gm/cm^3)	3.67	7.13	6.7	7.4	7.1	5.3	4.89
Effective atomic number (*Z*)	51	74	59	66	64	47	54
Linear attenuation coefficient (cm^{-1})	0.34	0.92	0.62	0.87	0.86	0.47	0.44
Light yield (% NaI[Tl])	100	15	30	75	75	160	5
Decay time (ns)	230	300	60–65	40	41	16	0.8
Hygroscopic	Yes	No	No	No	No	Yes	Slightly
Photoelectric effect (%)	17	40	25	32	33	13	12
Refractive index	1.85	2.15	1.85	1.82	1.81	1.88	1.56
Emission maximum (nm)	410	480	440	420	420	370	220

are accelerated, they collide with electrodes in the tube (known as dynodes) releasing additional electrons. This increased electron flux is then further accelerated to collide with succeeding electrodes, causing a large multiplication (by a factor of 10^5 or more) of the electron flux from its initial value at the photocathode surface. Finally, the amplified charge burst arrives at the output electrode (the anode) of the tube. The magnitude of this charge surge is proportional to the initial amount of charge liberated at the photocathode of the PMT; this is defined as the gain of the PMT.

Furthermore, by virtue of the physics of the photoelectric effect, the initial number of photoelectrons liberated at the photocathode is proportional to the amount of light incident on the PMT which in turn is proportional to the amount of energy deposited in the scintillator by the gamma ray (assuming no light loss from the scintillator volume). Thus, an output signal is produced that is proportional to the energy deposited by the gamma ray in the scintillation medium. However, the spectrum of deposited energies (even for a monoenergetic photon flux) is quite variable because of the occurrence of the photoelectric effect, Compton scattering, various scattering phenomena in the scintillation medium and statistical fluctuations associated with all of these processes.

1.9.4 Neutron Detectors

Neutrons are neutrally charged particles that maintain the nuclear binding stability by moderating the repulsion force exhibited by protons. The story of discovering neutrons by James Chadwich in 1932 and its properties is central to the extraordinary developments in atomic physics that took place in the early decades of the twentieth century. Neutrons are not essential part of daily practice for those who are working in nuclear medicine environment. However, it has some significant concerns in medical cyclotrons and shielding construction as well as in operation of nuclear reactors. The former is our focus, and therefore some information about neutron detectors can be useful to mention here. Neutrons are classified according to their energy into:

1. Thermal neutrons in energy range of 0.025 eV up to 0.2 eV at 20.44 °C
2. Slow neutrons with energy between 1 and 10 eV, sometimes up to 1 keV
3. Fast neutrons which have energy above 0.5 MeV

Due to the well-known fact that neutrons are uncharged particles, it is therefore cannot be detected in a direct way. It can be measured via their interactions with atoms to produce a kind of radiation that can be detected in one of the conventional methods. The most common nuclear reactions for thermal neutrons detection are through (n, α) or (n, p) reactions using ${}_5^{10}B$, ^{6}Li and ^{3}He. There are two other methods that depend on (n, fission) reactions and neutron activation. The former is based on fission fragments detection, while the latter utilizes the emissions of the radioactive produced nuclei to detect neutron flux.

Boron-trifluoride proportional counter is used in case of ^{10}B (n, α) reaction which uses BF_3 as proportional gas and neutron detection material. Boron has a high interaction cross section (4010 barns) for this reaction. The BF_3 gas is usually enriched in ^{10}B, and it has to be used at lower absolute pressures in order to get a good performance as a proportional gas.

Similarly, ^{3}He is used as a conversion target and proportional gas in the ^{3}He proportional counter. But ^{3}He(n, p) reaction shows low Q-value of almost 765 keV. As a result the discrimination of gamma rays is more difficult than with BF_3 counters, since secondary electrons only deposit a small amount of energy in the gas.

Instead of using the gas-filled proportional counter, Li has also a good interaction cross section for (n, α) reaction and has been used in a neutron scintillator detector in the form of europium (Eu)-doped lithium iodide crystal. Due to the density of enriched ^{6}LiI(Eu) crystals, a 10 mm-thick detector is almost 100 % efficient for neutrons ranging from thermal energies up to about 0.5 eV.

However, some modification in the neutron detection system should be considered in case of intermediate and fast neutrons such as adding moderator material to slowing down neutrons to energies where the detection efficiency is high. Materials such as polyethylene and paraffin are the most widely used moderators. The use of moderator in case of fast neutron is no longer effective, and thus fast neutron detection depends on elastic scattering with light nuclei. Therefore, fast neutrons incident on a hydrogen-containing scintillator will scatter elastically and give rise to recoil protons ranging in energy up to the full neutron energy. Fluorescence light is emitted as the recoil protons energy is absorbed by the scintillator. A series of spheres of different diameters were developed to thermalize neutrons of low, medium and higher energies. This method allows one to detect neutron energy flux of different energies or neutron energy spectrum.

1.9.5 Solid State Detectors

A semiconductor detector acts as a solid-state ionization chamber. Ionization will take place in the sensitive volume of the detector as ionized particle hit the detector. The charge produced by the photon interactions is then collected directly. The operation of semiconductor detector depends on having either excess electrons or holes which depend on the impurities added to pure semiconductor material. The sensitive volume in the detector is an electronically conditioned region (known as the depleted region) in which liberated electrons and holes move freely.

Germanium (Ge) and silicon (Si) are the most common semiconductor used to construct solid-state detectors. The detector functions as a solid-state proportional counter, with the ionization charge swept directly to the electrodes by the high electric field produced by the bias voltage. The early design of solid-state detector used lithium-drifted germanium [Ge(Li)] as the detection medium. The lithium served to inhibit trapping of charge at impurity sites in the crystal lattice during the charge collection process. Hyperpure germanium (HPGe) crystals were then used with no further doping, and detector operation became more simple. Cooling is one drawback of HPGe detector but serves to reduce thermal excitations of valence electrons. This makes the incident gamma radiation provide the energy necessary for the electrons to cross the band gap and reach the conduction band.

Recently, cadmium telluride (CdTe) and cadmium zinc telluride (CdZnTe or CZT) started to be used as solid-state detector in SPECT modalities as well as in prototype PET scanners. The former has density of 6.06 g/cm^3 and atomic number Z of 48. CZT is CdTe in which some of the Te atoms (typically 20 %) are replaced by zinc atoms. Average energy expended per electron-hole pair created is 4.4 eV, while the ionization energy for dry air is 34 eV. These measures make this type of detectors amenable

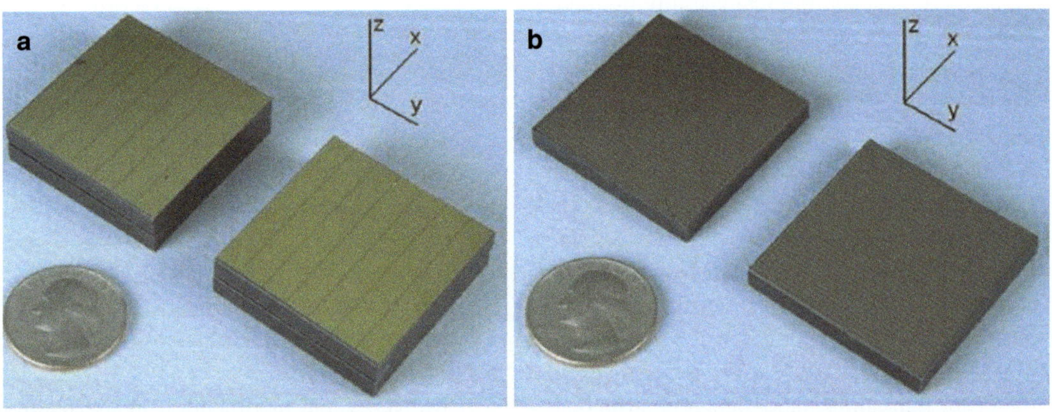

Fig. 1.23 Cross-strip of CZT detector with dimensions 4×4 mm×0.5 mm, cathode (**a**) and anode (**b**) (Reprinted from Gu et al. [20] with permission)

for good stopping efficiency against gamma radiations. In addition, it is featured by room temperature operation without excessive electronic noise. Due to some manufacturing limitations and cost-related issues, the use of CdTe and CZT is confined to small-sized counters or imaging systems, such as micro-PET imaging systems.

In small animal PET, the aim of CZT scanners is to improve system spatial resolution achieving almost 1 mm with recent submillimetre resolution in experimental setup using very small pitch pixelated detector. In general, the spatial resolution of a pixelated CZT detector is limited by the anode pixel size. In addition, the spatial resolution is also affected by the charge sharing between the neighbouring anode pixels that collect the electrons created after gamma ray interactions. Also, one of the major challenges in using pixelated CZT detectors is to read out the large number of channels of anode signals with high accuracy and efficiency.

CZT-based PET detector with 4 cm thickness introduces intrinsic detection efficiency exceeding 86 % for single 511 keV photons (>73 % for coincidence photons). Furthermore, CZT detector has superior energy resolution better than 3 % full width at half maximum at 511 keV. This feature allows one to design a system with significant reduction of scattered radiation, random events and better accuracy of event localization. However, the major drawback of CZT detector as PET detector is the poor timing performance due to variability in charge movement. Figure 1.23 shows cross-strip CZT detector.

References and Further Reading

1. Evans RD. The atomic nucleus. McGraw-Hill, New York; 1955.
2. Cherry SR, Sorenson JA, Phelps ME, editors. Physics in nuclear medicine. 4th ed. Philadelphia: W.B. Saunders; 2012.
3. Martin James E. Physics for radiation protection. 2nd ed. Weinheim: Wiley-VCH Verlag GmbH & Co. KGaA; 2006.
4. Khalil MM, editor. Basic sciences of nuclear medicine. Heidelberg/Dordrecht/London/New York: Springer; 2011.
5. Ahmed Syed N. Physics and engineering of radiation detection. Britain: Elsevier; 2007. ISBN 13: 978-0-12-045581-2.
6. Freeman LM, Biersack H-J, editors. Clinical nuclear medicine. Germany: Springer; 2007. 24/3150-543210.
7. Sharp PF, Gemmell HG, Murray AD, editors. Practical Nuclear Medicine. 3rd ed. Oxford University/Verlag/ London: Springer; 2005.
8. IAEA human health reports No.5. Status of computed tomography dosimetry for wide cone beam scanners. 2011.
9. AAPM REPORT NO. 181; The selection, use, calibration, and quality assurance of radionuclide calibrators used in nuclear medicine. Report of AAPM Task Group 181. 2012.
10. Madsen MT, Anderson JA, Halama JR, Kleck J, et al. AAPM Task Group 108: PET and PET/CT shielding requirements. Med Phys. 2006;33(1):4–15.
11. Mohr PJ, Taylor BN, Newell DB. CODATA recommended values of the fundamental physical constants: 2010. NIST.2012. p. 1–94.
12. Pillai MR, Dash A, Knapp Jr FF. Sustained availability of 99mTc: possible paths forward. J Nucl Med. 2013;54:313–23.
13. IPSM. Radiation protection in nuclear medicine and pathology. In: KE Goldstone, PC Jackson, MJ Myers, AE Simpson, editors. Report No 63, York: Institute of Physical Sciences in Medicine; 1991.
14. Saha GB. Fundamentals of nuclear pharmacy. 6th ed. New York/Heidelberg/Dordrecht/London: Springer; 2010.
15. Shankar V, editor. Molecular imaging: radiopharmaceuticals for PET and SPECT. Dordrecht/Heidelberg London/New York: Springer; 2009. ISBN 978-3-540-76734-3.
16. Basdevant JL, Rich J, Michel S. Fundamentals in nuclear physics. New York: Springer Science + Business Media, Inc.; 2004.
17. Sarah K, editor. Passive nondestructive assay of nuclear materials. Nuclear Regulatory Commission, Washington U.S., Springfield; 1991.
18. Dewan L. Design and construction of a cyclotron capable to accelerating protons to 2 MeV. Massachusetts Institute of Technology, Department of Nuclear Science and Engineering; 2007.
19. Friesel DL, Antaya TA. Medical cyclotrons. Cambridge: Massachusetts Institute of Technology; 2007.
20. Gu Y, Matteson JL, Skelton RT, Deal AC, Stephan EA, et al. Study of a high-resolution, 3D positioning cadmium zinc telluride detector for PET. Phys Med Biol. 2011;56:1563–84.
21. Baumann T. Minicourse on experimental techniques at the NSCL neutron detection & spectroscopy. National Superconducting Cyclotron Laboratory. Michigan State University, East Lansing, Michigan; 2001.
22. Smith DS, Stabin MG. Exposure rate constants and lead shielding values for over 1,100 radionuclides. Health Phys. 2012;102(3):271–91.
23. Podgorsak EB. Radiation physics for medical physicists. Germany: Springer; 2006.

2 Radiation Safety and CT Dosimetry in PET/CT Imaging

Debbie Peet and Sue Edyvean

Contents

2.1 **Introduction** 37

2.2 **Facility Design** 38
2.2.1 Shielding Calculations 40
2.2.2 Staff Exposure 42
2.2.3 Optimisation: Fixtures, Fittings and Accessories 43

2.3 **Staff Dose and Optimisation** 44

2.4 **CT Technology** 46
2.4.1 Basic Technology 46
2.4.2 Technology Developments 47
2.4.3 Factors Affecting Dose in CT Scanning 48
2.4.4 Dose Metrics in CT 49
2.4.5 Diagnostic Reference Levels (DRLs) and Optimisation in CT 59
2.4.6 Doses for Attenuation Scans and Whole-Body Scans in PET/CT 61
2.4.7 Quality Control of CT Scanners 61

Conclusions 62

References 63

Abstract

Some of the particular radiation safety challenges associated with PET/CT are described for those more familiar with working in conventional nuclear medicine departments. Facility design and shielding calculations are described and examples given. Challenges in keeping doses to the staff and public down are described with some of the approaches to keeping doses as low as reasonably achievable. Computed tomography (CT) technology and dose metrics are described in some detail, and some guidance on quality control checks and patient dose in CT and PET/CT is given with references to sources of information on these topics in this rapidly changing field.

2.1 Introduction

Nuclear medicine departments have historically been designed and operated with consideration of the workflow through the department and local shielding of sources and radioactive material. Less consideration of any structural shielding within the facility has been made in the past.

For traditional nuclear medicine studies, radionuclides are generally administered in the

D. Peet, MSc (✉)
University Hospitals of Leicester, Leicester, UK
e-mail: debbie.peet@nhs.net

S. Edyvean, MSc
Public Health England, Chilton, UK
e-mail: sue.edyvean@phc.gov.uk

M.M. Khalil (ed.), *Basic Science of PET Imaging*, DOI 10.1007/978-3-319-40070-9_2

department. Patients are then encouraged to leave the department during the uptake phase to both improve the uptake of the radiopharmaceutical and to minimise the radiation risk to the staff and the public from the gamma radiation emitted from the patient.

It was accepted practice for the staff to be in the same room as the patient during the scan on a gamma camera. The introduction of new technology in the form of SPECT/CT has caused a change to this approach, and it is now an accepted practice to have a separate shielded control room to protect the operator from the CT radiation scattered from the patient. It can also be seen from the whole-body monitoring data that this approach reduces staff exposure.

SPECT/CT has also required the nuclear medicine staff to learn new skills and acquire new knowledge around CT operation, dosimetry and quality control techniques. These will be covered later in this chapter.

PET/CT is different from conventional nuclear medicine. The energy of the gamma ray is higher, and patients spend longer in the department, thereby irradiating the staff to potentially significant levels.

The 511 keV gamma rays emitted as the electrons and positrons annihilate are more penetrating than the 140 keV gamma ray emitted by technetium-99 m (Tc-99m). The energy is the same for all radionuclides used, e.g. fluorine-18 (F-18) and carbon-11 (C-11). The half-lives of the different radionuclides can vary [1]. F-18 is most readily available and has a half-life of 110 min so that the radiopharmaceutical can be distributed some distance and travelling time from the point of manufacture. This means that PET/CT scanners can be installed in hospitals across a region with access to a single cyclotron.

The radionuclide is attached to a pharmaceutical as in conventional nuclear medicine. F-18 is commonly used as the radiolabel with FDG, although new agents are being introduced [2]. FDG is taken up in tissues in a similar way to glucose, and whilst it seemed a promising agent in neurological imaging, it is now widely used in tumour imaging for diagnosis, staging and monitoring of treatment.

As the uptake phase duration for this agent is typically 60 min and patients must rest in a quiet, warm environment to minimise uptake in muscles and then undergo a scan taking typically 20 min, the design of PET/CT facilities for F-18 FDG imaging has been a challenge to those used to conventional nuclear medicine.

This chapter will therefore consider some of the issues around this work that may be less familiar to those working in conventional nuclear medicine:

- Facility design
- Shielding calculations
- Staff exposure
- Optimisation of radiation protection in practice – fixtures fittings and accessories
- Optimisation of radiation protection in practice – staff dose
- CT technology
- Dosimetric quantities in CT
- Patient dose in CT
- CT quality control checks
- Patient dose in PET/CT

The patient flow through a PET/CT facility depends on the radiopharmaceutical, its form and means of administration (some are gaseous), the uptake phase, scan phase and discharge. The examples in this chapter will concentrate on F-18 FDG, but the principles can be extrapolated to other agents.

2.2 Facility Design

Standard building materials and hospital construction techniques may not provide sufficient protection for PET/CT facilities. The attenuation required may be greater than that afforded by brick or block construction, and scatter from the CT element of the test may require some shielding up to the underside of the soffit of the floor above; floors and ceilings may not afford sufficient protection from either the 511 keV gamma rays or the CT radiation.

The design of any facility should involve many professionals who have expertise in their individual areas – architects, estate experts, structural engineers, mechanical and electrical engineers, patient representatives and project managers. Input from clinical staff similarly needs to be multidisciplinary so that the patients can be at the centre of the design but that workflow and radiation safety can also be optimised at the design stage.

Input from the equipment suppliers can also help and inform the process. A number of factors are required to be assessed to enable a design to be developed:

1. Workload – patient numbers and examination types. This will dictate the number of uptake bays.
2. Location – space is usually allocated or set by the boundaries of a building. This may limit the size of the facility. Space constraints are a common issue.
3. Potential future developments – consideration of these may be needed to enable new techniques to be adopted. For some facilities this may be less important, and an efficient throughput may be the overriding design consideration.
4. Equipment specification – this will inform the choice of scanner room size, floor loadings, electrical provision, etc. Quality control phantoms and sources should also be considered within this space.
5. Preparation room – a good ergonomic design will improve workflow and help with staff morale. This room may or may not include an area/uptake for waste and a spill kit.
6. Administration areas – privacy and dignity should be considered alongside the workflow and safety issues.
7. Consultation rooms might be considered. The patient consent process can be lengthy and might result in lower staff dose if this area is not close to the uptake areas.
8. Discharge – consideration might be required for patient refreshment after the scan or for those who need to wait for transport away from the facility. The patient will still have some residual activity and be a radiation hazard.
9. WC – a hot toilet will be required. Staff and/or visitor facilities should also be considered.
10. Other facilities – office space, staff rest areas and changing facilities, storage, etc. These are sometimes overlooked at the design stage and will be difficult to incorporate later.
11. Injectors – if injectors [3, 4] and/or automatic dispensers are to be or may be used, then consideration at the design stage is recommended.
12. Patient flow (see Fig. 2.1) – the processes that are undertaken as the patient moves through the facility, the situations when shielding or other operational procedures are needed to minimise dose can help with the design. Flow of radioactive material can be considered in a similar way.

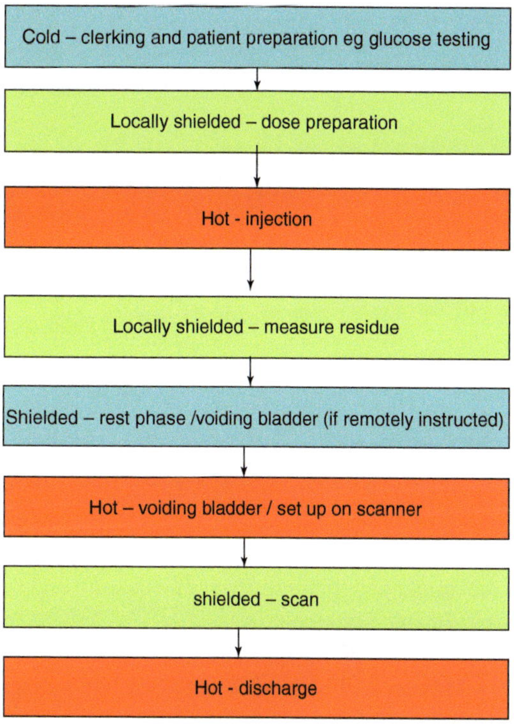

Fig. 2.1 Patient flow through the facility, highlighting hot, cold and shielded stages, and colour coded in proportion to the hazard

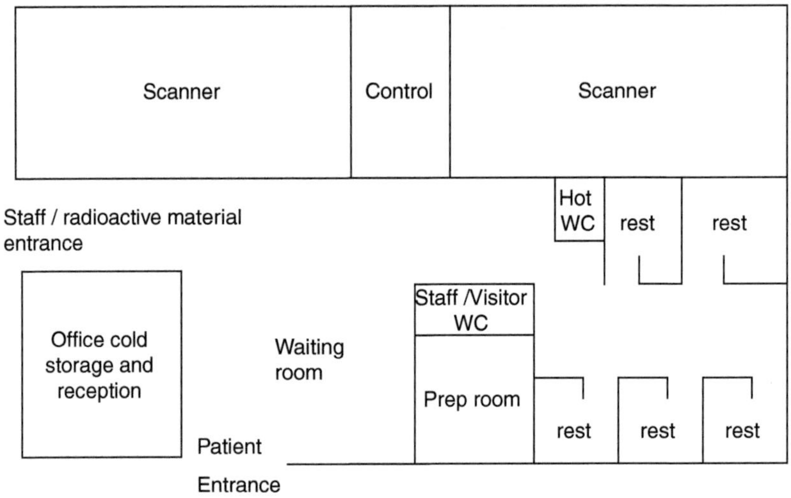

Fig. 2.2 An example of a well-designed facility

Consideration of the following points is recommended to minimise staff exposure and the cost of shielding materials:

1. Maximise the distance between hot patients and staff/members of the public.
2. Eliminate lines of sight between uptake bays and the operator console of the scanner (CCTV and intercoms can be built in cost-effectively at the design stage).
3. Use suitable local shielding for stock vials, syringes, waste, etc.
4. Consider the use of remote injectors and/or dispensers.
5. Consider the handling of QC sources.

The basic hazards to consider are:

- External dose rate hazard
- Contamination
- Emergency situations, e.g. a dropped vial

Standard radiation protection principles should be applied, i.e.:

- Distance
- Shielding
- Time

The inverse square law is very powerful and can dramatically reduce the level of shielding required.

Figure 2.2 shows a facility where there are no direct lines of sight between the rest bays and the control room where staff will spend most of their working time, i.e. there is always a barrier (which may be a wall) between the patient and the areas where staff spend significant periods of time. The preparation room is close to the rest bays and under supervision by staff in the control room and/or the office. The distance from the rest bays to high occupancy areas is maximised which will reduce the required shielding and minimise building costs. The hot WC(s) is/are close to the rest bays.

For maximum throughput with a single scanner, a minimum of three uptake bays are required. New scanners could increase throughput (or use reduced administered activity) which could impact on this choice.

Figure 2.3 shows a more challenging layout adopted on a number of mobile scanners, where staff in the control room are irradiated by patients in the uptake room and the scanner. The shielding required in this situation is much higher than for the facility in Fig. 2.2.

Further examples of design and layout are given in a number of publications [3, 5–8].

2.2.1 Shielding Calculations

Once the layout is established, shielding calculations are required to specify the thickness of

Fig. 2.3 Common layout for a mobile PET/CT scanner

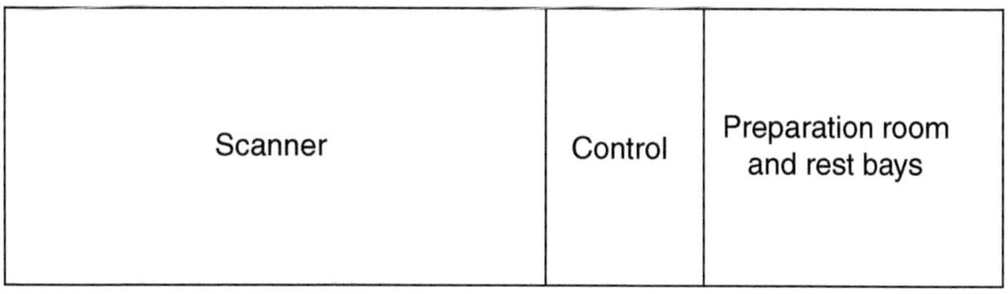

Table 2.1 Limiting TVLs for lead and concrete

Material	Limiting TVL (mm)
Lead	15
Concrete (density 2350 kg/m^3)	150

Table 2.2 Typical transmission factors for building materials

Thickness and material	Transmission F-18
2.24 mm Pb	0.738
4½″ brick	0.03
9″ brick	0.09
100 mm breeze block	0.66
100 mm solid concrete block	0.27
200 mm poured concrete	0.046

barriers around the facility. The choice of building/shielding material may be clear – but should be established.

Common bricks and blocks may be the cheapest materials to use, although some contractors prefer poured concrete. Lead may be the only solution particularly for mobile vans. As some barriers may have a considerable thickness (up to 300 mm poured concrete), this may impact on the design/space requirements. The attenuation properties of common shielding materials can be found in AAPM Report 108 and the BIR report on shielding in diagnostic x-ray [5, 6]. A simple methodology using limiting tenth value layers (TVLs) is used below. The values for lead and concrete are shown in Table 2.1.

The TVL for other materials such as concrete blocks can be extrapolated using the ratio of physical density, e.g. 176 mm for concrete blocks with density 2000 kg/m^3.

Typical transmission factors for common materials are shown in Table 2.2.

The air kerma rate immediately postinjection of 370 MBq of F-18 FDG has been reported to be 45 μGyh^{-1} at 1 m [9]. There is some self-absorption within the patient of over 30 % from the air kerma rate quoted [1]. Table 2.3 shows the instantaneous dose rates through typical barriers and shielding materials in diagnostic facilities.

It should be noted that for planning purposes, a lower value is used to include a correction for radioactive decay and for excretion during the procedure.

The following examples of layouts and shielding calculations will concentrate on F-18-FDG scanning assuming an administration of 370 MBq, a rest phase of 1 h and a scan time of 20 min.

The following should be established to enable the calculations to be performed:

1. Workload – this will dictate the time a hazard is present in a particular area, e.g. uptake bays, scanner and discharge area.

   At worst all uptake bays and the scanner might be occupied 100 % of the time.
2. Dose constraint – this is typically 0.3 mSv per annum to members of the public and 1 mSv to staff. Note it may be difficult to achieve 1 mSv to the staff in a mobile design [10]. It should be noted that the staff will also receive dose from their contact with patients during injection, set-up and discharge. Total dose per annum for a high throughput of patients can approach 6 mSv, so it is important to minimise the dose that the staff receive through the facility design.
3. Calculation points – areas where staff or members of the public may spend time or become close to patients:
   - Control room
   - Offices
   - Rest rooms
   - Areas above or below the facility
   - Corridors
   - Clinic rooms

Table 2.3 Instantaneous dose rate at 1 m from an injected patient through typical barriers

Thickness and material	Instantaneous dose rate postinjection (μGy/h)
2.24 mm Pb	33.2
4½″ brick	13.7
9″ brick	4.1
100 mm breeze block	29.8
100 mm solid concrete block	12.2
200 mm poured concrete	2.1

Occupancy in these areas will need to be estimated. Some common occupancy factors are described in the BIR publication [5] with a range quoted to enable local knowledge of the use of the area to be applied. The minimum occupancy that is recommended to be applied is 5 % for car parks and other transiently occupied areas. Corridors may be between 10 and 20 %, but if it is known that a corridor is very rarely used, a factor of 5 % could be applied. Potential changes in the use of such areas in the future needs to be considered particularly if a low occupancy factor is applied. The distance between the source and the calculation points should be assessed.

The following dose rates can be used for planning purposes. They include integrating the initial instantaneous dose rate over the 1 h uptake phase and include a factor for evacuation of the bladder and decay over a 20 min scan [5]:

- 37 μGyh^{-1} at 1 m for the uptake phase
- 24 μGyh^{-1} at 1 m for the scan phase

The values are slightly more conservative than those quoted by the AAPM [6].

The barrier thickness is calculated by considering the critical points around a room such as the uptake bay. If the adjacent room is an office which is occupied 100 % of the time, and the critical point, e.g. the office chair, is 2 m from the centre of the rest bed:

- Using this distance from the patient – 2 m.
- Air kerma rate at 1 m from the patient is 37 μGy/h.
- The kerma rate corrected for distance is 9.25 μGy/h.
- The dose per annum (over 2000 h) is 18.5 mSv.
- The chosen constraint is 0.3 mSv.
- The attenuation factor (AF) or transmission required is no more than 0.3/18.5 or 0.02.
- The number of TVLs to attenuate to this factor is $\log_{10}(1/AF)$.
- Therefore, 1.79 TVLs are required, i.e. 270 mm concrete or 30 mm lead.

This can be repeated many times over to look at all critical points around the facility. Some centres choose to look at the worst-case point and apply that barrier thickness to the whole room to minimise the chance of mistakes during construction.

However, individuals are likely to be irradiated from more than one source, and the doses from all should be considered and summed [5]. If the approach above is used, the dose constraint could be divided between all sources, or an iterative approach using different wall thicknesses to share the dose burden more equally can be used. A number of authors have described different approaches [11–13].

The resultant required wall thickness can vary, but 300 mm concrete will almost always be adequate. This is to protect persons around the facility and will normally only be required to be a height of 2200 mm above finished floor level. Areas above and below may need some consideration.

CT scatter requires shielding to the underside of the soffit [5]. This might be most cost-effectively achieved by fitting a minimum of 1.3 mm lead above the walls to the soffit. The walls below this height will normally be thicker than this to protect from the gamma rays. Consideration needs to be given to air conditioning and other service access into the room. The penetrations can be large and often in the worst place from a radiation protection perspective, e.g. over the doors, which is often the place where scatter is highest.

2.2.2 Staff Exposure

Staff exposure is potentially high as can be seen by the shielding calculations above. The member of the public dose limit is exceeded with 12 h at a metre from a patient during the uptake phase. Whole-body personal monitoring is recommended.

Finger dose can be exceptionally high with 500 mSv being reached within 3 h at a distance of 100 mm from a stock vial containing 10 GBq of activity. The inverse square law breaks down at closer distances, but it is clear that shielding and good technique are required. Finger dose monitoring is recommended for all staff manipulating radioactive sources in PET.

Eye doses may need to be considered in the light of the new dose limits [14] if whole-body doses are very high, but recent publications suggest that with adequate controls, dose limits should not be approached. However, radiation dose management in all hybrid imaging especially PET/CT can be a concern [15]. Direct reading dosemeters can be very useful devices to look at daily dose, to set alarms for staff who stand close to patients and can be used as an aid to audit.

2.2.3 Optimisation: Fixtures, Fittings and Accessories

Optimisation in terms of radiation protection is about keeping doses as low as reasonably achievable. The external dose rate hazard and the contamination risk both need to be considered. For the external dose rate hazard, the basic principles of operation in radiation protection apply:

- Distance
- Shielding
- Time

Distance is a powerful measure as the inverse square law comes into play. The basic design and layout can be used to maximise the distance between patients and staff, but there are times when staff need to be close to sources and the patient. The greatest hazard is from the stock vial which will need to be unpacked and measured. This could typically hold 10–80 GBq of activity. Simple handling tools can be used to maximise the distance between finger tips and the source

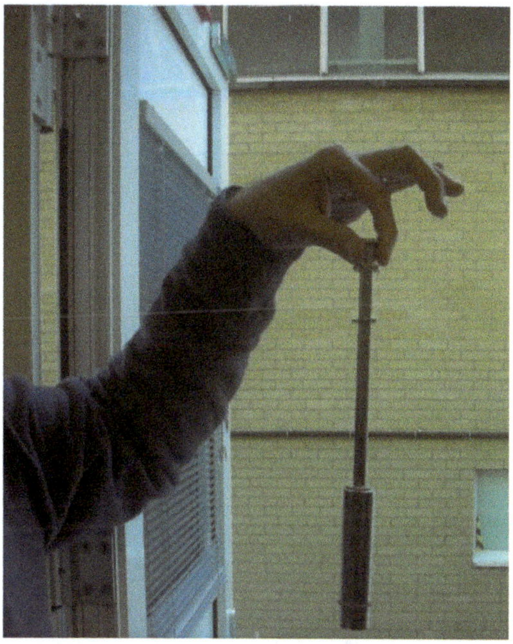

Fig. 2.4 Long-handled tool for handling stock vial

(Fig. 2.4). Long-handled forceps and other devices commonly used in nuclear medicine or radiotherapy can also be used.

The vial is generally placed into a dispensing unit which incorporates thick shielding (Fig. 2.5) and is designed to minimise exposure.

Automatic dispensing units are also commercially available and might be worth considering in high-throughput units. It is common practice to sink the dose calibrator into the preparation bench and to have a route to drop waste into a shielded waste bin. Bench top shields are recommended to protect the body and the eyes (Fig. 2.6).

All this local shielding is thicker than conventionally used in nuclear medicine. The weight may also need to be considered. Entry and exit portal monitors need careful consideration to eliminate background and to ensure contamination is not spread.

Plastic scintillators are used to detect beta emissions from the radionuclide although the gamma emissions are sufficient that some conventional sensitive scintillators may be adequate for contamination monitoring [16]. Storage and handling of sources used for quality control need

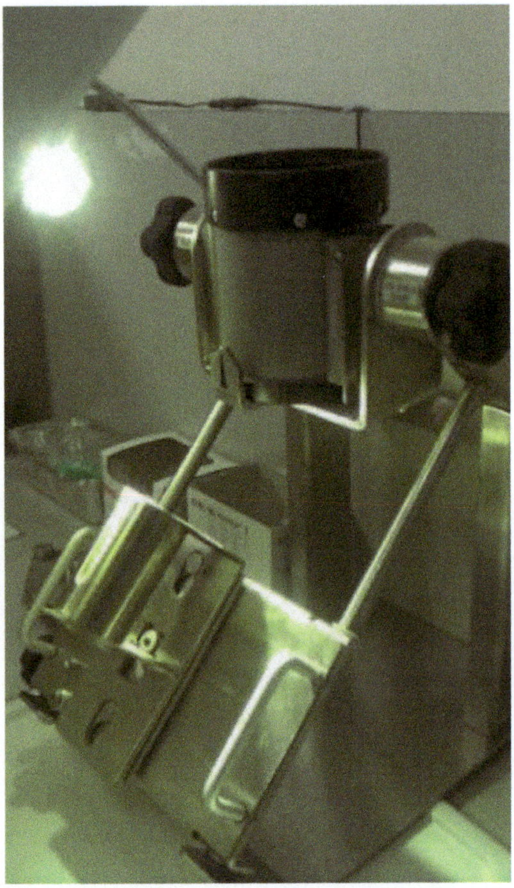

Fig. 2.5 Heavily shielded manual dispensing unit to hold the stock vial

to be considered. Sources should always be handled at the opposite end from where the activity is sited. Once doses have been dispensed, a syringe shield is required and the injection should be carried in a shielded box (Fig. 2.7).

There has been some debate as to whether Perspex or tungsten syringe shields reduce finger dose more effectively, but it is generally accepted that tungsten is more effective [17]. All syringe shields are bigger and more bulky than conventional shields, and staff should be initially trained to manipulate the radionuclide with inactive solutions. All surfaces must be easy to clean and decontaminate, flooring should be smooth without joints and cover up the wall and there needs to be space for decontamination kits and materials.

Risk assessments are essential to assess the level of protection required. High workload departments may need more automated accessories to keep doses low.

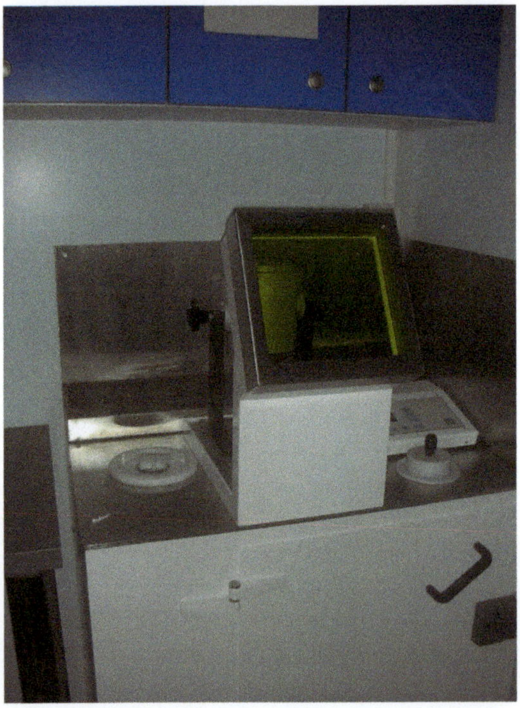

Fig. 2.6 Dispensing unit with bench top shield, sunken calibrator and waste route into shielded cupboard

Contingency plans must be prepared for all obvious problems – fire, flood, theft and contamination. The action to be taken in the event of a stock vial being broken or a single injection being dropped should be known and understood by all staff involved. Contingency plans should be practised. All staff should be experienced in clearing spills, but for training purposes, inactive materials should be used.

2.3 Staff Dose and Optimisation

Once the service is operational, further optimisation of doses is likely to be possible as staff become familiar with processes and local practices.

If the total whole-body dose results for all staff are plotted over time against the number of patients through the system graphs, such in Fig. 2.8 might be observed. This shows that as the

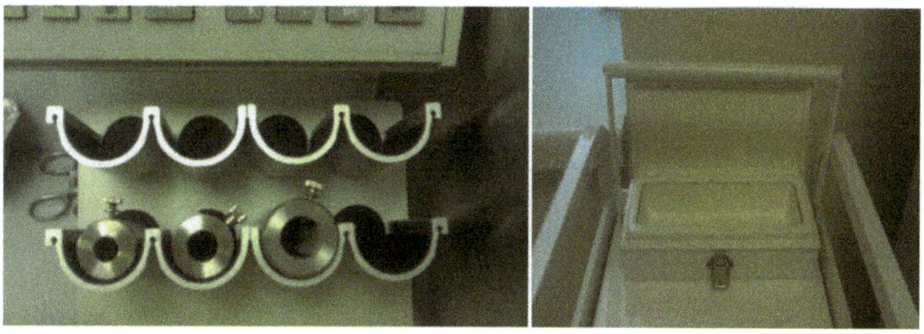

Fig. 2.7 Syringe shields and carrying boxes for individual injections

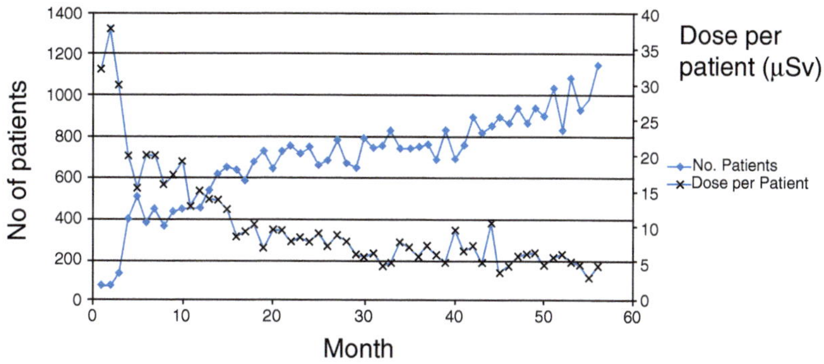

Fig. 2.8 Staff dose over time against increasing workload (Courtesy of InHealth Ltd)

workload increases, so does dose efficiency which plateaus out eventually.

The use of electronic personal dosemeters is advocated to monitor and help minimise dose for the whole procedure and individual parts of the procedure. A number of studies have been published showing the average dose per patient [18–22]. For a 370 MBq injection, the total dose per patient has been reported to be between 3.3 and 9.2 μSv.

Careful measurement of the doses recorded on electronic personal dosemeters can show the dose received during each stage of the process [22] as shown in Fig. 2.9.

Review of doses for individual members of staff can show that the doses vary by up to a factor of 5, giving further opportunity for optimisation and staff training. The opportunity to reduce these doses using automatic dispensers and injectors has been mooted [4]. There is some published data to suggest they can be successful, but it must be remembered they are in no way a substitute for excellent radiation protection in practice. Another tool advocated is to show areas where doses might be high within a facility – highlighting hot spots and

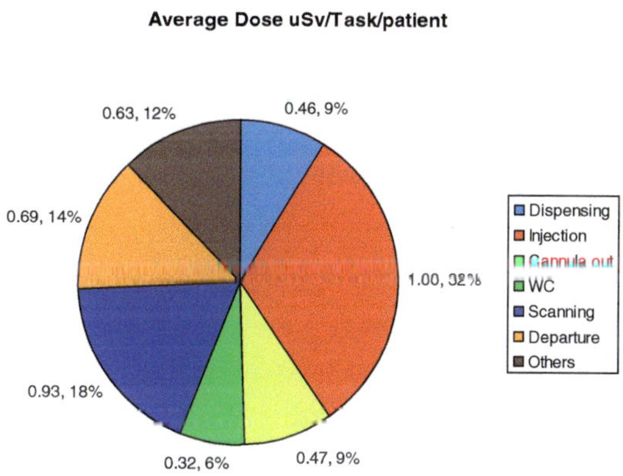

Fig. 2.9 Average dose for each part of the procedure (Republished with permission of British Institute of Radiology, from Peet et al. [22])

the safest places to spend time as shown in Fig. 2.10 [22].

It should also be noted that optimisation is an ongoing process. Success in reducing doses and keeping them at that level requires constant vigilance. The modality whilst having exciting clinical potential needs particular care around staff and public safety – finger doses and whole-body doses can be high and could without care approach dose limits.

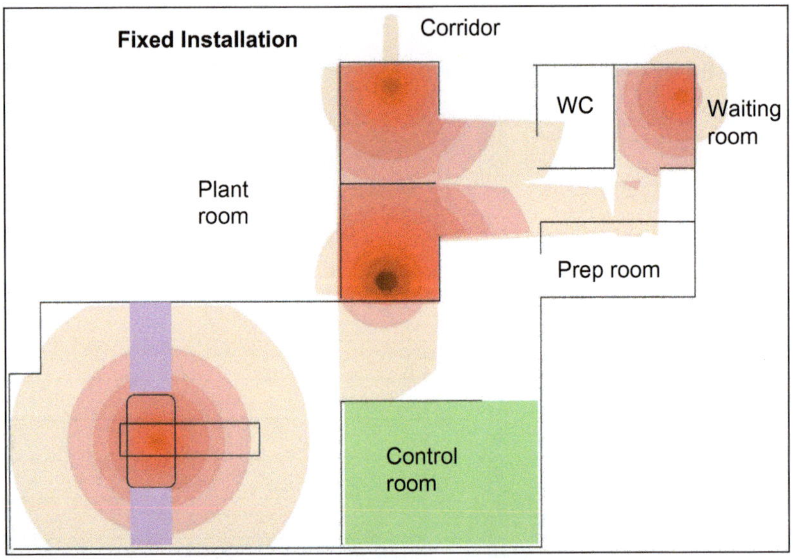

Fig. 2.10 Instantaneous dose rates plotted through the facility (Republished with permission of British Institute of Radiology, from Peet et al. [22])

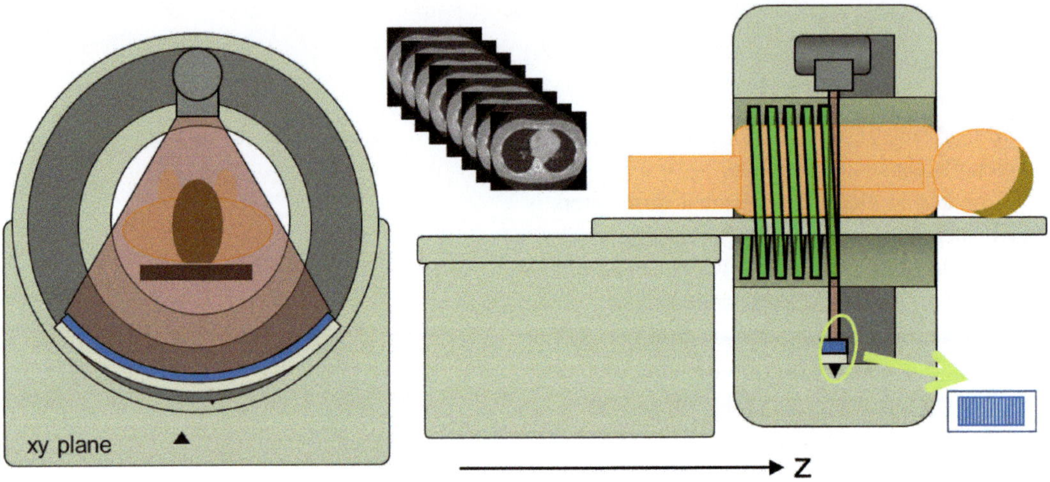

Fig. 2.11 Cross-sectional and lateral view of the CT scanner, with resultant images (Courtesy ImPACT)

2.4 CT Technology

2.4.1 Basic Technology

A CT scanner consists of a rotating gantry, a couch and an operator's console. The gantry, within an external housing, consists of an x-ray tube diametrically opposite to an arc of detectors, usually described as a detector row or rows. The whole construction rotates around a central point in space (the isocentre).

The patient lies on the couch whilst the x-ray tube and detectors are rotated around the patient, the x-ray source is activated for a scan and the detectors record the transmission of the x-ray beam through the patient. During this process, the couch can either be stationary, and the x-rays are switched off whilst the couch moves to the next position; this is called axial scanning. Alternatively the couch can be set to move continuously along the patient long axis, usually called the z-axis (Fig. 2.11), and this is called helical or spiral scanning.

The transmission data from the x-ray beam, attenuated by the patient, is collected by the detectors from many angles around the patient, and using either computerised 'back projection' or 'iterative' processes, a cross-sectional image of the patient is reconstructed.

The cross-sectional image presents maps of the x-ray attenuation properties of the tissues and organs. This can be used in PET/CT scanning to correct the PET image for the attenuation of the 511 keV gamma ray – known as attenuation scanning. This is in addition to the capability for anatomical localisation, as well as fully diagnostic anatomical information which can be acquired with or without contrast injection.

The exposure factors required for an accurate correction of attenuation are generally lower than those required for full diagnostic scanning where a less noisy image might be required. The dose the patient receives is related to these exposure factors, and this section describes the dose indices in common usage in CT and their relationship to effective dose (E).

2.4.2 Technology Developments

CT scanning has undergone many design changes since its inception. The introduction in 1985 of slip rings to transfer power and data, subsequently enabling helical scanning, could be regarded as a significant milestone and perhaps signals the design of modern scanners. In addition, since then, there have been numerous significant technological advances, and some of these need to be outlined to gain an understanding of the current dose indices.

It is not commonly remembered that the very first CT scanners in 1972 were dual-slice scanners, but this approach was very quickly dropped with a change in gantry design, and the single-slice design continued until 1991. Since then, over a period of 15 years, rapid developments in scanner technology have resulted in the transition from dual slice through 8, 16 and 64 'slice' and, in recent years, 320 detector row scanners.

Scanners are usually discussed, and sold, with respect to the competitive number of 'slices' that can be imaged in a single rotation. However, this can be extremely misleading. Any particular scanner model may reconstruct fewer (on older scanners) or more (on newer scanners) image slices per rotation than the number of detector rows. For example, an old 16-slice scanner may have 24 detector rows – the limitation at the time of their introduction being in terms of processing, cost of construction of thin detector elements and reconstruction capacity. Conversely a newer '64-slice' scanner may have 32 detector rows, a '640 slice' may have 320 rows or a '512 slice' 256 rows. This greater slice capability at a finer spacing than the actual detector rows is due to modern techniques in reconstruction and can be regarded as overlapping image slices. In terms of speed of coverage, therefore it is far more meaningful to categorise a scanner by the number of detector rows and the length of coverage along the patient axis by the whole detector bank, with consideration being given to the number of image slices acquired simultaneously (Fig. 2.12).

The time taken to undertake any particular examination scan is now shorter due to faster tube rotation times, longer detector arrays and more detector rows along the z-axis. Tube rotation times per revolution have been reduced to less than 0.5 s (of the order of 0.3 s to enable cardiac imaging). This together with the greater number of detector rows, and helical scanning, removes the need for breath-hold imaging in many circumstances. A large volume of the patient can therefore be scanned in a relatively short period of time (e.g. 20 s for the chest abdomen and pelvis). Radiation exposure must become a consideration both in terms of equipment design and operation of the scanner.

Image reconstruction has progressed from analytical filtered back projection methods to statistical iterative reconstruction techniques. On most modern scanners, both approaches are available. By the efficient use of the x-ray attenuation information, iterative techniques reduce image noise. Whilst this gives improved image quality, it also alternatively presents the operator an opportunity to lower the tube current (thus reducing the radiation dose), in order to restore the noise to the original level which had

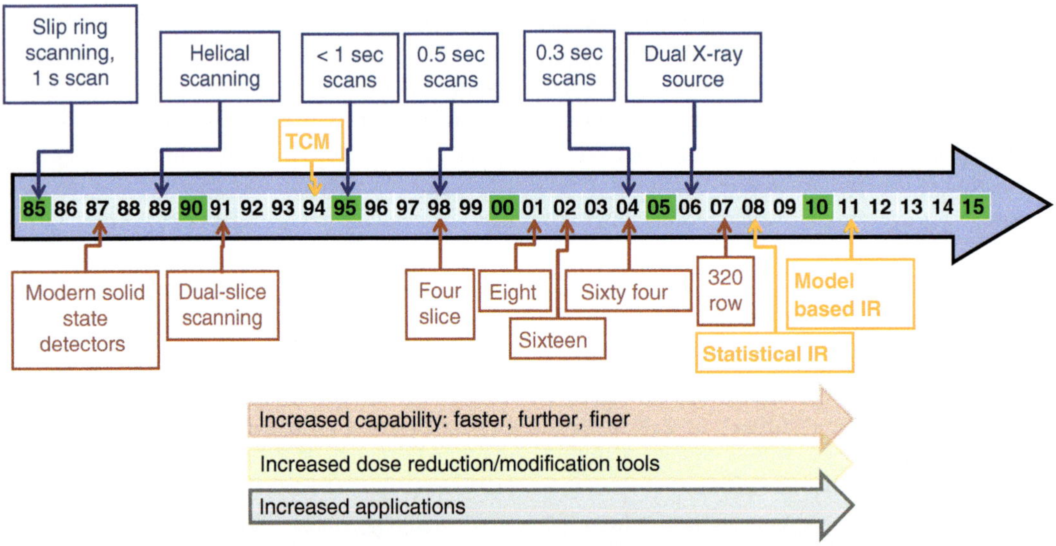

Fig. 2.12 CT technological advances 1985–2014

previously been accepted as suitable. A good description of CT technology and its evolution can be found in Kalendar's book [23].

2.4.3 Factors Affecting Dose in CT Scanning

The key parameters that affect patient (organ) dose are those that influence the photons delivered from the x-ray tube. Primarily therefore this is the tube voltage (kV), the tube current (mA) and the rotation time for one revolution(s).

There are also hardware features which are often built into the scan protocol, such as the x-ray beam-shaping filter which relates to patient body part (head or body) scanned (and sometimes patient size), and the x-ray tube focal spot which may be automatically adjusted according to tube current and imaged slice thickness.

In addition image reconstruction features may indirectly affect the dose. For example, the tube current may be set higher for a thinner reconstructed slice to allow enough photons for the required image quality. Reconstruction algorithms will affect the image noise, which also may require adjustment of the tube current.

The pitch in helical scanning may affect the dose, with a longer pitch reducing the average dose along the patient length. However, often the tube current is changed automatically to compensate.

The total dose imparted to the patient is governed by the site-specific (organ) dose, as well as by the scan length. A relevant aspect for consideration in helical scanning is that the total length of irradiation will be slightly longer than the resultant imaged volume, due to the interpolation of data in order to create planar images. This is of special relevance for shorter scan volumes, especially with wider beam widths, where the proportional increase in dose may be significant or where the end of the imaged volume is near organs of particular concern.

Most of the major manufacturers now have a 'dynamic collimation' that automatically, in real time, closes off the beam at the trailing and forward edges of the helical irradiation, i.e. at the beginning and end of the scan run, respectively. This ensures that unnecessary radiation is eliminated whilst keeping the appropriate transmission information in order to reconstruct the first and last images. Wider beam widths have the advantage of less penumbra proportionately and also faster scanner of a volume. Dynamic collimators allow the use of wider beam widths without the penalty of extra irradiation at either end of the scan run.

Automatic exposure control (AEC) functions are available for all scanners. They operate by adjusting the tube current in order to attempt to match the tube x-ray output to the attenuation of the patient – adjusting according to the whole size, the relative rotational dimensions or along the patient long axis.

Each manufacturer initially developed one or more of these features, but now all have software packages to allow all three dimensions of automatic exposure control at once. These systems operate in different ways, either aiming to match the estimated patient image noise to a given noise value or adjusting the tube current compared to a reference patient size. To achieve this, either the attenuation data from one or two initial scan projection radiograph(s) is used or the attenuation information acquired by the detectors in the previous 180° rotation. Some allow the user to specify a maximum or minimum tube current in order to limit the extent of the modulation of the tube current.

The AEC features may increase or decrease the tube current depending on the set-up. On balance they are generally used to normalise the dose distribution to the patient, and also to reduce unnecessary dose, but they may not necessarily do this – depending on the specific way these features are used.

Tube voltage modulation is also available to adapt the tube voltage most suitably to the size of the patient, especially with iodine contrast agents where a lower tube voltage will produce a better contrast between tissue and the contrast agent. This feature as an automatic function (with selectable levels) is currently available from one manufacturer where the process can change both the tube voltage and the tube current. The dose will therefore be affected.

There are other features such as iterative reconstruction which do not affect the tube current and dose directly, but these may result in the use of a lower tube current to achieve the same image quality. Often iteratively reconstructed images can be produced at significantly reduced dose to achieve the same noise as filtered back projection images. Images constructed with iterative reconstruction may present a different texture to the noise than with filtered back projection and may also demonstrate different trends with changing tube current on the normal image quality performance parameters (noise and spatial resolution) than with filtered back projection.

The manufacturers have tended to develop two approaches to iterative reconstruction. There is usually a simple image-based iterative process which builds on the first filtered back projection image, and then more recently, others have been developed which operate on the raw data through modelling the focal spot and detector sizes, and these require more computing processes and can take longer.

All of these examples, of the effect of scan and reconstruction parameters on radiation dose, illustrate the need to record the exact scanner settings used in any given protocol when quoting dose values.

2.4.4 Dose Metrics in CT

A range of metrics are used in CT (as shown in Table 2.4) and require some understanding to enable manufacturer's information, and claims, to be understood and also to be able to make comments on their interpretation.

In CT a cross section of the whole body is irradiated in a single rotation, rather than at one angle and with an area limited by the collimator position as in projection radiography (Fig. 2.13).

Furthermore, the distribution of the dose is complicated by the rotation of the x-ray tube around, and movement of the table along, the *z*-axis, thereby irradiating a volume of tissue and organs within the patient.

Table 2.4 Standard generic dose metrics in CT

CT does parameters	
MSAD	Multiple scan average does
CTDI	Computed tomography dose index
DLP	Does length product
E	Effective dose
SSDE	Size-specific dose estimate

In the scan plane, for body scanning, the resultant dose at the centre of the irradiated volume may be half that at the periphery; however, the distribution tends to be more uniform in the head (Fig. 2.14).

Along the *z*-axis things are no less complicated. The dose profile for a single irradiation consists of the primary beam and scattered radiation beyond the nominal beam width (Fig. 2.15).

For an examination, whether with axial or helical scanning, these individual dose profiles combine to give a net irradiation profile along the *z*-axis. The extensive scattered tails of the single-slice dose profile contribute to give an average maximum value of the total volume dose profile which is usually greater than that of an individual slice, depending on the slice spacing. This is often called the multiple slice average dose (MSAD) (Fig. 2.16). Whilst this is not a commonly used term, it presents a very useful concept.

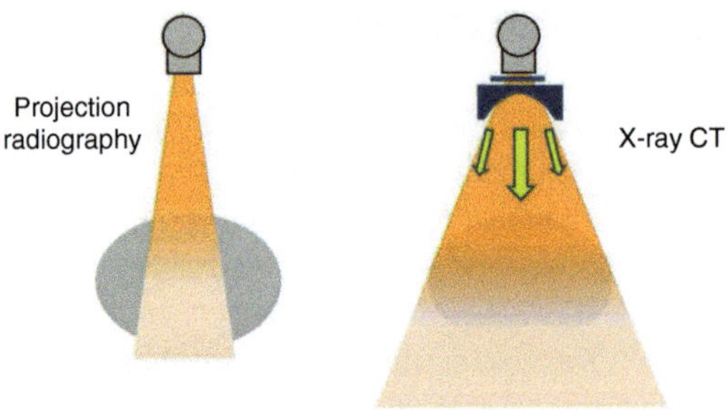

Fig. 2.13 Differences in dose distribution between conventional x-ray and CT – stationary beam (Courtesy ImPACT)

In helical scanning where the movement of the table, in one rotation of the tube, matches the beam width (pitch of 1), the dose pattern and transmission information are collected without any gaps along the *z*-axis. For faster relative table movement (a pitch greater than 1), or slower (a pitch less than 1), there will be subsequent gaps, or overlap, in the irradiation pattern along the *z*-axis. In all cases the data is interpolated to produce axial images.

The pitch also clearly has an impact on the average dose to the patient, with the average dose lower for higher pitch values, when other parameters such as the tube current remain the same. Many multi-slice scanners automatically adjust the tube current for changed pitch values, and in these situations, the dose remains constant.

The overall result of rotation and translation is a complex dose distribution as illustrated schematically in Fig. 2.17. The various dose indices have been developed to give simple approaches of measuring and expressing the average dose distribution.

2.4.4.1 Computed Tomography Dose Index (CTDI)

The CTDI is the standard dose index parameter used in CT. It is calculated from a single-slice measurement. It was originally designed to enable easy measurements to be made by a convenient method. Different forms of the CTDI have evolved with time and with scanner developments, and each depends on the specific use and application. A summary of the terminology for the current ones in use is given in Table 2.5.

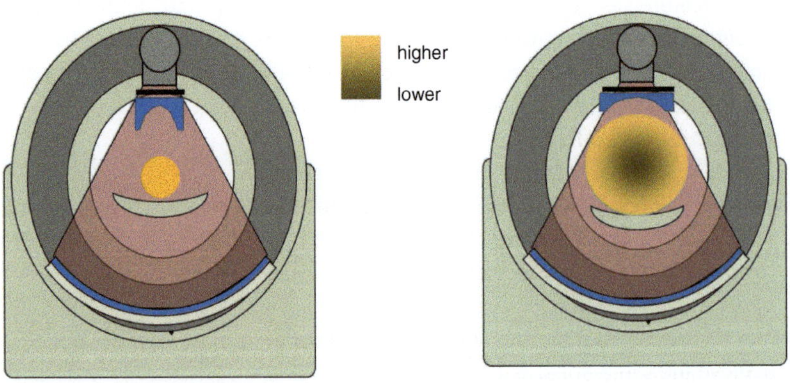

Fig. 2.14 Distribution of dose from a rotated beam – cross-sectional view. Periphery to centre ratio: head ~ 1:1, body ~ 2:1 (Courtesy ImPACT)

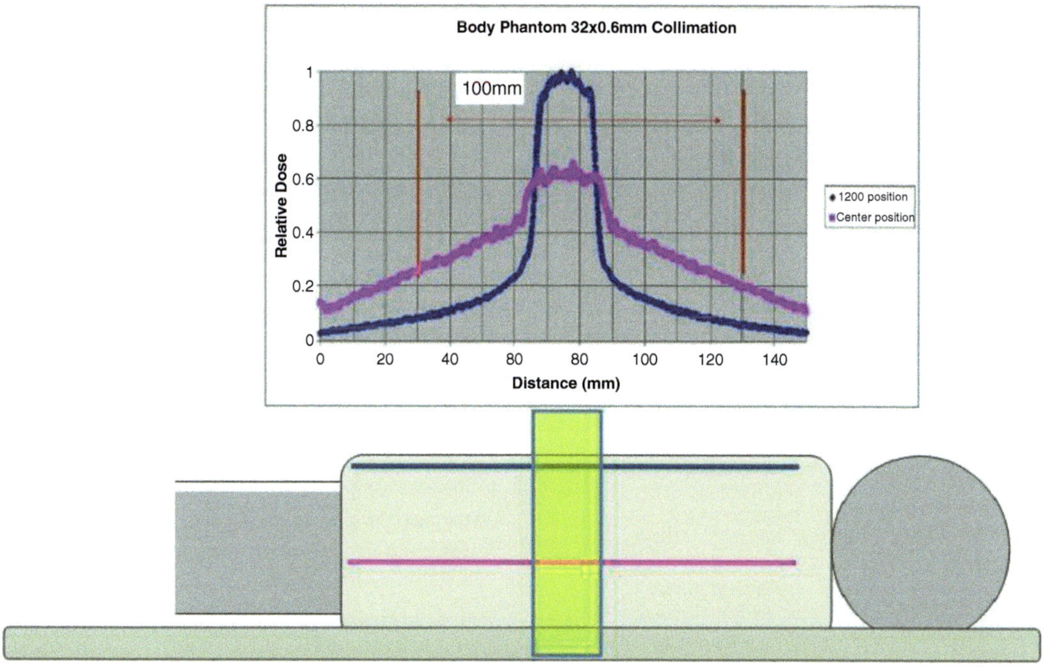

Fig. 2.15 Distribution of the single-slice dose profile along the z-axis, at the surface and centre of the patient or phantom (Courtesy ImPACT)

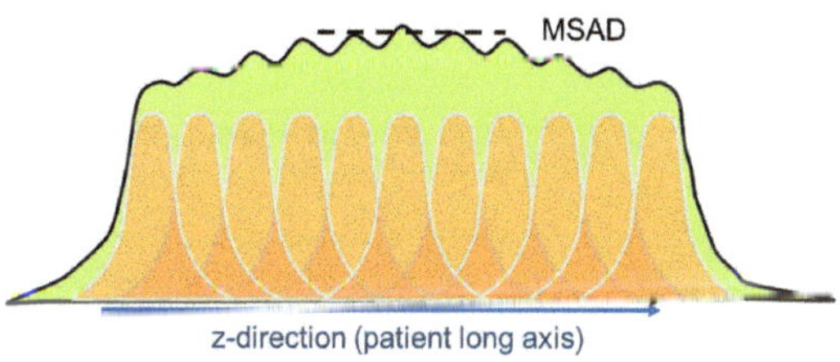

Fig. 2.16 A schematic view of an examination dose profile resulting from the contribution of scattered radiation from individual slices (Courtesy ImPACT). The MSAD (multiple scan average dose) is the value at the central region

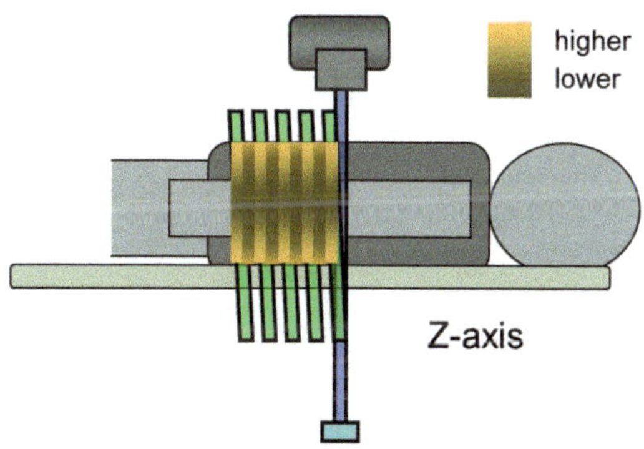

Fig. 2.17 Distribution of dose from a rotated beam along the z-axis: a complex radiation distribution (Courtesy ImPACT)

The general CTDI term consists of the integration of the single-slice profile, integrated over a given distance and essentially divided by the nominal beam width.

$CTDI_{100}$ is measured using a single rotation of the tube/detector, either in air or within standard polymethacrylate phantoms. The '100' in $CTDI_{100}$ refers to the length used from the single-slice dose profile. CT ionisation chambers for dose measurement are typically 100 mm, with a relatively small cross-sectional area (typically 1 cm^2).

The $CTDI_{100}$ is a calculation based on measuring the dose received to the chamber from the CT slice (including the primary and scattered beam) – essentially giving a value of dose that is averaged along the chamber length. By then dividing by the nominal beam width, it is essentially presenting an index whereby all the dose (primary and scattered) from the single slice is packaged within the nominal beam width (Fig. 2.18).

Though the CTDI is a calculation, based on the measurement from a single-slice irradiation, in concept it can be thought of as equivalent to the multiple slice average dose (MSAD), when measured in the same medium (air or phantom) and using the same length value. This is because both approaches take into account the scattered tails of the dose profile, the MSAD by measurement of the actual addition of scatter from neighbouring slices and the CTDI by the integration of dose profile, including scattered tails. Therefore, the $CTDI_{100}$ can also be interpreted as equivalent to the dose to the middle of a scanned length of 100 mm (Fig. 2.19).

Table 2.5 Standard generic dose metrics in CT

CTDI variations and terminology		
$CTDI_{100}$	CTDI one hundred	Calculated from a dose integral extending over 100 mm. Usually measured using a 100 mm pencil ionisation chamber
$CTDI_{air}$	CTDI in air	Measured in air
$CTDI_w$	Weighted CTDI	The weighted average of measurements at the periphery and centre of a standard phantom. Usually measured using a 100 mm pencil ionisation chamber
$CTDI_{vol}$	Volume-weighted $CTDI_w$	$CTDI_w$ adjusted for pitch in helical scanning
$CTDI_\infty$	CTDI infinity	Utilising the complete dose profile, including scattered radiation, integrated over 'infinite' distance

When the dose measurement is taken in air, the calculated $CTDI_{100}$ value is often referred to as $CTDI_{air}$, and this is very useful for quality control purposes. The weighted and volume CTDIs ($CTDI_w$ and $CTDI_{vol}$) result from measurements in standard-sized phantoms. They can also be used for quality control but are especially useful as indicators of relative patient dose when comparing protocols, scanners and values for similar-sized patients.

2.4.4.2 Weighted CTDI ($CTDI_w$)

$CTDI_w$ is calculated from $CTDI_{100}$ measurements undertaken in the standard 16 or 32 cm diameter polymethyl methacrylate (PMMA) phantom, which, being slightly longer than the standard CT ion chamber, is approximately 15 cm in length (Fig. 2.20).

The $CTDI_{100}$ is measured at the centre and periphery of the phantom to take into account the variation in dose across the phantom. This variation is more marked in the body as described earlier.

$$CTDI_{100} = \frac{1}{(N \times T)} \int_{-50}^{+50} D(z)\, dz$$

$$CTDI_{100} = \frac{\text{integral dose over 100 mm}}{\text{nominal beam width}}$$

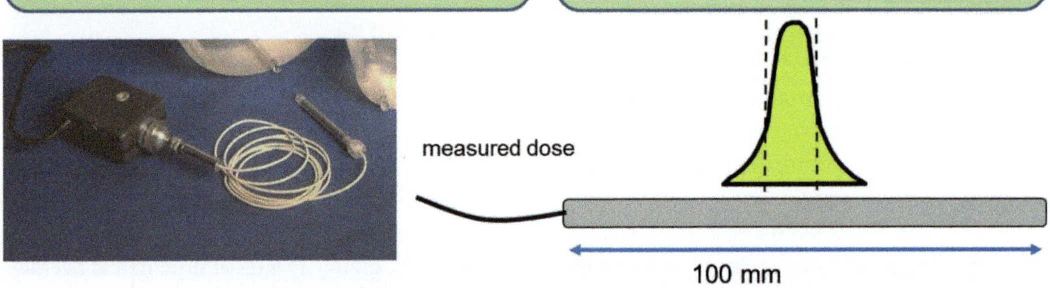

Fig. 2.18 The CTDI equation and presentation of an easy approach to remember it. D(*z*) is the single-slice dose profile, *N* is the number of image slices of thickness (*T*) that are acquired simultaneously and ($N \times T$) is usually equivalent to the nominal beam width. Also shown are the CT ionisation chamber (*left*) and an illustration (*right*) of a dose profile from a single slice including the scattered tails and the chamber. The dotted lines represent the nominal beam width (Courtesy ImPACT)

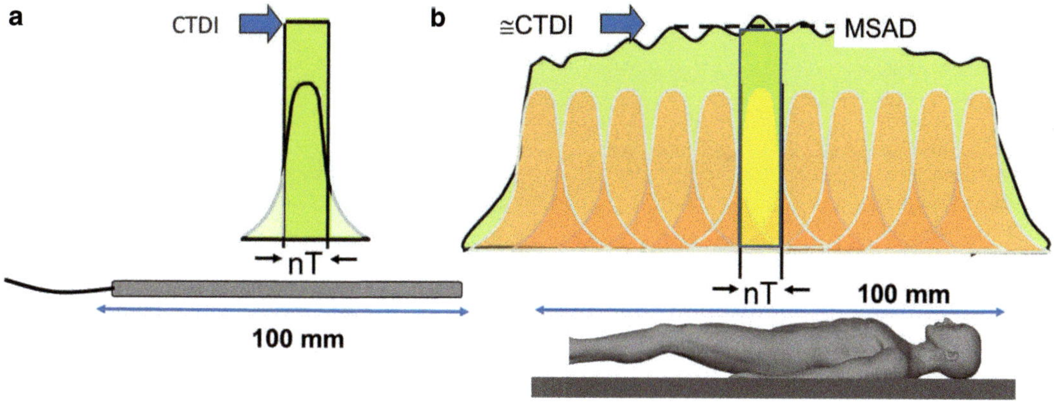

Fig. 2.19 Demonstrating the equivalence between the CTDI (**a**) and the MSAD (**b**) (Courtesy ImPACT)

Table 2.6 Conversion factors *K*, effective dose to DLP

Region of body	Conversion factor *K* = E/DLP (mSv mGy^{-1} cm^{-1})
Head and neck	0.0031
Head	0.0021
Neck	0.0059
Chest[a]	0.014
Abdomen and pelvis	0.015
Trunk	0.015

Ref. 2004 CT Quality Criteria (MSCT 2004) [24], also found at AAPM Report 96 [25]
[a]The chest value is a factor that must especially used with caution as it is sometimes quoted as 0.017

The definition is given as

$$CTDI_w = 1/3 CTDI_{100,c} + 2/3 CTDI_{100,p} \quad (2.1)$$

This gives a weighted average for the cross section of the phantom.

2.4.4.3 Volume CTDI ($CTDI_{vol}$)

Since the CTDI is a calculated dose index from a single-slice measurement, a correction must be applied to make it relevant for helical scanning. For example, where the helix of the primary dose beam is spread out, the resultant net dose will be averaged to be lower (unless other factors such as the tube current are adjusted to compensate). This spreading out of the helix is called the pitch and is defined by the relative table movement of the couch per tube rotation with respect to the nominal beam width:

$$\text{Pitch} = \text{table travel per rotation} / \text{nominal beam width} \quad (2.2)$$

A correction for the pitch is applied to the $CTDI_w$ to give the volume CTDI ($CTDI_{vol}$):

$$CTDI_{vol} = CTDI_w / \text{pitch} \quad (2.3)$$

A protocol with a pitch of 1 and a given $CTDI_w$ and $CTDI_{vol}$ would result in a halved $CTDI_{vol}$ for a pitch of 2, providing no other scan parameters were changed (Fig. 2.21).

The $CTDI_{vol}$ (or the $CTDI_w$ with older scanners) is presented on the operator console of the CT scanner (Fig. 2.22) as described in IEC 60601-2-44 3rd edition. The values will appear both prior to the scan as well as afterwards to reflect the actual value. This is particularly relevant where automatic exposure control has been used. In these cases either the maximum or the average value will be shown for the scan.

The $CTDI_{vol}$ values will also be given in the dose report, which presented as an image with the scan, and be populated into DICOM header information that will go to the PAC system. For those scanners that also support the DICOM Radiation Dose Structured Report (RDSR), more associated details are available with the $CTDI_{vol}$ data.

$CTDI_{vol}$ values are used for establishing local and national diagnostic reference levels (DRLs) as described in International Commission on Radiological Protection (ICRP) 105 and the UK

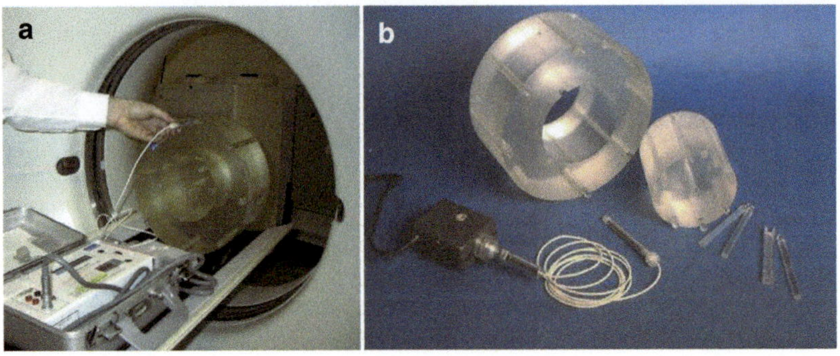

Fig. 2.20 Standard PMMA phantoms for the measurement of the CTDI. The head phantom fits inside the body annulus in this example of the phantoms. The standard CT ionisation chamber is also shown (Courtesy ImPACT)

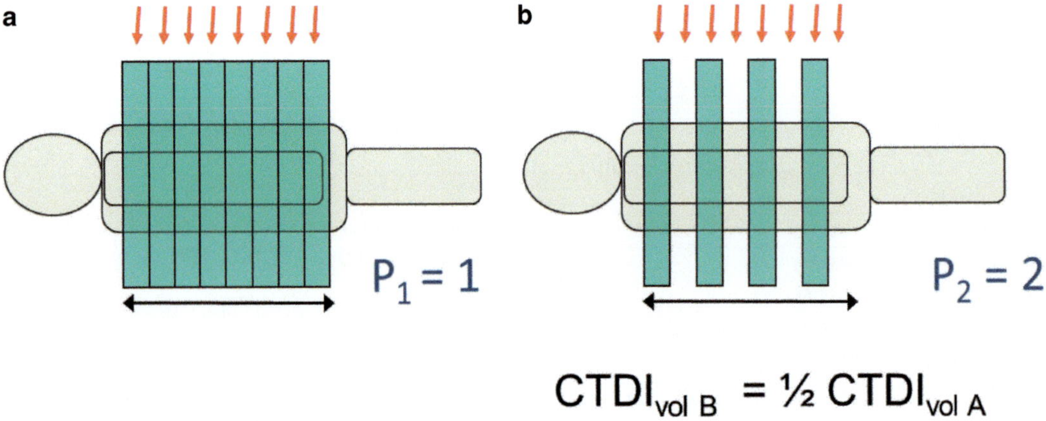

Fig. 2.21 Illustration of the effect of pitch on the calculation of $CTDI_{vol}$ (Courtesy ImPACT)

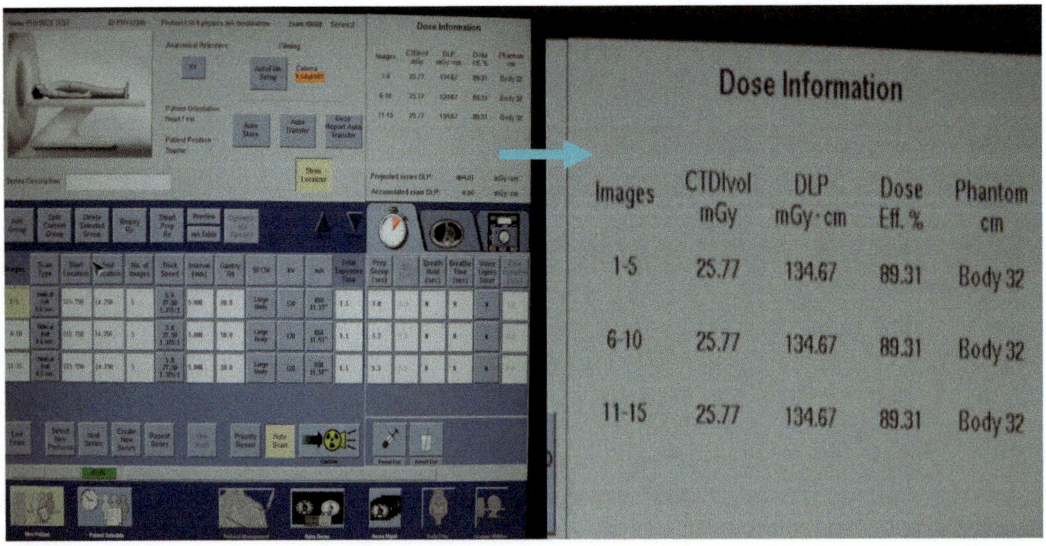

Fig. 2.22 Example of the presentation of the $CTDI_{vol}$ on the scanner console

IRMER regulations [27, 28]. DRLs will be discussed in more detail later in this chapter.

2.4.4.4 Dose Length Product (DLP)

Another metric can also be used to indicate dose taking account of the length of the scan – the dose length product. By utilising the $CTDI_{vol}$ as an indicator of 'dose per slice' and by taking into account the actual length scanned, a value can be calculated as an indicator to represent the total dose for the scan. This can then be considered to relate to radiation risk:

$$\mathrm{DLP} = \mathrm{CTDI}_{\mathrm{vol}} \times L(\mathrm{mGy.cm}) \quad (2.4)$$

L is the scanned length in centimetres.

It can easily be seen that a scan that is twice the length of another results in a doubling of the DLP (Fig. 2.23), where all other parameters are the same.

DLP values are used, in addition to the $CTDI_{vol}$, for establishing local and national DRLs [27, 28]. They can also be used to convert to an approximate effective dose for a given body region as described later in this chapter.

2.4.4.5 The Measurement of $CTDI_{vol}$ for Wide-Beam Scanners

Wide-beam scanners, with beams greater than 80 mm along the patient length, i.e. the z-direction (Fig. 2.24), present a problem for the practical measurement of the $CTDI_{100}$ (and thence the calculation of $CTDI_{vol}$) as they have a beam whose primary beam is close to, or exceeds, the length of the CT ionisation chamber length of 100 cm.

An IEC standard (Edition 3, Amendment 1) [26] has addressed this in a pragmatic approach, by redefining $CTDI_{vol}$ for beams greater than 40 mm. This approach ensures that the calculated $CTDI_{vol}$ is kept constant with all beam widths,

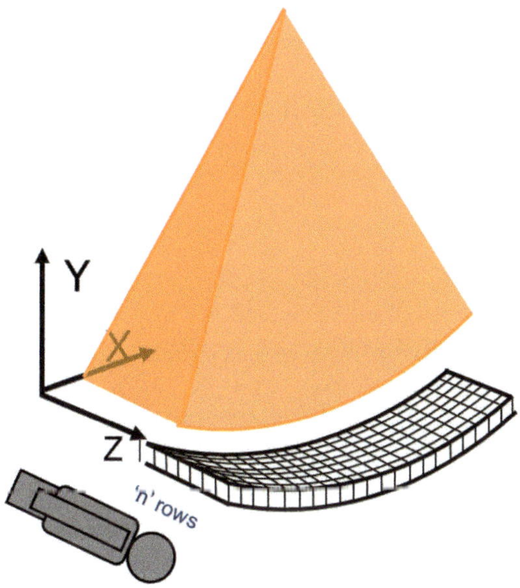

Fig. 2.24 Schematic view and photograph of the wide or cone beam and the axis orientation (Courtesy ImPACT)

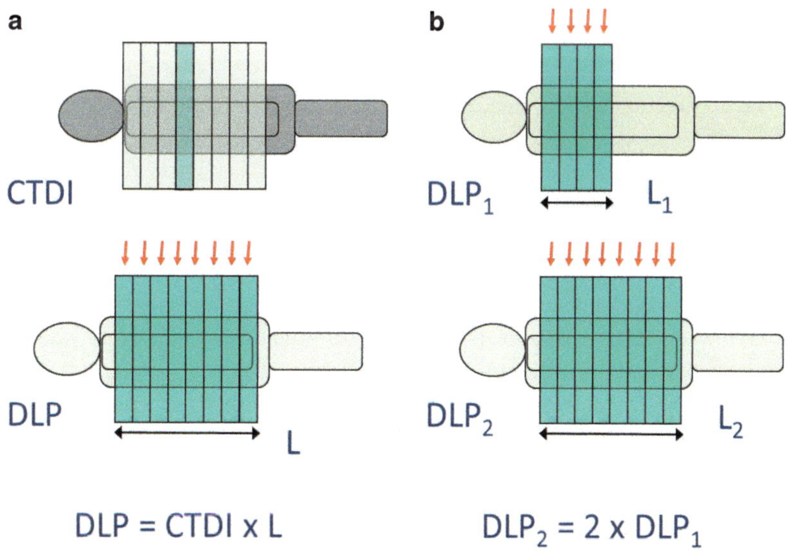

Fig. 2.23 Schematic view to demonstrate DLP and CTDI. In (**a**) the DLP is the length multiplied by the $CTDI_{vol}$. In (**b**) the DLP for length 2 (L_2) is twice that for scanned length 1 (L_1), whilst the CTDI is the same

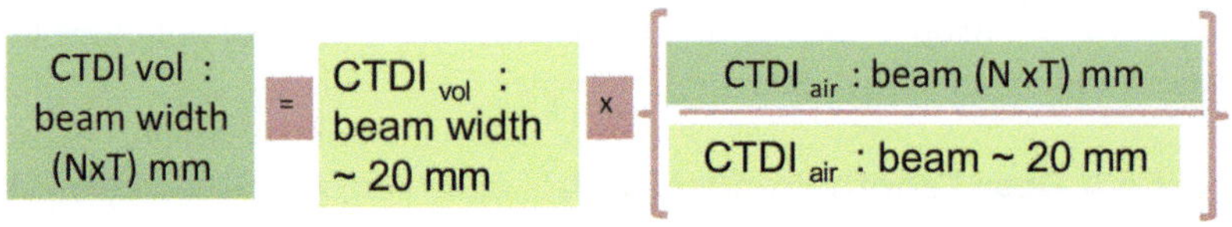

Fig. 2.25 IEC redefinition of $CTDI_{vol}$ for beams greater than 40 mm

despite the measurement tool (the CT ionisation chamber) being only 100 mm. This might seem an obvious approach for beams greater than 80 mm or indeed 100 mm; however, there are significant scatter considerations that also affect narrower beams; hence, the limit of 40 mm was chosen. The basic principle is to first undertake the measurements and calculations to obtain a $CTDI_{vol}$ for a suitable beam width of about 40 mm. A correction is then applied, based on the ratios of the $CTDI_{air}$ for the wide-beam width, relative to that at 40 mm (Fig. 2.25). $CTDI_{air}$ is easier to measure for wide beams due to the lack of scattered radiation, and this approach can be undertaken with existing equipment.

This pragmatic approach is clearly presented, with practical application in mind, in the IAEA report on wide-beam CT scanners [29], and further explored and presented in a paper in the British Journal of Radiology by Platten et al. [30].

These references also include some practical advice as to how to measure the integration of the dose profile (and thence the calculation of the $CTDI_{air}$).

2.4.4.6 Beyond $CTDI_{vol}$: Size-Specific Dose Estimate (SSDE)

The $CTDI_w$ and $CTDI_{vol}$ are dose indicators, and not patient dose values. They are highly valuable when used appropriately, such as comparing doses for different scan protocols and scanners as well as for establishing and comparing to National Diagnostic Reference Levels (NDRLs) which are based on standard patient sizes [28, 31].

However, these parameters cannot be used to compare actual patient scans unless the patients are of similar size. Patients come in many shapes and sizes, and the CTDI values only relate to a PMMA phantom of a fixed size.

Scanner settings generally should be adjusted to account for patient size, in order to give adequate dose to the detectors and thence a suitable image quality. This can happen either manually, through preset protocols, or on modern scanners with the use of automatic exposure control systems that adjust to meet a specified image quality.

In the scenario where the tube current has not been adjusted, the actual dose to a small patient, or child, would be greater than for a standard patient. However, the scanner would indicate the same phantom $CTDI_{vol}$ (Fig. 2.26). Similarly for a large patient, the actual dose would be less than for a standard-sized patient, but the scanner-indicated $CTDI_{vol}$ would be the same.

Conversely, by utilising tube current adjustment, it may mean that scans of two patients of different sizes, both resulting in similar image quality, will give an indication that one patient has a much higher $CTDI_{vol}$. The assumption might be that the larger patient received much higher dose; however, the actual dose delivered to the larger patient may be comparable to that of the smaller patient.

The AAPM have published two reports (AAPM 204 and 220 [32, 33]) giving correction factors that can be applied to the $CTDI_{vol}$ to give a dose indicator that takes into account the size of the scanned patient (Fig. 2.27). This revised dose metric is called the size-specific dose estimate (SSDE).

These correction factors were based on studies carried out by four different centres, using approaches based on measurements and Monte Carlo calculations on different sizes of 'CTDI'-type phantoms, elliptical anthropomorphic phantoms and voxel phantoms.

2.4.4.7 Beyond $CTDI_{vol}$: Scanned Length and Equilibrium Dose

$CTDI_{vol}$ is a dose index and as such is extremely valuable for quality control, scanner and protocol comparisons, as well as referencing to national

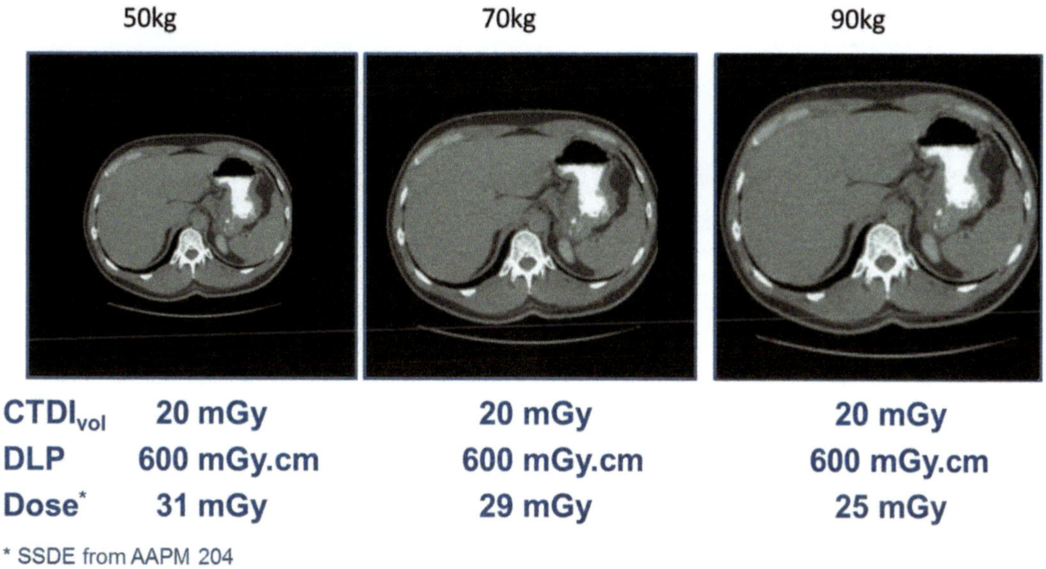

Fig. 2.26 Comparisons of $CTDI_{vol}$ (as measured for the 32 cm phantom) but presented for scans of different-sized patients and conversely an estimation of the actual relative dose received (using AAPM report 204)

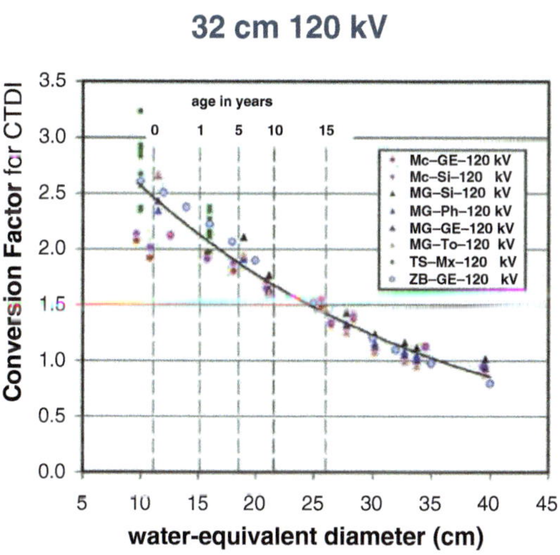

Fig. 2.27 Conversion factors based on the water equivalent diameter to apply to the $CTDI_{vol}$ to give an estimate of the SSDE (From AAPM report 204)

dose reference levels (National Diagnostic Reference Levels, NDRLS), as discussed later in this chapter.

However in a similar way to the endeavour to find a dose index that reflects patient size, there have been similar explorations to determine the relevance of the $CTDI_{vol}$ to the actual scanned length of an examination. The $CTDI_{vol}$ only utilises the scattered radiation over a total length of 100 mm, whereas the scattered tails of the single-slice dose profile have been shown to extend over a much greater distance. The term $CTDI_{infinity}$ is used for the limiting value of the generalised CTDI value where all the scattered radiation is considered. The issues are described in ICRU 87 [34] and AAPM 111 [35] and are likely to result in new phantoms and measurement methodologies in the future.

2.4.4.8 Effective Dose

Most people find the concept of effective dose the simplest as it enables a comparison of different scans and imaging modalities. However, it has to be used with caution and consideration given to derivation of values given.

Effective dose is based on utilising the radiation dose given to all organs in the body. Organ doses are calculated and weighted according to the sensitivity to radiation in terms of their statistical potential for the development of cancer (Fig. 2.28). The weighted doses are subsequently summed together. The resultant value gives an effective whole-body dose (effective dose, E). This value can be interpreted as the overall

Fig. 2.28 Organ weighting factors for effective dose (Factors from ICRP 103)

$$E = \sum w_T D_T$$

E = Effective dose (mSv)
D_T = mean dose to tissue (T) (mGy)
w_T = weighting factor according to tissue sensitivity

Weighting factors are derived for a whole population

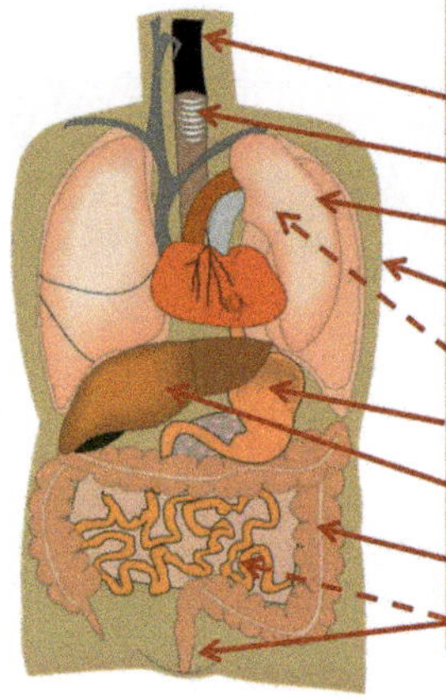

Organ (T)	W_T
Oesophagus	0.04
Thyroid	0.04
Lungs	0.12
Skin	0.01
Breast	0.12
Stomach	0.12
Liver	0.04
Colon	0.12
Gonads	0.08

potential risk of cancer development according to ICRP [31].

The organ weighting factors for the current ICRP report (2007) [31] have been updated with the major changes relating to the breast values (which have increased) and the gonad values (which have decreased).

Effective doses, and their associated risk estimates, are designed for a population and therefore do not take into account risk adjustments for age and gender. Effective dose should not be applied to individuals; if a situation requires some estimate of effective dose, then it must be used with caution, since it was not developed for this purpose.

When quoting effective dose (E), it is very important that the source of the weighting factors used is noted, whether the previous factors in ICRP 60 [30] or the current factors in ICRP 103 [31]. The phantom on which the calculation is made is also important. There are a number of phantoms that are widely used, and the ICRP has specified adult phantoms in their publication 110 [36]. It is not possible to make sensible comparisons of effective dose without this knowledge. If not noted, for example, this might be thought of as the equivalent of comparing two objects of the same length, one with a length value in centimetres and the other in inches. The numbers will be different, but they represent the same length of object.

The level of accuracy must also be borne in mind with these values, and therefore it may be possible to only consider broad estimates.

The impact of evolving International Commission on Radiological Protection (ICRP) recommendations concerning calculations of effective dose (E) are investigated by Shrimpton et al. [37], and their paper compares updated typical UK values for common CT examinations with previous data.

Organ doses, and thence effective dose, can be calculated using Monte Carlo techniques and with specific mathematical numerical or voxel (or hybrid) phantoms (Fig. 2.29).

Monte Carlo calculations are extensive calculations, where the x-ray source is mathematically described and used as the source for millions of mathematical generated photons. The path for each photon is followed through a statistical process with respect to its interactions with tissue. This process requires a number of elements, specialist knowledge of the x-ray tube and filtration, numerical or voxel versions of the phantoms, a Monte Carlo calculation package and often high computer processing power and/or time. There are many papers written in this field; a good overview paper is given in the references [24].

Effective dose can also be estimated from E/DLP factors (K-factors). These are specific factors which take the DLP value for specific regions of the body and where the effective dose has been calculated for the same scan parameters and body region.

There are a number of published sources. Sometimes the values are different depending on the examination region, the phantom and/or the ICRP report from which the underlying organ

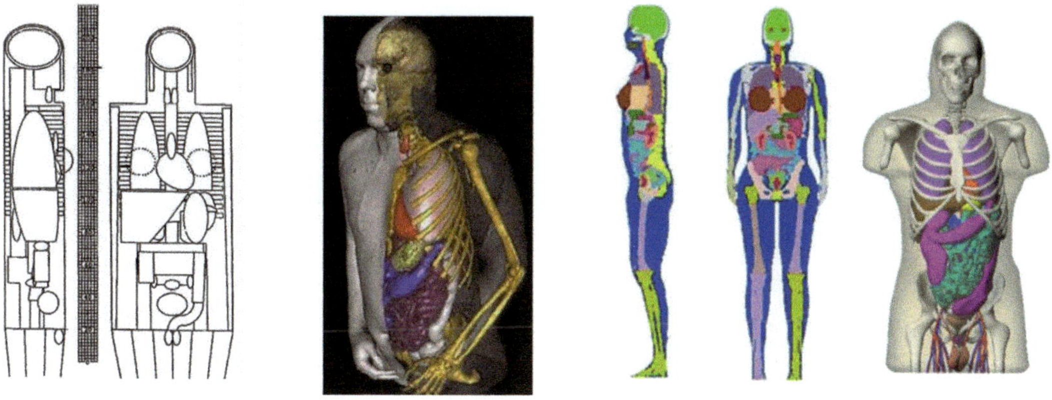

Fig. 2.29 A variety of phantoms used for Monte Carlo calculations

weighting factors are used. An example of published data is given in the 2004 CT Quality Criteria [25] (MSCT 2004) at http://www.msct.eu/CT_Quality_Criteria.htm# and the same values presented in AAPM 96 [38]. The chest value is a factor that must especially be used with caution as it is sometimes quoted as 0.017, compared to 0.014 in these references (Table 2.6).

Organ doses, DLP and effective dose, for specific examinations and scanner models, can also be calculated using commercially, or freely, available CT dosimetry software. One such is the ImPACT CT Calculator [39]. Others are also available [40, 41]. These utilise published organ dose data sets generated from Monte Carlo calculations. The examination and scanner can be selected easily, and conversions to adjust for newer scanner models can be made (Fig. 2.30).

2.4.5 Diagnostic Reference Levels (DRLs) and Optimisation in CT

DRLs are used as indicators of reasonable practice and are expressed in units of DLP or $CTDI_{vol}$. Much work has been done on assessing doses within CT. For example, the Public Health England Centre for Chemicals, Radiation and Environmental Hazards (CRCE), and its former affiliations (the Health Protection Agency, HPA and the National Radiation Protection Board, NRPB), has periodically published snapshots of CT scanner dose data from surveys of CT scanner practice in the UK. These surveys result in the quotation of typical $CTDI_{vol}$ and DLP for certain clinical examinations, as national reference doses, which are then formally adopted as the UK National Diagnostic Reference Levels (NDRLS).

The latest report, Doses from Computed Tomography (CT) Examinations in the UK (2011 review), was published in 2014 [42]. With repeat studies, these can show trends over time. Future national surveys should become easier with the introduction of automatic dose data collection systems; however, they can then present other difficulties due to the large volume of data.

The published data can help those working in PET/CT to see the range of doses for particular diagnostic examinations. Doses for attenuation scans are not as readily available from surveys such as these, but there is much information published from within individual centres particularly concentrating on optimising the scanning protocols used as described in the section below.

2.4.5.1 Optimisation in CT

Dose reduction has been discussed by Iball et al. [43] and can be used to optimise exposure factors in Table 2.7, to reduce doses without compromising the level of noise within an image. These concentrate on reducing the DLP and $CTDI_{vol}$ on individual scanners by understanding the functionality of the automatic exposure control (AEC) system in use on the CT scanner and by reviewing dose length product and image noise.

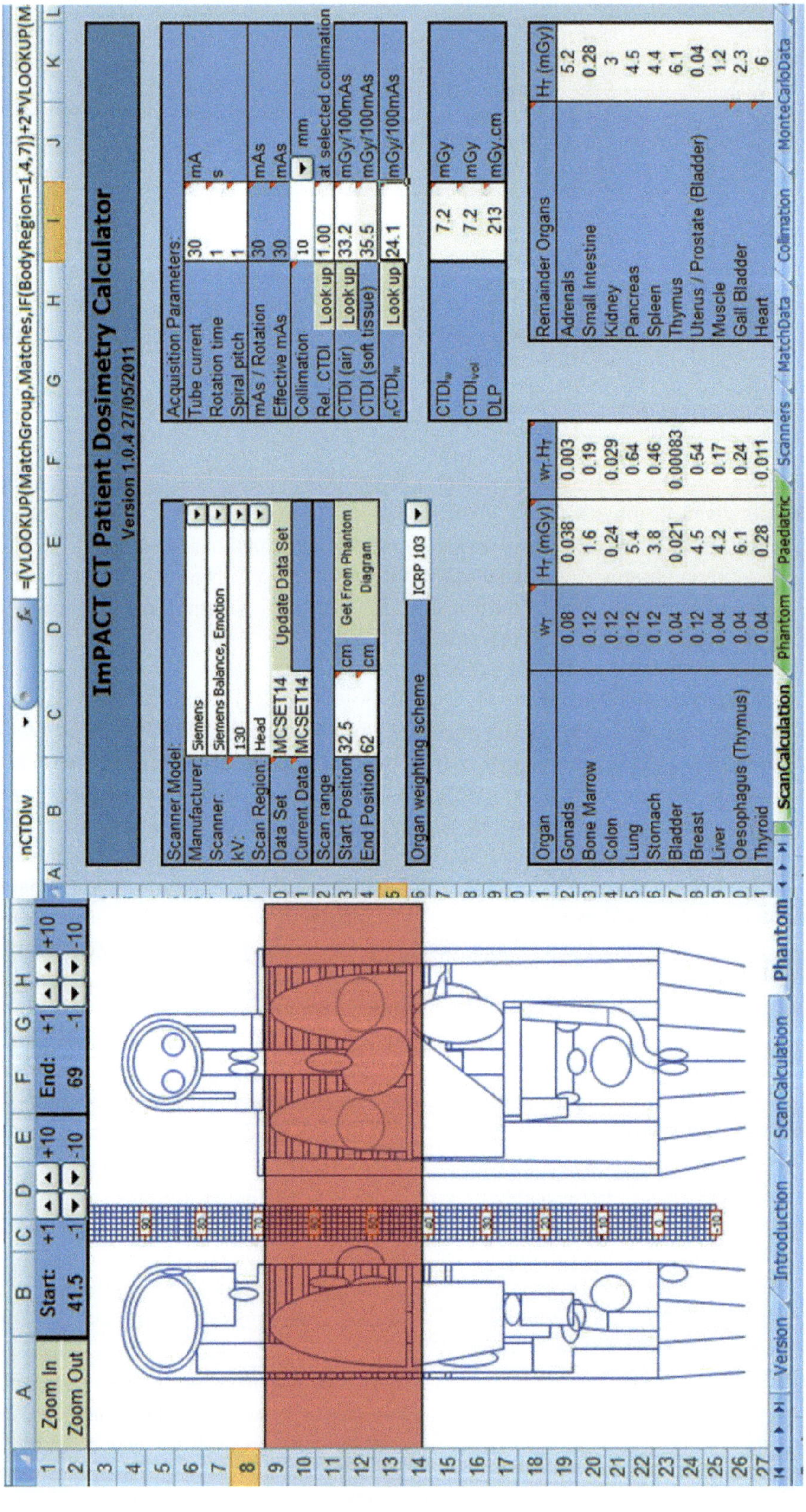

Fig. 2.30 The ImPACT Calculator

However, protocol review and optimisation is complex and requires a multidisciplinary approach as described in the AAPM guidelines [44].

2.4.6 Doses for Attenuation Scans and Whole-Body Scans in PET/ CT

Effective dose is the only way to compare the doses from the PET scan and the CT scan. The earlier sections demonstrated how much caution is required when comparing effective doses calculated using different methodologies in CT scanning. The radiation dose from the administration of the radiopharmaceutical is derived, for example, from ICRP 106 [45] or other sources as outlined in Chap. 3. This uses biokinetic models to generate coefficients of effective dose per MBq of administered activity (2×10^{-2} mSv/MBq), i.e. 8 mSv, for an administration of 400 MBq of F-18 FDG. Further caution must therefore be exercised when summing doses from PET and CT.

Furthermore, there are common descriptions of types of CT scan used in PET/CT. An attenuation scan is typically a low-dose, low mA scan. A diagnostic scan is typically described as a higher-dose scan which may also involve the use of contrast agents.

For whole-body PET/CT scans, doses of between 1.3 and 18.6 mSv are quoted for low-dose scans and diagnostic scans with contrast, respectively [46]. This results in a total examination dose of between 10 and 30 mSv. Effort and interest are going into minimising both CT dose and administered activity currently.

2.4.7 Quality Control of CT Scanners

As part of the life cycle of the equipment, safety checks, commissioning checks and routine quality control checks need to be carried out on the scanner. PET quality control checks are covered later in the book, but radiation safety and CT checks are included in the following section.

2.4.7.1 Commissioning Checks PET/CT

Checks should be carried out on the barriers installed within the facility. These can be assessed using a source of F-18 using the methodology described elsewhere [5]. Care needs to be taken in handling the source as a relatively high activity may be required to penetrate the barriers.

Further checks on safety signs and features should be made and recorded. A suggested list is shown in Table 2.8.

There is a full and rigorous testing programme for quality control that can be undertaken for all CT scanners (IPEM 91 [47], IPEM TGR 32 Part 3 [48], ImPACT Acceptance Testing [49], IAEA CT QA [50] and [51] IEC [52]).

Table 2.7 Scan parameters and impact on patient dose and image quality

Parameter	Impact on patient dose	Impact on image quality
kV	Increases with increasing kV ∞ kV^2 (approx.)	Noise decreases Contrast decreases
mA	Increases proportionally to mA	Noise decreases $\propto \sqrt{_{\text{mA}}}$
Rotation time (s)	Increases proportionally to time	Noise decreases $\propto 1/\sqrt{_{\text{sec}}}$
Pitch	Decreases as pitch increases (for constant mA)	Noise increases Depends on reconstruction algorithm and slice thickness
Beam collimation (beam width) (mm)	Decreases with increasing collimation	*Z*-axis resolution could decrease with wide beams for scanners with wider outer detector row elements
Detector collimation (mm) *z*-axis	Generally no effect	*Z*-axis resolution (image slice width) decreases with detector width
Scan length	Increases dose length product	No effect

The two most important measurements are dose and noise. The $CTDI_{air}$ is a valuable and quick test for quality control; in addition a full range of $CTDI_{vol}$ measurements for different scan conditions should be undertaken at acceptance and compared to the screen values. However, with the complexity of modern systems, a full test programme should be undertaken as listed in Table 2.9.

Table 2.8 Radiation safety checks for the PET/CT scanner and facility

Parameter
Room warning signs
Room warning lights: ready to emit radiation
Room warning lights: 'do not enter' prep/expose
Warning signals:
Mains on
Exposure light on control panel
Room protection:
General adequacy of protection
Adequate shielding of walls and doors
Surrounding dose rates meet design specification
Exposure switch
Labelling:
All controls clearly labelled
Focal spot position
Filtration/half value layer
Emergency off buttons
X-ray tube radiation leakage
Tube kilovoltage
Collimation x-ray to light beam and to detector

CT numbers are of interest to PET/CT scientists and should be included in any programme.

Conclusions

The design of PET/CT facilities has been described, considering some of the issues around working with PET radiopharmaceuticals that may be less familiar to those working in conventional nuclear medicine. The requirement for structural shielding around uptake bays and the scanner itself have been described, and a methodology outlined to calculate the thickness of barriers required to protect staff and members of the public within the facility and around it. The requirements to consider the external dose rate hazard, potential contamination and emergency situations are highlighted. The use of standard protection principles of distance shielding and time is emphasised and illustrated. Example calculations have been presented to help those unfamiliar with the methodology. The parameters required to perform the calculations have been summarised.

The potential for high staff dose is described, and approaches for assessment of whole-body dose finger dose have been discussed.

Fixtures, fittings and accessories within the facility have been explained with optimisation of radiation protection and minimisation of exposure and potential exposure described. Continued vigilance and review of staff dose have been advocated with some suggested

Table 2.9 CT quality control checks for the PET/CT scanner

Test	Comments	
CTDI in air	CT ion chamber/solid-state CT chamber	Compare with manufacturers specification
CTDI in phantom	CT ion chamber/solid-state CT chamber. IEC specified 16 cm and 32 cm phantoms	Calculate $CTDI_w$ Compare with specification
Image noise	Manufacturers phantom	Compare with manufacturers specification
Spatial resolution	Suitable phantom	Compare with manufacturers specification
CT number	Suitable phantom	0 for water −1000 for air Baseline for other materials
Imaged slice width	Suitable phantom	
Patient positioning vs. scan plane	Pins on surface of phantom	
Couch movement and position	Pins on surface of phantom	

methodologies to support keeping doses as low as reasonably achievable.

CT technology has been outlined in some detail to demonstrate the increase in speed and the number of detector rows between 1972 and the current day. The factors affecting dose in CT scanning – kV, mA and rotation time – have been illustrated. Image reconstruction, pitch, collimation and automatic exposure features have also been described. In order to fully understand each of these, a number of dose metrics have been defined and put into context against the technology and effective dose.

Diagnostic reference levels and optimisation of in CT have been discussed with the dose for attenuation scans and whole-body PET/CT scans.

The importance of quality control checks and references to support the checks required for CT have been supplied.

In conclusion, this chapter aims to supply sufficient information to support the safe design, operation and quality control of PET/CT scanners to those more familiar with conventional nuclear medicine.

References

1. Delacroix D, Guerre JP, Leblanc P, Hickman C. Radionuclide and radiation protection data handbook. Radiat Prot Dosimetry. 1998;76:24.
2. Royal College of Physicians and Royal College of Radiologists Evidence based indication for the use of PET-CT in the UK 2013. London: RCR; 2013.
3. IAEA Human Health Series No 11. Planning a Clinical PET centre. 2010. IAEA Vienna ISSN 2075–3772.
4. Lecchi M, Lucignani G, Maioli C, Ignelzi G, Sole A. Validation of a new protocol for 18F-FDG infusion using an automatic combined dispenser and injector system. Eur J Nucl Med Mol Imaging. 2012;39(11):1720–9.
5. Sutton DG, Martin CJ, Williams JR, Peet DJ. BIR working party, BIR, London. 2nd ed. 2012. ISBN –13 978-0-905749-74-x.
6. Madsen MT, Anderson JA, Halama JR, Kleck J, Simpkin DJ, Votaw JR, et al. PET and PET/CT shielding requirements AAPM task report 108. Med Phys. 2006;33:4–15.
7. Radiological Protection Institute of Ireland. The design of diagnostic medical facilities where ionising radiation is used. 2009. RPII Code of Practice.
8. IAEA Safety Report Series No 58. Radiation protection in newer medical imaging techniques PET/CT. 2008. STI/PUB/1343 ISBN 978-92-0-106808-8.
9. Benetar NA, Cronin BF, O'Doherty MJ. Radiation dose rates from patients undergoing PET: implications for technologists and waiting areas. Eur J Nucl Med. 2000;27:583–9.
10. L121 HSE. Work with ionising radiation. Approved code of practise and practical guidance on the Ionising Radiation Regulations 1999. London: HSE; 2000.
11. Pasciak AS, Jones AK. PShield: an exact three-dimensional numerical solution for determining optimal shielding designs for PET/CT facilities. Med Phys. 2012;39(6):3060–9.
12. Antić V, Stanković K, Vujisić M, Osmokrović P. Comparison of various methods for designing the shielding from ionising radiation at PET-CT installations. Radiat Protect Dosim. 2013;152(2):245–9.
13. Lo Meo S, Cicoria G, Campanella F, Mattozzi M, Panebianco AS, Marengo M. Radiation dose around a PET scanner installation: comparison of Monte Carlo simulations, analytical calculations and experimental results. Physica Medica. 2014;30(4):448–53.
14. Walsh C, O'Connor C, O'Reilly G. Eye dose monitoring of PET/CT workers. Br J Radiol. 2014. doi:10.1259/bjr.20140373.
15. Mattsson S, Soderborg M. Radiation dose management in CT, SPECT CT and PET/CT techniques. Radiat Protect Dosim. 2011;147(1–2):13–21. doi:10.1093/rpd/ncr261.
16. Burgess P. Guidance on the choice, use and maintenance of hand held radiation monitoring equipment NRPB-R326. 2001. ISBN 85951 461 7.
17. Kemerink GJ, Vanhavere F, Barth I, Mottaghy F. Extremity doses of nuclear medicine personnel: a concern. Eur J Nucl Med Mol Imaging. 2012;39:529–32.
18. Chiesa C. Radiation dose to technicians per nuclear medicine procedure: comparison between technetium-99m, gallium-67, and iodine-131 radiotracers and fluorine 18 fluorodeoxyglucose. Eur J Nucl Med. 1997;24(11).
19. Guillet B. Technologist radiation exposure in routine clinical practice with 18F-FDG PET. J Nucl Med Technol. 2005;33(3).
20. Roberts FO, Gunawardana DH, Pathmaraj K, Wallace A, Paul LU, Mi T, et al. Radiation dose to PET technologists and strategies to lower occupational exposure. J Nucl Med Tech 2005;33:44–7.
21. Seierstad T. Doses to nuclear technicians in a dedicated PET/CT centre utilising 18F fluorodeoxyglucose (FDG). Radiat Prot Dosimetry. 2007;123(2):246–9.
22. Peet DJ, et al. Radiation protection in fixed PET/CT facilities – design and operation. Br J Radiol. 2012; 85:643–6.
23. Kalendar WA. Computed tomography: fundamentals, system technology, image quality, applications. 3rd ed. Wiley, Erlangen; 2011. ISBN: 978-3-89578-317-3.
24. 2004 CT Quality Criteria (MSCT 2004) European Guidelines for Multislice Computed Tomography; Bongartz G, Golding SJ, Jurik AG, Leonardi M, van

Persijn van Meerten E, Rodríguez R, Schneider K, Calzado A, Geleijns J, Jessen KA, Panzer W, Shrimpton PC, Tosi, G. Funded by the European Commission, Contract number FIGM-CT2000-20078-CT-TIP. 2004. http://www.msct.eu/CT_Quality_Criteria.htm#. Download the 2004 CT Quality Criteria. Accessed July 2015.
25. Zhang Y, et al. Organ doses, effective doses, and risk indices in adult CT: comparison of four types of reference phantoms across different examination protocols. Med Phys. 2012;39(6):3404–23.
26. International Electrotechnical Commission Medical electrical equipment—Part 2–44, 3rd ed. Amendment 1: particular requirements for basic safety and essential performance of x-ray equipment for computed tomography. IEC-60601-2-44-am1. Geneva: International Electrotechnical Commission; 2012.
27. Annals of the ICRP 105 radiological protection in medicine. Ann ICRP. 2007;37(6):1–63.
28. IRMER the Ionising Radiation (Medical Exposure) Regulations 2000 SI1059. 2000.
29. International Atomic Energy Agency Status of computed tomography dosimetry for wide cone beam scanners. IAEA Human Health Report 5. Vienna: International Atomic Energy Agency; 2011.
30. Platten DJ, Castellano IA, Chapple C-L, Edyvean S, Jansen JTM, Johnson B, Lewis MA. Radiation dosimetry for wide-beam CT scanners: recommendations of a working party of the Institute of Physics and Engineering in Medicine. Br J Radiol. 2013;86(1027):20130089.
31. ICRP103. The 2007 Recommendations of the International Commission on Radiological Protection. ICRP Publication 103. Ann ICRP. 2007;37(2–4).
32. Report of AAPM TG 204: size-specific dose estimates (SSDE) in pediatric and adult body CT examinations Report of AAPM TG 204. 2011.
33. Report of AAPM TG220: use of water equivalent diameter for calculating patient size and Size-specific dose estimates (SSDE) in CT Report of AAPM TG220. 2014.
34. ICRU Report No. 87: radiation dose and image-quality assessment in computed tomography. International Commission on Radiation Units and Measurements. http://www.ncbi.nlm.nih.gov/pubmed/24158924. J ICRU. 2012;12(1):1–149. doi:10.1093/jicru/ndt007.
35. Report of AAPM TG111: comprehensive methodology for the evaluation of radiation dose in CT: the future of CT dosimetry AAPM TG111. 2010.
36. ICRP Publication 110 ICRP. Adult reference computational phantoms. ICRP Publication 110. Ann ICRP. 2009;39(2).
37. Shrimpton PC, Jansen JTM, Harrison JD. Updated estimates of typical effective doses for common CT examinations in the UK following the 2011 national review. Br J Radiol. 2016;89:1057.
38. AAPM 96 the Measurement, Reporting, and Management of Radiation Dose in CT AAPM Report 96. 2008.
39. ImPACT (Imaging Performance Assessment of CT scanners) (impactscan.org) http://www.impactscan.org/ctdosimetry.htm. Accessed May 2015.
40. CT-Expo. version 1.5; Medizinische Hochschule. Hannover.
41. ImpactDose. version 1.1; VAMP. Erlangen.
42. PHE – CRCE – 013 Doses from Computed Tomography (CT) Examinations in the UK – 2011 Review. 2011. https://www.gov.uk/government/publications/doses-from-computed-tomography-ct-examinations-in-the-uk.
43. Iball GR, Tout D. Computed tomography automatic exposure control techniques in F18-FDG oncology PET-CT scanning. Nucl Med Comms. 2014. doi:10.1097/MNM0000000000000064.
44. AAPM Guidelines. J Applied Clin Phys. 2013;14(5):2–12.
45. ICRP 106 radiation dose to patients from radiopharmaceuticals addendum 3 to ICRP 53. Ann ICRP. 2008;38:1–197.
46. Brix G, et al. Radiation exposure of patients undergoing whole-body dual modality F18-FDG PET/CT examinations. J Nucl Med. 2005;46(4):608–13.
47. IPEM Report 91 Recommended standards for the routine performance testing of diagnostic X-ray imaging systems. 2005. ISBN 1-903613-24-8.
48. IPEM Report No 32 Part III. 2nd ed. Measurement of the performance characteristics of diagnostic X-ray systems used in medicine. 2003. ISBN 0-904181-76-6.
49. ImPACT. http://www.impactscan.org/acceptance.htm.
50. http://www-pub.iaea.org/MTCD/Publications/PDF/Pub1557_web.pdf. IAEA Human Health Series Np 19. 2012.
51. Human Health series No. 1: quality assurance for PET and PET/CT systems. http://www-pub.iaea.org/MTCD/publications/PDF/Pub1393_web.pdf.
52. Evaluation and routine testing in medical imaging departments – Part 3–5: acceptance tests – imaging performance of computed tomography X-ray equipment IEC IEC 61223-3-5:2004.

Radiation Dosimetry of PET Imaging

3

Michael G. Stabin

Contents

3.1 **Introduction** 65
3.2 **Radiation Dose Calculations** 66
3.3 **Biokinetic Analyses** 66
3.4 **Example Dose Calculations** 71
3.5 **The Pregnant or Lactating Patient** 74
Conclusions 75
References 75

Abstract

The basics of internal dosimetry in nuclear medicine are reviewed. The design and execution of medical imaging studies are explained, for animal and human studies. Animal data extrapolation and data analysis for human imaging data are given by example. Dose quantities are explained and, again, given by example. Standardized doses, for general cases and for the pregnant or lactating female, are given.

3.1 Introduction

The majority of PET pharmaceuticals are used in diagnostic imaging. Radiation dosimetry is generally not evaluated on a daily basis for individual patients, unless a misadministration occurs or if a pregnant or potentially pregnant patient is imaged (in which case the dose to the embryo/fetus may be of concern). In order to get any radiopharmaceutical approved, however, a complete treatment of dosimetry is an essential part of the approval process. Systems of radiation dose calculations have been standardized for many years and now are greatly facilitated by standardized computer resources. The difficult task in establishing the dosimetry of a new PET agent lies in gathering the biokinetic data to use

M.G. Stabin, PhD, CHP
Department of Radiology and Radiological Sciences, Vanderbilt University, 1161 21st Avenue South, Nashville, TN 37232-2675, USA
e-mail: michael.g.stabin@vanderbilt.edu

M.M. Khalil (ed.), *Basic Science of PET Imaging*, DOI 10.1007/978-3-319-40070-9_3

in the dose calculations. Once these data are correctly gathered, the dose calculations may be performed in a matter of minutes using established computing resources. In this chapter, methods for designing and executing such studies will be outlined, some sample dose calculations will be shown, and dosimetry for a handful of PET agents will be provided.

3.2 Radiation Dose Calculations

The basic equation for calculating the radiation dose from one organ to another (or any organ to itself) is given as [1]

$$D_T = \frac{k\ \tilde{A}_s \sum_i n_i\ E_i\ \phi_i (T \leftarrow S)}{m_T}$$

where D_T = absorbed dose (Gy) in target organ T
$\tilde{A}_S$ = the number of nuclear transitions in a source organ S, sometimes referred to as the "cumulated activity" (MBq-s)
n_i = number of radiations with energy E_i emitted per nuclear transition
E_i = energy per radiation (MeV)
ϕ_i $f(T \leftarrow S)$ = fraction of energy emitted that is absorbed in target organ T from source organ S for radiation i
m_T = mass of target region (kg)
k = a proportionality constant (e.g., Gy-kg/MBq-s-MeV)

The term $\tilde{A}$ is the integral of the time-activity curve for a "source" organ, i.e., an organ that exhibits a significant uptake of the administered activity. As becquerel is the number of disintegrations per second that occur at a given time, the integral over time is Bq-s (MBq s was used above), which is the total number of disintegrations that occurred in the organ over the period of integration (almost always to infinite time). The activity at any given time is determined in the biokinetic analysis; data are obtained in animals or human subjects at specified times after administration of the radiopharmaceutical, and then these data are integrated over time to give $\tilde{A}$. First, a review of how to obtain the biokinetic data will be provided, and later we will return to show some actual sample dose calculations.

3.3 Biokinetic Analyses

(i) *Study design*
Time-activity curves for most organs are usually characterized by one or more exponential terms, i.e., $A(t) = A_1\ e^{-\lambda_1 t} + A_2\ e^{-\lambda_2 t} + \cdots$. The rate constants λ_1 and λ_2 describe the kinetics of removal of activity components A_1 and A_2; we can define half-times T_1 and T_2, by $\lambda = 0.693/T$; the half-time is the time needed for half of that component of activity to be removed from an organ. Each exponential term has two unknown variables; therefore, the time-activity curve has to have two data points for each phase of clearance for which we wish to define an exponential term. So, if a given time-activity curve is best characterized by two exponentials, an absolute minimum of four data points is needed to define the curve, with two points during each phase (i.e., not one during the first phase and three during the second). The starting point in a kinetic analysis is thus deciding on when to obtain samples, whether they are from a study involving animals or human subjects. For a completely new agent, this can obviously be a challenge, as the biokinetics are not yet known. An absolute limitation is the physical half-life of the radionuclide employed; F-18 has a half-life of 1.83 h, so data may be gathered over several hours after administration, but C-11 has a half-life of only 20 min, so data must be gathered much more quickly. Then, the biological clearance of the agent must be considered. The equation above with the exponential terms was not explicit, but the complete removal of activity from an organ or the body is due to both radioactive decay and biological clearance; this is characterized by a rate constant λ_e, an "effective rate constant," which is the sum of the biological rate constant (λ_b) and the physical rate

constant (λ_p). Some agents are cleared very quickly, others more slowly. So the study must be planned to get the needed number of data points taking into account both physical and biological clearance. Often experience with other similar agents can be helpful, or the data points can be spaced out over the range of times possible over several physical half-lives of the radionuclide, with several early time points and several later time points. There is not an exact formula for guiding the selection process of sampling times; care must be taken to provide enough data before spending the time and money on gathering the data so that the data collection process will be successful and the experiments will not have to be repeated. In addition to activity levels in organs and the body, an essential element of a biokinetic analysis is evaluation of the excretion of activity from the body (via the urinary or intestinal pathway). It is not uncommon for excretory organs to receive the highest doses of any other organ in the body, as often 100 % of the activity eventually passes through these organs (urinary bladder or intestines). For PET radiopharmaceuticals, excretion may be more limited than for other agents, due to their short physical half-lives. For C-11 compounds, for example, it is common to assume that there is no time for appreciable excretion from the body to occur, although activity might accumulate in the urinary bladder and decay there. So for studies using imaging data, if activity is seen in the urinary bladder, the activity levels may be quantified, and the activity may be integrated to get the number of disintegrations in the urinary bladder; collecting urine data is unlikely to provide any useful information. For F-18, it is common for there to be urinary excretion during the duration of the study, and the use of image data or urine collection may be helpful.

(ii) *Animal data*

Preclinical studies are required for any New Drug Application (NDA) to the US Food and Drug Administration (FDA). Most research is done with some rodent species, but any animal species in theory is acceptable. Some have an inclination to use primate species, with the idea that they may produce results more similar to humans. Extrapolation of animal data to humans has produced misleading information in many cases, in most any animal species [2]. So, this is a necessary step in the process of evaluating the dosimetry of a new radiopharmaceutical, but one should bear in mind that the real dosimetry will not be known until well-designed and executed studies using human subjects are performed. Time-activity curves for radiopharmaceuticals using animals may be established by administering the radiopharmaceutical and either sacrificing the animals, extracting tissue samples, and performing a radioassay or by small animal imaging studies.

(a) *Tissue extraction* – using a minimum of three animals per time point, individual samples of organs and tissues may be extracted from the animals after sacrificed and counted in any radiation detector system (e.g., sodium iodide scintillation, liquid scintillation). Collection of urine and/or fecal samples via the use of "metabolic cages" may characterize the excretion of the agent. Extrapolating the organ/tissue data to humans is not an exact science. One may assume that the percent of the administered activity seen in any organ at a given time will likely be the same concentration seen in humans; one may say that this is a "direct extrapolation." One may assume that the percent of administered activity per gram in an organ will be the same in humans; due to the normally considerable differences in body and organ masses, this is likely to produce erroneous results. Many have evaluated various extrapolation methods proposed in the literature. One method of extrapolating animal data that has been applied by many is the % kg/g method [3]. In this method, the animal organ data need to be reported as % of injected activity per gram of tissue, and this information plus knowledge of the animal whole body weight is employed in the following extrapolation:

$$\left(\frac{\%}{\text{organ}}\right)_{\text{human}} = \left[\left(\frac{\%}{\text{g}_{\text{organ}}}\right)_{\text{animal}} \times \left(\text{kg}_{\text{TB weight}}\right)_{\text{animal}}\right] \times \left(\frac{\text{g}_{\text{organ}}}{\text{kg}_{\text{TB weight}}}\right)_{\text{human}}$$

The percent uptake per gram of tissue is multiplied by the animal whole body weight in kg; the percent in any organ in humans is obtained by applying the corresponding organ and body masses of a reference adult human. A numerical example using this method was provided by Stabin [2] (Table 3.1): The animal whole body weight was 20 g (0.02 kg), and the source organ chosen had a mass of around 299 g. The human total body weight for the standard adult male of 70 kg was then applied in the transformation. For example:

$$\frac{38.1\ \%}{\text{g}}\ (\text{animal}) \times 0.020\ \text{kg} \times \frac{299\ \text{g}}{70\ \text{kg}} = \frac{3.26\ \%}{\text{organ}}\ (\text{human})$$

The idea of this method is that the percent in an organ is weighted for the fraction of total body mass that the organ comprises. As noted above, this is not a "gold standard" method by any means; it is an attempt to perform a reasonable extrapolation that avoids some pitfalls in other methods. Some also suggest adding a scaling in time, to account for the different metabolic rates of species of different size:

$$t_{\text{h}} = t_{\text{a}} \left[\frac{m_{\text{h}}}{m_{\text{a}}}\right]^{0.25}$$

where t_{a} is the time at which a measurement was made in an animal system, t_{h} is the corresponding time assumed for the human data, and m_{a} and m_{h} are the total body masses of the animal species and of the human. Again from Stabin [2], Table 3.2 shows an example case with data extrapolated from an animal species to the human using this time scaling approach:

Table 3.1 Animal data extrapolation example (mass extrapolation)

	Source organ				
Animal	1 h	3 h	6 h	16 h	24 h
%ID/organ	3.79	3.55	2.82	1.02	0.585
(%ID/g)	38.1	36.6	30.8	11.3	5.70
Human					
%ID/organ	3.26	3.12	2.63	0.962	0.486

Here, a human body mass of 70 kg was used, and the animal whole body mass was assumed to be 200 g. Sparks and Aydogan [4] studied the success of animal data extrapolation for several radiopharmaceuticals, using direct extrapolation, and mass and/or time extrapolation. They found that no particular method was superior to any other and that, in many cases, extrapolated animal data significantly underestimated observed uptakes in human organs. So, in conclusion, choice of an animal species and extrapolation method are areas of freedom in designing an animal study, and results obtained from animal studies must be recognized as only preliminary estimates of the dosimetry for any radiopharmaceutical.

(b) Small animal imaging

Small animal imaging techniques have greatly improved the science of drug

Table 3.2 Animal data extrapolation example (time extrapolation)

Animal time scale	5 min	15 min	30 min	60 min	1.5 h
Extrapolated human time scale	22 min	1.1 h	2.2 h	4.3 h	6.5 h

development. It has also allowed the characterization of radiopharmaceutical dosimetry in living animals, eliminating the need to sacrifice them. A drawback, however, is that the animals generally need to be anesthetized for the imaging session. Anesthetics may alter the distribution of the radiopharmaceutical, leading to inaccurate evaluation of organ uptakes and subsequent dosimetric analyses. Quantitative analyses of organ uptake at any imaging time are the same as those from human imaging studies. PET images are inherently quantitative; counts in a given voxel are easily related to absolute values of activity. Drawing volumes of interest (VOIs) over recognized organ regions provides values of activity in the organ that can be related to percentages or fractions of the administered activity, which is always known. Thus time-activity curves can be readily (but not easily!) developed from the image data and integrated to obtain the time-activity integrals needed for development of dose estimates. Organ and whole body biokinetics, combined with analyses of excretion, will allow development of a complete dosimetric analysis.

(c) *Small animal dosimetry*

Some researchers have expressed interest in calculating dose to animal organs. As with the development of human dosimetry phantoms, to be discussed below, early efforts involved animal dosimetry phantoms comprised of geometric shapes to describe organs and progressed to more realistic, image-based voxel phantoms. Yoriyaz and Stabin [5] constructed a geometric model of the mouse and generated dose factors (DFs) for a selected number of source and target pairs for ^{213}Bi and ^{90}Y. Muthuswamy et al. [6] developed a dosimetric model of mouse marrow and provided DFs for ^{131}I, ^{186}Re, and ^{90}Y. Konijnenberg et al. [7] developed a stylized representation of Wistar rats and performed Monte Carlo calculations to develop DFs for several radionuclides. With the advent of small animal imaging technologies, it became possible to move away from the use of stylized, equation-based body models and develop representations that more realistically define organ size, shape, and proximity. Kolbert et al. [8] used MR images of a female athymic mouse to develop realistic models of several organs and estimated self-dose and cross-dose values for these organs. Hindorf et al. [9] developed a model of a mouse using geometric shapes to define ten organs and then converted the model to a voxel format. Stabin et al. [10] segmented micro-CT images of a mouse and rat and developed specific absorbed fractions (SAFs) for photon and electron sources within the animal organs and DFs for several source and target regions. Keenan et al. [11] developed three mouse and five rat dosimetric models, using the MOBY and ROBY models developed by Segars and Tsui [12] and provided photon and electron absorbed fractions and dose factors for several radionuclides. These animal models have been incorporated into the OLINDA/EXM dosimetry code [13], thus facilitating dose calculations for these eight small animal types.

(iii) *Human data*

Imaging studies with either patients or healthy volunteers, required by the FDA for new drug approval (strict dose limits for new drugs do not exist, but dosimetry must be presented and is usually compared to other similar agents), need to be done according to the same requirements for number and spacing of time points as described above. The two basic imaging methods are planar imaging and tomographic imaging. For PET radiopharmaceuticals, tomographic methods are by far the most common approach, so an extensive description of planar methods will not be presented here. Briefly, anterior and posterior images are taken, regions of interest (ROIs) are drawn over recognized organs, and corrections for attenuation and scatter should be made [2]. Relating counts in an ROI to absolute values of activity is usually not straightforward, unless calibration factors have been developed from phantom image analysis, which is not common. Usually counts in the total body at the earliest imaging time, corrected for radioactive decay, are used to define 100 % of the administered activity, and counts in the body and organs at later times are related to this value. In tomographic images, as for animal studies, counts in voxels associated with an organ may be related to absolute values of activity via a calibration factor, and time-activity curves may be developed from this information. PET images are inherently quantitative, as PET analyses evaluate absolute levels of activity in organs and tumors (standardized uptake values, SUVs). In contrast, few centers practice quantitative analyses with single-photon emission computed tomography (SPECT); Dewaraja et al. [14] outlined the many steps required to obtain quantitative SPECT data for therapy dosimetry calculations, including choice of collimator, choice of energy windows, reconstruction methods, attenuation and scatter correction, dead time corrections, compensation for other image-degrading effects, choice of target regions, corrections for dose nonuniformities, and other aspects to be considered to obtain quantitative information in individual voxels used to define source and target regions.

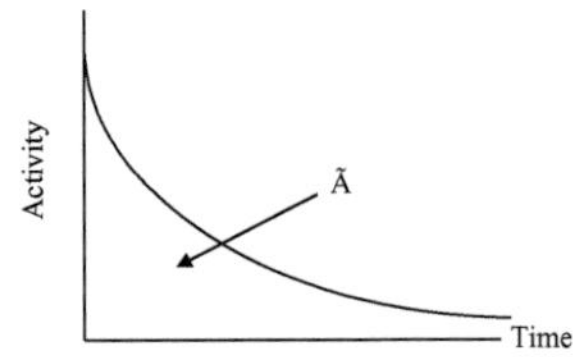

Fig. 3.1 Hypothetical time-Time abscissa curve

(iv) *Kinetic analyses*

The result of the biokinetic analyses described above is a series of values of percent or fraction of administered activity over time (Fig. 3.1). Values of doses for individual organs rely on the integration of these values over time. The most common method for performing this integration is to fit a function comprised of one or more exponential terms to the data. One may also integrate the data "directly," i.e., by a "trapezoidal" integration, simply directly calculating the area under the curve between any two time points and adding up the values. A drawback of this approach is that estimating the area under the curve after the last data point is complicated; various approaches include assuming only radioactive decay after the last point, using a straight line defined by the last two or three data points, and other approaches. When an exponential function is fit to the data, the time-activity integral is easily calculated. If the function is $A(t) = A_1\ e^{-\lambda_1\ t} + A_2\ e^{-\lambda_2\ t}$, and the values of λ are effective rate constants (including both radioactive decay and biological removal), the integral of this function to infinite time is just $A_1/\lambda_1 + A_2/\lambda_2$. If values of A are in MBq and values of λ have units of s^{-1}, then the integral has units of MBq-s or millions of disintegrations. These integrals are often normalized to the amount of activity administered (MBq), so that doses are developed per unit administered activity. The units of this normalized integral are thus MBq-s/MBq. It is tempting to think of this as having units of time (here s), but this is not any measure of time.

3.4 Example Dose Calculations

(a) *Organ doses*

Data from a kinetic study yield the following parameters for a new compound tagged to ^{18}F (the values of f are the fraction of administered activity observed with the noted half-times):

Liver	$f_1 = 0.35$	$T_{e1} = 0.9$ h
	$f_2 = 0.15$	$T_{e2} = 1.2$ h

Assuming a 1 MBq administration, the number of disintegrations would be

$$N = \frac{0.35\,\text{MBq} \times 3600\,s\,\text{h}^{-1}}{0.9\,\text{h}^{-1}} + \frac{0.15\,\text{MBq} \times 3600\,\text{s}\,\text{h}^{-1}}{1.2\,\text{h}^{-1}}$$

$$N = 1799\,\text{MBq} - \text{s} = 1.8 \times 10^9 \text{ disintegrations}$$

The dose factor from the liver to the liver for F-18 is 3.4E-05 mGy/MBq-s; the dose factor from the liver to the spleen is 5.54E-7 mGy/MBq-s. So given this input data, the dose to the liver and the spleen would be 1799 MBq-s × 3.4E-05 mGy/MBq-s = 0.061 mGy and 1799 MBq-s × 5.54E-07 mGy/MBq-s = 0.001 mGy, respectively. There would be many more source and target organs to consider in a real problem, of course. The OLINDA/EXM software code [13] facilitated and standardized the calculation of radiation doses from radiopharmaceuticals. Available dose factors have been based for years on "stylized" anthropomorphic phantoms for adults, children, and pregnant women (e.g., [15, 16]), but are now replaced with realistic, image-based voxelized models [17]. Monte Carlo studies establish absorbed fractions for electrons and photons for defined organ pairs; dose factors are developed using decay data and defined organ masses, as described above.

(b) *Effective dose*

The International Commission on Radiological Protection [18], in the context of radiation protection quantities and limits for radiation workers, defined a new dosimetry quantity, the "effective dose equivalent." The ICRP subsequently renamed this quantity "effective dose" in 1991 [19], and new weighting factors were given again in ICRP Publication 103 [20]. Certain organs or organ systems were assigned dimensionless weighting factors (Table 3.3), which are assumed to relate to their differing radiosensitivity for expressing fatal cancers or genetic defects.

Table 3.3 Weighting factors recommended by the ICRP for calculation of effective dose

Organ	ICRP 30 (1979)	ICRP 60 (1991)	ICRP 103 (2007)
Gonads	0.25	0.20	0.08
Red marrow	0.12	0.12	0.12
Colon		0.12	0.12
Lungs	0.12	0.12	0.12
Stomach		0.12	0.12
Bladder		0.05	0.04
Breasts	0.15	0.05	0.12
Liver		0.05	0.04
Esophagus		0.05	0.04
Thyroid	0.03	0.05	0.04
Skin		0.01	0.01
Bone surfaces	0.03	0.01	0.01
Brain			0.01
Salivary glands			0.01
Remainder	0.30	0.05	0.12

The assumed radiosensitivities were derived from the observed rates of expression of these effects in various populations exposed to radiation. Multiplying an organ's dose equivalent by its assigned weighting factor gives a "weighted dose equivalent." The sum of weighted dose equivalents for a given exposure to radiation is the effective dose:

$$E = \sum_T H_T \times w_T$$

An example calculation of the effective dose using the tissue weighting factors from ICRP

60 and assumed individual organ equivalent doses is shown here:

Organ	Weighting Factor	Equivalent Dose (mSv)	Weighted dose Equivalent (mSv)
Liver	0.05	0.59	0.0295
Kidneys	0.005	0.33	0.00165
Ovaries	0.20	0.25	0.050
Red marrow	0.12	0.42	0.0504
Bone surfaces	0.01	0.55	0.0055
Thyroid	0.05	0.15	0.0075
Total (effective dose)			0.145

The effective dose is meant to represent the equivalent dose that, if received uniformly by the whole body, would result in the same total risk as that actually incurred by a given actual nonuniform irradiation.

(c) *Standardized dose tables*
Dose tables for many PET radiopharmaceuticals have been generated by the OLINDA/EXM code [13]. Example tables are shown here (Tables 3.4 and 3.5):

(d) *Patient-individualized dosimetry in radiopharmaceutical therapy*
An extensive debate is ongoing regarding the role of patient-individualized dosimetry in therapeutic applications of radiopharmaceuticals. Stabin [21] addressed many of the objections raised by physicians and others to the use of dosimetry in radionuclide therapy, which is of course routine in external beam radiotherapy. Brans et al. [22] discussed the "quest for the 'Holy Gray,'" strengths and weaknesses of current models, and methods related to the development of clinical radiopharmaceutical dosimetry for individual subjects and concluded that "…only prospective, randomised trials with adequate methodology can provide the evidence that applied clinical dosimetry results in better patient outcome than is achieved with fixed activity dosing methods." Flux et al. [23] responded that " it is now time for a fundamental change in the way that radionuclide therapies are conducted. Individual treatment planning and assessment, based on accurate absorbed dose estimates, will prevent unnecessary therapies from being carried out, will significantly improve treatment efficacy and will provide the foundation for significant advances in radionuclide therapy." The discussion continues with considerable passion on both sides of the argument. In Europe, there is some movement toward advancing dosimetry into the nuclear medicine clinical environment, which will hopefully be reflected in other countries soon. Planning of individual therapies requires an evaluation of the biodistribution and biokinetics expected of the agent during the therapeutic regime.

Table 3.4 Sample dose estimates for selected PET radiopharmaceuticals in adults (mSv/MBq administered)

Target organ	F-18 FDG[a]	F-18L-DOPA[b]	C-11 acetate
Adrenals	1.16E-02	9.36E-03	3.27E-03
Brain	3.68E-02	6.79E-03	9.61E-04
Breasts	8.26E-03	6.40E-03	1.21E-03
Gallbladder wall	1.25E-02	1.00E-02	3.47E-03
LLI wall	1.34E-02	1.71E-02	1.33E-03
Small intestine	1.17E-02	1.23E-02	1.78E-03
Stomach wall	1.07E-02	9.10E-03	2.01E-03
ULI wall	1.14E-02	1.14E-02	1.88E-03
Heart wall	6.74E-02	8.56E-03	1.26E-02
Kidneys	1.03E-02	2.42E-02	5.33E-02
Liver	2.05E-02	8.73E-03	1.35E-02
Lungs	1.93E-02	7.61E-03	1.67E-03
Muscle	9.73E-03	9.53E-03	1.38E-03
Ovaries	1.35E-02	1.67E-02	1.44E-03
Pancreas	1.12E-02	9.73E-03	1.14E-02
Red marrow	9.59E-03	8.55E-03	1.47E-03
Osteogenic cells	1.45E-02	1.26E-02	1.82E-03
Skin	7.36E-03	6.71E-03	1.04E-03
Spleen	1.00E-02	8.96E-03	2.46E-03
Testes	1.05E-02	1.29E-02	1.05E-03
Thymus	1.10E-02	7.86E-03	1.48E-03
Thyroid	9.60E-03	7.81E-03	1.13E-03
Urinary bladder wall	1.32E-01	2.91E-01	1.27E-03
Uterus	1.79E-02	2.69E-02	1.43E-03
Total body	1.12E-02	9.43E-03	1.97E-03
Effective dose	1.79E-02	2.17E-02	2.75E-03

[a]Fluorodeoxyglucose
[b]L-3,4-dihydroxyphenylalanine

Table 3.5 Sample dose estimates for ^{18}FDG in adults and children (mSv/MBq administered)

	Adults	15-year-olds	10-year-olds	5-year-olds	1-year-olds
Adrenals	1.16E-02	1.46E-02	2.24E-02	3.54E-02	6.41E-02
Brain	3.68E-02	3.73E-02	3.92E-02	4.41E-02	6.09E-02
Breasts	8.26E-03	1.05E-02	1.66E-02	2.63E-02	5.00E-02
Gallbladder wall	1.25E-02	1.50E-02	2.29E-02	3.45E-02	6.30E-02
LLI wall	1.34E-02	1.60E-02	2.54E-02	3.81E-02	6.31E-02
Small intestine	1.17E-02	1.49E-02	2.36E-02	3.68E-02	6.65E-02
Stomach wall	1.07E-02	1.33E-02	2.05E-02	3.27E-02	6.03E-02
ULI wall	1.14E-02	1.40E-02	2.21E-02	3.53E-02	6.29E-02
Heart wall	6.74E-02	8.74E-02	1.35E-01	2.13E-01	3.78E-01
Kidneys	1.03E-02	1.29E-02	2.00E-02	3.26E-02	5.92E-02
Liver	2.05E-02	2.70E-02	4.00E-02	5.99E-02	1.10E-01
Lungs	1.93E-02	2.78E-02	3.93E-02	5.97E-02	1.15E-01
Muscle	9.73E-03	1.21E-02	1.90E-02	3.00E-02	5.55E-02
Ovaries	1.35E-02	1.71E-02	2.60E-02	3.98E-02	6.91E-02
Pancreas	1.12E-02	1.42E-02	2.22E-02	3.52E-02	6.49E-02
Red marrow	9.59E-03	1.20E-02	1.79E-02	2.76E-02	6.22E-02
Osteogenic cells	1.45E-02	1.87E-02	2.66E-02	4.06E-02	8.36E-02
Skin	7.36E-03	9.01E-03	1.43E-02	2.32E-02	4.40E-02
Spleen	1.00E-02	1.28E-02	1.97E-02	3.23E-02	5.96E-02
Testes	1.05E-02	1.37E-02	2.24E-02	3.41E-02	6.01E-02
Thymus	1.10E-02	1.38E-02	2.09E-02	3.24E-02	6.02E-02
Thyroid	9.60E-03	1.21E-02	1.91E-02	3.12E-02	5.85E-02
Urinary bladder wall	1.32E-01	1.68E-01	2.51E-01	3.45E-01	4.62E-01
Uterus	1.79E-02	2.18E-02	3.46E-02	5.14E-02	8.24E-02
Total body	1.12E-02	1.39E-02	2.20E-02	3.45E-02	6.39E-02
Effective dose	1.79E-02	2.30E-02	3.46E-02	5.17E-02	8.90E-02

Usually a small amount of the same radiopharmaceutical is administered, and subjects are imaged over several times, and the therapeutic administration may be monitored to confirm the behavior of the compound. Kobe et al. [24] significantly improved the first treatment efficacy of ^{131}NaI in treating hyperthyroidism with this approach. Flux et al. [25] stressed the importance of internal dose calculations for individual patients (many who are pediatric subjects) for the therapeutic use of ^{131}I-mIBG. Appropriate PET radiopharmaceuticals would be highly desirable for therapy planning, due to their superior resolution and inherent quantitative nature. "Surrogate" radiopharmaceuticals can be problematic to prove congruence (e.g., use of ^{111}In Zevalin to plan ^{90}Y Zevalin therapy for non-Hodgkin's lymphoma); the ideal situation is to use a positron emitting isotope of the same element, e.g., ^{124}I to plan ^{131}I therapies and ^{86}Y to plan ^{90}Y therapies. Blaickner and Baum [26] noted that "Individual organ dosimetry is also essential for critical organs in order to prevent radiotoxicities" and reviewed the clinical utility of using ^{86}Y-DOTATOC to plan ^{90}Y-DOTATOC therapy for neuroendocrine tumors, noting the advantages of spatial resolution and quantification and noting the drawback of the prompt gamma emissions and the short physical half-life. There are also issues of the availability of ^{86}Y in the marketplace. ^{90}Y has a very small positron component (0.003 %), but if therapeutic levels are administered, very nice PET images can be obtained for selective internal radiotherapy (SIRT) (e.g., [27]). Ga-68-labeled DOTA-peptides are useful in imaging and planning therapies for neuroendocrine tumors [28], but the short half-life (68 min) does not allow for characterization of some of the possible long-term retention components.

Because of the reluctance of physicians to gather data for dosimetry calculations, the database of information at present is sparse. Everyone agrees that a large clinical trial with and without a dosimetry component would settle the discussion about the relevance of dosimetry to radiopharmaceutical therapy, but no one seems willing to fund this effort. Many centers have established that clinical dosimetry can be done with good accuracy, with prediction of biological response. Still the resistance of most of the nuclear medicine community remains strong against realizing this component. PET radiopharmaceuticals will certainly have a role to play in this process, should it someday become routine.

3.5 The Pregnant or Lactating Patient

Dose to the embryo/fetus in the pregnant or potentially pregnant patient is an area of significant concern, due to the radiosensitivity of the unborn child. The distribution of the radiopharmaceutical in the pregnant patient is generally assumed to be the same as in the nonpregnant subject. Dose to the embryo/fetus is due to photon radiation coming from organs in the mother and photon and electron radiation from activity that may cross the placenta and enter the body of the embryo/fetus. There are some animal data regarding placental crossover of radiopharmaceuticals and sparse human data [29]. The pregnant female models of Stabin et al. [16], implemented in the OLINDA/EXM computer code [13], permit calculation of radiation dose to the embryo/fetus, including from the fetus itself, and activity in the placenta for the 6- and 9-month models. Again, data are difficult to obtain, but are available for some compounds. Particularly for ^{18}FDG, data have been obtained in both animal and human subjects. Russell et al. [30] reported dose estimates for ^{18}F-FDG with no consideration of placental crossover. Later, Stabin [31] revised the fetal doses throughout gestation using measured ^{18}FDG placental crossover in primates. Takalkar et al. [32] reported ^{18}FDG fetal uptakes in five pregnant subjects, using nuclear medicine imaging to quantify the uptakes. Their measured time-activity integrals and estimated doses were reasonably consistent with those of Stabin for different stages of gestation, but generally lower (0.007–0.02 mGy/MBq vs. 0.017–0.02 mGy/MBq reported by Stabin). Zanotti-Fregonara et al. [33] evaluated fetal uptake and dose in a 21-week pregnant subject. Their estimate of fetal dose was 0.0197 mGy/MBq administered to the mother.

Many radiopharmaceuticals are excreted in breast milk. Stabin and Breitz [34] discussed some of the many compounds and nutrients that are expressed in breast milk. Measuring activity in a milk sample is easier than quantitative imaging of the fetus in a pregnant subject, so a number of authors have presented data on measured concentrations at various times after radiopharmaceutical administration to a lactating mother. There are difficulties in assigning doses to the nursing infant, as most radiopharmaceutical dose estimates are based on injected, not ingested compounds. The measurements typically do not account for the chemical form that was in the breast milk. Calculated dose estimates generally assume that the ingested radioactivity quickly enters the infant's bloodstream and then is distributed and cleared from the body in the same manner as an injection to an adult subject, as this is probably a conservative way to treat the data and there are simply no data to support any other approach. A recent ICRP publication [35] reviewed the available data on breast milk excretion of radiopharmaceuticals using a dose criterion of 1 mSv effective dose to the infant to estimate recommended breast milk interruption times; they recommended that no breast feeding interruption is warranted for any PET compound that they evaluated.

Conclusions

Calculation of dose estimates for PET radiopharmaceuticals relies mostly on the gathering of high-quality biokinetic data. Data from animal studies are a necessary part, but are not highly reliable in predicting human dosimetry. Trials with human subjects are always the key step in understanding the dosimetry of a new agent. Once adequate biokinetic data are available, standardized dosimetry codes (i.e., OLINDA/EXM) can provide excellent tables of doses to organs and effective doses.

References

1. Stabin MG, Xu XG. Basic principles in the radiation dosimetry of nuclear medicine. Semin Nucl Med. 2014;44:162–71.
2. Stabin MG. Fundamentals of nuclear medicine dosimetry. New York: Springer; 2008.
3. Kirschner A, Ice R, Beierwaltes W. Radiation dosimetry of 131I-19-iodocholesterol: the pitfalls of using tissue concentration data, the author's reply. J Nucl Med. 1975;16(3):248–9.
4. Sparks R, Aydogan B. Comparison of the effectiveness of some common animal data scaling techniques in estimating human radiation dose. In: Proceedings of the sixth international radiopharmaceutical dosimetry symposium, Oak Ridge Institute for Science and Education; 1999, p. 705–16.
5. Yoriyaz H, Stabin M. Electron and photon transport in a model of a 30 g mouse. J Nucl Med. 1997; 38(Suppl):228P.
6. Muthuswamy MS, Roberson PL, Buchsbaum DJ. A mouse bone marrow dosimetry model. J Nucl Med. 1998;39:1243–7.
7. Konijnenberg MW, Bijster M, Krenning EP, de Jong M. A stylized computational model of the rat for organ dosimetry in support of preclinical evaluations of peptide receptor radionuclide therapy with 90Y, 111In, or 177Lu. J Nucl Med. 2004;45:1260–9.
8. Kolbert KS, Watson T, Matei C, Xu S, Koutcher JA, Sgouros G. Murine S factors for liver, spleen and kidney. J Nucl Med. 2003;44:784–91.
9. Hindorf C, Ljungberg M, Strand S-E. Evaluation of parameters influencing S values in mouse dosimetry. J Nucl Med. 2004;45:1960–5.
10. Stabin MG, Peterson TE, Holburn GE, Emmons MA. Voxel-based mouse and rat models for internal dose calculations. J Nucl Med. 2006;47:655–9.
11. Keenan MA, Stabin MG, Segars WP, Fernald MJ. RADAR realistic animal model series for dose assessment. J Nucl Med. 2010;51(3):471–6.
12. Segars W, Tsui B. 4D MOBY and NCAT phantoms for medical imaging simulation of mice and men. J Nucl Med. 2007;48(Supplement 2):203P.
13. Stabin MG, Sparks RB, Crowe E. OLINDA/EXM: the second-generation personal computer software for internal dose assessment in nuclear medicine. J Nucl Med. 2005;46:1023–7.
14. Dewaraja YK, Frey EC, Sgouros G, Brill AB, Roberson P, Zanzonico PB, Ljungberg M. MIRD pamphlet no. 23: quantitative SPECT for patient-specific 3-dimensional dosimetry in internal radionuclide therapy. J Nucl Med. 2012;53(8):1310–25.
15. Cristy M, Eckerman K. Specific absorbed fractions of energy at various ages from internal photons sources. ORNL/TM-8381 V1-V7. Oak Ridge: Oak Ridge National Laboratory; 1987.
16. Stabin M, Watson E, Cristy M, Ryman J, Eckerman K, Davis J, Marshall D, Gehlen K. Mathematical models and specific absorbed fractions of photon energy in the nonpregnant adult female and at the end of each trimester of pregnancy. ORNL report ORNL/TM-12907; 1995.
17. Stabin MG, Xu XG, Emmons MA, Segars WP, Shi C, Fernald MJ. RADAR reference adult, pediatric, and pregnant female phantom series for internal and external dosimetry. J Nucl Med. 2012;53:1807–13.
18. International Commission on Radiological Protection. Limits for Intakes of Radionuclides by Workers. ICRP Publication 30. New York: Pergamon Press; 1979.
19. International Commission on Radiological Protection. 1990 Recommendations of the International Commission on Radiological Protection. ICRP Publication 60. New York: Pergamon Press; 1991.
20. International Commission on Radiological Protection. Recommendations of the ICRP. ICRP Publication 103. Ann ICRP. 2007;37(2–3).
21. Stabin MG. The case for patient-specific dosimetry in radionuclide therapy. Cancer Biother Radiopharm. 2008;23(3):273 84.
22. Brans B, Bodei L, Giammarile F, Linden O, Luster M, Oyen WJG, Tennvall J. Clinical radionuclide therapy dosimetry: the quest for the "Holy Gray". Eur J Nucl Med Mol Imaging. 2007;34:772–86.
23. Flux G, Bardies M, Chiesa C, Monsieurs M, Savolainen S, Strand SE, Lassmann M. Letter to the editor, clinical radionuclide therapy dosimetry: the quest for the "Holy Gray". Eur J Nucl Med Mol Imaging. 2007;34:1699–700.
24. Kobe C, Eschner W, Sudbrock F, et al. Graves' disease and radioiodine therapy: is success of ablation dependent on the achieved dose above 200 Gy? Nuklearmedizin. 2007;47:13.
25. Flux GD, Chittenden SJ, Saran F, Gaze MN. Clinical applications of dosimetry for mIBG therapy. Q J Nucl Med Mol Imaging. 2011;55:116–25.
26. Blaickner M, Baum R. Relevance of PET for pretherapeutic prediction of doses in peptide receptor radionuclide therapy. PET Clin. 2014;9:99–112.

27. Werner MK, Brechtel K, Beyer T, et al. PET/CT for the assessment and quantification of (90)Y biodistribution after selective internal radiotherapy (SIRT) of liver metastases. Eur J Nucl Med Mol Imaging. 2010;37(2):407–8.
28. Breeman WA, de Blois E, Sze Chan H, et al. Ga-labeled DOTA-peptides and (68)Ga-labeled radiopharmaceuticals for positron emission tomography: current status of research, clinical applications, and future perspectives. Semin Nucl Med. 2011;41(4): 314–21.
29. Russell J, Stabin M, Sparks R. Placental transfer of radiopharmaceuticals and dosimetry in pregnancy. Health Phys. 1997;73(5):747–55.
30. Russell JR, Stabin MG, Sparks RB, Watson EE. Radiation absorbed dose to the embryo/fetus from radiopharmaceuticals. Health Phys. 1997;73(5):756–69.
31. Stabin M. Proposed addendum to previously published fetal dose estimate tables for 18F-FDG. J Nucl Med. 2004;45(4):634–5.
32. Takalkar AM, Khandelwal A, Lokitz S, Lilien DL, Stabin MG. 18F-FDG PET in pregnancy and fetal radiation dose estimates. J Nucl Med. 2011;52: 1035–40.
33. Zanotti-Fregonara P, Koroscil TM, Mantil J, Satter M. Radiation dose to the fetus from [18F]-FDG administration during the second trimester of pregnancy. Health Phys. 2012;102(2):217–9.
34. Stabin M, Breitz H. Breast milk excretion of radiopharmaceuticals: mechanisms, findings, and radiation dosimetry. Continuing Medical Education Article. J Nucl Med. 2000;41(5):863–73.
35. International Commission on Radiological Protection. ICRP Publication 106. Radiation Dose to Patients from Radiopharmaceuticals – Addendum 3 to ICRP Publication 53 ICRP Publication 106. Ann ICRP. 2008;38(1–2).

Part II

PET Chemistry and Regulation of PET Radiopharmaceuticals

Chemistry of PET Radiopharmaceuticals: Labelling Strategies

4

Stefano Boschi and Filippo Lodi

Contents

4.1	**Introduction**	79
4.2	**Positron Emission Tomography: Radionuclides for Labelling PET Radiopharmaceuticals**	80
4.3	**Radiolabelling with Fluorine-18**	81
4.3.1	Electrophilic Fluorination	82
4.3.2	Nucleophilic Fluorination	83
4.3.3	^{18}F-Labelling of Biomolecules	87
4.4	**Radiolabelling with Carbon-11**	90
4.4.1	^{11}C-Methylation Reactions	91
4.4.2	^{11}C-Carbonylation Reactions	92
4.4.3	Reactions with Organometallic Grignard Reagents	93
4.5	**Radiolabelling with Oxygen-15 and Nitrogen-13**	93
4.6	**Radiolabelling with Gallium-68**	94
References		98

Abstract

Positron emission tomography (PET) is an imaging technology developed to use compounds labelled with positron-emitting radioisotopes as molecular probes to image and measure biochemical processes of mammalian biology in vivo. Since this area is rapidly developing, the demand for rapid synthetic methods for radiolabelling the molecule of interest is one of the main challenges for the radiochemists. This chapter will provide information about the most common radiolabelling strategies as well as the more recent developments in the synthesis of PET radiopharmaceuticals labelled with fluorine-18, carbon-11, nitrogen-13 and oxygen-15. Since gallium-68 has gained enormous importance in radiopharmacy in the last 10 years, a chapter will highlight the important role of radiolabelling with gallium-68 in clinical radiopharmacy.

4.1 Introduction

Positron emission tomography (PET) is an imaging technology developed to use compounds labelled with positron-emitting radioisotopes as molecular probes to image and measure biochemical processes of mammalian biology in vivo. While imaging tests like X-rays can show

S. Boschi, PhD (✉) • F. Lodi, PhD
Department of Nuclear Medicine,
S.Orsola-Malpighi University Hospital,
Bologna, Italy
e-mail: stefanoboschi51@gmail.com;
filippo.lodi@aosp.bo.it

M.M. Khalil (ed.), *Basic Science of PET Imaging*, DOI 10.1007/978-3-319-40070-9_4

what the structures inside your body look like, a PET scan produces images that show how your organs work. For instance, a PET scan can show how blood flows to your heart, what areas of your brain are more active or less active and what lesion are metabolically altered or express a certain type of receptors.

These imaging techniques rely on the use of exogenous radioactive probes able to provide a detectable signal. These probes can be designed to be tissue- or receptor-specific and provide a detailed picture of the targeted structure or biological processes under study. Despite the great wealth of information that such probes can provide, the development of the exogenous probes represents an important challenge for organic chemists and radiochemists.

The aim of this chapter is to provide an overview of the most common chemical approaches for the synthesis of PET radiopharmaceuticals in clinical radiopharmacy, starting from the "classic" approach regarding ^{18}F and ^{11}C radiopharmaceuticals to the more recent development of ^{68}Ga and "metal-based" radiopharmaceuticals.

4.2 Positron Emission Tomography: Radionuclides for Labelling PET Radiopharmaceuticals

PET is a non-invasive molecular imaging technique that is used to study and visualise human physiology by the detection of probes labelled by positron-emitting radionuclides. Since some of the positron-emitting radionuclides are low atomic mass elements (e.g. C, N and O) found in biomolecules, it is possible to directly label molecules of interest without interfering with their biological activity. This ability differentiates PET from other techniques, which make use of relatively large molecule which, when attached to the targeting species, can modify its bioactivity.

The development of 2-deoxy-2-^{18}F-fluoro-D-glucose (FDG) for studying energy metabolism [1] together with the establishment of a reliable synthesis [2] and the subsequent demonstration of the high usefulness of FDG tracer to identify metastatic sites in cancer patients were major breakthroughs leading to the development of PET as an indispensable tool in clinical nuclear medicine. Since then, fluorine-18 ($t½$ = 110 min) is the most widely used radionuclide in PET, and it is often referred to as the "radionuclide of choice" because of its favourable physical and nuclear characteristics.

^{18}F can be produced by medical cyclotron in two different molecular forms: the elemental form, $^{18}F_2$, and the ionic form, ^{18}F-fluoride or $^{18}F^-$.

$^{18}F_2$ is obtained from the nuclear reactions of $^{20}Ne(d,\alpha)^{18}F$ or $^{18}O(p,n)^{18}F$ and represents the most common reagent for electrophilic fluorination. Nucleophilic $^{18}F^-$ is commonly produced by the nuclear reaction $^{18}O(p,n)^{18}F$ from enriched $H_2{}^{18}O$. Although nucleophilic fluorination is currently the most common synthetic approach for ^{18}F-radiolabelling, electrophilic fluorination has played an important and historic role in the development of ^{18}F-labelled molecules for PET imaging.

Carbon-11 is an attractive and important positron-emitting radionuclide for labelling molecules of biological interest because of the ubiquitous presence of carbon in natural products and drug compounds. ^{11}C is currently produced either by 11 or 18 MeV medical cyclotron. Production occurs by proton irradiation of pure ^{14}N, which emits an α particle to give ^{11}C, according to the nuclear reaction $^{14}N(p,\alpha)^{11}C$.

The two major ^{11}C precursors used in synthesis are $^{11}CO_2$ and $^{11}CH_4$, which are formed when either small amounts of oxygen or hydrogen, respectively, are present in the target.

Besides ^{11}C and ^{18}F, the radionuclides ^{15}O and ^{13}N are attractive choices for labelling since their stable isotopes are ubiquitous in biologically active organic molecules. The extremely short half-lives of ^{13}N ($t½$ = 10 min) and particularly ^{15}O ($t½$ = 2 min) have imposed limitations with regard to radiosynthetic methods for these two isotopes. ^{15}O is commonly produced in a cyclotron by the reaction $^{14}N(d,n)$ ^{15}O, whereby irradiation of N_2 with an O_2 content of less than 5 % gives the common precursor $^{15}O_2$.

^{13}N is produced in the cyclotron by the nuclear reaction $^{16}O(p,\alpha)^{13}N$. Since ^{13}N is available as nitrate or nitrite in water (^{13}NOx), subsequent reduction with Devarda's alloy yields the most commonly used ^{13}N source, $^{13}NH_3$ [3–5]. Direct in-target production of $^{13}NH_3$ is usually carried out by addition of ethanol as a scavenger to the target water [6] or the use of methane gas [7]. Using traditional PET isotopes, due to their often short half-lives and rapid clearance, only early time points are available for imaging, leaving the investigation of biological processes, which occur over the duration of hours or days, difficult to explore.

With the continuing development of biological targeting agents, such as proteins, peptides, antibodies and nanoparticles, which demonstrate a range of biological half-lives, the need to produce new radionuclides with half-lives complementary to their biological properties has increased. As a result, the production and radiochemistry of radiometals such as Zr, Y and Cu have been investigated as radionuclide labels for biomolecules since they have the potential to combine their favourable decay characteristics with the biological characteristics of the targeting molecule to become a useful radiopharmaceutical.

Different Cu radionuclides (^{60}Cu half-life, 0.4 h; ^{61}Cu half-life, 3.3 h; ^{64}Cu half-life, 12.7 h) can be cyclotron-produced by "p,n" nuclear reactions using the corresponding enriched Ni isotope(s) as target material: $^{60}Ni(p,n)$ ^{60}Cu, ^{61}Ni (p,n) ^{61}Cu and ^{60}Ni (p,n) ^{64}Cu. ^{86}Y (half-life 14,7 h) and ^{89}Zr can be produced by a cyclotron via "p,n" nuclear reactions as follows: $^{86}Sr(p,n)^{86}Y$ and $^{89}Y(p,n)^{89}Zr$. Besides radiometals, the radiohalogen ^{124}I can also be used in a variety of PET research applications, such as protein and antibody iodinations, as well as in the design and synthesis of new PET tracers because of its conveniently long half-life ($t½ = 4.2$ days), and well-established labelling chemistry is [8, 9].

An alternative production of positron-emitting radionuclides is via a generator. This is the case for radioisotopes such as ^{68}Ga, ^{82}Rb and ^{62}Cu, produced by $^{68}Ge/^{68}Ga$, $^{82}Sr/^{82}Rb$ and $^{62}Zn/^{62}Cu$ generators, respectively. Generators have the advantage of allowing clinical studies without an on-site cyclotron, or if cyclotron beam time is not available, and they may provide radionuclides and radioactive probes at any time on demand.

^{68}Ga is of great interest as a positron emitter because of some important advantages. It has a physical half-life of 67.71 min, which is compatible with the pharmacokinetics of most radiopharmaceuticals of low molecular weight such as peptides, antibody fragments, aptamers and oligonucleotides.

The impressive success of utilising ^{68}Ga-DOTA-octreotides and PET/CT [10, 11] for staging neuroendocrine tumours (NET) paved the way not only to the clinical acceptance of this particular tracer for imaging NET but also to the realisation of the great potential of the $^{68}Ge/^{68}Ga$ generator for modern nuclear medicine in general. The most important PET radionuclides produced both by cyclotron and generator are summarised in Table 4.1.

4.3 Radiolabelling with Fluorine-18

^{18}F is the most often used radionuclide for diagnostic PET imaging since the decay properties of ^{18}F provide significant advantages. Among the routinely produced positron emitters, the relatively longer half-life of ^{18}F ($T½ = 109.8$ min) poses less constraints on synthesis time and permits longer imaging protocols to investigate processes of slower tracer kinetic up to about 6 h.

Moreover, the relatively longer half-life of ^{18}F also permits the distribution of ^{18}F radiopharmaceuticals to clinical centres that can be reached within a few hours of transport. In recent years, however, there has been a huge increase in the number of biologically active fluoro-organic drugs; the reason for this is directly due to the beneficial effects of simple substitution of an H atom by an F atom on the physical and/or biological properties of the molecule.

Tagging a molecule with ^{18}F in place of a hydrogen atom often does not change its size or shape, and generally metabolically stable compounds are obtained. The unknown effects of introducing an "unnatural" fluorine atom, however,

Table 4.1 Positron-emitting radionuclides

Nuclide	Half-life	Nuclear reaction	Decay mode	$\beta^{\pm}_{mean}$ (KeV)	Target material	Product
Cyclotron-produced PET radionuclides						
^{18}F	109.8 m	$^{18}O(p,n)^{18}F$	β^+ (96.7 %) EC(3.3 %)	249.8	$H_2{}^{18}O$	$^{18}F^-$
		$^{20}Ne(d,\alpha)^{18}F$ $^{18}O(p,n)^{18}F$			Ne/F_2 $^{18}O_2$	$^{18}F_2$
^{11}C	20.33 m	$^{14}N(p,\alpha)^{11}C$	β^+ (99.77 %) EC(0,23 %)	386	N_2+O_2	$^{11}CO_2$
^{13}N	9.96 m	$^{16}O(p,\alpha)^{13}N$	β^+ (99.8 %) EC(0.2 %)	492	H_2O	$^{13}NH_3$
^{15}O	122.24 s	$^{14}N(d,n)^{11}C$	β^+ (99.9 %) EC(0.1 %)	735	N_2+O_2	$^{15}O_2$
^{60}Cu	23.7 m	$^{60}Ni(p,n)^{60}Cu$	β^+ (93 %) EC(7 %)	970	^{60}Ni	^{60}Cu
^{61}Cu	3.33 h	$^{61}Ni(p,n)^{61}Cu$	β^+ (61 %) EC(39 %)	500	^{61}Ni	^{61}Cu
^{64}Cu	12.7 h	$^{64}Ni(p,n)^{64}Cu$	β^+ (17.6 %) EC(43.9 %) β^-(38.5 %)	278 190	^{64}Ni	^{64}Cu
^{86}Y	14.74 h	$^{86}Sr(p,n)^{86}Y$	β^+ (31.9 %) EC(68.1 %)	660	$SrCO_3$	^{86}Y
^{89}Zr	78.41 h	$^{89}Y(p,n)^{89}Zr$	β^+ (22.74 %) EC(77.26 %)	396	Natural ^{89}Y	^{89}Zr
^{124}I	4.18 days	$^{124}Te(p,n)^{124}I$	β^+(22.7 %) EC(77.3 %)	820	^{124}TeO	$^{124}I_2$
Generator-produced PET radionuclides						
^{62}Cu	9.67 m	$^{62}Zn/^{62}Cu$ generator	β^+ (97.83 %) EC (2.17 %)	1319		
^{82}Rb	1.27 m	$^{82}Sr/^{82}Rb$ generator	β^+ (95.43 %)	1472		
^{68}Ga	67.71 m	$^{68}Ge/^{68}Ga$ generator	β^+ (88.91 %) EC(11.09 %)	829.5		

Data source: National Nuclear Data Centre, Brookhaven National Laboratory, based on ENSDF and the Nuclear Wallet Cards

render an analogous compound with potentially changed physicochemical properties and with possibly altered biochemical, pharmacological and toxicological features. This necessitates a careful evaluation of new ^{18}F-labelled compounds with respect to their anticipated use if they are not identical with drugs of known pharmacology [12].

With a few exceptions, radiofluorinations can be classified as either electrophilic or nucleophilic. The electrophilic reactions mainly use molecular fluorine ($^{18}F_2$) of moderately low specific radioactivity, or reagents prepared from it, and include additions to alkenes, reactions with carbanions and especially fluorodehydrogenation and fluorodemetallation. The nucleophilic reactions usually involve no-carrier-added (high specific radioactivity) fluoride ($^{18}F^-$) as its $K^{18}F$-K222 complex and include S_N2-type substitutions in the aliphatic series and S_NAr-type substitutions in the aromatic and heteroaromatic series.

4.3.1 Electrophilic Fluorination

There are *two* major processes for ^{18}F-electrophile production:

1. Historical method consists in using the $^{20}Ne(d,\alpha)^{18}F$ nuclear reaction [13, 14], where the target gas consists of natural abundance

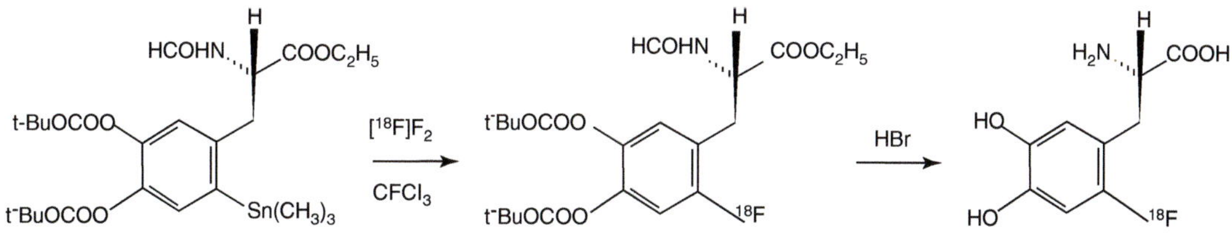

Fig. 4.1 Synthesis of 6-^{18}F-fluoro-L-DOPA

Ne containing 0.1–2 % F_2 as carrier. In this system, the carrier fluorine exchanges with ^{18}F produced by the nuclear reaction to yield ^{18}F-^{19}F molecules. Because of the large excess of $^{19}F_2$ molecules present, the resulting specific activity is very low.

Recovery from this target system is rather slow, ranging from about 50–70 % depending upon conditions such as beam current, length of irradiation and correlates with the carrier concentration. $^{18}F_2$ gas produced in the cyclotron can be directly used for electrophilic fluorination or alternatively be used as a progenitor of other fluorination reagents.

2. The two bombardment method, using $^{18}O(p,n)^{18}F$ nuclear reaction and O_2 gas for production of elemental fluorine $^{18}F_2$ [15], offers the opportunity to produce larger quantities, however, at the expense of being more complicated.

In this approach, the first bombardment is done on passivated nickel target charged with >95 % enriched O_2 and irradiated with 10 MeV protons to give ^{18}F. ^{18}F sticks to the target walls, while $^{18}O_2$ is recovered. Refilling the target with a noble gas (Ne or Kr)/$^{19}F_2$ mixture and a second irradiation allows radiolitically induced isotopic exchange reactions between the adsorbed ^{18}F and the molecular $^{19}F_2$ to generate the $^{18}F_2$. Specific activity is low and can be modulated by decreasing the $^{19}F_2$ concentration in the mixture which unfortunately leads to a decrease of $^{18}F_2$ yield.

Fluoride is a violently reactive gas that erratically reacts with organic molecules to give poor regioselectivity and mixtures of products that result from the addition across the double bond [16]. Considerable steps usually need to be taken to control the very reactive $^{18}F_2$ species. The use of fluorine diluted with an inert gas gives a more controllable reagent that can react selectively with organic compounds.

Another alternative for the use of the reactive $^{18}F_2$ electrophile is to convert it to the less reactive electrophilic moiety, acetyl hypofluorite (AcOF) [16, 17]. This method can be applicative for a direct labelling of small molecules [18] or peptides [17].

Other derivatives that have been used as electrophilic fluorinating reagents are ^{18}F Fluoropyridones [19, 20] and ^{18}F-fluoro-N sulfonamides [21]. These reagents can be used to fluorinate electron-rich substrates (such as alkenes and aryl compounds) by either direct electrophilic substitution or by demetallation reactions using organometallic reagents such as organomercury and organotin reagents. The widest use of ^{18}F-electrophile in clinical radiopharmacy is represented by the synthesis of ^{18}F-DOPA by regioselective, electrophilic fluorodestannylation reaction [22, 23] (Fig. 4.1).

$^{18}F_2$ gas with much higher specific activity can be produced with a "post-target" method developed by Bergman and Solin [24]. This could lead to three orders of magnitude higher improved specific activity of the tracer, but it is extremely difficult to implement in clinical radiopharmacy.

In conclusion, because of the relatively low specific activity caused by the carrier-added method of $^{18}F_2$ production and the poor specificity of labelling with electrophilic reagents, electrophilic ^{18}F-fluorinations are less favoured nowadays, and the general trend is to move to nucleophilic substitution reactions.

4.3.2 Nucleophilic Fluorination

Nucleophilic ^{18}F-fluorination reactions are routinely used to efficiently produce some of the most important PET radiotracers: virtually all

^{18}F-labelled radiopharmaceuticals used in clinical practice are obtained by this synthetic approach. Nucleophilic $^{18}F^-$ is commonly produced by the nuclear reaction $^{18}O(p,n)$ ^{18}F from enriched $H_2{}^{18}O$. The present technology for the production of $^{18}F^-$ consists of irradiating a small volume of enriched ^{18}O-H_2O in a metal target with protons of energies from near threshold (approximately 3 MeV) up to energy of the cyclotron, although energies above 13 MeV add little to yield while increasing the heat load on the target. Typical beam currents for research are on the order of 20–40 μA while beam currents for commercial production facilities are in the 60–100 μA range.

The new niobium target has proven to be a low maintenance target with reliable production and a good quality of $^{18}F^-$. Water targets in general can produce higher specific activity $^{18}F^-$ which is mandatory to achieve high specific activity tracers. Specific activities of 185 GBq/μmole or more (theoretical 63 TBq/μmol) have been achieved in routine production [25]. The choice of materials and careful handling are necessary to maintain high specific activity in the final product since stable fluorine can be found in many substances [26].

$^{18}F^-$ from the target is then trapped on an ion-exchange column which allows the recovery of $H_2{}^{18}O$. The trapped $^{18}F^-$ is then eluted from the ion-exchange resin using potassium carbonate in a water/acetonitrile solution. The aqueous $^{18}F^-$ obtained is, however, a poor nucleophile because of its high degree of solvation. The addition of the phase-transfer reagent kryptofix-222 (K222), followed by the removal of water has proven to be crucial in improving the reactivity of the ^{18}F fluoride ion for nucleophilic substitution reactions. The cryptand K222 forms a strong complex with the potassium cation (Fig. 4.2) and leaves the $^{18}F^-$ fluoride ion exposed (“naked”) and highly nucleophilic when dissolved in a polar non-protic solvent such as DMF, DMSO, or acetonitrile.

Tetrabutylammonium (TBA) is a phase transfer catalyst alternative to K222. Comparisons between the reactivity of the two catalysts seem to support the hypothesis that TBA fluoride gives greater yields of fluorinated products in short reaction times (<10 min) [27]. Conversely K222 could cope to metallic impurities from target better than tetraalkylammonium complexes [28].

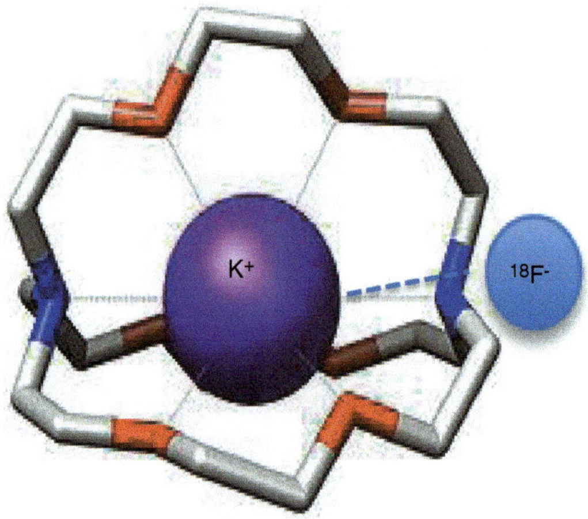

Fig. 4.2 Complexation of a potassium ion (*purple*) by the cryptand kryptofix-222 (K222); *light blue*: fluoride ion

In addition to ^{18}F-fluoride activation, the reacting precursor molecule is required to have a suitable leaving group and, in the case of aromatic rings, be suitably activated. In contrast to the wide variety of electrophilic reagents that have been developed and used with varying success, there is only one nucleophilic fluorinating reagent: fluoride ion. Nucleophilic fluorination can be performed both on aliphatic (S_N2) and aromatic compounds (S_NAr).

4.3.2.1 Aliphatic Nucleophilic Fluorination

Nucleophilic displacement that is usually used for aliphatic fluorination reactions involves the S_N2 substitution of ^{18}F ion and alkyl substrate containing good leaving groups such as halogens or sulfonic ester. Unlike aromatic substitution reactions, activating groups are not required.

Sulfonates are more reactive than halogens as a leaving group. There is a variety of sulfonate leaving groups available for aliphatic nucleophilic fluorination, such as p-toluenesulfonate (tosylate), methanesulfonate (mesylate), trifluoromethanesulfonate (triflate) and p-nitrosulfonate (nosylate). Among the sulfonates, reactivity increases from tosylate to mesylate and nosylate

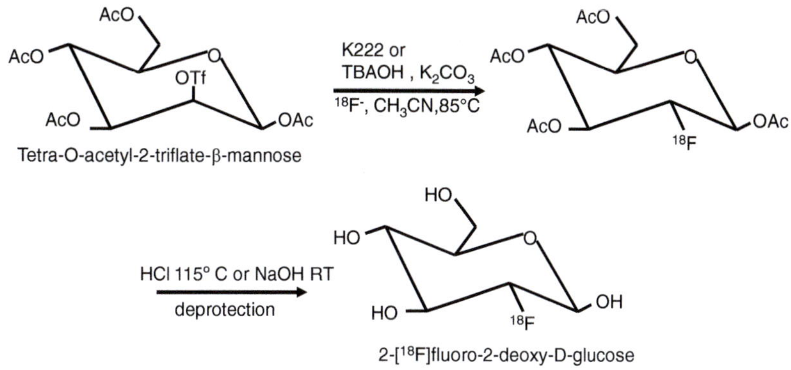

Fig. 4.3 Synthesis of ^{18}F-fluoro-2-deoxy-D-- glucose (^{18}F-FDG)

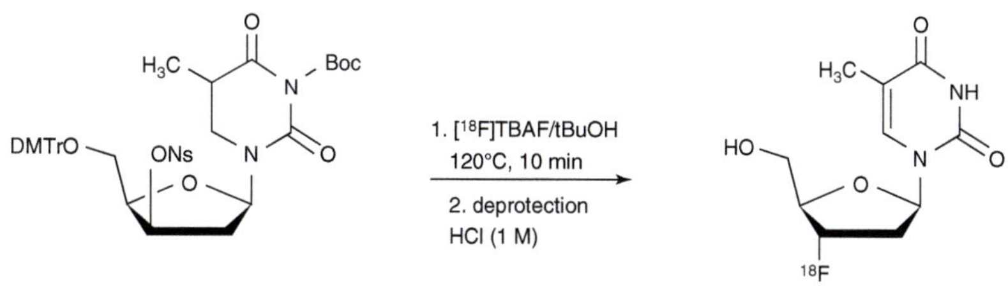

Fig. 4.4 Synthesis of ^{18}F-FLT by reaction in tert-butyl alcohol of the protected using [18F] TBAF as phase transfer catalyst

and to triflate that is the most reactive group for ^{18}F-labelling. Nevertheless, due to its high reactivity, triflate compounds may be unstable during the fluorination reaction temperatures; they cannot tolerate any water and are subject to side reaction such as elimination.

Depending on the stability of the precursor for labelling, the reactivity and simplicity of the incorporation, aliphatic fluorination can be formed by either direct labelling [2, 29] or formation of ^{18}F-fluoroalkyl agents [30, 31]. The main drawback of dirct labelling method is the need to protect any potentially competing sites of nucleophilic attack in the molecule (principally acid, alcohol or amine groups), thus resulting in additional synthesis and purification steps.

A good example of aliphatic nucleophilic ^{18}F substitution is the synthesis of ^{18}F-FDG [2] in which the acetyl-protected sugar tetra-O-acetyl-2-triflate-β-mannose is used during the direct ^{18}F-fluorination step. A deprotection of the ester groups completes the synthesis of ^{18}F-FDG. The synthesis of ^{18}F-FDG is now fully automated and can be achieved in approximately 30 min with radiochemical yields greater than 70 % (Fig. 4.3). A wide offer of synthesis modules, also equipped with disposable cassette that includes all the reagents, are available on the market.

Besides ^{18}F-FDG, many radiopharmaceuticals have been synthesised by S_N2 fluorination reactions involving aliphatic substitution such as ^{18}F-fluoro-3-deoxy-L-thymidine (^{18}F-FLT) [32, 33], ^{18}F-fluoroestradiol (^{18}F-FES) [34, 35], ^{18}F-fluoromisonidazole (^{18}F-FMISO) [36] and anti-1-amino-3-^{18}F-fluorocyclobutane-1-carboxylic acid (^{18}F-FACBC) [37], a promising tracer for staging prostate carcinoma.

Even if protic solvents, such as alcohols, are generally not used for nucleophilic substitution reactions because of their ability to solvate the nucleophile and retard its reactivity, the use of ionic solvents, such as tertiary alcohols, as a reaction media for the nucleophilic fluorination with alkali metal fluoride has been described [38, 39]. The protic medium is reported to suppress the formation of by-products and increase the rate of nucleophilic fluorination. An example is the significant improvement in the synthesis yield of ^{18}F-FLT [40] compared to previously described methods using ^{18}F-KF/K222 labelling procedure in aprotic solvents (Fig. 4.4).

^{18}F-fluoroalkyl agents are synthesised by S_N2 reaction of ^{18}F-fluoride with dihalo or disulfonate

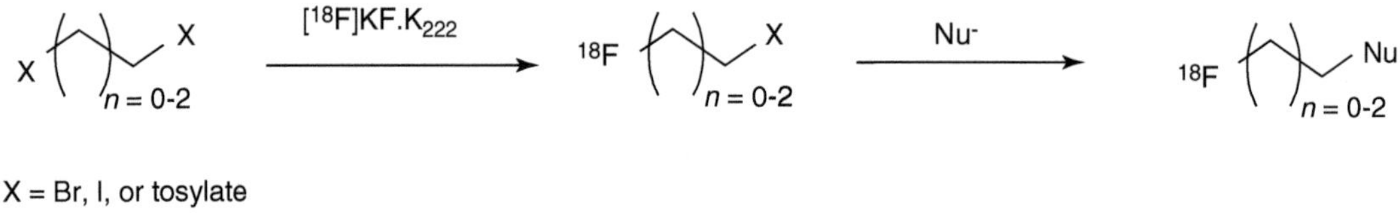

Fig. 4.5 Synthesis of a simple ^{18}F-fluoroaliphatic agents

alkyl starting materials with no-carrier-added fluoride ion in the presence of K_2CO_3/K222 complex or tetrabutylammonium hydroxide in organic solvents such as acetonitrile, o-dichlorobenzene or tetrahydrofuran [30, 31]. ^{18}F-fluoroalkylating agents with methyl, ethyl and propyl carbon backbones together with suitable leaving groups for reaction with nucleophilic species have been prepared (Fig. 4.5).

The large excess of the alkyl starting material compared to the $^{18}F^-$ allows exclusive formation of the mono ^{18}F-fluoroalkyl halide or sulfonate. After the formation of ^{18}F-fluoroalkyl agent, it can be used for the second alkylation reaction. ^{18}F-fluoroalkyl agents can be purified using gas chromatography separation or distillation from the reaction mixture into disposable C_{18} cartridges [31]. Purification of ^{18}F-fluoroalkyl agent before the next alkylation reaction provides more chemically and radiochemically pure product and eliminates non-volatile impurities, therefore increasing the radiochemical yield of the second alkylation reaction.

The most known aliphatic substitution reaction using ^{18}F-fluoroalkyl agents is the radiosynthesis of ^{18}F-fluorocholine, in which dibromomethane is fluorinated to generate ^{18}F-fluorobromomethane, which reacts with dimethylethanolamine to produce ^{18}F-fluorocholine [41]. In some cases, ^{18}F-fluorobromomethane can be converted to the more reactive synthon ^{18}F-fluoromethyltriflate, which would react more efficiently with 2-dimethylethanolamine to give ^{18}F-fluorocholine [31].

4.3.2.2 Aromatic Nucleophilic Fluorination

Introduction of no-carrier-added ^{18}F into aromatic ring is mostly limited to substitution on activated arenes. The presence of "activating" electron-withdrawing groups, such as cyano, trifluoromethyl, aldehydes, ketones and nitro, in the ortho and para positions on the aromatic ring decreases the electron density allowing for a sufficient activation for the nucleophilic substitution [16]. The leaving group most widely used in aromatic nucleophilic fluorination are nitro, quaternary trimethylammonium, alogens and sulphonates such as tosylate, mesylate and triflate. Due to low specific activity of the final product, isotopic exchange, ^{19}F-fluoride to ^{18}F-fluoride, is not used.

Direct aromatic nucleophilic fluorination has been used for obtaining high radiochemical yields and specific activities of ^{18}F-labelled compounds by a simple one-pot method [42]; however, not all the precursors for the labelling can handle high temperature and basic conditions of the fluorination; they may decompose during radiosynthesis. More often, the labelled compounds can be obtained by milder indirect ^{18}F-labelling methods. An example is the use of small ^{18}F-labelled reactive precursors bearing a reactive functional group that can form part of the intrinsic structure of the molecule or act as a "prosthetic label" to the molecule of interest such as proteins or other biomolecules. These ^{18}F-fluoroaromatic groups can be used as ^{18}F-precursor molecules by reacting rapidly and under mild conditions after the initial direct ^{18}F-fluorination step. A range of ^{18}F-fluoroaromatic precursors is shown in Fig. 4.6.

Nitrobenzene derivatives and ^{18}F-fluorobenzaldehydes are the most widely used precursors in the preparation of simple ^{18}F-fluoroaromatic compounds. The nitro group is both an activating group (in the ortho or para positions) and a leaving group under the right conditions. The strongly electron withdrawing nature of the nitrile group provide a high radiochemical yield of ^{18}F-fluorobenzonitrile precursors; moreover, the nitrile group can further be transformed

Fig. 4.6 ^{18}F-fluoroaromatic precursors synthesised by direct nucleophilic ^{18}F-substitution (*AG* activating group, *LG* leaving group, *X* I or Br)

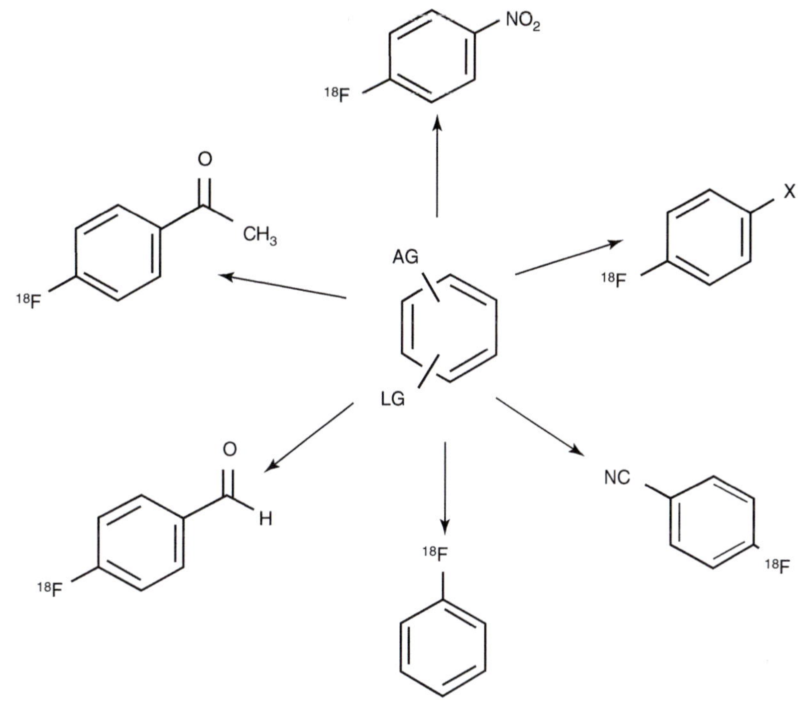

into reactive groups such as N-(4-^{18}F-fluorobenzyl)-2-bromoacetamide for the ^{18}F-labelling of peptides and oligonucleotides (see Sect. 4.3.3) [43].

The increased use and versatility of palladium-catalysed cross-coupling reactions in organic chemistry have had an important effect in the field of radiochemistry. The new chemical methods hold the unrealised potential of changing radiotracer design and development since the synthesis of relatively simple ^{18}F-fluoroaryl precursors has, until recently, been surprisingly quite problematic. Recently it has been described the process of the successful translation of a modern Pd-mediated fluorination reaction and the application to PET imaging. Transformation of ^{18}F-fluoride into an electrophilic fluorination reagent provides access to ^{18}F-aryl bonds that would be challenging to synthesise via conventional radiochemistry methods [44].

Aromatic nucleophilic substitution can also be done using diaryliodonium salts and, without the need of electron withdrawing groups, fluoride can be introduced into the arene. The introduction of ^{18}F-fluoride into dihomoaryliodonium salts precursor gives ^{18}F-fluoroarenes and the corresponding iodoarenes [45] and represents an extremely useful alternative for the synthesis of a range of simple ^{18}F-fluoroaromatic compounds in good radiochemical yields and in short reaction times that would be otherwise unobtainable by traditional methods. Very recently, it has been demonstrated that a novel synthetic approach to synthesise ^{18}F-DOPA via nucleophilic substitution of a diaryliodonium salt precursor with ^{18}F-fluoride [46] yielded a product with SA of three orders of magnitude higher than the product obtained by the traditional electrophilic destannylation with $^{18}F_2$ with comparable biological behaviour and imaging properties in neuroendocrine tumour model [47]. The simplicity of the synthesis method, compared with the conventional electrophilic approach along with the possibility of injecting a dose three orders of magnitude lower in comparison with the conventional product, thus dramatically reducing the risk of pharmacologic effects due to the co-administration of ^{19}F-DOPA, appears very promising.

4.3.3 ^{18}F-Labelling of Biomolecules

Biomolecules such as peptides, proteins, affibodies, antibodies and oligonucleotides can be labelled with fluoride-18 and evaluated for their potential as diagnostic imaging agents. Considering the relatively short ^{18}F half-life, labelling biomolecules with ^{18}F needs a careful consideration of the tracer kinetics since a fast clearance from the blood and high accumulation in target tissue should be required. Out of the biomolecules mentioned above, peptides fit these demands, with rapid clearance from the blood and high concentrations in target tissue. Moreover, the small size of peptides usually makes them relatively easy to synthesise with chemical modification, if needed, and they can often tolerate harsh chemical conditions for radiolabelling.

Larger biomolecules, such as antibodies, have slow pharmacokinetics (slow clearance from the blood) and high nonspecific binding, and they usually have lower uptake in target tissue and sometimes dependent on protein concentrations in the short time frame of the imaging.

Direct nucleophilic fluorination with ^{18}F-fluoride is not generally appropriate with larger peptides and proteins because of the high temperatures, organic solvents and basic conditions needed to obtain a good radiochemical yield. The strategy for labelling peptides and proteins for PET studies is based on the introduction of ^{18}F radionuclide by reaction with suitable prosthetic group under mild reaction condition. There is no general protocol for the synthesis of labelled peptides for PET, and often several labelling procedures need to be explored and optimised to find the best method for a particular peptide.

Many of these prosthetic ^{18}F-groups have been synthesised for targeting amino, carboxylic acid, or sulfhydryl functional groups within the peptide. N-terminal primary amino groups and lysine residues in proteins or peptides have received the greatest attention.

To date, the most common ^{18}F-prosthetic group for labelling biomolecules through the reactive amine group of lysine is the N-succinimidyl-4-^{18}F-fluorobenzoate (^{18}F-SFB) [48]. ^{18}F-SFB can be synthesised in different routes, starting from different precursors, but it requires a time-consuming three-step synthesis. Recently, however, significant advances have been taken to automate its synthesis [49]. Coupling of ^{18}F-SFB with peptides or proteins can be performed under mild pH and temperature conditions in aqueous media (pH 8–9). Acylation with ^{18}F-SFB was shown to be a convenient labelling method in terms of in vivo stability and radiochemical yield.

4-^{18}F-fluorobenzaldehyde (^{18}F-FBA) has also proven to be a versatile labelling reagent that is significantly easier to prepare than ^{18}F-SFB. Chemoselective ^{18}F-labelling, with high radiochemical yields and under mild reaction conditions, of peptides having an amino-oxyl functional group (via the formation of an oxime group) can be achieved using ^{18}F-FBA [50].

Another possible method involves labelling a thiol group (e.g. in cysteine) using ^{18}F-prosthetic group maleimide (^{18}F-maleimide) and its derivatives (^{18}F-FBABM) [51]. The radiosynthesis of ^{18}F-maleimide and its derivatives can also be done through the formation of other ^{18}F-prosthetic groups such as 4-^{18}F-fluorobenzaldehyde or ^{18}F-FBA that could be further reacted with different maleimide precursors to give various derivatives of ^{18}F-maleimide prosthetic groups [51]. 4-^{18}F-fluorobenzaldehyde is capable of forming bond with hydrazino group in the biomolecule, to form hydrazone [52].

^{18}F-glycosylation reactions of amino acids and peptides using chemoselective ^{18}F-fluoroglycosylated derivatives of ^{18}F-FDG have been reported to be an effective way of introducing an ^{18}F-label [53]. The glycosylation of biomolecules, such as peptides or proteins, has been frequently shown to improve the in vivo kinetics and stability in blood, to enhance bioavailability and BBB permeability and to accelerate the clearance of such glycoconjugates in vivo. Moreover, it has been shown by that glycosylation of peptides with subsequent radiolabelling opens the way to radiotracers with improved in vivo properties. The area of ^{18}F-glycosylation reactions has recently and comprehensively been reviewed [54].

The reaction of 1,3-dipolar cycloaddition (Huisgen reaction), flexible ^{18}F-labelling chemistry known as "click chemistry" and its use in radiochemistry were reported in 2006 [55] for the preparation of ^{18}F-labelled peptide fragments. Especially the Cu(I)-catalysed variant of the Huisgen 1,3-dipolar cycloaddition of terminal alkynes and azides (Cu-catalysed azide-alkyne cycloaddition, CuAAC) offers a very powerful reaction with high specificity and excellent yields under mild conditions [56].

^{18}F-labelled alkynes were prepared by the ^{18}F-nucleophilic substitution reaction of an alkyne tosylate. The large stoichiometric excess of the CuI catalyst and azide compared to the ^{18}F-alkyne results in good to excellent radiochemical yield for the conjugation step within 10 min at room temperature under basic conditions. The labelled compounds were obtained in high purity by using a simple purification method based on a C_{18} cartridge followed by evaporation of the eluent solvent and excess ^{18}F-fluoroalkyne. As a result, numerous PET tracers have been synthesised using CuAAC in a widespread spectrum of structural varieties of the prosthetic group within the last decade.

In 2007, it has been reported for the first time [57] ^{18}F-PEG derivatives as new ^{18}F-labelled prosthetic click groups. These compounds showed a reduced volatility and increased polarity compared with other ^{18}F-labelled prosthetic groups like ^{18}F-FEA or ^{18}F-fluoroalkynes. ^{18}F-labelled PEGylated prosthetic groups have been widely employed by for labelling peptides and nanoparticles [58–60]. ^{18}F-gluco derivatives for CuAAC-radiolabelling have been developed in order to improve the in vivo behaviour of peptides with respect to blood clearance and stability [54, 61].

However, the need of cytotoxic copper during CuAAC has led to the necessity of alternative fast and copper-free click reaction strategies for radiofluorination and additionally enabling pretargeting approaches in living systems. This has led to the development of copper-free click-labelling reactions which have been focused on derivatives of cyclooctynes and dibenzocyclooctynes [62] or on the possibility to perform Cu-free click reactions given by the inverse electron demand of the Diels-Alder cycloaddition between a cyclooctene and a tetrazine [63]. A detailed review on the development of click chemistry for ^{18}F-labelling has been recently published [64].

The field of click cycloadditions has a major impact in ^{18}F-labelling chemistry. Very mild reaction conditions, excellent efficiency and protection group chemistry not needed are particularly suitable for ^{18}F-labelling especially for complex and sensitive biomolecules such as peptide, proteins and oligonucleotides.

Silicon has a high affinity for F, allowing facile introduction of ^{18}F under mild conditions facilitating direct ^{18}F-labelling to Si-conjugated biomolecules. In silicon-based ^{18}F-fluoride acceptor (Si-FA) moieties, the Si atom is associated with an aromatic group, and ^{18}F-labelling of the Si is achieved by isotopic exchange or substitution of an OH group. The ^{18}F-Si-FA is then conjugated to the biomolecule. Since the side groups attached to the Si atom affect the stability of the ^{18}F-Si bond in the Si-FA moiety to hydrolysis, it has been demonstrated that tert-butyl groups dramatically improved the stability of the ^{18}F-Si complex in the labelling of peptide moieties [65, 66].

Efficient protein labelling by conjugation with ^{18}F-Si-FA has also been demonstrated [67, 68]. The authors [68] suggested that the ^{18}F-labelling of serum albumin for blood pool imaging procedure could be adapted to a simple kit method, avoiding time-consuming purification or toxic catalysts. The use of a boronic ester as a captor of aqueous ^{18}F-fluoride has been suggested as a means of labelling biomolecules in one step for PET imaging. Boroaryl compounds can form stable boron trifluorides, facilitating ^{18}F-fluorination of boronic acids or esters in the presence of ^{18}F-fluoride/KHF_2 mixtures. However, optimisation of radiolabelling conditions, as well as determination of the best electron-withdrawing substituents on the aromatic ring to achieve a practically applicable ^{18}F-labelling rate and tracers with ^{18}F-B bonds stable to hydrolysis, is strongly required. Further in vivo studies are needed to fully determine the potential of boron-based fluoride acceptor molecules for ^{18}F-labelling of macromolecules.

Radiolabelling of peptides and macromolecules with metal nuclides, for example, ^{68}Ga, ^{99m}Tc, ^{111}In, is carried out by a simple chelation step. These labelling procedures are easier than the ^{18}F and ^{11}C nucleophilic substitution reactions, do not require the use of the complex instrumentation and could be translated to a kit formulation.

A new method for ^{18}F-labelling was published by McBride et al. [69], which reported on the direct labelling of chelate-attached peptide with aluminium fluoride ($Al^{18}F$). Initially, ^{18}F-fluoride is attached to aluminium to form $Al^{18}F$, which is further reacted with peptides that contain macrocyclic chelator group such as NOTA (1,4,7-triaza cyclononane-1,4,7-triacetic acid), to form a stable complex of $Al^{18}F$-NOTA-peptide. This method is characterised by short synthesis time, aqueous environment, absence of toxic phase transfer catalysts and lower peptide concentration required for efficient labelling in comparison with ^{18}F-N-succinimidyl 4-(fluoromethyl) benzoate succinyl method [70].

^{18}F-fluoride should be purified with a QMA and the optimum pH adjusted with acetic acid to pH 4.0 and incubated with conjugated peptide at 100°. It has been also demonstrated [71] that ^{18}F-fluoride used directly without QMA purification produced similar labelling yields as QMA-purified ^{18}F-fluoride.

Optimisation of the factors that influence labelling yield including the Al^{3+}/peptide ratio, the presence of hydrophilic organic solvents and antioxidants allowed the translation of the labelling procedure to a kit form [72].

The aluminium fluoride approach has been applied to the labelling of several peptides such as RGD peptides for imaging of integrin $\alpha v\beta 3$ [73], bombesin derivatives [74], prostate-specific membrane antigen (PSMA) ligands [75], anti-CEA antibodies [76] and in vivo labelling of serum albumin for PET [77].

The chelation of $Al^{18}F$ with NOTA, NODA or other macrocyclic chelator-conjugated peptides represents the most promising novel approach for convenient ^{18}F-labelling of peptides and biomolecules since it is rather simple and can be developed in kit form, opening up the possibility of carrying out ^{18}F-labelling without the need for expensive PET chemistry facilities.

4.4 Radiolabelling with Carbon-11

Carbon-11 is an attractive PET radionuclide because is an ubiquitous element in biomolecules; thus, ^{11}C-labelled molecules will behave the same, chemically and biologically, as their unlabelled equivalent, preventing any doubts about the effect of introducing an "artificial" PET radionuclide (such as introducing an ^{18}F atom) may have on the biological properties of the compound of interest. Moreover, the possibility to choose from different labelling positions in the same molecule provides the possibility to refine the radiopharmaceutical in terms of metabolic stability and nonspecific background ratio [78]. The short life of ^{11}C also enables comparative PET studies with the same ^{11}C-tracer or with ^{11}C-tracer and ^{18}F-tracer (multitracer studies) in a short time frame with more favourable patient dosimetry [79].

On the other hand, the production of these radiopharmaceuticals must be performed in PET facilities with on-site cyclotrons and should be as fast as possible to reduce the loss of activity due to decay. Although the half-life of ^{11}C is rather short (20.4 min) and limits multistep synthesis, a diverse array of reactions has been applied and developed for the introduction of ^{11}C into target molecules.

One limitation is the small number of ^{11}C-precursors available that can be used directly in synthesis or converted into more reactive secondary precursors prior to the final radiolabelling step. $^{11}CO_2$ and $^{11}CH_4$, which are formed by $^{14}N(p,\alpha)^{11}C$ reaction (see Sect. 4.2) when either small amounts of oxygen or hydrogen, respectively, are present in the target, are the main ^{11}C-precursors used for the synthesis. Almost all ^{11}C-labelled compounds for PET are made from these two major synthons (Fig. 4.7).

$^{11}CO_2$ is produced using a mixture of nitrogen with trace amount to 2 % of oxygen, while $^{11}CH_4$ is produced using a mixture of nitrogen with 5–10 % of hydrogen as gas target. Another way to produce $^{11}CH_4$ is the reduction of $^{11}CO_2$ with hydrogen on a nickel catalyst at high temperature [80]. $^{11}CO_2$ can be recovered from cyclotron and purified by means of cryogenic trapping with liquid nitrogen or by trapping on molecular sieves [81]. $^{11}CH_4$ can be recovered and purified with a Porapak N trap [80]. The use of in-target-produced $^{11}CH_4$ improves the specific activity (SA) [82, 83] but requires a long time to reach

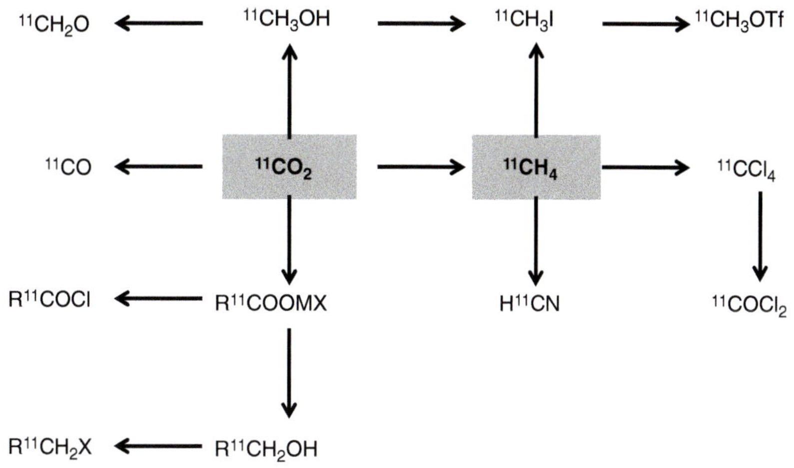

Fig. 4.7 Precursors used in the synthesis of ^{11}C-labelled compounds produced from the two major synthons $^{11}CO_2$ or $^{11}CH_4$

maximum yield, and, in general, total obtained activity is lower compared to $^{11}CO_2$ target [83].

The development of technology has had a pivotal role in the diffusion of ^{11}C tracers with relevant applications mainly in clinical oncology [84] and neurology. The use of fully automated synthesis modules [85–87] also combined with automated HPLC purification [88], microfluidic reactors [89, 90], "on-column" synthesis [91] and automated "loop" synthesis [92, 93] and other technological approaches, have enhanced the speed, efficiency, reliability and safety of radiosynthesis, leading to a final product characterised by pharmaceutical quality.

4.4.1 ^{11}C-Methylation Reactions

^{11}C-methylation leads to the incorporation of $^{11}CH_3$ methyl group into a target compound; it represents the most frequently used method for the introduction of ^{11}C into organic molecules.

^{11}C-methyl iodide ($^{11}CH_3I$) is the most commonly used methylating agent and can be prepared by using two different methodologies: the "wet chemistry", which is based on $^{11}CO_2$ reduction by $LiAlH_4$ and followed by iodination with hydroiodic acid [81, 94, 95], and the "gas-phase chemistry", which synthesises $^{11}CH_3I$ from radical iodination of $^{11}CH_4$ by molecular iodine [80, 96] (Fig. 4.8).

Compared to "gas phase chemistry", "wet chemistry" method generally provides $^{11}CH_3I$ in higher yields (almost twofold higher) and in shorter synthesis time. However, the use of reagents like HI and $LiAlH_4$ makes more difficult the management of the synthesis and cleaning procedures. Moreover, lower $^{11}CH_3I$ SA values are in general obtained since $LiAlH_4$ is a carrier of cold CO_2. Average SA values reached with this method are within 1–5 Ci/μmol decay corrected (DC) at the end of synthesis (EOS). Lowering $LiAlH_4$ amount, using freshly distilled solvent, low target volume and high purity gas are strongly recommended to increase $^{11}CH_3I$ SA [81].

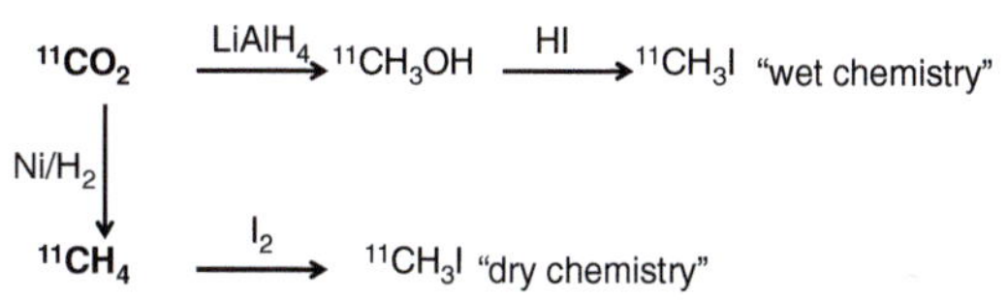

Fig. 4.8 Production of $^{11}CH_3I$ via $LiAlH_4$/HI method (*wet chemistry*) or via iodination of $^{11}CH_4$ (*dry chemistry*)

On the contrary, an advantage of the "gas phase chemistry" is the elimination of $LiAlH_4$, which contributes to the higher SA of $^{11}CH_3I$ (even more than 15 Ci/μmol DC at EOS [80]), a clear advantage of this method when higher SA radiopharmaceuticals are needed. Furthermore, elimination of $LiAlH_4$ and HI facilitates cleaning procedures and allows back-to-back syntheses of $^{11}CH_3I$ without adding or changing reagents.

The alternative methylating agent $^{11}CH_3$-methyl triflate ($^{11}CH_3OTf$) has become more important and more widely used in recent years because of its greater reactivity and volatility [97]; these properties make it ideally suited to rapid methylation reactions [98, 99].

^{11}C-methyl triflate is prepared by passing gaseous $^{11}CH_3$ through a column of silver triflate at 200 °C [97]. The introduction of the $^{11}CH_3$ group into a target molecule is generally carried out by nucleophilic substitution reactions of methyl iodide with a precursor amine, alcohol or thiol group to form the labelled primary or secondary amine, ether or thioether (N-, O- and S-methylation reactions). The synthetic methods used to carry out methylation reactions are relatively straightforward and usually involve simply trapping $^{11}CH_3I$ in a solution of the target precursor and heating for a short time. For some oncological tracers like ^{11}C-choline [91] or ^{11}C-methionine [100] that have an huge impact in clinical PET, methylation reactions are carried out also at room temperature using "on-column" approach.

The "loop" methods involve coating the inside surface of the loop with micromolar amounts of reagent precursor in a suitable solvent and then passing a gaseous stream of $^{11}CH_3I$ or $^{11}CH_3OTf$ through the stainless-steel or plastic/polymer loops as reaction chambers. This is an example of "captive method" where, as previously described in the "on-column" method, the solution of the target precursor is coated on a solid device and the $^{11}CH_3OTf$ is trapped. These methods have found increased use in simple ^{11}C-methylation reactions because of their ease of use, reproducibility and versatility.

The simplicity and speed of the methylation reaction has made it the primary method for the production of ^{11}C-labelled compounds. Many ^{11}C-methylation procedures have been reported not only for oncological tracers like ^{11}C-choline and ^{11}C-methionine but also for the production of ^{11}C tracers for imaging amyloid plagues (^{11}C-PIB [101]), dopamine receptors (^{11}C-raclopride [102], ^{11}C-*N*-methylspiperone [103]), opiate receptors (^{11}C-carfentanil [104]), benzodiazepine receptors (^{11}C-flumazenil [105]) and many others.

The dimethylamine functional group is a common component of the chemical structure of numerous drugs, thus representing an attractive moiety for ^{11}C-labelling. ^{11}C dimethylamine provides an attractive alternative method for the preparation of ^{11}C-methyl compounds with dimethylamine functional groups that avoid the direct use of ^{11}C-methyl iodide [106]. Many other reactions are used for ^{11}C-labelling particularly in research PET radiochemistry. Although the application of these labelling strategies in clinical radiopharmacy is still to be fully established, they should be briefly mentioned.

The vast developments in traditional synthetic chemistry where palladium catalysts are used for the formation of C-C, C-O and C-N bonds have led to a wider application of the palladium-catalysed reactions for C-C bond formation in the synthesis of ^{11}C compounds for PET. Palladium(0)-mediated Stille-type coupling reactions have been the most widely studied of the palladium coupling reactions for the introduction of ^{11}C methyl groups into organic molecules [107]. A review on the application of cross coupling reaction for the preparation of PET radiotracers has been published [108].

4.4.2 ^{11}C-Carbonylation Reactions

Labelling target molecules with ^{11}CO is an attractive strategy which came about for at least three reasons: first, the huge number of carbonyl-containing biologically interesting molecules that have the potential to be synthesised through carbonylation reactions; second, the use of ^{11}CO might be favourable because lower atmospheric concentration of stable carbon monoxide compared with carbon dioxide may result in higher SA of the tracer; third, the ready availability of ^{11}CO through the reduction of $^{11}CO_2$ over zinc or molybdenum.

The most widely applied ^{11}C-carbonylation method is the palladium-mediated carbonylation reaction [109]. Rhodium-mediated carbonylation reactions provide an alternative route for the introduction of ^{11}CO into organic molecules [110]. An exhaustive review of the ^{11}CO chemistry for the labelling of PET tracer covering all the aspects of transition-metal-catalysed carbonylation with ^{11}C has been published [111].

4.4.3 Reactions with Organometallic Grignard Reagents

$^{11}CO_2$ can be treated with organometallic Grignard reagents to form ^{11}C-carboxymagnesium halides and then transformed into ^{11}C-carboxylic acids. Acetate is an important metabolite in the synthesis of cholesterol and lipids. ^{11}C-acetate was initially employed for the study of myocardial metabolism [112, 113] and more recently in oncology for the imaging of prostate cancer [114, 115]. ^{11}C-acetate has been also employed in the study of hepatocarcinoma (HCC) [116, 117], lung cancer [118] and brain tumours [119].

^{11}C-acetate is synthesised by means of ^{11}C-carboxylation reaction of Grignard reagent methylmagnesium chloride or bromide (CH_3MgCl, CH_3MgBr) by cyclotron produced $^{11}CO_2$. Unlike ^{11}C-methylation reactions, the target product $^{11}CO_2$ is directly employed in the labelling step without any further chemical conversion. ^{11}C-carboxylation is then followed by hydrolysis and purification of the product. As regards the synthesis method, $^{11}CO_2$ can be bubbled directly in the Grignard reagent or can be flushed and reacted into a loop of different tubing materials containing methyl magnesium bromide coated onto the internal surface of the loop [93].

^{11}C-palmitate was identified as a valuable radiopharmaceutical for the assessment of myocardial metabolism and function [120]. A method for automated preparation on a commercial synthesis module of ^{11}C-palmitate and ^{11}C-acetate based on Grignard reaction has been described [121].

^{11}C-carboxylic acids obtained by reaction of $^{11}CO_2$ with Grignard reagents can also be converted into the more reactive acid chloride species and treated with amines to form [carbonyl-^{11}C] amides. This method has been used for ^{11}C-labelling at the carbonyl position of the $5HT_{1A}$ receptor ligand WAY100635 [122, 123].

4.5 Radiolabelling with Oxygen-15 and Nitrogen-13

Oxygen-15 and nitrogen-13 represent attractive choice for labelling since their stable isotopes are ubiquitous in biologically active organic molecules. Due to the extremely short half-lives, radiochemical syntheses of more than one reaction step are rarely performed. Simple chemical products such as $C^{15}O_2$, $H_2{}^{15}O$ and $^{13}NH_3$ can be obtained directly from the cyclotron target and used as such or rapidly converted into other simple products (e.g. $C^{15}O_2$ and $C^{15}O$).

$^{15}O_2$ is commonly produced in a cyclotron by the reaction $^{14}N(d,n)^{15}O$ by irradiation of N_2/O_2 mixture ($O_2 < 5\,\%$). $^{15}O_2$ could also be produced by the reaction $^{15}N(p,n)^{15}O$. This reaction could be used in any cyclotron, since it does not need deuterons option, but, on the other side, a ^{15}N recycling system to overcome the high cost of the enriched gas should be implemented. A common application of oxygen-15 is the study of regional cerebral blood flow by using ^{15}O-labelled water [124, 125]. ^{15}O-labelled water is obtained by conversion of $^{15}O_2$ into $H_2{}^{15}O$ by reduction over a platinum or palladium [126, 127] catalyst at high temperature. Other two ways to form ^{15}O-labelled water are available: (1) by the conversion of $^{15}O_2$ into $C^{15}O_2$, which is instantaneously converted after inhalation into $H_2{}^{15}O$ in the lungs by the carbonic anhydrase enzyme, and (2) by bombardment of $H_2{}^{16}O$ with protons according to the $^{16}O(p,pn)^{15}O$ nuclear reaction [128]. This yields $H_2{}^{15}O$ that can be administered intravenously.

The most commonly used ^{13}N source, $^{13}NH_3$, can be obtained by post target reduction of $^{13}NO_x$ (see Sect. 4.2) or by direct in-target production in presence of a scavenger such as ethanol (6) or methane (7). The 10-min half-life of ^{13}N precludes extensive synthetic reactions. In addition, the high positron range (maximum energy of 1.19 MeV, maximum range in water of 5.4 mm) usually leads to low resolution images, especially when compared with those obtained with ^{18}F-labelled radiotracers. Therefore, ^{13}N routine application in PET is limited to simple procedures, such as using ^{13}N-ammonia to measure myocardial blood flow [7, 129]. The developments in ^{13}N chemistry, including different production routes of primary precursors and their applications to the preparation of more complex ^{13}N-labelled molecules as well as current situation and future perspectives, have recently been reviewed [130].

4.6 Radiolabelling with Gallium-68

Fluorine-18, carbon-11, oxygen-15 and nitrogen-15 are radionuclides produced with a cyclotron and their use demands an on-site cyclotron. The half-life of the ^{18}F isotope is long enough to allow transportation of doses to sites several hours away.

An alternative production of positron-emitting radionuclides is via a generator. This is the case for radioisotopes such as ^{68}Ga, ^{82}Rb, ^{62}Cu (Tab.1.2); among them, ^{68}Ga has gained enormous importance in radiopharmacy in the last 10 years. The explosive growth of publications reflecting the success of ^{68}Ga applications is remarkable; rough estimation demonstrates that the number of ^{68}Ga-related scientific articles published during 2011–2012 stands for over 45 % of all publications since 1956 [131].

Gallium-68 is of great interest as a positron emitter because of some important advantages. It has a physical half-life of 67.71 min, which is compatible with the pharmacokinetics of most radiopharmaceuticals of low molecular weight such as antibody fragments, peptides, aptamers and oligonucleotides. ^{68}Ga decays to 88.91 % by positron emission and to 11.09 % via electron capture into stable ^{68}Zn. The average positron energy per disintegration is 829.5 keV (Tab.1.2) which is higher, for example, than that of ^{18}F and potentially leads to a somewhat lower resolution. Moreover, there is a well-established coordination chemistry of Ga^{3+} that allows the development of agents resistant to in vivo transchelation of Ga^{3+}.

The long half-life ($T½$.270.95 days) of the parent ^{68}Ge combined with the half-life of ^{68}Ga ($T½$.67.71 min) makes this pair almost ideal for a generator strategy. The development of the $^{68}Ge/^{68}Ga$ generator has been reviewed in several articles [132–135].

However, there are still some drawbacks for the direct use of the ^{68}Ga eluate in the preparation of radiopharmaceuticals. Among them are measurable activities of the long-lived ^{68}Ge (breakthrough), the high eluate volume and high HCl concentration. In addition, metallic impurities such as Zn^{2+}, generated from the decay of ^{68}Ga, Ti^{4+} or other residuals from the column material, as well as Fe^{3+}, could be present in the eluate. Thus, dedicated procedures to process the eluate from the radionuclide generator to remove the ^{68}Ge breakthrough, to purify from the metal impurities and to minimise the labelling volume of ^{68}Ga radiopharmaceuticals have been described. An anion exchange chromatography-based post-processing has been developed [136]. This strategy separates ^{68}Ge but does not allow for a direct loading of $^{68}Ga^{3+}$ on the anion exchange resin from 0.1 N HCl since it introduces an additional dilution step in 5.5 M HCl, and it does not provide purification of $^{68}Ga^{3+}$ from e.g. Zn^{3+} and Fe^{3+}. Another approach to overcome problems like eluate volume, acidic pH and content of ^{68}Ge and chemical impurities is to fractionate the initial generator eluate [137]. Contents of ^{68}Ge and metallic impurities are minimised because of the lower eluate volume used but in principle not chemically removed prior to the ^{68}Ga-labelling steps.

Cation exchange chromatography-based post-processing procedure consists in the direct transfer of the initial 0.1 N HCl ^{68}Ga eluate to a cation exchanger [138] and a selective elution with acetone/HCl mixtures. This procedure leads to almost complete removal of metallic impurities including ^{68}Ge breakthrough. More details on the purification of the $^{68}Ge/^{68}Ga$ generator eluate are extensively described in a recent review [134].

In aqueous solution, the only stable oxidation state of gallium is +3, where the free hydrated Ga^{3+} ion is stable only under acidic conditions. In the pH range of 3–7, it can hydrolyse to insoluble $Ga(OH)_3$, while at physiological pH, its solubility is high due to the almost exclusive formation of $[Ga(OH)_4]^-$ ions. Ga^{3+} is quite similar to the high spin Fe^{3+} ion with respect to its coordination chemistry; both are 3+ charged with similar ionic radii and the same major coordination number of six.

The Ga^{3+} ion is classified as a hard Lewis acid, forming thermodynamically stable complexes with ligands that are hard Lewis bases, containing oxygen, nitrogen and sulphur donor atoms, such as carboxylate, phosphonate, hydroxamate and amine but also softer functional groups, such as phenolate and thiol groups, were found to be appropriate. The main requirements for a Ga^{3+} chelate in order to be suitable as a radiopharmaceutical are the thermodynamic stability towards hydrolysis and the kinetic inertness during the period of clinical use in order to avoid ligand exchange with the blood serum protein transferrin. Human transferrin also has a high binding affinity for Ga^{3+} given by log $K_{ST}=20.3$ [139]. Thus, the complexes should be more stable than the Ga^{3+}-transferrin complex or kinetically inert in order not to exchange with this protein. On the other hand, hydrolysis and formation of the $Ga(OH)_3$ can be avoided in the presence of stabilising weak ligands such as acetate, citrate or HEPES, in the preparation of the complexes.

Several bifunctional chelators that present a functionality that allows covalent coupling to a targeting vector besides binding the metal cation have been proposed and coupled to biomolecules for gallium labelling. They should meet the following criteria:

1. They should chelate the radiometal rapidly and sufficiently when linked to a macromolecule.
2. The chelate should be kinetically stable to demetallation over a pH range of 4–8 and stable in the presence of other serum cations (Ca^{2+}, Zn^{2+}, Mg^{2+}).

One of the most known chelators used for radiometals in +3 oxidation state is the macrocyclic chelator 1,4,7,10-tetraazacyclododecane-1,4,7,10-tetraacetic acid (DOTA). DOTA and its derivatives are readily obtained from straightforward and convenient synthetic routes and available from commercial suppliers. Complexes obtained from DOTA, DO3A and its derivatives and DO2A and its derivatives have been shown to be sufficiently stable to avoid the loss of the Ga^{3+} core under physiological conditions.

Multiple applications of DOTA and its congeners have been reported in literature; a renaissance of ^{68}Ga radiopharmacy has come with the development of small tumour-affine peptides, most notably those targeting somatostatin receptors for the imaging of neuroendocrine tumours (NET) [136, 140].

The more promising compound was [^{68}Ga-DOTA,Tyr3]-octreotide (^{68}Ga-DOTA-TOC). It showed higher affinity for somatostatin receptor subtype 2 than [^{111}In/^{90}Y]-DOTATOC and also a 2.5-fold higher tumour uptake in a mouse model bearing the sst2-positive AR4-2 J tumour [141]. Other small molecules were labelled with ^{68}Ga, e.g. different somatostatin-based peptides, like DOTA-lanreotide [142], [^{68}Ga-DOTA,1-Nal3]octreotide (^{68}Ga-DOTA-NOC) [143, 144] and [^{68}Ga-DOTA, Tyr3, Thr8] octreotide (^{68}Ga-DOTATATE) [145]. Structural formulae of DOTA-TOC, DOTA-NOC and DOTA-TATE are showed in Fig. 4.9.

These compounds now represent the gold standard in the imaging of NET. It has been demonstrated that ^{68}Ga-DOTANOC PET/CT either affected stage or caused a therapy modification in more than half the patients, thus confirming the clinical role of PET in the management of NET [10]. Because of huge diffusion of these ^{68}Ga-labelled somatostatin analogues in clinical practice, specific guidelines to assist nuclear medicine physicians in recommending, performing, reporting and interpreting the results of somatostatin (SST) receptor PET/CT imaging using ^{68}Ga-DOTA-conjugated peptides have been published [11].

Though readily available and so widespread, DOTA is not intrinsically the most appropriate chelator for to Ga^{3+}, as its K_{ML} and pM values suggest. The thermodynamic stability constant of the Ga^{3+} complex of the tetraaza tetraacetic acid chelator DOTA is much lower (logK=21.33) [146] than that of the triaza triacetic acid chelator NOTA (logK=30.98) [147] due to the larger dimensions of its cavity. In contrast to DOTA, the smaller congener NOTA is much more suited for Ga, as its smaller 1,4,7triazacyclononane (TACN) ring apparently allows the formation of multiple five-membered chelate rings with one central Ga^{3+} core, without the intramolecular strain accompanied by the Ga-DOTA complex. NOTA forms slightly distorted octahedral complexes with Ga^{3+}; due to the facial arrangement of donors, the energetic barrier for complexation is significantly lower than with DOTA. Therefore, NOTA readily forms stable complexes with Ga^{3+} already at

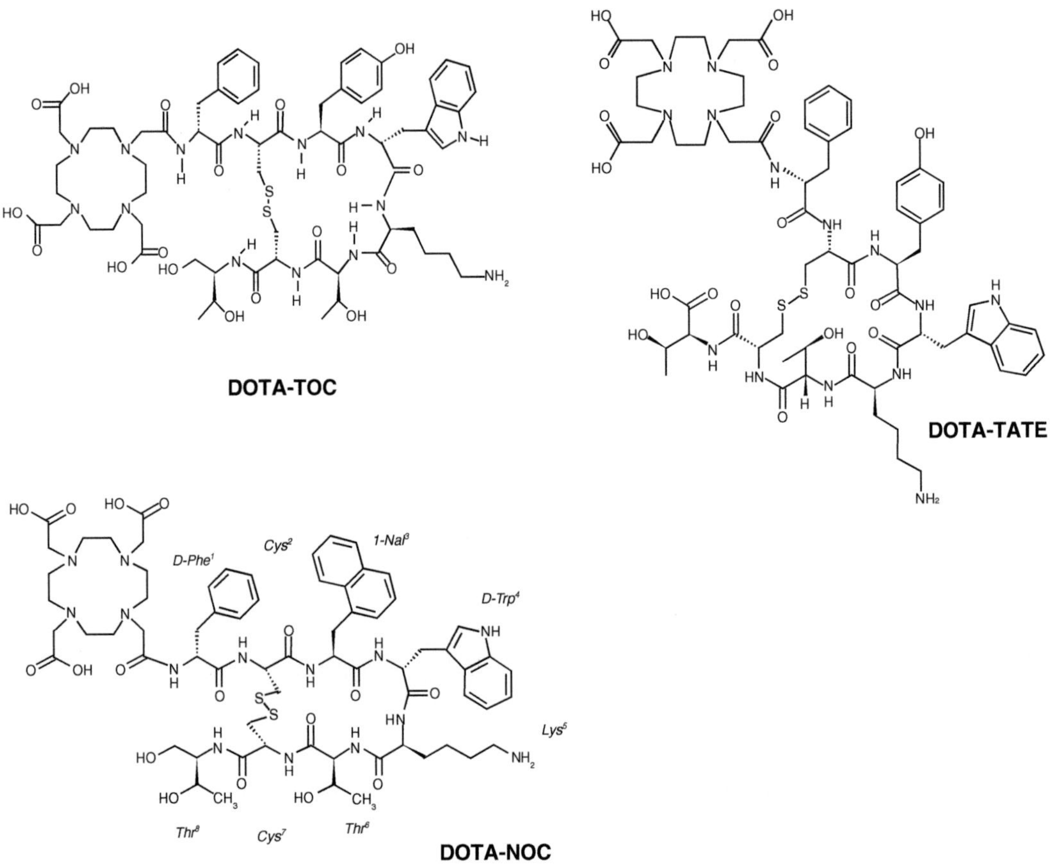

Fig. 4.9 Structural formulae of *DOTA-TOC*, *DOTA-NOC* and *DOTA-TATE*

moderate temperature while the formation of complex Ga-DOTA requires high temperature (80–100 °C) which can be dangerous for compounds like proteins and large molecular weight peptides.

NOTA does not offer the same opportunity of using a spare carboxylate or amine function for conjugation, thus needing chemical modifications to obtain bifunctional derivatives. Because of the huge potential of ^{68}Ga for medical application, several bifunctional derivatives of NOTA have been reported during the last decades [148–151] as well as the effect of different chelators in regard to pharmacokinetics, tumour uptake and retention [152].

Recently, it has been demonstrated that the chelators 1,4,7-triazacyclononane-1,4,7-tris [methyl(2-carboxyethyl)phosphinic acid] (TRAP-Pr) [153] and 1,4,7-triazacyclononane-1-[methyl(2-carboxyethyl) phosphinic acid]-4,7-bis[methyl(2-hydroxymethyl) phosphinic acid] (NOPO) [154] possess markedly improved affinity to Ga^{3+} and higher ^{68}Ga-labelling efficiency. Compared to DOTA and NOTA, quantitative incorporation of $^{68}Ga^{3+}$ into chelates requires smaller concentration of these chelators, thus obtaining TRAP and NOPO-based radiopharmaceuticals with extremely high specific activities [154, 155]. Furthermore, ^{68}Ga-labelling of triazacyclononane-triphosphinates can be performed at lower temperatures and over a broad pH range (0.5–5). Other factors influencing the performance of ^{68}Ga-labelling reactions should be taken into account. One of them is the presence of other metal ions in the $^{68}Ge/^{68}Ga$ generator eluate. These can compete with $^{68}Ga^{3+}$ for the chelator, thus diminishing the labelling yield, which is particularly problematic in view of the low concentration of the carrier-free $^{68}Ga^{3+}$ in the eluate. Structural

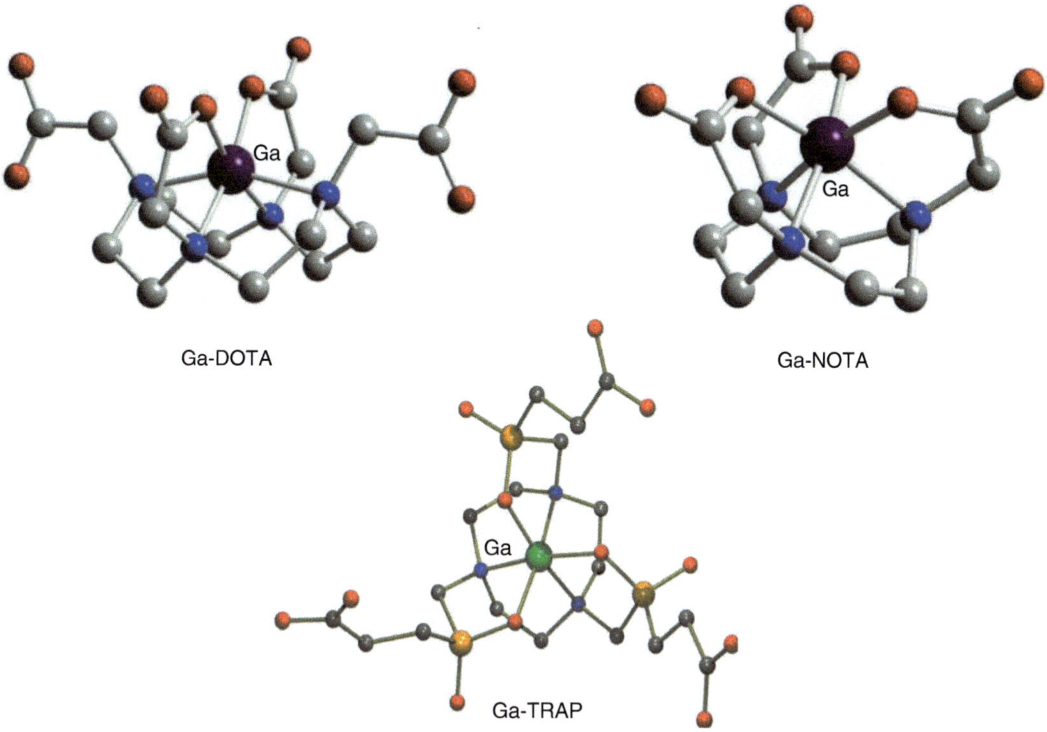

Fig. 4.10 Structural formulae of *Ga-DOTA*, *Ga-NOTA* and *Ga-TRAP* chelates

formulae of Ga-DOTA, Ga-NOTA and Ga-TRAP chelates are shown in Fig. 4.10

For example, the total amount of metal contaminants (Ga, Ge, Zn, Ti, Sn, Fe, Al and Cu) in the eluate of a SnO_2-based generator was reported to be <10 ppm (<3 ppm Zn^{2+}; <1 ppm for each of the other ions) [156]. The most remarkable feature of TRAP, triazacyclononane-phosphinate ligands, seems to rely in their selectivity for Ga^{3+}, rapid Ga^{3+} complexation kinetics with extraordinarily high thermodynamic stability and kinetic inertness of the respective ^{68}Ga chelates in comparison with other class of chelates. These compounds allow also preparation of ditopic Ga^{3+}/Gd^{3+} complex for application as bimodal imaging agent for PET/MRI [157]. Bifunctional derivatives of NOTA, TRAP and NOPO provide high potential for the development of ^{99m}Tc-kit-like formulations.

N,N′-Bis[2-hydroxy-5-(carboxyethyl)-benzyl]ethylenediamine- N,N′- diacetic acid (HBED-CC) was recently proposed as an efficient acyclic 68Ga chelator with fast complexing kinetics and a high in vitro as well as in vivo complex stability [158, 159].

Besides the efficient Ga^{3+} complexing characteristics, HBED-CC was selected because of its lipophilic nature. It was found that the "active binding site" of prostate specific membrane antigen (PSMA) is composed of two structural motifs, one representing a lipophilic pocket and the other interacting with urea-based inhibitors [160].

The simple replacement of HBED-CC by the prominent radiometal chelator DOTA was shown to dramatically reduce the in vivo imaging quality of the respective ^{68}Ga-labelled PSMA-targeted tracer proving that HBED-CC contributes intrinsically to the PSMA binding of the Glu-urea-Lys(Ahx) pharmacophore [161]. ^{68}Ga-labelled Glu-urea-Lys(Ahx)-HBED-CC ([68Ga]Ga-PSMA-HBED-CC) represents a successful novel PSMA inhibitor radiotracer which has recently demonstrated its relevance in the detection of prostate cancer [162, 163].

References

1. Gallagher BM, Ansari A, Atkins H, et al. Radiopharmaceuticals XXVII. 18F-labeled 2-deoxy-2-fluoro- D-glucose as radiopharmaceutical for measuring regional myocardial glucose metabolism in vivo: tissue distribution and imaging studies in animals. J Nucl Med. 1977;18:990–6.
2. Hamacher K, Coenen HH, Stöcklin G. Efficient stereospecific synthesis of no-carrier added 2-[18F]-fluoro-2-deoxy-D-glucose using aminopolyether supported nucleophilic substitution. J Nucl Med. 1986;27:235–8.
3. Vaalburg W, Kamphuis JA, Beerling-van der Molen HD, et al. An improved method for the cyclotron production of 13N-labelled ammonia. Int J Appl Radiat Isot. 1975;26:316–8.
4. Sobczyk DP, van Grondelle J, de Jong AM, et al. Production of chemically pure gaseous [13N]NH3 pulses for PEP studies using a modified DeVarda reduction. Appl Radiat Isot. 2002;57:201–7.
5. Suzuki K, Yoshida Y, Shikano N, et al. Development of an automated system for the quick production of 13N-labeled compounds with high specific activity using anhydrous [13N]NH3. Appl Radiat Isot. 1999;50:1033–8.
6. Berridge MS, Landmeier BJ. In-target production of [13N]ammonia: target design, products, and operating parameters. Appl Radiat Isot. 1993;44:1433–41.
7. Krasikova RN, Fedorova OS, Korsakov MV, et al. Improved [N-13] ammonia yield from the proton irradiation of water using methane gas. Appl Radiat Isot. 1999;51:395–401.
8. Koehler L, Gagnon K, McQuarrie S, et al. Iodine-124: a promising positron emitter for organic PET chemistry. Molecules. 2010;15:2686–718.
9. Belov VV, Bonab AA, Fischman AJ, et al. Iodine-124 as a label for pharmacological PET imaging. Mol Pharm. 2011;8:736–47.
10. Ambrosini V, Campana D, Bodei L, et al. 68Ga-DOTANOC PET/CT clinical impact in patients with neuroendocrine tumors. J Nucl Med. 2010;51:669–73.
11. Virgolini I, Ambrosini V, Bomanji JB, et al. Procedure guidelines for PET/CT tumour imaging with 68Ga-DOTA-conjugated peptides: 68Ga-DOTA-TOC, 68Ga-DOTA-NOC, 68Ga-DOTA-TATE. Eur J Nucl Med Mol Imaging. 2010;37:2004–10.
12. Krohn KA, Mankoff DA, Muzi M, et al. True tracers: comparing FDG with glucose and FLT with thymidine. Nucl Med Biol. 2005;32:663–71.
13. Casella V, Ido T, Wolf AP, et al. Anhydrous F-18 labeled elemental fluorine for radiopharmaceutical preparation. J Nucl Med. 1980;21:750–7.
14. Schlyer DJ. PET tracers and radiochemistry. Ann Acad Med Singapore. 2004;33:146–54.
15. Nickles RJ, Daube ME, Ruth TJ. An $^{18}O_2$ target for the production of $[^{18}F]F_2$. Int J Appl Radiat Isot. 1984;35:117–22.
16. Berridge MS, Tewson TJ. Chemistry of fluorine-18 radiopharmaceuticals. Int J Rad Appl Instrum A. 1986;37:685–93.
17. Ogawa M, Hatano K, Oishi S, et al. Direct electrophilic radiofluorination of a cyclic RGD peptide for in vivo alpha(v)beta3 integrin related tumor imaging. Nucl Med Biol. 2003;30:1–9.
18. Diksic M, Farrokhzad S, Yamamoto YL, et al. Simple synthesis of 18F-labelled 5-fluorouracil using acetylhypofluorite. Int J Nucl Med Biol. 1984;11:141–2.
19. Oberdorfer F, Hofmann E, Maier-Borst W. Preparation of ^{18}F-labelled N-fluoropyridinium triflate. J Label Compd Radiopharm. 1988;25:999–1005.
20. Oberdorfer F, Hofmann E, Maier-Borst W. Preparation of new fluorine-18-labelled precursor. Int J Rad Appl Instrum. 1988;39:685–8.
21. Satyamurthy N, Bida GT, Phelps ME, et al. Fluorine-18 labelled N-$[^{18}F]$ fluoro-N-alkylsulfonamides: novel reagents for mild and regioselective radiofluorination. Appl Radiat Isot. 1990;41:733–8.
22. Dolle F, Demphe S, Hinne F, et al. 6-[18F]Fluoro-L-DOPA by radiofluorodestannylation: a short and simple synthesis of a new labelling precursor. J Label Compd Radiopharm. 1998;41:105–14.
23. de Vries EFJ, Luurtsema G, Brüssermann M, et al. Fully automated synthesis module for the high yield one-pot preparation of 6-[18F]-Fluoro-L-DOPA. Appl Radiat Isot. 1997;51:389–94.
24. Bergman J, Solin O. Fluorine-18-labeled fluorine gas for synthesis of tracer molecules. Nucl Med Biol. 1997;24:677–83.
25. Cai L, Lu S, Pike VW. Chemistry with [18F]fluoride ion. Eur J Org Chem. 2008;2008:2853–73.
26. Berridge MS, Apana SM, Hersh JM. Teflon radiolysis as the major source of carrier in fluorine-18. J Label Compd Radiopharm. 2009;52:543–8.
27. Sun H, DiMagno SG. Fluoride relay: a new concept for the rapid preparation of anhydrous nucleophilic fluoride salts from KF. Chem Commun. 2007;5:528–9.
28. Tewson TJ. Procedures, pitfalls and solutions in the production of $[^{18}F]$2-deoxy-2-fluoro-D-glucose: a paradigm in the routine synthesis of fluorine-18 radiopharmaceuticals. Nucl Med Biol. 1989;16:533–61.
29. Kiesewetter DO, Eckelman WC, Cohen RM, et al. Syntheses and D2 receptor affinities of derivatives of spiperone containing aliphatic halogens. Int J Rad Appl Instrum A. 1986;37:1181–8.
30. Zhang MR, Suzuki K. [18F]Fluoroalkyl agents: synthesis, reactivity and application for development of PET ligands in molecular imaging. Curr Top Med Chem. 2007;7:1817–28.
31. Iwata R, Pascali C, Bogni A, et al. [18F]fluoromethyl triflate, a novel and reactive [18F]fluoromethylating agent: preparation and application to the on-column preparation of [18F]fluorocholine. Appl Radiat Isot. 2002;57:347–52.
32. Grierson JR, Shields AF. Radiosynthesis of 3′-deoxy-3′-[(18)F]fluorothymidine: [(18)F]FLT for imaging of cellular proliferation in vivo. Nucl Med Biol. 2000;27:143–56.
33. Pascali C, Bogni A, Fugazza L, et al. Simple preparation and purification of ethanol-free solutions of

3′-deoxy-3′-[18F]fluorothymidine by means of disposable solid-phase extraction cartridges. Nucl Med Biol. 2012;39:540–50.
34. Romer J, Fuchtner F, Steinbach J, et al. Automated production of 16alpha-[18F]fluoroestradiol for breast cancer imaging. Nucl Med Biol. 1999;26: 473–9.
35. Kiesewetter DO, Kilbourn MR, Landvatter SW, et al. Preparation of four fluorine-18- labeled estrogens and their selective uptakes in target tissues of immature rats. J Nucl Med. 1984;25:1212–21.
36. Grierson JR, Link JM, Mathis CA, et al. A radiosynthesis of fluorine-18 fluoromisonidazole. J Nucl Med. 1989;30:343–50.
37. McConathy J, Voll RJ, Yu W, et al. Improved synthesis of anti-[18F]FACBC: improved preparation of labelling precursor and automated radiosynthesis. Appl Radiat Isot. 2003;58:657–66.
38. Kim DW, Ahn DS, Oh YH, et al. A new class of SN2 reactions catalyzed by protic solvents: facile fluorination for isotopic labelling of diagnostic molecules. J Am Chem Soc. 2006;128:16394–7.
39. Kim DW, Jeong HJ, Lim ST, et al. Facile nucleophilic fluorination reactions using tert-alcohols as a reaction medium: significantly enhanced reactivity of alkali metal fluorides and improved selectivity. J Org Chem. 2008;73:957–62.
40. Lee SJ, Oh SJ, Chi DY, et al. Comparison of synthesis yields of 3′-deoxy-3′-[^{18}F]-fluorothymidine by nucleophilic fluorination in various alcohol solvents. J Label Compd Radiopharm. 2008;51:80–2.
41. De Grado TR, Baldwin SW, Wang S, et al. Synthesis and evaluation of 18Flabeled choline analogs as oncologic PET tracers. J Nucl Med. 2001;42:1805–14.
42. Kilbourn MR, Welch MJ, Dence CS, et al. Carrier added and no-carried added synthesis of [F-18]spiroperidol and [F-18]haloperidol. Int J Appl Radiat Isot. 1984;35:591–8.
43. Kuhnast B, Hinnen F, Boisgard R, et al. Fluorine-18 labelling of oligonucleotides: prosthetic labelling at the 5′-end using the *N*-(4-[^{18}F]fluorobenzyl)-2-bromoacetamide reagent. J Label Compd Radiopharm. 2003;46:1093–103.
44. Kamlet AS, Neumann CN, Lee E, et al. Application of palladium-mediated 18F-fluorination to PET radiotracer development: overcoming hurdles to translation. PLoS One. 2013;8(3):e59187.
45. Ross TL, Ermert J, Hocke C, et al. Nucleophilic 18F-fluorination of heteroaromatic iodonium salts with no-carrier added [18F]fluoride. J Am Chem Soc. 2007;129:8018–25.
46. Di Magno SG, inventor, Nutech Ventures, assignee. Fluorination of aromatic ring systems. US Patent 8,604,213 B2. December 10, 2013.
47. Kuik WJ, Kema IP, Brouwers AH, et al. In vivo biodistribution of no-carrier-added 6-18F-fluoro-3,4-dihydroxy-L-phenylalanine (18F-DOPA), produced by a new nucleophilic substitution approach, compared with carrier-added 18F-DOPA, prepared by conventional electrophilic substitution. J Nucl Med. 2015;56:106–12.
48. Vaidyanathan G, Zalutsky MR. Synthesis of N-succinimidyl 4-[18F]fluorobenzoate, an agent for labelling proteins and peptides with 18F. Nat Protoc. 2006;1:1655–61.
49. Mäding P, Füchtner F, Wüst F. Module-assisted synthesis of the bifunctional labelling agent N-succinimidyl 4-[(18)F]fluorobenzoate ([(18)F] SFB). Appl Radiat Isot. 2005;63:329–32.
50. Poethko T, Schottelius M, Thumshim G, et al. Two-step methodology for high-yield routine radiohalogenation of peptides: (18)F-labeled RGD and octreotide analogs. J Nucl Med. 2004;45:892–902.
51. Li X, Link JM, Stekhova S, et al. Site-specific labelling of annexin V with F-18 for apoptosis imaging. Bioconjug Chem. 2008;19:1684–8.
52. Chang YS, Jeong JM, Lee YS, et al. Preparation of 18F-human serum albumin: a simple and efficient protein labelling method with 18F using a hydrazone-formation method. Bioconjug Chem. 2005;16: 1329–33.
53. Prante O, Einsiedel J, Haubner R, et al. 3,4,6-Tri-O-acetyl-2-deoxy-2-[18F]fluoro glucopyranosyl phenylthiosulfonate: a thiol-reactive agent for the chemoselective 18F-glycosylation of peptides. Bioconjug Chem. 2007;18:254–62.
54. Maschauer S, Prante O. Sweetening pharmaceutical radiochemistry by (18)F-fluoroglycosylation: a short review. Biomed Res Int. 2014;2014:214748.
55. Marik J, Sutcliffe J. Click for PET: rapid preparation of [18F]fluoropeptides using CuI catalyzed 1,3-dipolar cycloaddition. Tetrahedron Lett. 2006;47: 6681–4.
56. Huisgen R. 1.3-dipolare cycloadditionen. Angew Chem. 1963;13:604–37.
57. Sirion U, Kim HI, Lee JH, et al. An efficient F-18 labeling method for PET study: huisgen 1,3-dipolar cycloaddition of bioactive substances and F-18-labeled compounds. Tetrahedron Lett. 2007;48:3953–7.
58. Li ZB, Wu Z, Chen K, et al. Click chemistry for 18F-labeling of RGD peptides and microPET imaging of tumor integrin α v β 3 expression. Bioconjug Chem. 2007;18:1987–94.
59. Gill HS, Marik J. Preparation of 18F-labeled peptides using the copper(I)-catalyzed azide-alkyne 1,3-dipolar cycloaddition. Nat Protoc. 2011;6:1718–25.
60. Lee CM, Jeong HJ, Kim DW, et al. The effect of fluorination of zinc oxide nanoparticles on evaluation of their biodistribution after oral administration. Nanotechnology. 2012;23:205102.
61. Maschauer S, Prante O. A series of 2-O-trifluoromethylsulfonyl- d-mannopyranosides as precursors for concomitant 18F-labeling and glycosylation by click chemistry. Carbohydr Res. 2009;344:753–61.
62. Hausner SH, Carpenter RD, Bauer N, et al. Evaluation of an integrin α v β 6-specific peptide labeled with [18F]fluorine by copper-free, strain-promoted click chemistry. Nucl Med Biol. 2013;40:233–9.
63. Li Z, Cai H, Hassink M, et al. Tetrazine-trans-cyclooctene ligation for the rapid construction of

18F labeled probes. Chem Commun. 2010;46: 8043–5.
64. Kettenbach K, Schieferstein H, Ross TL. 18F-labeling using click cycloadditions. Biomed Res Int. 2014;2014:361329.
65. Schirrmacher R, Bradtmoller G, Schirrmacher E, et al. 18F-Triorganofluorosilanes as tools for the development of silicon based 18F-radiopharmaceuticals: labelling chemistry for in vivo application. Angew Chem Int. 2006;45:6047–50.
66. Schirrmacher E, Wängler B, Cypryk M, et al. Synthesis of p-(Di-tert-butyl [18F]fluorosilyl) benzaldehyde ([18F]SiFA-a) with high specific activity by isotopic exchange: a convenient labeling synthon for the 18F-labeling of N-aminooxy derivatized peptides. Bioconjug Chem. 2007;18:2085–9.
67. Rosa-Neto P, Wangler B, Iovkova L, et al. [(18)F] SiFA-isothiocyanate: a New highly effective radioactive labeling agent for lysine-containing proteins. Chembiochem. 2009;10:1321–4.
68. Wangler B, Quandt G, Iovkova L, et al. Kit-like 18F-labeling of proteins: synthesis of 4-(ditert-butyl[18F]fluoro-silyl)benzenethiol (Si[18F]FA-SH) labeled rat serum albumin for blood pool imaging with PET. Bioconjug Chem. 2009;20:317–21.
69. McBride WJ, Sharkey RM, Karacay H, et al. A novel method of 18F radiolabeling for PET. J Nucl Med. 2009;50:991–8.
70. Lang L, Eckelmann WC. One-step synthesis of 18F labeled [18F]-N-succinimidyl 4-(fluoromethyl) benzoate for protein labeling. Appl Radiat Isot. 1994;45: 1155–63.
71. Lang L, Li W, Guo N, et al. Comparison study of [18F]FAl-NOTA-PRGD2, [18F]FPPRGD2, and [68Ga]Ga-NOTA-PRGD2 for PET imaging of U87MG tumors in mice. Bioconjug Chem. 2011;22: 2415–22.
72. Laverman P, D'Souza CA, Eek A, et al. Optimized labelling of NOTA-conjugated octreotide with F-18. Tumour Biol. 2012;33:427–34.
73. Liu S, Liu H, Jiang H, et al. One-step radiosynthesis of 18F-AlF-NOTA-RGD2 for tumor angiogenesis PET imaging. Eur J Nucl Med Mol Imaging. 2011;38:1732–41.
74. Varasteh Z, Aberg O, Velikyan I, et al. In vitro and in vivo evaluation of a (18)F-labeled high affinity NOTA conjugated bombesin antagonist as a PET ligand for GRPR-targeted tumor imaging. PLoS One. 2013;8(12), e81932.
75. Malik N, Zlatopolskiy B, Machulla HJ, et al. One pot radiofluorination of a new potential PSMA ligand [Al18F]NOTA-DUPA-Pep. J Label Compd Radiopharm. 2012;55:320–5.
76. Lütje S, Franssen GM, Sharkey RM, et al. Anti-CEA antibody fragments labeled with [(18)F]AlF for PET imaging of CEA-expressing tumors. Bioconjug Chem. 2014;25:335–41.
77. Niu G, Lang L, Kiesewetter DO, et al. In vivo labeling of serum albumin for PET. J Nucl Med. 2014;55: 1150–6.
78. Osman S, Lundkvist C, Pike VW, et al. Characterisation of the appearance of radioactive metabolites in monkey and human plasma from the 5-HT1A receptor radioligand, [carbonyl-11C]WAY-100635. Explanation of high signal contrast in PET and an aid to biomathematical modelling. Nucl Med Biol. 1998;25:215–23.
79. Antoni G, Kihlberg T, Langstrom B. Aspect on the synthesis of 11Clabelled compounds. In: Welch MJ, Redvanly CS, editors. Handbook of radiopharmaceuticals. Chichester: Wiley; 2003. p. 141–94.
80. Larsen P, Ulin J, Dahlstrom K, et al. Synthesis of [11C] Iodomethane by iodination of [11C]methane. Appl Radiat Isot. 1997;48:153–7.
81. Crouzel C, Langstrom B, Pike VW, et al. Recommendations for practical production of [11C] methyl iodide. Appl Radiat Isot. 1997;38:601–3.
82. Noguchi J, Suzuki K. Automated synthesis of the ultra high specific activity of [11C]Ro15-4513 and its application in an extremely low concentration region to an ARG study. Nucl Med Biol. 2003;30:335–43.
83. Andersson J, Truong P, Halldin C. In-target produced [11C]methane: increased specific radioactivity. Appl Radiat Isot. 2009;67:106–10.
84. Lodi F, Malizia C, Castellucci P, et al. Synthesis of oncological [11C]radiopharmaceuticals for clinical PET. Nucl Med Biol. 2012;39:447–60.
85. Matarrese M, Soloviev D, Todde S, et al. Preparation of [11C] radioligands with high specific radioactivity on a commercial PET tracer synthesizer. Nucl Med Biol. 2003;30:79–83.
86. Lodi F, Trespidi S, Di Pierro D, et al. A simple Tracerlab module modification for automated on-column [11C]methylation and [11C]carboxylation. Appl Radiat Isot. 2007;65:691–5.
87. Boschi S, Lodi F, Cicoria G, et al. Development of a modular system for the synthesis of PET [(11)C] labelled radiopharmaceuticals. Appl Radiat Isot. 2009;67:1869–73.
88. Lodi F, Carpinelli A, Malizia C, et al. Synthesis of [^{11}C]-Meta-Hydroxyephedrine ([^{11}C]MHED). In: Scott PJH, Hockley BG, Kilbourn MR, editors. Radiochemical syntheses, radiopharmaceuticals for positron emission tomography, vol. 1. Hoboken: Wiley; 2012. p. 191–8.
89. Kealey S, Plisson C, Collier TL, et al. Microfluidic reactions using [11C]carbon monoxide solutions for the synthesis of a positron emission tomography radiotracer. Org Biomol Chem. 2011;9:3313–9.
90. Audrain H. Positron emission tomography (PET) and microfluidic devices: a breakthrough on the microscale? Angew Chem Int. 2007;46:1772–5.
91. Pascali C, Bogni A, Iwata R, et al. [11C] methylation on a C18 Sep-Pak cartridge: a convenient way to produce [N-methyl-11C]choline. J Label Compd Radiopharm. 2000;43:195–203.
92. Iwata R, Pascali C, Bogni A, et al. Simple loop method for the automated preparation of [11C]raclopride from [11C] methyl triflate. Appl Radiat Isot. 2001;55:17–22.

93. Soloviev D, Tamburella C. Captive solvent [11C] acetate synthesis in GMP conditions. Appl Radiat Isot. 2006;64:995–1000.
94. Langstrom B, Lunquvist H. The preparation of [11C]methyl iodide and its use in the synthesis of [11C]methyl-L-methionine. Int J Appl Radiat Isot. 1976;27:357–63.
95. Marazano C, Maziere M, Berger G, et al. Synthesis of methyl iodide-11C and formaldehyde-11C. Int J Appl Radiat Isot. 1977;28:49–52.
96. Link JM, Clark JC, Larsen P, et al. Production of [11C]methyl iodide by reaction of [11C]CH4 with I2. J Label Compd Radiopharm. 1995;37:76–8.
97. Jewett DM. A simple synthesis of [11C]methyl triflate. Appl Radiat Isot. 1992;43:1383–5.
98. Dolle F, Emond P, Mavel S, et al. Synthesis, radiosynthesis and in vivo preliminary evaluation of [11C]LBT-999, a selective radioligand for the visualisation of the dopamine transporter with PET. Bioorg Med Chem. 2006;14:1115–25.
99. Nagren K, Halldin C, Müller L, et al. Comparison of [11C]methyl triflate and [11C]methyl iodide in the synthesis of PET radioligands such as [11C]beta-CIT and [11C]beta-CFT. Nucl Med Biol. 1995;22:965–79.
100. Pascali C, Bogni A, Iwata R, et al. High efficiency preparation of L-[S-methyl-11C]methionine by on-column [11C]methylation on C18 Sep-Pak. J Label Compd Radiopharm. 1999;42:715–24.
101. Klunk WE, Engler H, Nordberg A, et al. Imaging brain amyloid in Alzheimer's disease with Pittsburgh Compound-B. Ann Neurol. 2004;55:306–19.
102. Langer O, Nagren K, Dolle F, et al. Precursor synthesis and radiolabelling of the dopamine D-2 receptor ligand C-11 raclopride from C-11 methyl triflate. J Label Compd Radiopharm. 1999;42:1183–93.
103. Suzuki K, Inoue O, Tamate K, et al. Production of 3-N-[11C]methylspiperone with high specific activity and high radiochemical purity for PET studies: suppression of its radiolysis. Appl Radiat Isot. 1990;41:593–9.
104. Scott DJ, Stohler CS, Koeppe RA, et al. Time-course of change in [11C]carfentanil and [11C]raclopride binding potential after a nonpharmacological challenge. Synapse. 2007;61:707–14.
105. Pike VW, Halldin C, Crouzel C, et al. Radioligands for PET studies of central benzodiazepine receptors and PK (peripheral benzodiazepine) binding sites – current status. Nucl Med Biol. 1993;20:503–25.
106. Jacobson O, Mishani E. [11C]-dimethylamine as a labeling agent for PET biomarkers. Appl Radiat Isot. 2008;66:188–93.
107. Hosoya T, Sumi K, Doi H, et al. Rapid methylation on carbon frameworks useful for the synthesis of 11CH3-incorporated PET tracers: Pd(0)-mediated rapid coupling of methyl iodide with an alkenyltributylstannane leading to a 1-methylalkene. Org Biomol Chem. 2006;4:410–5.
108. Pretze M, Große-Gehling P, Mamat C. Cross-coupling reactions as valuable tool for the preparation of PET radiotracers. Molecules. 2011;16:1129–65.
109. Eriksson J, Aberg O, Langstrom B. Synthesis of [11C]/[13C] acrylamides by palladium-mediated carbonylation. Eur J Org Chem. 2007;2007:455–61.
110. Barletta J, Karimi F, Langstrom B. Synthesis of [^{11}C-*carbonyl*]hydroxyureas by a rhodium-mediated carbonylation reaction using [^{11}C]carbon monoxide. J Label Compd Radiopharm. 2006;49:429–36.
111. Langstrom B, Itsenko O, Rahman O. [11C]Carbon monoxide, a versatile and useful precursor in labelling chemistry for PET-ligand development. J Label Compd Radiopharm. 2007;50:794–810.
112. Brown MA, Myears DW, Bergmann SR. Validity of estimates of myocardial oxidative metabolism with carbon-11 acetate and positron emission tomography despite altered patterns of substrate utilization. J Nucl Med. 1989;30:187–93.
113. Sörensen J, Valind S, Andersson LG. Simultaneous quantification of myocardial perfusion, oxidative metabolism, cardiac efficiency and pump function at rest and during supine bicycle exercise using 11C-acetate PET—a pilot study. Clin Physiol Funct Imaging. 2010;30:279–84.
114. Yu EY, Muzi M, Hackenbracht JA, et al. C11-acetate and F-18 FDG PET for men with prostate cancer bone metastases: relative findings and response to therapy. Clin Nucl Med. 2011;36:192–8.
115. Albrecht S, Buchegger F, Soloviev D, et al. (11) C-acetate PET in the early evaluation of prostate cancer recurrence. Eur J Nucl Med Mol Imaging. 2007;34:185–96.
116. Park JW, Kim JH, Kim SK, et al. A prospective evaluation of 18F-FDG and 11C-acetate PET/CT for detection of primary and metastatic hepatocellular carcinoma. J Nucl Med. 2008;49:1912–21.
117. Huo L, Wu Z, Zhuang H, et al. Dual time point 11C-acetate PET imaging can potentially distinguish focal nodular hyperplasia from primary hepatocellular carcinoma. Clin Nucl Med. 2009;34:874–7.
118. Shibata H, Nomori H, Uno K, et al. 11C-acetate for positron emission tomography imaging of clinical stage IA lung adenocarcinoma: comparison with 18F -fluorodeoxyglucose for imaging and evaluation of tumor aggressiveness. Ann Nucl Med. 2009;23:609–16.
119. Liu RS, Chang CP, Guo WY, et al. 11C-acetate versus 18F-FDG PET in detection of meningioma and monitoring the effect of gamma-knife radiosurgery. J Nucl Med. 2010;51:883–91.
120. Machulla HJ, Stöcklin G, Kupfernagel C, et al. Comparative evaluation of fatty acids labeled with C-11, Cl-34m, Br-77, and I-123 for metabolic studies of the myocardium: concise communication. J Nucl Med. 1978;19:298–302.
121. Runkle AC, Shao X, Tluczek LJ, et al. Automated production of [11C]acetate and [11C]palmitate using a modified GE Tracerlab FX(C-Pro). Appl Radiat Isot. 2011;69:691–8.
122. Matarrese M, Sudati F, Soloviev D, et al. Automation of [11C]acyl chloride syntheses using commercially available 11C-modules. Appl Radiat Isot. 2002;57:675–9.

123. McCarron JA, Turton DR, Pike VW, et al. Remotely controlled production of the 5-HT1A receptor radioligand, [carbonyl11C]WAY-100635, via 11C-carboxylation of an immobilized Grignard reagent. J Label Compd Radiopharm. 1996;38:943–53.
124. Weber B, Westera G, Treyer V, et al. Constant-infusion H(2)15O PET and acetazolamide challenge in the assessment of cerebral perfusion status. J Nucl Med. 2004;45:1344–50.
125. Vakil P, Lee JJ, Mouannes-Srour JJ, et al. Cerebrovascular occlusive disease: quantitative cerebral blood flow using dynamic susceptibility contrast MR imaging correlates with quantitative H2[15O] PET. Radiology. 2010;266:879–86.
126. Berridge MS, Terris AH, Cassidy EH. Low-carrier production of [^{15}O]oxygen, water and carbon monoxide. Appl Radiat Isot. 1990;41:1173–5.
127. Clark JC, Crouzel C, Meyer GJ, et al. Current methodology for oxygen-15 production for clinical use. Appl Radiat Isot. 1987;38:597–600.
128. VanNaemen J, Monclus M, Damhaut P, et al. Production, automatic delivery and bolus injection of [15O]water for positron emission tomography studies. Nucl Med Biol. 1996;23:413–6.
129. Porenta G, Czernin J, Schelbert HR. Positron emission tomography of the heart. Bergmann SR, Sobel BE, editors. Mt. Kisco: Futura Publication; 1992, p. 153.
130. Gómez-Vallejo V, Gaja V, Gona KB, et al. Nitrogen-13: historical review and future perspectives. J Label Compd Radiopharm. 2014;57:244–54.
131. Velikyan I. Prospective of 68Ga-radiopharmaceutical development. Theranostics. 2014;4:47–80.
132. Lambrecht R, Sajjad M. Accelerator derived radionuclide generators. Radiochim Acta. 1988;43:171–9.
133. Mirzadeh S, Lambrecht R. Radiochemistry of germanium. J Radioanal Nucl Chem. 1996;202:7–102.
134. Roesch F, Riss PJ. The renaissance of the 68Ge/68Ga radionuclide generator initiates new developments in 68Ga radiopharmaceutical chemistry. Curr Top Med Chem. 2010;10:1633–68.
135. Rösch F. Past, present and future of 68Ge/68Ga generators. Appl Radiat Isot. 2013;76:24–30.
136. Meyer GJ, Mäcke HR, Schuhmacher J, et al. 68Ga-labelled DOTA-derivatised peptide ligands. Eur J Nucl Med. 2004;31:1097–104.
137. Breeman WAP, de Jong M, de Blois E, et al. Radiolabelling DOTA-peptides with 68Ga. Eur J Nucl Med. 2005;32:478–85.
138. Zhernosekov KP, Filosofov DV, Baum RP, et al. Processing of generator produced 68Ga for medical application. J Nucl Med. 2007;48:1741–8.
139. Harris WR, Pecoraro V. Thermodynamic binding constants for gallium transferrin. Biochemistry. 1983;22:292–9.
140. Maecke HR, Hofmann M, Haberkorn U. 68Ga-labeled peptides in tumor imaging. J Nucl Med. 2005;46:172S–8.
141. Antunes P, Ginj M, Zhang H, et al. Are radiogallium-labelled DOTA-conjugated somatostatin analogues superior to those labelled with other radiometals? Eur J Nucl Med Mol Imaging. 2007;34:982–93.
142. Traub T, von Guggenberg E, Kendler D, et al. First experiences with Ga-68-DOTA-lanreotide PET in tumor patients. Nuklearmedizin. 2005;44:A198.
143. Baum R, Schmucking M, Wortmann R, et al. Receptor PET/CT using the Ga-68 labelled somatostatin analog DOTA-1-Nal3-octreotide (DOTA-NOC): clinical experience in 140 patients. Nuklearmedizin. 2005;44:A57.
144. Hofmann M, Oei M, Boerner AR, et al. Comparison of Ga-68-DOTATOC and Ga-68-DOTANOC for radiopeptide PET. Nuklearmedizin. 2005;44:A58.
145. Win Z, Rahman L, Murrell J, et al. The possible role of 68Ga-DOTATATE PET in malignant abdominal paraganglioma. Eur J Nucl Med Mol Imaging. 2006;33:506.
146. Clarke ET, Martell AE. Stabilities of trivalent metal ion complexes of the tetraacetate derivatives of 12-, 13-, and 14-membered tetraazamacrocycles. Inorg Chim Acta. 1992;190:37–46.
147. Clarke E, Martell AE. Stabilities of the Fe(III), Ga(III) and In(III) chelates of N, N', N"triaza cyclononane triacetic acid. Inorg Chim Acta. 1991;181:273–80.
148. Eisenwiener KP, Prata MIM, Buschmann I, et al. NODAGATOC, a new chelator-coupled somatostatin analogue labeled with [67/68Ga] and [111In] for SPECT, PET, and targeted therapeutic applications of somatostatin receptor (hsst2) expressing tumors. Bioconjug Chem. 2002;13:530–41.
149. Kataky R, Matthes KE, Nicholson PE, et al. Synthesis and binding properties of amide-functionalized polyaza macrocycles. J Chem Soc Perkin Trans 2: Phys Org Chem. 1990;8:1425–32.
150. Andre JP, Maecke HR, Zehnder M, et al. 1,4,7-Triazacyclononane-1-succinic acid-4,7-diacetic acid (NODASA): a new bifunctional chelator for radio gallium labeling of biomolecules. Chem Commun. 1998;12:1301–2.
151. Riss PJ, Kroll C, Nagel V, et al. NODAPA-OH and NODAPA-(NCS)n: synthesis, 68Ga-radiolabelling and in vitro characterisation of novel versatile bifunctional chelators for molecular imaging. Bioorg Med Chem Lett. 2008;18:5364–7.
152. Fani M, Del Pozzo L, Abiraj K, et al. PET of somatostatin receptor-positive tumors using 64Cu- and 68Ga-somatostatin antagonists: the chelate makes the difference. J Nucl Med. 2011;52:1110–8.
153. Notni J, Hermann P, Havlícková J, et al. A triazacyclononane-based bifunctional phosphinate ligand for the preparation of multimeric 68Ga tracers for positron emission tomography. Chemistry. 2010;16:7174–85.
154. Simecek J, Zemek O, Hermann P, et al. A monoreactive bifunctional triazacyclononane phosphinate chelator with high selectivity for gallium-68. ChemMedChem. 2012;7:1375–8.
155. Notni J, Pohle K, Wester HJ. Comparative gallium-68 labeling of TRAP-, NOTA-, and DOTA-peptides: practical consequences for the future of gallium-68-PET. EJNMMI Res. 2012;2:28.

156. De Blois E, Chan HS, Naidoo C, et al. Characteristics of SnO2-based 68Ge/68Ga generator and aspects of radiolabelling DOTA-peptides. Appl Radiat Isot. 2011;69:308–15.
157. Notni J, Simecek J, Wester HJ. Phosphinic acid functionalized polyazacycloalkane chelators for radiodiagnostics and radiotherapeutics:unique characteristics and applications. ChemMedChem. 2014; 9:1107–15.
158. Eder M, Wangler B, Knackmuss S, et al. Tetrafluorophenolate of HBED-CC: a versatile conjugation agent for (68)Ga-labeled small recombinant antibodies. Eur J Nucl Med Mol Imaging. 2008; 35:1878–86.
159. Eder M, Knackmuss S, Le Gall F, et al. 68Ga labelled recombinant antibody variants for immuno-PET imaging of solid tumours. Eur J Nucl Med Mol Imaging. 2010;37:1397–407.
160. Kularatne SA, Zhou Z, Yang J, et al. Design, synthesis, and preclinical evaluation of prostate-specific membrane antigen targeted (99m)Tc-radioimaging agents. Mol Pharm. 2009;6:790–800.
161. Eder M, Schafer M, Bauder-Wust U, et al. 68Ga-complex lipophilicity and the targeting property of a urea-based PSMA inhibitor for PET imaging. Bioconjug Chem. 2012;23:688–97.
162. Afshar-Oromieh A, Zechmann CM, Malcher A, et al. Comparison of PET imaging with a (68) Ga-labelled PSMA ligand and (18)F-choline-based PET/CT for the diagnosis of recurrent prostate cancer. Eur J Nucl Med Mol Imaging. 2014;41:11–20.
163. Afshar-Oromieh A, Avtzi E, Giesel FL, et al. The diagnostic value of PET/CT imaging with the (68) Ga-labelled PSMA ligand HBED-CC in the diagnosis of recurrent prostate cancer. Eur J Nucl Med Mol Imaging. 2015;42:197–209.

Quality Control of PET Radiopharmaceuticals

5

Filippo Lodi and Stefano Boschi

Contents

5.1 **Introduction** 106

5.2 **Quality Control of PET Radiopharmaceuticals: Basic Concepts and Parameters** 106
5.2.1 Visual Inspection 107
5.2.2 pH Control 107
5.2.3 Radiochemical and Radionuclidic Identity 107
5.2.4 Radiochemical Purity 108
5.2.5 Radionuclidic Purity 108
5.2.6 Chemical Purity 108
5.2.7 Enantiomeric Purity 109
5.2.8 Sterility 109
5.2.9 Bacterial Endotoxin Test 110

5.3 **Analytical Techniques Used in Quality Control of PET Radiopharmaceuticals** 110
5.3.1 High-Performance Liquid Chromatography (HPLC) 111
5.3.2 Thin-Layer Chromatography (TLC) 112
5.3.3 Gas Chromatography (GC) 113
5.3.4 Gamma Spectrometry 114

5.4 **Validation of Analytical Procedures** 115
5.4.1 Specificity 116
5.4.2 Precision 116
5.4.3 Accuracy 116
5.4.4 Linearity and Range 116
5.4.5 Detection Limit (LOD) and Quantitation Limit (LOQ) 116
5.4.6 Robustness 117

5.5 **Quality Control of ^{18}F-Radiopharmaceuticals: ^{18}F-FDG** 117
5.5.1 Appearance 117
5.5.2 Radiochemical and Radionuclidic Identity 118
5.5.3 pH 119
5.5.4 Chemical Purity 119
5.5.5 Residual Solvents 120
5.5.6 Sterility 120
5.5.7 Bacterial Endotoxins (LAL Test) 120
5.5.8 Radionuclidic Purity 120
5.5.9 Radiochemical Purity 120

5.6 **Quality Control of ^{11}C-Radiopharmaceuticals: ^{11}C-Methionine** 121
5.6.1 Appearance 121
5.6.2 Radiochemical and Radionuclidic Identity 121
5.6.3 pH 122
5.6.4 Sterility 122
5.6.5 Bacterial Endotoxins (LAL test) 122
5.6.6 Chemical Purity 122
5.6.7 Residual Solvents 123
5.6.8 Radionuclidic Purity 123
5.6.9 Radiochemical Purity 123
5.6.10 Enantiomeric Purity 123

5.7 **Quality Control of ^{68}Ga-Radiopharmaceuticals: ^{68}Ga-Edotreotide (^{68}Ga-DOTATOC)** 123
5.7.1 Appearance 123
5.7.2 Radiochemical and Radionuclidic Identity 124
5.7.3 pH 125
5.7.4 Chemical Purity 125
5.7.5 Residual Solvents 125
5.7.6 Sterility 125
5.7.7 Bacterial Endotoxins (LAL Test) 125
5.7.8 Radionuclidic Purity 125
5.7.9 Radiochemical Purity 126

References 126

F. Lodi (✉) • S. Boschi
PET Radiopharmacy, Nuclear Medicine Unit, Azienda Ospedaliero Universitaria di Bologna, Policlinico S. Orsola-Malpighi, Policlinico St. Orsola-Malpighi, Bologna, Italy
e-mail: filippo.lodi@aosp.bo.it; stefanoboschi51@gmail.com

M.M. Khalil (ed.), *Basic Science of PET Imaging*, DOI 10.1007/978-3-319-40070-9_5

Abstract
PET radiopharmaceuticals are unique medicinal formulations administered to patients for diagnostic purposes in nuclear medicine. Quality control of these radiopharmaceuticals is important to assure the safety of the product before the release for clinical use. For this reason, efficient and quick tests have been adopted to check the quality of radiopharmaceutical preparations and specific procedures have been published in each country or regions such as found in the European Pharmacopoeia (EP), United States Pharmacopeia, and British Pharmacopoeia. In this chapter the parameters, the analytical techniques and the validation of analytical methods commonly employed in the quality control testing of PET radiopharmaceuticals are reported. Specific sections about the quality control of ^{18}F, ^{11}C, and ^{68}Ga radiopharmaceuticals according to EP monographs are also provided as example for the routine testing of these preparations.

5.1 Introduction

PET radiopharmaceuticals are unique medicinal formulations containing PET radionuclides administered to patients as intravenous injections for diagnostic purposes. In the clinical application of PET radiopharmaceuticals, it is essentially important to assure the safety of the product. Quality control testing is the part of quality assurance concerned with routine sampling, testing and release of materials and finished products. Quality control of PET radiopharmaceuticals is important for the pharmaceutical and radioactive characteristics of these preparations. Therefore, pharmaceutical and radioactive parameters are considered during the quality control testing of PET radiopharmaceuticals: pharmaceutical parameters are designed to ensure that no microbiological, pyrogenic, or particulate contamination can be present in the final preparation. Radioactive parameters are designed to ensure that the intended radiation exposure of patients is kept to a minimum by confirming that no radioactive or radionuclidic impurities may affect the biodistribution of the injected radiopharmaceutical and consequently the radiation dose to the patient.

In contrast to ordinary pharmaceuticals, PET radiopharmaceuticals have to be manufactured and quality control tested and then administered to patients within a short period of time due to the short half-life of the radionuclides. By these reasons several efficient and quick tests have been adopted to check the quality of radiopharmaceutical preparations before they are released for clinical use in nuclear medicine. Specific procedures for quality control of PET radiopharmaceuticals have been published in each country or regions such as found in the European Pharmacopoeia (EP), United States Pharmacopeia (USP), and British Pharmacopoeia (BP). In this chapter the parameters, the analytical techniques and the validation of analytical methods commonly employed in the quality control testing of PET radiopharmaceuticals are reported. Specific sections about the quality control of ^{18}F, ^{11}C, and ^{68}Ga radiopharmaceuticals according to EP monographs are also provided as example for the routine testing of these preparations.

5.2 Quality Control of PET Radiopharmaceuticals: Basic Concepts and Parameters

Quality control of PET radiopharmaceuticals involves several specific test and measurements to ensure product purity, identity, efficacy and biological safety. The quality control tests for several PET radiopharmaceuticals are reported in specific monographs or general monograph about radiopharmaceutical preparation in pharmacopoeias [1] and can be divided into chemical tests, physical tests, and biological tests. The chemical and physical tests include the control of pH, the visual inspection, and the radiochemical, chemical and radionuclidic purity determination, whereas biological tests establish sterility and bacterial endotoxins content.

5.2.1 Visual Inspection

Since injectable solutions should be free from particle contaminations, a visual inspection of the radiopharmaceutical solution should be performed before clinical use. The color and clarity of each radiopharmaceutical preparation should be checked as well. The appearance characteristics are reported in the monograph of the radiopharmaceutical. In general, only a clear and colorless solution should be used for injection.

5.2.2 pH Control

PET radiopharmaceutical must be formulated at appropriate pH. Individual monographs provide the acceptable pH range for PET radiopharmaceuticals, but in general, due to the blood's high buffer capacity, the range 4.5–8.5 is considered to be acceptable. The pH of a preparation can be checked using a properly calibrated pH meter or using a pH paper indicator strips.

5.2.3 Radiochemical and Radionuclidic Identity

Radiochemical identity may be defined as the molecular structure of the compound that contains the positron-emitting radionuclide. The radiochemical identity of a positron-emitting radiopharmaceutical should be determined by using a not radioactive analogue, which is commonly referred to as the "cold standard." The standard and the radiopharmaceutical are then chromatographically analyzed. The identical response in terms of retention time (HPLC) or retardation factor (R_f) (TLC) of the two compounds demonstrates the structural identity of the radiopharmaceutical. Using the example of ^{18}F-fluorodeoxyglucose (^{18}F-FDG) monograph in EP, the principal peak in the radio-chromatogram obtained with HPLC analysis of the sample must be similar in retention time to the principal peak in the chromatogram obtained with reference solution of a "cold" FDG. Regarding the radionuclidic identity, PET radionuclides are generally identified by half-life or by gamma-ray spectrometry or by both, as prescribed in the pharmacopoeia monographs.

5.2.3.1 Half-Life Determination

The half-life of a radionuclide ($T_{½}$) is the time in which the amount of radioactivity decreases to one half of its original value.

Radioactivity decays at an exponential rate with a decay constant characteristic of each radionuclide. The curve of exponential decay (decay curve) is described by the equation:

$$A(t) = A_0 e^{-\lambda t} \tag{5.1}$$

$A(t)$ = the radioactivity at time t.
A_0 = the radioactivity at time $t = 0$.
λ = the decay constant characteristic of each radionuclide.
e = the base of Napierian logarithms.

The half-life ($T_{1/2}$) is related to the decay constant (λ) by the equation:

$$T_{1/2} = \text{In}2 / \lambda \tag{5.2}$$

The half-life is measured with a suitable detection apparatus such as an ionization chamber, a Geiger–Müller counter, and a scintillation counter to determine chronological changes in radioactivity under the same measuring or geometrical conditions. The radioactivity chosen, having regard to experimental conditions, must be of a sufficiently high level to allow detection within a suitable period of time.

5.2.3.2 Gamma-Ray Spectrum Determination

In general gamma-ray spectrometry is used to obtain the characteristic spectrum of a radionuclide that emits gamma rays such as positron emission radionuclides. The gamma spectrum is unique to that nuclide and is characterized by the number of photons of particular energies emitted according to decay scheme. This property contributes to the identification of radionuclides present in a radiopharmaceutical preparation and to their quantification. Furthermore, gamma spectroscopy allows the estimation of the degree of radionuclidic impurity by detecting peaks other than those expected.

5.2.4 Radiochemical Purity

Radiochemical purity is defined as the ratio, expressed as a percentage, of the activity of the radionuclide concerned which is present in the radiopharmaceutical preparation in stated chemical form, to the total radioactivity of that radionuclide present in the radiopharmaceutical preparation. Since the radiochemical form of the radiopharmaceutical determines its biodistribution, the control of radiochemical impurities is important to avoid the patient unnecessary radiation exposure because the radiochemical impurities could have a different biodistribution and not specific uptake which may affect and invalidate the clinical outcome of PET imaging studies. The nature of contaminants will depend on the radionuclide production and on the production process of the radiopharmaceutical as well as the impurity profile of the starting material employed. Radiochemical impurities may also originate from the chemical changes of radiopharmaceutical during storage. Measurement of radiochemical purity requires the use of a method to separate the different labeled chemical species which may be present in the radiopharmaceutical preparation. Chromatographic methods are commonly used in radiochemical determination because they can effectively separate and quantify the radioactive species in the sample. For ^{18}F-FDG preparation, radiochemical impurities include $^{18}F^-$ fluoride ion or radiolabeled intermediates and by-products derived from the synthesis process, such as ^{18}F-2-fluoro-2-deoxy-D-mannose (^{18}F-FDM) and partially or fully acetylated derivatives of ^{18}F-FDG.

5.2.5 Radionuclidic Purity

The radionuclidic purity is defined as the ratio, expressed as a percentage, of the radioactivity of the radionuclide concerned to the total radioactivity of the radiopharmaceutical preparation. Radionuclidic impurities can contribute significant effects on the patient's overall radiation dose as well as impact the image quality. Radionuclidic impurities can originate from secondary nuclear reactions during the target irradiation as a result of isotopic impurities present in the irradiated material as well as in the target body. The specific monographs prescribe the required radionuclidic purity and may set limits for specific radionuclidic impurities. The most generally used method for radionuclidic purity testing is the gamma spectrometry. For example, the control of radionuclidic purity in ^{18}F-radiopharmaceutical EP monographs prescribes the determination of the amount of ^{18}F and radionuclidic impurities with a half-life longer than 2 hours. The preparation to be examined is retained for at least 24 hours to allow the ^{18}F to decay to a level that permits the detection of such impurities.

5.2.6 Chemical Purity

Chemical purity addresses to not radioactive materials in the PET radiopharmaceutical, including by-products, solvents, and other residual components used in the production process. not radioactive materials (e.g., stabilizers, additives, etc.) that are intentionally added to the PET radiopharmaceutical may also be included in this category. Chemical impurities are considered all not radioactive substances that can either affect radiolabeling or directly produce adverse biological effects in patients. In monographs, chemical purity is controlled by specifying limits on chemical impurities.

To characterize and determine the quantity of potential chemical contaminants in the final product, several methods may be used, including gas chromatography (GC), HPLC, or TLC. Using the example of ^{18}F-FDG, a colorimetric test for the detection of Kryptofix 2.2.2 has been developed. With this test, one can interpret whether the level of Kryptofix 2.2.2 is within the acceptable regulatory limits in the EP monograph for ^{18}F-FDG. Another example of chemical purity determination is in EP monograph of ^{11}C-methionine where is reported the HPLC method for testing the chemical impurities L-homocysteine thiolactone and from DL-homocysteine which derive from the synthesis of this radiopharmaceutical.

5.2.6.1 Residual Solvents

The determination of residual solvents in PET radiopharmaceutical preparations is also a part of the chemical purity testing. Residual solvents are defined as organic volatile chemicals that are used or produced in the manufacture of drug substances or excipients or in the preparation of drug products. The residual solvents are present at trace levels in pharmaceutical substances and their products. These solvents may be the result of the radiopharmaceutical synthesis or from packaging and storage. PET radiopharmaceutical preparations should contain low levels of residual solvents. The EP residual solvent chapter reported the concentration limit and the classification for each solvent set in the International Conference of Harmonization of Technical Requirements for Registration of Pharmaceuticals for Human Use guideline for residual solvents (ICH Q3C R5) [2] which describes the solvents grouped in three classes according to their toxicity:

- Class 1 solvents to be avoided in the manufacturing process because of their known unacceptable toxicities or deleterious environmental effects.
- Class 2 solvents to be limited because they are associated with less severe toxicity.
- Class 3 solvents with low toxic potential and lower risk to human health.

Other solvents for which no adequate toxicological data were found are classified. The residual of these solvents in the radiopharmaceutical preparation should be justified.

Residual solvents are usually determined by chromatographic techniques such as gas chromatography (GC).

5.2.7 Enantiomeric Purity

Enantiomers are either of a pair of optical isomers that are mirror images of each other. Enantiomers exhibit stereoisomerism because of the presence of one or more chiral centers. In the clinical use of chiral radiopharmaceutical, high enantiomeric purity is important since the biological inactive enantiomer could become a disturbing background source of radiation that interferes with interpretation of the signal of active enantiomer. For this reason the enantiomeric purity has to be verified where appropriate. The limit for each enantiomeric impurity is reported in the pharmacopoeia monograph of the radiopharmaceutical: for example, the limit for D-^{11}C-methionine is 10 % of the total radioactivity of the ^{11}C-methionine batch.

5.2.8 Sterility

PET radiopharmaceutical preparations must be prepared using precautions designed to exclude microbial contamination and to ensure sterility. The test for sterility [3] is carried out under aseptic conditions by inoculating the sample in two culture media Soybean-Casein Digest Medium and Fluid Thioglycollate Medium and by incubating for not less than 14 days. Soybean-Casein Digest Medium is a culture media for aerobic bacteria and fungi, while Fluid Thioglycollate Medium is primarily intended for the culture of anaerobic bacteria. Growth promotion tests should be performed by incubating reference bacteria in the two media. Bacterial growth should be visible within the period of incubation. Results of the growth promotion would indicate that both Soybean Casein Digest Medium and Fluid Thioglycollate Medium are capable of supporting bacterial growth; hence, results of the sterility test are reliable. A system suitability test should be performed using two methods: by transferring the solution to be tested in a membrane and by adding to the final portion of sterile diluents used to rinse the filter an inoculum of a small number of viable microorganism (the same used for growth promotion test) (membrane filtration) or by transferring the solution to be tested to the culture medium and by adding to the medium an inoculum of a small number of viable microorganism (the same used for growth promotion) (direct inoculation). The solutions are then incubated for not more than five days. If clearly visible growth of microorganism is obtained after incubation, visually comparable to that in the control vessel without product, the product possesses no antimicrobial activity under the conditions of the test so the test for sterility may then be carried out without further modifications. If clearly visible growth is not obtained, the conditions should be modified in order to eliminate antimicrobial activity of the product, and the system suitability should be repeated.

5.2.9 Bacterial Endotoxin Test

Bacterial endotoxins (pyrogens) are polysaccharides from bacterial gram-negative membranes which are water-soluble, heat stable, and filterable. Their presence in a radiopharmaceutical preparation can cause fever and also leukopenia in immunosuppressed patients. To minimize the presence of pyrogens, it is important that preparations are manufactured and dispensed under aseptic conditions. The test for bacterial endotoxins is used to quantify endotoxins, and it is based on the blood-clotting reaction that occurs when bacterial endotoxins activate the blood cell component Limulus amebocyte lysate (LAL) derived from horseshoe crabs (*Limulus polyphemus* or *Tachypleus tridentatus*). The test may be conducted with one of the following techniques reported in the EP chapter for bacterial endotoxins [4]:

- Gel-clot technique
- Turbidimetric technique
- Chromogenic technique

The limit for bacterial endotoxins is indicated in the individual monograph.

5.2.9.1 Gel Clot Technique

The gel-clot technique is based on clot formation in the reaction between endotoxins and LAL. The gel-clot method involves the use of a clotting protein that is cleaved by an activated clotting enzyme, at which point the insoluble cleavage products coalesce by ionic interaction to form the gel. Although the entire reaction has not been determined, it is understood that the reaction leading to clot formation involves a cascade of enzyme activation steps.

5.2.9.2 Turbidimetric Technique

This technique observes the changes in turbidity associated with the clotting protein formed in the reaction between endotoxins and LAL. Endotoxin concentration can be determined by the quantitative relationship between endotoxin concentration and turbidity (absorbance or transmission) of the reaction mixture at the end of incubation period (end-point-turbidimetric test) or by measuring the time needed for the reaction mixture to reach a predetermined absorbance or transmission or the rate of turbidity (kinetic-turbidimetric test).

5.2.9.3 Chromogenic Technique

This technique uses a chromogenic peptide which releases a chromophore (e.g., p-nitroaniline (pNA)) by the reaction of endotoxins with LAL. In the presence of endotoxin, the components of LAL are activated in a proteolytic cascade that results in the cleavage of a colorless artificial peptide substrate. Proteolytic cleavage of the substrate liberates p-nitroaniline (pNA), which has an absorbance of 405 nm. Endotoxin concentration can be determined by the quantitative relationship between the endotoxin concentration and the amount of chromophore released at the end of incubation period (end-point-chromogenic test) or by measuring the time needed for the reaction mixture to reach a predetermined absorbance or the rate of color (kinetic-chromogenic test).

5.3 Analytical Techniques Used in Quality Control of PET Radiopharmaceuticals

Chromatographic separation methods are commonly employed in the quality control of PET radiopharmaceuticals. Chromatography is an analytical technique based on the separation of two or more compounds by the distribution between two phases, a stationary and a mobile phase. These two phases can be solid–liquid, liquid–liquid, or gas–liquid. Chromatographic separation methods are used to separate radioactive or not radioactive species in the sample followed by their identification and quantification and are commonly

Table 5.1 Chromatographic methods employed in radiochemical, chemical, and enantiomeric purity determination in some PET radiopharmaceuticals described in EP monographs. *NR* not required

	Radiochemical purity		Chemical purity			Enantiomeric purity	
Radiopharmaceutical	TLC	HPLC	TLC	HPLC	GC	TLC	HPLC
^{18}F-FDG	X	X	X	X	X	NR	NR
^{11}C-methionine	X	X	–	X	X	X	-
^{11}C-acetate	–	X	–	X	X	NR	NR
^{18}F-NaF	–	X	–	X	NR	NR	NR
^{18}F-FLT	X	X	X	X	X	NR	NR
^{18}F-FDOPA	X	X	–	X	X	X	–
^{18}F-FMISO	X	X	X	X	X	NR	NR
^{68}Ga-Edotreotide	X	X	X	X	X	NR	NR

employed in radiochemical, chemical, and enantiomeric purity determinations. The most used chromatographic methods are high-performance liquid chromatography (HPLC), thin-layer chromatography (TLC), and gas chromatography (GC) (Table 5.1).

5.3.1 High-Performance Liquid Chromatography (HPLC)

High-performance liquid chromatography (HPLC) is a type of liquid chromatography used to separate and quantify compounds that have been dissolved in solution. HPLC utilizes a column that holds packing material (stationary phase), a pump that moves the mobile phase through the column, an injector to introduce the sample in a small volume, and a detector that shows the retention times of the molecules for identification and quantification. Retention time varies depending on specific chemical or physical interactions between the stationary phase, the molecules being analyzed, and the solvent used as a mobile phase. Types of HPLC generally depend on phase system used in the process. Following types of HPLC are commonly used in the quality control of radiopharmaceuticals:

1. Normal-phase chromatography (NP-HPLC)
2. Reversed-phase chromatography (RP-HPLC)
3. Ion-exchange chromatography

NP-HPLC separates analytes based on polarity. NP-HPLC uses a polar stationary phase and a not polar mobile phase. The polar analyte interacted with and is retained by the polar stationary phase. RP-HPLC has a not polar stationary phase and an aqueous, moderately polar mobile phase. RP-HPLC operates on the principle of hydrophobic interactions, which result from repulsive forces between a polar eluent, the relatively not polar analyte, and the not polar stationary phase. In ion-exchange chromatography, retention is based on the attraction between analyte ions and charged sites bound to the stationary phase. Ions of the same charge are excluded and eluted with the mobile phase. There are different types of detectors that can be used for HPLC. The detector is used to detect the presence of a compound passing through and to provide an electronic signal to a data-acquisition device. In HPLC analysis of PET radiopharmaceuticals, radio-detectors are used such as NaI scintillator or BGO radiodetector to determine the radiochemical purity. Radioactivity may be measured by integration using an automatic-plotting instrument or a digital counter. The ratios of the areas under the peaks give the ratios (or percentage) of the radioactive concentration of the compounds (Fig. 5.1). Moreover, the retention time of each compound allows radiochemical identification by comparison with solutions of the same not radioactive chemical substances (cold standard) using a suitable detection method. Ultraviolet (UV–VIS), electrochemical, conductivity, and refractive index (RI) detectors are commonly connected to radiodetectors in order to determine the radiochemical identity of the radiopharmaceuticals and the amount and identification of chemical impurities.

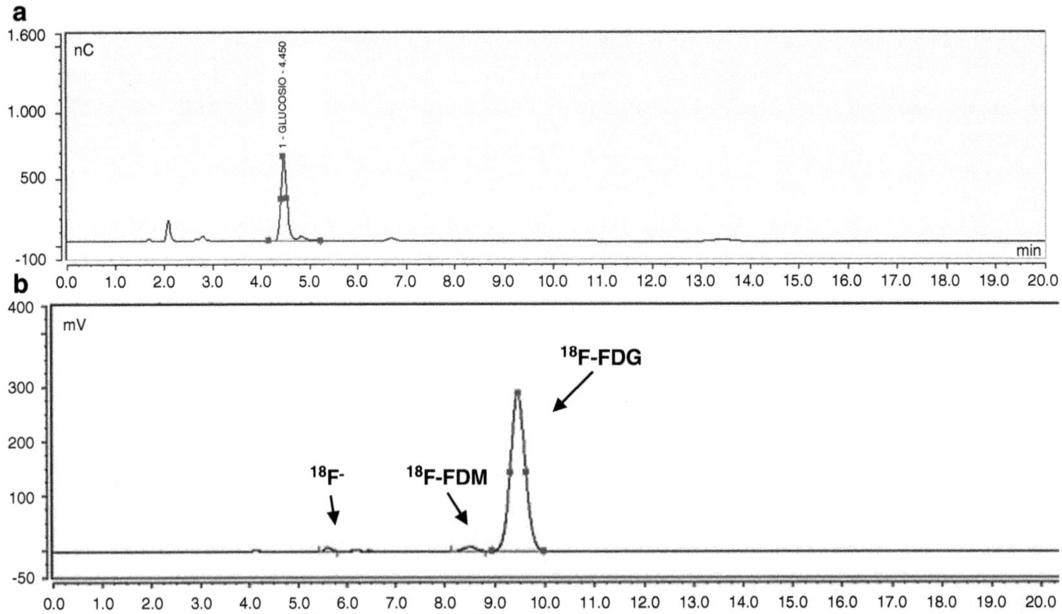

Fig. 5.1 (**a**) ECD-PAD chromatogram of ^{18}F-FDG preparation, (**b**) radio-chromatogram: $^{18}F^-$, free ion fluoride; ^{18}F-FDM, ^{18}F-2-fluoro-2-deoxy-D-mannose. HPLC conditions: stationary phase CarboPac PA10 column, mobile phase NaOH 0.1 M, and flow rate 1 ml/min

5.3.2 Thin-Layer Chromatography (TLC)

Thin-layer chromatography (TLC) is a solid–liquid form of chromatography where the stationary phase is normally a polar absorbent and the mobile phase can be a single solvent or combination of solvents. TLC technique can be used to determine the number of components in a mixture or to verify a substance's identity. In thin-layer chromatography, the stationary phase is a polar absorbent, usually finely ground alumina or silica particles. For enantiomeric purity determination, a chiral reagent absorbed to an inert support is used. This absorbent is coated on a glass slide or plastic sheet creating a thin layer of the particular stationary phase. Almost all mixtures of solvents can be used as the mobile phase. The TLC plate is marked at the origin and at the front distance. The sample of radiopharmaceutical is spotted to the origin in volume equal or less than 10 μl with microsyringes or micropipettes, and the TLC plate is transferred to the development chamber filled with a small amount of mobile phase (Fig. 5.2a, b). The solvent, which is in the bottom of the chamber, travels up the layer of adsorbent by capillary action, passes over the spot, and, as it continues up, moves the compounds in the mixture up the plate at different rates. The result is the separation of the compounds due to the differences in their affinity to the stationary phase and because of differences in solubility in the solvent. Once the solvent has run to the front mark, the plate is removed.

After development, the support is dried, and the position of radioactive spots is detected by autoradiography or by measurement of radioactivity over the length of the chromatogram using suitable collimated counters. Radioactivity may be measured by integration using an automatic-plotting instrument or a digital counter. The ratios of the areas under the peaks give the ratios of the radioactive concentration of the chemical substances to determine the radiochemical purity (Fig. 5.2c). TLC can also provide a chromatographic measurement known as an R_f value. The R_f value is the "retardation factor" or the "ratio-to-front" value expressed as a decimal fraction. The R_f value can be calculated as:

$$R_f = \text{distance travelled by compounds} / \text{distance travelled by solvent front}$$

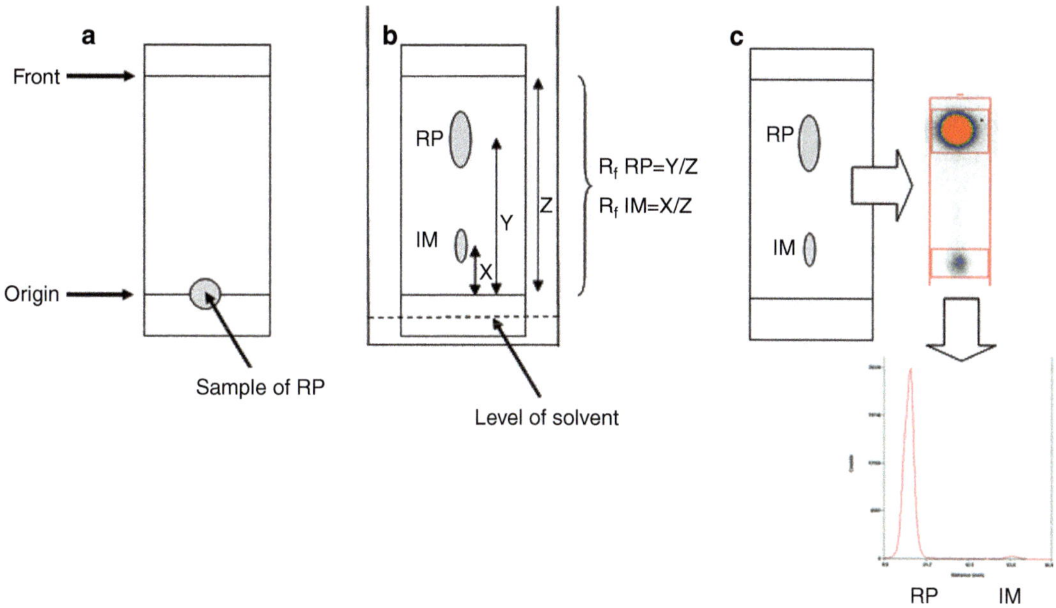

Fig. 5.2 TLC analysis of PET radiopharmaceutical. (**a**) Sample spotting, (**b**) development, (**c**) detection and integration. *RP* radiopharmaceutical, *IM* impurity

R_f calculation of the spots or areas allows chemical identification by comparison with solutions of the same not radioactive chemical substances (cold standard) using a suitable detection method.

5.3.3 Gas Chromatography (GC)

Gas chromatography (GC) is a gas–liquid chromatography which involves a sample being vaporized and injected onto the head of the chromatographic column. The sample is transported through the column by the flow of inert, gaseous mobile phase. Separation of each sample component is achieved by repeated distribution between two phases. Commonly used mobile phases are N_2, He, or Ar. GC columns can be packed or capillary. Packed columns contain a finely divided, inert, solid support material (commonly based on diatomaceous earth) coated with liquid stationary phase, while capillary columns can be wall-coated open tubular (WCOT) or support-coated open tubular (SCOT). Wall-coated columns consist of a capillary tube whose walls are coated with liquid stationary phase. In support-coated columns, the inner wall of the capillary is lined with a thin layer of support material such as diatomaceous earth, onto which the stationary phase has been adsorbed. Transport of the analytes is achieved in the gas phase; separation is accomplished in the stationary phase.

The quality of a separation depends on how long the components to be separated stay in the stationary phase and on how often they interact with this phase. The type of interaction between component and phase is determined by the functional groups. The polarity of the phase is a function of stationary phase substituents. The temperature of the column can be varied during the analysis improving the separation. The time taken for a particular compound to travel through the column to the detector is known as its retention time. This time is measured from the sample injection to when a maximum peak height for that compound is displayed. There are several different types of detectors in use. The flame ionization detector (FID) is the most commonly used.

Headspace gas chromatography (HSGC) is a GC technique where the liquid sample is set in a closed vessel until the volatile components reach equilibrium between the sample and the gas volume above. An aliquot of the gas volume (headspace) is sampled and introduced into a GC column for analysis. Direct injection of analytes evaporated through equilibration between liquid phase and gas phase minimized GC system contamination and column deterioration. In addition, the automation of equilibrium and injection procedure reduces analysis time and improves reproducibility. Due to the volatility of organic solvents, GC is commonly used to identify and quantify the presence of residual solvents in radiopharmaceutical preparations.

5.3.4 Gamma Spectrometry

Gamma-ray determination measures gamma photons emitted from radionuclides. Gamma-ray spectrometers use the direct proportionality between the energy dissipated by incoming gamma radiation into the detector and the pulse amplitude at the output of the detector. After amplification and digitization, the pulse amplitudes are analyzed, and the output of the spectrometer is an energy spectrum of detected radiation. Since individual radionuclides emit specific gamma-ray energies, gamma-ray spectra can be used to perform a qualitative analysis of a sample, identifying the radionuclides present. This requires a calibration of the system as a function of energy. Quantitative analysis is also possible, by measuring the areas of specific peaks and correcting for the system efficiency and other factors. The calibration in energy and efficiency must be made for the specific energies of interest or in a range of energies (e.g., 50–2000 keV). To this end, certified sources supplied by an accredited laboratory are used; these sources have specified level of accuracy and are traceable to the international system of measurement [5]. Gamma-ray spectrometry is used in the radiopharmaceutical field for:

- The identification of gamma-emitting radionuclides
- The accurate measurement of the activity
- The detection and assessment of gamma-emitting radionuclidic impurities
- The estimation of the upper limit for the potential presence of an impurity that has not been possible to detect

5.3.4.1 Identification of radionuclides and Radionuclide Impurities

This test is performed by analyzing the spectral distribution of gamma radiation absorbed in the detector, in order to detect any peak. The energies of peaks are then evaluated, by using the energy calibration of the system. Samples of a radiopharmaceutical solution may present several peaks; moreover, peaks of impurities present in very low activity levels may not be easily detected at a visual inspection of the spectrum. Dedicated and relatively sophisticated software are used in the analysis for the spectrum, in order to automate the radionuclide identification.

It has to be noticed that in some cases there is more than one single radionuclide emitting gamma radiation at a given value of energy. In the case of PET radionuclides, all can be detected by detection of the annihilation photons at 511 keV (Fig. 5.3). The energy analysis is then not sufficient in some cases to make an unequivocal identification. In

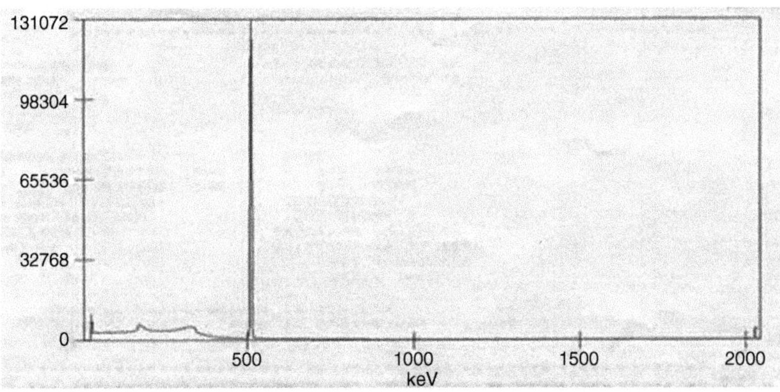

Fig. 5.3 Gamma spectrum of a solution of ^{18}F-FDG with the peak due to annihilation photons at 511 keV

these cases, the repetition of several acquisitions during time and the consequent measurement of the decreasing peak area make possible to evaluate the half-life of the radionuclide and confirm the identification.

5.3.4.2 Determination of Radionuclide Radioactivity

This test is basically made by measuring the area of specific peaks obtained in the spectra of the sample and comparing with the peak area produced by a reference standard of the same radionuclide with known activity. In this case, the activity can simply be calculated according to equation:

$$A_{\text{sample}} = A_{\text{standard}} \cdot \frac{C_{\text{sample}}}{C_{\text{standard}}} \frac{D_{\text{sample}}}{D_{\text{standard}}} \cdot G \quad (5.3)$$

where:

A_{standard} is the known activity of the reference standard.
C_{sample} are net counts (i.e., corrected for the background) in the peaks of the sample.
C_{standard} are net counts (i.e., corrected for the background) in the peaks of the standard.
D symbols are indicated as the respective dilution factors.
G is an eventual geometrical correction factors.

In many cases, however, it is not possible to have a certified standard for comparison; this in particular is the case of short-lived radionuclides. In these situations, a full calibration of the spectrometry system in energy and efficiency is necessary. This is typically performed using so called "multi-gamma" solutions, mixtures of calibration radionuclides with well-spaced peaks in a wide range of energies. A typical calibration solution covers the energy range 59–1836 keV. Sophisticated software algorithms make possible to obtain for this spectral distribution the efficiency calibration in the same interval of energies. Once the peak of a radionuclide is detected, its energy is accurately calculated, on the basis of the energy calibration; the nuclide can be identified, and the efficiency value at that level of energy is gathered from the efficiency calibration. At this point, the activity of radionuclide can be calculated by

$$A = \frac{A_n}{t \cdot \varepsilon(E) \cdot y} \cdot f_g \quad (5.4)$$

where:

A_n is the net (background corrected) area of the peak.
t is the time of acquisition of the spectra.
$\varepsilon(E)$ is the peak efficiency at the specific energy E of interest.
y is the tabulated yield of emission of the peak from the radionuclide.
f_g is an eventual correction factors.

5.4 Validation of Analytical Procedures

The validation of analytical procedures is required to demonstrate that the methods are suitable for their intended purpose. All the methods used during quality control of PET radiopharmaceuticals should be validated in order to provide assurance of quality to the process. The reference for this topic is the guideline produced by the International Conference of Harmonization of Technical Requirements for Registration of Pharmaceuticals for Human Use and Validation of analytical procedures, text, and methodology (ICH Q2 R1) [6] where the methods and the analytical techniques are separated in four most common types such as:

- Identification tests
- Quantitative tests for impurities' content
- Limit tests for the control of impurities
- Quantitative tests of the active moiety in samples of drug substance or drug product or other selected component(s) in the drug product

The type of method or analytical procedure used will determine the nature and extent of the validation studies required. The validation of analytical method is performed by considering a number of characteristics:

- Specificity
- Precision
- Accuracy
- Linearity and range
- Detection limit
- Quantitation limit
- Robustness

5.4.1 Specificity

Specificity is the ability to assess the desired component in its intended formulation, in the presence of components which may be expected to be present including impurities, by-products, additives, etc. A chromatographic method is specific if it can separate the component of interest from other components in the formulation. An example of specificity in PET radiopharmaceuticals quality control is the HPLC method for the determination of ^{18}F-FDG radiochemical purity in EP monograph. In this case, the method should separate ^{18}F-FDG from other radiolabeled impurities such as ion fluoride $^{18}F^-$and ^{18}F-2-fluoro-2-deoxy-D-mannose (^{18}F-FDM). In order to demonstrate specificity, it is necessary to prepare each component and to inject a mixture of the components to the HPLC analysis. Separation of the individual components demonstrates the specificity of the method.

5.4.2 Precision

The precision of a method is the closeness of agreement between a series of measurements. Precision should be a quantitative measure of the repeatability of the method under the same operating conditions over a short interval of time. The precision of an analytical procedure is usually expressed as the variance, standard deviation, or coefficient of variation (CV) of a series of measurements. An example of precision determination should be applied to analysis of residual solvents in ^{18}F-FDG solution with GC method. In order to demonstrate the precision of this method, it is necessary to perform multiple analyses of acetonitrile solutions at different concentration. CV values less than 10 % demonstrate the precision of the method.

5.4.3 Accuracy

The accuracy of a method is the degree of agreement between the test result and the value which is accepted as a conventional true value or an accepted reference value. Accuracy is the ability of the method to provide the correct answer. Accuracy may be measured by the analysis of a known standard and comparison of the measured value to the actual value.

5.4.4 Linearity and Range

Linearity may be defined as the method ability to obtain test results which are directly proportional to the concentration (amount) of analyte in the sample within a given range. The range of the method defines the region where the response is linear. A linear relationship exists if the detector response is directly proportional to the amount of analyte in the sample. The linearity of the GC method for quantification of residual solvents in PET radiopharmaceutical solution may be determined by the analysis of standards containing different known concentrations of solvents. The method is linear if the solvents' peak areas increase proportionately with increasing standard concentrations. The range is the interval between the upper and lower concentration of analyte in the sample (including these concentrations) for which it has been demonstrated that the analytical procedure has a suitable level of precision, accuracy, and linearity. The linear range of the GC method should cover the concentrations of solvents found in routine quality control measurements.

5.4.5 Detection Limit (LOD) and Quantitation Limit (LOQ)

The detection limit (LOD) is the lowest amount of analyte that can be detected. The quantitation limit (LOQ) is defined as the lowest amount of analyte which can be quantitatively determined with suitable precision and accuracy. LOD and LOQ can be determined by using several approaches. The signal-to-noise ratio approach is performed by comparing measured signals from samples with known low concentrations of analyte with those of blank samples and by establishing the minimum concentration at which the analyte can be reliably detected and quantified. Signal-to-noise ratios between 3 or 2:1 for LOD and 10:1 for LOQ are generally considered acceptable for estimating these characteristics. Other approach is based on the standard deviation of the response and the slope where the detection limit (LOD) may be expressed as

$$\mathrm{LOD} = 3.3\sigma / S \tag{5.5}$$

where:

σ = the standard deviation of the response.
S = the slope of the calibration curve.

The quantitation limit (LOQ) may be expressed as

$$\mathrm{LOQ} = 10\sigma / S \tag{5.6}$$

where:

σ = the standard deviation of the response.
S = the slope of the calibration curve.

The slope S may be estimated from the calibration curve of the analyte, while σ may be estimated by the calibration curve or by blank.

These characteristics are most important in chemical and radiochemical impurity determination and quantification in the quality control of PET radiopharmaceuticals.

5.4.6 Robustness

Robustness is the ability of a method to remain unaffected by small, deliberate changes in method parameters. A method is robust if the results remain unaffected by small variations of pH in a mobile phase, variations of temperature, mobile phase composition, flow rate, different columns (different lots and/or suppliers), etc.

The validation characteristics that should be applied for different types of analytical method as well as the minimum requirement for the number of determinations and replicates are provided by ICH guidelines. Once the validation characteristics have been identified, the validation protocol should be assessed. This protocol should include the details of analytical method to be validated, the validation characteristics which will be investigated, the experimental procedure, the equipment and the reference material which will be used, the obtained results, the acceptance criteria, and the responsibilities. Finally, the results and statistics associated with each validation characteristics should be interpreted and compared with the acceptance criteria in order to decide if the method meets the validation requirements.

5.5 Quality Control of ^{18}F-Radiopharmaceuticals: ^{18}F-FDG

^{18}F-FDG is the mostly used PET radiopharmaceutical, and it is designed to study glucose metabolism of cancer cells in vivo. Approximately 95 % of all clinical PET studies in oncology are performed with ^{18}F-FDG.

The quality requirements of ^{18}F-FDG are set out in several pharmacopoeias. Different countries adopt a different set of standards and methods. For example, the determination of the radiochemical purity of ^{18}F-FDG by USP is made by TLC, while EP prescribes both HPLC and TLC methods. The EP standard is described in this chapter [7], and the quality control tests are listed in Table 5.2. Due to short half-life of ^{18}F-FDG, not all the listed tests can be completed before the release of the ^{18}F-FDG product. The EP allows the ^{18}F-FDG to be released before radionuclidic purity, residual solvents, bacterial endotoxin, and sterility tests are finished.

5.5.1 Appearance

The appearance of ^{18}F-FDG solution is reported in EP monograph. The product should be observed behind adequate shielding. ^{18}F-FDG product should be clear and colorless or slightly yellow solution.

Table 5.2 Quality control tests for ^{18}F-FDG listed in EP

QC test	Method	Acceptance criteria
Appearance	Not specified	Clear and colorless or slightly yellow solution
Radiochemical and radionuclidic identity	Examine the HPLC chromatogram peak from radiochemical purity test	The retention time of principal peak in the radio-chromatogram is similar to that obtained with reference standard solution of FDG
	Gamma spectroscopy	Photon energy of 0.511 MeV and the sum peak at 1.022 MeV
	Half-life measurement	105–115 min
pH	Not specified	4.5–8.5
Chemical purity	HPLC (FDG and CDG)	The areas under the peaks of FDG and CDG in the test solution are not greater than the areas of the reference standard peaks (0.5 mg/V)
	TLC (Kryptofix 2.2.2)	The spot due to the test solution shows a less intense color than that of the spot due to reference solution (2.2 mg/V)
	UV/VIS spectrophotometry (4-(4-methylpiperidin-1-yl) pyridine)	Absorbance at 263 nm showed by test solution should not be more than that obtained with reference standard (0.02 mg/V)
	HPLC (TBA)	The area under the peak of the test solution is not greater that the area of the TBA reference standard peak (2.6 mg/V)
Residual solvents	Not specified	According to limits reported on Residual solvents EP chapter
Sterility	Sterility test according to EP	No bacterial growth
Bacterial endotoxin	According to EP	Less than 175/V (maximum recommended dose in ml) IU/ml
Radionuclidic purity	Gamma spectroscopy	Photon energy of 0.511 MeV and the sum peak at 1.022 MeV
		Radionuclidic impurities: maximum 0.1 % of the total radioactivity (after at least 24 hours)
Radiochemical purity	HPLC	^{18}F-FDG and ^{18}F-FDM: not less than 95 % of the total radioactivity ^{18}F-FDM: maximum 10 % of the total radioactivity
	TLC	^{18}F-FDG and ^{18}F-FDM: not less than 95 % $^{18}F^-$ and partially or fully acetylated derivatives: maximum 5 %

5.5.2 Radiochemical and Radionuclidic Identity

In EP, the tests for radionuclidic identity and radiochemical identity are included in the tests for radionuclidic purity and radiochemical purity, respectively. The radionuclidic identity can be confirmed both by obtaining a gamma spectrum and measuring the half-life of the product. The photon energy should be 0.511 MeV and the sum peak at 1.022 MeV which is typical for positron emitter radionuclides. Measurement of the half-life can be carried out by measuring the same test solution in a dose calibrator with the same geometry condition by no fewer than three measurements. The half-life is then calculated by plugging the results into the radioactivity decay equation. The EP does not specify the time interval between each measurement, but it should be long enough to allow a significant decay (e.g., 30 min). The obtained result to confirm the presence of ^{18}F should be within 105–115 min.

The radiochemical identity can be confirmed by HPLC method. The mobile phase is a solution of sodium hydroxide in carbon dioxide-free water (4 g/L), and the stationary phase is a strongly basic anion exchange resin. The prescribed detector is a suitable one for carbohydrates such as pulse amperometric detector (PAD) connected in series with radioactivity detector (for radiochemical purity determination), and the flow rate is 1 ml/min. Since sodium hydroxide absorbs carbon dioxide from the environment, the HPLC should be equipped with a system to prevent the contact of mobile phase with air (e.g., under inert gas pressure). The identification includes HPLC injection of a reference standard solution of cold FDG followed by the test solution. The acceptance criterion is that the retention time of principal peak in the radiochromatogram obtained with the test solution is similar to that of principal peak in the chromatogram obtained with reference standard solution of FDG.

5.5.3 pH

The EP specifies the pH value range of ^{18}F-FDG solution that should be 4.5–8.5. However, the monograph does not specify the method for testing pH.

5.5.4 Chemical Purity

The EP specifies the test for FDG and the impurity 2-chloro-deoxyglucose (CDG) that could be present in the product if acidic hydrolysis is used during the synthesis. The chemical purity is determined by HPLC with the same analytical conditions described in the radiochemical identity. The test protocol includes the injection of a reference standard solutions of FDG (0.5 mg/V) (the same used for the radiochemical identity) and CDG (0.5 mg/V) corresponding to the maximum admitted concentration diluted to the maximum recommended dose in ml (V), followed by the test solution. The acceptance criterion is that the area under the FDG and CDG peaks of the test solution should be less than those of the reference solutions. Furthermore, the EP monograph prescribes the injection of a standard solution of 2-fluoro-2-deoxy-D-mannose (FDM) mixed with FDG reference standard to check the resolution between the 2 peaks that should be minimum 1.5. This is for system suitability and for the determination of the radiochemical impurity ^{18}F-FDM described in the radiochemical purity section.

Other chemical purity tests described in EP monograph are for the residual concentration of the phase transfer catalysts used during the synthesis such as Kryptofix 2.2.2 and tetrabutylammonium hydroxide (TBA). The test for Kryptofix 2.2.2 involves spotting the test solution and the reference standard with the maximum admitted concentration diluted to the maximum recommended dose in ml (2.2 mg/V) on a TLC silica gel plate with the adsorbed iodoplatinate reagent for aminopolyether test [8]. The central portion of the spot due to the test solution should show a less intense color than that of the spot due to reference solution.

The content of TBA is determined by HPLC with a mobile phase of a solution of toluenesulfonic acid (0.95 g/L) and acetonitrile 25:75 (V/V) and octadecylsilyl silica as a stationary phase. The detector is UV/VIS (254 nm) absorption spectrophotometer and the flow rate is 0.6 ml/min. The test involves the injection of a reference standard of TBA corresponding to the maximum admitted concentration diluted to the maximum recommended dose in ml (2.6 mg/V), followed by the test solution: the peak showed by this solution should not be more than the area of the corresponding peak in the chromatogram obtained with reference standard.

Other chemical impurity test is for 4-(4-methylpiperidin-1-yl) pyridine, determined by ultraviolet and visible absorption spectrophotometry. The test involves the absorbance measurement at 263 nm of a reference standard corresponding to the maximum admitted concentration diluted to the maximum recommended dose in ml (0.02 mg/V), followed by the test solution: the absorbance showed by this solution should not be more than that obtained with reference standard.

5.5.5 Residual Solvents

Residual solvents should be limited according to the principles defined in general chapter of residual solvents of EP. The monograph prescribes that the preparation may be released for use before completion of the test. The EP does not specify the test method, although the description implies that a GC should be used. Acetonitrile is a class 2 solvent which is commonly used during the synthesis, and the residual should be controlled. The limit for this solvent is 4.1 mg/day (410 ppm). Ethanol is also used in ^{18}F-FDG synthesis, but the low toxic potential (class 3 solvent) increases the limit value to 50 mg/day (5000 ppm).

5.5.6 Sterility

The control of sterility of ^{18}F-FDG preparation can be done after the release of the preparation for clinical use. As reported in the EP monograph of radiopharmaceutical preparation, the test is performed by incubating the sample with both Soybean Casein Digest Medium and Fluid Thioglycollate Medium for 14 days. Soybean Casein Digest Medium is a culture media for aerobic bacteria and fungi, while Fluid Thioglycollate Medium is a media for anaerobic bacteria. The product should be sterile.

5.5.7 Bacterial Endotoxins (LAL Test)

The control of bacterial endotoxins of ^{18}F-FDG preparation can be done after the release of the preparation for clinical use. The monograph does not prescribe a specific method to detect the endotoxins among those reported in the EP general chapter. As reported in the ^{18}F-FDG monograph, the limit for endotoxins is less than 175 IU/V with V being the maximum recommended dose in milliliters.

5.5.8 Radionuclidic Purity

The EP prescribes two methods to determine the radionuclidic purity of a ^{18}F-FDG preparation. One method is the same employed for the determination of the radionuclidic identity by obtaining a gamma spectrum of the product, and the photon energy should be 0.511 MeV and the sum peak at 1.022 MeV. The EP monograph prescribes also the determination of the amount of ^{18}F and radionuclidic impurities with a half-life longer than 2 hours which can be done after the release of the preparation for clinical use. For the detection and quantification of impurities, an aliquot of ^{18}F-FDG preparation should be retained and analyzed with gamma spectrometry after at least 24 hours in order to allow the fluorine-18 to decay to a level that permits the detection of impurities. The limit for such radionuclidic impurities is 0.1 % of the total radioactivity.

5.5.9 Radiochemical Purity

The EP prescribes both HPLC and TLC methods for the determination of radiochemical purity. These two methods allow the detection of different radiochemical impurities; therefore, they should be carried out together before the release of preparation for clinical use. HPLC method has been described in radiochemical and radionuclidic identity section and is used to detect radiolabeled impurities such as free ion fluoride $^{18}F^-$ and ^{18}F-2-fluoro-2-deoxy-D-mannose (^{18}F-FDM). The last impurity derives from an epimerization reaction of ^{18}F-FDG in alkaline condition and during steam sterilization [9, 10]. The limit for ^{18}F in the form of ^{18}F-FDG and ^{18}F-FDM is minimum 95 % of the total radioactivity, and the limit for ^{18}F-FDM is maximum 10 % of the total radioactivity due to ^{18}F-FDG and ^{18}F-FDM. The TLC method is used to detect free ion $^{18}F^-$ and the partially or fully acetylated derivatives of ^{18}F-FDG and ^{18}F-FDM. TLC silica gel plate is used as stationary phase, and the mobile phase is acetonitrile/water (95:5 V/V). The R_f of $^{18}F^-$, ^{18}F-FDG and ^{18}F-FDM, and acetylated ^{18}F-FDG are about 0.0, 0.45, and 0.8 to 0.95, respectively. The limit for ^{18}F in the form of ^{18}F-FDG and ^{18}F-FDM is minimum 95 % of the total radioactivity, and the limit for $^{18}F^-$ and partially or fully acetylated derivatives is maximum 5 % of the total radioactivity.

5.6 Quality Control of ^{11}C-Radiopharmaceuticals: ^{11}C-Methionine

Among ^{11}C-radiopharmaceuticals, ^{11}C-methionine is one of the most widely used in clinical PET with important applications in oncology. ^{11}C-methionine is a labeled analogue of the essential amino acid methionine, and it is used since tumor cells present an enhanced expression of amino acid transporter systems as well as protein synthesis [11]. Due to the very short half-life of ^{11}C (20.4 min), the synthesis and the quality control of this radiopharmaceutical should be as faster as possible. The tests reported in EP monograph are described in this chapter as example of ^{11}C-radiopharmaceutical quality control [12], and they are listed in Table 5.3.

5.6.1 Appearance

The solution of ^{11}C-methionine, observed behind adequate shielding, should be clear and colorless.

5.6.2 Radiochemical and Radionuclidic Identity

As for ^{18}F-FDG, the test for radiochemical identity is included in the test radiochemical purity,

Table 5.3 Quality control tests for ^{11}C-methionine listed in EP

QC test	Method	Acceptance criteria
Appearance	Not specified	Clear and colorless solution
Radiochemical and radionuclidic identity	Examine the HPLC chromatogram peak from radiochemical purity test	The retention time of principal peak in the radio-chromatogram is similar to that obtained with reference standard solution of methionine
	Gamma spectroscopy	Photon energy of 0.511 MeV and the sum peak at 1.022 MeV
	Half-life measurement	19.9–20.9 min
pH	Not specified	4.5 –8.5
Sterility	Sterility test according to EP	No bacterial growth
Bacterial endotoxin	According to EP	Less than 175/V (maximum recommended dose in ml) IU/ml
Chemical purity	HPLC	The areas under the peaks of methionine, L-homocysteine thiolactone, and DL-homocysteine in the test solution are not greater than the areas of the reference standard peaks (2.0 mg/V, 0.6 mg/V, 2 mg/V)
Residual solvents	Not specified	According to limits reported on residual solvents EP chapter
Radionuclidic purity	Gamma spectroscopy	Minimum 99 %. Photon energy of 0.511 MeV and the sum peak at 1.022 MeV
	Half-life measurement	19.9–20.9 min
Radiochemical purity	HPLC	Not less than 95 % of the total radioactivity
Enantiomeric purity	TLC	Not less than 95 % of the total radioactivity (D-^{11}C-methionine and L-^{11}C-methionine) D-^{11}C-methionine maximum 10 % of the total radioactivity

while the test for radionuclidic identity is the same for radionuclidic purity. The radionuclidic identity can be confirmed both by obtaining a gamma spectrum and measuring the half-life of the product. The photon energy should be 0.511 MeV and the sum peak at 1.022 MeV. The spectrum of the solution should be compared with a standardized ^{18}F solution spectrum from which should not differ significantly. Measurement of the half-life can be carried out by measuring the same test solution in a dose calibrator, and the obtained result should be within 19.9–20.9 min.

The radiochemical identity can be confirmed by HPLC method. The mobile phase is a solution of potassium dihydrogen phosphate (1.4 g/L) and the stationary phase octadecylsilyl silica gel. The prescribed detectors are UV/VIS (225 nm) and radioactivity detector (for radiochemical purity determination) connected in series, and the flow rate is 1 ml/min. The identification includes the HPLC injection of a reference standard solution of methionine followed by the test solution. The acceptance criterion is that the retention time of the principal peak in the radio-chromatogram obtained with the test solution is similar to that of principal peak in the chromatogram obtained with reference standard solution.

5.6.3 pH

The EP specifies the pH value range of ^{11}C-methionine solution that should be 4.5–8.5. However, the monograph does not specify the method for testing pH.

5.6.4 Sterility

The control of sterility of ^{11}C-methionine preparation can be done after the release of the preparation for clinical use following the tests prescribed in the EP radiopharmaceutical preparation chapter.

5.6.5 Bacterial Endotoxins (LAL test)

The control of bacterial endotoxins of ^{11}C-methionine preparation can be done after the release of the preparation for clinical use. The monograph does not prescribe a specific method to detect the endotoxins among those reported in the EP general chapter. The limit for endotoxins is less than 175/V IU/mL with V being the maximum recommended dose in milliliters.

5.6.6 Chemical Purity

The chemical purity is determined by HPLC with the same analytical conditions described in the radiochemical identity. The EP specifies the test for methionine and the impurities L-homocysteine thiolactone and DL-homocysteine which derives from the synthesis. The test protocol includes the injection of a reference standard solution of methionine (2 mg/V), L-homocysteine thiolactone hydrochloride (0.6 mg/V), and DL-homocysteine (2 mg/V) corresponding to the maximum admitted concentration diluted to the maximum recommended dose in ml, followed by the test solution (Fig. 5.4). The acceptance criterion is that the area under the methionine and impurities peaks of the test solution should be less than these of the reference solution.

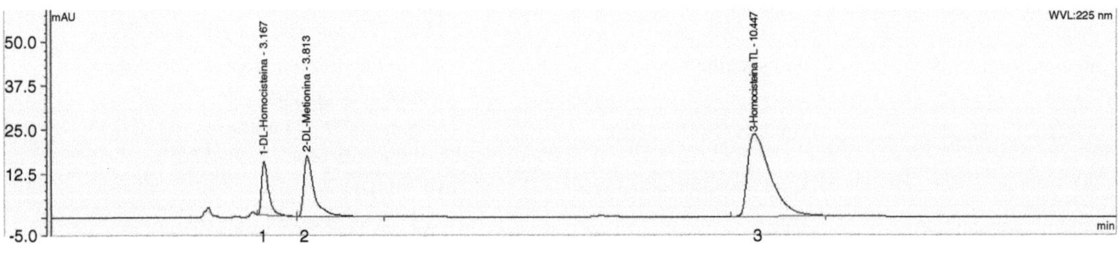

Fig. 5.4 HPLC chromatogram of standard solution for chemical purity of ^{11}C-methionine: 1: DL-homocysteine, 2: DL-methionine and 3: L-homocysteine thiolactone

5.6.7 Residual Solvents

Residual solvents should be limited according to the principles defined in general chapter of residual solvents of EP. The monograph prescribes that the preparation may be released for use before completion of the test. The EP does not specify the test method, although the description implies that a GC should be used.

5.6.8 Radionuclidic Purity

Radionuclidic purity method is the same employed for the determination of the radionuclidic identity, and the preparation may be released for use before completion of the test. The radionuclidic purity of ^{11}C should be minimum 99 %.

5.6.9 Radiochemical Purity

The method to assess the radiochemical purity is the same employed for the determination of the radiochemical identity. The acceptance criterion is minimum 95 % of the total radioactivity for D-^{11}C-methionine and L-^{11}C-methionine. The monograph also reported the radiolabeled impurities that may be present in the preparation as the oxidation by-products S-oxide and S,S-dioxide of the methionine [13].

5.6.10 Enantiomeric Purity

EP monograph prescribes this control since the ^{11}C-methionine is a chiral radiopharmaceutical with two different enantiomers L- and D-form (Fig. 5.5). The L-form is the preferable enantiomer which should be present in the preparation for clinical use with high purity because it is directly involved in protein synthesis. A TLC method is described to perform the enantiomeric purity test using an octadecylsilyl silica gel plate for chiral separations as stationary phase and methanol: water (50:50 V/V) as mobile phase. The procedure involves spotting the test solution and the reference standard solutions with

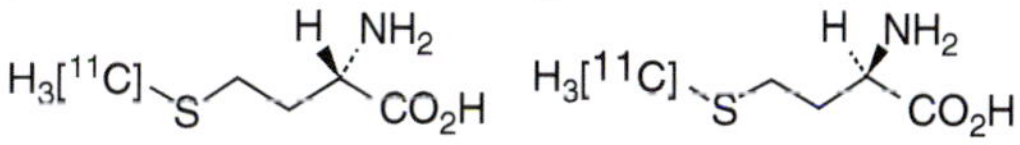

Fig. 5.5 L (**a**) and D (**b**) ^{11}C-methionine enantiomers

L-methionine and DL-methionine on a TLC silica gel plate. After developing, the plate is sprayed with a solution of ninhydrin in ethanol and heated at 60 °C for 10 min in order to visualize the spots and to show the separation of L- and D-enantiomers in the standard solution. TLC should be read by radio TLC scanner. R_f of L-^{11}C-methionine and D-^{11}C-methionine are about 0.58 and 0.51, respectively. The limit for D-^{11}C-methionine is 10 % of the total radioactivity and for the sum of D-^{11}C-methionine and L-^{11}C-methionine is 95 %. The preparation may be released for use before completion of the test.

5.7 Quality Control of ^{68}Ga-Radiopharmaceuticals: ^{68}Ga-Edotreotide (^{68}Ga-DOTATOC)

^{68}Ga-edotreotide (^{68}Ga-1,4,7,10-tetra-azacyclododecane-1,4,7,10-tetraaceticacid-D-Phe1-Tyr3 octreotide) (^{68}Ga-DOTATOC) is DOTA-labeled somatostatin analogue labeled with ^{68}Ga and used in PET imaging of somatostatin receptors for the diagnosis and characterization of neuroendocrine tumors (NETs). ^{68}Ga is produced by decay of ^{68}Ge in commercially available ^{68}Ge/^{68}Ga generators without using cyclotron. In this chapter ^{68}Ga-edotreotide EP monograph tests [14] are reported as example of quality control of PET radiopharmaceutical labeled with a generator-produced radionuclide (Table. 5.4).

5.7.1 Appearance

The appearance of ^{68}Ga-edotreotide solution is reported in EP monograph. The product should be observed behind adequate shielding. ^{68}Ga-edotreotide solution should be clear and colorless solution.

Table 5.4 Quality control tests for ^{68}Ga-edotreotide listed in EP

QC test	Method	Acceptance criteria
Appearance	Not specified	Clear and colorless solution
Radiochemical and radionuclidic identity	Examine the HPLC chromatogram peak from radiochemical purity test	The retention time of principal peak in the radio-chromatogram has a relative retention of 1.3 with reference to standard solution of edotreotide
	Gamma spectroscopy	Photon energy of 0.511 MeV and 1.077 MeV and the sum peak at 1.022 MeV
	Half-life measurement	62–74 min
pH	pH indicator strip	4.0–8.0
Chemical purity	HPLC (edotreotide, metal complexes of edotreotide, and other related substances)	The sum of the areas of the peaks in the test solution with a relative retention with reference to edotreotide between 0.8 and 1.4 is less than that of the edotreotide standard solution (50 μg/V) The area under the peak of each unspecified impurity is less than that of the edotreotide standard solution (disregarding any peak with a relative retention with reference to edotreotide of 0.5 or less)
	TLC (HEPES buffer)	The spot due to the test solution shows a less intense color than that of the spot due to HEPES reference solution (200 μg/V)
Residual solvents	Gas chromatography	Ethanol: 10 % (V/V) and maximum 2.5 g per administration
Sterility	Sterility test according to EP	No bacterial growth
Bacterial endotoxin	According to EP	Less than 175/V (maximum recommended dose in ml) IU/ml
Radionuclidic purity	Gamma spectroscopy	Minimum 99.9 % of the total radioactivity
		^{68}Ge and other radionuclidic impurities: maximum 0.001 % of the total radioactivity (after at least 48 hours)
Radiochemical purity	HPLC	^{68}Ga-Edotreotide: not less than 91 % of the total radioactivity $^{68}Ga^{3+}$: maximum 2 % of the total radioactivity
	TLC	^{68}Ga in colloidal form: maximum 3 % of the total radioactivity

5.7.2 Radiochemical and Radionuclidic Identity

The test for radiochemical identity is included in the test radiochemical purity. The radiochemical identity can be confirmed by HPLC method. The stationary phase is base-deactivated octadecylsilyl silica gel with a gradient mobile phase water/acetonitrile with trifluoroacetic acid (99.9:0.1 V/V). The detectors are spectrophotometer (220 nm) and radioactivity detector (for radiochemical purity determination) connected in series, and the flow rate is 0.6 ml/min. The identification includes the HPLC injection of a reference standard solution of edotreotide followed by the test solution. The acceptance criterion is that the retention time of the principal peak in the radio-chromatogram obtained with the test solution has a relative retention of 1.3 with reference to the principal peak in the chromatogram obtained with standard solution.

The radionuclidic identity can be confirmed either by obtaining a gamma spectrum and measuring the half-life of the product. The spectrum photon energies should be 0.511 MeV and 1.077 MeV and the sum peak at 1.022 MeV which may be observed. Measurement of the half-life can be carried out by measuring the same test solution in a dose calibrator; the result should be within 62–74 min.

5.7.3 pH

The monograph specifies the pH value range of ^{68}Ga-edotreotide solution that should be 4.0–8.0 measured by pH indicator strip.

5.7.4 Chemical Purity

The monograph specifies the test for edotreotide, metal complexes of edotreotide, and other related substances. The chemical purity is determined by HPLC with the same analytical conditions described in the radiochemical identity. The test protocol includes the injection of a reference standard solution of edotreotide (the same used for the radiochemical identity) corresponding to the maximum admitted concentration diluted to the maximum recommended dose in ml (50 μg/V), followed by the test solution. The acceptance criterion is that the sum of the areas of the peaks in the test solution with a relative retention with reference to edotreotide between 0.8 and 1.4 should be less than that of the edotreotide standard solution. Furthermore, the EP monograph prescribes the limit for each unspecified impurities present in the test solution: the area under the peak of each impurity should be less than that of the edotreotide standard solution.

Other chemical purity test is a TLC method to assess the residual concentration of HEPES buffer, if used during the labeling reaction of the peptide with ^{68}Ga. TLC silica gel F_{254} with aluminum plate is used as stationary phase and a standard solution of HEPES corresponding to the maximum admitted concentration diluted to the maximum recommended dose in ml (200 μg/V), and the test solution are spotted. TLC is developed with a mobile phase of acetonitrile/water (75:25 V/V) and detected by exposing to iodine vapor. R_f of HEPES is 0.3 and the spot due to the test solution should show a less intense color than that of the spot due to reference solution.

5.7.5 Residual Solvents

The monograph prescribes the test for the residual ethanol by using GC. The limit reported in the monograph for this solvent is 10 % (V/V) and maximum 2.5 g per administration.

5.7.6 Sterility

The control of sterility of ^{68}Ga-edotreotide preparation can be done after the release of the preparation for clinical use following the tests prescribe in the EP radiopharmaceutical preparation chapter.

5.7.7 Bacterial Endotoxins (LAL Test)

The control of bacterial endotoxins of ^{68}Ga-edotreotide preparation can be done after the release of the preparation for clinical use. The monograph does not prescribe a specific method to detect the endotoxins among those reported in the EP general chapter. The limit for endotoxins is less than 175/V IU/mL with V being the maximum recommended dose in milliliters.

5.7.8 Radionuclidic Purity

EP prescribes two tests to determine the radionuclidic purity of ^{68}Ga-edotreotide by using gamma spectrometry. One test prescribes that the peaks in the gamma spectrum of the product corresponding to photon energy different from 0.511 MeV, 1.077 MeV, 1.022 MeV, and 1.088 MeV should represent not more than 0.1 % of the total radioactivity. The second test, which can be done after the release of the preparation for clinical use, prescribes the determination of the amount of ^{68}Ge and other radionuclidic impurities with a half-life longer than 5 hours. For the detection and quantification of such impurities, an aliquot of test solution should be retained and analyzed with gamma spectrometry after at least 48 hours in order to allow the ^{68}Ga to decay to a level that permits the detection of impurities since ^{68}Ge does not emit gamma radiation and can be detected indirectly as a decay product ^{68}Ga. The limit for ^{68}Ge and other radionuclidic impurities is 0.001 % of the total radioactivity.

5.7.9 Radiochemical Purity

TLC and HPLC methods are reported for the determination of radiochemical purity. These two methods allow for the detection of different radiochemical impurities; therefore, they should be carried out together before the release of preparation for clinical use. The TLC method is used to detect the impurity ^{68}Ga in colloidal form. TLC silica gel plate is used as stationary phase, and the mobile phase is ammonium acetate (77 g/L)/methanol 50:50 (V/V). The R_f of ^{68}Ga in colloidal form and ^{68}Ga-edotreotide are 0.0–0.1 and 0.8–1.0, respectively. The limit for ^{68}Ga in colloidal form is maximum 3 % of the total radioactivity. HPLC method has been described in radiochemical and radionuclidic identity section and is used to detect radiolabeled impurities such as free ion $^{68}Ga^{3+}$ and other radiochemical impurities. The limit for $^{68}Ga^{3+}$ is maximum 2 % of the total radioactivity. The radiochemical purity of ^{68}Ga-edotreotide should be minimum 91 % and it is assessed by the formula:

$$(100 - \mathrm{A}) \times T \quad (5.7)$$

where A is the percentage of the radioactivity due to ^{68}Ga in colloidal form determined by TLC method and T is the proportion of the area of the peak due to ^{68}Ga-edotreotide relative to the total areas of the peaks in the chromatogram obtained with HPLC method.

References

1. European Pharmacopoeia. General monographs: radiopharmaceutical preparations. 8th ed. Strasbourg: European Directorate for the Quality of the Medicines and Healthcare; 2014. p. 759–63.
2. International Conference of Harmonization of Technical Requirements for Registration of Pharmaceuticals for Human Use guideline for residual solvents (ICH Q3C R5). Current step 4 version dated. 4 Feb 2011.
3. European Pharmacopoeia. 2.6 Biological test: 2.6.1 Sterility. 8th ed. Strasbourg: European Directorate for the Quality of the Medicines and Healthcare; 2014. p. 175–8.
4. European Pharmacopoeia. 2.6 Biological test: 2.6.14 Bacterial Endotoxins. 8th ed. Strasbourg: European Directorate for the Quality of the Medicines and Healthcare; 2014. p. 194–8.
5. Debertin K, Helmer RG. Gamma and X-ray spectrometry with semiconductor detectors. North – Holland: Elsevier Science Pub. Co.; 1988.
6. International Conference of Harmonization of Technical Requirements for Registration of Pharmaceuticals for Human Use Validation of analytical procedures (ICH Q2 R1). Current step 4 version dated. Nov 2005.
7. European Pharmacopoeia. Fludeoxyglucose [^{18}F] injection. 8th ed. Strasbourg: European Directorate for the Quality of the Medicines and Healthcare; 2014. p. 3957–9.
8. European Pharmacopoeia. 4.1.1 Reagents: iodoplatinate reagent. 8th ed. Strasbourg: European Directorate for the Quality of the Medicines and Healthcare; 2014. p. 477.
9. Meyer GJ, Matzke KH, Hamacher K, Fuchtner F, Steinbach J, Notohamiprodjo G, Zijlstra S. The stability of 2-[^{18}F]Fluoro-deoxy-D-glucose towards epimerisation under alkaline conditions. Appl Rad Isot. 1999;51:37–41.
10. Karwath P, Sartor J, Gries W, Wodarski C, Dittmar C, Biersack HJ, Guhlke S. Steam sterilization and automatic dispensing of [^{18}F]fludeoxyglucose (FDG) for injection. Appl Rad Isot. 2005;62:577–86.
11. Ishiwata K, Vaalburg W, Elsinga PH, Paans AMJ, Woldring M. Comparison of L-[1-^{11}C]methionine and L-methyl-[^{11}C]methionine for measuring in vivo protein synthesis rates with PET. J Nucl Med. 1988; 29:1419–27.
12. European Pharmacopoeia. L-Methionine([^{11}C] Methyl) injection. 8th ed. Strasbourg: European Directorate for the Quality of the Medicines and Healthcare; 2014. p. 1073–4.
13. Bogni A, Bombardieri E, Iwata R, Cadini L, Pascali C. Stability of L-[S-methyl-^{11}C]methionine solutions. J Radioanal Nucl Chem. 2003;256(2):199–203.
14. European Pharmacopoeia. Gallium(^{68}Ga)Edotreotide injection. 8th ed. Strasbourg: European Directorate for the Quality of the Medicines and Healthcare; 2014. p. 4847–8.

Regulation of PET Radiopharmaceuticals Production in Europe

6

James R. Ballinger and Jacek Koziorowski

Contents

6.1 **Introduction** 128
6.1.1 Development of Pharmaceutical Regulations 128
6.1.2 Regulatory Agencies 128
6.1.3 Pharmaceutical Inspection Cooperation Scheme (PIC/S) 129
6.1.4 The European Pharmacopoeia (*Ph. Eur*) 129
6.1.5 International Conference on Harmonisation (ICH) 130
6.1.6 Qualified Person (QP) 130

6.2 **Regulatory Framework** 130
6.2.1 Manufacturing Authorisation (MA) 131
6.2.2 Clinical Trial 131
6.2.3 Magistral Approach/Extemporaneous Preparation 131
6.2.4 Documentation 131

6.3 **Drug Development and Approval** 132
6.3.1 Stages of Drug Development 132
6.3.2 Data Needed for Submission 134

6.4 **Scientific Writing** 135

6.5 **Good Manufacturing Practice (GMP)** 136
6.5.1 Components of GMP 136
6.5.2 Challenges for PET 137

6.6 **Future Directions** 138
6.6.1 New European Clinical Trials Regulations .. 138
6.6.2 Recognition of Special Status of Radiopharmaceuticals 138
6.6.3 Risk Assessment Approaches 139
6.6.4 Quality by Design (QbD) 140

Conclusion 141

References 141

Abstract

Radiopharmaceuticals are a unique species of pharmaceuticals, containing both a drug and a radionuclide. This distinctive character can be challenging from a regulatory point of view as both pharmaceutical good manufacturing practice (GMP) and radiation safety aspects have to be balanced against each other. As a consequence of this, the production of PET radiopharmaceuticals must comply with both GMP and local radiation safety rules. This chapter describes some of the regulatory framework that covers the human use of PET radiopharmaceuticals in Europe. For preclinical applications there are no regulations on production, apart from the local/national animal rights rules. The different approaches which may be used to obtain permission to use the PET radiopharmaceutical in humans are described. For "first in human" use in a clinical trial, the content of the Investigational Medicinal Product Dossier is described, also

J.R. Ballinger
Division of Imaging Sciences and Biomedical Engineering, King's College London, London, UK
e-mail: jim.ballinger@kcl.ac.uk

J. Koziorowski (✉)
Department of Radiation Physics and Department of Medical and Health Sciences, Linköping University, Linköping, Sweden
e-mail: jacek.koziorowski@regionostergotland.se

M.M. Khalil (ed.), *Basic Science of PET Imaging*, DOI 10.1007/978-3-319-40070-9_6

an approach to minimise the very costly toxicological studies. The essentials of GMP and quality management systems are explained. The chapter ends with some future directions and convenient GMP approaches.

6.1 Introduction

Radiopharmaceuticals are a unique species of pharmaceuticals, containing both a drug and a radionuclide. This distinctive character can be challenging from a regulatory point of view as both pharmaceutical good manufacturing practice (GMP) and radiation safety aspects have to be balanced against each other. As a consequence of this, the production of PET radiopharmaceuticals must comply with both GMP and local radiation safety rules. This chapter describes some of the regulatory framework that covers the human use of PET radiopharmaceuticals in Europe. For preclinical applications there are no regulations on production, apart from the local/national animal rights rules. This chapter starts with a brief history of GMP and pharmaceutical regulations and some of the regulatory organisations involved. The different approaches which may be used to obtain permission to use the PET radiopharmaceutical in humans are described. For "first in human" use in a clinical trial (CT), the content of the Investigational Medicinal Product Dossier (IMPD) is explained with respect to content, procedures and writing, also an approach to minimise the very costly toxicological studies. Next, the essentials of GMP and quality management systems (QMS) are explained. The chapter ends with some future directions and convenient GMP approaches.

6.1.1 Development of Pharmaceutical Regulations

The first pharmaceutical regulations in Europe were published in 1965 in response to thalidomide and other drugs which produced unexpected effects with tragic results [1]. However, it was more than 20 years before radiopharmaceuticals were considered as drugs [2–4]. Since then, regulations have become increasingly strict, as has their enforcement, though there are variations between countries [5]. Regulatory compliance now constitutes as significant proportion of the work in a centre which produces PET radiopharmaceuticals for clinical use. In addition to pharmaceutical regulations, which are addressed here, there is a range of other regulations, some of which conflict, which must be addressed. These include radiation protection of workers, patients and the public, radioactive waste handling and transport of radioactive materials. All in all, radiopharmacy is arguably the most highly regulated health profession. Managing this complexity is of utmost importance when planning and designing a PET radiopharmacy. Both GMP and radiation protection must be considered at all stages. If possible, meeting with both the medicines and radiation protection authorities in the early planning phase is highly recommended in order to achieve an efficient and compliant PET radiopharmacy. Environmental monitoring and control systems, such as air handling and other ancillary components, must be designed for heat dissipation, adequate humidity and temperature control, air quality and filtration systems, maintenance of room classes and provision of gas lines.

In many countries, PET radiopharmaceuticals are covered in the monographs of pharmacopoeias. A pharmacopoeia is a book containing directions and information on the identification and properties of drugs. A monograph is detailed information on purity criteria and tests to be used for a particular drug. If there is no national or regional pharmacopoeia available, the World Health Organization's International Pharmacopoeia (http://apps.who.int/phint/en/p/about/) may be used. Quality control of PET tracers is discussed in Chap. 5.

6.1.2 Regulatory Agencies

The practice of pharmacy and manufacturing of radiopharmaceuticals is regulated at a national level, with each country having a regulatory body or "competent authority". In 1995 the European Union (EU) set up the European Medicines Agency (EMEA, later EMA; www.ema.europa.eu) to provide a framework for a single approval which would apply throughout the EU. However, submission of all products to the EMA was not compulsory, except for certain classes of pharmaceuticals, and national approvals are still possible [6]. The advantage of EMA route (*centralised procedure*) is a single approval which applies throughout the EU. However, the disadvantages include higher application fees, the cost of providing product information and labelling in all EU languages and the lack of a sufficient market in all nations. Only a small number of radiopharmaceuticals have EMA approval, but that number will continue to increase as central approval is the only route for therapeutic radiopharmaceuticals. At the time of writing, the only PET radiopharmaceuticals with EMA approval are the three amyloid imaging agents: florbetapir (Amyvid), florbetaben (NeuroCeq) and flutemetamol (Vizamyl). With its commitment to transparency, the EMA publishes detailed assessment reports, with only commercially sensitive material withheld. It may seem strange that the most widely used PET tracer, ^{18}F-fluorodeoxyglucose (FDG), is not approved by the EMA; however, it is a generic drug with local or regional production and there are no pan-European manufacturers.

Submission to individual countries is still possible, and most products which were licensed before the EMA was established are still regulated nationally. Once a product is accepted in one country, there is a *mutual recognition procedure* via which a product can be approved in another country without full separate evaluation. A third route is the *decentralised procedure* under which the product is submitted for approval in several countries at the same time with one country named as the reference country which carries out the full evaluation; this is a cheaper alternative to EMA approval.

It is only in recent years that the manufacture of PET radiopharmaceuticals began to be highly regulated and there are still differences between countries [7]. Some countries require all manufacturing of widely used tracers such as FDG to be performed under a licence, albeit with an abridged application as described in Sect. 6.2.1. The United Kingdom is unique in having a "specials" licence under which a wide range of products that are not commercially viable can be manufactured. It has the additional advantages that products do not need to be released by a qualified person (see Sect. 6.1.6) and prior approval of new products is not required.

Pharmaceutical regulations were intended for the pharmaceutical industry and commercial scale manufacturing. Full compliance with GMP is difficult in small facilities producing short-lived radiotracers because of the small number of personnel, half-life constraints on analysis and rapid reuse of shared equipment (see Sect. 5.2). The first official recognition of the special status of radiopharmaceuticals came in the EU Clinical Trials Regulations of 2014, wherein it was acknowledged the clinical trials of diagnostic radiopharmaceuticals did not fall within the regulations [8, 9]. This opens the door to the use of risk assessment as a tool for interpretation of legislation [7].

6.1.3 Pharmaceutical Inspection Cooperation Scheme (PIC/S)

Although inspections of pharmaceutical manufacturing facilities are carried out by the national authorities, the Pharmaceutical Inspection Convention has a cooperation scheme, PIC/S, under which there is a degree of harmonisation of inspection standards throughout Europe (www.picscheme.org). Of most relevance is the guide to good practices for the preparation of medicinal products in healthcare establishments, which now has an annex on radiopharmaceuticals [10]. Although PIC/S aims to harmonise inspection standards, each national authority retains full responsibility.

6.1.4 The European Pharmacopoeia (*Ph. Eur*)

Although most countries have their own pharmacopoeia, there is also a European Pharmacopoeia (http://online.edqm.eu/EN/entry.htm) which has legal status in all nations. It contains general monographs on classes of drugs such as radiopharmaceuticals or parenteral preparations as well as methods of analysis. Recently a general chapter on extemporaneous preparation of radiopharmaceutical preparations has been added.

Monographs on individual radiopharmaceuticals, at the time of writing approximately 70, specify such aspects as chemical and radionuclidic identity, tests for parameters such as pH, radionuclidic impurities and chemical and radiochemical impurities as well as setting limits for each. Importantly, the specifications are for the end product and do not dictate the route of synthesis except for its impact on the impurity profile. The remit of the *Ph. Eur* is drug quality; inclusion in the pharmacopoeia is independent of licensing status or clinical utility.

Radiopharmaceutical monographs are written ("elaborated") by Group 14, composed of academic, commercial and regulatory specialists. Once a monograph has been drafted, it is circulated for comment by national authorities, professional bodies and other concerned parties before final revision and acceptance.

Increasingly the *Ph. Eur* is being seen as the route forward for introduction of new compounds. The short half-lives of PET radiopharmaceuticals limit their market to local distribution; thus only extremely high-volume products will be manufactured commercially. However, once a radiopharmaceutical has a *Ph. Eur* monograph, it can be prepared locally to accepted quality standards under the magistral approach described in Sect. 6.2.3. The tests in the monographs are usually (1) identification, by gamma-ray spectrometry, half-life or high-pressure liquid chromatography (HPLC); (2) pH determination; (3) radionuclidic purity, by gamma-ray spectrometry or half-life; (4) chemical purity, by HPLC; (5) radiochemical purity, by HPLC with a radioactivity detector or by TLC and radioactivity scanner; (6) residual solvents, by gas chromatography; (7) sterility; (8) bacterial endotoxins; and (9) radioactivity, by measurement in an ionisation chamber ("dose calibrator"). See Chap. 5.

6.1.5 International Conference on Harmonisation (ICH)

The International Conference on Harmonisation of Technical Requirements for Registration of Pharmaceuticals for Human Use (ICH) brings together the regulatory authorities and pharmaceutical industry to discuss scientific and technical aspects of drug registration. It was established in 1990 and has gradually evolved to respond to the increasingly global face of drug development, so that the benefits of international harmonisation for better global health can be realised worldwide. The mission of ICH is to achieve greater harmonisation to ensure that safe, effective and high-quality medicines are developed and registered in the most resource-efficient manner (http://www.ich.org/home.html).

6.1.6 Qualified Person (QP)

The EU pharmaceutical directive of 2001 [5] designates the status of *qualified person* (*QP*) who is authorised to release products for clinical use under a manufacturing licence or clinical trial licence. To be eligible to be a QP, the individual must be a registered pharmacist, chemist or biologist who has sufficient experience in a manufacturing environment and who has passed an exam conducted jointly by the professional registration body and the national authority.

6.2 Regulatory Framework

There are three main routes to get a radiopharmaceutical into the clinic for human use: (1) marketing authorisation, (2) clinical trial and (3) the "magistral approach".

A marketing authorisation is very expensive ($$$$$) and takes years to obtain. A clinical trial is less expensive ($$$) and takes at least a year. In contrast, the "magistral approach" is the least expensive ($) and can take only a matter of months. A marketing authorisation may be used for both established and new tracers. A clinical trial is mainly for novel tracers ("first in human" studies) and for new or additional uses of an already established tracer. The magistral approach is for known radiopharmaceuticals that have been previously tested in man, and preclinical data, such as safety, efficacy, toxicology and dosimetry, is available.

6.2.1 Manufacturing Authorisation (MA)

A manufacturing authorisation may be issued by the EMA or by a national authority. The documentation which must be submitted is extensive, as described in Sect. 6.3.2. If it is a novel tracer, the evidence of efficacy and safety will have been obtained from a clinical trial, as described in Sect. 6.2.2.

Because of the cost of obtaining an MA, this route will only be taken if there is a commercial market for a tracer or if a national authority requires an MA even for local use. This mainly applies to widely used tracers such as FDG.

For generic tracers (i.e. no longer under patent) with well-established use, an abridged application may be submitted where literature references are used for the non-clinical and clinical data. This applies if the tracer has been in use for 8–10 years [article 10 of reference 5]. The manufacturer only needs to present data on product quality. This is discussed in Sect. 6.3.2.

6.2.2 Clinical Trial

Volume 10 of Eudralex contains all the information needed for clinical trials [11]. Trials are conducted under the guidelines of the International Conference on Harmonisation (ICH) of pharmaceutical trials [12]. The quality data to be submitted is similar to that required for a manufacturing authorisation.

In addition to the quality and safety of the product, trials must be performed according to good clinical practice (GCP) which ensures the quality of the data obtained from the trial and safeguards the human subjects who take part in trials. This too is enshrined in Eudralex [11]. In addition to the inspections of manufacturing facilities, there are also GCP inspections which assess the systems and data kept at clinical research sites. It is required that every employee who is involved in a clinical trial receives GCP training with updates at 2–3 year intervals. Thus, radiochemists who provide data which will be part of the clinical trial must undergo this training.

6.2.3 Magistral Approach/Extemporaneous Preparation

A less formal system is the magistral approach. A *magistral formula* is a pharmaceutical compound prepared by the pharmacist or someone under his/her direction for a given patient according to a prescription and following the technical and scientific standards of the pharmaceutical art. An *official preparation* is a pharmaceutical compound developed or prepared by a pharmacist or someone under his/her direction which is listed and described by the national formulary. The two ancient terms provide a means for the small-scale production of PET tracers essentially under the practice of pharmacy rather than a manufacturing authorisation. In the United Kingdom, this is termed a Sect. 10 exemption from the Medicines Act.

6.2.4 Documentation

The general requirements for the approval of tracers include process validation, product quality (chemical purity, radiochemical purity, stability, sterility, bacterial endotoxins, bioburden) and analytical method validation according to ICH guidelines (specificity, repeatability, precision, sensitivity, linearity, accuracy) [13].

There must be a written application which includes description and composition of the drug product, description of the manufacturing process and process controls, control of reagents and excipients (including the quality and purity of precursor) and control of drug product (specifications, analytical methods, stability).

The formats for manufacturing authorisation and clinical trial are identical, with the exception on the numbering. It may be advisable to use the same format for the magistral approach as the assessors are familiar with it. Use all the points in the template and write "not applicable" or "N/A" in the fields where it is so.

6.3 Drug Development and Approval

6.3.1 Stages of Drug Development

The process of drug development can be broadly divided into two stages: preclinical and clinical. Each of these can then be subdivided into multiple parts.

6.3.1.1 Preclinical Studies

The preclinical development of a drug begins with chemistry, whether a novel compound or a variant on a known synthetic or natural compound. With radiopharmaceuticals there is the added problem of where to put the radioactive atom on the molecule. Among the factors in this choice is ease of chemistry to perform the radiolabelling in high yield, generally as the final step of synthesis to avoid losses due to radioactive decay during subsequent synthetic steps. The location of the label should not significantly change the biological properties of the molecule, particularly if it is designed to mimic a natural substance and bind to a receptor. Furthermore, the label should be metabolically stable so as not to complicate image interpretation or mathematical modelling.

Once the chemistry has been established, though not necessarily optimised, the chemical and in vitro biological properties of the labelled molecule can be established. These include stability in a biological milieu, such as incubation with human serum at 37 °C. There may be in vitro binding assays which can be performed to characterise the binding affinity and selectivity of the compound.

If a potential radiotracer shows appropriate in vitro properties, it can be evaluated in small animals, generally mice or rats. Increasingly, transgenic species are being used in which human tumours can be grown or human diseases mimicked. In recent years, preclinical PET/CT and SPECT/CT scanners have become widely available which provide excellent spatial resolution (~1 mm) and allow longitudinal studies in the same animal, which is particularly important with expensive transgenic rodents [14, 15]. With only a small number of animals, it can be established whether the radiotracer does indeed target the desired lesion and whether uptake in adjacent organs interferes with visualisation of the target. These studies also give an idea of the route (s) of excretion of the radiotracer. In the past, imaging studies were only semi-quantitative, but quantitative values can be obtained by tissue biodistribution studies following sacrifice of the animal. Individual organs are dissected, placed in pre-weighed counting tubes, weighed and assayed in a gamma well counter along with a known dilution of the dose. This allows determination of the % dose per organ and % dose per gramme of each organ and calculation of target to background ratios. With current preclinical PET/CT and SPECT/CT systems, absolute quantification can be performed on imaging studies alone. Displacement studies can be performed with a nonradioactive drug which competes with the radiotracer for binding to the same target site. These animal studies allow prediction of human radiation dosimetry of the radiotracer. See Chaps. 3 and 14 for further details on PET dosimetry and PET kinetic modelling, respectively.

6.3.1.2 Toxicological Studies

There is also a need for preclinical safety, toxicology and dosimetry data. The toxicology is generally the most expensive part of the preclinical data. Normally for radiopharmaceuticals, biodistribution and dosimetry data from preclinical studies is often available, including imaging, autoradiography and direct measurement of radioactivity in harvested tissues and organs. Such studies may give detailed quantitative data on accumulation and elimination in tissues and excretion pathways. Using this data the design of extended single-dose toxicity studies may be focused on high-risk organs and tissues, thereby reducing the requirement for histopathological data in all organs, but focusing on main organs where the radiopharmaceutical accumulates.

If amounts are minute (in the microgram range), the Threshold of Toxicological Concern (TTC) approach may be used. Medicinal products such as radiopharmaceuticals may be exempt from toxicological studies when (single) doses up to 120 μg are used [16]. The ICH has also recently adopted the TTC approach in the assessment of DNA reactive mutagenic impurities in pharmaceuticals [17]. For larger molecules, such as peptides and monoclonal antibodies, one can argue that the molar amount is of importance. The adopted/assumed molecular weight for the medicinal product is set to 300 g/mol. For larger molecules such as proteins, FDA guidance sets the limit to <30 nanomoles. "Due to differences in molecular weights as compared to synthetic drugs, the maximum dose for protein products is ≤30 nanomoles" [18]. This corresponds to <100 μg of a drug having a molecular weight of 300.

6.3.1.3 Clinical Studies

If the chemical, in vitro and small animal studies are promising, the decision can be taken to evaluate the potential radiotracer in humans. In the past this was quite informal, with the initial volunteers often being the researchers themselves or graduate students in their departments. However, now this is highly regulated [19–21].

Traditionally, clinical studies of drugs proceed through Phase I, Phase II and Phase III before regulatory approval. However, with radiopharmaceuticals an initial step called Phase 0, pre-Phase I, microdosing (Europe) or exploratory Investigational New Drug (IND, USA) is often employed. Microdosing is defined as the administration of no more than 100 micrograms of the tracer and no more than 1/100 of the dose producing a pharmacological effect, which is often achievable with radiopharmaceuticals, particularly with PET agents [22, 23]. The toxicity testing for microdosing studies is much less rigorous than for later studies. Only an extended single-dose acute toxicity study in one species, generally a rodent, is required, with sacrifice of animals after 1 and 14 days followed by necroscopy. A microdosing study in 5–10 subjects will give a good indication of whether the radiotracer shows the same properties in humans that it did in animals and informs the decision on whether to proceed with product development.

A new potential radiopharmaceutical is classed as an investigational medicinal product (IMP). One of the documents required in support of a clinical study is an IMP Dossier (IMPD) which describes how the radiotracer will be produced and tested and summarises the information available about the compound. The Radiopharmacy Committee of the European Association of Nuclear Medicine has published guidance on the preparation of IMPDs for radiopharmaceuticals [24]. An important part of the IMPD is the criteria for release of a product for clinical use. The dossier addresses such aspects as radiochemical purity, pH, specific activity and content of residual solvents, as well as sterility and apyrogenicity.

There must also be an Investigator's Brochure (IB) which contains some of the same information but has a more clinical viewpoint.

Phase I studies are generally carried out in small numbers (<10) of normal volunteers, though with oncology tracers, sometimes patients are used. The main aim of Phase I is safety, though with the small chemical quantities of radiotracers, this is rarely a real concern. Usually whole-body images are obtained at different time points to allow calculation of radiation dosimetry in humans.

Phase II studies are proof of principle to demonstrate targeting of the intended organ or disease process. With radiotracers, Phase II is also used to determine the optimal imaging protocol which will be used in subsequent studies.

Phase III studies are the definitive efficacy studies required for receipt of a marketing authorisation. With radiopharmaceuticals the number of patients required is much smaller than for therapeutic drugs. However, the regulatory authorities prefer to see two independent Phase III studies. It may be necessary to perform multicentre studies in order to accrue a sufficient number of patients. Each phase must be approved by the medicines agency before the next is undertaken.

6.3.2 Data Needed for Submission

The clinical trial application to a national authority or to the EMA consists of several sections [25]:

1. Module I contains administrative information relevant to the authority to which the application is being made. The remainder of the application is called the Common Technical Document (CTD) and consists of modules II through V. The CTD was introduced by ICH in 2003 and standardises the presentation of data to regulatory authorities.
2. Module II contains summaries of quality data, preclinical studies and clinical studies, while modules III through V contain the details of those three aspects. The quality data includes the chemistry, manufacturing and controls (CMC), in the same format as was presented in the IMPD. The preclinical section includes toxicity studies which must be performed to Good Laboratory Practice (GLP) standards.

The structure of the CTD is shown in Fig. 6.1. For generic or well-established tracers, an abridged application may be submitted [article 10 of reference 5]. The red circle in Fig. 6.1 indicates which sections are included in the abridged application. The non-clinical and clinical trial data normally required for an application may be replaced by appropriate scientific literature. This kind of application is also known as a bibliographic application.

Many radiopharmaceuticals are manufactured directly to the final drug product; i.e. the drug substance or active pharmaceutical ingredient (API) is not isolated before formulation. This has some consequences for the CTD. Section "6.3.2. P Drug Product (Name, Dosage Form)" will be essentially the same as Sect. "6.3.2. S Drug

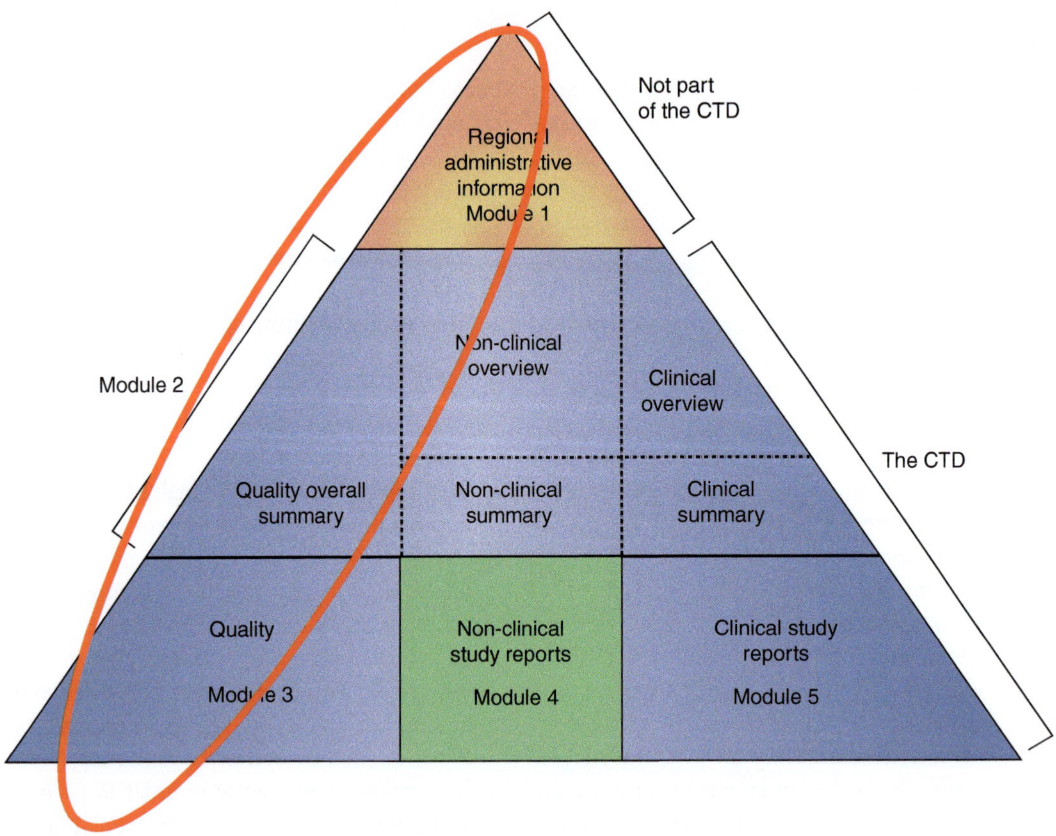

Fig. 6.1 The structure of the Common Technical Document (*CTD*) pyramid. *Module 1* is region specific and *modules 2*, *3*, *4* and *5* are intended to be common for all regions. The topics within the *red circle* are the components of the abridged application (From http://www.ich.org/products/ctd.html)

Substance (Name, Manufacturer)" [24]. Copy and paste these sections; do not use different wording as this may confuse the assessor at the regulatory body. There will more about the language for applications in "scientific writing" section.

For each marketed product, there must be a Summary of Product Characteristics (SPC or SmPC) which presents information about the product, including dosimetry and instructions for its use. The EMA is developing standard SPCs for generic products [26].

6.4 Scientific Writing

> My words fly up, my thoughts remain below;
> Words without thoughts never to heaven go
> (Claudius in Shakespeare's "Hamlet", Act III, scene iii).

Any application submitted to a regulatory body or competent authority must be very stringent and sober in both structure and language. It is, unquestionably, not a scientific paper to pass a peer review, but a description of drug manufacturing and quality control. Not all assessors are experts on radiopharmaceuticals and will thus react to any ambiguous or unclear wording.

Example: How Not to Write

Radionuclidic impurities

Radioactive oxygen-14 and nitrogen-13 may form as a result of minor side reactions in the cyclotron target: $^{14}N(p,n)^{14}O$ and $^{16}O(p,\alpha)^{13}N$. N-13 and O-14 are both positron-emitting radionuclides. The presence of O-14 in the drug substance may be ruled out as a significant contaminant because it has an ultrashort half-life of O-14 ($T_{1/2}=70.6$ s); thus in the course of synthesis ca 25 min, it will decay to 4.7×10^{-7} of its original amount. N-13 can appear in the form of gaseous ^{13}N-labelled oxides (e.g. $[^{13}N]NO$, $[^{13}N]NO_2$, etc.). The presence of ^{13}N would alter the measured half-life of the drug substance and would be seen as a radiochemical impurity during chromatographic analyses. This has not yet been observed. It is worth noting that ^{11}C in its process from starting material $[^{11}C]CO_2$ to the final product undergoes several chemical transformation steps with intermediate purifications. Therefore the probability for unwanted N-13 and O-14 species to survive through the same pathway as C-11 and end up in the final formulation is expected to be very low.

This is lengthy and confusing. Stating "not yet been observed" implies that it may be observed. Similarly, "the probability for unwanted" implies that there is a probability.

Example: How to Write

Radionuclidic impurities

Radioactive nitrogen-13 may form as a result of a minor side reaction in the cyclotron target: $^{16}O(p,\alpha)^{13}N$. N-13 can appear in the form of gaseous ^{13}N-labelled oxides (e.g. $[^{13}N]NO$, $[^{13}N]NO_2$, etc.). However, contamination of the final product with ^{13}N is not possible because the chemistry of nitrogen oxides is different from that of the starting material, $[^{11}C]CO_2$, which undergoes multiple chemical transformation steps with intermediate purifications.

This is short and sweet. By saying "is not possible", there is no doubt that it cannot be present. The language should be concise and formal, not verbose and/or sounding like a scientific investigation.

Example: "The product is purified by means of XXX and no impurities have been found" rather than "The product is purified by means of XXX, the possible impurity YYY which can potentially be produced by.....has so far not been detected".

Example: "All batches passed the sterility test", not "All batches passed the sterility test. However..."

Example: "The product is thus safe for human use", not "The product is thus safe for human use, yet some investigations have found..."

Have enough data/information to make a clear statement. It is better to spend a few hours extra in the laboratory than spending a few months in discussions with the competent authority.

6.5 Good Manufacturing Practice (GMP)

6.5.1 Components of GMP

The goal of pharmaceutical GMP is to ensure a consistent high-quality product which is appropriate for its intended use and which meets the specifications of its marketing authorisation. Because standards are constantly changing, the term current good manufacturing practice, cGMP, is often used. The three main components of GMP are facilities and equipment, personnel and procedures and documentation, all carried out within a quality management system. European rules for GMP are described in Eudralex volume 4 [27] with specific reference to radiopharmaceuticals in annex 3 [28] and investigational medicinal products in annex 13 [29].

6.5.1.1 Facilities and Equipment

The design and construction of facilities must afford a clean environment. Surfaces must be impervious and able to withstand regular cleaning. Activities must be segregated with interlocking doors to prevent cross-contamination. There must be a cascade of filtered air pressure from the cleanest area to the exterior to minimise the ingress of particles. This is achieved by heating, ventilation and air conditioning system (HVAC) with high-efficiency particulate air (HEPA) filters. Similarly, there must be a regimen of gowning up to prevent staff from carrying contaminants into the clean areas. Materials are sanitised and then transferred in via hatches with interlocking doors. Aseptic processes must be carried out within an appropriate environment of filtered air. Generally, radiosynthesis can be carried out in Grade C, but sterile filtration and dispensing must be carried out in Grade A. These are generally achieved with a hot cell, pharmaceutical isolator or laminar airflow cabinet. All equipment must be kept in good working order with regular checks of performance and records of maintenance undertaken. Proper operation of the facility must be documented by routine environmental and microbiological monitoring. This includes a combination of measurements of air flows and air change rates, active air sampling and particle counting and routine microbiological monitoring including agar settle plates, contact plates and finger dab plates. All of this is covered by the site master file (SMF).

6.5.1.2 Personnel

Personnel must be adequately trained in any procedures they carry out, with a training record. The training record must indicate that the member of staff has read the SOP and has demonstrated competence with evidence of a certain number of monitored activities. The responsibilities and authorities of each grade of staff must be specified. Persons who perform aseptic procedures must undergo periodic revalidation of their competence. If production facilities are shared with a research institution, the research personnel must be adequately trained in GMP regulations, and the quality controller (see below) must review and approve the research activities to ensure that they do not pose any hazard to the manufacturing of radiopharmaceuticals.

There must be a person designated as production manager, sometimes called responsible person. This person is responsible for the routine operation of the facility to ensure that the radiopharmaceuticals are produced to GMP standards. This includes ensuring that there are sufficient numbers of suitably trained staff available on a daily basis. This person makes sure that all documentation is complete before products are passed on to the quality assurance department.

There must be another independent person designated as quality controller. This person takes ultimate responsibility for the quality of the radiopharmaceuticals produced, though the act of release may be delegated to a suitable trained person. In some situations the quality controller might also be a qualified person.

6.5.1.3 Procedures and Documentation

All Standard Operating Procedures (SOPs) must be written down, approved and reviewed at regular intervals. There must be contemporaneous manufacturing records which document the adherence to SOPs and record the identities and quantities of all materials used and any in-process checks, all of which must be initialled or signed by the operator and checker. Quality assurance results must include evidence that the analytical equipment had been properly calibrated. There must be a Validation Master Plan (VMP).

One of the underpinning features of GMP is the quality of starting materials. Precursors must be obtained from approved vendors. There must be a process for auditing or inspecting vendors. It may be possible for a single such audit to be performed on behalf of a number of PET centres in the same country. All chemicals which remain in the final formulation must be obtained from certified pharmaceutical suppliers. In particular, active pharmaceutical ingredients (API) must be obtained from a certified GMP source.

6.5.1.4 Quality Management System (QMS)

In recent years, inspectors have placed increasing emphasis on the quality management system [30]. Indeed, this chapter was revised in 2013. Quality management is a wide-ranging concept, encompassing all matters which individually or collectively influence the quality of a product. The components of a QMS include the following. Product and process knowledge is managed throughout all life cycle stages. Managerial responsibilities are clearly specified. Arrangements are made for the manufacture, supply and use of the correct starting and packaging materials, the selection and monitoring of suppliers and verifying that each delivery is from the approved supply chain. Processes are in place to assure the management of outsourced activities. The results of product and process monitoring are taken into account in batch release, in the investigation of deviations and with a view of taking preventive action to avoid potential deviations occurring in the future. All necessary controls on intermediate products and any other in-process controls and validations are carried out. Where the true root cause (s) of the issue cannot be determined, consideration should be given to identifying the most likely root cause (s) and to addressing those in order to assess which might be responsible. Where human error is suspected or identified as the cause, this should be justified having taken care to ensure that process, procedural or system-based errors or problems have not been overlooked. Appropriate corrective actions and/or preventative actions (CAPAs) should be identified and taken in response to investigations in a timely manner. The effectiveness of such actions should be monitored and assessed, in line with quality risk management principles. There is a process for self-inspection and/or quality audit, which regularly appraises the effectiveness and applicability of the pharmaceutical QMS.

6.5.2 Challenges for PET

There are two separate challenges for the application of GMP to the manufacture of PET radiopharmaceuticals. The first is dictated by the short half-lives of most radionuclides used in PET, e.g. ^{18}F, 109 min; ^{11}C, 20 min; ^{13}N, 10 min; and ^{15}O, 2 min. There is no time for all quality parameters to be assessed before release for clinical use. Following risk assessment it must be specified which parameters can be determined retrospectively. This would include sterility testing and determination of levels of residual solvents. If at all possible, endotoxin testing, as a surrogate of sterility testing, should be performed before release, while sterility testing is performed post release. Endotoxins are heat-stable toxins released from the cell wall of gram-negative bacteria; thus, the absence of endotoxins suggests that the product does not contain bacteria. Before a new product is introduced, there must be a number of validation runs with full analysis to establish the quality of the product and its reproducibility.

The second challenge is the small-scale production, usually only a few doses at a time, in relation to the number of members of staff who would be required for implementation of full GMP. There should be segregation of responsibilities for production and quality control, and there should be independent release. Moreover, this small-scale production of a range of products is carried out with a small number of automated synthesis units. In the past this often involved reusable apparatus for which there had to be a validated cleaning procedure between operations and a strict regime of segregation.

Nowadays sterile single-use cassettes are available for many products, making production more reliable and less risky [31]. The Radiopharmacy Committee of the European Association of Nuclear Medicine has published guidance on good radiopharmacy practice (cGRPP) for the preparation of radiopharmaceuticals on a small scale [32].

6.6 Future Directions

6.6.1 New European Clinical Trials Regulations

The implementation of the European Clinical Trials Directive of 2001 had the unintended effect of reducing the number of clinical trials carried out in Europe [33]. Following consultation, the Directive was amended and reintroduced as a regulation [8]. Even though this regulation entered into force on 16 June 2014, it will apply no earlier than 28 May 2016. As a result of lobbying during the revision process, the special status of radiopharmaceuticals has been recognised, and there has been a relaxation of several requirements for radiopharmaceuticals [9].

Article 61, paragraph 5, states that the requirement for an investigational medicinal product (IMP) manufacture authorisation will *not* apply to "preparation of radiopharmaceuticals used as diagnostic investigational medicinal products where this process is carried out in hospitals, health centres or clinics, by pharmacists or other persons legally authorised in the Member State concerned to carry out such process, and if the investigational medicinal products are intended to be used exclusively in hospitals, health centres or clinics taking part in the same clinical trial in the same Member State". There are two important points within this statement. Firstly, it only applies to diagnostic radiopharmaceuticals, not therapeutic. Secondly, it only applies to small-scale preparation in hospitals and affiliated centres but does allow for supply to other centres taking part in the same clinical trial but lacking facilities for preparation of radiopharmaceuticals.

It is further stated in article 63, paragraph 2, the full requirements of GMP will not be applied to preparation of radiopharmaceuticals under this exemption. This will reduce the regulatory burden on PET centres but will not compromise the quality of the radiopharmaceuticals produced.

Finally, article 68 simplifies the labelling requirements for containers used to hold radiopharmaceuticals, recognising that it is a challenge to fit all the components required for an IMP product label onto a small square of adhesive paper.

It is anticipated that this precedent may be built upon in future revisions of European pharmaceutical legislation which affects PET radiopharmaceuticals.

6.6.2 Recognition of Special Status of Radiopharmaceuticals

Following on from the recognition of radiopharmaceuticals in the Clinical Trials Regulation [8], the relatively new PIC/S guidance document with annex 3 on radiopharmaceuticals contains some useful tips and ideas for the non-commercial "in-house" manufacturing of radiopharmaceuticals [10]. In this document, for example, the use of risk assessment can justify less stringent requirements for the environment that is written in annex 1 of Eudralex [27].

There can be a conflict in the requirements of GMP and radiation protection regulations as the former consider only the patient's safety and the latter only the worker's safety. In a case where the two regulations cannot be met, a decision based on a risk assessment should be made in order to determine which is of higher impact. Weighting should be applied based on the probability, risk and danger for the employees versus the patients, e.g. number of employees exposed to risk × probability of an incident × impact of incident to be compared with number of patients exposed to risk × probability of an incident × impact of incident.

An example of the use of risk assessment is the GMP requirement for an integrity test of the sterile filter after use: the filter contains residual radioactivity and thus poses a radiation risk. If many filters (>10) have been tested and the product has been demonstrated to be sterile each time or if the sterile filter is removed and the product is tested for bioburden (the microbial/bacterial load before sterile filtration) and is low (<1 CFU/10 mL; CFU – colony-forming unit) each time, one can make a risk assessment in order to avoid doing the sterile filter integrity test until the radioactivity has decayed.

6.6.3 Risk Assessment Approaches

As already mentioned in Sect. 6.6.2, risk assessment can be used to justify less stringent environment for the manufacturing of radiopharmaceuticals. Two of the most frequent approaches to risk assessment in the manufacturing of tracers are FMEA (failure modes and effects analysis) and FMECA (failure mode, effects and criticality analysis). Both approaches provide an evaluation of potential failure modes for processes and their likely effects. They investigate the probability of occurrence (O), degree of severity of the consequences (S), and the detectability (D). The occurrence, severity and detectability are placed in a matrix and then the Risk Priority Number (RPN) is calculated as O × S × D. RPN is a method to determine the criticality.

An example of a three-level FMEA/FMECA matrix:

Parameter	Level	Score	Description
Probability of occurrence (O)	Low	1	Very unlikely to occur
	Medium	2	Moderately likely to occur
	High	3	High probability of occurrence
Severity (S)	Low	1	Expected to have little or brief negative influence
	Medium	2	Expected to have a medium negative influence with possible minor long-term harm
	High	3	Expected to have a harmful or hazardous impact, including long-term effects with possible catastrophic or fatal effect
Detectability (D)	High	1	All failures are expected to be detected and the consequences avoided
	Medium	2	Some but not all failures are expected to be detected and the consequences avoided
	Low	3	None of the failures are expected to be detected and the consequences avoided

6.6.3.1 Risk Evaluation

(Sub) System	Function	Failure mode	Failure cause	Consequences	O	S	D	RPN	Action

Continue analysing the problem and fill out the schedule above and calculate RPN for each subsystem. Find suitable action levels depending on the character of the problem, for example:

RPN ≥12	High risk, unacceptable, action needed
5< RPN <12	Medium risk, further investigations to decide actions
RPN <5	Low risk, acceptable

Document the actions decided and their outcome.

Risk Control One way to control the risks is to create a risk matrix.

6.6.3.2 Risk Matrix

Probability (OxD)

		Low		Medium		High	
Severity (S)	Low	1	2	3	4	6	9
	Medium	2	4	6	8	12	18
	High	3	6	9	12	18	27

Level 1 = Acceptable	Level 2 = ALARP (As Low As Reasonably Practical)	Level 3 = Intolerable

To construct this matrix, the probability and detectability parameters are multiplied together and tabulated against the severity parameter. Standard risk classification is used to discriminate between levels of risk.

The ALARP level will be determined according to the kind of problem being assessed. You will also have to consider regulatory requirements and other demands stated by authorities, for example, marketing authorisations. Further information can be found in the ICH Q9 guideline [34].

6.6.4 Quality by Design (QbD)

Quality by design can be seen as an approach similar to parametric release. All critical parameters and set points are evaluated, normally using multivariate analysis. Once this is done, the knowledge space and design space are assigned (see Fig. 6.2a). As long as the set points and parameters are within the design space (see Fig. 6.2b), the finished product will meet the specifications and may be released. This approach may demand more in-process controls but should demand less or less frequent, quality control, thus enabling easier and faster release of radiopharmaceuticals. Further information can be found in the ICH Q8(R2) guideline [35].

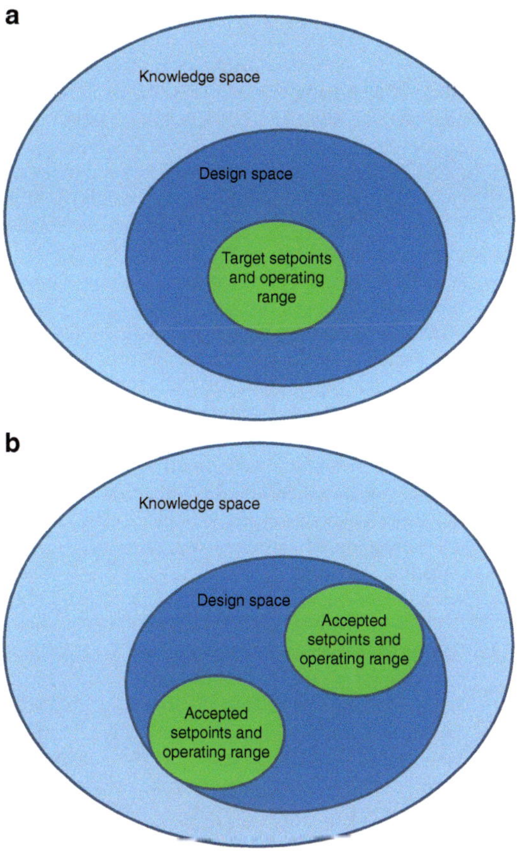

Fig. 6.2 (**a**) The QbD spaces. (**b**) Accepted set points and operating ranges within the QdB spaces

Conclusion

All in all, GMP is here to stay. It started as a reactive process to the inconsistencies in drugs and the manufacture thereof but is slowly and steadily changing towards being a proactive approach for the manufacturing of drugs. Globalisation pushes the different regions and countries to harmonise their regulations for medicinal products, and radiopharmaceuticals are becoming recognised as a special breed of drugs. In the near future, it may become easier to gain approval for the use of PET radiopharmaceuticals in humans as the special status of radiopharmaceuticals is recognised.

References

1. Council of the European Economic Community. Directive 65/65/EEC of 26 Jan 1965 on the approximation of provisions laid down by law, regulation or administrative action relating to medicinal products. OJ L No 22, 9 Feb 1965, p. 369–73.
2. Council of the European Communities. Directive 87/22/EEC of 22 December 1986 on the approximation of national measures relating to the placing on the market of high-technology medicinal products, particularly those derived from biotechnology. OJ L 015, 17 Jan 1987, p. 38–41.
3. Council of the European Communities. Directive 89/343/EEC of 3 May 1989 extending the scope of Directives 65/65/EEC and 75/319/EEC and laying down additional provisions for radiopharmaceuticals (89/343/EEC). OJ L142, 25 May 1989, p. 16.
4. Fallais CJ, Sivewright S, Ogle JR. The radiopharmaceutical industry and European Union regulations. Eur J Nucl Med. 1997;24:77–9.
5. European Parliament and the Council of the European Union. Directive 2001/83/EC of 6 November 2001 on the community code relating to medicinal products for human use. OJ L 311, 28 Nov 2001. p. 67–128.
6. Decristoforo C. Regulation of radiopharmacy practice in Europe. In: Theobald T, editor. Sampson's textbook of radiopharmacy. 4th ed. London: The Pharmaceutical Press; 2011. p. 483–93.
7. Lange R, Ter Heine R, Decristoforo C, Peñuelas I, Elsinga PH, van der Westerlaken MM, Hendrikse NH. Untangling the web of European regulations for the preparation of unlicensed radiopharmaceuticals: a concise overview and practical guidance for a risk-based approach. Nucl Med Commun. 2015;36:414–22.
8. European Parliament and the Council of the European Union. Regulation (EU) no 536/2014 of 16 April 2014 on clinical trials on medicinal products for human use, and repealing Directive 2001/20/EC. OJ, 27 May 2014, L 158/1.
9. Decristoforo C, Penuelas I, Elsinga P, Ballinger J, Winhorst AD, Verbruggen A, Verzijlbergen F, Chiti A. Radiopharmaceuticals are special, but is this recognized? The possible impact of the new Clinical Trials Regulation on the preparation of radiopharmaceuticals. Eur J Nucl Med Mol Imaging. 2014;41:2005–7.
10. Pharmaceutical Inspection Convention. PIC/S guide to good practices for the preparation of medicinal products in healthcare establishments. PE 010-4. 1 Mar 2014.
11. European Commission. Eudralex – Vol 10. Clinical trials guidelines. http://ec.europa.eu/health/documents/eudralex/vol-10/index_en.htm.

12. International conference on harmonisation of technical requirements for registration of pharmaceuticals for human use. Guidance on nonclinical safety studies for the conduct of human clinical trials and marketing authorisation for pharmaceuticals. ICH M3(R2). 17 Jul 2008. http://www.ich.org/fileadmin/Public_Web_Site/ICH_Products/Guidelines/Multidisciplinary/M3_R2/Step4/M3_R2__Guideline.pdf.
13. International conference on harmonisation of technical requirements for registration of pharmaceuticals for human use. Validation of analytical procedures: text and methodology. ICH Q2(R1). Nov 2005. http://www.ich.org/fileadmin/Public_Web_Site/ICH_Products/Guidelines/Quality/Q2_R1/Step4/Q2_R1__Guideline.pdf.
14. Koba W, Jelicks LA, Fine EJ. MicroPET/SPECT/CT imaging of small animal models of disease. Am J Pathol. 2013;182:319–24.
15. Franc BL, Acton PD, Mari C, Hasegawa BH. Small-animal SPECT and SPECT/CT: important tools for preclinical investigation. J Nucl Med. 2008;49:1651–63.
16. European Medicines Agency. Questions and answers on the "Guideline on the limits of genotoxic impurities". EMA/CHMP/SWP/431994/2007 Rev. 3. 23 Sep 2010. http://www.ema.europa.eu/docs/en_GB/document_library/Scientific_guideline/2009/09/WC500002907.pdf.
17. International conference on harmonisation of technical requirements for registration of pharmaceuticals for human use. Assessment and control of DNA reactive (mutagenic) impurities in pharmaceuticals to limit carcinogenic risk. ICH M7. 23 Jun 2014. http://www.ich.org/fileadmin/Public_Web_Site/ICH_Products/Guidelines/Multidisciplinary/M7/M7_Step_4.pdf.
18. Food and drugs administration. Guidance for industry, investigators and reviewers: exploratory IND studies. Jan 2006. http://www.fda.gov/downloads/drugs/guidancecomplianceregulatoryinformation/guidances/ucm078933.pdf.
19. Verbruggen A, Coenen HH, Deverre JR, Guilloteau D, Langstrom B, Salvadori PA, Halldin C. Guideline to regulations for radiopharmaceuticals in early phase clinical trials in the EU. Eur J Nucl Med Mol Imaging. 2008;35:2144–51.
20. Salvadori PA. Radiopharmaceuticals, drug development and pharmaceutical regulations in Europe. Curr Radiopharm. 2008;1:7–11.
21. Fleming IN, Whelan M, Baxendale R, Gilbert FJ, Matthews PP, Aigbirhio FI. Positron emission tomography radiopharmaceutical studies in humans: a guide to regulations for academic researchers. Nucl Med Commun. 2012;33:899–906.
22. European Medicines Agency. ICH guideline M3(R2) on non-clinical safety studies for the conduct of human clinical trials and marketing authorisation for pharmaceuticals. EMA/CPMP/ICH/286/1995. Dec 2009. http://www.ema.europa.eu/docs/en_GB/document_library/Scientific_guideline/2009/09/WC500002720.pdf.
23. Wagner CC, Langer O. Approaches using molecular imaging technology – use of PET in clinical microdose studies. Adv Drug Deliv Rev. 2011;63:539–46.
24. Todde S, Windhorst AD, Behe M, Bormans G, Decristoforo C, Faivre-Chauvet A, Ferrari V, Gee AD, Gulyas B, Halldin C, Peitl PK, Koziorowski J, Mindt TL, Sollini M, Vercouillie J, Ballinger JR, Elsinga PH. EANM guideline for the preparation of an Investigational Medicinal Product Dossier (IMPD). Eur J Nucl Med Mol Imaging. 2014;41:2175–85.
25. International conference on harmonisation of technical requirements for registration of pharmaceuticals for human use. Organisation of the common technical document for the registration of pharmaceuticals for human use. ICH M4(R3). 13 Jan 2004. http://www.ich.org/fileadmin/Public_Web_Site/ICH_Products/CTD/M4_R3_Organisation/M4_R3__organisation.pdf.
26. European Medicines Agency. Implementation plan of the summary of product characteristics (SmPC) guideline. EMA/655980/2008. 19 Feb 2009. http://www.ema.europa.eu/docs/en_GB/document_library/Other/2013/01/WC500137101.pdf.
27. European Commission. Eudralex – Vol 4. Good manufacturing practice (GMP) guidelines. http://ec.europa.eu/health/documents/eudralex/vol-4/index_en.htm.
28. European Commission. Eudralex – Vol 4. Annex 3. Manufacture of radiopharmaceuticals. 1 Mar 2009. http://ec.europa.eu/health/files/eudralex/vol-4/2008_09_annex3_en.pdf.
29. European Commission. Eudralex – Vol 4. Annex 13. Manufacture of investigational medicinal products. 31 Jul 2010. http://ec.europa.eu/health/files/eudralex/vol-4/2009_06_annex13.pdf.
30. European Commission. Eudralex – Vol 4. Chapter 1. Pharmaceutical quality system. 31 Jan 2013. http://ec.europa.eu/health/files/eudralex/vol-4/vol4-chap1_2013-01_en.pdf.
31. Aerts J, Ballinger JR, Behe M, Decristoforo C, Elsinga PH, Faivre-Chauvet A, Mindt TL, Kolenc Peitl P, Todde SC, Koziorowski J. Guidance on current good radiopharmacy practice for the small-scale preparation of radiopharmaceuticals using automated modules: a European perspective. J Label Compd Radiopharm. 2014;57:615–20.
32. Elsinga P, Todde S, Penuelas I, Meyer G, Farstad B, Faivre-Chauvet A, Mikolajczak R, Westera G, Gmeiner-Stopar T, Decristoforo C, Radiopharmacy Committee of the EANM. Guidance on current good radiopharmacy practice (cGRPP) for the small-scale preparation of radiopharmaceuticals. Eur J Nucl Med Mol Imaging. 2010;37:1049–62.
33. Hartmann M. Impact assessment of the European Clinical Trials Directive: a longitudinal, prospective, observational study analyzing patterns and trends in clinical drug trial applications submitted since 2001 to regulatory agencies in six EU countries. Trials. 2012;13:53.

34. International conference on harmonisation of technical requirements for registration of pharmaceuticals for human use. Quality risk management. ICH Q9. 9 Nov 2005. http://www.ich.org/fileadmin/Public_Web_Site/ICH_Products/Guidelines/Quality/Q9/Step4/Q9_Guideline.pdf.

35. International conference on harmonisation of technical requirements for registration of pharmaceuticals for human use. Pharmaceutical development. ICH Q8(R2). Aug 2009. http://www.ich.org/fileadmin/Public_Web_Site/ICH_Products/Guidelines/Quality/Q8_R1/Step4/Q8_R2_Guideline.pdf.

Regulatory Aspects of PET Radiopharmaceutical Production in the United States

7

Joseph C. Hung

Contents

7.1	**Introduction**	146
7.2	**PET Drug**	147
7.2.1	Is PET Drug for Imaging or Therapy or Both?	147
7.2.2	Definition of PET Drug	147
7.2.3	PET Drug Versus PET Drug Product	147
7.2.4	Compounded and Noncompounded PET Drugs	147
7.2.5	PET Drug Production Versus Practice of Pharmacy	148
7.3	**CGMP for PET Drugs**	148
7.3.1	Unique Aspects of PET Drug Production	148
7.3.2	Part 212 Versus Parts 210 and 211	149
7.3.3	Application of Part 212	149
7.3.4	QA and QC	150
7.3.5	Personnel and Resources	150
7.3.6	QA	151
7.3.7	Facilities and Equipment	151
7.3.8	Control of Components, Containers, and Closures	152
7.3.9	Production and Process Controls	153
7.3.10	Laboratory Controls	154
7.3.11	Finished Drug Product Controls and Acceptance Criteria	155
7.3.12	Packaging and Labeling	158
7.3.13	Distribution	158
7.3.14	Complaint Handling	159
7.3.15	Records	159
7.4	**USP <823>**	159
7.4.1	Flexibility in USP 32nd <823>	159
7.4.2	More Flexibility in Part 212 and the Guidance	160
7.4.3	Revised USP <823>	161
7.5	**Inspection on the PET Drug Production Facility**	166
7.5.1	Types of FDA Inspections	166
7.5.2	Selection of Inspection Coverage	167
7.5.3	Major Issues Identified in 2013/2014 PET Drug Inspections	167
	References	169

J.C. Hung, PhD, BCNP, FASHP, FAPhA
Department of Radiology, Mayo Clinic,
200 First Street SW, Rochester,
MN 55905-0001, USA
e-mail: jhung@mayo.edu

Abstract

The Food and Drug Administration (FDA) Modernization Act (the Modernization Act) of 1997 directed FDA to establish current good manufacturing practice (CGMP) requirements for positron emission tomography (PET) drugs. As directed by the US Congress in the Modernization Act, the costly CGMP regulations which the FDA applies to large pharmaceutical manufacturers are not appropriate for the PET drugs due to the unique properties of these drugs mainly the short half-lives. In consideration of the unique nature of PET drugs and PET drug production, FDA instituted specific CGMP requirements in 21 Code of Federal Regulations

M.M. Khalil (ed.), *Basic Science of PET Imaging*, DOI 10.1007/978-3-319-40070-9_7

(CFR) part 212. Sections 1 and 2 of this book chapter illustrate the significant different aspects and the rationales for such differences between part 212 and parts 210/211 which are the CGMP requirements for non-PET drugs. The PET drug CGMP regulation found in part 212 also provides a more flexible regulatory framework for investigational PET drugs for human use produced under an investigational new drug application (IND) in accordance with part 312 and PET drugs produced with the approval of a Radioactive Drug Research Committee (RDRC) in accordance with part 361. The PET CGMP requirements for these PET drugs can be met either by compliance with part 212 or by producing such drugs in accordance with the 32nd edition of the United States Pharmacopeia (USP) General Chapter <823>, "Radiopharmaceuticals for Positron Emission Tomography – Compounding," which was published in 2009. In 2012, USP revised and renamed this General Chapter <823>, "Positron Emission Tomography Drugs for Compounding, Investigational, and Research Uses." FDA is currently considering whether to amend the PET CGMP regulations to incorporate this revised chapter into part 212. Section 4 describes format/content of the revised USP General Chapter <823> which is very much in line with part 212 and offers more flexible requirements than the <823> in 32nd USP.

FDA expects to perform a CGMP surveillance inspection of each PET facility once every 2 years on average, but may visit some sites more than once every 2 years when warranted, such as when the site is named in an application for a new type of PET drug product or has undergone substantial change. As part of the drug approval process, a preapproval inspection (PAI) will be performed by the FDA inspector(s) to provide assurance that a PET drug production facility that is named in a drug application is capable of producing the PET drug in accordance with CGMPs and that the submitted application data are reliable, accurate, and complete. Section 5 summarizes the major deficiencies identified by the FDA inspectors during their 2013 and 2014 inspection programs at various PET drug production facilities in the United States.

7.1 Introduction

Positron emission tomography (PET) radiopharmaceuticals are unique among radiopharmaceuticals because of their short half-lives. There are four positron-emitting radioisotopes that are considered the biologic tracers, carbon-11, nitrogen-13, oxygen-15, and fluorine-18. ^{11}C ($t_{½}$=20.4 min), ^{15}O ($t_{½}$=2.1 min), and ^{13}N ($t_{½}$=10 min) are referred to as the essentials of life. They can be easily substituted directly into biomolecules without changing the properties of the molecule. ^{18}F ($t_{½}$=110 min) is not a normal constituent of biological molecules but can often be substituted for a hydroxyl group as in the case of deoxyglucose or can be substituted for a hydrogen atom in a molecule or placed in a position where its presence does not significantly alter the biological behavior of the molecule. Fluorodeoxyglucose (^{18}FDG) is currently the most widely used PET radiopharmaceutical in clinical oncology in addition to its clinical applications in cardiology and neurology. ^{18}FDG is one of the important factors for the wide acceptance of PET imaging in clinical practice. The application of PET in clinical oncology is increasing since many molecular targets relevant to cancer can be labeled with positron emitter radionuclides.

The concept of PET and the design and construction of PET scanners were initiated in the United States back in the late 1950 [1–3]. However, the benefits of PET imaging were not widely available to American patients for many years due to "lack of reimbursement and inappropriate and costly regulations promulgated by FDA" [4]. The same current good manufacturing practice (CGMP) requirements that FDA typically applies to large drug manufacturers were also placed on the production of PET radiopharmaceuticals without taking into consideration the special properties of these drugs (e.g., short half-lives). In order to make PET imaging technology more accessible to the US patients at reasonable cost, the US Congress establishes a new regulatory framework for PET drugs within the Food and Drug Administration Modernization Act of 1997 (FDAMA) which was signed by President Bill Clinton on November 21, 1997 [5].

Specifically, section 121(c)(1)(A) of 1997 FDAMA directed FDA to establish CGMP requirements for PET drugs [5]. In the Federal Register (FR) of September 20, 2005 (i.e., 70 FR 55038), FDA published a proposed rule to establish CGMP requirement for PET drugs [6]. On December 10, 2009, FDA issued a final rule in 74 FR 65409 [7] and an accompanying guidance document to establish specifically "tailored" CGMP requirements for PET drugs [8].

These requirements are codified in the Title 21 of the Code of Federal Registrations (CFR) part 212 (part 212) [7]. The deadline for this regulation to become effective was originally set on December 12, 2011 [7]. Two years later, with the deadline looming, FDA received numerous requests for extending the submission deadline. FDA was concerned about preventing access to the PET drugs, and therefore this deadline was extended by the FDA to June 12, 2012 [9].

7.2 PET Drug

7.2.1 Is PET Drug for Imaging or Therapy or Both?

"PET drug" as defined in part 212 is "a radioactive drug that exhibits spontaneous disintegration of unstable nuclei by the emission of positrons and is used for providing dual photon positron emission tomographic *diagnostic* images" (emphasis added) [10]. Under section 121(a) of the FDAMA (codified as section 201(ii)(1)(A) of the Food, Drug, and Cosmetic Act [FD&C]) [5, 11], a compounded PET drug is defined as a drug that "exhibits spontaneous disintegration of unstable nuclei by the emission of positrons and is used for the purpose of providing dual photon emission tomographic *diagnostic* image" (emphasis added). The word "diagnostic" in each of these two definitions appears to indicate that part 212 [10] and the provisions of the FDAMA concerning PET drugs [5] do not apply to PET drugs used for therapeutic purposes.

7.2.2 Definition of PET Drug

The definition of PET drug as stated in part 212 specifically includes any nonradioactive reagent, reagent kit, ingredient, nuclide generator, accelerator, target material, electronic synthesizer, or other apparatus or computer program to be used in the preparation of a PET drug [10]. Once again, this definition closely parallels the definition of PET drug in section 121(a) of the FDAMA [5].

It seems that the inclusion of these "ancillary" components and equipment (e.g., nuclide generator, accelerator, electronic synthesizer, etc.) is overly broad and not appropriate within the practical and technical definition of a drug. However, since these items were included in definition of "compounded PET drug" as stated in the section 121 (a) of the FDAMA [5], FDA felt that the definition of "PET drug" in the final rule should include these items as well [7]. Thus, these "ancillary" items are also subject to the same CGMP requirements for PET drugs as stipulated in part 212 [10].

7.2.3 PET Drug Versus PET Drug Product

Part 212 defines "PET drug product" as a finished dosage form of a PET drug, and it is included in the FDA definition for "PET drug" [10]. As such, the CGMP requirements for PET drugs do apply to PET drugs, as well as PET drug products.

7.2.4 Compounded and Noncompounded PET Drugs

The FDAMA does not have separate regulations for compounded PET drugs and noncompounded PET drugs [5]. In fact, section 121(b) of the

FDAMA states that 4 years after the date of enactment of the FDAMA or 2 years after the FDA establishes approval procedures and CGMP requirements for PET drugs, whichever is longer, the CGMP requirements established by the FDA for PET drugs will apply to compounded or non-compounded PET drugs [5]. In other words, once the aforementioned condition is met, all PET drugs (including compounded PET drugs) would be subject to PET drug CGMP requirements.

During either of these two time frames, section 121(b) of the FDAMA indicated that a compounded PET drug was not adulterated if it was compounded, processed, packed, or held in conformity with the PET compounding standards and official monographs of the United States Pharmacopeia (USP) [5].

7.2.5 PET Drug Production Versus Practice of Pharmacy

Although part 212 defines "production" of a PET drug as the manufacturing, compounding, processing, packaging, labeling, reprocessing, repacking, relabeling, and testing of a PET drug [10], FDA has traditionally deferred the dispensing of a patient-specific dose and the use of the drug product to state and local authorities. As such, these postproduction activities are regarded by the FDA as the practice of medicine and pharmacy. Consequently, a guidance – a version marked on the front cover with *Small Entity Compliance Guide* – issued by the FDA in 2011(Guidance) stated that production includes all operations only to the point of final release of a finished dosage form [12]. In general, a routine FDA inspection to ensure compliance with CGMP would focus on activities up to and including the point of final release of a PET drug product [12].

7.3 CGMP for PET Drugs

CGMP is a minimum standard that ensures that a drug meets the requirements of safety, as well as it has the identity, strength (or potency), quality, and purity characteristics as it is represented to possess. CGMP is demonstrated through written documentation of procedures and practices.

After visiting several PET drug production sites, FDA concluded that a PET drug producer's status as either a not-for-profit or for-profit entity does not and should not have any significant bearing on the safety, identity, strength, quality, and purity of PET drugs that it produces and distributes for administration to patients. The same conclusion goes to the methods, facilities, and controls that a PET drug production facility needs to ensure product's safety, identity, strength, quality, and purity. Instead, FDA believes production, and CGMP differences among PET drug producers are primarily a function of the size, scope, and complexity of their production operations.

Consequently, FDA approach to the CGMP regulation for PET drugs has been shaped largely by the statutory and the imperatives of product's safety, identity, strength, quality, and purity, rather than commercialization or reimbursement concerns. In fact, FDA found that implementing certain production standards and controls could further ensure the production of suitable PET drugs, regardless of differences among the various PET drug production facilities. FDA believes that the welfare of a patient undergoing a PET scan should not depend on where a particular PET drug was produced.

7.3.1 Unique Aspects of PET Drug Production

PET drug manufacturing procedures differ in a number of important ways from those associated with the manufacture of conventional drug products, mainly due to the short half-lives of PET radioisotopes. These unique aspects are as follows:

- Because of the short physical half-lives of PET radioisotopes, prolonged manufacturing time significantly would erode the useful clinical life of PET drugs. Likewise, the produced PET drug product is administered to the patient usually within a matter of hours. Due to a relatively small number of patients per day, PET drug production facilities generally manufacture the products in response to daily demand. Thus, a maximum of only a few lots are manufactured per day, with one lot equaling one multiple-dose vial.

- Because one lot equals one multiple-dose vial containing a homogeneous solution of a PET drug product, results from end product testing of samples drawn from the single vial have the maximum possible probability of being representative of all the doses administered to patients from that vial. This special characteristic of the produced PET drug prevents sampling or testing error.
- An entire lot may be administered to one or several patients, depending upon the radioactivity remaining in the container at the time of administration. Consequently, the administration of the entire quantity of a lot to a single patient should be anticipated for every lot manufactured. This is an important consideration when establishing the testing limits for certain attributes such as endotoxins and impurities.
- PET drugs usually do not enter a general drug distribution chain. Rather, the entire lot (one vial) is usually distributed directly from the PET drug production facility either to a single medical department or physician for administration to patients or to a nuclear pharmacy for dispensing. Distribution may occur to other PET centers when the geographic proximity will allow for distribution and use within the PET drug product's half-life parameters.
- The quantities of radioactive active ingredients contained in each lot of a PET drug generally vary from nanogram to milligram amounts, depending upon various product parameters.

7.3.2 Part 212 Versus Parts 210 and 211

In consideration of these unique natures of PET drugs and PET drug production, FDA recognized that application of certain provisions of the CGMP regulations in parts 210 and 211 [13, 14] to the manufacture of PET drugs might result in unsafe handling or be otherwise inappropriate [7]. Thus, part 212 differs in many significant ways from the CGMP requirements for non-PET drugs found in the regulations of parts 210 and 211[12–14].

Included among these differences are the following (to be described in more details later):

- Fewer required personnel with fewer organizational restrictions consistent with the scope and complexity of operations
- Allowance for multiple operations (or storages) in the same area as long as organization and other controls are adequate
- Streamlined requirements for aseptic processing consistent with the nature of the production process
- Streamlined quality assurance (QA) requirements for components
- Self-verification of significant steps in PET drug production consistent with the scope and complexity of operations
- Same-person oversight of production, review of batch production and control records (please refer to the section titled "Production and Process Controls" for the distinction between master production and control record and batch production and control record), and authorization of product release consistent with the scope and complexity of operations
- Greater flexibility in approaches to determining whether PET drug products conform to their specifications
- Specialized QA requirements for PET drugs produced in multiple sub-batches (sub-batch means a quantity of PET drug having uniform character and quality, within specified limits, that is produced during one succession of multiple irradiations, using a given synthesis and/or purification operation) [10]
- Simplified labeling requirements consistent with the scope and complexity of operations

7.3.3 Application of Part 212

The regulations in part 212 apply only to the production, quality control (QC), holding, and distribution of PET drugs [10]; human drugs that do not meet the definition of a PET drug must be manufactured in accordance with the CGMP requirements in parts 210 and 211 [13, 14]. Part 212 regulations are designated to be sufficiently flexible to accommodate the unique aspects of PET drugs [10].

However, section 212.5(b) also gives producers of PET drugs under the review of an investigational new drug application (IND) or under a Radioactive Drug Research Committee (RDRC) the option of following the CGMP regulations in part 212 *or* producing PET drugs in accordance with General Chapter <823> (USP <823>) of the 32nd edition of the USP *Radiopharmaceuticals for Positron Emission Tomography – Compounding* [10, 15].

Originally developed in 1990, USP <823> sets forth requirements for PET drug production, including control of components, materials, and supplies, verification of procedures, stability testing and expiration dating, QC, and sterilization and sterility assurance [15]. The 1997 FDAMA stipulates that a compounded PET drug is adulterated unless it is produced in conformity with the USP compounding standards (including USP <823>) and official monographs for PET drugs [5].

The main reason that the FDA allows USP <823> to constitute CGMP standards for IND and RDRC PET drugs is to "allow more flexibility during the development of these drugs" [12]. Although the provisions in USP <823> [15] are generally less specific and explicit than the requirements in part 212 [10], FDA believes that provisions in USP <823> are "adequate to ensure that investigational and research PET drugs are produced safely under appropriate conditions" and are "appropriate CGMP requirements for the investigational and research stage of development" [12]. FDA also recognizes that the majority of these investigational and research PET drugs do not have commercial potential [12], and, therefore, it is not necessary to subject these drugs under the stipulations of part 212, which is more geared to approved or to-be-approved PET drugs [10].

Better compliance outcome is another reason that FDA permits producers of IND and RDRC PET drugs to choose USP <823> as an alternative standard for meeting CGMP requirements [12]. FDA stated that because "most PET drug producers are very familiar with the requirements in Chapter <823>, allowing producers to meet the CGMP requirements for investigational and research PET drugs by following Chapter <823> should greatly facilitate producers' compliance with the CGMP requirements" [12].

Nevertheless, once a PET drug producer intends to seek marketing approval for a PET drug or a new indication, the production of the PET drug to be used in phase 3 study should be conducted in accordance with the CGMP requirements for PET drugs as stipulated in part 212 which is mainly designated as CGMP requirements for *approved* PET drugs [8].

7.3.4 QA and QC

On the initiative taken by the FDA, the term "quality control" was replaced with "quality assurance" [8]. Nevertheless, the term "quality control" still appears in the definition of the term "batch production and control record" [10]. The Guidance lists the term "quality control" in the document seven times [12]. Please refer to the section titled "Revised USP <823>" for the definitions of "quality control" and "quality assurance."

7.3.5 Personnel and Resources

Section 212.10 requires a PET drug production facility to have a sufficient number of personnel with the necessary education, background, training, and experience to enable them to perform their assigned functions correctly [10]. Each site also must provide adequate resources, including equipment and facilities, to enable their personnel to perform their functions. This section only addresses personnel issues whereas the resources aspects (facilities and equipment) are discussed in section titled "Facilities and Equipment."

A small PET drug production operation is not properly characterized in part 212 [10]; however, it is stated in the Guidance as one that produces only one or two batches each day (or week) of a single PET drug [12]. As such, it may be adequate to employ only a few employees (typically at least two persons) to accomplish all production and QA functions. The Guidance further elaborates that one individual can be designated to perform the production as well as QA functions, provided this person is highly qualified in the performance of all such functions [12]. Self-checks in such a PET drug production facility are also permissible as indicated in the Guidance [12]. This is not allowed under current part 211 in which second-person checks are required at various stages of productions as well as test verification [15].

7.3.6 QA

Section 212.20 requires PET drug production facilities to establish and follow written QA procedures for production operations, materials, specifications and processes, and production records to ensure drug.

The Guidance recommends each PET drug production facility to establish a QA function which consists of execution and oversight activities related to QA requirements [12]. It further suggests the following activities to be handled by the execution and oversight of QA function, respectively [12]:

Execution activities of QA function include the following:

- Examine and evaluate each lot of incoming material before use to ensure that the material meets its established specifications.
- Review the production batch records and laboratory control records for accuracy, completeness, and conformance to established specifications before authorizing the final release or rejection of a batch or lot of a PET drug.
- Ensure that deviations from normal procedures are documented and justified.

Oversight activities of QA functions include the following:

- Approve procedures, specifications, process, and methods.
- Ensure that personnel are properly trained and qualified, as appropriate.
- Ensure that PET drugs have adequately defined identity, strength, quality, and purity.
- Ensure that all errors are reviewed. When it is determined that an investigation is appropriate, document the investigation and take corrective action(s) to prevent the recurrence of the errors.
- Conduct periodic audits to monitor compliance with established procedures and practices.

For PET drug production facilities currently producing one or two PET drugs, the Guidance indicates that employees located at the facility can perform both the daily execution and oversight functions [12]. On the other hand, a PET drug production organization managing multiple production facilities may designate the oversight duties to an internal QA department or an outside consultant to achieve a more objective and efficient management [12].

7.3.7 Facilities and Equipment

7.3.7.1 Facilities

Section 212.30(a) requires a PET drug production facility to have adequate facilities to ensure the orderly handling of materials and equipment, the prevention of mix-ups, and the prevention of contamination of equipment or product by substances, personnel, or environmental conditions that could reasonably be expected to have an adverse effect on product quality [10].

For the potential sources of contamination, the Guidance points out that they include particulate matter, chemical, and microbiological materials [12]. The general principles for preventing mix-ups as suggested by the Guidance are equipment to be appropriately located, work areas to be organized and proximally located, components to be properly labeled and kept separate according to the classifications (i.e., quarantined, approved, or rejected), and access these aforementioned items to be restricted to authorized personnel [12].

Section titled "Facility Design and Environmental Control" in USP General Chapter

<797> *Pharmaceutical Compounding – Sterile Preparations* is a good reference for a proper setup of an aseptic processing area [16]. Some precautions suggested by the Guidance should be followed to help maintain the appropriate air quality of the aseptic workstation [12]:

- Sanitize the aseptic workstation before each operation.
- Keep items within a laminar airflow aseptic workstation to a minimum and do not interrupt the airflow.
- Have operators wear clean lab coats and sanitized gloves when conducting an aseptic manipulation within the aseptic workstation.
- Frequently sanitize gloved hands or frequently change gloves when working in the aseptic workstation. Examine gloves for damage (tears or holes) and replace them if they are damaged.
- Sanitize the surface of non-sterile items (e.g., test tube rack, the overwrap for sterile syringes, filters) and wipe with an appropriate disinfectant (e.g., sterile 70% isopropyl alcohol) before placing them in the aseptic workstation.

7.3.7.2 Equipment

Section 212.30(b) requires the implementation of procedures to ensure that all equipment that would reasonably be expected to adversely affect the identity, strength, quality, or purity of a PET drug, or give erroneous or invalid test results when improperly used or maintained, is clean, suitable for its intended purposes, properly installed, maintained, and capable of repeatedly producing valid results [12]. Activities in accordance with these procedures must be documented [12]. Section 212.30(c) stipulates the equipment to be constructed and maintained so that surfaces that contact components, in-process materials, or drug products are not reactive, additive, or absorptive so as to alter the quality of the PET drug [10].

For any newly installed equipment, the Guidance recommends a three-step process – installation qualification (IQ), operational qualification (OQ), and performance qualification (PQ) – to qualify the new equipment before its first use in order to ensure it was installed correctly, was operated adequately, and is capable of producing the anticipated results [12].

Normally, the equipment vendor verifies that the equipment is installed correctly (IQ) and operates according to specifications, OQ. Before the equipment is used for production, personnel in the PET drug production facility should verify that the equipment, when operated under actual production parameters or selected method, produces consistent results within established specifications – PQ [12].

Representative equipment is discussed in the Guidance to illustrate how it should be controlled [12]. Some examples are listed below:

- The provisions contained in the USP General Chapter <1015> *Automated Radiochemical Synthesis Apparatus* can help ensure proper functioning of a synthesis apparatus [17].
- Microbiological monitoring (e.g., using settle plate) in the aseptic workstation should be conducted during sterility testing and critical aseptic manipulation.
- In order to make sure that a gas chromatograph (GC) or a high-performance liquid chromatograph (HPLC) system is functioning correctly, a suitability testing should be conducted. At least one injection of the standard preparation (reference standard or internal standard) should be done before the injection of test samples into a GC or HPLC system.

7.3.8 Control of Components, Containers, and Closures

Section 212.40(a) and (b) requires PET drug production facilities to establish, maintain, and follow written procedures for the control (i.e., receipt, log-in, identification, storage, handling, testing, and acceptance and/or rejection) of components, containers, and closures. Appropriate written specifications for the components, containers, and closures must be established [10]. Section 212.40(c) establishes the minimum standards for controlling components, containers, and closures from receipt to consumption [10]. Any incoming lot must be appropriately designated as quarantined, accepted, or rejected. One must use a reliable supplier for each component, container, and closure [10]. Section 212.40(d) requires that components, containers, and closures be handled and stored in a manner that prevents contamination, mix-ups, and deterioration [10]. Section 212.40(e) requires that PET drug production facilities keep a record of each shipment of each lot of components, containers, and closures that they receive [10].

The Guidance defines "reliable vendor" as "qualified vendors," and a vendor is qualified when there is evidence to support its ability to supply a material that consistently meets all quality specifications [12]. It is preferable as suggested by the Guidance to have more than one qualified vendor for a component [12].

For acceptance testing, the specific identity test is only required if the finished-product testing does not ensure that the correct components have been used or if an inactive ingredient (e.g., 0.9 % sodium chloride solution) was prepared on site from a component that is not subject to finished-product testing [10, 12]. Otherwise, examination of a certificate of analysis (COA) provided by the supplier should be sufficient [10].

7.3.9 Production and Process Controls

Section 212.50 requires adequate production and process controls to ensure consistent production of a PET drug that meets the applicable standards for identity, strength, quality, and purity [10].

7.3.9.1 Master Production and Control Record and Batch Production and Control Record

Section 212.50(b) requires PET drug production facilities to have master production and control records that document all steps in the PET drug production process [10]. Master production and control record (or master record) is a principal document that describes how a drug product is made. It is used to derive an individual batch record (i.e., batch production and control record) and specifies how each batch is to be produced. Since the master record is a compilation of detailed step-by-step instructions, it has been suggested, during the comment period for the final rule, to change the term "control record" to "control procedure" [7]. However, FDA did not accept it because "control record" is a standard term used in the production of drugs [7].

Section 212.50(c) requires that a batch production and control record (i.e., batch record) be created for each new batch of a PET drug [10]. The batch record provides complete traceability and accountability for production and control of each batch of drug product.

7.3.9.2 Radiochemical Yield Limit

Section 212.50(b)(1) through (b)(6) listed certain items of information that would be required in a master record [10]. One of these required information, as described in section 212.50(b)(6), is a statement of acceptance criteria on radiochemical yield [10]. In the 2005 proposed rule, section 212.50(b)(6) described this statement as *acceptance criteria* on radiochemical yield (i.e., the minimum percentage of yield beyond which investigation and corrective action are required) (emphasis added) [7].

During the comment period of the 2005 proposed rule, one comment suggested the deletion of this requirement [7]. The comment indicated that radiochemical yields could have significant variations even in a well-controlled PET manufacturing operation and that many factors could affect the yield [7]. The comment maintained that radiochemical yield is not a significant predictor of product quality [7]. According to the comment, discarding useful quality product and having to produce another lot based on arbitrary radiochemical yield increase radiation exposure [7].

FDA's response to this comment was that although a low radiochemical yield would not necessarily require the rejection of a batch, low radiochemical yield can be a useful predictor of control of the production process for a PET drug [7]. FDA further articulated that a low radiochemical yield might result from a leak in the production system that introduces an extraneous substance, resulting in a contaminated product that might not be easily purified [7].

As such, FDA concluded that repeated occurrences of low radiochemical yield or a downward trend in radiochemical yield should prompt an investigation and, if necessary, corrective action [7]. Nevertheless, FDA did revise section 212.50(b)(6) to require a statement of *action limits*, rather than *acceptance criteria*, on radiochemical yield, because not meeting the radiochemical yield limits would require investigation and corrective action but not necessarily rejection of the batch [10]. This is one good example to illustrate the openness and willingness of FDA to work with the PET community during the establishment of PET drug CGMP regulations.

Another example – one comment suggested that it is not necessary to record date and time of each production step. The comment maintained that recording the date once is sufficient since the majority of PET drug productions only take a few hours at most. The comment also recommended that recording the time be limited to critical steps due to the importance of these processes [7]. Although FDA did not accept their suggestion for the removal of date-recording requirement, FDA adopted their recommendation of recording time for each critical production step (e.g., start of irradiation, beginning and end of synthesis) [7, 10].

7.3.9.3 Process Verification

Section 212.50(f)(2) requires that when the results of the production of an entire batch of a PET drug are not fully verified through finished-product testing or when only the initial sub-batch in a series is tested, the PET drug producer must demonstrate that the process for producing the PET drug is reproducible and is capable of producing a drug product that meets the predetermined acceptance criteria [10]. If each entire batch of a PET drug undergoes full finished-product testing to ensure that the product meets all specifications, section 212.50(f)(1) indicates that process verification as described in section 212.50(f)(2) is not required [10].

For the process verification under section 212.50(f)(2), the Guidance recommends that if a PET drug production facility has an established history of PET drug production, the process verification can be accomplished using historical batch records, provided that there is adequate accumulated data to support a conclusion that the current process yields batches meeting predetermined acceptance criteria [12].

The Guidance also recommends that new processes or significant changes to existing processes be shown to reliably produce PET drugs meeting the predetermined acceptance criteria before any batches are distributed [12]. This verification should be conducted according to a written protocol and generally include at least three *consecutive* acceptable production runs [12].

Because of the unique characteristics of PET drug production, a PET drug producer may decide to evaluate the reliability of a new process or a significant change to an existing process to produce a PET drug by meeting the predetermined acceptance criteria *concurrently* with the distribution of the batch, provided that this approach is consistent with the product's approved application [12]. Such a decision should be justified in writing, subjected to QA procedures, and performed according to a written protocol [12]. Each batch should be processed in strict adherence to the written procedures, fully tested (except sterility testing), and found to comply with all procedural and quality test requirements prior to final release [12].

For computer control, the Guidance indicates that the operation of the computer program be verified before first use or any subsequent changes or upgrades made to the computer program [12]. PET drug production facilities can rely on a certification by the software or system vendor that the specified software was verified under its operating condition [12].

7.3.10 Laboratory Controls

Section 212.60 requires the establishment and implementation of procedures for testing components, in-process materials, and finished PET drug products [10]. All necessary tests of materials and products must be documented [10]. Each laboratory must have sampling and testing procedures designed to ensure that components, drug product containers and closures, in-process materials, and PET drug products conform to appropriate standards [10]. Analytical methods and test equipment must be suitable for their intended uses [10]. Reagents, solutions, and supplies used in testing procedures must be adequately controlled [10]. The preventive maintenance, calibration, and procedures to make sure that the equipment is functioning properly must be documented [10]. A complete record of all tests related to the production of a PET drug must be kept to ensure compliance with established specifications and standards, including examinations and assays [10].

For reference standards used in analyses, the Guidance states that if a primary reference standard is obtained from an officially recognized source (e.g., USP), acceptance testing of the material is not required [12]. However, if the reference standard is not available from the official source, the identity and purity of the substituted material must be fully confirmed [12].

7.3.10.1 Stability Testing

Section 212.61 requires the establishment of a written stability testing program for each PET drug product [10]. This program must be used to establish suitable storage conditions as well as expiration dates and times [10].

PET drugs have extremely short shelf lives due to their short half-lives; it might seem to be pointless to evaluate and establish the stability of PET drugs. However, the Guidance indicates that stability concerns for PET drugs are well grounded because of radiation-related radiolysis [12]. As such, appropriate stability parameters such as radiochemical identity and purity (including levels of radiochemical impurities), appearance, pH, stabilizer or preservative effectiveness, and chemical purity should be evaluated to establish and document the stability of PET drug products under proposed storage conditions [12].

Stability testing of the PET drug product should be performed at the highest radioactive concentration, and the whole batch volume in the intended container/closure should be stored [12]. At least three production runs of the final product should be studied for a time period equal to the labeled shelf life of the PET drug product [12].

7.3.11 Finished Drug Product Controls and Acceptance Criteria

Section 212.70 requires that specifications be established for each PET drug product batch (or sub-batches) including identity, strength, quality, purity, sterility, and apyrogenicity [10]. Except as conditional final release (section 212.70(f)), section 212.70(c) requires an appropriate laboratory determination be conducted to ensure that each batch (or sub-batches) of a PET drug product conforms to specifications, except for sterility, before final release [10].

However, due to the very short half-life of certain PET drug (e.g., ^{13}N-ammonia), the release of subsequent sub-batches can be qualified if the initial sub-batch meets all acceptance criteria as per the Guidance [12]. This exception is only permissible provided that a sufficient number of sub-batches (beginning, middle, and end) have been demonstrated to produce a product meeting the predetermined acceptance criteria [12]. In certain cases, it may be appropriate to include testing each sub-batch for certain attributes prior to release (e.g., for pH determination in ^{13}N-ammonia production method using Devarda's alloy catalyst) [12].

7.3.11.1 Finished-Product Testing

If finished-product testing alone is used, each batch of PET drug should be tested for conformance to all specifications [10]. Otherwise, the Guidance suggests that the following approaches might be employed to achieve the same objective [12]:

- In-process testing – in-process testing might involve the use of an online test to measure an attribute that is equivalent to finished-product testing, provided that the relevant attribute does not change during the production of the finished product.

- Continuous process monitoring of an attribute with statistical process controls – this process involves comprehensive testing of an attribute using online monitoring and corresponding adjustments to prevent an upward or downward drift in batch-to-batch measurements of the attribute.
- Some combination of these approaches:

Although section 212.70(c) addresses conformance to specifications [10], there might be certain QC attributes for a PET drug product that are not as significant as those included in the specifications [12]. Examples of these *noncritical* QC attributes might include radionuclidic purity (when potentially contaminating radionuclides, do not impact the safety or effectiveness of the drug product), certain low-level nontoxic impurities, and class 3 residual solvents [12, 18].

FDA indicated that a PET drug producer may conduct a periodic quality indicator test (PQIT) on a particular noncritical QC attribute [12]. A PQIT can be performed at predetermined intervals (similar to the skip-testing concept) rather than on a batch-to-batch basis. The selection of noncritical QC attribute(s), as well as the determination of testing frequency, should be set by each PET drug producer to fit within its internal quality system. The PQIT's QC attribute(s), analytical method(s), limit(s), and frequency should be included in an approved application before implementation.

Under section 212.70(d) when it is determined that all acceptance criteria have been met, the PET drug production facility should then provide a notice of final release to the receiving facility so that the dose may be given to the patient [10].

7.3.11.2 Sterility Testing

Section 212.70(e) requires that sterility testing be started within 30 h after the completion of PET drug production; however, the 30 h requirement may be exceeded due to a weekend or holiday [10]. The regulation states that if the sample for sterility testing is held longer than 30 h, the PET drug producer must demonstrate that the longer period does not adversely affect the sample and the test results obtained will be equivalent [10]. Tested samples must be from individual batches and not pooled [10]. If the product fails to meet a criterion for sterility, all facilities that received the product must be *immediately* notified (emphasis added) with the test results [10].

During the public comment period for the 2005 proposed rule, FDA received several comments objected to the proposed requirement to notify receiving facilities immediately if a PET drug product fails the sterility test [6]. The reasons of these comments against the immediate notification include detection of a growth in an inoculated media does not necessarily equate to sterility failure; only confirmed non-sterility rather than technical error should be notified; a sterility test failure might not be known for 2–4 weeks; the observation of any sterility testing failure would occur several days after administration of the drug product and critical data, such as species identification, would not be available; and immediate, unqualified notification would be alarming and unproductive [6].

In FDA response it stated that "[w]e understand that initial results from conventional sterility tests are not definitive, and we appreciate that it takes some time to investigate a failed test. However, we believe that it is important to convey to the clinician the potential risks to a patient when a PET drug product initially fails to meet a criterion for sterility." [7].

The Guidance recommends that the samples should be stored appropriately (e.g., under refrigeration) [12]. Verification of equivalent results can be accomplished by inoculation of a USP indicator organism (e.g., *E. coli*) and should demonstrate that there is little, if any, loss in viability of the inoculated microorganism [12].

7.3.11.3 Conditional Final Release

When one of the required finished-product tests cannot be completed due to a malfunction involving analytical equipment, the product may still be released for human use under the conditions stated in section 212.70(f) [10]. This is another initiative took by the FDA during the establishment of the CGMP requirements for PET drugs [7].

Breakdown Versus Malfunction Initially the 2005 proposed rule limited the conditional final release to a circumstance of a complete *breakdown* of analytical equipment [6]. However, the feedback that FDA received during the public comment period indicated that equipment *malfunction* might be a more appropriate term to depict the circumstance for conditional release [7]. An equipment malfunction might cause atypical test result(s); however, other indicators may show that release of raw materials, production, and purification process events have occurred as expected. For example, a PET drug producer might observe a baseline drift in an HPLC analysis for a product, but if the peak shape is similar to what is normally seen and the production and purification events have progressed as expected, it might be reasonable to conclude that there is an equipment malfunction, rather than that the product is contaminated.

Clearly equipment breakdown as originally mentioned in the 2005 proposed rule [6] might still be an adequate circumstance for meeting the conditional release criteria. In this instance, the term "equipment malfunction" does encompass this situation.

Reserve Sample Under section 212.70(f)(1)(iii)(iv), which was another FDA's initiative, a reserve sample of the conditionally released batch of drug product should be retained [10]. The malfunction of analytical equipment should be promptly corrected, and then the omitted test should be completed using the reserve sample [10].

Public comments that FDA received on this particular subject disagreed with this requirement [7]. They argued that, depending on when analytical equipment is repaired, the PET drug producer might not be able to obtain meaningful data for testing (e.g., radionuclidic identity or purity) because the radioactivity of the radionuclide might be decayed to background level [7]. In the response [7], FDA was in agreement that some critical tests would not able to be performed at a later time (i.e., after correction of an analytical equipment malfunction) because of the short half-life of a product.

However, FDA did not think that radionuclidic identity, of which a dose calibrator is required for testing, would be impacted. If the dose calibrator is not functioning properly, FDA indicated that the dose of the product would not be accurately measured [7]. Even if a dose calibrator is malfunctioning and the activity of a product could not be assayed, a sample of known dilution could still be counted using other equipment, and the activity concentration could be determined by correcting for counting efficiency and dilution [7]. As for radionuclidic purity, FDA believed that it is possible to conduct the test on a decayed sample of the product [7].

Overall, FDA recommended that PET drug producers develop alternate tests for specifications for which they conclude it is not possible to conduct a particular test after an analytical equipment malfunction has been corrected [7].

Notification of an Incomplete Testing or an Out-of-Specification Result Initially the immediate notification was required when the incomplete product testing is noted [6]. Several comments indicated that the personnel at the receiving facility might not be knowledgeable of the conditional final release allowance and lack the expertise to interpret the meaning of such a release in the context of patient safety and product efficacy [7]. The comments stated that the notification in these circumstances would cause uncertainty and undue apprehension, which would not serve the best interest of patients [7]. FDA agreed with these comments and subsequently deleted this requirement from the section 212.70(f)(1) [7, 10].

Nevertheless, section 212.70(f)(1)(iv) requires the PET drug producer to immediately notify the receiving facility *if an out-of-specification (OOS) result is obtained when testing the reserve sample* (emphases added) [10]. Notifying receiving facilities of OOS results so that personnel can take appropriate action, usually to prevent administration of the drug, is consistent with the intent of CGMP to ensure that patients receive appropriate

PET drugs. This differs from the conditional release situation involving notification of incomplete product testing under proposed section 212.70(f)(1)(iii), in which it is still possible that the batch may actually conform to specifications and therefore be appropriate for administration to patients [10].

Radiochemical Identity/Purity and Specific Activity Under section 212.70(f)(2), conditional final release of a PET drug product cannot be permitted if a PET drug producer could not perform a radiochemical identity/purity test on a PET drug product or could not determine the product's specific activity [10]. The determination of the product's specific activity is vital in particular for a PET drug product with mass-dependent target localization and/or potential to elicit a physiological effect, where the specific activity limit is quantitatively expressed.

Releasing of Another Batch Section 212.70(f)(3) stipulates that the PET drug producers may not release another batch of PET drug product until the aforementioned conditions (i.e., correction of the malfunction problem and completion of the omitted test) are met [10].

FDA felt that these changes would not impose a significant additional burden on PET drug producers because many medical facilities that produce and administer PET drugs might be able to obtain PET drugs for their patients from other PET drug producers while they were correcting an equipment malfunction [7]. Clearly this provision does present a patient-care issue when PET drugs are not readily available from other source(s) due to the very short half-lives of these drug products (e.g., ^{11}C- or ^{13}N-labeled PET drugs).

Rejection and Reprocessing Under section 212.71(a), a batch of a PET drug product that fails to meet established specifications must be rejected, and procedures must be established to identify and segregate the product [10]. Section 212.71(b) requires that documentation of the investigation of a nonconforming product includes the results of the investigation and final disposition of any rejected product [10]. Section 212.71(c) requires corrective action be taken for any identified problems to prevent recurrence of a nonconforming product or other quality problems [10].

Under section 212.71(d), a drug product can be reprocessed if procedures stated in the product's approved application are followed and the finished product conforms to specifications (except for sterility) before final release [10]. When the option for reprocessing is exercised, FDA recommended that the event be documented and conditions be described in a brief deviation report [12]. Examples of reprocessing could include a second passage through a purification column to remove an impurity or a second passage through a filter if the original filter failed the integrity test [12].

7.3.12 Packaging and Labeling

Because of radiation exposure concern, the Guidance states that it is a common practice to prepare much of the labeling in advance [12]. For example, an empty product vial can be prelabeled with partial information (e.g., product name, batch number, date) prior to filtration of the radioactive product, and upon completion of a QC test, the outer shielded container can be labeled with the required information (e.g., radioactivity). Alternatively, a string label can be used to label the immediate container provided that there is a way to associate the label with the vial if the label were to come off. Different approaches can be used as long as the approach ensures that the required information is available on the label.

7.3.13 Distribution

Section 212.90 requires the development of procedures to ensure that shipment will not adversely affect the product [10]. PET drug production facilities must maintain distribution records for PET drug products. The Guidance further recommends that a system be put in place by which the chain of distribution of each batch of PET drug product can be readily determined to permit its recall if necessary [12]. A recall should consist of notifying the receiving facility, the pharmacist, and the patient's physician, if known [12].

7.3.14 Complaint Handling

Section 212.100 states that a PET drug product that is returned because of a complaint or for any other reason may not be reprocessed and must be destroyed in accordance with applicable federal and state law [10].

7.3.15 Records

Section 212.110 requires all records be reasonably accessible to responsible officials of the facility and FDA investigators and all records be kept for at least 1 year from the date of the final or conditional final release of a PET drug product [10]. The Guidance indicates that verification reports should be kept as long as the systems are in use [12].

7.4 USP <823>

USP <823> provides QA standards for PET drugs that are produced for compounding, investigational, or research purposes in the United States. USP <823> was originally published in 1998 in the *US Pharmacopeia 23 – National Formulary 18* (USP 23–NF 18), Eighth Supplement [19]. Monographs for individual drugs and dosage forms as well as general chapter guidelines are also published in USP–NF in different formats (i.e., print, USB flash drive, or online subscription).

Under a long-standing provision of the FD&C [20], drugs recognized in USP–NF must comply with compendial identity standards, as well as compendial standards for strength, quality, and purity, as set forth in applicable USP monographs and General Chapters. This is described in FD&C 501(b) [20]. However, the USP has no role in enforcement, which is the responsibility of FDA and other government authorities.

Although the provisions in USP 32nd <823> [15] are generally less specific and explicit than the requirements in part 212 [10], FDA believes that they are adequate to ensure that RDRC and IND PET drugs are produced safely under appropriate conditions, consistent with section 501(a)(2)(B) of the FD&C [20], and are appropriate CGMP requirements for the RDRC or IND stage of development.

7.4.1 Flexibility in USP 32nd <823>

Only the major flexible items in USP 32nd <823> [15] are listed here:

- The post-filtration integrity test is not required prior to the release of the batch of ^{15}O water for human use.
- The unacceptable QC test result after investigation is not required to be notified to the receiving facilities [15].
- Less demanding on microbiologic testing of aseptic workstations – the Guidance stipulates that this testing "be performed during sterility testing and critical aseptic manipulations" [12], whereas USP 32nd <823> requires only that testing be performed periodically ("e.g., weekly") [15].
- More liberal in verification of the identities of components, containers, and closures, allowing the identities of these items to be verified by "defined procedures, tests, and/or documented certificates of analysis, as appropriate" [15]. Part 212 stipulates that identity testing must be conducted on an active or inactive ingredient if the finished-product testing cannot "ensure that the correct components have been used" [10].
- Unlike part 212 and the Guidance [10, 12], a sterility test is not required to be performed on every batch of PET drug: "After a record of successful sterility tests is established for a particular PET drug, only the first lot prepared each day shall be subject to a sterility test

using cultivation methods. However, when a different PET drug is made at the facility or a new lot of sterile components (for example, filter or final product container) is substituted, then the first daily lot of that PET drug is tested for sterility" [15].

7.4.2 More Flexibility in Part 212 and the Guidance

In general, CGMP requirements as stated in part 212 and its associated Guidance [10, 12] are for approved PET drugs, and the "less specific and explicit" USP 32nd <823> [15] constitutes the minimum CGMP requirements for investigational and research PET drugs [10]. However, it is interesting to note that several provisions in part 212 and the Guidance [10, 12] are more liberal and accommodating than the requirements in USP 32nd <823> [15]; only significant examples are described here:

- Production procedure is not required to be reviewed and verified at a minimum of once a year.
- Copies of outdated production procedures or computer software programs do not need to be retained.
- The evaluations for chemical purity do not have to include analyses for the presence of starting materials, known intermediates, by-products, and known degradation products.
- Terminal sterilization is an acceptable method for producing sterile PET drugs [12].
- Only one injection, rather than five or six replicate injections as per USP General Chapter <621> *Chromatography* [21], of the standard preparation is required for checking system suitability before injection of test samples into either a GC system or a HPLC system [12]. The standard preparation for the system suitability evaluation can be either the officially recognized reference standard (e.g., USP) or internal standard where an official standard is not available or if a PET drug production facility establishes its own reference standard [12].
- Process verification is not required if (a) the results of the production of an entire batch of a PET drug are fully verified through finished-product testing and (b) established historical batch records show that "there is adequate accumulated data to support a conclusion that the current process yields batches meeting predetermined acceptance criteria" [12].
- "PET drug production facilities can rely on a certification by the software or system vendor that the specified software was verified under its operating conditions" [12].
- Stability parameters required for testing include "radiochemical identity and purity (including levels of radiochemical impurities), appearance, pH, stabilizer or preservative effectiveness, and chemical purity" [12]. However, USP 32nd <823> stipulates that a PET drug under the stability testing "must meet all acceptance criteria" [15].
- The initiation time for the sterility testing is 30 h (FDA guidance 2011) rather than 24 h as required in USP 32nd <823> [15]. Furthermore, this 30-h requirement can be extended because of an intervening weekend or holiday [10].
- To ensure that each batch of PET drug meets its established acceptance criteria (except for sterility) before final release, the Guidance allows an appropriate laboratory determination to include not only the traditional finished-product testing but also in-process testing, continuous process monitoring of an attribute with statistical process controls, and some combination of these approaches [12].
- PQIT – a PQIT is a noncritical QC test performed at predetermined intervals rather than on a batch-to-batch basis [12]. Examples of these noncritical QC attributes might include "radionuclidic purity (when potentially contaminating radionuclides do not impact the safety or effectiveness of the drug product), as well as certain low-level nontoxic impurities and class 3 residual solvents" [12].
- If the required finished-product tests (with the exception of radiochemical identity/purity test and specific activity test) cannot be completed because of a malfunction of analytical equipment, the related PET drug could still be released for human use under the "conditional final release" provision [10].

- Reprocessing of a batch of a PET drug that does not conform to specifications is allowable [10].

7.4.3 Revised USP <823>

At the time the monographs and general chapters for PET drugs were published by USP in the 1990s, most PET drugs were produced and used within research or medical institutions. Since then, the environment where PET drugs are produced and used has changed significantly. Today, research or medical institutions continue to produce and use PET drugs for investigational and research purposes. In addition, commercial producers supply most PET drugs used in routine diagnostic imaging procedures. PET imaging agents also have attracted the interest of pharmaceutical companies as potential tools to accelerate and reduce the cost of traditional drug-discovery efforts. Finally, numerous efforts are underway to develop new routine diagnostic imaging agents for use in cardiology, oncology, and neurology. Thus, the use of PET imaging agents today spans discovery, research, clinical development, and routine diagnostic imaging procedures. The diversification of PET during the past 15–20 years has resulted in new requirements for the PET environment, including a greater number of PET drugs, higher production levels, shorter synthesis times, shorter quality control times, more complex syntheses, and increased regulatory oversight.

To understand these changes, USP jointly sponsored two symposia with the Society of Nuclear Medicine (SNM) during SNM's annual meetings in 2008 and 2009. USP staff and members of the USP Expert Committee on Radiopharmaceutical and Medical Imaging Agents (RMI EC) presented talks and led discussions about historical trends and changes in the PET environment. One goal of these symposia was to describe issues related to USP General Chapters for PET drugs and to gather feedback from the PET community. The USP–SNM joint symposia and regulatory requirements led USP RMI EC to conclude that USP 32nd <823> must be revised.

Deficiencies in the USP 32nd <823> [15] were identified as follows:

- Differences in the organization of USP 32nd <823> compared to FDA's final rule and Guidance on CGMP for PET drugs [10, 12]
- Further enhancement of USP <823>'s flexible provisions by incorporating items such as PQIT, a 30-h initiation time frame for sterility testing, and conditional final release according to FDA's CGMP requirements for PET drugs [10, 12]
- The need for consistency with other revision efforts for USP General Chapters
- Inappropriate methodologies for system suitability and quantitative analysis in current chromatographic tests
- Lack of defined frequency for certain QC tests
- Lack of discussion about the timing of the completion of certain QC tests relative to product release
- Lack of requirements for OOS investigations for quality control tests

7.4.3.1 The Revision Process for USP <823>

To address these deficiencies, USP RMI EC proposed the establishment of an Ad Hoc Advisory Panel (Advisory Panel) composed of academic and industrial members of the PET community. The goal of the USP Advisory Panel was to advise RMI EC about suitable revisions to USP 32nd <823> in accordance with USP's mission. The formation of the USP Advisory Panel was completed in late 2008, and beginning of July 2009, the USP Advisory Panel met or teleconferenced numerous times. The outcome of this effort is summarized here.

7.4.3.2 Organization of the Revised USP <823>

To reflect the new role of the revised USP <823> in part 212 [10] and to uphold PET compounding practice, the title of the revised USP <823> has been changed to *Positron Emission Tomography – Drugs for Compounding, Investigational, and Research Uses* [22].

By means of compounding, pharmacists (or other qualified individuals working under the authority and supervision of a physician), according to state-regulated practice of medicine and pharmacy, fulfill an essential health-care need – providing patients with medications tailored to their needs. In some cases compounding pharmacists provide a drug that is not commercially available. In other cases the patient may be allergic to certain ingredient(s) of the drug, or the dosage form may not be suitable for administration to the patient. In addition to giving patients access to otherwise unavailable or more appropriate PET drugs, compounding may also be used for teaching or QC purposes.

In FDA's view, part 212 covers both compounded and noncompounded PET drugs and thus believes that these two types of PET drugs should be within the scope of FDA's authority in accordance of part 212 [7]. However, USP is not addressing the extent of FDA's regulatory authority, and therefore, by its terms, USP <823> should apply to compounding of PET drugs for human use whether such compounding is or is not subject to federal regulation.

To streamline USP General Chapters related to PET drugs, the USP Advisory Panel decided to consolidate key standards and requirements stated in USP <1015> [17] into the revised USP <823>. Consequently, USP <1015> will be deleted from USP. In addition, a new proposed general chapter numbered <1823>, "Positron Emission Tomography Drugs-Information" [23], has recently been developed to supplement <823>. This new general chapter describes concepts, technologies, and procedures for the preparation of PET drugs and QA. These supplemental descriptions are more suitable for an informational general chapter. This is consistent with USP's General Chapter Design Project, which is an effort to exclude nonenforceable information from general chapters numbered less than 1000 (USP General Chapter Project Team 2009).

The following are the sections in the revised USP <823> [22]:

- Definitions
- Adequate Personnel and Resources
- QA
- Facilities and Equipment
- Control of Components, Materials, and Supplies
- Process and Operational Controls
- Stability
- Controls and Acceptance Criteria for Finished PET Drugs
- If a PET Drug Does Not Conform to Specifications
- Reprocessing
- Labeling and Packaging

7.4.3.3 Definitions

The definitions discussed below are different from those defined in the final rule:

Batch Versus Lot Part 212 uses the terms *batch* and *lot* interchangeably [10]. In addition, part 212 appears to use *lot* synonymously with *sub-batch* [10]. These definitions and usages may be confusing to the PET community. To differentiate the specific meaning of each term, the USP Advisory Panel and RMI EC propose that the definition of *batch* applies explicitly to the PET drug and that the definition of *lot* applies only to components used in the preparation (including QC) of a PET drug. As defined in the revised USP <823>, the term *lot* means a quantity of materials (e.g., reagents, solvents, gases, purification columns, and other auxiliary materials) that have uniform character and quality within specified limits and are used to make a PET drug product [22].

PET Drug The definition of *PET drug* in the part 212 [10] includes "any non-radioactive reagent, reagent kit, ingredient, nuclide generator, accelerator, target material, electronic synthesizer, or other apparatus or computer program to be used in the preparation of a PET drug." USP feels that nonradioactive reagents, reagent kits, ingredients, and target materials are components used to produce a PET drug and that radionuclide generators, accelerators, electronic synthesizers, and computer programs are ancillary items used in the production of PET drugs. As such, the revised USP <823> defines *PET drug* as "a finished form of a radioactive drug that exhibits spontaneous disintegration of unstable nuclei by the emission of positrons and is intended for human administration in diagnosis or therapy" [22].

FDAMA defines the "compounded" PET drug to be used for diagnostic images [5]. As such, therapeutic PET drugs are explicitly excluded from part 212 [10]. However, USP believes that the revised USP <823> should apply to any PET drug whether it is for diagnostic or therapeutic use. Therefore, the definition of *PET drug* in the revised USP <823> includes "therapeutic" use (e.g., tumor therapy) [22].

QA Versus QC QA and QC are commonly used interchangeably in the PET community even though the terms have fundamental differences. As per the revised USP <823>, QA and QC are defined as follows [22]:

QA: A planned system for ensuring that a PET drug product possesses defined identity, strength, quality, and purity required for its intended purpose by procedures, tests, and analytical methods.

QC: A system for testing the quality of components, materials, supplies, and PET drug products by procedures, tests, analytical methods, and acceptance criteria.

Thus, QC is a subset of QA that deals with testing materials and products to determine if they meet acceptance criteria.

Strength Part 212 defines *strength* as radioactivity on a volume or weight basis [10]. USP believes that this definition risks confusing *strength* and *specific activity* because it is not clear if weight refers to the cold mass of the active pharmaceutical ingredient or the overall weight of the solution.

In addition, it is common practice in PET to define strength on a volume basis. Therefore, *strength* is defined in the revision of USP 32nd <823> strictly based on volume (e.g., mCi/mL or MBq/mL) which is the same as *specific concentration*.

Validation Versus Verification Part 212 has a definition of *verification*; however, it does not define the term *validation* [10]. Although the terms *validate*, *validated*, and *validation* are used in the Guidance [12], these terms are also not defined there.

Validation and verification are essential and complementary elements in the CGMP process. The revised USP <823> defines *validation* as the "establishment of documented evidence that a method, process, or system accomplishes its intended requirements" [22]. In addition, *verification* is defined as "confirmation that an established method, process, or system meets predetermined acceptance criteria" [22]. It is helpful to think of validation as "building the right thing," and verification as "building it right."

7.4.3.4 Adequate Personnel and Resources

Adequate personnel and resources are addressed in several sections of the 32nd version of USP <823> [15], including *Compounding Procedure Verification*, *PET Radiopharmaceutical Compounding for Human Use,* and *Quality Control.* The revised revision of USP <823> includes a separate section titled *Adequate Personnel and Resources,* which requires a sufficient number of personnel with appropriate education and training and indicates that the number of personnel depends on the size and complexity of the facility [22]. This section of the revised USP <823> reflects the layout of part 212 addressing personnel and resources as the first topic [10, 22].

7.4.3.5 QA

This section of the revised USP <823> describes the difference between QA and QC in the production of PET drugs [22]. QA covers all matters that influence the product's identity, strength, purity, and quality. QC is a subset of QA that deals with testing materials and products to determine if they meet acceptance criteria. The QA function typically consists of oversight activities and the QC function consists of execution activities [24]. According to the Guidance, QA function in a PET drug production facility consists of oversight and execution activities [12].

7.4.3.6 Facilities and Equipment

The revised USP <823> requires the certification (i.e., integrity testing of the high-efficiency particulate air [HEPA] filter) of the aseptic workstation be performed at least annually [22] when the Guidance requires this every 6 months [12]. As for the microbiological monitoring (e.g., using swab or contact/settle plate) in the aseptic workstation, revised USP <823> requires it be assessed after use and each day of use [22], whereas the Guidance requires it be conducted during sterility testing and critical aseptic manipulation [12].

Cleaning Equipment and Components The 32nd USP <823> describes the cleaning of equipment but does not specifically address cleaning between batches of PET drugs [15]. As a result, there has been confusion about the acceptability of cleaning between batches. The revised USP <823> addresses this deficiency by describing requirements for cleaning equipment between multiple batches or one of more PET drugs [22]. This approach is consistent with the equipment cleaning requirements described in the Guidance [12].

System Suitability for QC Equipment The Guidance states that at least one injection of a standard is required for system suitability [12]. The Guidance does not address reproducibility as a part of system suitability but instead references USP <621> which describes system suitability requirements (resolution, replicate injections, and tailing factor) [12, 21].

Although these requirements are important for chromatography systems used in PET drug production, the number of injections required for replicate injections in USP <621> (i.e., five injections for reproducibility if the relative standard deviation is 2.0 % or less and six injections if the relative standard deviation is more than 2.0 %) may not be practical because of the nature (i.e., half-life) and number of different PET drugs and/or the number of batches prepared at a typical academic or commercial PET facility [21]. Consequently, the revision of USP <823> describes two acceptable system suitability approaches that can be used for chromatographic systems [22].

The first approach is the construction of a calibration curve that can be used for an extended period of time. In routine use, the injection of a known standard is used to verify that the calibration curve is appropriate for use in subsequent sample injections. The second approach is the use of a single-point calibration created from two injections of a known standard at the beginning of each testing cycle. In each case, the requirement for replicate injections is met by comparison of multiple injections, either within a single testing cycle or over an extended period of time. Together, the approaches described in the revised USP <823> provide more flexibility and clarity than does the Guidance [12, 22].

Other chromatographic parameters such as signal-to-noise ratio, limit of detection, and limit of quantitation can be determined as part of routine system suitability testing [22]. System suitability tests also may be appropriate for other QC equipment, including dose calibrator, radio-thin layer chromatography, and multichannel analyzer [22].

7.4.3.7 Control of Components, Materials, and Supplies

If growth media used in the sterility testing of PET drug products are obtained from commercial sources, the revised USP <823> requires a growth promotion testing that uses a suitable single species of organism be performed on initial qualification of the supplier and periodically (e.g., quarterly) thereafter [22]. This is not required by part 212 or the Guidance if the manufacturer of the growth media provides COA that contains the results of the growth promotion testing [10, 12].

7.4.3.8 Process and Operational Controls

This section of the revised USP <823> covers the "Production and Process Controls" and "Laboratory Control" sections as described in part 212 and the Guidance [10, 12, 22].

Acceptance criteria must be established in the master record for each PET drug, and if a USP monograph exists, USP standards are the minimum acceptable requirements unless there are acceptance criteria specified in an FDA-approved IND or RDRC protocol [22].

Aseptic Operation The revision of USP <823> allows the preparation of multiple PET drug vial assemblies in a single aseptic operation cycle [22]. It also allows the sterility testing with the use of a septum-sealed sterility test tube be carried out in a shielded area that does not contain an HEPA filter [22]. This provision is to address radiation shielding requirements when inoculating radioactive samples for sterility test [22]. USP felt that the flexibility is necessary since many hot cells used for this purpose do not have laminar airflow and the use of a media tube with a septum cap provides adequate protection from accidental contamination during the inoculation process. If media tubes have a screw cap opening, inoculations must be performed in the aseptic workstation. The Guidance does not differentiate inoculation requirements for screw cap or septum cap media tubes [12].

Process Verification Documented studies must be performed to ensure that the process described in the master record yields a PET drug that meets the defined acceptance criteria.

The revised USP <823> indicates that the process verification must be completed on three batches that do not have to be consecutive [22]. This allowance was added to account for a batch that may not be completed because of factors that are not relevant to the quality characteristics of the PET drug (e.g., cyclotron malfunction, hardware malfunction, and so on). This allows the completion of process validation without the potential losses that could occur with three consecutive batches stipulated in the Guidance [12].

As per part 212, process verification is required if an entire batch of a PET drug is not fully verified through finished-product testing or when only the initial sub-batch in a series is tested [10]. The Guidance allows the use of historical batch records to substitute the process verification provided that there is adequate accumulated data to support the current process that would yield batches meeting the predetermined acceptance criteria [12]. Due to the unique characteristics of PET drug production, FDA allows the distribution of the batch of PET drug under process verification if the produced PET drug met the predetermined acceptance criteria [12].

Based on these statements, USP should consider adding similar requirements in USP <823> to clarify when the process verification is or is not required to be performed.

7.4.3.9 Stability

The revised USP <823> [22] is consistent with the Guidance [12] in the evaluation parameters and test conditions to establish and document the stability profile of PET drug products under proposed storage conditions.

7.4.3.10 Controls and Acceptance Criteria for Finished PET Drug Products

The 32nd USP <823> permits a reduction in the frequency of sterility tests after a record of successful sterility tests is established for a particular PET drug [15]. Because sterility testing and bacterial endotoxins test (BET) are both biological assessments, the revised USP <823> includes a reduction in the frequency of the BET [22]. Similar to the sterility test, the BET must be performed on the first batch of each PET drug prepared each day [22].

The 32nd USP <823> describes an in-process 20-min endotoxin test [15]. USP believes that this test is out of date and is too prescriptive (i.e., a 20-min process and "incorporating positive controls in the range of 5 EU per mL to 175 EU/*V*, where *V* is the maximum volume of injection"). Therefore, the revision of USP <823> does not include the 20-min in-process test [22].

If a PET Drug Does Not Conform to Specifications If a PET drug does not conform to specifications, the first action generally is to investigate the QC process. Such investigations typically are known as OOS investigations which are not addressed in the USP 32nd <823> [15].

The guidance for OOS investigations of traditional pharmaceuticals [25] does not apply well to short-lived PET drugs. Section 212.71 addresses the question, "What actions must I take if a batch of PET drug does not conform to specifications?" [10] This section requires the rejection of PET drugs that do not meet specifications but does not discuss OOS investigations and the possibility of analytical error as a cause of OOS results. The result is that none of the FDA documents adequately address OOS investigations for PET drugs. To resolve these shortcomings, the revised USP <823> includes a description of OOS investigations [22].

The focus of an OOS investigation is to determine if the OOS QC finding is the result of an analytical error or a true product failure. If the investigation determines that the OOS result is caused by analytical error, the original test results are invalidated. Thus, an OOS result does not necessarily mean that the batch fails and must be rejected. However, if the investigation determines that the OOS result indicates a true product failure, the batch must be rejected, and the cause of the failure must be investigated. However, the revised USP <823> does not address the notification requirements to the receiving facilities.

When a sterility test for a PET drug product shows signs of microbial growth, revised USP <823> indicates that the test result is an OOS and should be investigated [22]. Upon completion of the investigation, immediately notify all receiving facilities if the product fails to meet the criterion for sterility, including the microbiological findings from the investigation [22]. According to part 212, if the PET drug product fails the sterility test, immediate notification to all receiving facilities must be initiated and provide these facilities with the test results, as well as any appropriate recommendations [10]. Upon completion of an investigation, the findings must be immediately notified to all receiving facilities [10].

7.4.3.11 Reprocessing

Depending on the nature of the failure, the rejected PET drug product may be reprocessed according to preestablished written procedures [22].

7.4.3.12 Labeling

Labeling requirements for PET drugs are not described in the 32nd USP <823> but are included in a separate section in the proposed revision [15]. The section in the revised USP <823> is divided into information required on the immediate container for PET drugs and on the immediate shielding during storage and use [22].

The revised USP <823> does not list the "Distribution" and "Complaint Handling" sections [22]. This is probably due to the fact that the revised USP <823> only addresses PET drugs for compounding, IND, and RDRC which are most likely not distributed to outside of the facility. The "Records" section described in part 212 and the Guidance [10, 12] is also not included in the revised USP <823> as the record requirements (e.g., composition and quality of the PET drug product, process and production records, and OOS results, etc.) are placed in the related sections of the revised USP <823> [22].

7.5 Inspection on the PET Drug Production Facility

FDA inspects manufacturers or processors of FDA-regulated products to verify that they comply with relevant regulations. In general, a routine FDA inspection to ensure compliance with CGMP would focus on activities up to and including the point of final release of a PET drug product.

7.5.1 Types of FDA Inspections

There are three types of FDA inspections on drug production facilities:

- Preapproval inspection (PAI) – this is for new NDAs and ANDAs. The purpose of a PAI is to verify existence of the raw data included in the submission (often the focus here will be on laboratory results for lot release and stability as well as validation) and confirm that the facility is capable of manufacture (e.g., correct scale qualified equipment, process validation, etc.). Yes, there will be an overall CGMP evaluation, but the stated purpose of the PAI (in response to the generic scandal of the 1980s) is focused on those two items. The outcome is a recommendation for approval or not. If the site has no approved products, FDA cannot issue a warning letter, but they will block approval of the product until such time as remediation occurs and has been confirmed by a reinspection.

- Routine surveillance CGMP inspection – periodically (every 2–3 years generally as resources and priorities allow), the FDA will perform an unannounced CGMP inspection for manufacturers who make commercial products. FDA generally does not inspect clinical manufacturing sites unless there are known issues, such as unexpected deaths in a clinical trial that may be linked to method of manufacture. This can cover all CGMP systems or can be a more limited (abbreviated) inspection.
- Compliance inspection – this is either a follow-up inspection post of a regulatory action (e.g., warning letter, untitled letter, regulatory meeting, etc.) or an inspection on a for-cause basis (i.e., when FDA becomes aware of a potential safety concern related to the production of an investigational or research drug). Similar to inspection of production facilities for non-PET investigational drugs, FDA generally will only conduct for-cause inspections of facilities that produce investigational or research PET drugs.

A full inspection covers at least four items, whereas an abbreviated inspection consists of at least two items of the inspection systems listed below:

- Quality system with aseptic sterility controls
- Facilities and equipment system
- Materials system
- Production system
- Laboratory control system
- Packaging and labeling system

The first item "quality system and aseptic sterility controls" is mandatory for both full and abbreviated inspections.

7.5.2 Selection of Inspection Coverage

According to an FDA talk titled "PET Drug Inspection," which was presented at the 2014 Society of Nuclear Medicine and Molecular Imaging (SNMMI) annual meeting [25], in 2013 100 % of all FDA inspections on PET drug production facilities were full inspection (at least four systems to be inspected) conducted due to any of the following circumstances:

- Firm has never been inspected.
- Follow-up to regulatory action.
- Significant manufacturing changes.
- Microbial contamination or cross-contamination.
- Poor compliance history – initial inspection conducted in 2012.

In 2014 (as of June 9, 2014, when this presentation was given), FDA indicated that approximately 10 % facilities might get abbreviated inspection (at least two systems to be inspected) for any of the following reasons [26]:

- Adequate compliance history.
- Firm has been inspected for similar class of product.

7.5.3 Major Issues Identified in 2013/2014 PET Drug Inspections

This FDA report at the 2014 SNMMI meeting [25] revealed several major deficiency issues during their inspections carried out in 2013 and up to June 2014:

- Lack of appropriate training and QA oversight
- Inadequate aseptic techniques and environmental monitoring
- Analytical assay methods not validated or verified for intended use
- Inappropriate controls of equipment and materials

- Deficiencies in production and process controls (including the inadequate media fill control process)
- Deficiencies in laboratory controls
- Lack of adequate finished drug product controls and acceptance criteria (including lack of proper "out-of-specification" investigations)
- Lack of appropriate record keeping

The more specific deficiencies for each of the abovementioned six major issues are listed as follows [25]:

7.5.3.1 Deficiencies in Appropriate Training and QA Oversight

Failure to train employees, identify as deviation and conduct investigation, review batch record for release, review records in a timely manner, reject batches with OOS result, maintain on-site software, follow established procedures, document handling of nonconformance, and establish a change control procedure.

7.5.3.2 Aseptic Operation Deficiencies

Identified deficiencies of aseptic operation are:

- The use of an overcrowded laminar flow hood
- The use of non-sterile disinfectants
- Dilution of drug product in unclassified area
- Frequency of environmental monitoring not reflecting manufacturing operation
- Storage of bulk product vial in non-sterile bag
- Out of limit personnel monitoring results
- No record of aseptic area been cleaned
- Lack of documentation on the qualification of personnel conducting aseptic operation

7.5.3.3 Inappropriate Controls of Equipment and Materials

- Inadequate qualification of chemical synthesizer
- Cleaning not adequate for multiproduct equipment
- Failure to fully evaluate all materials received for use in production

7.5.3.4 Deficiencies in Production and Process Controls

These deficiencies in production and process controls are:

- Master record does not contain complete instruction of production, sampling, and testing (use of sticky notes).
- Written procedures not specific enough (corporate standard operation procedure).
- No determination to conduct investigation when errors occurred.
- Deficiencies in batch record:
  - Failure to record manufacturer's name and/or expiration dates of material utilized in production
  - Does not include actual weights or volumes of the components used in the process
  - Ensuring all portions are complete before final quality approval
- Verification not performed to ensure consistency of the process upon process change
- Revalidation not done on computer-based programmable logic controller

7.5.3.5 Media Fills Deficiencies

Media fills did not simulate production: bulk product vial hold was not the worst case, dilution step not simulated, manufacturing process flow not matched, and withdrawal of QC samples not simulated, and there was no positive control and negative control. Also, media does not come into contact with all interior surface, and not all production personnel participate in media fills.

7.5.3.6 Deficiencies in Laboratory Controls

The reported deficiencies in laboratory controls are listed below:

Analytical Method Validation Failure to validate methods which deviate from USP test method

Analytical Equipment Qualification Failure to qualify equipment for intended use and failure to maintain and calibrate equipment – dose calibration not calibrated for linearity to cover the range being test, multichannel analyzer not recalibrated, and thin-layer chromatography scanner. No audit trail for GC, HPLC, and allowed ability to delete raw electronic test data

System Suitability GC and HPLC – number of injections: one vs. three. Lack of documentation on daily system suitability. Deficient in analytical balance accuracy verification and pH indicator range

Expiry of Reagent, Reference Standards No justification for expiration dating of ^{18}F-fludeoxyglucose reference solution, Kryptofix, buffers, and mannose triflate

7.5.3.7 Lack of Adequate Finished Drug Product Controls and Acceptance Criteria

Several deficiencies in this area were releasing drug that did not pass specification, releasing without calculating or reporting the radiochemical purity in the batch record, failure to conduct all QC tests for release, and releasing multiple lots under conditional release.

Lack of Proper "Out-of-Specification" Investigations OOS test averaged to generating passing results and not retaining raw test data.

7.5.3.8 Lack of Appropriate Record Keeping

Failure to retain raw analytical data, no documentation that sterility test was conducted and the lot was released and equipment maintenance log missing sufficient details

References

1. Ter-Pogossian MM, Phelps ME, Hoffman EJ, Mullani NA. A positron-emission transaxial tomograph for nuclear imaging (PETT). Radiology. 1975;114:89–98.
2. Phelps ME, Hoffman EJ, Mullani NA, Ter-Pogossian MM. Application of annihilation coincidence detection to transaxial reconstruction tomography. J Nucl Med. 1975;16:210–24.
3. Sweet WH, Brownell GL. Localization of brain tumors with positron emitters. Nucleonics. 1953;11:40–5.
4. Congress. Report 105-43 Food and Drug Administration modernization and accountability act of 1997. 1997. http://www.gpo.gov/fdsys/pkg/CRPT-105srpt43/pdf/CRPT-105srpt43.pdf. Accessed 19 Aug 2015. p. 52–3.
5. Food and Drug Administration. Section 121 Positron emission tomography. Food and Drug Administration Modernization Act of 1997. 1997. http://www.fda.gov/downloads/RegulatoryInformation/Legislation/FederalFoodDrugandCosmeticActFDCAct/SignificantAmendmentstotheFDCAct/FDAMA/FullTextofFDAMAlaw/UCM089145.pdf. Accessed 25 Aug 2015.
6. Food and Drug Administration. 21 CFR Parts 210, 211, and 212 current good manufacturing practice for positron emission tomography drugs [proposed rule]. 2005. http://www.fda.gov/ohrms/dockets/98fr/05-18510.pdf. Accessed 25 Aug 2015.
7. Food and Drug Administration. 21 CFR Parts 210, 211, and 212 current good manufacturing practice for positron emission tomography drugs [final rule]. 2009. http://www.gpo.gov/fdsys/pkg/FR-2009-12-10/pdf/E9-29285.pdf. Accessed 30 June 2015.
8. Food and Drug Administration. Guidance PET drugs – current good manufacturing practice (CGMP) (small entity compliance guide). 2009. http://www.fda.gov/downloads/drugs/guidancecomplianceregulatoryinformation/guidances/ucm070306.pdf. Accessed 20 Aug 2015.
9. Food and Drug Administration. Guidance FDA oversight of PET drug products questions and answers. 2012. http://www.fda.gov/downloads/drugs/guidancecomplianceregulatoryinformation/guidances/ucm290024.pdf. Accessed 25 Aug 2015.
10. Food and Drug Administration. 21 CFR Part 212 current good manufacturing practice for positron emission tomography drugs. 2015. http://www.accessdata.fda.gov/scripts/cdrh/cfdocs/cfCFR/CFRSearch.cfm?CFRPart=212. Accessed 1 July 2015.
11. Food and Drug Administration. Food, drug, and cosmetic act section 201(ii)(1)(A) (U.S. Code: Title 21 – food and drugs 321(ii)(1)(A)) definitions; generally. 2015. http://www.gpo.gov/fdsys/pkg/USCODE-2010-title21/pdf/USCODE-2010-title21-chap9-subchapII-sec321.pdf. Accessed 25 Aug 2015.
12. Food and Drug Administration. Guidance PET drugs – current good manufacturing practice (CGMP) (small entity compliance guide). 2011. http://www.fda.gov/downloads/Drugs/GuidanceComplianceRegulatoryInformation/Guidances/UCM266640.pdf. Accessed 25 Aug 2015.
13. Food and Drug Administration. 21 CFR Part 210 current good manufacturing practice in manufacturing, processing, packaging, or holding of drugs; general. 2015. http://www.accessdata.fda.gov/scripts/cdrh/cfdocs/cfcfr/CFRSearch.cfm?CFRPart=210. Accessed 1 July 2015.

14. Food and Drug Administration. 21 CFR Part 211 current good manufacturing practice for finished pharmaceuticals. 2015. http://www.accessdata.fda.gov/scripts/cdrh/cfdocs/cfcfr/CFRSearch.cfm?CFRPart=211. Accessed 1 July 2015.
15. United States Pharmacopeia. <823> Radiopharmaceuticals for positron emission tomography-compounding. 2009. http://www.pharmacopeia.cn/v29240/usp29nf24s0_c823.html. Accessed 1 July 2015.
16. United States Pharmacopeia. <797> Pharmaceutical compounding-sterile preparations. 2015. http://www.uspnf.com/uspnf/pub/index?usp=38&nf=33&s=1&officialOn=August1,2015. Accessed 25 Aug 2015 (online access with paid subscription).
17. United States Pharmacopeia. <1015> Automated radiochemical synthesis apparatus. 2015. http://www.uspnf.com/uspnf/pub/index?usp=38&nf=33&s=0&officialOn=May1,2015. Accessed 1 July 2015 (online access with paid subscription).
18. United States Pharmacopeia. <467> Residual solvents. 2015. http://www.uspnf.com/uspnf/pub/index?usp=38&nf=33&s=0&officialOn=May1,2015. Accessed 1 July 2015 (online access with paid subscription).
19. United States Pharmacopeial Convention. Frequently asked questions: <823> Radiopharmaceuticals for positron emission tomography (PET) – compounding, investigational, and research uses. 2015. http://www.usp.org/frequently-asked-questions/radiopharmaceuticals-positron-emission-tomography-pet-compounding-investigational-and-research-uses. Accessed 25 Aug 2015.
20. Food and Drug Administration. Food, drug, and cosmetic act section 501(b) (U.S. code: title 21 – food and drugs 351(b)) adulterated drugs and devices. 2015. http://www.gpo.gov/fdsys/pkg/USCODE-2010-title21/pdf/USCODE-2010-title21-chap9-subchapV-partA-sec351.pdf. Accessed 25 Aug 2015.
21. United States Pharmacopeia. <621> Chromatography. 2015. http://www.uspnf.com/uspnf/pub/index?usp=38&nf=33&s=0&officialOn=May1,2015. Accessed 1 July 2015 (online access with paid subscription).
22. United States Pharmacopeia. <823> Positron emission tomography drugs for compounding, investigational, and research uses. 2015. http://www.uspnf.com/uspnf/pub/index?usp=38&nf=33&s=0&officialOn=May1,2015. Accessed 1 July 2015 (online access with paid subscription).
23. United States Pharmacopeia. <1823> Positron emission tomography drugs-information. 2015 [proposal]. http://www.usp.org/sites/default/files/usp_pdf/EN/USPNF/key-issues/general-chapter-1823-proposed-revision.pdf. Accessed 19 July 2016.
24. Zigler SS, Breslow K, Nazerias M. A quality system for PET: an industry perspective. Nucl Instrum Methods Phys Res B. 2005;241:645–8.
25. Food and Drug Administration. Guidance for industry investigating out-of-specification (OOS) test results for pharmaceutical production. 2006. http://www.fda.gov/downloads/Drugs/Guidances/ucm070287.pdf. Accessed 25 Aug 2015.
26. Ghosh K. PET drug inspection [PowerPoint presentation in PDF format]. 2014. http://www.fda.gov/downloads/Drugs/ScienceResearch/ResearchAreas/Oncology/UCM403790.pdf. Accessed 1 July 2015.

Part III

PET Physics and Instrumentation

PET Physics and Instrumentation

8

Srilalan Krishnamoorthy, Jeffrey P. Schmall, and Suleman Surti

Contents

8.1 **Introduction** 174
8.1.1 Positron Annihilation 174
8.1.2 Coincidence Logic and Electronic Collimation 174
8.1.3 Types of Events Detected by a PET Scanner 175
8.1.4 Time-of-Flight PET 176

8.2 **PET Instrumentation** 176
8.2.1 Scintillation Detectors 176
8.2.2 Photosensors 178
8.2.3 PET Detector Designs 178
8.2.4 PET Data Acquisition and Signal Processing 180
8.2.5 PET System Design and Geometry 180

8.3 **PET System Characteristics** 180
8.3.1 Sensitivity 180
8.3.2 Spatial Resolution 180
8.3.3 Energy Resolution 181
8.3.4 Coincidence Timing Resolution 181
8.3.5 Count-Rate Performance 182

8.4 **Multimodality PET/CT** 183
8.4.1 Motivation and Review of Fusion Imaging 183
8.4.2 Hardware-Based Multimodality PET/CT 183
8.4.3 Attenuation Correction 184
8.4.4 Scatter Correction 186
8.4.5 Randoms Correction 187
8.4.6 Limitations and Issues with PET/CT Imaging 187
8.4.7 Low-Dose CT 187

8.5 **Time-of-Flight PET** 190
8.5.1 Simplified Mathematical Approach to SNR Improvement with Time of Flight 190
8.5.2 Instrumentation Advances Leading to the Reemergence of TOF-PET 190
8.5.3 Benefits of TOF Information for Clinical PET Imaging 191

8.6 **Advances and Future Directions** 193
8.6.1 Silicon Photomultiplier and Its Impact 193
8.6.2 Multimodality PET/MR 193
8.6.3 Organ-Specific Imaging 194
8.6.4 Direct Conversion Detectors 194

8.7 **Summary** 194

References 194

S. Krishnamoorthy, PhD • J.P. Schmall, PhD
S. Surti, PhD (✉)
Department of Radiology, Perelman School of Medicine at the University of Pennsylvania, 156B John Morgan Building, 3620 Hamilton Walk, Philadelphia, PA 19104, USA
e-mail: srilalan@mail.med.upenn.edu; schmall@mail.med.upenn.edu; surti@mail.med.upenn.edu

Abstract

The design of instrumentation for positron emission tomography (PET) scanners has vastly progressed over the past ~30 years. In this chapter, we focus on the motivations and technical advancements that lead to the development of multimodality imaging systems, including the integration of PET and CT into combined PET/CT scanners for whole-body imaging. We also provide a review of recent advances in time-of-flight (TOF) PET, ending with a description of current state-of-the-art TOF-PET/CT imaging systems. We begin with

M.M. Khalil (ed.), *Basic Science of PET Imaging*, DOI 10.1007/978-3-319-40070-9_8

an overview of PET detector design and explore the trade-offs associated with the choice of scintillator, photodetector, and their arrangement. Next, PET data correction approaches, including attenuation correction, for PET/CT are discussed along with a technical description of PET/CT system hardware. Specific concepts and instrumentation aspects of TOF-PET are then reviewed, ending with a brief discussion on the outlook and future directions for PET instrumentation research. This chapter highlights recent advances in PET instrumentation and describes their impact and contribution to the improvement in clinical PET imaging.

8.1 Introduction

The idea for positron annihilation coincidence imaging can be traced to the early days of radionuclide imaging when it was initially explored by Hal Anger [1] and Gordon Brownell [2]. The early instrumentation efforts utilized dual planar stationary detectors that produced longitudinal tomographic images. Subsequently, with the development of transverse section image reconstruction algorithms [3, 4] and the arrival of relatively cost-effective computers in the early to mid-1970s, there was a push toward the development of PET systems providing transverse section images. The system design, therefore, evolved from stationary, dual planar detectors to circular or full angular coverage systems [5–13]. The primary detector design in all these systems utilized scintillation detectors directly coupled to a photomultiplier tube (PMT). Due to PMT sizes, this significantly limited the spatial resolution of these early PET systems. Since then, PET system design has evolved toward higher resolution detectors that are suitable for imaging not only humans but also small animals such as mice.

8.1.1 Positron Annihilation

The signal that is measured in PET originates from unstable neutron-deficient isotopes, which can undergo nuclear decay emitting a positron and a neutrino in the process. The positron has the same mass as an electron but has the opposite charge—it is a form of antimatter that will combine with a free electron resulting in a matter-antimatter annihilation. The probability of positron annihilation and the mean positron energy will vary depending on the specific isotope. The annihilation event transfers the energy mass of the positron, and any residual kinetic energy, to simultaneously create two photons, whose direction is ~180° apart, each having an energy of 511 keV. This may be obvious, but it represents an important distinction: the PET scanner is designed to detect the annihilation photons, not the positron itself, only a signature of its existence. These fundamental characteristics, the simultaneous emission of two, antiparallel, 511 keV photons, form the basis of the detection logic employed by all PET scanners.

8.1.2 Coincidence Logic and Electronic Collimation

Shown in Fig. 8.1 is a schematic of two detectors operating in coincidence mode 180° apart, with a positron source in between them. A coincidence is made when both detectors detect a 511 keV photon at the same time; this tells us that somewhere along a line connecting the two detectors, an annihilation event occurred—we call this coincidence logic. A PET scanner is a scaled-up version of this simple two-detector system, to a full ring of detectors, with each detector able to form coincidences with another detector in the ring. Unlike single-photon emission computed tomography (SPECT), which uses a physical collimator, localization of events in PET is done by electronically collimating events using multiple detector pairs; coincidence combinations within the ring of detectors allow for complete angular and radial sampling of the imaging field of view. Electronic collimation is one of PET's greatest advantages and is a primary reason for PET's high sensitivity. The physical collimation used in SPECT attenuates much of the signal incident on the detector surface; this makes the sensitivity of

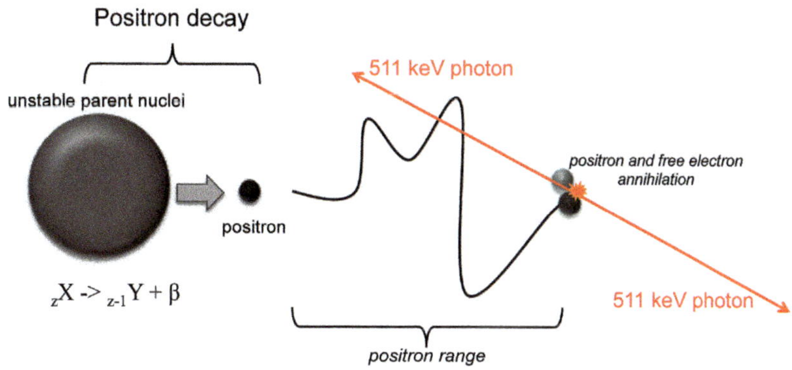

Fig. 8.1 Schematic of positron decay: the unstable parent nuclei decay emitting a positron in the process. The positron travels some distance (referred to as positron range) while losing its kinetic energy through interactions with surrounding molecules before combining with an electron causing an annihilation event to occur. The annihilation results in the emission of two 511 keV photons emitted 180° apart (±0.25°)

Fig. 8.2 Types of events detected in coincidence. A true event would provide correct localization of the annihilation site; if one or both of the annihilation photons undergo Compton scatter in the tissue and change direction, the event is considered scattered; a random event occurs when two separate decays each contribute a photon to be detected

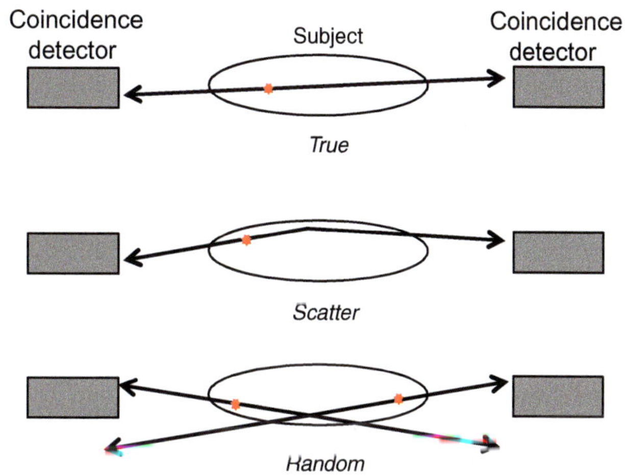

PET many times higher than SPECT for a comparable midplane resolution.

8.1.3 Types of Events Detected by a PET Scanner

Events from coincidence detection can be categorized into three groups: trues (signal), scatter (background), and randoms (background). Figure 8.2 shows a diagram of a positron source emitting inside of a scattering medium. Ideally, during the detection process, two separate annihilation events would not overlap in time, and photons would not scatter within the body—events meeting these criteria would be considered true events. If either of the two annihilation photons undergoes a Compton scatter interaction before reaching the detector, the event is designated a scattered event. If two decays occur close in time, each contributing at least one photon to be detected, the event is considered a random. Unlike true events, which do not scatter within the body or overlap in time, scatter and random events reduce image quality by adding background signal to the image and reducing contrast.

Because photons lose energy when they scatter and, in theory, there is a very low probability that two events happen at exactly the same time (within ~10^{-12} s), coincidence logic can perfectly distinguish all true events. The detector's ability to perform coincidence detection is characterized by its energy resolution and timing resolution—parameters that quantify the uncertainty in measuring the photon energy and its time of arrival.

The detector works by creating an electronic pulse when a photon hits the detector. The electronic pulse is then integrated to calculate the total energy deposited. If the detected energy is not 511 keV, the event is typically discarded. Another specialized electronic circuit is used to assign a digital "time stamp" to each detected event. The time stamp is then sent to a coincidence processor, which looks for overlapping coincidences in opposing detectors. If an overlapping time stamp from another detector is found, the event is kept; if no time stamp is found, the event is discarded. A detector with perfect energy resolution and timing resolution would be able to identify all true coincidences and discard any scattered or random events; however, because of the detector's finite resolution, this is not possible in practice.

8.1.4 Time-of-Flight PET

It is possible to measure additional parameters of the positron decay with coincidence detection when using detectors with extremely good timing resolution. A very accurate measurement of the time difference between interactions occurring in the two detectors allows for time-based information to be used to localize the event, as shown in Fig. 8.3. This technique is referred to as time-of-flight PET. The time difference (Δt), between the arrival times of the two coincidence photons, can be related to the location of the annihilation (Δx), with respect to the midpoint between the two detectors, using Eq. 8.1, where c is the speed of light:

$$\Delta x = (\Delta t \times c) / 2 \tag{8.1}$$

A time difference of zero corresponds to the annihilation occurring at the midpoint. The measurement of Δt will have some uncertainty (determined by the detector timing resolution), limiting the precision of Δx. In theory, with perfect timing resolution, image reconstruction would not be needed as all events could be localized in three dimensions with the timing and spatial information from each coincidence detector. As will be discussed later, current clinical whole-body PET scanners achieve a timing resolution of ~375–600 ps, corresponding to a localization uncertainty of about 5.6–9.0 cm; a timing resolution of ~30 ps would be needed for a direct formation of the image without reconstruction. Over the last 10 years, TOF-PET/CT has vastly improved PET imaging quality and capabilities, with all commercial manufacturers offering a TOF-PET/CT scanner model.

8.2 PET Instrumentation

8.2.1 Scintillation Detectors

As described earlier, a PET scanner is designed to detect antiparallel pairs of 511 keV photons originating from positron annihilations and typically consists of a ring of detectors surrounding the imaging subject. The typical role of a detector is to measure the position and energy of the incoming 511 keV photon. Since PET relies on detecting 511 keV photons that occur near in time, PET detectors also need to measure arrival times of the two coincident photons.

The standard PET detector utilizes an inorganic scintillation crystal coupled to a photosensor. The scintillation crystal converts the energy of the ionizing radiation into optical photons that are subsequently detected by the photosensor and converted into an electrical signal. The 511 keV photons interact within the scintillator primarily via photoelectric or Compton interactions and generate electron-hole pairs that transfer this energy to luminescent centers in the scintillator. The process results in the emission of many scintillation (light) photons within a very short time frame (<1 μs). Birks [14] provides a more detailed explanation of this process. An important property of the scintillator is its ability to respond proportionally to the energy deposited by the 511 keV photon, i.e., the number of scintillation photons produced is directly proportional to the

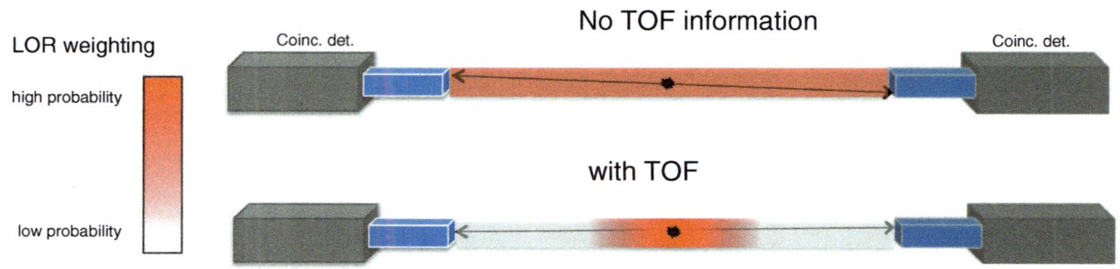

Fig. 8.3 The time-of-flight (*TOF*) information measured through the recorded time difference between the two detectors is incorporated into the image reconstruction model, limiting the event localization probability along the line of response (*LOR*). Without TOF there is a uniform probability applied along the LOR

energy deposited by the 511 keV photon. An ideal PET scintillator should have (i) high density and large atomic number to efficiently stop 511 keV photons with the least amount of scintillator material, (ii) the scintillation light pulse should have fast response to provide high count-rate capability and good timing resolution for rejecting random coincidences, and (iii) high light output and good energy resolution to identify the scattered photons. In addition, the scintillation material should be optically transparent, mechanically rugged, nonhygroscopic, affordable, and easy to produce. While the search for an ideal scintillator is still ongoing [15], amongst currently available scintillators, lutetium-based scintillators such as LSO and LYSO are widely used as they have the best overall characteristics. Their high density (7.1 g/cm^3), high light output (32,000 photons/MeV), and fast response time (decay time = 41 ns) make them appropriate for use in PET [16].

8.2.2 Photosensors

Photomultiplier tubes (PMTs) are the most common photosensor used in scintillation PET detector designs. The PMT is used to convert the scintillation photons into a proportional electrical signal. PMTs are vacuum devices and offer excellent signal-to-noise characteristics for detecting optical photons from scintillators. They are fast, linear, stable, mature, low-noise devices having very high gain (10^6–10^7). While single-channel PMTs have been the standard photosensor used in clinical PET scanners for a long time, these PMTs do not easily permit design of a high spatial resolution detector required for small animal PET. In this scenario, multi-anode (MA) or position-sensitive (PS) PMTs and avalanche photodiodes (APD) provide viable alternatives. In a MA-PMT, a single PMT is segmented into multiple smaller channels with independent anode readout for each channel (N channels along each direction leading to a total of N^2 channels). To decrease the complexity and cost associated with reading out all individual channels of a MA-PMT, a charge-resistive readout network integrated with the PMT anode outputs is sometimes used to encode the interaction position with fewer electronic channels. On the other hand, PS-PMTs utilize a 2D arrangement of cross wired anodes to readout and decode the gamma-ray interaction location. While the MA-PMT has '$N \times N$' readout channels, the PS-PMT only has '$N + N$' readout channels. Unlike PMTs, APDs are solid-state photosensors that are compact, have high quantum efficiency, offer low gamma attenuation, and are insensitive to magnetic fields. APDs are particularly interesting, as they can be made very small and close packed, opening up the possibility of one-to-one coupling of crystal to photosensor that may be needed for developing higher spatial resolution PET detectors.

8.2.3 PET Detector Designs

The first SPECT camera designed by Hal Anger comprised of a single continuous scintillator slab viewed by an array of PMTs and position decoding performed by using a weighted centroid algorithm [17]. Some of the early large-area PET scanners borrowed the same design, albeit with a more appropriate thicker scintillator for PET (Fig. 8.4a). This design is more practical in comparison with the first PET scanners that used a one-to-one coupling scheme with a single PMT to read out a single scintillation crystal [18, 19]. Since then the major detector designs used for clinical PET have relied on using some form of light sharing to decode the gamma-ray interaction location. One approach modifies the original Anger detector to read out an array of pixelated scintillators [20] (Fig. 8.4b). The "block detector" developed in the mid-1980s [21] is another popular design that relies on coupling a scintillator block to four PMTs. Cuts are introduced in the scintillator, and the block is segmented in a careful manner to induce sharing of light between the four PMTs (Fig. 8.4c). A modified version of the block detector concept which uses larger PMTs that overlap adjoining block detectors is known as the quadrant-sharing detector [22]. Higher

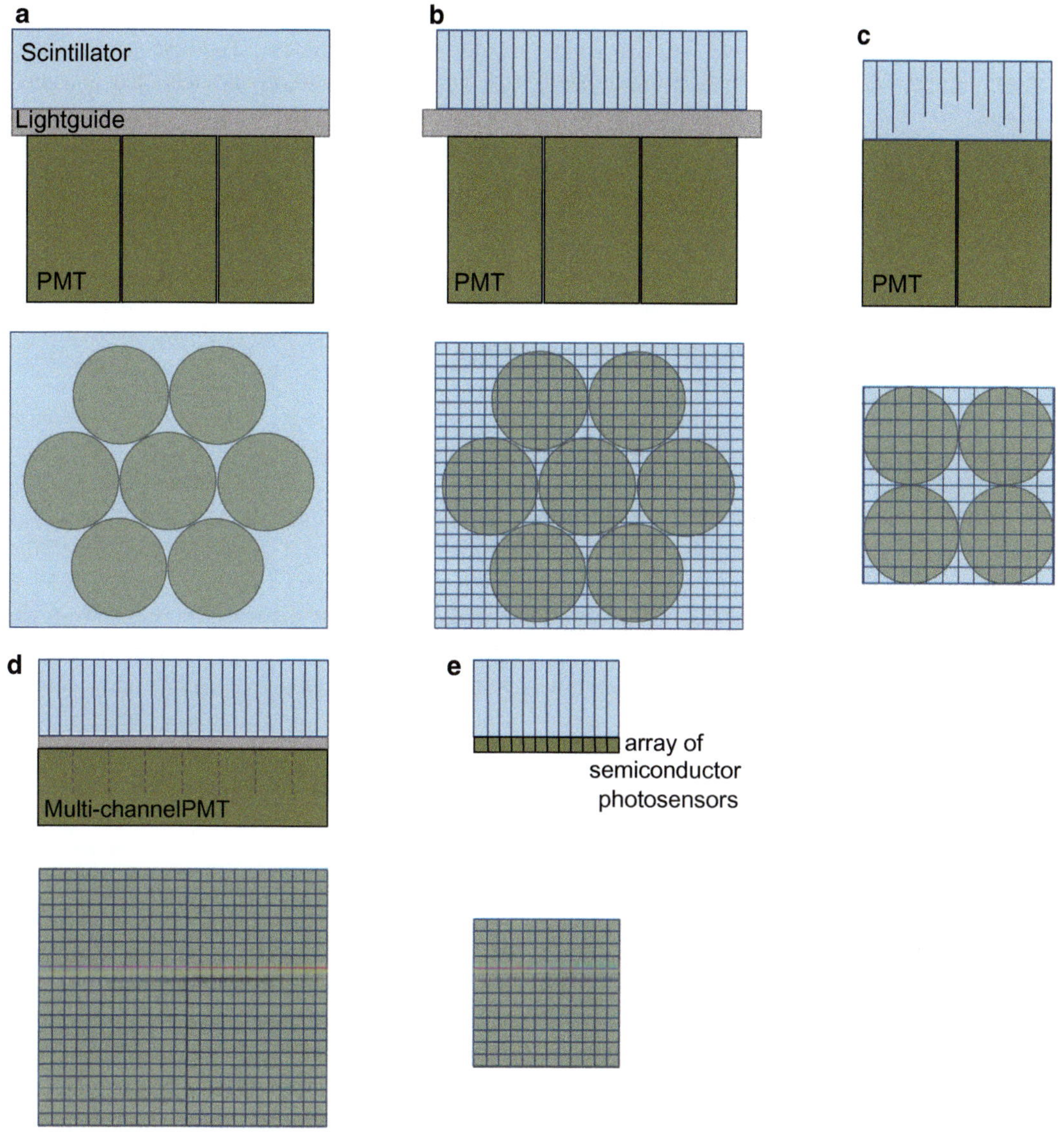

Fig 8.4 Illustration of commonly used PET detector designs used in clinical and preclinical PET scanner designs: (**a**) continuous crystal light-sharing detector, (**b**) pixelated light-sharing detector, (**c**) block detector, (**d**) pixelated light-sharing detector with a multi-anode or position-sensitive PMT, and (**e**) one-to-one coupling detector with an array of solid-state photosensors

spatial resolution detectors required for small animal PET, on the other hand, typically utilize multi-anode or position-sensitive PMTs and APDs in a light-sharing (Fig. 8.4d) or one-to-one coupling design (Fig. 8.4e) configuration [23–29]. Each of the above detector designs has their own merits and trade-offs, but they all provide a practical technique for designing a clinical scanner. Continuous crystal detectors have lower manufacturing costs and offer continuous position sampling, but have limited count-rate capability. The one-to-one or direct coupling detector offers the best count-rate performance but requires a larger number of photosensors and readout electronics, which can increase the scanner complexity and cost. Pixelated light-sharing detectors offer a compromise between count-rate performance and cost. Current whole-body PET/CT scanners typically use pixelated detectors with 4 mm wide crystals, while small animal scanners use 1.5–2 mm wide crystals.

8.2.4 PET Data Acquisition and Signal Processing

The electrical pulse produced by the PET detector undergoes signal conditioning and processing before being handled by the data acquisition system. The PMT outputs are routed to an amplifier and shaper first, before being digitized by an analog to digital convertor (ADC). Since the timing resolution is very sensitive to the scintillation pulse rise time, separate energy (slow) and timing (fast) pathways are typically employed. A sum of all PMT signals belonging to the full or some predetermined portion of the detector is used to determine event energy and time of arrival, while a weighted centroid algorithm is used to compute the interaction position of the 511 keV photon. The calculated interaction position is mapped to scanner coordinates via a pre-computed look-up table that is generated in a separate scanner calibration step. To efficiently use data acquisition transfer rates and decrease scanner dead time, coincidence detection is followed by energy thresholding (via analog or digital energy discriminators). Only coincidences depositing a predefined minimum energy (typically 300–400 keV) are handled. The position, energy, and TOF information for all valid events are stored by the data acquisition and are used later for performing data corrections and PET image generation.

8.2.5 PET System Design and Geometry

While some of the early generation PET systems made use of flat-panel detectors that were rotated around the patient to collect full tomographic data, these designs eventually evolved to using a stationary ring of detectors. Current whole-body PET scanners have an ~90 cm ring diameter and 16–22 cm axial field of view (FOV). All scanners operate in fully 3D mode and require good energy resolution to discard the scattered radiation and fast scintillators to keep up with the expected count rate in these systems. Lutetium-based scintillators like LSO/LYSO are thus attractive and preferred in current PET/CT scanners.

8.3 PET System Characteristics

8.3.1 Sensitivity

PET scanner sensitivity is defined as the fraction of positron annihilation events that are detected in the scanner. The PET scanner is essentially a photon counter, and the statistical noise is inversely proportional to the square root of the number of coincident events it detects. Hence, scanner sensitivity plays an important role in determining image noise or activity concentrations at which imaging can be performed. A high sensitivity scanner would reduce imaging time and/or permit imaging at lower activity concentration, thereby decreasing the injected activity and/or radiation dose. It would also permit dynamic scans with short-lived isotopes and repeated longitudinal studies without exaggerating concerns over administered dose. Scanner sensitivity is determined by two factors: scanner geometric coverage, also referred to as solid angle, and the scintillator stopping power and thickness. Clinical whole-body scanners use 20–30 mm long crystals with ~20 % angular coverage and typically have ~5–6 % sensitivity for a point source at the center. Small animal scanners use 10–15 mm long crystals with ~40 % scanner angular coverage and achieve typical sensitivity values in the range of ~2–7 % for a point source at the center.

8.3.2 Spatial Resolution

Spatial resolution determines the smallest structure that can be clearly visualized, and a scanner with the highest spatial resolution is necessary to resolve the finest details in an object. Two physic processes that arise from positron decay limit spatial resolution in PET scanners: positron range and annihilation photon acollinearity. The positron emitted by the radionuclide has some kinetic energy and therefore travels a short distance from the emission point before annihilating with an electron. This positron range is related to its kinetic energy; for ^{18}F (maximum positron energy = 0.635 MeV), the root mean square value of distanced traveled in water is 0.2 mm, while for ^{82}Rb (maximum positron energy = 3.4 MeV), it is 2.6 mm [30, 31]. Annihilation photon acollinearity arises from the conservation of momentum during the electron-positron annihilation process. Instead of being emitted at exactly 180°, there is a small deviation of ±0.25° on account of some residual kinetic energy the positron-electron pair possesses at the time of annihilation. While the deviation is small, its contribution to the spatial resolution degradation is dependent on the scanner diameter, i.e., the larger the diameter of the scanner, the larger its contribution. For whole-body PET scanners having a diameter of 90 cm, the degradation is ~2 mm, while for small animal scanners with an 18 cm ring diameter, the contribution is ~0.4 mm. In addition to the limits from fundamental positron decay physics, PET scanner spatial resolution is also dependent upon the spatial resolution of the detector. The spatial resolution in pixelated-detector designs is limited by the cross section (width) of the individual crystals used in the PET detector. While a theoretical spatial resolution of half the crystal width can be achieved (for events at the center of the scanner), the finite detector sampling over the FOV often degrades it [32]. There are additional contributions from Compton scattering of the 511 keV photon in the detector and the error in interaction position determination due to the use of light-sharing techniques in the detector. Currently clinical PET scanners for whole-body imaging have a spatial resolution in the range of 4–6 mm [33–35], while small animal scanners have a spatial resolution of 1.5–2 mm [36], both of which are primarily determined by the scintillation crystal widths used in the detector.

An additional source of spatial resolution degradation is from parallax error. Events that occur away from the center of the scanner result in the 511 keV photons no longer traveling perpendicular to the scintillator entrance face. Depending on the scintillator depth at which the 511 keV photon interacts, there is an error in determining the correct line of response (LOR). This LOR mispositioning error is known as parallax error (Fig. 8.5) and degrades the overall spatial resolution as a function of the distance from the center of the scanner. Parallax error is particularly evident in small animal scanners since they make use of small ring diameters and long crystals to improve sensitivity. Clinical whole-body scanners have ~90 cm ring diameter and ~50 cm FOV, making them less susceptible to parallax errors.

8.3.3 Energy Resolution

Energy resolution determines the accuracy with which the scanner can measure the energy of the 511 keV photon interactions and affects the ability to reject scatter coincidences where at least one of the two 511 keV photons has incident energy <511 keV. Current clinical whole-body PET scanners using LSO/LYSO scintillators have ~12 % energy resolution that allows the use of a high event energy acceptance threshold (up to 440 keV), thereby collecting all true coincidences with a small fraction of scattered coincidences as well. The importance of energy resolution is less significant for small animal PET where object scatter from the animal is small relative to that observed in clinical whole-body imaging.

8.3.4 Coincidence Timing Resolution

Since a PET scanner relies on collecting coincident pairs of 511 keV photons, the coincidence detection mechanism is an essential component of a PET scanner. In addition to measuring the interaction location and energy, the PET detector also measures time of arrival for both the coincident 511 keV photons. The time within which coincidence pairs are identified is called the coincidence timing window (τ). A smaller τ

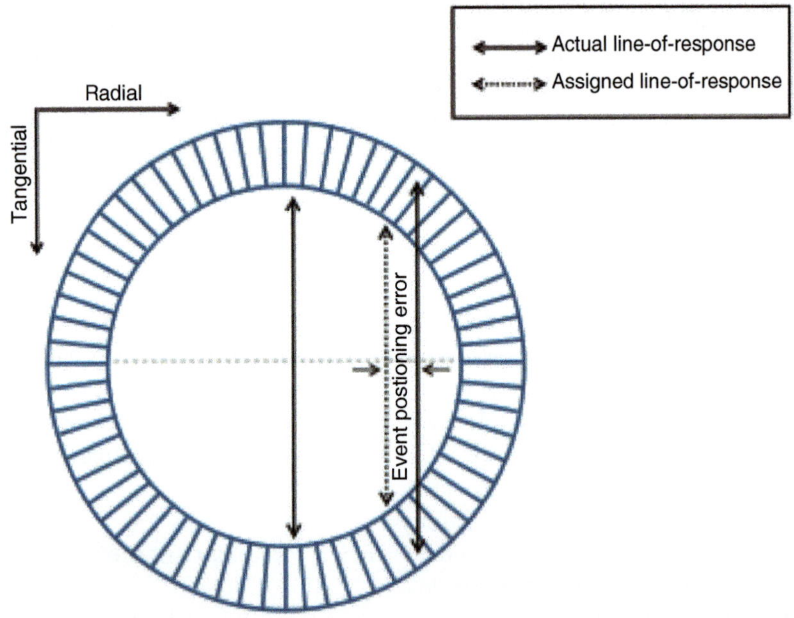

Fig 8.5 Parallax error in a PET scanner: for off-center positron annihilations, there is an error in determining the correct line of response, which degrades the overall spatial resolution of the scanner

will reduce the number of random coincidences collected by the scanner. While the time-of-arrival measurement is fundamentally limited by the timing accuracy of the detector (timing resolution), there is also the path length of the photon to keep in mind. For an annihilation occurring near one detector surface, one of the two 511 keV photon possibly needs to travel much longer before it reaches the detector. In a clinical scanner with ~90 cm ring diameter, it takes the photon ~3 ns to travel this distance. Also, depending on the scanner readout design, either of the two 511 keV photons can be detected first.

8.3.5 Count-Rate Performance

With all scanner designs, there is a minimum amount of time necessary for the scanner to process the event before it is ready to accept another event. This minimum time is referred to as "dead time" and defines the maximum rate at which the scanner can operate. A lower dead-time value (less time in processing events) translates into a higher count-rate capability. While the scanner dead time has contributions from the readout electronics and coincidence processing, it is typically the scintillator conversion process within the detector that primarily limits the overall count-rate performance. A short scintillator signal decay time will allow higher count-rate capability. LSO has an ~40 ns decay time and can provide an average count-rate capability of ~10 million counts/s. Dead time is classified as being either non-paralyzable or paralyzable. A non-paralyzable system will not accept any additional events for processing when it is busy processing an earlier event, and hence all events arriving during this time are simply lost. A paralyzable system on the other hand will process all the events as a single event, increasing the dead time as a result. Dead time arising due to readout electronic limitations is typically non-paralyzable, while scintillator dead time is paralyzable. The count-rate measurement for a scanner is characterized by plotting the measured scanner count rate with a known amount of activity in its FOV. Whatever the mechanism, a scanner with the highest count-rate capability is desirable and remains a priority for PET system designs.

8.4 Multimodality PET/CT

8.4.1 Motivation and Review of Fusion Imaging

Imaging techniques like computed tomography (CT) and magnetic resonance imaging (MRI) offer excellent spatial resolution better than 1 mm and produce exquisite three-dimensional anatomical images. They help in identifying abnormalities based on structural and anatomic changes in the body. While they are well established and are routinely used in the clinic, they provide limited or no physiological information. PET, on the other hand, can measure many different physiological parameters, such as glucose metabolism with ^{18}F-FDG that can help differentiate between malignant and nonmalignant tissue. However, the relatively limited spatial resolution of PET makes it difficult to accurately localize such lesions, especially ones that occur in heterogeneous regions like the abdomen or at organ boundaries. To make the best use of their individual strengths, clinicians in the past viewed images acquired from both modalities separately. Differences in the system spatial resolutions, image pixel sizes, and slice thicknesses limited the accuracy with which information from both modalities could be correlated. Several techniques, such as the use of external fiducial markers and stereotactic methods, were developed to correlate the data with other image sets or to an image atlas [37]. Dedicated fusion software that performed co-registration in a semiautomatic or automatic manner was also devised [38–40]. These techniques improved co-registration accuracy, and software fusion found a larger role, especially in brain imaging, as the brain is a sufficiently rigid organ unaffected by organ motion. For whole-body imaging, these techniques were often laborious and sometimes unfeasible. The longer duration for PET imaging meant that whole-body PET images were inconsistent and their resolution affected due to patient breathing. Involuntary internal organ motion and variability/mismatch in patient positioning due to patient transfer and scanner availability constraints added to their troubles. Subsequently, software-based fusion PET/CT found limited success in routine whole-body PET.

8.4.2 Hardware-Based Multimodality PET/CT

The problems encountered by the software-based approach were addressed by a hardware approach to combine them, one that could provide a fully co-registered PET/CT image in a single imaging session. In PET/CT scanners, the PET and CT data are acquired sequentially on a common bed requiring no additional software alignment. While acquiring the two datasets with a single scanner would have been ideal, it engenders several technological challenges that need to be overcome. Apart from improving the scanner readout electronics and count-rate performance, the most important challenge lies in designing a common detector that would work efficiently for both imaging modalities. The very first multimodality nuclear-imaging scanner was designed in the early 1990s and made use of a single high-purity germanium detector to integrate CT with single-photon emission computed tomography (SPECT) [41]. While the prototype scanner demonstrated single detector feasibility, there were some performance compromises, and it was more challenging to adapt for PET/CT. As opposed to the 511 keV photons emitted by PET tracers, the most commonly used SPECT tracer, i.e., Technetium-99 (^{99m}Tc), generates 140 keV photons, close to the X-ray energies used for CT imaging (40–140 keV). The use of a single detector for a PET/CT scanner necessitates compromises for either or both modalities.

It was not until the late 1990s that the first design for a combined PET/CT scanner was presented [42]. It combined an existing partial-ring PET scanner and an existing CT scanner into a single-gantry scanner with a single bed. Independent consoles were used for scanner control, data acquisitions, and image reconstructions. The PET/CT scanner could be operated either independently (i.e., PET or CT) or in a combined mode with the CT assisting PET imaging. After image reconstruction both the images were sent to a workstation for fused viewing. During normal operation patients were scanned sequentially, first in the CT and then PET. The primary goal of the prototype was to demonstrate the value of a combined scanner providing accurately co-registered PET/CT images. Numerous studies were successfully performed with this prototype that provided sufficient proof of its diagnostic powers and also generated sufficient interest in the clinic [43–47]. Whilst the prototype scanner design was not optimized, it was a significant milestone that spurred the design of next generation PET/CT scanners. Medicare reimbursement approval for certain whole-body FDG-PET scans in 1999 provided further impetus to the utilization and popularity of PET/CT scanners.

By the early 2000s there was enough enthusiasm and clinical evidence for whole-body PET that all major PET vendors began manufacturing and selling PET/CT scanners. Excluding for some variations in the gantry design from each vendor, the commercial PET/CT scanners essentially all include fixed full-ring PET and CT scanners that are melded into a common gantry housing (Fig. 8.6). The individual PET and CT scanners have minimal modifications to potentially offer full performance PET and CT scans, as if they were sold individually. There is typically a gap between the two scanner rings in order to accommodate the scanner readout electronics as well as to minimize the interference (e.g., temperature variations) from each scanner. Care is also taken to match the patient-port sizes for patient comfort. The scanner control and acquisition hardware have better integration than the first prototypes. A common patient couch that traverses the entire axial field of view (FOV) with minimum deflection is key to acquiring accurately co-registered images between the two scanners. Imaging sequences comprise of a short CT scout scan to position the patient within the FOV followed by the CT scan. At the end of the CT scan, the patient couch is translated to the PET FOV and PET imaging begins. Image reconstruction occurs on separate hardware for the PET and CT, each of which is optimized for fast image reconstruction. Proprietary dedicated software to visualize the PET and CT images as overlaid [49–52] or separate images, image analysis, and measurement tools are also provided with the scanner. Figure 8.7 shows an example image acquired with a clinical whole-body PET/CT scanner. As can be seen, the fused PET/CT image improves anatomic localization of lesion within the body.

8.4.3 Attenuation Correction

In PET, the 511 keV photon can interact within the patient and get absorbed or scattered. The linear attenuation coefficient defines this probability of interaction per unit length and is material and photon energy dependent. It increases with the density of the material and decreases with the photon energy. The attenuation probabilities for 511 keV photons is not only dependent on material but also on the object size, i.e., a larger-sized object presents a higher probability of interaction, and the probability is higher for single events near the center than toward its periphery. Attenuation estimation in PET is simplified by the fact that it relies on the detection of both the 511 keV photons that are emitted antiparallel. Let us consider a positron annihilation occurring at depth x in an object with diameter D and linear attenuation μ at 511 keV. The probability (P) that both photons reach the detector is given by the product of their individual transmission probabilities:

$$P = e^{-\mu x} e^{-\mu(D-x)} = e^{-\mu D} \tag{8.2}$$

Thus the total probability is independent of the emission location and only depends on the total path length. The attenuation coefficients for a single LOR can be measured by simply collecting data along that LOR from a known external source placed around the patient. If uncorrected for, attenuation effects produce a nonuniform representation of the true activity distribution, typically observed by a reduced activity in the center of large objects. It can also impair lesion detectability, particularly in heavier patients, as shown in Fig. 8.8.

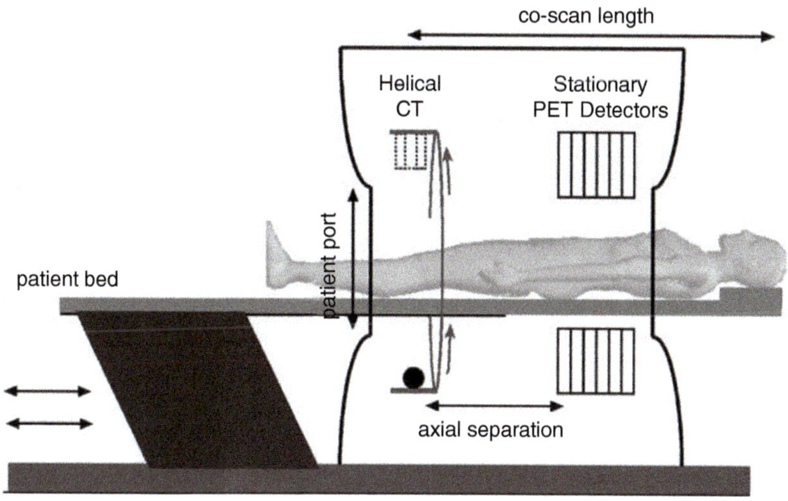

Fig. 8.6 Illustration of current commercial PET/CT scanner designs (Figure reprinted with permission from Alessio et al. [48])

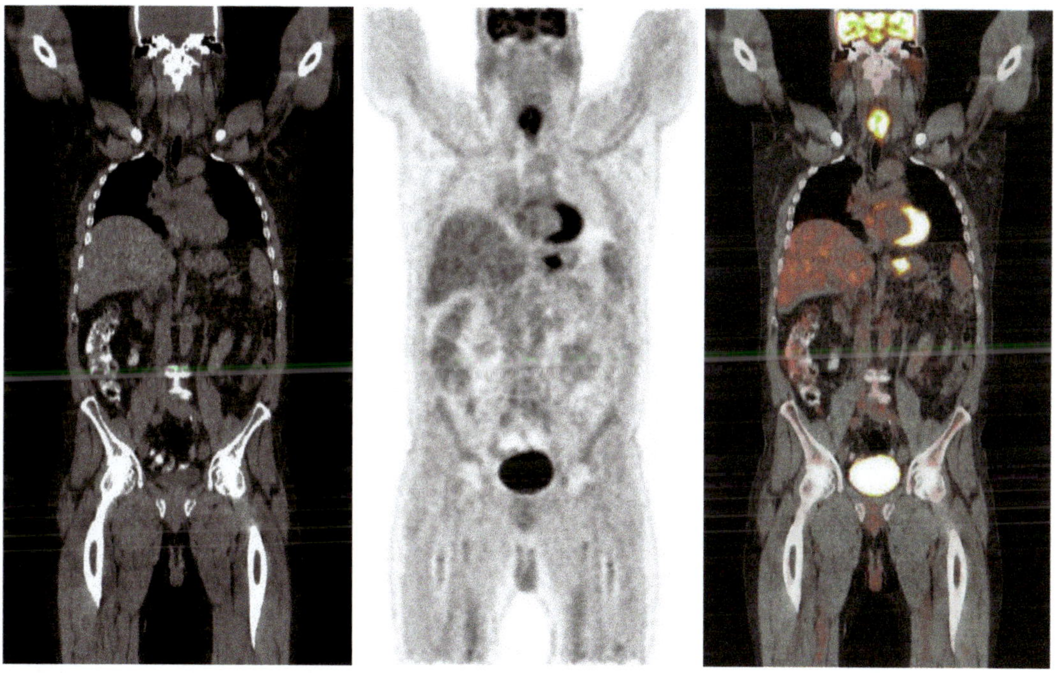

Fig. 8.7 Clinical ^{18}FDG scan images from a whole-body PET/CT scanner. Shown are CT (*left*), PET (*middle*), and fused PET/CT (*right*) images

One of the many advantages offered by multimodality CT is its use for attenuation correction in nuclear-emission imaging. Hasegawa et al. were the first to demonstrate this with their prototype SPECT/CT scanner [41], wherein two separate energy windows were used to collect emission and transmission data simultaneously without interference. The ability to measure attenuation of PET data via CT has even greater significance. Prior to the arrival of PET/CT, PET attenuation was measured by making use of transmission-based methods. A separate

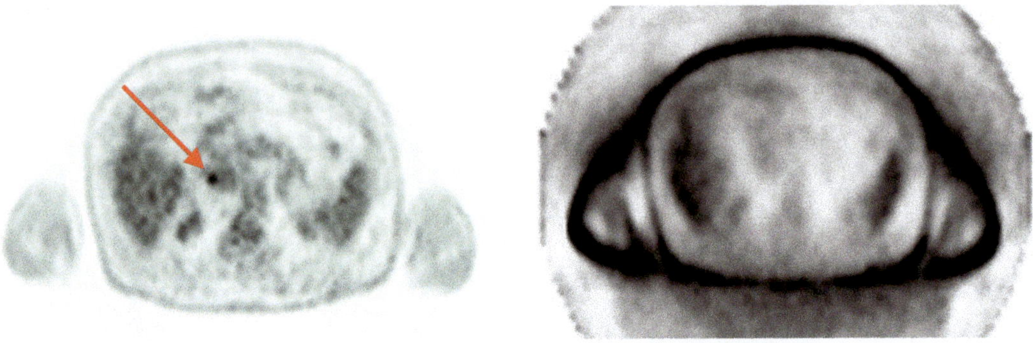

Fig. 8.8 Importance of attenuation correction in PET: Shown are transverse images from a whole-body ^{18}FDG PET scan, with attenuation correction (*left*) and without attenuation correction (*right*). If uncorrected for, attenuation effects can impair lesion detectability (highlighted by the *red arrow*). Images acquired courtesy of the Hospital of the University of Pennsylvania PET Center

transmission scan was measured with a rotating positron or gamma source with the patient laying in the FOV [53, 54]. While each of those techniques had their own merits, the use of a rotating positron source generated the most accurate attenuation map but also introduced statistical noise (on account of counting statistics) into the image reconstruction process. Further reduction of the noise from attenuation estimation required increasing the overall scan time. The availability of CT provides a fast and virtually noise-free alternative to measure the attenuation map. The main concern regarding the use of CT data for PET attenuation lies in the mismatch of energies used for the two measurements. CT scanners use a range of X-ray energies (40–140 keV), and the attenuation values for PET need to be scaled to energy of 511 keV photons. However, at low energies photoelectric interactions dominate, and the CT-measured attenuation depends on both material density and composition. At 511 keV, Compton interactions dominate, and attenuation is primarily dependent on material density alone. Thus a simple scaling of the measured CT attenuation can introduce bias and should not be used for PET. Several techniques using a linear scale factor [55] and a two-layer segmentation and scaling technique [56, 57] have been devised to demonstrate the accuracy in determining attenuation factors from CT [58, 59]. Today, PET/CT scanners are no longer equipped with a rotating source for transmission scanning, and the use of CT for attenuation correction is a standard practice routinely used in clinical PET.

8.4.4 Scatter Correction

The primary mode of interaction for 511 keV photons in the patient is Compton scatter. Compton scattering not only changes the energy of the photon but also alters its direction. The energy and direction of the scattered photon are described by the following equation:

$$E' = \frac{E_\gamma}{1 + \frac{E_\gamma}{m_0 c^2}\left(1 - \cos\theta\right)} \tag{8.3}$$

where E_γ and E' are the energies of the incident (511 keV) and scattered photon, respectively, θ is the scattering angle, and m_0c^2 is the rest mass energy of the electron (511 keV). One or both of the coincident 511 keV photons can undergo single or multiple scattering. If uncorrected, the scattered photons add a background signal to the true activity distribution, lowering image contrast and affecting image quantitation capabilities. Scatter correction techniques can be broadly classified under tail fitting, convolution subtraction, energy based, Monte Carlo, and analytical methods [54]. Amongst them, Monte Carlo-based simulations provide the most accurate estimate but are also very computationally intensive and impractical to implement on a clinical scanner. The most popular and clinically feasible is a model-based technique called the "single scatter simulation" (SSS) [60–64]. The algorithm assumes single scatter (only one of the two coincident photon scatters and it scatters once) to be the most dominant source of degradation and is a reasonable assumption given the improved energy resolution of current PET scanners allowing higher energy threshold (≥400 keV). In this technique, the initial emission activity distribution is based on the uncorrected emission image, and scatter points are distributed within the measured (i.e., patient specific) attenuation image. For each of the scatter points, the Klein-Nishina equation [65] is used to compute its scatter contribution to each of the LORs in the scanner. The scatter estimate for each LOR is a summation of the computed scatter estimate from all scatter points. The absolute scatter distribution is typically derived by using the tails of the emission data to scale the above estimated scatter distribution. Since the initial emission image will be a poor approximation of the actual activity distribution (uncorrected for scatter), this process is repeated iteratively until a stable scatter distribution is achieved.

8.4.5 Randoms Correction

As described earlier, a random coincidence event is an event wherein two uncorrelated photons arrive within the coincidence time interval (τ). The randoms rate (R) in a scanner can be described by

$$R = 2\tau S_1 S_2 \qquad (8.4)$$

where S_1 and S_2 are the single-photon count rates in the two coincident detectors. Randoms correction can be performed based on the single-photon count-rate information (Eq. 8.4) along each LOR. This method called the "singles-based" estimation however requires an accurate knowledge of scanner dead time and detector count rates along each LOR. An alternate technique that is more commonly used for correction of randoms is called the "delayed window technique." In addition to looking for coincidences using the normal coincidence window (τ), it also looks for coincidences using a window that is significantly delayed with respect to the normal coincidence window. Since random coincidences are formed due to random temporal correlation, there should be no true coincidences in the delayed coincidence window (τ_d). While the technique is accurate and simpler for real-time implementation on a scanner, the relatively fewer number of counts can possibly introduce statistical noise in the emission image. Random coincidences are usually stored separately for use during the reconstruction process [54].

8.4.6 Limitations and Issues with PET/CT Imaging

While the improved anatomical localization of lesions, confidence in interpreting scans, and increased clinical throughput have played a significant role in making PET/CT routine, it also has its share of challenges which require attention. Patient movement during the CT scan or in between the CT and PET scans can lead to attenuation correction mismatch and cause artifacts in the PET image. Differences in the respiratory breathing patterns for CT (fast scan performed typically with breath-hold) and PET (longer scan) another area of concern. The use of contrast agents (Fig. 8.9), presence of metallic implants (Fig. 8.10), and areas with significant calcification can generate incorrect attenuation correction factors if not taken into consideration. CT truncation artifacts caused by mismatch between the CT and PET FOV and bias in the CT image caused by beam-hardening effects can also affect the PET data.

8.4.7 Low-Dose CT

Since the dawn of PET/CT, the focus has always been on improving PET scanner performance. With advances in PET detector technology and

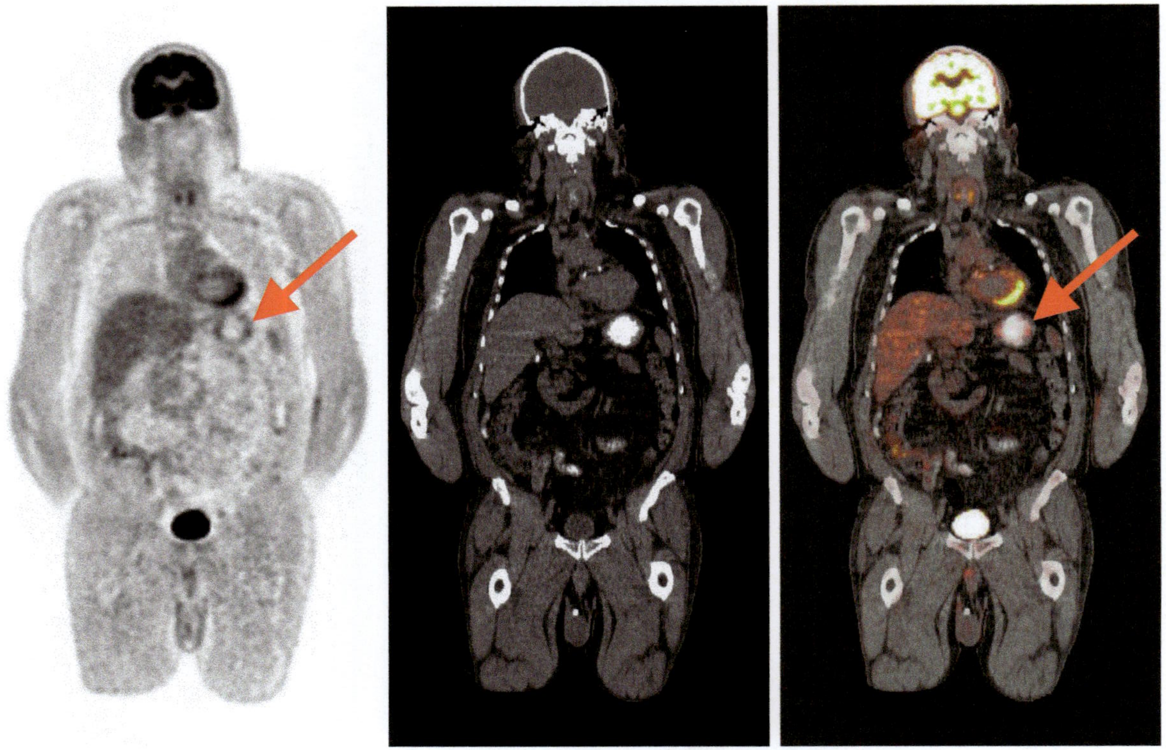

Fig. 8.9 PET artifacts from the use of CT contrast agents in PET/CT: incorrect identification of regions with CT contrast can result in erroneous attenuation correction factors that can affect the PET image. Shown are PET (*left*), CT (*middle*), and fused PET/CT (*right*) images correlating area of CT contrast uptake with radioactivity overestimation (*red arrow*) resulting from IV contrast use. Images acquired courtesy of the Hospital of the University of Pennsylvania PET Center

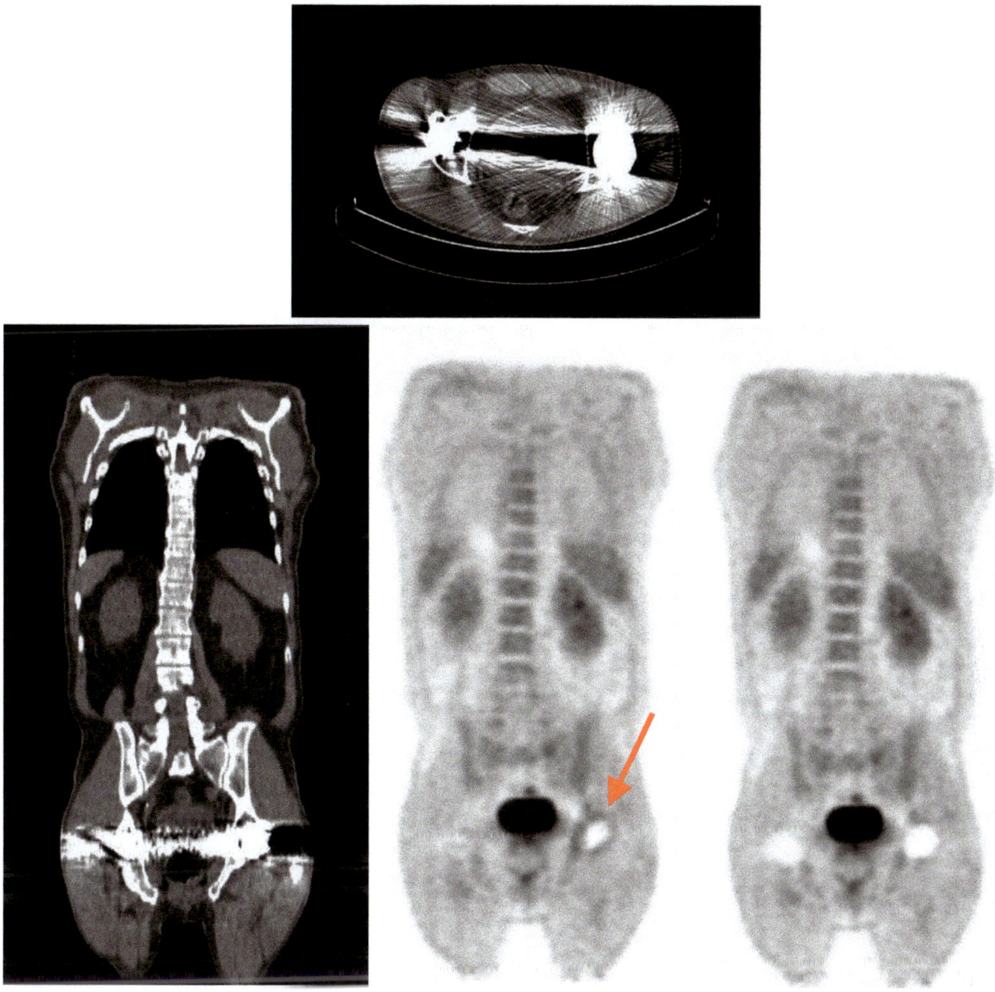

Fig. 8.10 Presence of metallic implants can generate streaking artifacts in CT images, as shown in the transverse (*top*) and coronal (*bottom row left*) CT images from a patient with a hip implant. These artifacts can lead to incorrect estimation of patient attenuation correction factors, and unless corrected for (*bottom row right*), it can lead to incorrect estimation of radioactivity distribution (highlighted by *red arrow* in *bottom row middle*) in the PET image. Images acquired courtesy of the Hospital of the University of Pennsylvania PET Center

scanner design, scan times and image quality have improved significantly. The popularity and effectiveness of PET/CT has led to it being widely used, especially in oncology. The popularity, coupled with the emergence of other multimodality PET devices, has raised concern about the cancer risks associated from receiving additional radiation exposure from CT. The PET improvements have been accompanied by hardware and software improvements in CT that not only improve image quality but also aim to reduce patient dose. Features such as tube current modulation, automatic exposure control, and adaptive collimation lower dose and are now available on many scanners [66–69]. Iterative reconstruction that was impractical previously is now feasible and sufficiently lowers dose without affecting image quality. A full diagnostic CT delivers significantly more dose than one acquired for only assisting the PET. Not only are clinicians making a careful choice here but scanner vendors are also proactively providing options. While the additional dose from CT cannot be completely eliminated, studies have demonstrated that a task-based optimization of imaging parameters can greatly reduce dose without affecting the clinical outcome [70–73].

8.5 Time-of-Flight PET

8.5.1 Simplified Mathematical Approach to SNR Improvement with Time of Flight

The resurgence of TOF-PET imaging, with the current generation of lutetium-based scanner designs, has provided one of the greatest leaps forward in PET imaging capability and image quality to date. The idea of using TOF information in the reconstruction has been around since the very early days of PET. However, TOF detector designs at the time proved to have a large design trade-off in system performance, most notably poor system spatial resolution that was limited by size of the PMT used in the one-to-one coupled detector. Another big issue at the time was the complexity and stability of the system TOF electronics. Both of these factors led to the use of non-TOF, BGO-based scanners that were commercially manufactured from the late 1980s through the early 2000s—though at least one major manufacturer still sells BGO-based PET/CT systems [74]. In the early 1990s, researchers began to investigate new scintillation materials that could provide excellent timing resolution as well as good stopping power. LSO has been the most widely used, but other materials capable of TOF were discovered [75], such as $LaBr_3$ for which a prototype TOF-PET scanner has been constructed [76].

Many studies have now shown that incorporating TOF information into the reconstruction process improves the quality of the PET data. It is perhaps best to conceptualize this improvement by thinking about the back projection and forward projection processes used in tomographic reconstructions. TOF will limit the probability of localization to an area much less than the entire length of the LOR. Overall, this leads to a reduction in image variance as noise will be spread over fewer image voxels, and also by this same assumption, signal will be more tightly confined. Rigorous mathematical approaches to quantifying the improvement in image SNR with TOF have been attempted [77, 78]. However there are limitations in the mathematical definitions used for the source distribution. Ideally one would use source activities and distributions that are typically encountered during clinical imaging, as what we are really interested in is the clinical improvement in TOF-PET imaging. The approximation that is generally accepted to provide the closest correlation with TOF SNR improvement is well described in Budinger [79]. Assuming you have a uniform distribution of activity in a cylinder of diameter D, the image SNR gain near the center is related to the system timing resolution by $\sqrt{\frac{D}{t}}$, where Δt is the system timing resolution.

Because of the Poisson count statistics nature of PET data, one can also view this SNR gain by considering that SNR is proportional to the square root of the total number of events, and therefore an increase in SNR^2 is equivalent to an increase in the number of counts (increase in sensitivity). For this reason, the TOF benefit is often referred to as a sensitivity gain and has been used as an approximate measure to motivate reducing total scan times or lowering patient dose by using a lower amount of injected activity.

8.5.2 Instrumentation Advances Leading to the Reemergence of TOF-PET

There have been several important instrumentation advances that led to the resurgence of TOF: the introduction of LSO as a scintillator used in PET, advances in the system electronics, and improvements in PMT technology. The timing resolution of a scintillator depends on the scintillation pulse temporal characteristics and its total light output. Soon after the discovery of LSO, it was realized that its high light output, short decay time, and fast rise time would allow for a timing resolution comparable to BaF_2 (the scintillator used in first-generation TOF-PET scanners), without sacrificing other performance characteristics, such as sensitivity and spatial resolution, which are critical for PET [80].

By the late 1990s, bench-top measurements from various research groups had shown that coincidence timing resolution on the order of ~400 ps could be achieved with LSO crystals coupled to commonly used single-channel PMTs [81]. During this time, LSO was also being pursued for use in fully 3D PET, and in 2001 the first commercial whole-body PET scanner was introduced. It was shown that LSO has a clear advantage over BGO in fully 3D PET; however, the system achieved a timing resolution of ~3 ns [82]—an improvement over BGO systems but not capable of TOF reconstruction. Though the scintillation light pulse from LSO was capable of resolutions needed for TOF, the system electronics of the PET scanner could not process events to that degree of timing accuracy. Over the next several years (2001–2006), significant upgrades to the PET system electronics were made allowing the full benefit of LSO timing properties to be used [33]. New PMT technology was also implemented into the later TOF scanner designs, which focused on improved timing performance of the PMT itself and better quantum efficiency [83]. It is also worth mentioning, that even though the fundamental detector module design did not drastically change, a crystal-by-crystal timing correction was implemented, as well as methods for system timing calibration [84–86].

8.5.3 Benefits of TOF Information for Clinical PET Imaging

It is perhaps most straightforward to quantify the TOF benefit in phantom studies where the source distributions are simple, having known locations and activity concentrations. Based on results from these experiments, it is obvious that TOF has improved the quality of the data. However, the more important and relevant question is to understand the degree of this improvement in clinical imaging studies—this is a much more difficult problem [87, 88]. No single metric, such as the SNR gain discussed previously, can describe the benefit of TOF-PET in clinical studies; primarily because clinical imaging tasks are different from imaging uniform phantoms, and the use of iterative reconstruction algorithms, which have become standard in clinical imaging, have varying parameter settings and trade-offs that need to be considered.

In clinical use, TOF information independently improves several components of the PET imaging process—from reducing the impact of errors in data correction to improving the detection and quantification of lesions in oncology imaging and lowering patient dose. It has been observed that TOF-PET data, compared to non-TOF-PET data, is much more robust and less sensitive to errors in applied data corrections, such as attenuation, scatter, and normalization [89]. As an example, Fig. 8.11 shows a comparison of TOF vs non-TOF reconstructions with a shifted attenuation correction map. Artifacts are produced in the non-TOF image due to the mismatch between emission data and the attenuation map. However, with TOF information, these incorrect areas of increased or decreased uptake are reduced.

Another important benefit of TOF-PET data for clinical imaging is the improved convergence observed in iterative reconstruction methods. Shown in Fig. 8.12 are contrast recovery coefficients for lesions using reconstruction algorithms with and without TOF information. Though an absolute quantification of the lesion is difficult, and will vary from patient to patient, the improved convergence of the TOF reconstruction generally provides a better trade-off between lesion contrast and noise [87].

Improved lesion contrast and noise trade-off with TOF-PET naturally results in improved oncology imaging where the primary task of PET is to detect and quantify the uptake of cancer lesions [90]. This was demonstrated for clinical studies by Surti et al. [91] using a lesion insertion technique, to create artificial images from clinical patient data mixed with known lesion locations and activities, and human observes to quantify the impact of TOF-PET on whole-body oncologic studies over non-TOF-PET. The methodology was then extended to study the improvement in accuracy and precision of lesion uptake with

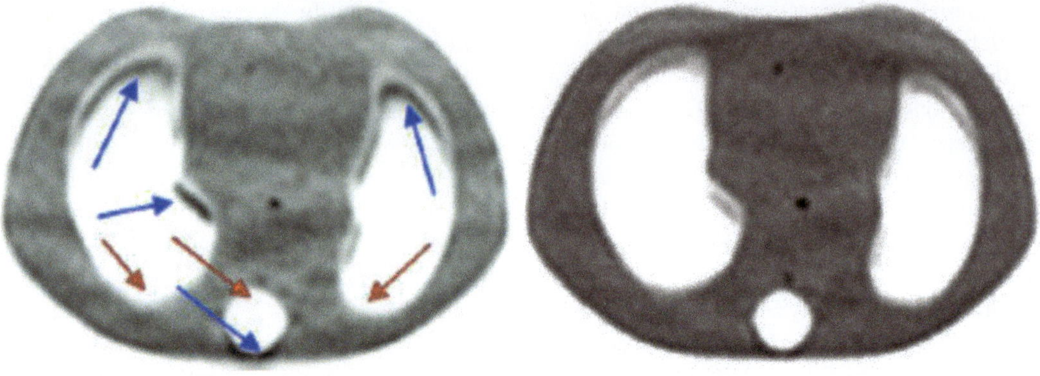

Fig. 8.11 Non-TOF (*left*) and TOF (*right*) images of a thorax phantom using a shifted attenuation correction map. *Arrows* in the non-TOF image indicate incorrect areas of increased and decreased counts (Figure reprinted with permission from [89])

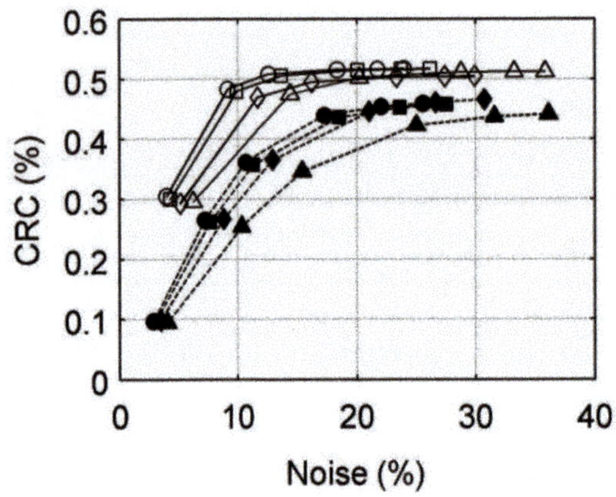

Fig. 8.12 CRC vs noise curves for 17-mm hot spheres with 6:1 contrast in a 35-cm diameter cylinder. Scan times were 2 (σ), 3 (υ), 4 (ν), and 5 (λ) min (35-cm phantom) with closed symbols for non-TOF and open symbols for TOF reconstruction as a function of number of iterations (1, 2, 5, 10, 15, and 20) (Figure reprinted with permission from [87])

TOF-PET [92] and also demonstrated further improvement with better TOF resolution of the scanner.

Another benefit of TOF-PET in clinical imaging is the improvement observed in reconstructed images of larger body mass index (BMI) patients, as shown in Fig. 8.13. This is important because TOF-PET, compared to non-TOF-PET, provides a more uniform clinical performance over a wide range of patient sizes leading to more consistent image quality in all studies. This result is also consistent with the expected SNR gain due to TOF being proportional to $\sqrt{\frac{D}{t}}$.

The TOF gain in larger patients will be higher, and this offsets the effects of increased scatter and attenuation in these patients, which roughly equates to the image quality observed in average size patients.

Lastly, except for benefits in data corrections, the improvement from TOF-PET can generally be replicated by increasing the number of counts used in the reconstruction; without TOF this can only be done by either increasing the scan time or increasing the injected activity—both of these are undesirable in the clinical application of PET. Conversely, while keeping image quality constant, improving TOF will allow for reduced scan times and injected activities leading to a higher patient throughput and lower patient dose. Most clinical imaging protocols using TOF-PET already benefit from lower scan times and resulting in better patient throughput. Further improvement in scanner TOF resolution will yield higher gains in patient throughput. It is anticipated that new generations of TOF-PET scanners with timing resolutions ranging from 350–400 ps will therefore use their improved TOF capability to lower patient dose. In [93], a more detailed summary of the benefits of TOF imaging for clinical imaging is provided.

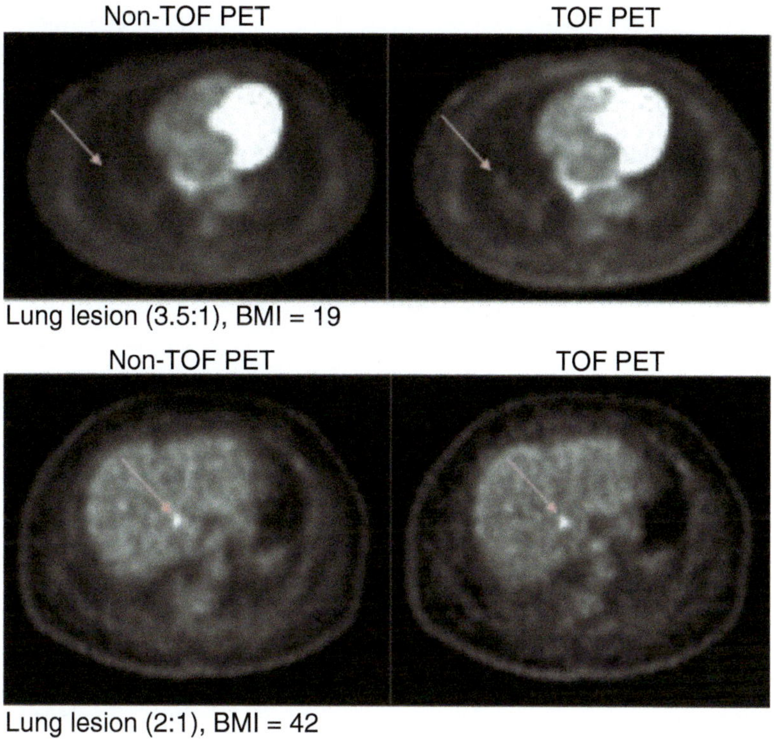

Fig. 8.13 "Lesion present" (*arrow*) transverse slices showing a lung lesion in a subject patient with normal BMI = 19 (*top*) and a liver lesion (*2:1*) in a patient with a BMI = 42 (*bottom*) (Figure reprinted with permission from [90])

8.6 Advances and Future Directions

8.6.1 Silicon Photomultiplier and Its Impact

Basic PET detector design has not changed significantly in more than two decades. However, advances in scintillator, photosensor technology, and data acquisition/electronics design have made clinical PET imaging faster and of higher image quality. While PMT technology continues to improve and is the standard photosensor used in clinical PET, solid-state photosensor technology is also maturing rapidly. An exciting development over the last decade has been the introduction of silicon photomultipliers (SiPMs). SiPMs are solid-state devices that combine the best properties of PMTs and APDs. They are compact, fast, high gain, low noise, and insensitive to magnetic fields [94, 95]. Hence they allow design of fast, high spatial resolution PET detectors that are not only TOF capable but can also operate in high-strength magnetic field. In recent years, a number of research scanners that utilize the advantages of SiPMs in a light-sharing detector design or 1:1 coupling (Fig. 8.4) have been developed [96]. In fact, SiPM-based whole-body PET scanners having system timing resolution of 300–400 ps are already commercially available [97, 98].

8.6.2 Multimodality PET/MR

The complementary information collected from PET and other established imaging modalities such as CT and MRI has always attracted a multimodality approach to combining them. While PET/MR was envisioned before PET/CT, the rapid success of combined PET/CT reinvigorated scientists into looking at ways to combine PET and MRI into a single imaging modality. While a detailed description of the challenges, strategies, and applications of multimodality PET/MR is provided in Chap. 9, it is important to note that unlike PET/CT, PET/MR was first made available for preclinical use [96]. It was not until the mid-2000s when APD technology matured that it became available, first for dedicated brain imaging [99] and then a few years later for whole-body PET/MR imaging [100]. Due to the noise properties of APDs, these APD-based PET/MR scanners are not TOF capable. However, rapid adoption of SiPM technology has now enabled development of clinical TOF-PET/MR scanners and made them commercially available [98].

8.6.3 Organ-Specific Imaging

Current whole-body PET has a spatial resolution of about 4–6 mm. This is a serious limitation, especially for imaging smaller organs where one often encounters smaller structures and lesions. The use of a dedicated scanner offers several benefits. Due to the size of the organs, the scanner diameter can be reduced. The lower amount of scintillator reduces scanner cost, and the larger geometric coverage increases the scanner sensitivity. While the smaller diameter can cause parallax errors, there is also a decrease in contribution from positron acollinearity. Overall, a dedicated scanner can improve image quality and quantitation by offering higher spatial resolution and sensitivity at lower cost. Dedicated PET scanners were first developed for brain imaging [101–104], but the introduction of dedicated or multimodality PET/MRI [99] has reduced enthusiasm for stand-alone brain PET scanners. Dedicated breast PET however has continued to garner attention with a few research scanners demonstrating better and accurate lesion detection, especially in patients with dense breasts [105].

8.6.4 Direct Conversion Detectors

While scintillators are more efficient in stopping the 511 keV photons, direct gamma-ray conversion detectors making use of cadmium telluride (CdTe) or cadmium zinc telluride (CZT) are now also more widely available. They offer excellent energy resolution (~3 % at 511 keV) and can be highly segmented to offer high (<1 mm) spatial resolution. Although the technology has not been translated for whole-body clinical PET, they appear promising for small animal PET due to the potential for achieving very high and uniform spatial resolution [106–109].

8.7 Summary

PET instrumentation and system design have seen a continuous evolution ever since the first systems were conceived. System spatial resolution has improved by an order of magnitude for clinical imaging. In parallel, system sensitivity has increased with the scanner designs utilizing longer axial coverage and higher-efficiency detectors. Reintroduction of TOF imaging in recent years without any performance trade-offs in terms of system spatial resolution and sensitivity has further transformed the performance of these systems. Combined with a CT scanner, modern TOF-PET/CT produces very high quality and quantitative images in imaging times of <10 min. New technical developments are ongoing that promise further gains not only in PET performance but also opening of new imaging areas.

References

1. Anger HO. Gamma-ray and positron scintillation camera. Nucleonics. 1963;21:10–56.
2. Brownell GL, et al. New developments in positron scintigraphy and the application of cyclotron produced positron emitters In: Medical Radioisotope Scintigraphy; 1969; IAEA (Proceedings Series), Vienna. p. 163–76.
3. Kuhl DE, Edwards RQ. Cylindrical and section radioisotope scanning of the liver and brain. Radiology. 1964;83(5):926–36.
4. Cormack AM. Representation of a function by its line integrals, with some radiological applications. J Appl Phys. 1963;34(9):2722–7.
5. Phelps ME, et al. Design considerations for a positron emission transaxial tomograph (PET III). IEEE Trans Nucl Sci. 1976;23(1):516–22.
6. Cho ZH, Farukhi MR. Bismuth germanate as a potential scintillation detector in positron cameras. J Nucl Med. 1977;18(8):840–4.
7. Terpogossian MM, et al. Design considerations for a positron emission transverse tomograph (pett-V) for

imaging of brain. J Comput Assist Tomogr. 1978; 2(5):539–44.
8. Bohm C, Eriksson L, Bergstrom M, Litton J, Sundman R, Singh M. A computer assisted ring detector positron camera system for reconstruction tomography of the brain. IEEE Trans Nucl Sci. 1978;NS-25:624–37.
9. Thompson CJ, Yamamoto YL, Meyer E. Positome II: a high efficiency positron imaging device for dynamic brain studies. IEEE Trans Nucl Sci. 1979; 26(1):583–9.
10. Derenzo SE, et al. Imaging properties of a positron tomograph with 280-Bgo-crystals. IEEE Trans Nucl Sci. 1981;28(1):81–9.
11. Cho ZH, et al. High-resolution circular ring positron tomograph with dichotomic sampling: Dichotom-I. Phys Med Biol. 1983;28(11):1219–34.
12. Wong WH, et al. Performance characteristics of the University of Texas TOF PET-I camera. J Nucl Med. 1984;25(5):46–7.
13. Burnham CA, Bradshaw J, Kaufman D, Chesler DA, Brownell GL. Positron tomograph employing a one dimension BGO scintillation camera. IEEE Trans Nucl Sci. 1983;30:661–4.
14. Birks JB. The theory and practice of scintillation counting. London: Pergamon Press; 1964.
15. Derenzo SE, et al. The quest for the ideal inorganic scintillator. Nucl Instrum Methods Phys Res Sect A: Accelerators Spectrometers Detectors and Associated Equipment. 2003;505(1-2):111–7.
16. Saint-Gobain Crystals. LYSO/Prelude420 datasheet. 2015. Available from: http://www.crystals.saint-gobain.com/uploadedFiles/SG-Crystals/Documents/PreLude420datasheet.pdf.
17. Anger HO. Scintillation camera. Rev Sci Instrum. 1958;29(1):27–33.
18. Ter-Pogossian MM, et al. A positron-emission transaxial tomograph for nuclear imaging (PETT). Radiology. 1975;114(1):89–98.
19. Hoffman EJ, et al. Design and performance-characteristics of a whole-body positron transaxial tomograph. J Nucl Med. 1976;17(6):493–502.
20. Surti S, et al. Optimizing the performance of a PET detector using discrete GSO crystals on a continuous lightguide. IEEE Trans Nucl Sci. 2000;47:1030–6.
21. Casey ME, Nutt R. A multicrystal two dimensional BGO detector system for positron emission tomography. IEEE Trans Nucl Sci. 1986;33(1):460–3.
22. Wong W-H, et al. A 2-dimensional detector decoding study on BGO arrays with quadrant sharing photomultipliers. IEEE Trans Nucl Sci. 1994;41(4):1453–7.
23. Lightstone AW, et al. A Bismuth Germanate-avalanche photodiode module designed for use in high resolution positron emission tomography. IEEE Trans Nucl Sci. 1986;33(1):456–9.
24. Watanabe M, et al. A high resolution PET for animal studies. IEEE Trans Med Imaging. 1992;11:577–80.
25. Watanabe M, et al. A compact position-sensitive detector for PET. IEEE Trans Nucl Sci. 1995;42(4): 1090–4.
26. Cherry SR, et al. MicroPET: a high resolution PET scanner for imaging small animals. IEEE Trans Nucl Sci. 1997;44:1161–6.
27. Lecomte R, et al. Design and engineering aspects of a high-resolution positron tomograph for small animal imaging. IEEE Trans Nucl Sci. 1994;41(4): 1446–52.
28. Ziegler SI, et al. A prototype high-resolution animal positron tomograph with avalanche photodiode arrays and LSO crystals. Eur J Nucl Med. 2001; 28(2):136–43.
29. Vaska P, et al. RatCAP: miniaturized head-mounted PET for conscious rodent brain imaging. IEEE Trans Nucl Sci. 2004;51(5):2718–22.
30. Derenzo SE. Mathematical removal of positron range blurring in high-resolution tomography. IEEE Trans Nucl Sci. 1986;33(1):565–9.
31. Levin CS, Hoffman EJ. Calculation of positron range and its effect on the fundamental limit of positron emission tomography system spatial resolution. Phys Med Biol. 1999;44(3):781–99.
32. Brooks RA, et al. Sampling requirements and detector motion for positron emission tomography. IEEE Trans Nucl Sci. 1979;NS-26:2760–3.
33. Surti S, et al. Performance of Philips Gemini TF PET/CT scanner with special consideration for its time-of-flight imaging capabilities. J Nucl Med. 2007;48(3):471–80.
34. Bettinardi V, et al. Physical performance of the new hybrid PET/CT discovery-690. Med Phys. 2011;38(10):5394–411.
35. Jakoby BW, et al. Physical and clinical performance of the mCT time-of-flight PET/CT scanner. Phys Med Biol. 2011;56(8):2375–89.
36. Goertzen AL, et al. NEMA NU 4-2008 comparison of preclinical PET imaging systems. J Nucl Med. 2012;53(8):1300–9.
37. Bergstrom M, et al. Determination of object contour from projections for attenuation correction in cranial positron emission tomography. J Comput Assist Tomogr. 1982;6(2):365–72.
38. Hill DL, et al. Medical image registration. Phys Med Biol. 2001;46(3):R1–45.
39. Hutton BF, Braun M. Software for image registration: algorithms, accuracy, efficacy. Semin Nucl Med. 2003;33(3):180–92.
40. Slomka PJ. Software approach to merging molecular with anatomic information. J Nucl Med. 2004;45: 36S–45.
41. Lang TF, et al. Description of a prototype emission-transmission computed tomography imaging system. J Nucl Med. 1992;30(10):1881–7.
42. Beyer T, et al. A combined PET/CT scanner for clinical oncology. J Nucl Med. 2000;41(8):1369–79.
43. Charron M, et al. Image analysis in patients with cancer studied with a combined PET and CT scanner. Clin Nucl Med. 2000;25(11):905–10.
44. Kluetz PG, et al. Combined PET/CT imaging in oncology. Impact on patient management. Clin Positron Imaging. 2000;3(6):223–30.

45. Meltzer CC, et al. Whole-body FDG PET imaging in the abdomen: value of combined PET/CT. J Nucl Med. 2001;42(5):35p.
46. Meltzer CC, et al. Combined FDG PET/CT imaging in head and neck cancer: impact on patient management. J Nucl Med. 2001;42(5):36p.
47. Yeung HW, Schoder H, Larson SM. Utility of PET/CT for assessing equivocal PET lesions in oncology-initial experience. J Nucl Med. 2002;43:32P.
48. Alessio AM, et al. PET/CT scanner instrumentation, challenges, and solutions. In: Alavi A, editor. PET imaging I. Philadelphia: W. B. Saunders Company; 2004. p. 1017–32.
49. Rhem K, et al. Display of merged multimodality brain images using interleaved pixels with independent color scales. J Nucl Med. 1994;35(11):1815–21.
50. Hutton BF, et al. Image registration: an essential tool for nuclear medicine. Eur J Nucl Med. 2002;29(4):559–77.
51. Stokking R, Zubal G, Viergever MA. Display of fused images: methods, interpretation, and diagnostic improvements. Semin Nucl Med. 2003;33(3):219–27.
52. Baum KG, Helguera M, Krol A. Fusion viewer: a new tool for fusion and visualization of multimodal medical data sets. J Digit Imaging. 2008;21(1):59–68.
53. Bailey DL. Transmission scanning in emission tomography. Eur J Nucl Med. 1998;25(7):774–87.
54. Valk PE, et al., editors. Positron emission tomography: basic science and clinical practice. London: Springer; 2003.
55. LaCroix KJ, et al. Investigation of the use of X-ray CT images for attenuation compensation in SPECT. IEEE Trans Nucl Sci. 1994;41(6):2793–9.
56. Kinahan PE, et al. Attenuation correction for a combined 3D PET/CT scanner. Med Phys. 1998; 25(10):2046–53.
57. Kinahan PE, Hasegawa BH, Beyer T. X-ray-based attenuation correction for positron emission tomography/computed tomography scanners. Semin Nucl Med. 2003;33(3):166–79.
58. Nakamoto Y, et al. PET/CT: comparison of quantitative tracer uptake between germanium and CT transmission attenuation-corrected images. J Nucl Med. 2002;43(9):1137–43.
59. Burger C, et al. PET attenuation coefficients from CT images: experimental evaluation of the transformation of CT into PET 511-keV attenuation coefficients. Eur J Nucl Med Mol Imaging. 2002;29(7):922–7.
60. Ollinger JM. Model-based scatter correction for fully 3D PET. Phys Med Biol. 1996;41(1):153–76.
61. Watson CC, Newport D, Casey ME. A single scatter simulation technique for scatter correction in 3D PET. Three-Dimens Image Reconstr Radiol Nucl Med. 1996;4:255–68.
62. Accorsi R, et al. Optimization of a fully 3D single scatter simulation algorithm for 3D PET. Phys Med Biol. 2004;49(12):2577–98.
63. Werner ME, Surti S, Karp JS. Implementation and evaluation of a 3D PET single scatter simulation with TOF modeling. In: 2006 IEEE Nuclear Science Symposium and Medical Imaging Conference, San Diego; 2006.
64. Watson CC. Extension of single scatter simulation to scatter correction of time-of-flight PET. IEEE Trans Nucl Sci. 2007;54(5):1679–86.
65. Knoll GF. Radiation detection and measurement. 4th ed. Hoboken: Wiley; 2010.
66. Kalender WA, Wolf H, Suess C. Dose reduction in CT by anatomically adapted tube current modulation. II phantom measurements. Med Phys. 1999;26(11):2248–53.
67. McCollough CH, Bruesewitz MR, Kofler JM. CT dose reduction and dose management tools: overview of available options. Radiographics. 2006;26(2):503–12.
68. Tzedakis A, et al. The effect of z overscanning on patient effective dose from multidetector helical computed tomography examinations. Med Phys. 2008;32(6):1621–9.
69. Deak PD, et al. Effects of adaptive section collimation on patient radiation dose in multisection spiral CT. Radiology. 2009;252(1):140–7.
70. Elstrom RL, et al. Combined PET and low-dose, noncontrast CT scanning obviates the need for additional diagnostic contrast-enhanced CT scans in patients undergoing staging or restaging for lymphoma. Ann Oncol. 2008;19(10):1770–3.
71. Alessio AM, et al. Weight-based, low-dose pediatric whole-body PET/CT protocols. J Nucl Med. 2009;50(10):1570–7.
72. Xia T, et al. Ultra-low dose CT attenuation correction for PET/CT. Phys Med Biol. 2012;2012(57):2.
73. Tonkopi E, Ross AA, MacDonald A. CT dose optimization for whole-body PET/CT examinations. Am J Roentgenol. 2013;201(2):257–63.
74. Lewellen TK, Time-of-flight PET. Semin Nucl Med. 1998;28(3):268–75.
75. Conti M, et al. Comparison of fast scintillators with TOF PET potential. IEEE Trans Nucl Sci. 2009; 56(3):926–33.
76. Daube-Witherspoon ME, et al. Imaging performance of a $LaBr_3$-based time-of-flight PET scanner. Phys Med Biol. 2010;55:45–64.
77. Tomitani T. Image reconstruction and noise evaluation in photon time-of-flight assisted positron emission tomography. IEEE Trans Nucl Sci. 1981;28(6):4582–9.
78. Surti S, et al. Investigation of time-of-flight benefit for fully 3-D PET. IEEE Trans Med Imaging. 2006;25(5):529–38.
79. Budinger TF. Time-of-flight positron emission tomography – status relative to conventional PET. J Nucl Med. 1983;24(1):73–6.
80. Moses WW. Time of flight in PET revisited. IEEE Trans Nucl Sci. 2003;50(5):1325–30.
81. Moses WW, Derenzo SE. Prospects for time-of-flight PET using LSO scintillator. IEEE Trans Nucl Sci. 1999;46(3):474–8.

82. Spinks TJ, Bloomfield PM. A comparison of count rate performance for 15O-water blood flow studies in the CTI HR+ and Accel tomographs in 3D mode. In: IEEE Nuclear Science Symposium and Medical Imaging Conference, Norfolk; 2002.
83. Moszynski M, et al. New Photonis XP20D0 photomultiplier for fast timing in nuclear medicine. Nucl Instrum Meth A. 2006;567(1):31–5.
84. Thompson CJ, Camborde M-L, Casey ME. A central positron source to perform the timing alignment of detectors in a PET scanner. IEEE Trans Nucl Sci. 2005;52(5):1300–4.
85. Perkins AE, et al. Time of flight coincidence timing calibration techniques using radioactive sources. In: 2005 IEEE Nuclear Science Symposium and Medical Imaging Conference, San Juan; 2005.
86. Lenox MW, et al. Digital time alignment of high resolution PET Inveon block detectors. In: IEEE Nuclear Science Symposium and Medical Imaging Conference, San Diego; 2006.
87. Karp JS, et al. Benefit of time-of-flight in PET: experimental and clinical results. J Nucl Med. 2008;49(3):462–70.
88. Lois C, et al. An assessment of the impact of incorporating time-of-flight information into clinical PET/CT imaging. J Nucl Med. 2010;51:237–45.
89. Conti M. Why is TOF PET reconstruction a more robust method in the presence of inconsistent data? Phys Med Biol. 2011;56:155–68.
90. El Fakhri G, et al. Improvement in lesion detection with whole-body oncologic TOF-PET. J Nucl Med. 2011;52:347–53 (* joint first authors).
91. Surti S, et al. Impact of time-of-flight PET on whole-body oncologic studies: a human observer lesion detection and localization study. J Nucl Med. 2011;52(5):712–9.
92. Daube-Witherspoon ME, et al. Determination of accuracy and precision of lesion uptake measurements in human subjects with time-of-flight PET. J Nucl Med. 2014;55:602–7.
93. Surti S. Update on time-of-flight PET imaging. J Nucl Med. 2015;56(1):98–105.
94. Buzhan P, et al. Silicon photomultiplier and its possible applications. Nucl Inst Methods Phys Res A. 2003;504(1–3):48–52.
95. Degenhardt C, et al. The digital Silicon Photomultiplier — A novel sensor for the detection of scintillation light. In: 2009 IEEE Nuclear Science Symposium Conference Record (NSS/MIC), Orlando; 2009.
96. Vandenberghe S, Marsden PK. PET-MRI: a review of challenges and solutions in the development of integrated multimodality imaging. Phys Med Biol. 2015;60:R115.
97. Miller M, et al. Initial characterization of a prototype digital photon counting PET system. Soc Nucl Med Ann Meet Abstr. 2014;55:658.
98. Levin C, et al. Initial results of simultaneous whole-body ToF PET/MR. Soc Nucl Med Ann Meet Abstr. 2014;55(Supplement 1):660P.
99. Schmand M, et al. BrainPET: first human tomograph for simultaneous (functional) PET and MR imaging. Soc Nucl Med Ann Meet Abstr. 2007;48(Supplement 2):45P.
100. Delso G, et al. Performance measurements of the Siemens mMR integrated whole-body PET/MR scanner. J Nucl Med. 2011;52(12):1914–22.
101. Freifelder R, et al. Design and performance of the head PENN-PET scanner. IEEE Trans Nucl Sci. 1994;41(4):1436–40.
102. Wienhard K, et al. The ECAT HRRT: performance and first clinical application of the new high resolution research tomograph. IEEE Trans Nucl Sci. 2002;49(1):104–10.
103. Watanabe M, et al. A new high-resolution PET scanner dedicated to brain research. IEEE Trans Nucl Sci. 2002;49(3):634–9.
104. Karp JS, et al. Performance of a brain PET camera based on anger-logic gadolinium oxyorthosilicate detectors. J Nucl Med. 2003;44(8):1340–9.
105. Surti S. Radionuclide methods and instrumentation for breast cancer detection and diagnosis. Semin Nucl Med. 2013;43:271–80.
106. Ishii K, et al. First achievement of less than 1 mm FWHM resolution in practical semiconductor animal PET scanner. Nucl Instrum Methods Phys Res, Sect A. 2007;576(2-3):435–40.
107. Drezet A, et al. CdZnTe detectors for small field of view positron emission tomographic imaging. Nucl Instrum Methods Phys Res, Sect A. 2007;571(1-2): 465–70.
108. Mitchell GS, et al. CdTe strip detector characterization for high resolution small animal PET. IEEE Trans Nucl Sci. 2008;55(3):870–6.
109. Vaska P, et al. Ultra-high resolution PET: A CZT-based scanner for the mouse brain. J Nucl Med. 2009;50(2):293.

PET/MR: Basics and New Developments

9

Magdy M. Khalil

Contents

9.1 **Introduction** 200

9.2 **PET/CT** 200

9.3 **PET/MR: System Design** 201
9.3.1 PET/MR Technical Challenges 203
9.3.2 What Is the Solution Then? 206
9.3.3 PET Detector in PET/MR 207
9.3.4 Crystal 207
9.3.5 Photodetectors 207

9.4 **MR System Technology** 210
9.4.1 Magnetic Shielding 211

9.5 **Small Animal PET/MR** 212

9.6 **Attenuation Correction** 213
9.6.1 Template-Based Attenuation Correction 215
9.6.2 Atlas-Based Attenuation Correction 215
9.6.3 Image Segmentation 216

9.7 **Data Acquisition** 218
9.7.1 Imaging Workflow 218
9.7.2 Motion in PET/MR 220

9.8 **Opportunities, Challenges, and Future** 221

References 224

M.M. Khalil, PhD
Medical Biophysics, Department of Physics, Faculty of Science, Helwan University, Cairo, Egypt
e-mail: magdy_khalil@hotmail.com

Abstract

It has become evident that hybrid modalities are one of the most important technical and clinical achievements in clinical imaging over the last two decades. This has impacted significantly many aspects of patient diagnosis, stratification, prognosis, and treatment strategies. After the advent of SPECT/CT and PET/CT to the clinical arena, PET/MR was introduced shortly afterward with real simultaneous capabilities and additional features mainly characterized by the inherent differences between MR and CT imaging techniques. In this chapter, objectives were made to describe the technical challenges behind the hybridization of PET and MR in one imaging system especially if the aim is to produce a simultaneous data acquisition. Different commercially available PET/MR systems were also described along with their specific characteristics, geometry, and design. The use of new PET detector technology was one of the reasons beyond the success of hybrid PET/MR. Thus, some details were provided for different types of crystals and light photosensors along with other interfering variables with MR detector components. Attenuation and motion correction in PET/MR imaging were reviewed with recent tips on approaches devised and their relative merits. Small animal PET/MR was outlined as well. Challenges, opportunities, and future directions were highlighted at the end of the chapter.

M.M. Khalil (ed.), *Basic Science of PET Imaging*, DOI 10.1007/978-3-319-40070-9_9

9.1 Introduction

In the last two decades, there was a large interest in multimodality hybrid imaging. The combination of functional imaging with anatomical imaging modalities was so attractive to the nuclear medicine community on both clinical and technical levels. The functional imaging is provided by nuclear medicine imaging techniques that include single-photon emission computed tomography (SPECT) and positron emission tomography (PET), while the latter is the main focus of morphological diagnostic imaging such as x-ray computed tomography (CT) and magnetic resonance imaging (MRI). The advent of hybrid multimodal SPECT/CT, PET/CT, and PET/MR and introduction into the clinic were so close in time such that we can call the last two decades the age of hybrid imaging.

The rationale behind that interest was to gain the strength of each imaging modality, to reveal the maximum information about human diseases in one imaging session, to shorten the diagnostic workup, and to accelerate the treatment decision-making process. This obviously has several features and advantages in patient management and clinical outcome. The morphological modalities have several quality parameters such as high spatial and contrast resolution providing high anatomical details of patient morphology. Nuclear medicine and molecular imaging techniques, on the other hand, have much better molecular sensitivity but poor spatial resolution in comparison to the structural modalities. The tracer or radiopharmaceutical can be injected in nano- or picomolar molar concentration without disturbing the physiological system or molecular/cellular pathways [1–3]. PET tracers lie in a wide range library, and tailoring new probes able to decipher a biological question or investigate a particular molecular pathway can be designed. The advent of PET/CT and SPECT/CT to the clinical arena and their wide spread in routine practice have encouraged researchers to copy the same experience in introducing PET/MR imaging systems into the clinic.

First attempts to combine PET with MR were focused on preclinical system model in the 1990s, whereas it was not until 2006 that the first integral simultaneous PET/MR (BrainPET, Siemens Healthcare, Inc.) imaging of the brain took place [4]. Combining PET with MRI in the same scanner has several diagnostic benefits and clinical advantages. A great soft tissue contrast can be achieved with MRI sequences avoiding the use of ionizing radiation imparted by CT imaging procedures. MRI has also a functional part but with sensitivity significantly lower than PET; it is in the range of 10^{-5} mol/L, while for molecular PET imaging lies in the range of 10^{-9}–10^{-12} mol/L. MRI can provide functional information such as tissue perfusion, diffusion, and spectroscopy in addition to other benefits such as motion correction and anatomy-based image reconstruction as well as reduction of positron range effects and improvement in spatial resolution [5].

There are many technical and operational differences between PET/CT and PET/MR, and this obviously comes from the different underlying principles of CT and MR imaging components. These are but not limited to image acquisition, data reconstruction and processing, clinical examinations and data flow, contrast agents and contraindications, scan speed and patient throughput, radiation exposure to patients and staff and some other variables that include reimbursement and examination fees, etc. [6]. PET/MR examinations have successfully been introduced into the clinic, and extensive research work is being carried out to assess its effectiveness in routine practice of medical diagnosis. Nevertheless, the clinical utility of simultaneous PET/MR may be seen more effective in organ-specific, disease-specific, and pediatric-related applications or in those patients where their follow-up would be of important clinical value [7]. Eventually, the marathon of PET/CT and PET/MR has started trying to address some questions such as whether PET/MRI will be able to provide incremental diagnostic accuracy, an incremental impact on management, or an incremental impact on patient outcome compared with PET/CT [8].

9.2 PET/CT

One of the ideal design goals of a hybrid imaging modality is to acquire diagnostic information at the same time without compromising patient comfort or prolonging acquisition times with little or no mutual interference of one system to another. Up to the moment of writing this chapter, there is no commercial hybrid system able to acquire PET signal as well as CT or MRI information at the same time using the same detector module. However, the commercial designs available so far are built on the notion of simultaneously acquiring the different diagnostic signals using two different detector systems or sequentially acquiring one after the other. The first PET/CT design has incorporated a single-slice spiral CT scanner (Somatom AR.SP; Siemens Medical Solutions, Forchheim, Germany) and a rotating ECAT ART scanner (CTI PET Systems, Knoxville, TN) [9]. The PET scanner consisted of two opposing detector banks leaving a physical gap between the two detectors. This gap was suggested to be a useful space for incorporating a CT scanner so that anatomical information can be obtained. While this idea was not practically applicable due to the heavy elements of CT imaging system, it was inspiring to design a hybrid PET/CT such that both can be located side by side [10].

The first PET/CT prototype was funded by the National Institutes of Health (NIH) and designed such that the CT and PET components rotated as a single assembly acquiring CT and PET data sequentially. The entire rotating assembly was housed within a single gantry cover. This prototype became operational in 1998 and subsequently clinically evaluated at the University of Pittsburgh [9].

An increased radiation dose especially for repeated measurements of therapy monitoring is one of the PET/CT drawbacks that might have a potential risk implication. This is particularly critical in pediatric patients and response monitoring. Poor soft tissue contrast is also a limitation in some clinical examinations such as brain, prostate, abdomen, and breast imaging that may require an injection of contrast agents. Similarly, PET/CT in small animal research has some limitations as increased dose to the animal may contribute to the total radiation burden, creating a confounding or interfering effect to the drug under investigation. The poor soft tissue contrast provided by CT especially in the era of developing new specific radiotracers that need clear anatomical details is also a clear drawback in animal research. Physics and instrumentation of PET and PET/CT are described in Chap. 8.

9.3 PET/MR: System Design

Attempts to manufacture PET/MR imaging systems were based on two distinct designs, sequential versus concurrent (or simultaneous) data acquisition. The main difference in both systems is the way how the two detector systems are located in relation to each other. Sequential design is straightforward, is less integrated, is not temporally correlated, and requires less hardware modifications, and two major vendors have adopted that design.

One design was implemented by Philips Healthcare (The Ingenuity TF PET/MR, Cleveland, OH) and fabricated such that the PET and MR scanners are located in the same imaging room and able to perform a time of flight (TOF) data acquisition [11]; see Fig. 9.1. The PET and MR scanners are axially aligned at opposite ends of a linearly translating bed and the centers of the scanners are 4.2 m apart. The room dimension requirement is relatively large measuring 4.5 × 13 m. The chance of patient motion between the two scans still exists, and the acquisition time is also compromised and varies according to the clinical question. The PET detector ring is surrounded by additional shielding (i.e., laminated steel shield), and each photomultiplier is inserted in a mu-metal case [12].

The other sequential system was adopted by GE Healthcare (Milwaukee, USA) where two scanners, one hybrid (PET/CT) and one standalone (MR), are separated and installed in two different rooms as shown in Fig. 9.2. The two separate systems have the same imaging table that can be transferred from one room to another achieving a multimodality sequential PET/CT and MR diagnostic examination [13]. This system has minimal if no mutual interference between the two scanning units, and therefore image quality and quantitative accuracy are maintained. While this approach provides more flexibility to use the two imaging systems separately and independently and can be optimized to select those patients who

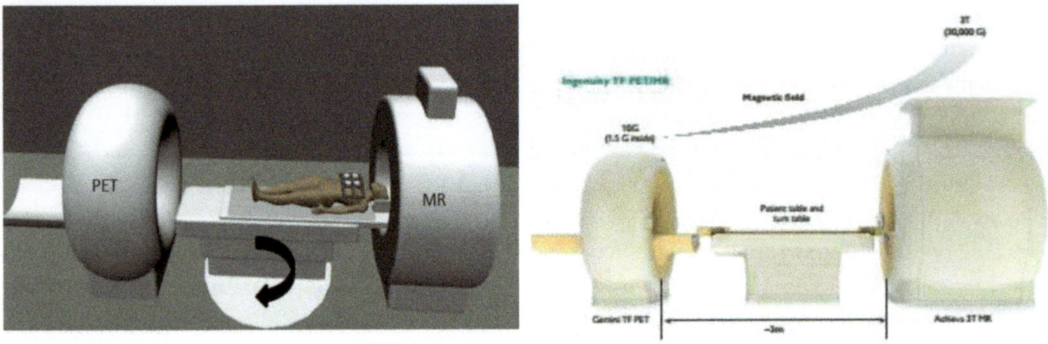

Fig. 9.1 The model implemented in Philips PET/MR system. The two modules are located at adequate far distant apart, minimizing mutual interference between the two systems, and data are acquired in a sequential mode (Image is courtesy of Philip Health Care, Inc.)

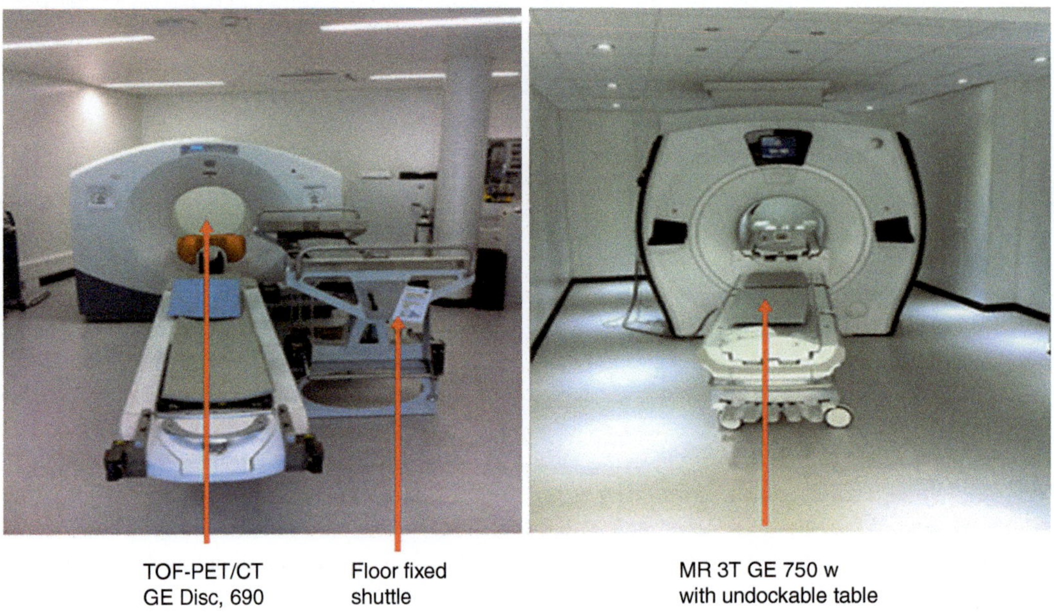

Fig. 9.2 First PET/CT/MR version adopted by GE Healthcare using 3 T MRI system and a TOF-PET/CT in two rooms directly adjacent to each other (Taken from Ref. [14] with permission)

need PET/CT or a combination of PET/CT/MR, it remains an additional source of radiation due to CT part of the examination besides likelihood of patient motion that causes undesired imaging artifacts [13].

On the other hand, the concurrent PET/MR systems provide a simultaneous data acquisition preserving the temporal and spatial correlation between the two data sets. This approach is either a PET insert located inside the magnet bore or alternatively a PET detector fully integrated into an MR scanner [14–16]. Initial attempts were focused on the insert type to reduce positron range and thus improved spatial resolution of the PET data. However, some challenges are needed to be tackled due to the presence of PET scintillator and associated electronics within the MR field of view. Magnetic susceptibility of the PET components needs to be minimized; otherwise, a deleterious influence on the static field would impact data acquisition and image quality. Therefore, shielding of the magnetic-sensitive components would be essential to maintain field homogeneity and minimize cross talk interference. Alternatively, using magnetic insensitive PET components or placing the PET electronics outside the fringe field would be an alternative option. Size constraints would impact negatively on PET detection sensitivity as the axial extent would be limited as well.

The insert-type PET/MR provides a reduced total acquisition time, minimizes likelihood of patient motion, and doesn't require major modifications in the MR magnet configurations. The PET insert design is successful in scanning small objects like small animals' imaging, brain, and extremities but of limited feasibility in whole-body PET/MR due to space limitations that created in the magnet bore. In addition, removing the insert would make the MR to work as a single imaging module providing a cost-effective less integrated option [6, 17].

In comparison to PET/CT, the integrated design is a unique feature that characterizes PET/MR over PET/CT in providing a perfect intrinsic co-registration. Reduction of the total acquisition time is also another advantage provided by simultaneous PET/MR systems in comparison to sequential design. However, integrated design is more challenging and expensive and requires major changes and modification when compared to separate scanning units. The first hybrid whole-body PET/MR scanner (Biograph mMR, Siemens Healthcare) was installed in 2010. It is based on the Siemens Verio 3-T MRI scanner using avalanche photodiode with water cooling mechanism. The bore has been reduced due to this integration from 70 to 60 cm and the PET detector was placed behind the RF coil [14] (Fig. 9.3).

Note that larger-bore magnet is also challenging because the gradient system pays a steep price and performance penalty for its increased size as power requirements go steeply with radius and manufacturing tolerances for gradient shielding become much more demanding [18]. Having the PET detector behind the RF coils allows for reduction of interference with excitation pulses, but temperature and other gamma rays' attenuation and photon scatter need to be addressed. A split magnet is an approach that also permits PET detector integration and facilitates coupling of the processing electronics, rendering the signal more robust to interference [19].

The other simultaneous PET/MR system recently reported by GE Healthcare is the Signa TOF-PET/MR. The MR component is based on the GE 3-T Discovery 750w MRI system which has an inner bore of 70 cm diameter. The PET scanner has a transverse FOV of 60 cm and an axial extent of 25 cm (89 slices) and comprises of five rings of 112 detector blocks. Each block consists of 4 × 9 array of lutetium based with similar density to LYSO crystal [3.95 mm (transverse) × 5.3 mm (axial) × 25 mm^3 (depth)] coupled to 1 × 3 arrays of SiPM devices [20]. The PET detectors' modules are centered inside the MR gradient set and mounted on the outside of the RF body coil that provides additional space to accommodate the PET detector ring with a 60-cm patient bore. The PET detector relies on SiPM photodetector technology and uses a custom-made ASIC for readout, which permits gain adjustment on the individual pixel level.

Preliminary system performance showed 4-mm spatial resolution (using line source), 10.5 % energy resolution, 22.5 kcps MBq^{-1} system sensitivity based on NEMA measurements, and 215 kcps at 17 kBq/ml activity concentration [21]. Initial evaluation resulted in roughly more than 50 % of dose reduction can be clinically achieved [22]. The relatively high sensitivity is owing to large axial extent (25 cm), detector depth, and recovery of events occurred by Compton interactions within the detector [23]. The system is shown in Fig. 9.4. The three major vendors of PET/MR systems are summarized in Table 9.1.

9.3.1 PET/MR Technical Challenges

Allocation of the PET detector within the magnetic bore and removing mutual interference with MRI components are the two initial but major issues that need to be tackled before realizing an integrated hybrid PET/MR system. The magnetic field has its well-known degrading effect on the photomultiplier tube (PMT). The vacuum of the PMT

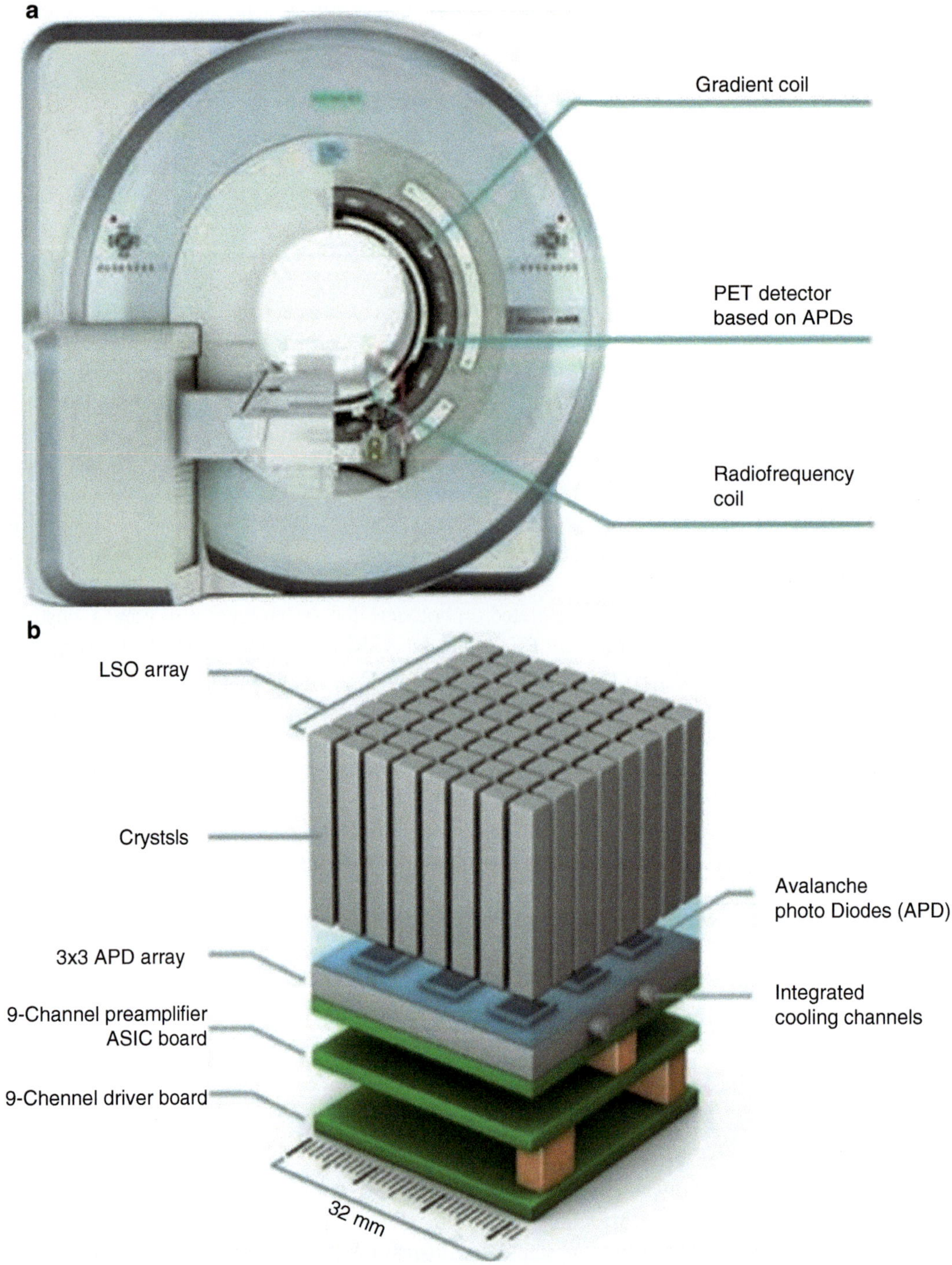

Fig. 9.3 (**a**) Cross section of the Siemens fully integrated PET/MR (Biograph mMR, Siemens Healthcare, Inc.). (**b**) PET detector module showing the segmented LSO crystal coupled to APD with the integrated cooling system (Images are courtesy of Siemens Healthcare)

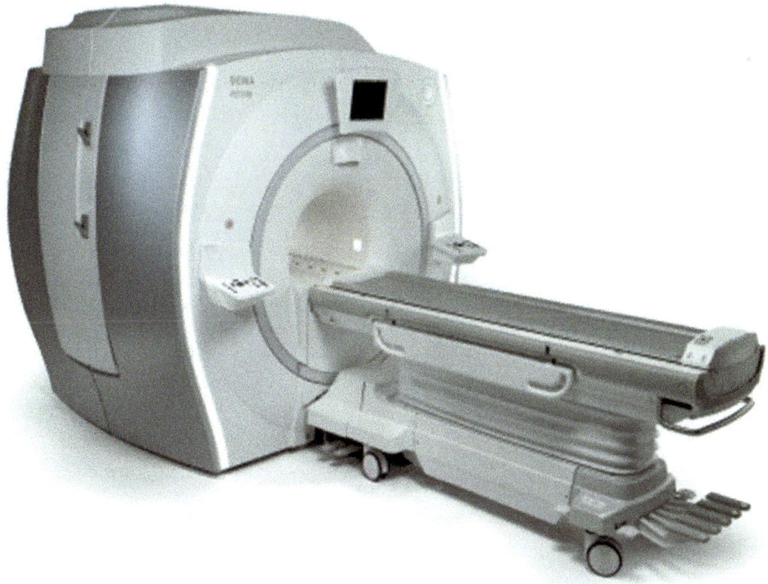

Fig. 9.4 GE Healthcare TOF-PET/MR integrated system (i.e., Signa) that simultaneously acquires PET and MR signals. It combines simultaneous data acquisition from GE's latest 3.0 T MR750w and SiPM-based PET technology

Table 9.1 Summary of the PET/MR systems released by the three major manufacturers

PET/MR system	Biograph mMR (Siemens)	Ingenuity TF (Philips)	Discovery PET/CT 690 + MR 750 (GE)
PET system			
Crystal material	LSO	LYSO	LYSO
Crystal elements dimension	4 × 4 × 20 mm³	4 × 4 × 22 mm³	4.7 × 6.3 × 25 mm³
Photomultipliers	No, 4032 APDs	420	1024
Ring diameter	65.6 cm	90.3 cm	88.6 cm
Transaxial FoV	59.4 cm	67.6 cm	70 cm
Axial FoV	25.8 cm	18.0 cm	15.7 cm
Energy window	430–610 keV	460–665 keV	425–650 keV
Coincidence window	5.9 ns	6 ns	4.9 ns
Time of flight	No	Yes	Yes
MR system			
Field strength	3 Tesla	3 Tesla	3 Tesla
Bore diameter	60 cm	60 cm	60 cm
Max FoV	50 × 50 × 45 cm³	50 × 50 × 45 cm³	48 × 48 × 48 cm³
Field homogeneity (40 cm³)	0.25 ppm	0.5 ppm	0.25 ppm
PET/MR			
Acquisition	Simultaneous	Sequential (same room)	Sequential (2 separate rooms)
PET attenuation correction	MR-based	MR-based	CT-based

Namely, Biograph mMR from Siemens, Ingenuity TF from Philips, and the trimodality hybrid system from GE Healthcare that consists of Discovery PET/CT and MR 750 [24]. The GE Healthcare Signa PET/MR system is described in the text

has several accelerating dynodes of varying potential difference. The photoelectrons emitted from the tube cathode are amplified through this process which is very sensitive to magnetic fields. The existence of PMT-based PET detector in the MRI magnetic fields results in a potential signal deterioration and distorted PET image. Another undesired feature of the PMT is the bulky structure that doesn't facilitate an easy integration inside the magnet core.

The strong static magnetic field and abrupt changes in the gradient magnetic field in addition to the radio-frequency pulse are major MRI elements that influence the PET detector system. Furthermore, the radio frequency and its rapidly changing pulses create eddy currents in any conductive material present in the field in addition to mechanical and vibrational noise [25–27]. Eddy current is a phenomenon created when a time-varying magnetic flux through a closed circuit produces an electromotive force proportional to its rate of change in a close proximity conductive material. It results from the excitation RF pulse and the rapidly changing gradient coil and could have several imaging drawbacks like a spatially variant phase change of the resonance signal, or the associated field will alter the spatial encoding of the signal leading to a distortion of the reconstructed images [24].

The presence of PET electronics in the magnetic field of the MR system has also its own drawbacks. It is important to maintain the magnetic field homogeneity avoiding any source that affects this uniform pattern. PET electronics including crystal, front-end electronics, any RF or radiation shielding, and particularly ferromagnetic components could potentially affect field homogeneity and linearity of the coil gradient system. Therefore, the shielding material should be carefully selected and optimized for data acquisition and elimination of imaging artifacts and data distortion [28].

In terms of image quantitation, attenuation correction is one of the major challenges that need to be properly tackled in order to achieve reliable (absolute or relative) quantitative measures. Other aspects that are tightly associated with MR imaging are the presence of metallic components and bony structures that have no significant information on the MR images. MR hardware is also critical in photon attenuation and could compromise correction techniques. These points will be discussed later.

9.3.2 What Is the Solution Then?

To solve the aforementioned problems, there were two major but different approaches that were taken into consideration. One of them was to keep the PMT at adequate distance away from the MR interfering signal. The distance was calculated such that the fringe magnetic field drops below 10 mT and the scintillation light was transmitted through lines of optical fibers. The first simultaneous preclinical prototype was built analogous to that way and consisted of a ring of forty eight $2\times2\times10$ mm^3 lutetium oxyorthosilicate (LSO) crystals of 38-mm inner diameter, implementing a one-to-one pixel coupling to three multichannel PMTs (MC-PMT) connected via (2 mm diameter and 4 m long) double clad optical fibers [29].

Shielding the PMT using steel or mu-metal is effective in weak magnetic field but fails in the strong fields used in MRI imaging systems. Using long optical fibers was not a perfect solution and showed some drawbacks such as loss of light signal (five to tenfold), deterioration of energy resolution, as well as degradation of timing resolution [30]. However, recent work on this area has also been extended to use a 90° light guide to transfer the light from the crystal to the optical fibers permitting the PMT to be placed in a magnetic-shielded region of 0.3 mT behind the yoke [31]. A reduction of light loss was achieved by newly developed flexible optical fiber bundle-based block detectors, employing them in a high-resolution integrated PET⁄MRI system [31].

The other solution was to use solid-state semiconductor photodetector such as avalanche photodiode (APD) or silicon photomultiplier (SiPM) that are insensitive to high magnetic field of the MR scanner [32, 33]. Avalanche photodiodes can operate in MR magnetic field without apparent distortion and have been successfully coupled to bismuth germinate (BGO) or cerium-doped lutetium oxyorthosilicate (LSO) crystals. The size of the APD is very small, and thus a compact PET/MR design can be manufactured using this type of solid-state photodetectors. The timing resolution in the range of nanoseconds and thus TOF is not possible. However, SiPM has been emerging as a potential and better candidate due to its signal-to-noise (SNR) ratio, higher gain, and timing resolution in the range of sub-nanosecond, and thus time of flight can be realized [34]. Further details on those types of photodetectors are discussed in Sect. 9.2.5.

9.3.3 PET Detector in PET/MR

The current generation of PET imaging systems relies on the full ring design that provides a simultaneous data acquisition of all projection angles at the same time. So detector rotation is eliminated and count sensitivity is greatly improved in comparison to older versions such as partial ring or single ring design. As discussed in Chap. 8, the block detector is the conventional and most adopted standard detector design used in PET imaging scanners. The scintillator block is viewed from the backside normally by 4 PMT that read out the light signal converting it into electric current for further processing and event spatial, temporal, and energy determination.

TOF-PET scanners do utilize the new advances in scintillation crystals, electronics, and computer technology by exploiting the full potential of PET in improving SNR [35]. TOF was not the only feature, but in the last decade, there were several developments in PET imaging such as an improved detector technology, electronic circuitry, data acquisition boards, processing and computer workstations, image reconstruction, and modeling of image-degrading factors, and all of these resulted in overall improved system performance and diagnostic accuracy.

9.3.4 Crystal

Scintillation crystal is the first component that receives the coincidence photons during the scanning process. The crystal role is to shift the wavelength of the incident energy into higher values that permit further downstream signal processing. This is because the light quanta emitted from the crystal have lower energy (higher wavelength) than the incident radiation beam. BGO crystal was the conventional detector material used for many years in PET systems due to its efficient stopping power and nonhygroscopic properties in comparison to Na(Tl) crystal. The scintillation crystal in PET/MR system should be carefully selected so that any magnetic susceptibility must be avoided (i.e., the degree of magnetization of a material in response to an applied magnetic field) [36]. BGO, LSO, and LYSO crystals were found to have lower magnetic susceptibility, but GSO and LGSO are not appropriate and can cause MRI artifacts. The former group is the most common in the current PET/CT and PET/MR systems. Currently, the most preferred crystal type is the LSO-type crystals due to high light output, good detection efficiency, and short decay constant that permits TOF applications.

9.3.5 Photodetectors

9.3.5.1 Photomultiplier Tube (PMT)

The most commonly used photosensors in gamma camera and PET imaging systems are the PMTs due to its high gain that lie in the range of 10^5–10^7 in addition to the fast timing characteristics. It is manufactured in wide range of geometries, sizes, and designed base on vacuum tube technology that improved significantly over the years. Some of these improvements are better timing performance, enhanced quantum efficiency, and developments of multichannel and position-sensitive PMT [34]. PMT has two major undesired properties that make its integration in PET/MR systems indeed difficult. These are the sensitivity to magnetic field and the relatively large structure that impedes its easy integration inside the magnetic bore. Keeping the PMT tube at a distance from the magnetic field fringe below 500 μT has been reported in simultaneous preclinical PET/MR system. However, this configuration results in great reduction of scintillation light (90 %) leading to a degraded energy resolution [31].

9.3.5.2 Avalanche Photodiode (APD)

One of the major transitions in the field of PET/MR detector technology is the use of semiconductor photosensors in PET detector design [32]. APD operates below the breakdown voltage, and the signal produced is proportional to the ion pair created and to the energy deposited by the coincident photons interacted with the crystal. APDs also have an advantage over PMTs in not requiring high bias voltages to operate. At reverse bias, a volume close to the junction is depleted of

Table 9.2 Comparison of three major photodetectors used in clinical or preclinical PET/MR imaging systems[a]

Characteristic	PMT	APD	SiPM
Active area (mm^2)	1–2000 cm^2	1–100 mm^2	1–10 mm^3
Gain	10^5–10^7	100	10^5–10^7
Rise time	<1 ns	2–3 ns	~1 ns
Dark current/count rate	<0.1 nA/cm^2	1–10 nA/mm^2	0.1–1 MHz/mm^2
Capacitance (pF/mm^2)	9	2–10	>30
Quantum efficiency @ 420 nm (%)	25	60–80	<40[a] [~25–75] Photon detection efficiency
After pulsing	Yes	No	Yes
Bias voltage (V)	1000–2000	~200–1500	~50 [30–80]
Power consumption	100 mW/ch	10 μW/mm^2	<50 μW/mm^2
Temperature coefficient (%/°C)	<1 %/°C	2–3 %/°C	3–5 %/°C
Bias coefficient	<1 %/V	10 %/V	~100 %/V
Magnetic susceptibility	Very high (mT)	No (up to 9.4 T)	No (up to 15 T)
Price/channel ($) in 2010	>200	~100	~50

[a]Taken from [41, 44]

free charge carriers. The charge carriers created in the depleted region drift in the electric field toward corresponding electrodes and, while traversing this region, acquire enough energy to produce electron-hole pairs by impact ionization. The newly created charge carriers may create new ones and so on. Thus, there is an avalanche of electrons and holes moving through the detector. An external circuit then detects these current pulses [37].

The quantum efficiency reaches 70–80 %, and when coupled to LSO crystal (peak wavelength 420 nm), the timing resolution lies in the range of few nanosecond. Avalanche photodiodes provide great advantages in terms of dimension and subsequent detector design compactness. The small size provided by APD is a positive characteristic toward an improved spatial resolution that matches small crystal dimensions and high packing fraction. The insensitivity to magnetic field was central property that made APD an acceptable alternative to PMT in PET/MR systems [38]. APD coupled to LSO crystal in preclinical 9.4 T magnet showed stable performance with no dependence in gain and energy resolution (14.4 % at 511 keV) of APD on the magnetic field. There was also no effect of changes in the orientation of the APD electric field with respect to the main magnetic field lines (parallel vs. perpendicular), hence proving the feasibility of operating such a PET detector module inside an MRI [39].

However, APD has a number of limitations that requires special attention in the detector system. It has low internal gain (10^2–10^3) and requires charge-sensitive preamplifiers to convert electron charge to a measurable voltage signal. Charge integration occurs over several nanoseconds to achieve high conversion factors, and pulse pileup takes place at high counting rates. APD needs advanced front-end electronics to meet the lower gain, and therefore special and application-specific integrated circuits are used [40]. Noise and time variation in electron drift during multiplication process are factors that restrict using the APD in time of flight applications [41]. The gain is sensitive to changes in temperature and voltages applied, and thus special measures are required to control these technical factors. Thus, temperature sensitivity of APD imposes special constraint on the design of PET/MR such that a well control over the solid-state detector should be maintained and eddy current, if not minimized, would affect the gain of the electron avalanche due to increased collision with semiconductor lattice [36, 37]; see Table 9.2.

APD can be coupled directly to the scintillator but also can be located at a short distance using optical fibers, depending in large part on system configuration including space allocated for PET module inside the magnet and minimizing the interference between the two subsystems [15, 42]. The advent of APD to the medical arena has been attractive for large academic institutions to build their own hybrid PET/MR systems. It has been successful in initial attempts made to construct simultaneous hybrid systems with further investigations performed to optimize the design and improve the quality of either systems [43]. The first insert-type PET detector was a prototype released by Siemens (BrainPET, Siemens Healthcare, Inc.) providing an opportunity to acquire a simultaneous PET/MR on human brain [17, 43] as mentioned earlier. The insert was integrated with a standard 3-T MRI scanner (Magnetom TIM Trio; Siemens Healthcare, Inc.), and proof-of-principle simultaneous data acquisition was demonstrated. In addition, the BrainPET can be docked at the back of the magnet without obstructing the bore so that the MR scanner can be used in standalone mode [17, 43].

9.3.5.3 Silicon Photomultiplier (SiPM)

Geiger-mode avalanche photodiode (AVP) or SiPM (also called multi-pixel photon counter) is made of arrays of small APD (e.g., 50 × 50 μm) and operated beyond the voltage breakdown in the Geiger counting mode [44]. The compact size permits also an easy incorporation in small animal PET/MR systems and implementation in depth of interaction-based scanners [31]. In this solid-state photodetector, the high electric field in a very small space that collects the ion pair allows for better quantum efficiency and provides good resistance to magnetic field in contrary to those effects seen in PMT. It was shown that SiPM can tolerate a magnetic field of 7 T [45]. Coupling of the SiPM to scintillation needs some attention especially one-to-one coupling as it increases the number of photodetector in the magnet substantially; however, it eliminates light sharing and improves spatial resolution [31, 41].

Like APD, low temperature is also an important prerequisite for operating SiPM, and variation in temperature can lead to alteration of the breakdown voltage and subsequent variation of photodetection efficiency, dark current, and gain [27]. Each cell in SiPM photodetector works independently, and the charge created from the ion pair is no longer proportional to the energy deposited, but the summed output from all cells is proportional to the energy deposited in the scintillator. It is therefore important to maintain good energy linearity as photodetector outputs need to be compared in crystal identification schemes [11]. While the quantum efficiency of APD is nearly 80% (as mentioned above), the photodetection efficiency of SiPM is below 40% when coupled to LSO crystal. Proper eddy current management, cooling system, and accounting for residual inaccuracies in system calibration are measures taken to tackle heat generation and associated problems.

Based on the above discussion, the SiPM has a high gain similar to that revealed from PMT, resistance to high magnetic field, and low bias voltage when compared to APD. The emerging digital SiPMs have shown improved performance and low temperature sensitivity. It also provides a good timing, energy and spatial resolution, as well as good temperature stability, making it a promising candidate concerning their MR compatibility. However, they tend to generate digital electromagnetic noise patterns which might degrade the MR image quality; a design measure that needs to be taken into consideration [46]. Table 9.1 compares the three commonly used photodetectors used in PET/MR.

As previously mentioned, the Signa PET/MR from GE Healthcare utilizes the SiPM technology. This new digital detector is characterized by its enhanced sensitivity; it is up to three times more sensitive than GE Healthcare's Discovery 690 PET/CT. SiPM photosensor is also being adopted in the European Hyperimage collaboration to build a small animal PET insert inside a clinical 3 T MR system of a ring diameter of 20 cm and axial field of view of 9 cm. Each detector comprises a 22 by 22 array of 1.3 × 1.3 × 10 mm^3 LYSO crystals coupled to an 8 × 8 array of 4 × 4 mm^2 SiPM where the signal is immediately digitized using application-specific integrated circuit (ASIC) that release digital energy,

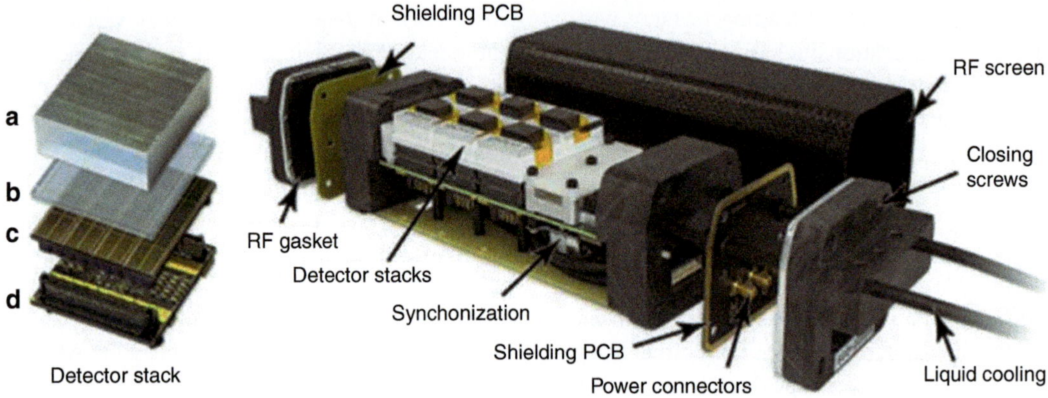

Fig. 9.5 Digital silicon photomultiplier (dSiPM)-based detector stack (*left*) with scintillation crystal array (**a**), light guide (**b**), sensor (**c**), and interface board (**d**). On the right side of the figure, the single detection module (SDM) contains up to six detector stacks. The carbon fiber shield is pushed over the module and the RF screen is closed on both sides by shielding plates (From Ref. [48] under Creative Commons Attribution 3.0 License)

timing, and channel information [46, 47]. This last feature is substantial as it reduces and could eliminate the interference that affects connection and transmission cables between photodetectors and signal processing circuitry. See Fig. 9.5.

9.4 MR System Technology

An MR imaging system has several major components that interplay to acquire an image. The most important parts are static magnetic field, gradient magnet, and radio-frequency coil. The magnetic field magnetizes the human body once the patient is inside the magnet bore. Most of the imaging interest in MR is the hydrogen atom (i.e., protons) due to its plenty and large abundance in human tissues and cells. Under the strong magnetic field applied by the static magnet, the protons are aligned into two directions: parallel and antiparallel. Majority of protons are aligned in parallel with the magnetic field (B_0) in comparison to those protons aligned antiparallel as the former is a lower energy state compared to high energy state of the antiparallel direction. A net magnetization is therefore produced in parallel to the magnetic field (B_0) and takes place along the z-direction. In addition, a precession or rotational motion of the protons is created that precess with frequency proportional to the magnetic field. In clinical setting, 1.5 and 3 T static magnet is used, but higher strength (e.g., 7 and 9.4 T) is used for more advanced application. It is important to maintain the homogeneity of the static magnetic field, and any component of magnetic susceptibility (a property of a material to be magnetic when exposed to magnetic field) must be avoided or adequately isolated within the field of view to keep image quality with minimal distortion.

The gradient coil has an important role in providing a spatial localization of the MR signal by varying the static field strength in the three orthogonal planes in a linear fashion. Gradients are loops of wire or thin conductive sheets on a cylindrical shell lying just inside the bore of an MR scanner. When current is passed through these coils, a secondary magnetic field is created. This *gradient field* slightly distorts the main magnetic field in a predictable pattern, causing the resonance frequency of protons to vary as a function of position. The primary function of gradients, therefore, is to allow a spatial encoding of the MR signal. Gradients are also critical for a wide range of "physiologic" techniques, such as MR angiography, diffusion, and perfusion imaging [49].

The second important part is the transmission coil which sends uniform radio-frequency excitation at the Larmor frequency over the field of view. Local receive coil or surface coil is placed over the region of interest to improve the magnetic sensitivity and hence signal-to-noise ratio. This coil is also affected by distance such that the sensitivity decreases appreciably beyond a distance equal to the diameter of the coil. Upon relaxation and switching off the RF signal, the information received is processed using a reconstruction algorithm from 2D to 3D images of the resonance signal [27].

Most commercial MRI scanners are superconducting high-field strength magnets because of their faster scanning ability, higher magnetic field homogeneity, higher SNR, and wider range of applications. In a superconducting magnet, a magnetic field is generated by a current that runs through a loop of wire. The wire is surrounded with a coolant, such as liquid helium, to markedly reduce the electric resistance of the wire. Once a system is energized, it maintains its magnetic field [50]. Early work on PET/MR systems was specially focused on manufacturing an MR-compatible PET detector with modifications made to the PET detector system. Recent approaches taken are to modify aspects of the MRI in order to achieve close integration and minimize interactions between the two systems within the magnet bore [25].

9.4.1 Magnetic Shielding

The presence of PET front end electronics and data transmission cables inside the magnet bore represents one of the major challenges in hybrid simultaneous PET/MR systems. A proper but effective shielding system should be implemented to reduce to an acceptable level the interferences that come from the gradient as well as radio-frequency pulse and able not to disturb the main magnetic field uniformity [51]. Signal reflection and absorption together with material skin depth are important physical measures of the shield. Moreover, magnetic susceptibility, gamma rays' attenuation coefficient, and eddy currents are factors to be considered in the candidate shield material. Connection and transmission cables need also a sort of attention as it needs to be masked from the above interferences sources.

Reflection loss is proportional to material conductivity and inversely proportional to permeability, while absorption loss is proportional to conductivity, permeability, and thickness of the shield [27]. In electromagnetism, permeability is the measure of the ability of a material to support the formation of a magnetic field within itself. Hence, it is the degree of magnetization that a material obtains in response to an applied magnetic field. Skin depth, however, is inversely proportional to permeability, electrical conductivity, and signal frequency. One skin depth is defined as the required thickness of a metal to reduce the RF to 37 % of its original strength. The smaller the skin depth, the thinner the material is used for shielding to a particular level. Gradient switching typical in MRI sequences can result in count losses in the particular PET detector design studied. Moreover, the magnitude of this effect depends on the location of the detector within the magnet bore and which MRI gradient is being switched. This information is substantial in the design of PET shielding in MR environment [43].

Aluminum (Al), copper (Cu), and carbon (C) are different materials that can be used for shielding. High conductive materials, e.g., copper, show excellent radio-frequency (RF) shielding properties, but have negative impact on the MRI image quality due to induced eddy currents. However, carbon fiber composites are less conductive for low frequencies and thus can minimize MRI gradient-induced eddy currents. Furthermore, they show good RF shielding properties for higher frequencies. First prototypes using carbon fiber have shown excellent eddy current performance, good RF shielding properties, and superior mechanical robustness in a preclinical simultaneous PET/MRI insert in a clinical 3-T scanner [52].

In a different setting of 7-T PET/MR preclinical scanner (RF at Larmor frequency of 300 MHz, 81 kHz from gradient power supply), placing the PET detector module between two carbon fiber tubes and grounding the inner carbon fiber tube to the PET detector module ground reduced the RF and the eddy currents. Further reductions were achieved by adding thin copper (Cu) foil on the outer carbon fiber case and electrically grounding the PET detector module so that all three components had a common ground [43].

9.5 Small Animal PET/MR

As outlined earlier, initial incentives on PET/MR imaging were on developing small animal hybrid system. This has several advantages in terms of superb soft tissue contrast provided by MRI and wide range of MRI sequences that address anatomical and functional questions in biomedical imaging research [53]. Radiation dose reduction is also another important advantage provided by PET/MR when compared to PET/CT due to the great reduction of cumulated radiation dose over several sessions as occurs in longitudinal studies. Small animal imaging has become a substantial tool in development of new diagnostic biomarkers and drug and essential step in translational medicine. Hybrid PET/MR should have a superb spatial and contrast resolution in order to meet small structure challenges posed by rodents such as mice and rats during in vivo animal imaging. In addition to the difficulties placed by the integration of the PET and MR scanners into one hybrid system, the spatial and temporal resolution together with system sensitivity should also be enhanced.

Small animal hybrid PET/MR systems vary substantially in terms of design parameters that include but not limited to magnet strength, scintillator-photodetector coupling method, type of photodetectors and associated electronics, arrangement of the front-end electronics, and configuration and positioning of the gradient and RF coils. Also, there are some variations in PET detector ring dimensions (axial and transaxial field of views), shielding of the PET electronics, and methods of reducing mutual interferences between the two subsystems. The PET detector is mostly LSO-based scintillator with different array size and segmentation and also whether it is positioned at distance or in direct coupling to readout photodetector.

The use of position-sensitive APD (PSAPD) has become attractive for some reasons such as less contact terminals and hence less connection lines. It consist of a continuous layer of detector material with output terminals positioned such that the relative intensity of the avalanche signal at these contacts serves to determine the exact location of the photon interaction [42]. This easily permits incorporation of PET system electronics within the magnet bore while maintaining the same spatial resolution provided by the conventional APD, as well as it helps reducing costs and complexity of system design. Depth of interaction or parallax error is a potential source of resolution degradation due to radial shift of radioactivity from detector center within the PET ring. The small solid angle and increased crystal thickness are desired detector properties in small animal PET systems but unfortunately serve to increase this parallax error that can be mitigated with the use of PSAPD [54].

Two nonstandard designs employed by different research groups are split magnet and field-cycled PET/MR systems. The former was devised and employed in Cambridge small animal PET/MR model in which the microPET Focus 120 was inserted in a gap of 80 mm between a split 1-T superconducting magnet (Fig. 9.6). The magnet and the PMT were appropriately shielded producing a net magnetic field below 1 mT around the PMT. Furthermore, the gradient was also split with little impact on static field homogeneity and gradient performance [55]. A novel set of gradient and shim coils has been specially designed for this split MRI scanner to include an 110-mm gap from which wires are excluded so as not to interfere with annihilation detection [55].

Field-cycled MRI systems use two independent, actively controlled resistive magnets to polarize a sample and to provide the magnetic field environment during data acquisition producing comparable quality to clinical superconducting systems [56]. The static magnet is split so that the PET block detectors can be placed but with less shielding to the detector and without the use of optical fibers. However, the gradient magnet is not split in this design [57].

Mediso nanoScan® PET/MRI scanner consists of PET scanner (LYSO coupled to 256 channel position-sensitive PMT) in sequential mode with 1 T static magnet [59]. The PET component of the instrument is based on the PET ring of the NanoPET/CT scanner [60]. The PET detector consists of 12 modules, each comprising a 39 × 81 (tangential x axial) array of 1.12 × 1.12 × 13.00 mm

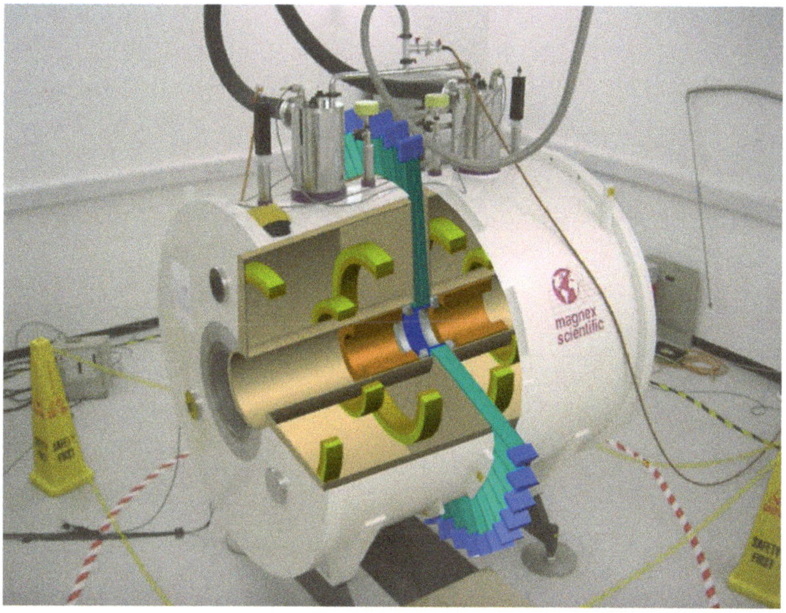

Fig. 9.6 The preclinical PET/MR Cambridge model where 1 T actively shielded superconducting magnet with 80-mm gap to accommodate a multi-ring PET detector array is shown. The PET detectors and MR imager view the same region in space, which facilitates simultaneous MRI and PET acquisition (Reprinted from Ref. [58] with permission)

LYSO crystal on a pitch of 1.17 mm, and the system matrix is monitored by two position-sensitive photomultipliers (PSPMT). The MR imaging component of the instrument is based on the M2 system by Aspect Imaging. The 1-T vertical field, horizontal-bore permanent magnet has better than 5-ppm homogeneity in the central 60-mm-diameter region and a fringe field below 13 mT anywhere on the magnet surface. It features built-in gradient coils used for shimming and an internal radio-frequency cage. The gradient can deliver 450 mT/m pulses with a 250-μs ramp time. It was shown that system integration had no adverse effect on the PET performance with acceptable system spatial resolution and sensitivity [59].

A recent report highlighting the use of digital SiPM coupled to LYSO assembled in MRI-compatible PET insert has been published [48]. Digital SiPM from Philips Digital Photon Counting (PDPC) was used to develop a preclinical PET/RF gantry as an insert for clinical MRI scanners. The scintillation arrays were made from 30×30 12-mm-long LYSO crystal applying 1-mm crystal pitch and optical isolation. With three exchangeable RF coils, the hybrid field of view has a maximum size of 160 × 96.6 mm (transaxial x axial). Depending on the coil, MRI SNR is decreased by 13 or 5% by the PET system. PET performance measures such as count rates, energy resolution (12.6% full width at half maximum, FWHM), and spatial resolution (0.73 mm^3) were not affected by applied MRI sequences. PET time resolution of 565 ps (FWHM) is degraded by 6 ps during an echo planar imaging [48]. See Fig. 9.7.

9.6 Attenuation Correction

Photon attenuation is the major source of errors in SPECT and PET imaging [61]. Photoelectric effect and Compton scattering are the two main interactions that serve to produce suboptimal quantitative results and deteriorated image quality. The former results in photon absorption and complete loss of the 511 keV photons energy, while the latter interaction serves to reduce photon energy by imparting part of the incident energy to the orbital electrons. When considering the total attenuation length that varies from small range as in patient skull or more longer as in chest area, there is approximately 5–22% of the PET signal that is recoded by the scanner accounting for attenuation factors of 18 and 4.5, respectively. These measures indicate that small errors or erroneous values may lead to a

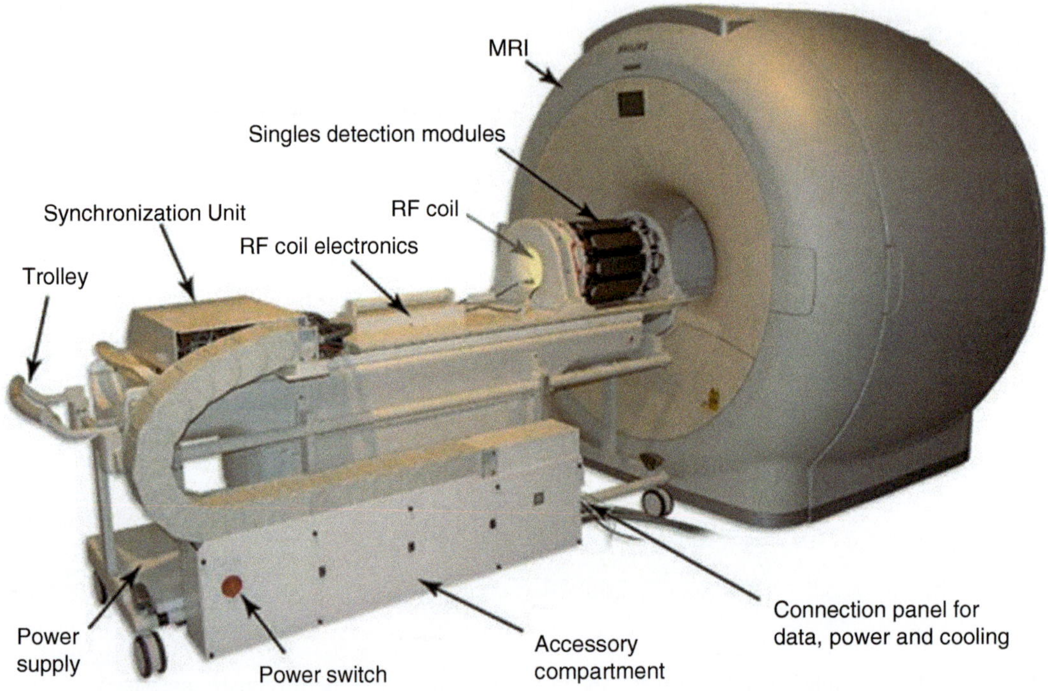

Fig. 9.7 The PET/RF insert "Hyperion II^{D}" mounted on the patient table of a clinical 3 T MRI system (gantry cover removed). The single detector module is described in Fig. 9.4 (Reprinted from Ref. [48] under Creative Commons Attribution 3.0 License)

significant deterioration of image quantitative accuracy [62].

The traditional way of attenuation correction in the past and still used in small percentage of old PET scanners is the use of radioactive transmission sources such as Cs-137 or Co-60 [63, 64]. After the advent of the PET/CT and introduction of the CT as complementary component in the diagnostic process, it has become so feasible to use the Hounsfield units to get the μ-values of individual image pixels. This permits to derive the attenuation correction factors by forward projecting the μ-map produced from the CT scan. Low dose, diagnostic, or contrast-enhanced CT images (with treatment of increased area of contrast concentration) can be used for CT-based attenuation correction using the most common method of bilinear transformation. In this algorithm, HU units below zero are considered as combination of water and air, while values above zero are considered as combination of the bone and soft tissue. This assumption allows one to produce a two regression lines intersecting at HU of zero with different regression slopes [65, 66]. However, two important steps need to be considered while correcting for photon attenuation in CT. The first is pixel down-sampling due to small size of the pixels of the CT image in comparison to PET image. The second is the energy conversion of the μ-values produced from the CT energy photons (around 50 keV for 120 kV tube voltage) to the corresponding value at 511 keV [65].

For the purpose of relative and absolute quantitative PET imaging, correction of photon attenuation is a fundamental prerequisite to achieve better image quality and acceptable quantitative accuracy. MRI data set, on the other hand, has an essential drawback in which the images reflect protons' density and longitudinal (T1) and transverse (T2) magnetization relaxation properties of the tissue of interest. These parameters unfortunately don't reflect the electron density and attenuation properties of the human tissues, and this is exemplified in bone- and air-containing tissues such as the skeletal system and lung tissues, respectively. Both tissues have similar MRI signal output and greatly influence the correction process. Therefore, correction of photon attenuation in PET/MR is not a straightforward process, and some maneuvers are required to tackle this issue. Various approaches have been developed such as those based on templates, atlas information, direct segmentation of T1-weighted MR images, or segmentation of images from special MR sequences, as well as methods relying on PET emission data and MR anatomic information to obtain attenuation map [67].

9.6.1 Template-Based Attenuation Correction

In this technique, an MR template image and co-registered attenuation correction map are generated. The MR template can be produced from MR T1-weighted images and the attenuation map can be derived from transmission scan [68, 69]. The MR template is initially warped to fit the patient MR image using nonlinear registration, and the transformation parameters are used to align the attenuation map template to the PET data of the same patient. This process allows one to produce an individual attenuation map for a given patient study. The incorporation of bone tissues into the correction is relatively easy, but the algorithm suffers from misalignment errors caused by nonlinear registration due to inter-patient anatomical variations. Variants of this method include gender specific or combination of both male and female to generate attenuation map template or produce an average template based on spatial normalization of the individual MR images and the associated co-registered measured attenuation maps [70]. Template-based methods are common only in brain studies.

9.6.2 Atlas-Based Attenuation Correction

Atlas-based approaches are implemented using global anatomical knowledge derived from a representative intensity-based or segmented reference data set into the attenuation correction process. Atlas-based methods have been devised to account for bone attenuation in the PET/MR hybrid images using the bone tissue density revealed from co-registration with CT template [71]. The idea is to utilize a standard CT atlas or a combination of MR and CT atlas data sets and co-register with the patient MR data set to come up with information regarding the transformation parameters. This information is then used to produce a pseudo or synthetic CT data set valid for attenuation correction [67, 72].

One approach is to deform one representative CT data to co-register with patient MR image, and then the newly deformed CT is used for PET data attenuation correction. The registration is carried out through a multistep process that include rigid, B-spline, and optical flow [73]. Another approach utilizes a pair of CT and MR atlas to produce the pseudo-CT data set. In this algorithm, the MR atlas is co-registered with the patient MR, and the transformation parameters are then applied to the CT atlas to produce individualized CT attenuation map. The pseudo-CT data set is weighted sum from each co-registered atlas data set [71, 74].

Advantages of atlas-based methods are the possibility of providing attenuation maps with continuous linear attenuation coefficients eliminating issues associated with the use of single tissue values that do not account for tissue heterogeneities [75]. However, shortcomings of these algorithms include limitations in identifying pathologic lesion using the atlas data set, lung density variations among different patients, and metallic implants. Performance of atlas-based algorithms can be enhanced by the incorporation of the pattern recognition, multiple sequences to improve tissue classification, modifying the registrations method, and artifact detection [71, 76–79].

A relatively recent study compared four different methods in MR attenuation correction in relation to CT-based attenuation correction [76]. Namely:

1. Two segmentation-based methods that do not account for the bone.
2. An atlas and pattern recognition method and accounted for the bone.

3. A hybrid method that combined both approaches, atlas-based and segmentation. It accounted for the bone tissues such that the attenuation map in areas where the bone is likely to occur was predicted with atlas and pattern recognition, whereas a segmentation-based method was used for the rest of the body.

For soft tissue lesions, none of the methods revealed a significant difference, whereas for bone lesions, underestimation of PET standardized uptake values was found for all methods with minimized error for the atlas-based approaches. There were also underestimations of lower magnitude observed in lesions near to bony structure. For lesions affected by MR susceptibility artifacts, quantification errors could be reduced using the atlas-based artifact correction [76].

9.6.3 Image Segmentation

Image segmentation is the process of classifying or clustering every similar group of pixels into a distinct category. In MR segmentation, image intensity is the most common way that enables to classify the human body into air, water, and fats. However and as mentioned earlier, areas that contain air or bone structures have poor MR signal and thus imposing great difficulties on segmentation and classification algorithms. The algorithm works such that every group of pixels that have the same MR signal would be assigned the same tissue properties and hence will be given corresponding attenuation coefficients.

Direct segmentation methods depend on MR T1-weighted sequence routinely acquired in patient examinations. Segmentation methods have been applied to brain as well as whole-body PET/MR imaging procedures. Approaches like the use of fuzzy clustering and anatomical knowledge combined with neural network-based tissue classification have been reported. These methods require further processing tools to segment, for example, lung tissues, bone structures, or outlining the body boundaries [80–84].

Specific MR sequences combined with segmentation algorithms are the most common approach employed in clinical practice of attenuation correction in PET/MR imaging systems [75]. It is based on the two-point Dixon gradient echo sequence that enables separation of water and fat tissues by using the chemical shift of fat relative to that of water. This allows one to segment the MR images into individual different tissue types including either 3-class (air, lung, soft tissue) or 4-class segmentation (air, lung, soft tissue, and fat). The former has no distinction between water-equivalent and fat tissues, while the latter provides water and fat distinction using Dixon MRI sequence [81, 83, 85, 86]. Figure 9.8 shows the attenuation map derived from different methods.

One major drawback of image segmentation using this approach is that every individual tissue is given a specific value ignoring tissue heterogeneities. Another drawback is the absence of bone signal, and its similarity to air-containing structures serves to confound the attenuation correction process. The deviation of the quantitative results relies on the location of the pathology and areas of osseous lesions [82, 84].

It is not only the location and type of tissues but quantitative results could also be negatively impacted by the composition of the bone lesions. An underestimation of more than 20 % of tracer concentration was found in the brain cortex when inaccurate assessment of bone attenuation was performed while not identifying the internal cavities resulted in more than 20 % overestimation of the adjacent structures [87]. In the same report, ignoring the RF coil in the attenuation correction process leads to up to 50 % underestimation of the reconstructed PET images.

In whole body, the situation is relatively different as bone segmentation is not so influential, especially in body regions located at distance from bone tissues, as in brain-based applications. There were some directions to perform segmentation without bone classification in areas of the body that are not adjacent to bone structure without a trade-off in quantification accuracy or image interpretation [83]. Another issue is lung segmentation which appears with low signal in conventional MR sequences in addition to inter-patient variability in tissue density. The utilization of

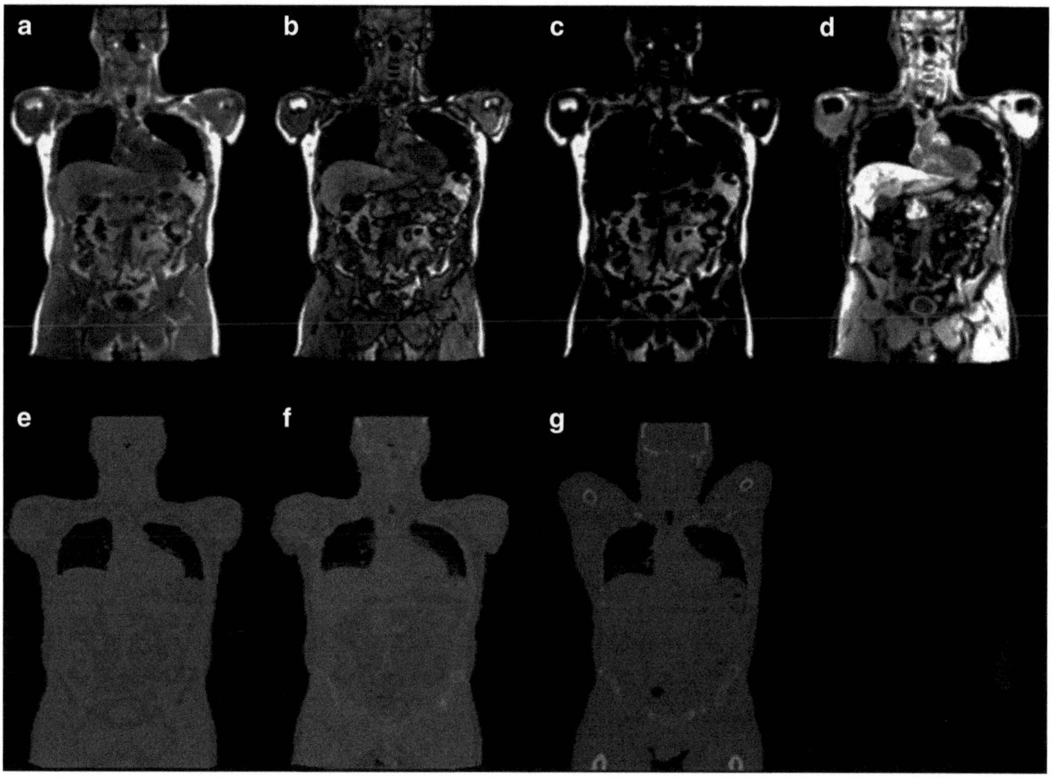

Fig. 9.8 Upper row: a sample MR data set acquired with a T1-weighted 3D gradient echo sequence with 2-point Dixon fat and water separation. (**a**) In-phase, (**b**) opposed phase, (**c**) fat, and (**d**) water images. Lower row: attenuation maps created from the MR data using (**e**) the segmentation method based on Martinez-Möller [83] and (**f**) the atlas- and pattern recognition-based method described in Hofmann et al. [71]. (**g**) The corresponding CT slice from the same patient (Reproduced from Ref. [88] with permission)

ultrashort echo time (UTE) or zero echo time (ZTE) sequences may benefit this problem by preserving signal within the lung parenchyma and therefore allows better differentiation of diseased or consolidated lung with possible incorporation of these values into tissue classifications [89]. The latter sequence was successfully implemented in skull attenuation correction when compared to corrections derived from CT data. The segmentation results show better bone depiction and separation from air cavities and collagenous tissue than previously reported methods; however, further work would be interesting to show its feasibility in chest and cardiac imaging [86].

The UTE sequence enables an improved signal of the bone tissue due to the low T2 relaxation times of the bone. This when combined with an image of longer echo time where bone signal is significantly low can produce an improved segmentation outcome of bone structures. Recently, this approach has been adopted to synthesize a brain CT image (or μ-map) from dual echo UTE images using reference or training data while avoiding the step of co-registering the reference atlas with the subject MR [90]. This algorithm (GENErative Sub-Image Synthesis, GENESIS) matches patches between the reference images and subject images based on a statistical model. It has three major features which are as follows: (1) it does not require any segmentation of the MR images, (2) it does not require the reference images to be registered to the subject images, and (3) it utilizes the MR images to determine the optimal matching patches in the reference data as well as the reference CT image [90].

UTE time sequences have also some limitations like increased acquisition time and induced artifacts when the field of view is increased. In whole-body PET/MR, it will be time-consuming to use UTE. An underestimation down to 40% and overestimation up to 11% were recorded in brain PET quantitation using UTE sequence when compared to CT-based attenuation correction at the same location [91, 92]. Further improvement of UTE in clinically adopted PET/MR system has been suggested due in part to bone misclassification and in adequate performance in the neck and nasal/face area [93].

Joint estimation of radioactivity and attenuation from the emission data using a constrained maximum likelihood reconstruction of attenuation and activity has been also proposed to determine the attenuation map which improves by the inclusion of time of flight information [94]. Time of flight capabilities were found to improve the accuracy of attenuation correction especially when attenuation correction is not accurate [25, 95].

9.7 Data Acquisition

PET/MR imaging systems vary in their approach in data acquisition. Image acquisition may start by acquiring a short sequence for anatomical referencing and attenuation correction. Oncologic application is generally lengthier than non-oncologic studies and may extend to 60 or 70 min in simultaneous data acquisition. However, in sequential PET/MR examinations, the scan length may go up to 90 min [96]. PET data acquisition is simple in comparison to MRI since the former is a time-based acquisition system, and once the collected information is thought to satisfy the diagnostic task, nothing needs to be added. MRI sequences are various but longer and reveal different information and often the primary cause of prolonging the acquisition time.

Before starting looking at the appropriate protocol for a given patient study, a number of steps need to be taken into consideration. Patient preparation, instructions, positioning, and setup are some of those that should be viewed not only from one modality perspective but also from other diagnostic angles. In PET, physiologic parameters such as glucose levels or other safety concerns that are related to pregnancy or pediatric examinations will need to be properly assessed. In MR, some precautions need to be checked as well like metallic implants and patient claustrophobia, while patient motion remains an issue in both imaging techniques. Patient centering on the couch and positioning of the surface coils in addition to time taken to perform these tasks are important parameters to avoid imaging artifacts and reduce technologist radiation exposure [97]. Patient preparation in PET/MR studies shouldn't be different in terms of plasma glucose level, fasting conditions, hydration, pregnancy, and uptake period void of any muscular activity that also need to be potentially minimized 24 h before the commence of the study. MR patient precautions are different and include MR-incompatible implants and contraindications from injecting contrast agents.

9.7.1 Imaging Workflow

Imaging workflow is an essential element in the diagnostic workup and of considerable interest in patient throughput. It is controlled and managed through a number of variables such as the organ or disease under investigation, type of hybrid PET/MR scanner, patient indications, partial or whole-body scan, and other imaging logistics [12, 96, 97].

Workflow is platform dependent. Simultaneous systems provide about 10–15-min saving due to the fact that patient is positioned and removed only once [98]. Apart from acquisition time reduction, patient comfort, and other logistics, the clinical rationale behind simultaneous PET/MR needs to be fully exploited and demonstrated similar to its biomedical applications where several biological or physiological questions can be answered. However, one of the major goals is to maintain the total acquisition time as low as possible while achieving the required diagnostic accuracy. Another feature provided by simultaneous hybrid PET/MR is the ability of acquiring complex imaging workflow and multiple MR sequence acquisitions with different contrasts during the PET data acquisition [7, 8].

In cardiac and neurologic applications, one-bed position might be sufficient to address a particular clinical question, and the total acquisition time is determined by the modality that would stay longer. Multiple bed positions might be needed, and this largely depends on scanner axial extent and the organ or disease under examination.

In oncology-based studies, the imaging protocol might differ significantly as different parts of the body may require different MR sequences and accordingly different time frames. For the same purpose, the acquisition time may be extended longer due to more elaborate examinations required such as those used in advanced molecular imaging applications and MR spectroscopy analysis [8]. Similar to stand-alone MR scanner, surface coils in PET/MR are used to increase MRI image quality and reduce imaging time. However, because the surface coils may cause additional photon attenuation of the 511-keV photons, only dedicated coils approved for PET/MRI should be used [8, 96].

In the trimodality imaging systems proposed by GE Healthcare as well as in tandem-based hybrid PET/MR introduced by Philips Company, imaging session can start in the MR module at approximately 25 min postinjection, and this permits to exploit the rest of the uptake time (around 30–35 min, usually 60 min uptake time) in performing the required MR sequences. Once the MR examination is carried out, then the patient can be moved to the PET/CT or PET portion of the imaging scanner [12, 13].

Whole-body PET/MR imaging protocol is significantly different than other organ-based protocols such as cardiac or neurological disorders. A scout or topogram initial image is performed outlining the axial extent of the patient under examination. This MR localizer is similar to the CT scout image normally taken in commencing PET/CT imaging procedures. The acquisition of PET data is taken in a step-and-shoot mode with bed acquisition time of 2–5 min, but it may extend for longer exploiting the time demanding feature of MR sequences [96]. Time of flight helps reduce the acquisition time or the injected dose further, but overall the acquisition time of PET is determined based on many factors such as clinical preferences and experience, system performance, and the adopted standard protocol [22].

In integrated PET/MR, the attenuation correction 2-point Dixon volume-interpolated breath-hold examination (VIBE) is performed first before the desired MR protocol for each bed position; VIBE takes 19 s. This is followed by the simultaneous acquisition of the PET and the desired MR sequence [99]. A number of diagnostic MRI sequences may be variably and flexibly selected based on body region and clinical indications but usually at a minimum include a T1-weighted and a T2-weighted sequence [97]. After completion of a whole-body scan, a dedicated MR imaging confined to one-bed position is started with or without simultaneous PET data acquisition. The dedicated MR imaging includes standard anatomic sequences and multiparametric MR sequences such as diffusion-weighted imaging (DWI), perfusion-weighted imaging (PWI), and dynamic contrast-enhanced (DCE) MR sequences, depending on the diagnostic purposes [18, 96].

In a similar fashion, in sequential design adopted by Philips Company, a specific MR sequence (i.e., MRAC) is run prior to PET acquisition. The MRAC sequence is acquired only with the integrated body coil of the MR scanner, matches the PET dimensions, and allows both anatomical detail and attenuation correction. The MRAC image is then segmented into three tissue classes (air, soft tissue, and lungs), and predetermined linear attenuation coefficients are assigned to each class (0, 0.095 and 0.022 cm^{-1}, respectively). An attenuation template of the patient table and MR coils (provided by system manufacturer) is incorporated into the attenuation correction map [100, 101].

To show data acquisition and imaging workflow provided in sequential PET/MR systems, one approach is to perform all the diagnostic MR acquisitions at the beginning, followed by attenuation correction dedicated sequences and then starting PET. For instance, this imaging scenario could be an indication to assess response to treatment or in head and neck cancer surgery planning [12, 50]. The acquisition time of MR sequences has been an issue as it works against patient comfort and low throughput imaging rate and is vulnerable to imaging artifacts due to likelihood of patient motion. New technologies are attempting to tackle this issue by developing fast pulse sequence in addition to parallel acquisition with multiple coil elements and also the use of parallel transmission [44].

9.7.2 Motion in PET/MR

Object motion in photography is generally an undesired feature that results in image blurring but in medical imaging is a crucial source of image quality degradation and impaired quantitative accuracy. Patient motions either voluntary or involuntary are among those degrading sources that need special attention in routine clinical practice. Consequences are loss of sharp edges and difficulties in outlining pathologic lesions in addition to less confidence in image interpretation [56, 102].

This resulting image blurring is simply due to the lack of timing information about the moving object in relation to stationary assumptions of the detection process or absence of an accurate motion model in the iterative reconstruction scheme. Patient motion and associated imaging artifacts in PET/CT are discussed in details in Chap. 16. Although the scanning period of MR sequences is relatively lengthy and might appear that it could be in temporal matching with those images from PET scanning, the data acquired with time-averaging process by MR are not comparable to the same average process in PET data acquisition [11]. However, the MR data which are used for attenuation correction produce an image from an average of fewer respiratory cycles but carrying a lot of motion compared to CT.

Voluntary (cardiac and respiratory) and involuntary motion artifacts need to be addressed before an accurate image interpretation takes place. Organ or lesion motion causes a count smearing effect over an area larger than the actual size of the lesion and hence causes volume inaccuracy determination and loss of quantitative accuracy. Acquiring the images at small time interval using the conventional "freezing" or gating approach has been effective in eliminating many of the motion-related diagnostic artifacts, but still suffers from low sensitivity and high image noise with low statistical quality due to the short scan time. In case of static cardiac imaging and free-breathing conditions, the heart moves in the range of 4.9–9 mm due to heartbeat and respiration, together with changes in myocardial shape and density. ECG gating, however, helps to acquire multiple frames representing heart motion intervals from diastole to systole, and hence motion-related artifacts can be removed.

In an attempt to match the two data sets and improve attenuation correction in cardiac PET/MR, a specific pulse sequence (two-dimensional fast spoiled gradient-recalled echo (SPGR)) has been applied to obtain an average MR image of patient under free-breathing conditions [103]. MR images were converted into PET attenuation maps using a three-class tissue segmentation method. In the myocardium, the voxel-by-voxel differences and the differences in mean slice activity between the attenuation MR-corrected PET data and the average CT-corrected PET data were found to be small (less than 7 %). The use of MR-derived attenuation images in place of CT-based attenuation correction did not also affect the summed stress score [103].

In principle, an accurate attenuation correction map is obtained if the CT- or MR-derived attenuation coefficients have the same static or dynamic phase as the acquired PET data. Diaphragmatic motion (i.e., 7–28 mm excursion) is a major source of image spatial resolution loss and degraded quantitative accuracy such as SUV measurements. It is of particular importance in oncological studies where the lung and upper abdomen are involved in a number of different tumor types. In similar fashion to cardiac gating, the respiratory signal can be acquired over short time bins (i.e., respiratory gating), and this approach was found successful in part solving motion-associated artifacts. It also prolongs the acquisition time affecting patient comfort and reduce patient throughput. Nevertheless, gating methods are the most widely used in motion correction strategies in the clinic. Realignment of the PET image bins after reconstruction into a single reference image is also a proposed solution but denatures the Poisson characteristics of the PET data [104, 105].

Using the list-mode PET data to derive motion estimates based on elastic deformation from simulated respiratory gating phantom has been proposed [106, 107]. Comparison of corrected and uncorrected respiratory motion average frames suggests that an affine transformation in the list-mode data prior to reconstruction can produce significant improvements in accounting for respiratory motion artifacts in the lungs and heart [104]. On the other hand, list-mode-based and model-based image reconstruction where motion information is incorporated, similar to other image-degrading factors, in the framework of image reconstruction has shown to be superior in improving the temporal sampling as well as a reduction in the effects of irregular respiratory motion [106, 108].

The simultaneous nature of some hybrid PET/MR opened new avenues for researchers to use the MRI information to address the issue of organ motion by either using simple methods such as T2-weighted imaging during free breathing and T1-weighted imaging using either shallow end expiration or free breathing using a radial acquisition scheme [105, 109]. More advanced approaches are to use motion-sensitive MRI imaging sequences such as velocity-encoded phase contrast MRI (VEPC-MRI) or MRI tagging technique [105, 110]. MRI-based motion correction has not demonstrated robust translation into the clinic because of signal to noise and/or field of view problems within the larger human. The most promising techniques proposed with human applications include a T1-weighted approach that utilizes navigator echoes combined with either a 2D multi-slice gradient echo technique [111] or a steady-state free precession (SSFP) [104] in order to both track the respiratory excursion and create a motion tracking field that is utilized in the PET processing algorithm [109].

Tagged MR uses a special pulse sequence to create temporary features (tags) in tissue, which deform and can be tracked in images as the anatomy deforms. Another recent approach has been devised such that no external hardware exist to provide a respiratory signal and no change to the imaging examination except for the addition of a short PET/MR sequence after the clinical acquisition [112]. The authors hypothesized that sufficient data for respiratory correction can be acquired in just 1 min. The acquisition was used to build a patient-specific respiratory motion model and then used to motion correct the clinical PET data of any duration. The method used only standard MR sequences and image registration techniques. The PET-derived signal was used to drive a motion model formed by nonrigid registration of MR slices acquired rapidly after the main scan. This motion was then incorporated into the PET reconstruction. An increase in SUV measurements has been reported, and sharpness of count profiles drawn over some lesions was observed. However, further work is requested to investigate the technical feasibility in clinical setting and to prove significant lesion detectability over large patient population [112].

An MR self-gating method was also applied to perform respiratory gating of the MRI data and simultaneously acquired PET raw data [113]. The MRI sequence allows for retrospective self-gating without the need for additional MRI navigator echoes or sensors attached to the patient. After gated PET reconstruction, the MRI motion model is used to fuse the individual gates into a single, motion-compensated volume with high SNR. The MRI motion model is utilized for motion-corrected PET image reconstruction according to the post-reconstruction registration scheme [113]. The motion model yielded a reduced motion blur and improved quantification accuracy compared to static reconstructions and in higher SNR compared to conventional gated reconstructions.

Figure 9.9 shows PET data acquired in a simultaneous mode with MR signal integrating motion correction, attenuation correction, and point spread function modeling into a single PET reconstruction framework. A dedicated MRI pulse sequence (denoted "NAV-TrueFISP") was used allowing an accurate measurement of respiratory motion in the lower abdomen. It is composed of two-dimensional (2D) multi-slice steady-state free precession MRI acquisitions ("TrueFISP") interleaved by pencil-beam navigator echoes.

9.8 Opportunities, Challenges, and Future

PET/MR provides a significant number of technical and clinical advantages to the current state of molecular and morphologic imaging. These features can be exploited to improve the overall perfor-

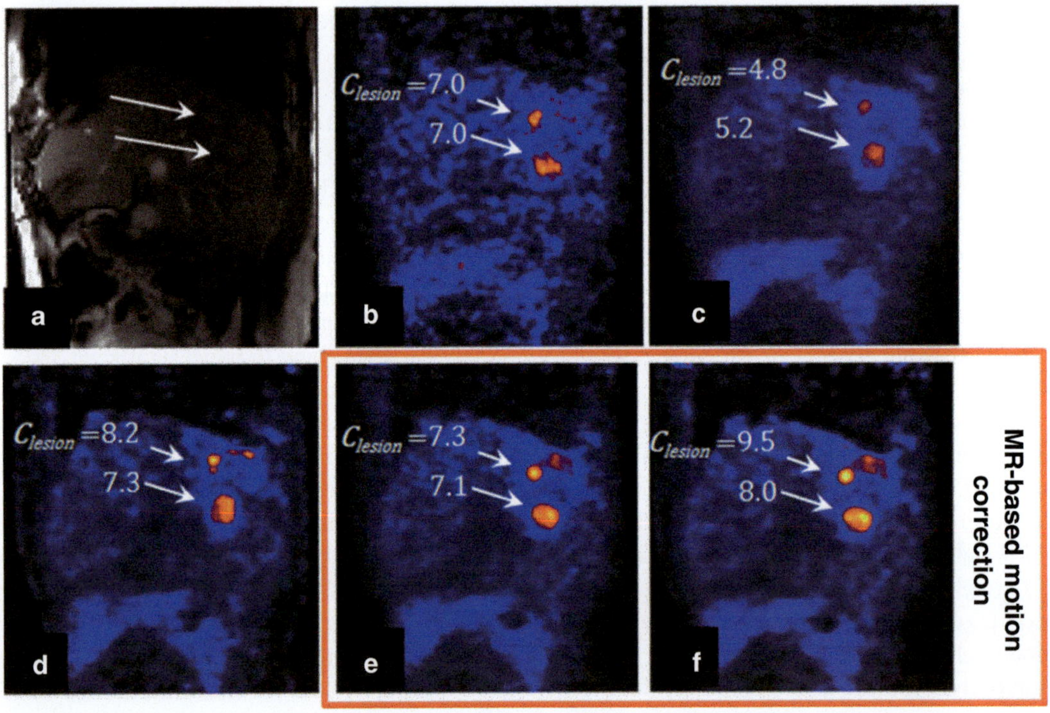

Fig. 9.9 Sagittal MRI (**a**) and corresponding PET slices reconstructed using (**b**) respiratory gating (OP-OSEM "gated"), (**c**) no motion correction (OP-OSEM), (**d**) no motion correction with PSF modeling (PSF-OP-OSEM), (**e**) MR-based motion correction (MC-OP-OSEM), and (**f**) motion and PSF corrections ("MC-PSF-OP-OSEM"). The gated volume was reconstructed using PET counts detected at end exhalation (approximately one-seventh of the total number of events). As can be seen, the proposed reconstruction methods (**e**, **f**) substantially improved hepatic lesion contrast and structure delineation as compared to the conventional uncorrected reconstruction method (**c**). *OP-OSEM* ordinary Poisson ordered-subset expectation, maximization, *PSF* point spread function (Reprinted from Ref. [114] with permission)

mance of hybrid PET/MR imaging systems in patient diagnosis, therapy, and management. The well-known improved soft tissue contrast characterizing MR imaging is a unique feature when compared to CT-based examinations. This characteristic is essential in brain studies, head and neck, abdomen, pelvis, and other soft tissue abnormalities. Furthermore, it will be beneficial in breast, liver, musculoskeletal, and urogenital imaging [115]. The lack of ionizing radiation in image acquisition is also an important asset in pediatric age group, pregnant women, and repeated acquisitions in patient follow-up and therapy monitoring. A recent work looking at diagnostic risk of medical exposure to CT scans in pediatric patients showed a probable triple risk of leukemia after a cumulative CT dose of 50 milligray (mGy), and a dose of 60 mGy might nearly triple the risk of brain tumors [116].

The simultaneous hybrid PET/MR imaging would in principle maximize the amount of information for real and direct benefit to patient management. MR can be very instrumental in synergizing the quality and quantitative accuracy of PET in terms of using the MR as guide to image reconstruction and incorporation of partial volume and/or attenuation correction in time of flight PET/MR systems [117–120]. MR-based motion correction and derivation of arterial input function are also potential applications that undergo significant research interest. Accurate determination of arterial input function is essential to obtain accurate physiologic parameter estimation when attempts are made to quantify tracer kinetics in absolute fashion. The MR component can help provide a way to determine blood flows such that partial volume correction and blood vessel contribution to PET signal can be accounted for in the kinetic model. Realizing this last benefit would enhance the dynamic PET applications in routine practice in addition to eliminating the complications associated with arterial catheterization and serial blood sampling [121, 122].

In addition to superior contrast resolution among different types of soft tissue, MRI allows physiological (e.g., dynamic contrast-enhanced MRI), metabolic (e.g., MR spectroscopy), and molecular (e.g., diffusion-weighted imaging) besides functional MRI (fMRI) phenomena to be observed [123, 124]. MRI has a multitude of image pulse sequence that can flourish the diagnostic process, and when combined with PET data, particularly when using newly developed specific tracers, the amount of diagnostic information would be enormous and very supportive in clinical decision-making. For example, tumor perfusion using blood-oxygen-level-dependent (BOLD) imaging and correlating the results with O15-water or hypoxia-based tracers could substantially enhance the diagnostic interpretation [16, 125, 126]. Furthermore, the study of tumor uptake and dynamics with dual-labeled or more functionalized nanoparticle contrast agents and simultaneous PET/MRI monitoring of disease pharmacokinetics or pharmacodynamics are new avenues utilizing this multimodality imaging system [127].

PET/MR proved useful in a number of malignancies such as head and neck where improved soft tissue contrast is required. This can be represented by providing information about tumor extent and involvement of bony structures and bone marrow. Tissue reactions such as distortion, scarring, and fibrosis that appear posttreatment surveillance can obscure early detection of recurrence by conventional follow-up [128, 129]. It has also potential in evaluating pelvic malignancies such as gynecologic, rectal, and prostatic cancers because of its improved soft tissue discrimination compared with CT [130]. In breast imaging, specific breast MRI sequences permit high diagnostic accuracy for local tumor staging, and whole-body MRI can also be of great use in distant staging, especially when combined with F18-FDG-PET which has a high diagnostic performance for the detection of distant metastases [131]. FDG-PET/MR has an evolving role in breast cancer management, for example, in the detection of liver metastases and in the research setting for treatment monitoring [132].

In malignancies involving liver disease where metastases can occur from different sites, MR imaging has good diagnostic performance for lesions smaller than <10 mm; however, FDG-PET has some limitation such as heterogeneous uptake in the normal liver, its low sensitivity to lesions smaller than 10 mm, and the concomitant decrease in sensitivity in patients with underlying liver disease, including cirrhosis and nonalcoholic fatty liver disease [133, 134]. In bone marrow imaging, whole-body MR imaging has been proposed for detecting infiltrative focal bone marrow lesions and was demonstrated to have higher sensitivity than a skeletal survey for this task. It can also have potential in therapy monitoring or in the development of new therapies [129].

The role of PET/MR in neurology and psychiatry is one of the motivating aspects for developing such kind of devices due to the long-term experience of PET methodology and tracers in studying brain biochemistry. This has included a number of critical disorders that require early detection and response monitoring and even go beyond to stratify drugs in early stage of development. Anatomical and functional MRI information when combined with PET would have a definite incremental value to the diagnostic process in brain studies [135, 136]. In neuro-oncology, while gadolinium-enhanced MRI remains standard of care for brain tumor management (i.e., diagnosis, treatment, and posttreatment response assessment), other advanced MR techniques could be valuable in difficult cases providing key pathways into improved diagnostics. Different PET tracers such as F18-FLT, F18-FMISO, C11-Met, F18-FDOPA, and F18-FET can also assist in characterizing different aspects of tumor biology, and the availability of simultaneous PET/MR would facilitate investigations that look at improved patient management [135–137].

In cardiovascular diseases, PET imaging has unique capabilities in quantifying myocardial blood flow and flow reserve and is considered the gold standard for assessing myocardial viability [see Chap. 19 for further details]. MR can be used to assess ventricle function, structural changes, perfusion, and tissue viability. It can also evaluate cardiac anatomy and detailed tissue characterization. Functional MR images and dynamic assessment of myocardial perfusion from transit of intravascular contrast medium can provide useful criteria for identifying areas of decreased myocardial perfusion or for assessing tissue viability from late contrast enhancement of scar tissue [138].

High temporal resolution cine image sequences have been devised to capture high-resolution images of the cardiac cycle. Blood flow can be visualized and measured via velocity-encoded cine sequences. Spectroscopic techniques, T1 mapping, and sequences capable of measuring myocardial strain are advanced MR techniques that can be integrated in the diagnostic scheme. Other utilities can be seen in detection of inflammation and characterizing atherosclerotic plaques and differentiate with a high risk of rupture from stable plaques. With the development of new tracers, there will be good opportunities in evaluating myocardial remodeling and in assessing the kinetics of stem cell therapy in myocardial infarction. New tracers will also provide new means for evaluating alterations in cardiac innervation, angiogenesis, and even the assessment of reporter gene technologies [138, 139].

Multimodal hybrid imaging in general and PET/MR in particular provide a great opportunity for understanding tumor pathophysiology and tackling biomedical questions that may arise from diagnostic or treatment clinical practices. The wide range of responses among patients suggests that further studies of individual responses to therapy, correlating structural and functional imaging, metabolic imaging, and clinical findings, will not only be helpful in understanding the mechanism of action of novel therapeutic agents but also support the new trend of precision medicine [129]. PET/MR could help in this dilemma by providing a one-stop-shop hybrid imaging platform that would eventually improve patient diagnosis and treatment outcomes. Extensive work has been and is being performed to elicit the several advantages of these systems in order to build up significant amount of evidences able to locate the hybrid PET/MR into its real clinical position in the near future.

References

1. Phelps ME. PET: the merging of biology and imaging into molecular imaging. J Nucl Med. 2000;41: 661–81.
2. Chatziioannou AF. Molecular imaging of small animals with dedicated PET tomographs. Eur J Nucl Med Mol Imaging. 2002;29:98–114.
3. Jones T. Molecular imaging with PET – the future challenges. Br J Radiol. 2002;75:S6–15.
4. Yeh SH, Lin CF, Kong FL, et al. Molecular imaging of nonsmall cell lung carcinomas expressing active mutant EGFR kinase using PET with [(124)i]-morpholino-IPQA. Biomed Res Int. 2013;2013:549359.
5. Hammer BE, Christensen NL, Heil BG. Use of a magnetic field to increase the spatial resolution of positron emission tomography. Med Phys. 1994;21: 1917–20.
6. Gaertner FC, Furst S, Schwaiger M. PET/MR: a paradigm shift. Cancer Imaging. 2013;13:36–52.
7. Jadvar H, Colletti PM. Competitive advantage of PET/MRI. Eur J Radiol. 2013;83:84–94.
8. Martinez-Moller A, Eiber M, Nekolla SG, et al. Workflow and scan protocol considerations for integrated whole-body PET/MRI in oncology. J Nucl Med. 2012;53:1415–26.
9. Beyer T, Townsend DW, Brun T, et al. A combined PET/CT scanner for clinical oncology. J Nucl Med. 2000;41:1369–79.
10. Townsend DW. Combined positron emission tomography-computed tomography: the historical perspective. Semin Ultrasound CT MR. 2008;29:232–5.
11. Zaidi H, Del Guerra A. An outlook on future design of hybrid PET/MRI systems. Med Phys. 2011;38: 5667–89.
12. Kalemis A, Delattre BM, Heinzer S. Sequential whole-body PET/MR scanner: concept, clinical use, and optimisation after two years in the clinic. The manufacturer's perspective. MAGMA. 2012;26:5–23.
13. Veit-Haibach P, Kuhn FP, Wiesinger F, Delso G, von Schulthess G. PET-MR imaging using a tri-modality PET/CT-MR system with a dedicated shuttle in clinical routine. MAGMA. 2012;26:25–35.
14. Delso G, Furst S, Jakoby B, et al. Performance measurements of the Siemens mMR integrated whole-body PET/MR scanner. J Nucl Med. 2015;52:1914–22.
15. Judenhofer MS, Catana C, Swann BK, et al. PET/MR images acquired with a compact MR-compatible PET detector in a 7-T magnet. Radiology. 2007;244: 807–14.
16. Judenhofer MS, Wehrl HF, Newport DF, et al. Simultaneous PET-MRI: a new approach for functional

and morphological imaging. Nat Med. 2008;14:459–65.
17. Schlemmer HP, Pichler BJ, Schmand M, et al. Simultaneous MR/PET imaging of the human brain: feasibility study. Radiology. 2008;248:1028–35.
18. Yoo HJ, Lee JS, Lee JM. Integrated whole body MR/PET: where are we? Korean J Radiol. 2015;16:32–49.
19. Hawkes RC, Fryer TD, Siegel S, Ansorge RE, Carpenter TA. Preliminary evaluation of a combined microPET-MR system. Technol Cancer Res Treat. 2010;9:53–60.
20. Levin CGG, Deller T, McDaniel D, Peterson W, Maramraju SH. Prototype time-of-flight PET ring integrated with a 3T MRI system for simultaneous whole-body PET/MR imaging. J Nucl Med. 2013;54 Suppl 2:148.
21. Levin CFJ, Deller T, Maramraju SH and Lagaru A. Performance of a high sensitivity time-of-flight PET ring operating simultaneously within a 3T MR system Proceeding of 3rd conferences on PET-MR and SPECT-MR. Kos Island, 19–21 May 2014. 2014.
22. Queiroz MA, Delso G, Wollenweber S, et al. Dose optimization in TOF-PET/MR compared to TOF-PET/CT. PLoS One. 2015;10:e0128842.
23. Wagadarikar I, Dolinsky M. Sensitivity improvement of time-of-flight (ToF) PET detector through recovery of compton scattered annihilation photons. IEEE Trans Nucl Sci. 2014;61:121–5.
24. Balyasnikova S, Lofgren J, de Nijs R, et al. PET/MR in oncology: an introduction with focus on MR and future perspectives for hybrid imaging. Am J Nucl Med Mol Imag. 2012;2:458–74.
25. Keereman V, Mollet P, Berker Y, Schulz V, Vandenberghe S. Challenges and current methods for attenuation correction in PET/MR. MAGMA. 2012;26:81–98.
26. Carrio IR, Pablo R, editors. PET/MRI: methodology and clinical applications. Heidelberg: Springer; 2014.
27. Delso G, Ziegler S. PET/MR system design. In: Ignasi C, Pablo R, editors. PET/MRI: methodology and clinical applications. Heidelberg: Springer; 2014. p. 1–19.
28. Wu Y, Catana C, Farrell R, et al. PET performance evaluation of an MR-compatible PET insert. IEEE Trans Nucl Sci. 2009;56:574–80.
29. Shao Y, Cherry SR, Farahani K, et al. Simultaneous PET and MR imaging. Phys Med Biol. 1997;42:1965–70.
30. Shao Y, Cherry SR, Farahani K, Slates R, Silverman RW, Meadors K, Bowery A, Siegel S, Marsden PK, Garlick PB. Development of a PET detector system compatible with MRI/NMR systems. IEEE Trans Nucl Sci. 1997;44:1167–71.
31. Yamamoto S, Imaizumi M, Kanai Y, et al. Design and performance from an integrated PET/MRI system for small animals. Ann Nucl Med. 2010;24:89–98.
32. Pichler BJ, Judenhofer MS, Catana C, et al. Performance test of an LSO-APD detector in a 7-T MRI scanner for simultaneous PET/MRI. J Nucl Med. 2006;47:639–47.
33. Del Guerra A DN, Bisogni MG, Corsi F, Foresta M, et al. Silicon photomultipliers (SiPM) as novel photodetectors for PET. Nucl Instrum Methods Phys. Res. A. 2011;648:S232–5
34. Roncali E, Cherry S. Application of silicon photomultipliers to positron emission tomography. Ann Biomed Eng. 2011;39:1358–77.
35. Surti S. Update on time-of-flight PET imaging. J Nucl Med. 2014;56:98–105.
36. Yamamoto S, Kuroda K, Senda M. Scintillator selection for MR-compatible gamma detectors. IEEE Trans Nucl Sci. 2003;50:1683–5.
37. Zaidi HE. Molecular imaging of small animals: instrumentation and applications. New York: Springer; 2014.
38. Khalil M. Positron emission tomography (PET): basic principles. In: Khalil M, editor. Basic sciences of nuclear medicine. Berlin/Heidelberg: Springer; 2011. p. 179–209.
39. Pichler B, Lorenz E, Mirzoyan R, et al. Performance test of a LSO-APD PET module in a 9.4 tesla magnet. IEEE Nuclear Science Symposium Conference Record of the IEEE Nuclear Science Symposium and Medical Imaging Conference Piscataway. IEEE; 1998. p. 1237–9.
40. Disselhorst JA, Bezrukov I, Kolb A, Parl C, Pichler BJ. Principles of PET/MR imaging. J Nucl Med. 2014;55:2S–10.
41. Spanoudaki V, Levin C. Photo-detectors for time of flight positron emission tomography (ToF-PET). Sensors (Basel). 2010;10:10484–505.
42. Catana C, Wu Y, Judenhofer MS, et al. Simultaneous acquisition of multislice PET and MR images: initial results with a MR-compatible PET scanner. J Nucl Med. 2006;47:1968–76.
43. Peng BJ, Wu Y, Cherry SR, Walton JH. New shielding configurations for a simultaneous PET/MRI scanner at 7T. J Magn Reson. 2014;239:50–6.
44. Beyer T, Mawlawi O, Harald Q. PET/MR instrumentation. In: Ratib O, Scwaiger M, Beyer T, editors. Atlas of PET/MR imaging in oncology. Berlin/New York: Springer; 2013.
45. España S, Fraile L, Herraiz J, Udías J, Desco M, Vaquero J. Performance evaluation of SiPM photodetectors for PET imaging in the presence of magnetic fields. Nucl Instrum Methods Phys Res A. 2010;613:308–16.
46. Wehner J, Weissler B, Dueppenbecker P, et al. PET/MRI insert using digital SiPMs: investigation of MR-compatibility. Nucl Instrum Methods Phys Res A. 2014;734:116–21.
47. Ay MR, Mehranian A, Abdoli M, Ghafarian P, Zaidi H. Qualitative and quantitative assessment of metal artifacts arising from implantable cardiac pacing devices in oncological PET/CT studies: a phantom study. Mol Imaging Biol. 2011;13:1077–87.
48. Weissler B, Gebhardt P, Duppenbecker P, et al. A digital preclinical PET/MRI insert and initial results. IEEE Trans Med Imaging. 2015;34:2258–70.
49. http://mri-q.com/gradient-coils.html. Accessed Nov 2015.

50. Shah SN, Huang SS. Hybrid PET/MR imaging: physics and technical considerations. Abdom Imaging. 2015;40:1358–65.
51. Truhn D, Kiessling F, Schulz V. Optimized RF shielding techniques for simultaneous PET/MR. Med Phys. 2011;38:3995–4000.
52. Duppenbecker PM, Wehner J, Renz W, et al. Gradient transparent RF housing for simultaneous PET/MRI using carbon fiber composites. In: Nuclear Science Symposium and Medical Imaging Conference (NSS/MIC). IEEE; 2012. p. 3478–80.
53. Wolf G, Abolmaali N. Preclinical molecular imaging using PET and MRI. Recent Results Cancer Res. 2012;187:257–310.
54. Yang Y, Wu Y, Qi J, et al. A prototype PET scanner with DOI-encoding detectors. J Nucl Med. 2008;49: 1132–40.
55. Poole M, Bowtell R, Green D, et al. Split gradient coils for simultaneous PET-MRI. Magn Reson Med. 2009;62:1106–11.
56. Vandenberghe S, Marsden PK. PET-MRI: a review of challenges and solutions in the development of integrated multimodality imaging. Phys Med Biol. 2015;60:R115–54.
57. Bindseil GA, Gilbert KM, Scholl TJ, Handler WB, Chronik BA. First image from a combined positron emission tomography and field-cycled MRI system. Magn Reson Med. 2011;66:301–5.
58. Lucas AJ, Hawkes RC, Ansorge RE, et al. Development of a combined microPET-MR system. Technol Cancer Res Treat. 2006;5:337–41.
59. Nagy K, Toth M, Major P, et al. Performance evaluation of the small-animal nanoScan PET/MRI system. J Nucl Med. 2013;54:1825–32.
60. Szanda I, Mackewn J, Patay G, et al. National Electrical Manufacturers Association NU-4 performance evaluation of the PET component of the NanoPET/CT preclinical PET/CT scanner. J Nucl Med. 2011;52:1741–7.
61. Marshall HR, Stodilka RZ, Theberge J, et al. A comparison of MR-based attenuation correction in PET versus SPECT. Phys Med Biol. 2011;56: 4613–29.
62. Teuho J, Johansson J, Linden J, et al. Quantitative bias in PET/MR from attenuation correction and reconstruction: a comparison with PET and PET/CT with an anatomical brain phantom and Hoffman brain phantom. In, Nuclear Science Symposium and Medical Imaging Conference (NSS/MIC). IEEE; 2013. p. 1–8.
63. Meikle SR, Bailey DL, Hooper PK, et al. Simultaneous emission and transmission measurements for attenuation correction in whole-body PET. J Nucl Med. 1995;36:1680–8.
64. deKemp RA, Nahmias C. Attenuation correction in PET using single photon transmission measurement. Med Phys. 1994;21:771–8.
65. Kinahan PE, Townsend DW, Beyer T, Sashin D. Attenuation correction for a combined 3D PET/CT scanner. Med Phys. 1998;25:2046–53.
66. Blankcspoor SC HB, Brown JK, Heanue JA, Gould RG, Cann CE, Dae MW. Development of an emission-transmission CT system combining X-ray CT and SPECT. Conference Record of the 1994 IEEE Nuclear Science Symposium and Medical Imaging Conference. 1994. p. 1758–61.
67. Wagenknecht G, Kaiser HJ, Mottaghy FM, Herzog H. MRI for attenuation correction in PET: methods and challenges. MAGMA. 2012;26:99–113.
68. Malone IB, Ansorge RE, Williams GB, et al. Attenuation correction methods suitable for brain imaging with a PET/MRI scanner: a comparison of tissue atlas and template attenuation map approaches. J Nucl Med. 2011;52:1142–9.
69. Ashburner J, Friston KJ. Nonlinear spatial normalization using basis functions. Hum Brain Mapp. 1999;7:254–66.
70. Kops R, Herzog H. Alternative methods for attenuation correction for PET images in MR-PET scanners. Nuclear Science Symposium Conference Record. Vol 6. NSS'07 IEEE;2007. p. 4327–30.
71. Hofmann M, Steinke F, Scheel V, et al. MRI-based attenuation correction for PET/MRI: a novel approach combining pattern recognition and atlas registration. J Nucl Med. 2008;49:1875–83.
72. Hofmann M, Bezrukov I, Mantlik F, et al. MRI-based attenuation correction for whole-body PET/MRI: quantitative evaluation of segmentation- and atlas-based methods. J Nucl Med. 2011;52:1392–9.
73. Schreibmann E, Nye JA, Schuster DM, et al. MR-based attenuation correction for hybrid PET-MR brain imaging systems using deformable image registration. Med Phys. 2010;37:2101–9.
74. Hofmann M, Pichler B, Scholkopf B, Beyer T. Towards quantitative PET/MRI: a review of MR-based attenuation correction techniques. Eur J Nucl Med Mol Imaging. 2009;36 Suppl 1:S93–104.
75. Visvikis DMF, Bert J, Hatt M, Fayad H. PET/MR attenuation correction: where have we come from and where are we going? Eur J Nucl Med Mol Imaging. 2014;41(6):1172–5.
76. Bezrukov I, Schmidt H, Mantlik F, et al. MR-based attenuation correction methods for improved PET quantification in lesions within bone and susceptibility artifact regions. J Nucl Med. 2013;54:1768–74.
77. Burgos N, Cardoso MJ, Modat M, et al. Attenuation correction synthesis for hybrid PET-MR scanners. Med Image Comput Assist Interv. 2014;16:147–54.
78. Burgos N, Cardoso MJ, Thielemans K, et al. Attenuation correction synthesis for hybrid PET-MR scanners: application to brain studies. IEEE Trans Med Imaging. 2014;33:2332–41.
79. Lois C, Bezrukov I, Schmidt H, et al. Effect of MR contrast agents on quantitative accuracy of PET in combined whole-body PET/MR imaging. Eur J Nucl Med Mol Imaging. 2012;39:1756–66.
80. Zaidi H, Montandon ML, Slosman DO. Magnetic resonance imaging-guided attenuation and scatter corrections in three-dimensional brain positron emission tomography. Med Phys. 2003;30:937–48.

81. Schulz V, Torres-Espallardo I, Renisch S, et al. Automatic, three-segment, MR-based attenuation correction for whole-body PET/MR data. Eur J Nucl Med Mol Imaging. 2010;38:138–52.
82. Akbarzadeh A, Ay MR, Ahmadian A, Alam NR, Zaidi H. MRI-guided attenuation correction in whole-body PET/MR: assessment of the effect of bone attenuation. Ann Nucl Med. 2012;27:152–62.
83. Martinez-Moller A, Souvatzoglou M, Delso G, et al. Tissue classification as a potential approach for attenuation correction in whole-body PET/MRI: evaluation with PET/CT data. J Nucl Med. 2009;50:520–6.
84. Kim JH, Lee JS, Song IC, Lee DS. Comparison of segmentation-based attenuation correction methods for PET/MRI: evaluation of bone and liver standardized uptake value with oncologic PET/CT data. J Nucl Med. 2012;53:1878–82.
85. Steinberg J, Jia G, Sammet S, et al. Three-region MRI-based whole-body attenuation correction for automated PET reconstruction. Nucl Med Biol. 2010;37:227–35.
86. Delso G, Wiesinger F, Sacolick LI, et al. Clinical evaluation of zero-echo-time MR imaging for the segmentation of the skull. J Nucl Med. 2015;56:417–22.
87. Catana C, van der Kouwe A, Benner T, et al. Toward implementing an MRI-based PET attenuation-correction method for neurologic studies on the MR-PET brain prototype. J Nucl Med. 2010;51:1431–8.
88. Bezrukov I, Mantlik F, Schmidt H, Scholkopf B, Pichler BJ. MR-Based PET attenuation correction for PET/MR imaging. Semin Nucl Med. 2013;43:45–59.
89. Gibiino F, Sacolick L, Menini A, Landini L, Wiesinger F. Free-breathing, zero-TE MR lung imaging. MAGMA. 2014;28:207–15.
90. Roy S, Wang WT, Carass A, et al. PET attenuation correction using synthetic CT from ultrashort echo-time MR imaging. J Nucl Med. 2014;55:2071–7.
91. Keereman V, Fierens Y, Broux T, et al. MRI-based attenuation correction for PET/MRI using ultrashort echo time sequences. J Nucl Med. 2010;51:812–8.
92. Berker Y, Franke J, Salomon A, et al. MRI-based attenuation correction for hybrid PET/MRI systems: a 4-class tissue segmentation technique using a combined ultrashort-echo-time/Dixon MRI sequence. J Nucl Med. 2012;53:796–804.
93. Aasheim LB, Karlberg A, Goa PE, et al. PET/MR brain imaging: evaluation of clinical UTE-based attenuation correction. Eur J Nucl Med Mol Imaging. 2015;42:1439–46.
94. Rezaei A, Defrise M, Bal G, et al. Simultaneous reconstruction of activity and attenuation in time-of-flight PET. IEEE Trans Med Imaging. 2012;31:2224–33.
95. Conti M. Focus on time-of-flight PET: the benefits of improved time resolution. Eur J Nucl Med Mol Imaging. 2011;38:1147–57.
96. Torigian DA, Zaidi H, Kwee TC, et al. PET/MR imaging: technical aspects and potential clinical applications. Radiology. 2013;267:26–44.
97. Bashir U, Mallia A, Stirling J, et al. PET/MRI in oncological imaging: state of the art. Diagnostics (Basel). 2015;5(3):333–57.
98. von Schulthess GK, Veit-Haibach P. Workflow considerations in PET/MR imaging. J Nucl Med. 2014;55:19S–24.
99. Drzezga A, Souvatzoglou M, Eiber M, et al. First clinical experience with integrated whole-body PET/MR: comparison to PET/CT in patients with oncologic diagnoses. J Nucl Med. 2014;53:845–55.
100. Schramm G, Langner J, Hofheinz F, et al. Quantitative accuracy of attenuation correction in the Philips Ingenuity TF whole-body PET/MR system: a direct comparison with transmission-based attenuation correction. MAGMA. 2013;26:115–26.
101. Izquierdo-Garcia D, Sawiak SJ, Knesaurek K, et al. Comparison of MR-based attenuation correction and CT-based attenuation correction of whole-body PET/MR imaging. Eur J Nucl Med Mol Imaging. 2014;41:1574–84.
102. Nehmeh SA, Erdi YE. Respiratory motion in positron emission tomography/computed tomography: a review. Semin Nucl Med. 2008;38:167–76.
103. Ai H, Pan T. Feasibility of using respiration-averaged MR images for attenuation correction of cardiac PET/MR imaging. J Appl Clin Med Phys. 2015;16(4):5194.
104. Petibon Y, Huang C, Ouyang J, et al. Relative role of motion and PSF compensation in whole-body oncologic PET-MR imaging. Med Phys. 2014;41:042503.
105. Guerin B, Cho S, Chun SY, et al. Nonrigid PET motion compensation in the lower abdomen using simultaneous tagged-MRI and PET imaging. Med Phys. 2011;38:3025–38.
106. Lamare F, Ledesma Carbayo MJ, Cresson T, et al. List-mode based reconstruction for respiratory motion correction in PET using non-rigid body transformations. Phys Med Biol. 2007;52:5187–204.
107. Rahmim ABP, Houle S, Lenox M, Michel C, Buckley KR, Ruth TJ, Sossi V. Motion compensation in histogram-mode and list-mode EM reconstructions: beyond the event-driven approach. IEEE Trans Nucl Sci. 2004;51(5):2588–96.
108. Reyes M, Malandain G, Koulibaly PM, Gonzalez-Ballester MA, Darcourt J. Model-based respiratory motion compensation for emission tomography image reconstruction. Phys Med Biol. 2007;52:3579–600.
109. Attenberger U, Catana C, Chandarana H, et al. Whole-body FDG PET-MR oncologic imaging: pitfalls in clinical interpretation related to inaccurate MR-based attenuation correction. Abdom Imaging. 2015;40:1374–86.
110. Bryant D, Payne J, Firmin D, Longmore D. Measurement of flow with NMR imaging using a gradient pulse and phase difference technique. J Comput Assist Tomogr. 1984;8:588–93.
111. Würslin CSH, Martirosian P, Brendle C, Boss A, Schwenzer NF, Stegger L. Respiratory motion correction in oncologic PET using T1-weighted MR

imaging on a simultaneous whole-body PET/MR system. J Nucl Med. 2013;54(3):464–71.
112. Manber R, Thielemans K, Hutton BF, et al. Practical PET respiratory motion correction in clinical PET/MR. J Nucl Med. 2015;56:890–6.
113. Grimm R, Furst S, Souvatzoglou M, et al. Self-gated MRI motion modeling for respiratory motion compensation in integrated PET/MRI. Med Image Anal. 2014;19:110–20.
114. Ouyang J, Petibon Y, Huang C, et al. Quantitative simultaneous positron emission tomography and magnetic resonance imaging. J Med Imaging (Bellingham). 2014;1:033502.
115. Bagade S, Fowler KJ, Schwarz JK, Grigsby PW, Dehdashti F. PET/MRI evaluation of gynecologic malignancies and prostate cancer. Semin Nucl Med. 2015;45:293–303.
116. Pearce MS, Salotti JA, Little MP, et al. Radiation exposure from CT scans in childhood and subsequent risk of leukaemia and brain tumours: a retrospective cohort study. Lancet. 2012;380:499–505.
117. Bai B, Li Q, Leahy RM. Magnetic resonance-guided positron emission tomography image reconstruction. Semin Nucl Med. 2012;43:30–44.
118. Mehranian A, Zaidi H. Emission-based estimation of lung attenuation coefficients for attenuation correction in time-of-flight PET/MR. Phys Med Biol. 2015;60:4813–33.
119. Mehranian A, Zaidi H. Clinical assessment of emission- and segmentation-based MR-guided attenuation correction in whole-body time-of-flight PET/MR imaging. J Nucl Med. 2015;56:877–83.
120. Fei B, Yang X, Nye JA, et al. MRPET quantification tools: registration, segmentation, classification, and MR-based attenuation correction. Med Phys. 2012;39:6443–54.
121. Fluckiger J, Li X, Whisenant J, et al. Using dynamic contrast-enhanced magnetic resonance imaging data to constrain a positron emission tomography kinetic model: theory and simulations. Int J Biomed Imaging. 2013;2013:576470.
122. Su Y, Blazey T, Snyder A, et al. Quantitative amyloid imaging using image-derived arterial input function. PLoS One. 2015;10:e0122920.
123. Wehrl HF, Hossain M, Lankes K, et al. Simultaneous PET-MRI reveals brain function in activated and resting state on metabolic, hemodynamic and multiple temporal scales. Nat Med. 2013;19:1184–9.
124. Sander CY, Hooker JM, Catana C, et al. Neurovascular coupling to D2/D3 dopamine receptor occupancy using simultaneous PET/functional MRI. Proc Natl Acad Sci U S A. 2013;110:11169–74.
125. Bruehlmeier M, Roelcke U, Schubiger PA, Ametamey SM. Assessment of hypoxia and perfusion in human brain tumors using PET with 18F-fluoromisonidazole and 15O-H2O. J Nucl Med. 2004;45:1851–9.
126. Rauscher I, Eiber M, Souvatzoglou M, Schwaiger M, Beer AJ. PET/MR in oncology: non-18F-FDG tracers for routine applications. J Nucl Med. 2014;55:25S–31.
127. Yang X, Hong H, Grailer JJ, et al. cRGD-functionalized, DOX-conjugated, and (6)(4) Cu-labeled superparamagnetic iron oxide nanoparticles for targeted anticancer drug delivery and PET/MR imaging. Biomaterials. 2011;32:4151–60.
128. Covello M, Cavaliere C, Aiello M, et al. Simultaneous PET/MR head-neck cancer imaging: preliminary clinical experience and multiparametric evaluation. Eur J Radiol. 2015;84:1269–76.
129. Catana C, Guimaraes AR, Rosen BR. PET and MR imaging: the odd couple or a match made in heaven? J Nucl Med. 2013;54:815–24.
130. Lee SI, Catalano OA, Dehdashti F. Evaluation of gynecologic cancer with MR imaging, 18F-FDG PET/CT, and PET/MR imaging. J Nucl Med. 2015;56:436–43.
131. Catalano OA, Nicolai E, Rosen BR, et al. Comparison of CE-FDG-PET/CT with CE-FDG-PET/MR in the evaluation of osseous metastases in breast cancer patients. Br J Cancer. 2015;112:1452–60.
132. Gaeta CM, Vercher-Conejero JL, Sher AC, et al. Recurrent and metastatic breast cancer PET, PET/CT, PET/MRI: FDG and new biomarkers. Q J Nucl Med Mol Imaging. 2013;57:352–66.
133. Floriani I, Torri V, Rulli E, et al. Performance of imaging modalities in diagnosis of liver metastases from colorectal cancer: a systematic review and meta-analysis. J Magn Reson Imaging. 2009;31:19–31.
134. Niekel MC, Bipat S, Stoker J. Diagnostic imaging of colorectal liver metastases with CT, MR imaging, FDG PET, and/or FDG PET/CT: a meta-analysis of prospective studies including patients who have not previously undergone treatment. Radiology. 2010;257:674–84.
135. Barthel H, Schroeter ML, Hoffmann KT, Sabri O. PET/MR in dementia and other neurodegenerative diseases. Semin Nucl Med. 2015;45:224–33.
136. Drzezga A, Barthel H, Minoshima S, Sabri O. Potential clinical applications of PET/MR imaging in neurodegenerative diseases. J Nucl Med. 2014;55:47S–55.
137. Fink J, Muzi M, Peck M, Krohn KA. Multi-modality brain tumor imaging – MRI, PET, and PET/MRI. J Nucl Med. 2015;56:1554–61.
138. Ratib O, Nkoulou R. Potential applications of PET/MR imaging in cardiology. J Nucl Med. 2014;55:40S–6.
139. Nappi C, El Fakhri G. State of the art in cardiac hybrid technology: PET/MR. Curr Cardiovasc Imaging Rep. 2013;6:338–45.

PET Calibration, Acceptance Testing, and Quality Control

10

Magnus Dahlbom

Contents

10.1 **Introduction** 230

10.2 **PET Instrumentation and Dataflow** 230
10.2.1 Detector Flood Maps 231
10.2.2 Sinogram 233

10.3 **Detector and System Calibration** 236
10.3.1 Tube Balancing and Gain Adjustments 237
10.3.2 Energy Calibration 237
10.3.3 Timing Calibration 237
10.3.4 System Normalization 238
10.3.5 Activity Calibration 240

10.4 **Acceptance Testing** 240
10.4.1 Spatial Resolution 241
10.4.2 Scatter Fraction 241
10.4.3 Count Rate Performance and Correction Accuracy 243
10.4.4 Sensitivity 244
10.4.5 Systems with Intrinsic Background 245
10.4.6 Image Quality 245
10.4.7 Other Tests 246

10.5 **Routine Quality Assurance** 249
10.5.1 Daily Tests 249
10.5.2 Monthly/Quarterly Tests 251
10.5.3 Annual Tests 251
10.5.4 Tests for Clinical Trials 251

10.6 **Summary** 253

References 254

M. Dahlbom, PhD, DABR
UCLA Ahmanson Translational Imaging Division,
Department of Molecular and Medical Pharmacology,
David Geffen School of Medicine at UCLA,
University of California,
Los Angeles, CA 90024, USA
e-mail: MDahlbom@mednet.ucla.edu

PET/CT is a routinely performed diagnostic imaging procedure. To ensure that the system is performing properly and produces images of best possible quality and quantitative accuracy, a comprehensive quality control (QC) program should be implemented. This should include a rigorous initial acceptance test of the system, performed at the time of installation. This will ensure the system performs to the manufacturer's specifications and also serves as a reference point to which subsequent tests can be compared to as the system ages. Once in clinical use, the system should be tested on a routine basis to ensure that the system is fully operational and provides consistent image quality. To implement a successful and effective QC program, it is important to a have an understanding of the basic imaging components of the system. This chapter will describe the basic system components of a PET system and the dataflow that will aid a user in identifying potential problems. Acceptance tests and QC procedures will also be described and explained, all designed to ensure that a consistent image quality and quantitative accuracy are maintained. As will be discussed, an effective QC program can be implemented with a few relatively simple routinely performed tests.

M.M. Khalil (ed.), *Basic Science of PET Imaging*, DOI 10.1007/978-3-319-40070-9_10

10.1 Introduction

PET/CT imaging has for several years been an accepted and a routine clinical imaging procedure. To ensure that the imaging system is operating properly and is providing the best possible image quality, a thorough acceptance testing of the system should be performed. The purpose is to ensure that that the system is performing as specified by the manufacturer and also to ensure that the system is fully functional before being taken into clinical use. Following the initial testing, the system should be tested on a routine basis to ensure that the system is operational for patient imaging and will provide consistent image quality. These tests are not as rigorous as the initial acceptance testing, but should provide the user with enough information to decide if the system is operational or is in the need of service.

This chapter will describe various tests that are used in an acceptance test of a PET scanner. The various aspects of quality control (QC) procedures will be discussed as well as the different elements of a QC program.

10.2 PET Instrumentation and Dataflow

To develop tests for a PET system, it is important to have a basic understanding of the detector and data acquisition system used in a PET scanner. Although the specific design differs between manufacturers, the overall designs are fairly similar [1, 2]. A schematic of the dataflow in a PET system is shown in Fig. 10.1. The detector system typically consists of a large number of scintillation detector modules with associated front-end electronics, such as high voltage, pulse-shaping amplifiers, and discriminators. The outputs from the detector modules are then fed into processing units or detector controllers that determine which detector element was hit by a 511 keV photon, how much energy was deposited, and information about when the interaction occurred. This information is then fed into a coincidence processor, which receives information from all detectors in the system. The coincidence processor determines if two detectors were registering an event within a predetermined time period (i.e., the coincidence time window). If this is the case, a coincidence has been recorded, and the information about the two detectors and the time of when the event occurred are saved. This information is later used for image reconstruction. Since the events are saved as they occur as a stream or long list of events, this method of data storage is sometimes referred to as list mode. Events can also be sorted into projection data or sinograms on the fly, which is a convenient method of organizing the data prior to image reconstruction. Data are subsequently stored on disk and later reconstructed.

In the most recent generation of PET systems, time-of-flight (TOF) information is also recorded. The TOF information that is recorded is the difference in time of arrival or detection of a pair of photons that triggered a coincidence. In the case of a system with infinite time resolution (i.e., there is no uncertainty in time when the detector triggered and the actual time the photon interacted in the detector), the event could be exactly localized to a point along the line connecting the two detectors [3]. This would allow the construction of the activity distribution without the need of an image reconstruction algorithm. However, all detector systems used in modern PET systems have a certain finite time resolution, which translates into an uncertainty in positioning of each event [3]. Currently the fastest detectors available have a time resolution of a few hundred picoseconds, which translates into a positional uncertainty of several centimeters. This time resolution is clearly not good enough to eliminate the need for image reconstruction. However, the TOF information can be used in the image reconstruction to reduce the noise in the reconstructed image. Since systems having TOF capability need to detect events to an accuracy of a few hundred picoseconds, compared to tenths of nanoseconds in conventional PET systems, these systems require a very accurate timing calibration and stable electronics [see Chap. 8 for further details on TOF technology].

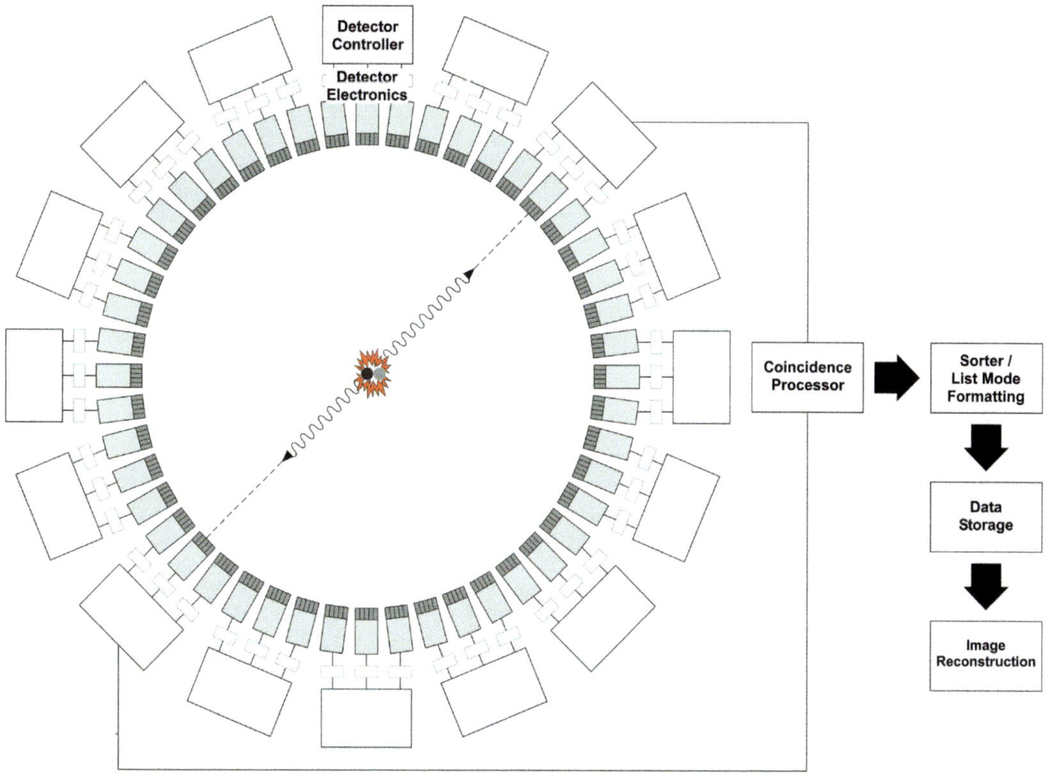

Fig. 10.1 Schematic of the dataflow in a PET system. The detector system consists of a large number of detector modules with associated front-end electronics. The outputs from the detector models are then fed into processing units or detector controllers that determines in which detector element a 511 keV photon interaction occurred. This information is then fed into a coincidence processor, which receives information from all detectors in the system. The coincidence processor determines if two detectors were registering an event within a predetermined time period (i.e., the coincidence time window). If this is the case, a coincidence has been recorded and the information about the two detectors and the time of when the event occurred are saved

10.2.1 Detector Flood Maps

The detector system used in all modern commercial PET systems is based on scintillation detectors coupled to some sort of photodetector readout. One of the most commonly used detector designs is the block detector [4]. In this design, an array of scintillation detector elements is coupled to a smaller number of PMTs, typically four, via a light guide. An example of a block detector is illustrated in Fig. 10.2. The light generated in scintillator following an interaction by a 511 keV photon is distributed between the PMTs in such a way that each detector element produces a unique combination of signal intensities in the four PMTs. To assign the event to a particular detector element, the signals from the PMTs are used to generate two position indices, X_{pos} and Y_{pos}:

$$X_{pos} = \frac{PMT_A - PMT_B + PMT_C - PMT_D}{PMT_A + PMT_B + PMT_C + PMT_D}$$
$$Y_{pos} = \frac{PMT_A + PMT_B - PMT_C - PMT_D}{PMT_A + PMT_B + PMT_C + PMT_D} \quad (10.1)$$

where PMT_A, PMT_B, PMT_C, and PMT_D are the signals from the four PMTs.

This is similar to the positioning of events in a conventional scintillation camera; however, the X_{pos} and Y_{pos} values do not directly translate into a spatial position or a location of the individual detector elements in the block detector. Each module therefore has to be calibrated to allow an

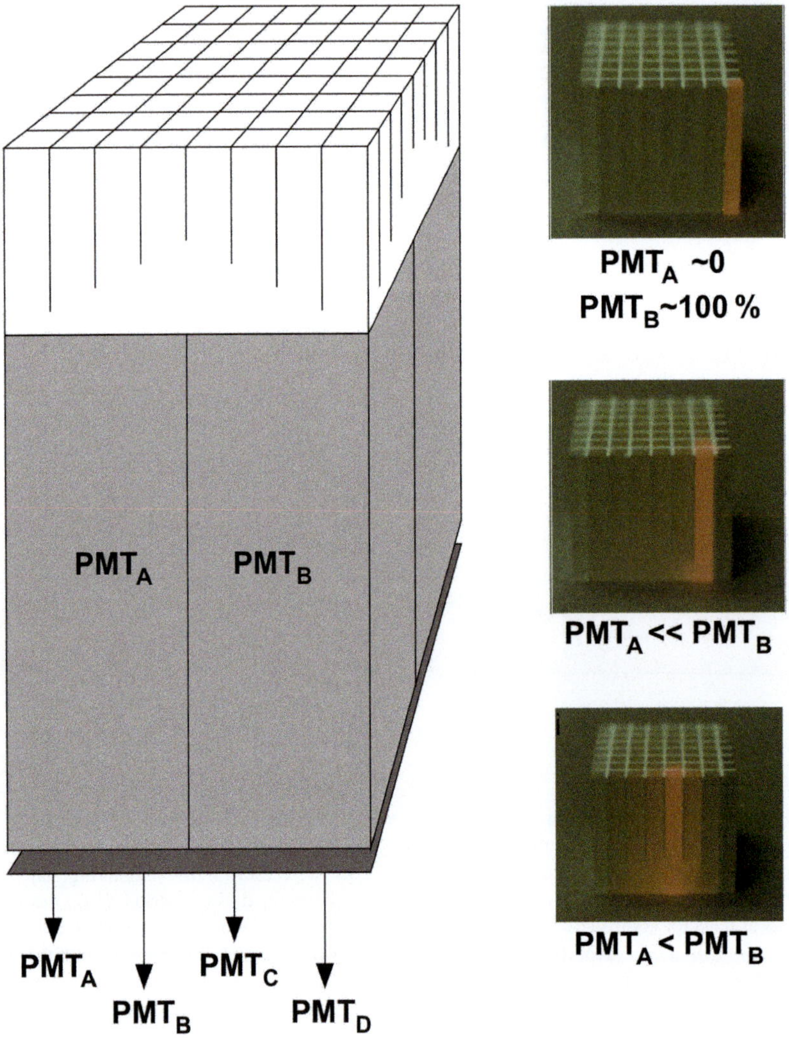

Fig. 10.2 Schematic of a block detector module used in modern PET systems. The array of scintillator detector elements is coupled to the four PMTs via a light guide. The light guide can be integral (i.e., made of the scintillator material) or a non-scintillating material (e.g., glass). The purpose of the light guide is to distribute the light in the detector elements to the four PMTs in such a way that a signal amplitude pattern unique to each detector element is produced. Three examples are illustrated. Top: almost all of the light is channeled to PMT_B and almost no light is channeled to the three other PMTs. This uniquely identifies the corner detector. Middle: In the next element over, most of the light is channeled to PMT_B and a small amount is channeled to PMT_A. By increasing the light detected by PMT_A, this allows this scintillator element to be distinguished from the corner element. Bottom: In the central detector element, light is almost equally shared between the PMT_B and PMT_A, but since the element is closer to PMT_B, this signal amplitude will be slightly larger compared to the signal in PMT_A. How well the elements can be separated depends on how much light is produced in the scintillator/photon absorption (more light allows better separation). Increasing the number of detector elements in the array makes it more challenging to accurately identify each detector element

accurate detector element assignment following an interaction of a photon in the detector. The distribution of X_{pos} and Y_{pos} can be visualized if a block detector is exposed to a flood source of 511 keV photons. For each detected event, X_{pos} and Y_{pos} are calculated using an equation [1] and are then histogrammed into a 2-dimensional matrix which can be displayed as a gray-scale image. An example of this is shown in Fig. 10.3. As can be seen in this figure, the distribution of

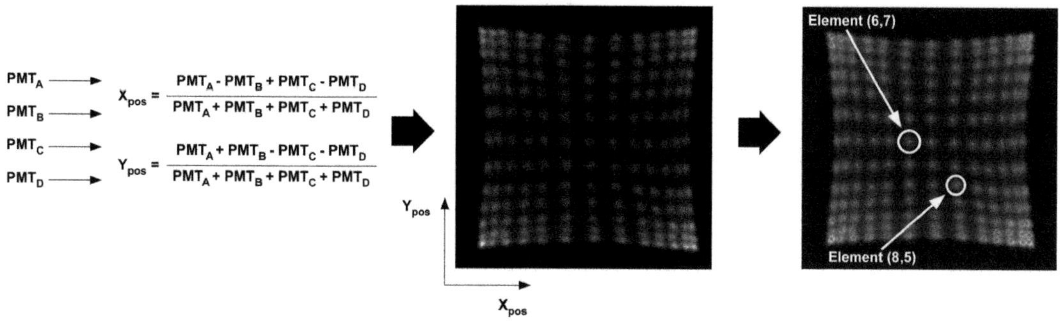

Fig. 10.3 The detector elements in a block detector are identified using a flood map. The flood map is generated by exposing the block detector to a relatively uniform flood of 511 keV photons. For each energy-validated detected event, the position indices X_{pos} and Y_{pos} are calculated from the PMT signals (PMT_A, PMT_B, PMT_C, and PMT_D). The X_{pos} and Y_{pos} values are histogrammed into a 2-D matrix, which can be displayed as a gray-scale image. The distribution of X_{pos} and Y_{pos} values is not uniform but is instead clustered around specific values, which corresponds to specific detector elements. The peak and the area of X_{pos} and Y_{pos} values around it are then assumed to originate from a specific detector element in the block detector, as illustrated in the figure. From the flood map and the peak identification, a look-up table is generated which rapidly identifies each detector element during an acquisition

X_{pos} and Y_{pos} is not uniform, but instead the events are clustered around specific positions. These clusters are the X_{pos} and Y_{pos} values that correspond to a specific detector element in the array. As can be seen from the flood image, the location of the clusters does not align on an orthogonal or linear grid. Instead, there is a significant pincushion effect due to the nonlinear light collection versus the position of the detector elements. To identify each element in the detector block, a look up table is generated based on a flood map like the one shown in Fig. 10.3. First, the centroid of each peak is localized (i.e., one peak for each detector element in the array). Then a region around each peak is generated that will assign the range of X_{pos} and Y_{pos} values to a particular element in the array. During a subsequent acquisition, the values of X_{pos} and Y_{pos} are calculated for each event; then the look-up table is used to assign the event to a specific detector element. Also associated with the positioning, look-up table is an element-specific energy calibration, which will accept or reject the event if it falls within or outside the predefined energy range.

To ensure that the incoming events are assigned to the correct detector element, the system has to remain very stable. A small drift in the gain in one or more of the PMTs would cause an imbalance and would affect the locations of the clusters in the flood map. This would in the end result in a misalignment between the calculated X_{pos} and Y_{pos} and the predetermined look-up table [5], which will result in a mispositioning of the events. As will be discussed below, to check gain balance between the tubes is one of the calibration procedures that need to be performed regularly.

10.2.2 Sinogram

The line connecting a pair of detector is referred to as a coincidence line or line of response (LOR). If the pair of detectors is in the same detector ring, this line can be described by a radial offset r from the origin with an angle θ. A set of LORs that all have the same angle (i.e., they are all parallel to each other), but they all have different radial offsets; these then form a projection of the object to be imaged at that angle. For instance, all lines with $\theta=0°$ would produce a lateral projection, whereas all lines with a $\theta=90°$ would produce an anterior-posterior view.

A complete set of projections necessary for image reconstruction would consist a large number of projections collected between 0° and 180°. If all the projections between these angles are organized in a 2-dimensional array, where the

1st dimension is the radial offset r and the 2nd dimension is the projection angle θ, then this arrangement or matrix forms a sinogram, as illustrated in Fig. 10.4. A sinogram is a common method of organizing the projection data prior to image reconstruction. The name sinogram comes from the fact that a single point source located at an off-center position in the field of view (FOV) would trace a sine wave in the sinogram. The visual inspection of a sinogram also turns out to be a very useful and efficient way to identify detector or electronic problems in a system.

Consider a one particular detector in the system and the coincidence lines it forms with the detectors on the opposite side in the detector ring (Fig. 10.4, right). In a sinogram, this fan of LORs would follow a diagonal line across the width of the FOV. By placing a symmetrical positron emitting source such as a uniform-filled cylinder with ^{68}Ge or ^{18}F, at the center of the FOV of the scanner, all detectors in the system would be exposed to approximately the same photon flux. If all detectors in the system had the same detection efficiency, then each detector would record

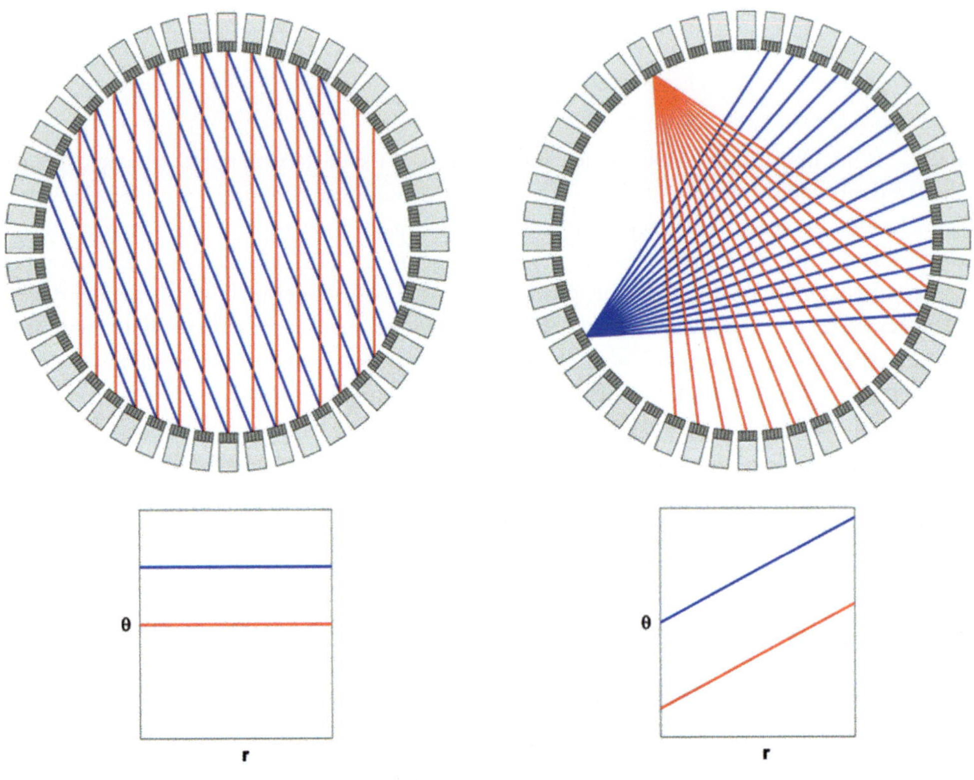

Fig. 10.4 A sinogram is a convenient of histogramming and storing the events along the coincidence lines or LORs in a tomographic study. In its simplest form, a sinogram is a 2-D matrix where the horizontal axis is the radial offset r of a LOR and the vertical axis is the angle θ, of the LOR. If one considers all LOR that are parallel to each other, these would fall along a horizontal line in the sinogram. In the left figure, this is illustrated for two different angles of LOR. If one considers all the coincidences or LOR between one specific detector and the detectors on the opposite side in the detector ring, these will follow a diagonal line in the sinogram, as illustrated in the right figure. The sum of all the counts from the fan of coincidence lines or LOR is sometimes referred to as a fan sum. These fan sums are used in some systems to generate the normalization that corrects for efficiency variations and can also be used to detect drifts and other problems in the detector system. In multi-ring systems, there will be a sinogram for each detector ring combination. In a TOF system each time bin will also have its own sinogram. A sinogram can therefore have up to five dimensions (r, θ, z, ϕ, t) depending on the design of the system

the same number of counts per second in this source geometry. In this source geometry, the summation of all the coincidences between a particular detector element and its opposing detector element is sometimes referred to as fan sum. The fan sums are used in some systems to derive the normalization correction that is used to correct for efficiency variations between the detector elements in the system. The fan sums can also be used to detect problems in the detector system

Figure 10.5 shows a normal sinogram of a uniform cylinder phantom in a PET system. In addition to the noise originating from the counting statistics, it contains a certain amount of a more structured noise or texture. The observed variation seen in the sinogram is normal and originates primarily from the fact that all detectors in the system do not have the same detection efficiency. There are several additional factors that contribute to this, such as variation in how energy thresholds are set, geometrical differences, differences in physical size of the each detector element, etc. These variations are removed using a procedure that is usually referred to as normalization, which is discussed later in this chapter.

One thing that is clearly noticeable in the sinogram is the "crosshatch" pattern, which reflects the variation in detection efficiency as discussed above. As mentioned, it is expected to observe a certain amount of normal variation in detection efficiency. This can under most circumstances be calibrated or normalized out as long as the system is stable in there is no drift in the gain of the detector signals. Since a certain amount of electronic drift is inevitable, a normalization calibration needs to be performed at regular intervals. The frequency depends on the manufacturers specifications but can be as frequent as every single day as part of the daily QC or done monthly or quarterly.

If a detector drifts enough or fails, this is typically very apparent by a visual inspection of the sinogram. A detector failure of a PET detector block can either result in that the detector does not respond at all when exposed to a source or

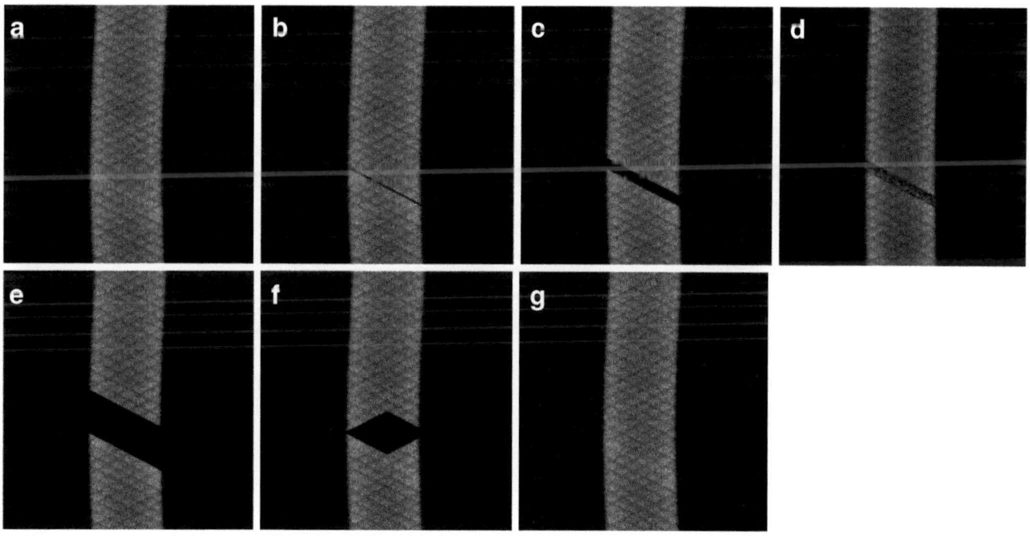

Fig. 10.5 Illustration of how the sinogram can be used to identify detector problems in a PET system. (**a**) A normal sinogram of a uniform cylinder phantom placed near the center of the FOV of the system. The crosshatch pattern reflects the normal variation in efficiency between the detector elements in the system. (**b**) The *dark diagonal line* indicates a failing detector element in the system (no counts generated). (**c**) The *broad dark diagonal* line indicates that an entire detector module is failing in. (**d**) Example of when a detector module is generating random noise. (**e**) Example of when the receiver or multiplexing board of the signals from a group of the detector modules is failing. (**f**) Example of problems in the coincidence processing board. In this case, the signals from two groups of opposite detector modules are lost. (**g**) Example of problems in the histogramming memory, where random numbers are added to the valid coincidences in the sinogram

that the detector constantly produces event even when no source is present (i.e., noise). The cause of a detector failure could be many, ranging from simple problems such as a loose cable, which usually results in a nonresponding detector, to more complex problems as a faulty PMT, drift in PMT gains, and drift in set energy threshold. The latter issues may result in either a nonresponding detector or that a detector is producing an excessive count rate.

Examples of failing detectors or associated electronics are also illustrated in Fig. 10.5. A failing single detector element in the detector module would appear as a single dark diagonal line in the sinogram (Fig. 10.5b). This problem was fairly common in older PET systems where each detector element was coupled to its own PMT. A common cause of this type of failure was either a failing PMT or the associated electronics (e.g., amplifiers). In the case of a system that uses block detectors, a single dark line may also occur if the detector tuning software had difficulties identifying all detector elements in the detector array. This could be caused by poor coupling of the detector element to the light guide and/or the PMTs or poorly balanced PMTs.

Since the PMTs and associated electronics are shared by many detector elements in block detector, a failure in these components will affect a larger number of detector channels. This is then seen as a wider diagonal band across the sinogram, as illustrated in Fig. 10.5c. Another common detector problem is illustrated in Fig. 10.5d. In this case one of the detectors is generating a large number of random or noise pulses. This could be caused by an energy threshold that is set too low, which, for instance, could be caused by a failing or weak PMT.

As described above, the signals from a larger group of detector blocks are typically multiplexed into what is sometimes referred to as a detector controller. In the case of a failure of the detector controller, the signals from the entire detector group might be lost, which in the sinogram is visualized as an even broader band of missing data (Fig. 10.5e). A problem further downstream in the signal processing chain such as in the electronics determining coincidences may result in a problem illustrated in Fig. 10.5f. Here the signals from two entire detector groups are lost in the coincidence processor, which in this case is seen as a diamond-shaped area in the sinogram. A final example of a hardware failure is shown in Fig. 10.5g. In this case there is a problem with the histogramming system, where random counts are added to the sinogram in addition to the normal data.

There are naturally a large number of variations in other artifacts or patterns in the sinograms that are specific to the design or a particular system, but the sinogram patterns related to the front electronics as described in this section are common for most modern PET systems.

Thus, by a visual inspection of the sinograms from a phantom scan, it is possible to relatively quickly identify whether the system is operational or not. By looking at the patterns in the sinogram, it is also possible to figure out where in the signal chain a problem is occurring. A complete failure is very apparent in the sinogram and makes it easy to make the determination that the system is in need of repair. However, many times there are more subtle problems, such as a slow drift in the system that is not easily detected by visual inspection. Some systems therefore provide a numerical assessment that gives the user some guidance whether the system is operational or not. These tests usually require that the user acquires data of a phantom, such as a ^{68}Ge-filled cylinder every day at the same position in the FOV for a fixed number of counts. The daily QC scan is then compared to a reference scan (e.g., a scan acquired at the time of the most recent calibration or tuning). By comparing the number of counts acquired by each detector module in the QC scan to that in the reference scan, it is possible to determine if a drift has occurred in the system and the system needs to be retuned and recalibrated.

10.3 Detector and System Calibration

The purpose of the detector and system calibration is to make sure that the recorded events are assigned to the correct detector element in the detector module. An energy validation is performed such that only events within a certain energy range are passed on to the subsequent event processing. In addition to positioning and energy calibration of each detector module, each module has to be time calibrated to make sure that coincidence time windows between all detector modules are aligned.

10.3.1 Tube Balancing and Gain Adjustments

As described earlier, the assignment of the events to individual detector elements in the block is based on the comparison of the signal output from the four PMTs. The first step in the calibration of the front-end detector electronics is to adjust the gain of the amplifiers such that the signal amplitude from the four PMTs is on the average and is about the same. This usually entails exposing the detectors to a flood source of 511 keV photons, and the gains are adjusted until an acceptable signal balance is achieved.

Following the tube balancing, detector flood histograms are acquired and generated (as described earlier) to make sure that each detector element in each detector block can be identified. A look-up table is then generated from the flood histogram that is used to assign a particular combination of X_{pos} and Y_{pos} values to a particular detector element.

10.3.2 Energy Calibration

Once all detector elements in the block have been identified, the signal originating from each detector element has to be energy calibrated. Independent of the design of the detector block, it is very likely that signal from each detector element will vary in terms of amplitude, primarily due to differences in light collection by the photodetectors. A detector positioned right above a PMT is very likely to produce a stronger signal compared to a detector located at the edge of a PMT. This is similar to what is observed in conventional scintillation cameras. When comparing energy spectra from the individual elements in a block detector, the location of the photopeak will vary depending on the light collection efficiency of the light.

For the energy calibration, energy spectra are acquired for each detector element, and the calibration software will search for the photopeak in each spectrum. A simple energy calibration is then typically performed where it is assumed that the photopeak corresponds to 511 keV (provided that the source is emitting 511 keV photons and zero amplitude corresponds to zero energy).

10.3.3 Timing Calibration

Coincidence measurements only accept pairs of events that occur within a narrow time window of each other. In order to ensure that most true coincidences are recorded, it is imperative that all detector signals in the system are adjusted to a common reference time. How this is done in practice is dependent of the manufacturer and the system design. The general principle is to acquire timing spectra between all detector modules in the system when a positron emitting source is placed at the center of the system by recording differences in the time of detection of annihilation photon pairs. For a non-calibrated system, the timing spectrum has approximately a Gaussian distribution, centered around an arbitrary time. The distribution around the mean is caused by the timing characteristic of scintillation detectors and the associated electronics and the location of centroid caused by variation in time delays in PMTs, cables, etc. In the timing calibration, this time delay is measured for each detector, and time adjustments are introduced such that the centroid of all timing spectra is aligned. It is around this centroid where the coincidence time window is placed. For non-TOF PET systems, the timing calibration has to be calibrated to an accuracy of around a few nanoseconds. For TOF system, the calibration has to be accurate to below 100 picoseconds.

A modern PET system consists of several tens of thousands of detector elements and requires very accurate and precise calibration. The outcome of the calibration steps many times depends on each other and some of the processes are iterative. Due to the complexity of the system, manufacturers have developed highly automated procedures for these calibration steps. It used to be that a trained on-site physicist or engineer had access to the manufacturer's calibration utilities, which allowed recalibration or retuning of parts or the entire system. However, in recent years the general trend among manufacturers is that the user does not have access to the calibration utilities, and these tasks are only performed by the manufacturer's service engineers. Fortunately, PET scanners today are very stable, and the need for recalibration and retuning is far less compared to systems that were manufactured 10–20 years ago.

10.3.4 System Normalization

After a full calibration of the detectors in a PET system, there will be a significant residual variation in both intrinsic and coincidence detection efficiency of the detector elements. There are several reasons for this, such as imperfections in the calibration procedures, geometrical efficiency variations, imperfections in manufacturing, etc. These residual efficiency variations need to be calibrated out to avoid the introduction of image artifacts. This process is analogous to the high-count flood calibration used in SPECT imaging to remove small residual variation in flood-field uniformity. In PET this process is usually referred to as the normalization, and the end result is usually a multiplicative correction matrix that is applied to the acquired sonograms as illustrated in Fig. 10.6. The effects of the normalization on the sinogram and the reconstruction of uniform cylinder phantom are shown in Fig. 10.6. If the normalization is not applied, there is a subtle but noticeable artifact in the image such as the ring artifacts and the cold spot in the middle of the phantom. The origin of the ring artifacts comes from a repetitive pattern in detection efficiency variation across the face of the block detector modules, where the detectors in the center have a higher detections efficiency compared to the edge detectors. Once the normalization is applied, these artifacts are greatly reduced. It should also be noted that the normalization is a volumetric correction as can be noted by the removal of the "zebra" pattern in the axial direction when the normalization is applied (Fig. 10.6).

Normalization is usually performed after a detector calibration. There are several approaches on how to acquire the normalization. The most straightforward method is to place a plane source filled with a long-lived positron emitting isotope, such as ^{68}Ge in the center of the FOV. This allows a direct measurement of the detection efficiencies of the LORs that are approximately perpendicular to the source [6]. The source typically has to be rotated to several angular positions in the FOV to measure the efficiency factors for all detector pairs in the system. However, there are several drawbacks of this method. First of all, it is very time consuming to acquire enough counts at each angular position to ensure that the emission data are not contaminated with statistical noise from the normalization. This problem can to a certain degree be alleviated by the use of variance-reducing data processing methods [7].

The most common method for determining the normalization is the component-based method [8, 9]. This method is based on the combination of efficiency factors that are less likely to change over time, such as geometrical factors and other factors that are expected to change over time due to drifts in detector efficiency or due to settings of energy thresholds. This method typically only requires a single measurement that estimates the individual detector efficiency. This is usually done with a uniform cylinder phantom placed at the center of the FOV. The measured detector efficiencies are then combined with the factory-determined factors to generate the final normalization

It is usually not necessary to generate a new normalization, unless there is some noticeable detector drift, which most of the time would require detector service. Some manufacturers have found that by acquiring the normalization more frequently or even to be included in the

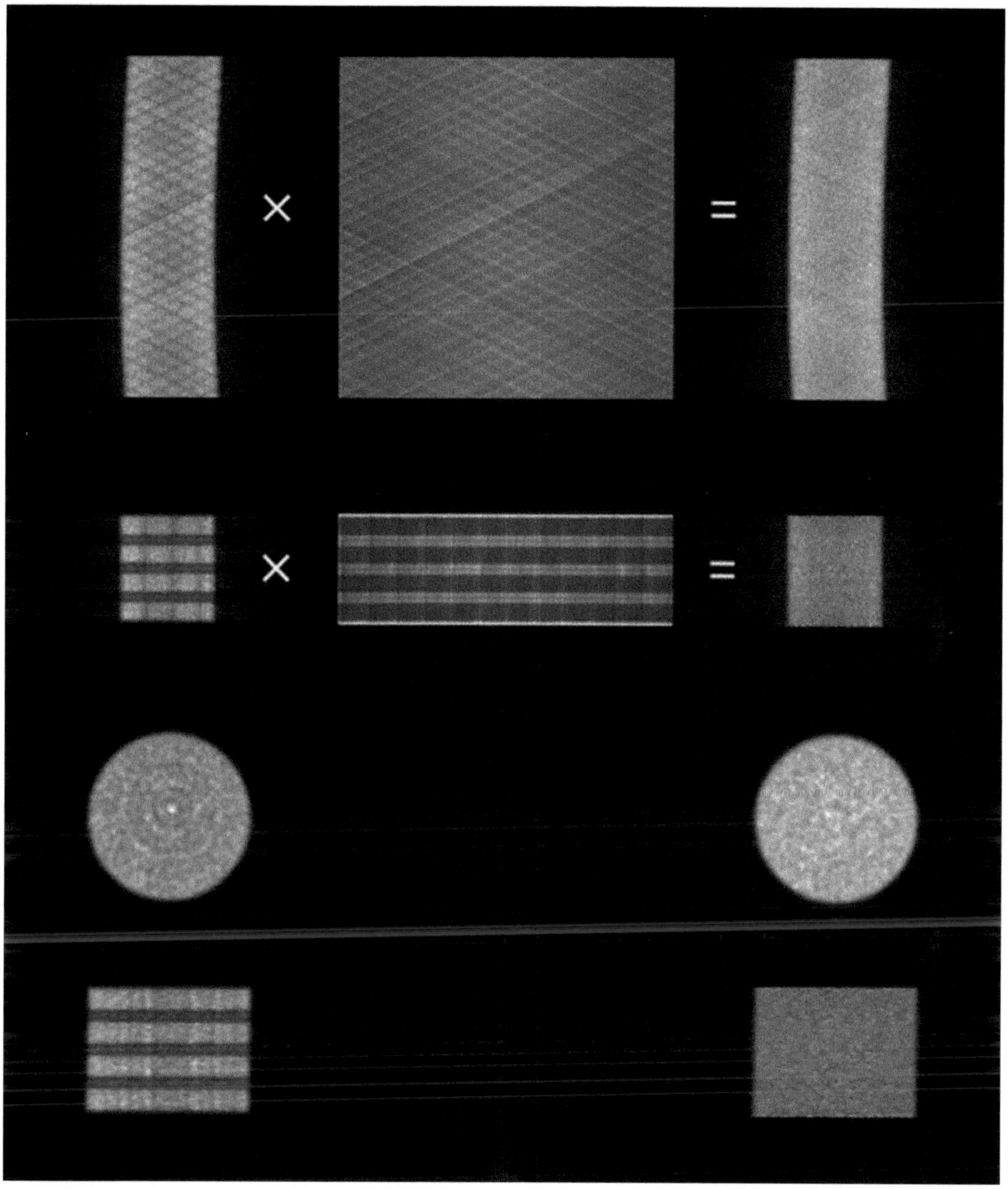

Fig. 10.6 *1st row*: The sinogram to the left is a normal uncorrected sinogram of a uniform cylinder phantom. The crosshatch pattern reflects the normal variation in efficiency between the detector elements in the system. The normalization matrix (*middle*), which is multiplicative, corrects for this and produces a corrected sinogram (*right*), where the efficiency variations have been greatly reduced. *2nd row*: Illustration of the effect of the normalization in the axial direction of the system. The efficiency variation is typically greater in the z-direction compared to the in-plane variation. *3rd and 4th rows*: Illustration of the effect of the normalization on a reconstructed image. The transaxial image to the left in the 3rd row shows ring artifacts due to the lack of normalization. These are eliminated when the normalization is applied (*right image*). The axial cross section of the reconstructed cylinder in the 4th row reflects the efficiency variation axially in a "zebra pattern" when the normalization is not applied (left image). These artifacts are greatly reduced when the normalization is applied (*right*)

daily QC, a better stability in image quality and quantification is achieved.

10.3.5 Activity Calibration

The final step in the calibration of a PET system is to perform an activity calibration. When the acquired emission data are reconstructed with all corrections applied, including normalization, scatter, and attenuation correction, the values in the resulting images are proportional to the activity concentration, but are typically not quantitative (i.e., in units of Bq/ml). It is therefore necessary to acquire a calibration scan in order to produce images that are quantitative and allow quantitative measurements. This is usually done by acquiring scan of a uniform cylinder phantom, filled with a known amount of activity. ^{18}F and ^{68}Ge are the most commonly used isotopes for this purpose. Images of the phantom are then reconstructed, with all corrections applied (normalization, scatter, attenuation, isotope decay). A volume of interest of the reconstructed phantom is then placed well within the borders of the phantom. This is used to determine the average phantom concentration expressed in arbitrary units (counts per second). Since the activity concentration is known from either the manufacture of the ^{68}Ge cylinder or by a careful assay of the ^{18}F dose in a dose calibrator, knowing the volume of the phantom used in the calibration, the calibration factor can then be calculated from

$$\text{Act.Cal.Factor} = \frac{\text{Phantom Activity}/\text{Phantom Volume}}{\text{VOI Counts/s}/\text{ROI Volume}} \tag{10.2}$$

It is important that the branching fraction of the isotope used in the calibration is included in the calculation of the calibration factor as well as the branching fraction of the isotope used in subsequent measurements.

It should be mentioned that a common source of error in the determination of the calibration factor comes from the activity in the phantom. If ^{18}F is used, the activity is usually determined using a dose calibrator. Studies have shown that there can be a large variation in the determination of the calibration factors which can be traced back to how well the dose calibrator itself is calibrated and how the dose is assayed [10] [11]. In the past, the activity concentration in ^{68}Ge cylinders had a relatively large uncertainty due to the lack of available NIST traceable standards of ^{68}Ge for dose calibrators. In recent years, NIST traceable standards have become available, which allow a more accurate calibration of the PET system [12]. The accuracy of the activity calibration is of great importance in multicenter trials, where data of subjects imaged on several different PET systems at different sites are used in quantitative studies for the evaluation of, for instance, response to new therapies. A large variation in the system calibration between the different systems could potentially mask out an actual physiological response when the data from the subjects are pooled together for analysis. As will be discussed later in this chapter, there are additional QC steps needed when using PET in multicenter trials.

10.4 Acceptance Testing

Acceptance testing is the rigorous testing a user would perform of a system when it has been installed and handed over to the user for clinical use. The purpose of the acceptance testing is to make sure that the system is fully operational and is performing to the manufacturer's specifications. The test results from the acceptance test should also be used as a reference for future testing (e.g., annual performance testing) to make sure the system performance has not degraded since the time of installation.

NEMA has in collaboration with scientists and manufacturers of PET scanners developed guidelines and a set of tests that are used to specify the performance of a PET system. These standardized tests were initially developed to allow a relatively unbiased comparison of the performance of PET systems of different designs. These tests have also become the core of the tests that are performed in the acceptance test of a newly installed system.

As PET systems have evolved over the years, so have the NEMA specifications and the latest document is the NEMA NU 2–2012 [13]. These tests include a series of tests that are described in the sections below. For a more detailed description of each test, the reader is referred to the NEMA NU-2 document.

Although most PET systems manufactured today are hybrid systems such as PET/CT and PET/MRI systems, NEMA has chosen to only specify tests for the PET component and not for the system as a whole. Some suggested additional measurements are included below which tests the system as a whole. Chapter 2 covers some details about the CT component.

10.4.1 Spatial Resolution

Unlike a scintillation camera, the spatial resolution is not expected to degrade due to the aging of the scintillation crystal itself since the crystal materials used in PET systems are not hygroscopic. However, other components of the block detectors do age over time, such as the PMTs, which may result in a loss in spatial resolution. It is therefore important to have a reference of the spatial resolution, which can be used as indicator of detector degradation as the system ages.

The spatial resolution measurements as specified by NEMA represent the lower limit of the resolution that can be achieved on the system and do not represent the resolution of clinical images. Since the spatial resolution of PET system varies across the FOV, measurements of the resolution are performed at different positions in the FOV (see Fig. 10.7). The measurements are performed with a set of point sources of ^{18}F with a physical extent of less than 1 mm in diameter (radially and axially). The sources used for these measurements are made by filling the tip of a capillary tube (1 mm inner diameter and 2 mm outer diameter) such that the axial extent of the source is less than 1 mm. Measurements of the source should be performed at 1, 10, and 20 cm horizontal or vertical offsets, where the 1 cm offset represents the center of the FOV. It is worth mentioning that the locations of the point source measurements have changed since the previous NEMA 2–2007 document [14], where the resolution measurements were limited to within 10 cm of the central FOV. Extending the measurements out to a radial offset of 20 cm adds a measure of the spatial resolution toward the edge of the FOV where there is a significant degradation in resolution, which is relevant for whole body imaging.

Two sets of measurements should be acquired, where the source is positioned at the center of axial FOV and at 3/8 offset from center of the axial FOV (or 1/8 of the axial FOV from the edge of the FOV). In order to minimize secondary effects on the spatial resolution (e.g., pulse pile-up), the activity in the source should induce less than 5 % dead-time and the randoms rate should be less than 5 % of the total event rate. For each data point, enough counts should be acquired at each position to ensure that a smooth and well-defined point-spread function can be generated from the acquired data. Typically at least 100,000 counts should be acquired.

The data acquired from the point sources are then reconstructed using filtered back projection (FBP) without any filtering, to ensure that the measurements as close as possible reflect the intrinsic resolution properties of the scanner. Resolution measurements in all three spatial directions (radial, tangential, and axial) are derived from orthogonal profiles through the point source in the reconstructed images and are reported as FWHM and FWTM. The NEMA specifications state very specifically how these measurements should be performed. The axial, radial, and tangential spatial resolutions for the three radial positions, averaged over the two axial positions, are reported as the system spatial resolution.

10.4.2 Scatter Fraction

The scatter fraction (SF) is a measure of the contamination of the coincidence data by photons that have scattered prior to being detected. If not corrected for, the scattered events will result in a

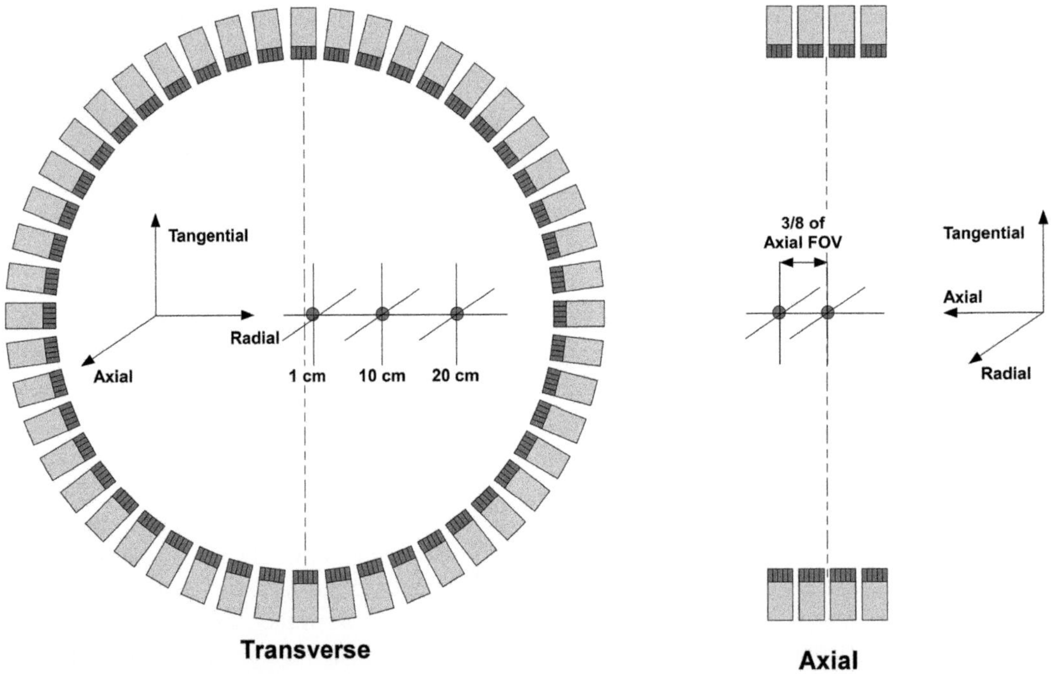

Fig. 10.7 NEMA spatial resolution measurements. The NEMA protocol specifies that the spatial resolution of a PET system should be measured at six different points in the system. The measurements should be taken at three radial offsets: 1 cm, 10 cm, and 20 cm at the axial center of the FOV (left figure). These measurements are then repeated at a 3/8 offset of the axial FOV

loss in image contrast. Although scattered events can be corrected for, this usually results in an increase in image noise and/or bias. The SF is highly dependent on the source geometry and scattering environment as well as instrumentation parameters such as system geometry, shielding, and energy thresholds. To measure the SF according to the NEMA specifications, a catheter source is placed at 4.5 cm vertical offset inside a 20 cm diameter and 70 cm long polyethylene phantom, which is placed at the center of the FOV. The SF is defined as the number of scattered to total events measured and is estimated from the sinogram data of the line source. It is important that the data is acquired at a low count rate to minimize the influence of dead time and random coincidences on the estimate. In the analysis of the projection data, only data within the central 24 cm of the FOV is considered. A summed projection profile of the line source is generated from all the projection angles in the sinogram. Prior to summation, the projection at each angle has to be shifted in such a way that the pixel with the highest intensity is aligned with the central pixel in the sinogram (see Fig. 10.8). From the summed projection, the scatter is estimated by first determining the counts at 20 mm of either side of the peak (Fig. 10.8). These two values are then used to create a trapezoidal region under the peak. Scatter is defined as the total counts outside the 20 mm central region and area of the trapezoidal region under the peak. The SF is then simply the scatter counts divided by the total counts in the summed profile. This calculation is performed for each slice of the system and for the system as a whole. If data are acquired in 3-D, the sinograms have to be binned into 2-D data sets using single-slice rebinning (SSRB) [19] prior to the analysis.

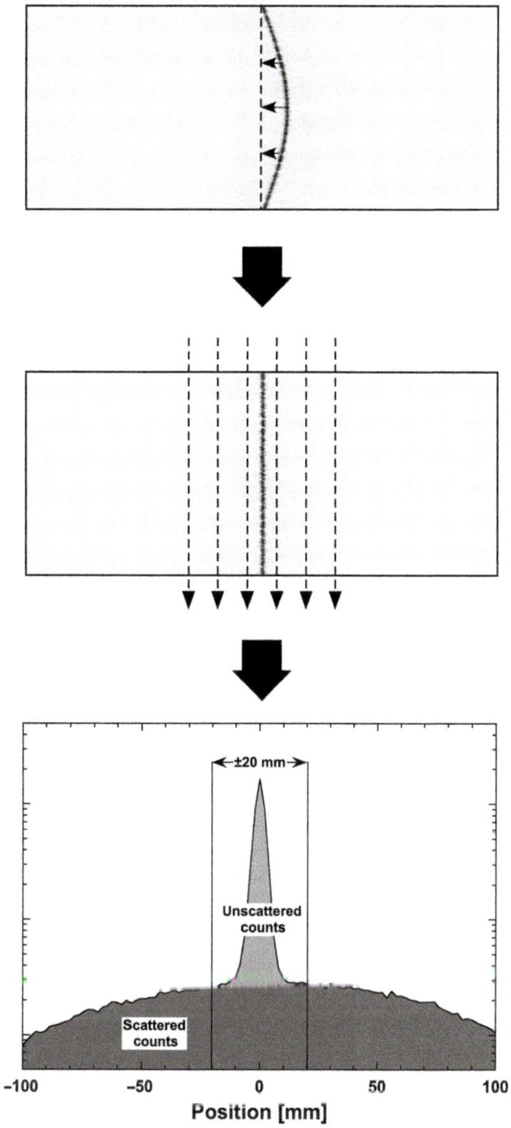

Fig. 10.8 The NEMA protocol specifies that the scatter fraction is measured with a line source placed at a 4.5 cm vertical offset inside a 20 cm diameter and 70 cm long cylindrical polyethylene phantom, placed at the center of the FOV. A typical sinogram of the line source is shown in the top figure. Each row or projection line in the sinogram is shifted in such a way that the pixel with the highest intensity is aligned with the central pixel in the sinogram. All the rows are then summed to form a summed projection profile. The scatter counts are all the counts outside the 40 mm central region plus the trapezoidal section under the peak. The scatter fraction is the scatter counts divided by the total counts

10.4.3 Count Rate Performance and Correction Accuracy

The count rate performance of a PET system is a measurement that determines the count rate response of the system at different activity levels in the FOV. For this measurement, the same phantom used for the scatter fraction measurements is used (i.e., a 20 cm diameter and 70 cm long polyethylene phantom). The catheter is filled with a known amount of ^{18}F, carefully assayed in a dose calibrator, and the total length of the source should be 70 cm. The amount of activity in the source at the start of the measurement should be high enough so that the peak count rate of the system is exceeded. Count rate data are then collected at regular time points as the source decays until the dead-time losses in the true event rate is less than 1 %. Data should be collected frequent enough so that the peak count rate can be accurately determined. If possible, the acquisition should be configured in such a way that random coincidences are acquired separately from the prompt coincidences, which allows for a more straightforward analysis of the count rates. If not possible, the NEMA documents provide an alternative approach.

From the collected data, count rate curves should be generated, which includes the system true count rate (T), system random count rate (R), system scatter count rate (S), system total count rate (TOT), and system noise equivalent count rate (NEC). The NEC [15] is calculated using

$$\mathrm{NEC} = \frac{T^2}{T + S + kR}$$

where k is 1 for a system that acquires randoms separate from prompt coincidences and 2 for system that subtracts the randoms directly during the acquisition. The NEC is a valuable performance metric that has been shown to be proportional to the signal-to-noise ratio of the reconstructed images [16, 17]. From the count rate curves, the following metrics should be derived: maximum true count rate and at what activity this is reached and maximum NEC rate and at what activity this is reached.

The count rate data is also used to determine how accurately the system can correct for dead time at high activity levels in the FOV. The dead-time correction is typically incorporated as part of the numerous correction applied to the data before and during the image reconstruction. For each image slice and time frame, the average count rate (R_{image}) is determined within a 180 mm diameter regions of interest (ROI). This value is compared to a "true" average count rate (R_{true}), which is determined from an average of image count rates at activity concentrations less than or equal to where the peak NEC is reached. The relative count rate error is then derived for image slice and frame:

$$\%\text{error} = 100\left(\frac{R_{\text{image}}}{R_{\text{true}}} - 1\right)$$

The maximum error or bias below the activity at which the maximum NEC is reached should be reported.

10.4.4 Sensitivity

The sensitivity of the PET scanner is the count rate of the system for a given amount and distribution of activity in the FOV. According to the NEMA specifications, the sensitivity of the PET system should be measured with a 70 cm long thin catheter filled with activity. The activity in the source should be low enough to minimize any dead time in the system (preferably less than 1 % and a random rate less than 5 % of the true coincidence rate). The sensitivity is calculated as the total count rate of the system divided by the activity in the catheter. To ensure that all positrons annihilate near the location of the radioactive decay, the catheter source has to be placed inside a sleeve such as an aluminum sleeve that stops all positrons. This sleeve will unfortunately also attenuate some of the annihilation photons, which prevents a direct measurement of the sensitivity in air. To estimate the attenuation-free sensitivity in air, NEMA has adopted the method first described by Bailey et al. [18]. By successive measurement of the count rate, using sleeves of known thickness, the attenuation-free sensitivity in air can be estimated by exponentially extrapolating the count rate to zero sleeve thickness (see Fig. 10.9).

The measurement of sensitivity is performed both at the center and at a 10 cm radial offset and reported for the system as a whole (i.e., total counts acquired by the system). The individual plane sensitivity should also be reported and is derived from the data acquired at the center position. For a system acquiring data in 2-D, the plane sensitivity is straightforward to determine since the data are directly sorted into individual planes. The plane sensitivity is simply the total count rate in each plane divided by the activity in the 70 cm long source. For a system acquiring data in 3-D, the plane sensitivity is determined by first sorting the 3-D sinograms into 2-D sinograms using SSRB. The plane sensitivity is then calculated from the rebinned sinograms.

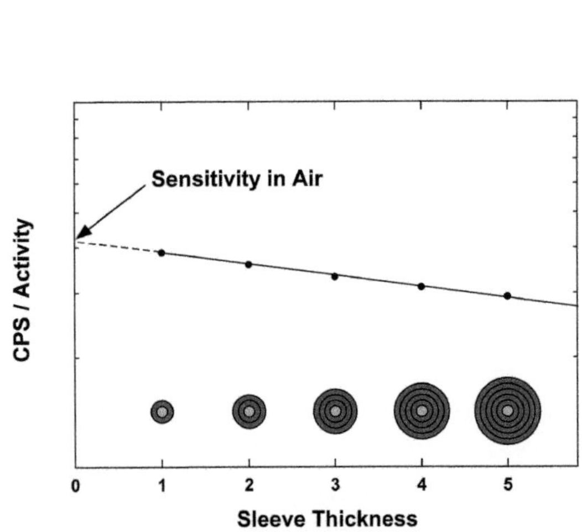

Fig. 10.9 NEMA sensitivity (extrapolation back to zero thickness). The sensitivity according to the NEMA protocol is determined from successive measurements of a 70 cm line source of known activity placed inside aluminum sleeves of known thickness. To estimate the attenuation-free count rate in air is estimated by exponentially extrapolating the measured count rates back to zero sleeve thickness. The sensitivity is then the attenuation-free count rate divided by the activity in the line source

10.4.5 Systems with Intrinsic Background

The detector materials used in the latest generation of PET systems are lutetium-based scintillators. LSO was the first lutetium-based scintillator and was discovered in 1992 [20]. LSO is an almost ideal detector material for PET in that it is dense, bright, and fast scintillator. Since the initial discovery, lutetium-based scintillators with similar properties as LSO have been manufactured, such as LYSO and LGSO. The lutetium-based scintillators have allowed the manufacturers to produce PET systems that allow 3-D and TOF acquisition. One of the slight drawbacks of all lutetium-based scintillator is that they all contain a natural background radioactivity originating from ^{176}Lu. The decay of ^{176}Lu results in a significant intrinsic background coincidence count rate in the system, which is not observed in systems using traditional PET scintillators such as BGO. The background coincidence count rate is primarily due to randoms, but there is also a small contribution of true coincidences. These are produced by coincidences between a beta particle absorbed in the local detector and the absorption in a distant detector of a gamma that is also emitted in the beta decay of ^{176}Lu. The distribution of these events is uniform across the FOV, and the count rates from these are on the order of 1000 cps, without any objects in the FOV. This count rate is dependent on the energy window used, and with attenuating objects in the FOV, the contribution from these events will be attenuated. The contribution of these events in clinical imaging can in general be considered negligible since the contribution from emission counts of the patient in the FOV is several orders of magnitude higher [21]. Nevertheless, the presence of the coincidences generated by ^{176}Lu background makes it necessary to modify the original NEMA procedure in order to minimize the influence of the background on the results.

The procedure for estimating the scatter fraction states that the measurement is measured as part of the count rate performance test, using data from the test where the randoms to true count rate is less that 1 % (i.e., a near randoms free condition). For a system with lutetium-based scintillator, this condition is impossible to achieve due to the background radiation. Using the original NEMA protocol for estimating the scatter fraction would result in an overestimation of the scatter fraction, due to the randoms rate from the ^{176}Lu background [22]. It is therefore suggested that the protocol is modified in such a way that the prompts and randoms are both measured and stored. Randoms free data (i.e., net trues) can then be produced by subtracting the measured random coincidences from the prompt coincidences. This data can then be used to estimate the scatter fraction. Since this is part of the count rate performance test, this method allows the estimation of the scatter fraction as a function of count rate.

For the sensitivity measurements, it is necessary to correct the prompt coincidences in the same manner as described above. It may also be necessary to correct the true coincidence data for the true coincidences produced by ^{176}Lu background since the background may not be negligible compared to the count rate from the line source. To perform the correction, a blank scan is acquired without phantom or source in the FOV. This count rate is then subtracted from the count rate in the line source measurements.

A more complete discussion of the concerns and special considerations for NEMA performance testing of scanners using lutetium-based scintillators can be found in [21]. Detailed results and discussion from a modified NEMA performance test of a system using LSO scintillators can be found in [23].

10.4.6 Image Quality

The NEMA document also specifies an image quality test, which serves to provide an overall assessment of the imaging capabilities of the system under similar conditions as a clinical whole body scan. This test uses a chest-like phantom, sometimes referred to as the NEMA image quality phantom or IEC phantom, which contains six fillable spheres with diameters between 10 and 37 mm and a 50 mm diameter low-density cylindrical insert to simulate the lower attenuation of the lungs. This test also uses the 20 cm diameter and 70 cm long phantom used in the count rate and scatter fraction test. This phantom is placed adjacent to the chest phantom with activity in the catheter that serves as a source of out-of-field background activity as one would expect in clinical whole body imaging conditions. The phantom should be filled with a background activity concentration of 5.3 kBq/ml (0.14 μCi/ml) of ^{18}F, which corresponds to typical whole body injection of 370 MBq (10 mCi) into a 70 kg patient. The line source in the 70 cm long phantom should be filled with 116 MBq (3.08 mCi) of ^{18}F, which yields approximately the same activity concentration as in the chest phantom.

The two largest spheres should be filled with cold water to allow an evaluation of cold lesion imaging. The remaining spheres should be filled with an activity concentration that is four times the background concentration for evaluation of hot lesion imaging. NEMA also recommends that this test also should be performed at 8:1 lesion to background ratio. The acquisition time of the phantom should be selected to simulate a whole body scan covering 100 cm in 30 min. Because of the relatively high noise levels in the resulting image, it is recommended that three replicate scans are acquired of the phantom, where the scan time in each replicate is adjusted for the decay of the isotope.

The acquired data is then reconstructed using the standard protocol that a site uses for routine whole body imaging. The images are then evaluated in terms of:

- Hot sphere contrast (four values)
- Cold sphere contrast (two values)
- Background variability for each sphere (four values)
- Attenuation and scatter correction (one value for each image slice)

NEMA describes in great detail how the phantom is to be analyzed, including placement and dimensions of ROIs for the derivation of these values, and the reader is referred to the NEMA document to the details.

The manufacturers of PET systems do not specify the values or ranges of expected values of the parameters derived from the image quality test for a specific scanner. One of the reasons for this is the large number of factors that will influence the values, especially acquisition and reconstruction parameters, which are specific to each imaging site. However, one of the primary values in this test is that it provides a baseline imaging performance values that can be used for comparison as the system ages. Due to the complexity of the test, it is of great importance that all imaging parameters, such as phantom activities, acquisition times, and reconstruction parameters, are well documented so the test can be reproduced at a later time.

The image quality test is also a good starting point to optimize existing or develop new imaging protocols. Using the acquired data sets, the effect of reconstruction parameters in contrast and noise can be evaluated.

10.4.7 Other Tests

In addition to the NEMA tests described above, there are a number of other tests a user might perform on the system. The purpose of these tests is to determine that the system is operational and to check that corrections applied to the data are producing images that are free of artifacts and also are quantitatively accurate. These tests may also be used as a reference for the long-term evaluation of the system and may be used as part of an annual performance testing.

10.4.7.1 Image Uniformity

Uniformity was part of the first NEMA specifications for the performance testing of PET scanner [24]. This test was for various reasons dropped in later revisions of the NEMA specification, but the tests still have some merits in terms of testing an individual PET scanner, since it can reveal problems in the processing chain of generating an image. This test involves imaging of a uniform phantom (typically 20 cm diameter and 20 cm or longer axially). At least 20 million counts/slice should be acquired and then reconstructed with FBP without filtering, but with all corrections applied (i.e., scatter, attenuation, and normalization). The high number of counts is necessary in order to better visualize any subtle problems in the corrections that otherwise might be masked by statistical noise.

The images can either be evaluated by visual inspection or quantitatively as described in [24]. During a visual inspection, any signs of concentric ring artifacts are typically a sign of issues in the normalization. This type of artifact could also originate from detector pileup if the amount of activity in the phantom is too high. It is therefore important that this test is performed at an activity level that does not produce more than 10–20 % dead time in the system.

It is also suggested that horizontal and vertical profiles through the phantom are generated to ensure that activity profile is flat and uniform. Any asymmetries may be the result of an incorrect attenuation correction (e.g., misalignment of the CT-generated attenuation correction and the emission data). Any increase or decrease in the activity profile toward the center may be the result from a problem in the scatter correction or the attenuation correction.

10.4.7.2 Overall Imaging Performance

As an alternative to the NEMA method, to evaluate the overall imaging performance of the system is to use a phantom like the Jaszczak phantom. Using this phantom, the lesion contrast, uniformity, and spatial resolution can be fairly quickly evaluated semiquantitatively. The phantom should be filled with an activity concentration that is close to what is used on the system clinically. The phantom should then be imaged and reconstructed using typical clinical imaging protocols (e.g., whole body and brain). This test would show the typical expected imaging performance during routine imaging.

A high statistic scan may also be useful to evaluate "best possible" imaging performance. This may also reveal artifacts from corrections that otherwise might be masked by statistical noise. Both the typical and high statistic images can then be used as reference images when evaluating the imaging performance as the system ages.

10.4.7.3 Quantification

Since most sites use the data from a PET scanner to generate quantitative values such as the standardized uptake value or SUV [25], it is important that the quantitative accuracy of the system is tested. This is done by imaging a uniform phantom, of known volume, filled with a known amount of activity. Images of the phantom are then reconstructed with all corrections applied. The images are analyzed by drawing regions of interest (ROIs) on each image slice, typically a centrally placed circular region with a diameter that is well within the edge of the phantom. The measured activity concentration from the ROI analysis is then compared with the calibrated activity concentration, decay corrected to the same reference time as the phantom scan (typically scan start time). Most workstations designed for the analysis of PET images provide values in SUV, and this test may also reveal issues in the calculation of the SUV or more likely issues in data entry of relevant parameters (calibrated activity, time of calibration, and phantom weight or volume) when the scan was acquired. If all parameters were entered correctly, then the SUV values should not deviate from 1.0 more than 5–10 % for a properly calibrated system.

10.4.7.4 Bed Motion

Since most PET/CT system is used for whole body imaging, the bed motion should be tested to make sure the movement and assembly of the multiple data sets do not introduce artifacts. This test can be performed with a uniform cylinder phantom that is placed in such a way in the FOV that is necessary to image the phantom in two or more axial bed position. Once the images have been reconstructed and assembled into a whole body image set, the images are visually inspected for artifacts. In addition, an axial count profile from a centrally placed ROI in the images of the cylinder can also be helpful to reveal problems in the assembly of the multiple bed position. Any problem with the bed movement would be manifested in an increased nonuniformity in the region where the adjacent image sets are assembled.

A phantom with internal structures, such as the Jaszczak phantom, can also be useful in detecting problems in the bed motion assembly of the image sets. In this case the phantom has to position in such a way that the structures to be evaluated are in the part of the FOV where the adjacent bed positions overlap. Any issues with the bed motion would be seen as distortions such as discontinuities in the coronal and sagittal views of the final assembled images.

One manufacturer recently introduced a continuous bed motion as an alternative to the conventional step-and-shoot bed motion [26]. To verify that this bed motion is working properly, one could image a phantom with a resolution pattern such as the Jaszczak or Derenzo phantom. In this case the axis of the phantom has to be rotated 90° to the axis of the scanner so the resolution pattern is visualized in the coronal view of the final images. In this case the images would be inspected for potential losses in resolution and image distortions and should be compared to corresponding images acquired as a single static bed position.

10.4.7.5 Image Registration

Most modern PET systems are multimodality systems such as PET/CT systems and in recent years PET/MRI systems where the images from the two modalities are fused in the diagnostic readout. It is therefore important that the images from the two modalities are spatially registered. Another reason image registration is of importance is that the images from the CT (or MRI) are used to generate the attenuation correction and any mis-registration could introduce image artifacts and quantitative errors. There are several methods for performing the image registration calibration and how to check the registration. One manufacturer uses a set of angled line sources that are imaged on both the PET and CT systems. From the reconstructed PET and CT images, a transformation matrix (three translations and three rotations) is generated to which is used to register the two image sets. Another manufacturer uses a set of distributed glass spheres imbedded in a foam phantom that is imaged the PET and the CT systems. In this case the PET scanner generates a transmission image by using a built-in rotating pin source. Similarly, from the two reconstructed image sets, a transformation matrix is generated that allows the registration of subsequent image acquisitions.

Under normal circumstances, the transformation matrix should not change over time if since the image gantries are fixed relative each other. However, during service of a system, the gantries are usually physically separated, and the calibrations need to be repeated once the system is reassembled. Although the calibration procedure for the registration calibration is very robust, it is recommended that the registration is checked from time to time. One method is to image a series of point sources placed at different positions in the FOV. It is important that the sources can be visualized on both the PET and CT systems, which can be accomplished by using, for instance, ^{68}Ge or ^{22}Na source mixed with iodine. The position of each source in FOV of the PET and CT images can then be calculated using, for instance, a center of mass calculation, and the position of each source is then compared between the two image sets. For a well-calibrated system, the error should not be more than about a millimeter. Since point sources mixed with iodine may not be readily available, a registration check can also be performed using a phantom with some built-in structures such as spheres. This could, for instance, be a Jaszczak phantom with fillable spheres or the NEMA image quality phantom. The spheres in these phantoms can then be filled with a mixture of ^{18}F and iodine contrast and imaged on the system. The registration of the two image sets can then either be checked visually by fusing the PET images with the contrast-enhanced CT images or by calculating the center of mass of each sphere in the two image sets, and the registration error can be quantified.

10.4.7.6 PET/MRI

Combined PET and MRI systems have been recently developed by all major manufacturers of PET systems [27, 28]. The tests for these systems are basically the same as the test performed on a PET/CT (e.g., NEMA test, image/gantry registration, quantification). One of the main challenges in combined PET/MRI systems is the derivation of an accurate attenuation map for the object to be imaged. Unlike CT images, the MRI images do not provide information regarding the photon attenuation properties of the object. Although in many situations the use of appropriate pulse sequences together with sophisticated segmentation techniques using a priori information about the imaged object, fairly accurate attenuation maps can be generated. However, a major complication arises when an object does not produce a signal in the MRI scanner such as bone in patients and the plastic used in phantom. These objects will appear as voids in the MRI image, and as a consequence, most algorithms for producing an attenuation map would incorrectly consider these objects to have zero attenuation. This will result in an undercorrection of the emission data and will result in an underestimation of the activity concentration in the reconstructed PET images. In the worst scenario, this may also lead reconstruction artifacts.

For phantoms, the amount of attenuation from the container or other solid structures can be added to the MRI-generated attenuation map by using data from separately acquired CT images. In order to avoid reconstruction artifacts, the attenuation map derived from CT images has to be accurately registered to the MRI images.

Another source of attenuation in PET/MRI scanners is the presence of transmission and receiver coils, which are essential in the acquisition of the MR images. These coils are typically placed in close vicinity of the object that is imaged and are therefore inside the FOV of the PET scanner. Since these coils are not visualized in the MRI images, they would not contribute to an MRI-derived attenuation map. The amount of attenuation of these coils would cause depends on the design and materials used in the construction of the coil. Some of the coils used for whole body imaging are very thin and are made of low attenuating materials and therefore have almost a negligible amount of attenuation. If the coil has produced a significant amount of attenuation, a CT-derived attenuation map of the coil can be added to the MRI-derived attenuation map. This requires that the coil is rigid and is placed at a fixed and known position during the scan (e.g., a head coil).

10.5 Routine Quality Assurance

Routine quality assurance tests are performed to verify that the system is operational for routine imaging. It will also ensure that a consistent image quality is maintained and that image quantification is reliable and accurate. These tests are designed to give the operator an overall assessment of the status of the system and whether it can be used for imaging or not. Although the particulars of these routine QC tests are manufacturer specific, the basic test are in general very similar and common to all systems.

10.5.1 Daily Tests

Common for all PET systems, independence of manufacturer is a test of the detector system that should be performed every day, prior to scanning the first patient. This is analogous to the daily flood image that is acquired on a conventional scintillation camera. Depending on the manufacturer, this test is either performed with a uniform cylinder source or a built-in rotating line source filled with a long-lived positron emitter such as ^{68}Ge. The idea is to expose all detectors in the system to a uniform flux of annihilation photons. The collected data are then presented to the user either as a series of sinograms or a display of the counts collected by each detector element (i.e., fan sum). An example of this is shown in Fig. 10.10, where four out of the total 109 sinograms of a uniform ^{68}Ge are shown in the upper half of the figure. The lower part of the same figure shows the fan-sum counts for all of

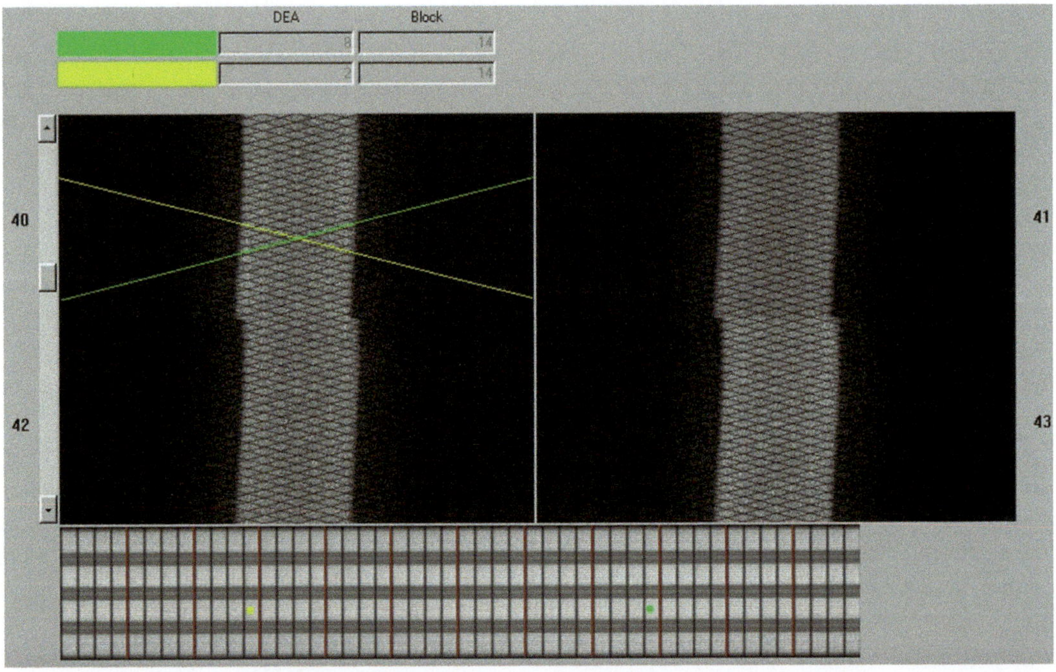

Fig. 10.10 Example of the presentation of the sinograms (4 out of 109) and the fan-sum counts displayed as a grayscale image (*bottom*) from a normal QC scan of a cylinder phantom. The yellow and green diagonal lines indicate two specific detector elements in the system and are also indicated with their corresponding locations in the fan-sum display. Any detector problem would be seen in the sinogram as illustrated in Fig. 10.5, with corresponding dark or hot spots in the fan-sum image (Note: the repetitive pattern or dark diagonal lines are normal for this particular system)

the detectors in the systems, shown as a grayscale image. The diagonal lines in green and yellow in the sinogram are the fan sums for a pair of detectors in the system. The locations of these detectors are also indicated in the fan-sum count image. This figure illustrates a fully functional system. The dark diagonal lines seen in the sinograms are normal for this system and are not an indication of failing detector elements. The variation in the fan sums is also normal for this system. This particular system has four rings of block detectors with 48 blocks in each ring, and the efficiency of the detector elements at the edge tends to be less efficient compared to the centrally located elements. This drop in efficiency is the explanation for the lower number of counts between each detector module and detector ring.

As described earlier in this chapter, this will give the operator a quick feedback whether the system is operational or not and whether there are some apparent deficiencies in the system such as a failing detector module. A trained operator may also detect more subtle changes in the system such as a drift in the energy thresholds or detector gains by changes in patterns in the sinograms (e.g., appearances of cold or hot diagonal streaks). The daily flood test performed on most PET system is very sensitive in detecting the most common problem seen in a PET system (i.e., detector failures).

One manufacturer uses a calibrated ^{68}Ge cylinder source as the source for the daily QC. This source is placed at the center of the FOV, and a fixed number of true coincidence counts are acquired every day. This data set is used not only to check that all the detectors are operational but also to generate a new normalization file and calibration factor every day. By generating a new normalization every day, small drifts in the detector system can be corrected for without the need of any detector adjustments or tuning. Measuring the calibration factor every day allows the long-term stability of the system to be tracked, and any large change may indicate that the system is in the need of retuning or might possibly be a sign of a hardware failure (e.g., failing high-voltage supply).

Figure 10.11 shows the output from a successful QC scan. The top window tells the operator that the system has passed all the QC tests. A more detailed report of the results of the test can also be generated which is shown in the bottom window. In case of a failure, this report will tell the user what part of the QC test that failed. This will provide guidance whether the problem can be easily resolved (e.g., repeat the QC scan after repositioning the phantom) or whether the system is in need of service.

10.5.2 Monthly/Quarterly Tests

Since a PET system is used to provide quantitative images, the quantitative accuracy should be tested. Most modern PET systems tend to be very stable in terms of detector drifts; this test is typically only necessary to perform quarterly. It is recommended that quantitative accuracy is tested after a major service or detector adjustments. As described earlier, this is tested with a uniform cylinder phantom filled with a known amount of activity. ROI analysis is then used to compare the activity concentration in the reconstructed images to the actual assayed activity concentration. It is important to point out that this test should not be performed with the same phantom used for the determination of the calibration factor (e.g., the ^{68}Ge phantom used in the daily QC) since this would not reveal any problems in the quantitative accuracy.

10.5.3 Annual Tests

It is recommended that a more thorough test is performed on the system on an annual basis. In the US, this is required by the ACR as part of PET scanner accreditation. The main purpose of the annual test is to ensure that the imaging properties of the system have not degraded. The annual test does not have to be as rigorous as the acceptance test, but it is a good idea to perform at least a subset of these tests. An overall imaging performance test using, for instance, a Jaszczak phantom or ACR accreditation phantom allows for a quick evaluation of the spatial resolution, contrast, and uniformity. This test should be performed using the same phantom and under similar conditions as the acceptance testing. This allows a comparison of the performance since the time of installation and could reveal any degradation in imaging performance.

It is also recommended to perform the spatial resolution, sensitivity, and scatter fraction tests. Any significant changes in the measured values over time may be an indication that the system may be in the need of a readjustment of detector LUTs and energy thresholds.

A count rate performance test is a good way to ensure that the whole system is operational under somewhat extreme count rate conditions. In a way, it can be seen as a stress test of the system, since it requires that the whole system is fully functional from the front-end detectors, through the processing electronics to the final data storage.

10.5.4 Tests for Clinical Trials

Quantitative PET imaging is becoming increasingly important in various clinical trials in the evaluation of new cancer therapies. The most commonly used semiquantitative index in PET imaging is the SUV, which is a simplified measure of glucose metabolism. The SUV has been used extensively to characterize lesions and to differentiate between malignant and benign lesions and for the assessment of therapy response [29–33]. The SUV is defined as the tissue concentration of the tissue activity divided by the activity injected per body weight:

$$\mathrm{SUV} = \frac{\mathrm{VOI}\ [\mathrm{Bq/ml}]}{A_{\mathrm{injected}}\ [\mathrm{Bq}] / \mathrm{Body\ Weight}\ [\mathrm{kg}]}$$

where VOI is the activity within a volume of interest and A_{injected} is the total injected activity decay corrected to the time same as the VOI

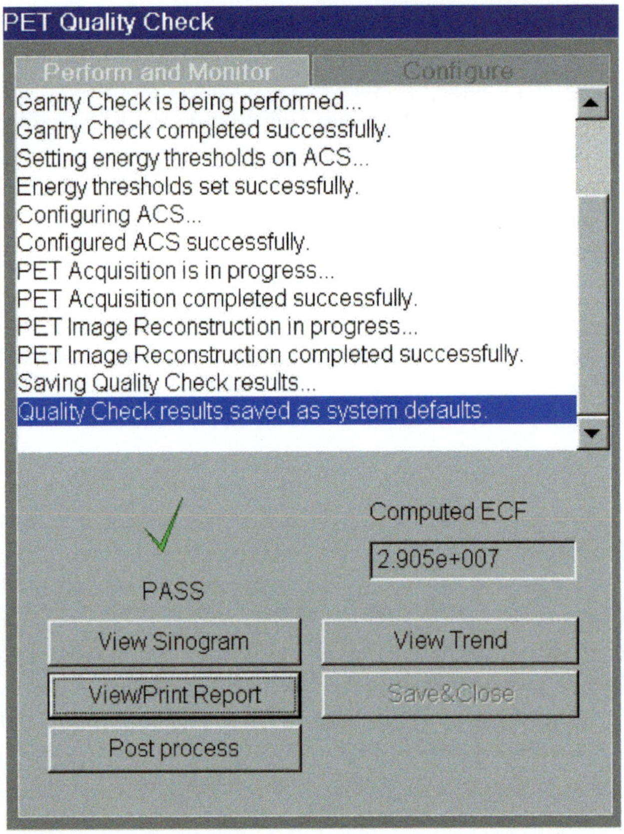

Results	
System Quality Results	Passed
QC Phantom Activity	Passed
QC succesfully completed. All values are within valid ranges.	
QC Phantom has remaining activity greater than 0.5 mCi.	

Detailed System Quality Report				
Item	Upper Bound	Lower Bound	Value	Decision
Block Noise	3 [crystal]	0 [crystal]	0 Blocks out of range	Passed
Block Efficiency	120 [%]	80 [%]	0 Blocks out of range	Passed
Measured Randoms	115 [%]	85 [%]	102 [%]	Passed
Scanner Efficiency	47.32 [cps/Bq/cc]	25.48 [cps/Bq/cc]	40.4 [cps/Bq/cc]	Passed
Scatter Ratio	35.2 [%]	28.8 [%]	31.6 [%]	Passed
Scanner efficiency correction factor (ECF)	4e+007 [Bq*s/ECAT counts]	2e+007 [Bq*s/ECAT counts]	2.905e+007 [Bq*s/ECAT counts]	Passed
Image Plane Efficiency	5 [%]	-5 [%]	0 Planes out of range	Passed
Block Timing Offset	0.5 [bin]	0 [bin]	0 Blocks out of range	Passed
Block Timing Width	5 [bin]	0 [bin]	0 Blocks out of range	Passed
Time Alignment Residual	2 [mm]	0 [mm]	1.3 [mm]	Passed
Time Alignment Fit (x / y)	2 [mm]	0 [mm]	0.8 [mm] / 0.2 [mm]	Passed

Fig. 10.11 Example of the results of reports from the daily QC from a Siemens PET/CT system. The top figure tells the user that the system passed all the daily QC tests and that the systems are operational. A more detailed report is also produced which would provide information what test(s) did not pass and could also give insight to what might cause the QC to fail

measurement. Using the SUV as a quantitative index is very attractive from a practical point of view since it eliminates the complexities of traditional quantitative study protocols used in PET. These studies involve applying a pharmacokinetic model to the dynamically acquired PET data. These types of studies are typically limited to single organ studies and are typically length and labor intensive to perform. On the other hand, the SUV is very sensitive to a number of factors that may introduce unacceptable large errors. For instance, it is very important that all clocks used to record relevant time points (i.e., dose assay time, injection time, and scan start time) are synchronized. Furthermore, the SUV has been shown to be very sensitive to the uptake time where the SUV in lesions tend to increase over time. The blood glucose level is another factor that will affect the SUV value.

In a clinical trial, a subject is typically scanned prior to the start of treatment. The subject is then imaged in one or more PET imaging sessions, either during or after the treatment. The change in SUV in a lesion is then used as an indicator of the efficacy of the drug.

In addition to keeping the imaging condition close to identical at each imaging session, it is also of great importance to maintain the quantitative accuracy and stability in quantification of the PET system over time. Large studies are typically performed as multicenter trials, where the subjects are imaged at different institutions and imaging centers. Although each individual patient is imaged at a specific imaging center and on the same scanner, the entire subject population is very likely to have been imaged on a range of different systems, each with its own specific imaging characteristics. A major challenge in these multicenter trials is therefore to ensure that data acquired on these different systems are quantitatively accurate and comparable.

There are a multitude of factors that could affect the quantitative accuracy when collecting data from multiple systems [11]. Each system has its own imaging characteristics, such as spatial resolution, sensitivity, and image reconstruction algorithm used which all will affect quantification. The calibration accuracy and long-term stability of the system may differ between systems. There are numerous technical parameters that may affect the quantification, such as synchronization of clocks (i.e., scanner time and dose assay time) and cross calibration between the dose calibrator and the scanner.

To make sure data acquired at the different sites are comparable, it is therefore important that all the steps involved in performing a quantitative scan is standardized between imaging sites [34]. This includes patient preparation, assay techniques, uptake times, and imaging conditions. In addition, the image reconstruction and processing of the acquired data at the different sites should produce images that have comparable spatial resolution. This will ensure similar partial volume effects and SUV recovery, independent of imaging system. To achieve this, a phantom allowing recovery coefficient measurements is scanned on all systems used in the trial. A set of reconstruction parameters is determined that will produce a recovery curve that is approximately the same for all systems. These scanner-specific reconstruction parameters are then used for all the subjects imaged on that specific scanner.

It is also important that the quantitative accuracy of the systems used in the trial is monitored at regular intervals. At a minimum, this should be done quarterly with a uniform cylinder phantom filled with a known amount of activity. To repeat the measurement of the recovery coefficients is typically not necessary since these are not likely to change over time, unless there is a major change to the reconstruction software.

10.6 Summary

Performing routine performance and QC tests on PET and PET/CT systems is important to ensure that the imaging system is operating properly and that the system is producing images of highest possible image quality. A thorough standardized acceptance test of the system, such as the NEMA tests, at the time of installation provides a reference point to which later tests can be compared to. By performing routine testing of the system as the system ages, any degradation in performance and image and image quality can hopefully be caught and immediately rectified. As discussed in this chapter, an effective QC program can be implemented with a few relatively simple daily and less frequent (quarterly and annual) phantom scans. A routine and thorough QC program will ensure consistent image quality and stable quantitative accuracy is maintained.

References

1. Dent HM, Jones WF, Casey ME. A real time digital coincidence processor for positron emission tomography. IEEE Trans Nucl Sci. 1986;33:556–9.
2. Moses WW, Buckley S, Vu C, Peng Q, Pavlov N, Choong WS, Wu J, Jackson C. OpenPET: a flexible electronics system for radiotracer imaging. IEEE T NUCL SCI. 2010;57:2532–7.
3. Moses WW. Recent advances and future advances in time-of-flight PET. Aip Conf Proc. 2009; 1204:119–25.
4. Casey ME, Nutt R. A multicrystal two dimensional BGO detector system for positron emission tomography. IEEE Trans Nucl Sci. 1986;NS-33:460–3.
5. Dahlbom M, Hoffman EJ. An evaluation of a two-dimensional array detector for high-resolution PET. IEEE Trans Med Imag. 1988;7:264–72.
6. Hoffman EJ, Guerrero TM, Germano G, Digby WM, Dahlbom M. PET system calibration and corrections for quantitative and spatially accurate images. IEEE Trans Nucl Sci. 1989;NS-36:1108–12.
7. Casey ME, Hoffman EJ. Quantitation in positron emission computed tomography: 7. A technique to reduce noise in accidental coincidence measurements and coincidence efficiency calibration. J Comput Assist Tomogr. 1986;10:845–50.
8. Casey ME, Gadagkar H, Newport D. A component based method for normalisation in volume PET. In Proc. 3rd Int. Meeting on fully three-dimensional image reconstruction in radiology and nuclear medicine. France: Aix-les-Bains; 1995. p. 67–71.
9. Badawi RD, Marsden PK. Developments in component-based normalization for 3D PET. Phys Med Biol. 1999;44:571–94.
10. Lockhart CM, MacDonald LR, Alessio AM, McDougald WA, Doot RK, Kinahan PE. Quantifying and reducing the effect of calibration error on variability of PET/CT standardized uptake value measurements. J Nucl Med. 2011;52:218–24.
11. Boellaard R. Standards for PET image acquisition and quantitative data analysis. J Nucl Med. 2009;50 Suppl 1:11S–20.
12. Zimmerman BE, Cessna JT. Development of a traceable calibration methodology for solid (68)Ge/(68)Ga sources used as a calibration surrogate for (18)F in radionuclide activity calibrators. J Nucl Med. 2010;51:448–53.
13. NEMA. 2013. NEMA NU 2–2012 performance measurements of positron emission tomographs. National Electrical Manufacturers Association, Rosslyn, VA
14. NEMA. 2007. NEMA NU 2–2007 performance measurements of positron emission tomographs. National Electrical Manufacturers Association, Rosslyn, VA.
15. Strother SC, Casey ME, Hoffman EJ. Measuring PET scanner sensitivity: relating count rates to image signal-to-noise ratios using noise equivalent counts. IEEE Trans Nucl Sci. 1990;NS-37:783–8.
16. Dahlbom M, Schiepers C, Czernin J. Comparison of noise equivalent count rates and image noise. IEEE T Nucl Sci. 2005;52:1386–90.
17. Watson CC, Casey ME, Bendriem B, Carney JP, Townsend DW, Eberl S, Meikle S, Difilippo FP. Optimizing injected dose in clinical PET by accurately modeling the counting-rate response functions specific to individual patient scans. J Nucl Med. 2005;46:1825–34.
18. Bailey DL, Jones T, Spinks TJ. A method for measuring the absolute sensitivity of positron emission tomographic scanners. Eur J Nucl Med. 1991;18:374–9.
19. Daube-Witherspoon M, Muehllehner G. Treatment of axial data in three-dimensional PET. J Nucl Med. 1987;28:1717–24.
20. Melcher C, Schweitzer J. Cerium-doped lutetium oxyorthosilicate: a fast new scintillator. IEEE Trans Nucl Sci. 1992;NS-39:502–5.
21. Watson CC, Casey ME, Eriksson L, Mulnix T, Adams D, Bendriem B. NEMA NU 2 performance tests for scanners with intrinsic radioactivity. J Nucl Med. 2004;45:822–6.
22. Eriksson L, Watson CC, Wienhard K, Eriksson M, Casey ME, Knoess C, Lenox M, Burbar Z, Conti M, Bendriem B, Heiss WD, Nutt R. The ECAT HRRT: an example of NEMA scatter estimation issues for LSO-based PET systems. IEEE T NUCL SCI. 2005;52:90–4.
23. Erdi YE, Nehmeh SA, Mulnix T, Humm JL, Watson CC. PET performance measurements for an LSO-based combined PET/CT scanner using the National Electrical Manufacturers Association NU 2–2001 standard. J Nucl Med. 2004;45:813–21.
24. Karp JS, Daube-Witherspoon ME, Hoffman EJ, Lewellen TK, Links JM, Wong WH, Hichwa RD, Casey ME, Colsher JG, Hitchens RE, et al. Performance standards in positron emission tomography. J Nucl Med. 1991;32:2342–50.
25. Huang SC. Anatomy of SUV. Standardized uptake value. Nuclear Med Biol. 2000;27:643–6.
26. Dahlbom M, Reed J, Young J. Implementation of true continuous bed motion in 2-D and 3-D whole-body PET scanning. IEEE Trans Nucl Sci. 2001;NS-48:1465–9.
27. Schlemmer HP, Pichler BJ, Krieg R, Heiss WD. An integrated MR/PET system: prospective applications. Abdom Imaging. 2009;34:668–74.

28. Zaidi H, Ojha N, Morich M, Griesmer J, Hu Z, Maniawski P, Ratib O, Izquierdo-Garcia D, Fayad ZA, Shao L. Design and performance evaluation of a whole-body ingenuity TF PET-MRI system. Phys Med Biol. 2011;56:3091–106.
29. de Geus-Oei LF, van der Heijden HF, Corstens FH, Oyen WJ. Predictive and prognostic value of FDG-PET in nonsmall-cell lung cancer: a systematic review. Cancer. 2007;110:1654–64.
30. Borst GR, Belderbos JS, Boellaard R, Comans EF, De Jaeger K, Lammertsma AA, Lebesque JV. Standardised FDG uptake: a prognostic factor for inoperable non-small cell lung cancer. Eur J Cancer. 2005;41: 1533–41.
31. Avril NE, Weber WA. Monitoring response to treatment in patients utilizing PET. Radiol Clin North Am. 2005;43:189–204.
32. Weber WA. Use of PET for monitoring cancer therapy and for predicting outcome. J Nucl Med. 2005;46:983–95.
33. Larson SM, Schwartz LH. 18F-FDG PET as a candidate for "qualified biomarker": functional assessment of treatment response in oncology. J Nucl Med. 2006;47:901–3.
34. Boellaard R, O'Doherty MJ, Weber WA, Mottaghy FM, Lonsdale MN, Stroobants SG, Oyen WJ, Kotzerke J, Hoekstra OS, Pruim J, Marsden PK, Tatsch K, Hoekstra CJ, Visser EP, Arends B, Verzijlbergen FJ, Zijlstra JM, Comans EF, Lammertsma AA, Paans AM, Willemsen AT, Beyer T, Bockisch A, Schaefer-Prokop C, Delbeke D, Baum RP, Chiti A, Krause BJ. FDG PET and PET/CT: EANM procedure guidelines for tumour PET imaging: version 1.0. Eur J Nuclear Med Mole Imaging. 2010;37:181–200.

Part IV

PET Image Reconstruction, Processing and Quantitation

PET Image Reconstruction: Methodology and Quantitative Accuracy

11

Bing Bai and Evren Asma

Contents

11.1	**Introduction**	259
11.2	**Analytic Image Reconstruction**	260
11.2.1	PET Data Formation and Storage	260
11.2.2	Filtered Backprojection	261
11.2.3	Reconstruction of 3D PET Data	263
11.3	**Model-Based Statistical Reconstruction**	264
11.3.1	Noise Model	265
11.3.2	System Model	266
11.3.3	Maximum Likelihood Estimation Methods	267
11.3.4	Maximum-a-Posteriori Estimation Methods	269
11.3.5	Analysis of Image Properties	273
11.4	**PET Image Quantitation**	275
11.4.1	PET Data Corrections	275
11.4.2	PET Image Calibration	277
11.5	**Recent Developments**	277
11.5.1	Time of Flight PET	277
11.5.2	Parametric Image Reconstruction	279
Conclusions		280
References		281

Abstract

This chapter reviews the techniques developed for positron emission tomography (PET) image reconstruction and image property analysis. Both mathematical theory and practical considerations are introduced. We focus on the commonly used methods on commercial PET scanners, in particular model-based statistical reconstruction methods. We also briefly describe data corrections necessary for PET image reconstruction, which are important for reducing artifacts and improving quantitative accuracy. Finally some recent developments are described, including the reconstruction of time-of-flight (TOF) PET data and direct parametric image reconstruction.

11.1 Introduction

The theory of image reconstruction from projections has been developed since the early twentieth century [1] and flourished after the introduction of x-ray computed tomography (CT) [2]. Many methods have been proposed and implemented successfully for various imaging techniques including CT, positron emission tomography (PET), single-photon emission computed tomography (SPECT), and magnetic resonance imaging (MRI).

B. Bai, PhD (✉)
Toshiba America Medical Systems, Inc.,
2441 Michelle Drive, Tustin, CA 92780, USA
e-mail: bing.bai@toshiba.com

E. Asma, PhD
Toshiba Medical Research Institute USA, Inc.,
706 N Deerpath Drive, Vernon Hills, IL 60061, USA
e-mail: easma@tmriusa.com

M.M. Khalil (ed.), *Basic Science of PET Imaging*, DOI 10.1007/978-3-319-40070-9_11

Image reconstruction techniques can be broadly grouped into two categories: analytic and statistical methods. Analytic image reconstruction methods model the PET data as line integrals through the image. An exact or approximate formula is sought to invert the x-ray transform [3]. Despite the fact that the line integral model is only a very rough approximation to the underlying physics in PET and the fact that the statistical nature of measured data is ignored, analytic image reconstruction methods have been used extensively in clinical practice due to their speed. In the last 10 years, the rapid increase of computational power has also made model-based statistical reconstruction methods feasible for routine clinical studies. These methods employ system models to describe the scanner geometry and the data acquisition physics and statistical noise models to account for noise in the data. They use iterative numerical optimization algorithms to maximize a chosen cost function to obtain the final reconstructed image. As a result of these physical and statistical models, images reconstructed using model-based statistical methods have less noise and higher resolution compared to analytic reconstruction methods. All recent commercial PET scanners have model-based statistical reconstruction packages, and many clinics have switched to them for their routine clinical applications.

PET data acquisition involves counting of photon pairs as the radioactive isotope decays, which is a complex random process, and the data is usually very noisy. The spatial resolution of the data is limited due to the finite size of the detectors and other physical factors including positron range and noncollinearity of the photon pair. In general it is not possible to achieve the best image resolution and minimize noise at the same time. Thus one important goal of image reconstruction is to optimize the tradeoff between image noise and resolution.

This chapter reviews the techniques developed for PET image reconstruction and image property analysis. We introduce both mathematical theory and practical considerations, focusing on the methods commonly used on commercial PET scanners. We also briefly describe data corrections necessary for PET image reconstruction, which are important for reducing the artifacts and improving quantitative accuracy. The details of these corrections can be found in other chapters. Finally some recent developments are given, including the reconstruction of time-of-flight (TOF) PET data and direct parametric image reconstruction.

11.2 Analytic Image Reconstruction

11.2.1 PET Data Formation and Storage

In order to understand the theory of PET image reconstruction, let us first describe briefly how PET data is acquired and stored.

PET scanners are typically composed of multiple detector rings. Historically PET data was acquired in 2D mode with lead or tungsten septa inserted between detector rings to only allow for coincidences within the same or neighboring rings to be recorded and to reduce the number of scattered events. Figure 11.1 shows one ring of a typical PET gantry. When two photons are detected in the scanner, they are processed through electronics to check for various criteria such as whether each photon has the right amount of energy (typically between 350 and 650 keV) or whether the photons have arrived almost simultaneously (within 5–6 ns or less of each other). If all criteria are satisfied, then the two photons are recorded as a coincidence event. Each coincidence event can be stored separately as is the case with "list-mode" data, or alternatively, the total number of events detected at each detector pair can be stored. Usually such data is stored in a two-dimensional array for 2D PET indexed by radial element and view angle coordinates and is called a sinogram because measurements from a point source are concentrated on a sinusoid curve.

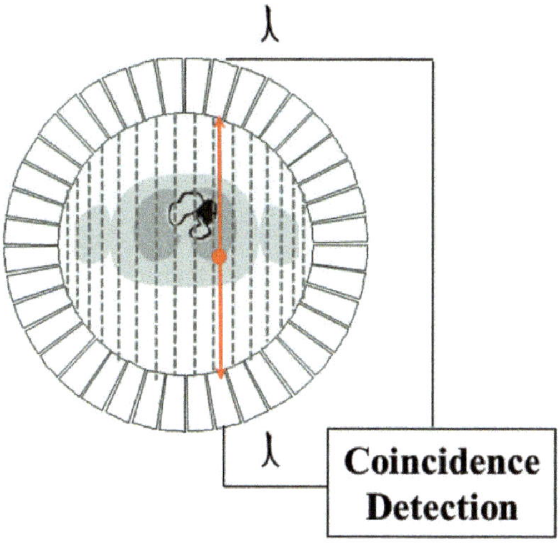

Fig. 11.1 One ring of a typical PET scanner and data processing

In modern PET scanners, the septa were removed for 3D data acquisition to improve the system sensitivity. For 3D PET, the data can be stored either as projections indexed by (x_r, y_r, θ, ϕ) or equivalently as stacks of sinograms indexed by (s, ϕ , z, θ), as shown in Fig. 11.2. Data on 3D PET scanners are typically stored in the stacked sinogram format and sometimes compressed by adding the neighboring angles or sinograms together.

11.2.2 Filtered Backprojection

11.2.2.1 Line Integral Model and Central Slice Theorem

A simple model for PET data assumes that the number of events detected at each detector pair is proportional to the integral of the radioactivity along the line connecting the centers of the two detectors. This is the basis upon which analytic image reconstruction algorithms are developed. Here we illustrate the line integral model for the 2D case.

Mathematically, the spatial distribution of the tracer is represented by a 2D continuous function $f(x,y)$. Measured projection data can then be approximated by the discrete samples of the x-ray transform of $f(x,y)$, which is defined by

$$p(s,\phi) = \int_{-\infty}^{\infty} f(s\cos\phi - t\sin\phi, s\sin\phi + t\cos\phi)\,dt \tag{11.1}$$

where s is the distance of the projection line to the center and ϕ is the projection angle, as shown in Fig. 11.2b.

An important result that underlies analytic image reconstruction is the central slice theorem. In 2D, the central slice theorem relates the 2D Fourier transform of the image to the 1D Fourier transform of its x-ray transform $p(s,\phi)$, as illustrated in Fig. 11.3:

$$F(\omega_s\cos\phi, \omega_s\sin\phi) = P(\omega_s;\phi) \tag{11.2}$$

where the 1D and 2D Fourier transforms are defined by

$$F(\omega_x,\omega_y) = \iint f(x,y)e^{-2\pi i(\omega_x x+\omega_y y)}dxdy$$
$$P(\omega) = \int p(s)e^{-2\pi i\omega s}ds \tag{11.3}$$

This relationship shows in 2D that the Radon transform uniquely describes any Fourier transformable image and that the image can be reconstructed by forming its 2D Fourier transform according to (Eq. 11.2) and taking an inverse 2D Fourier transform. Although this is a straightforward way of reconstructing 2D images, it requires the interpolation of the image's 2D Fourier transform onto a rectangular grid, and reconstructed image quality depends on the accuracy of the interpolation. As a result, direct Fourier reconstruction methods are not commonly used.

11.2.2.2 Backprojection Filtering

An image can be formed by integrating all the projections passing through a point and assigning the value of the integral to the point. This linear operation is called backprojection and can be expressed mathematically as:

$$b(x,y) = \int_0^{\pi} p(x\cos\phi + y\sin\phi, \phi)\,d\phi \tag{11.4}$$

Fig. 11.2 3D PET data stored in (**a**) projection and (**b**) sinogram format

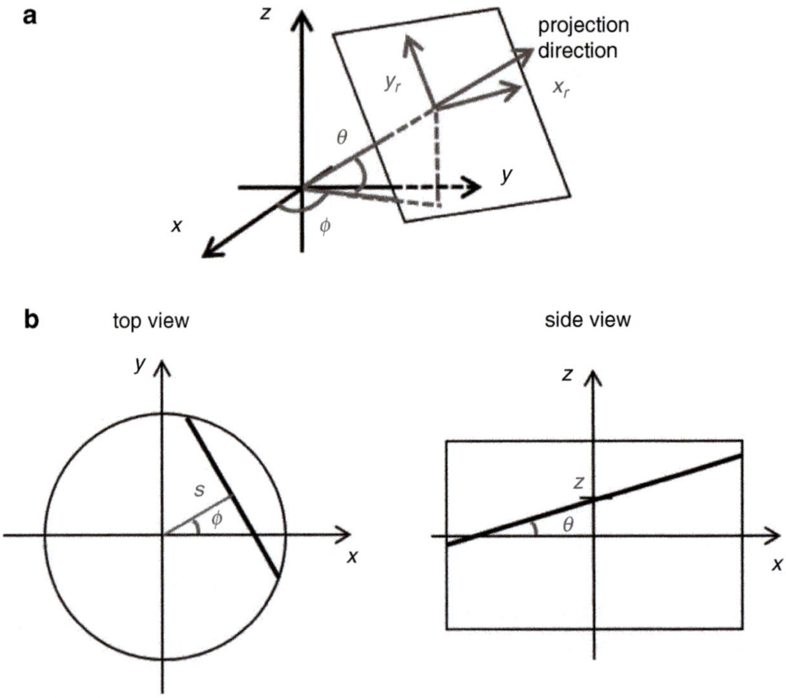

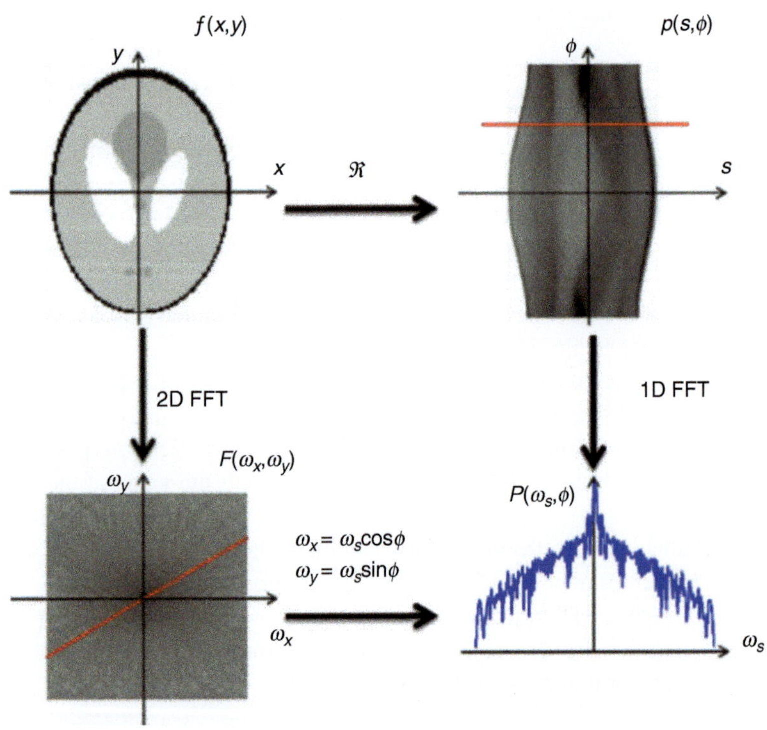

Fig. 11.3 2D central slice theorem

It can be shown that this backprojected image corresponds to the original image smoothed by the "1/r" blurring in Fourier transform domain:

$$B(\omega_x,\omega_y) = F(\omega_x,\omega_y) / \sqrt{\omega_x^2 + \omega_y^2} \quad (11.5)$$

In order to recover the original image $f(x)$, we can filter this backprojected image, and the overall approach is known as backprojection filtering (BPF). A common approach is to switch the order of the linear backprojection and filtering operations and to apply filtering to the 1D projection data (usually by convolution with the filter function in projection space) before backprojection, thus called filtered backprojection or FBP [4]. As shown in (Eq. 11.5), the reconstruction filter has a frequency response of $|\omega|$. This so-called ramp filter amplifies high-frequency noise; therefore, in practice, a windowed ramp filter is used in FBP reconstruction and frequency components above a threshold (cutoff frequency) are set to zero. Frequently used window functions in 2D FBP include Shepp–Logan, Butterworth, and Hann windows [5, 6]. Figure 11.4 shows FBP images of a simulated NCAT phantom using different window functions.

11.2.3 Reconstruction of 3D PET Data

The 2D central slice theorem can be extended to 3D PET, resulting in the derivation of 3D FBP [7]. However, due to the limited axial coverage of PET scanners, not all oblique projections are recorded, and therefore some oblique projections through the imaging volume are missing. As a result, a typical 3D PET scanner corresponds to a shift–variant system where FBP cannot be directly applied to reconstruct the data. Figure 11.5 shows a direct line of response (LOR) which is acquired in 2D PET, an oblique LOR acquired in 3D PET and a missing oblique LOR in 3D PET that is not measured because the LOR does not intersect the detector surface.

One solution to the missing data problem is to estimate the truncated projections before applying 3D FBP. The 3D reprojection (3DRP) algorithm was proposed to estimate the missing data and has been a standard analytic reconstruction algorithm for 3D PET [8]. In 3DRP, unmeasured data is estimated by calculating the line integrals along the LORs through an initial image estimate obtained by applying 2D FBP to the non-oblique sinograms.

We note that 3DRP is based on the fact that 2D data is sufficient for reconstruction (e.g., 2D images reconstructed from line integrals on parallel planes can be stacked to form the final 3D image), and the goal of using additional 3D data is to improve the statistical properties of reconstructed images. While 2D and 3D reconstructions would be identical for reconstructions from noiseless data, at typical clinical data noise levels, by including the events detected by two detectors on different rings, 3D reconstructions significantly improve the signal-to-noise ratio (SNR) of the image.

Another way to reconstruct 3D PET data is to explore the redundancy in the data and to reduce it to a 2D dataset. Such a process is called rebinning. Since the computational cost of rebinning is negligible compared to the computational cost of image reconstruction, the resulting reconstruction speed is almost the same as that of 2D reconstructions.

A simple way to rebin 3D PET data is through the process called single slice rebinning (SSRB) [9] where a stack of 2D sinograms are created by placing detected events on the plane perpendicular to the scanner axis (z) and lying in the middle of the line connecting the two detectors that detected the event. Mathematically we have

$$p(s,\phi,z) = \sum_{\frac{z_1+z_2}{2}=z} p(s,\phi,z_1,z_2) \quad (11.6)$$

where s and ϕ are the coordinates of the line of response projected onto the x–y plane and z_1 and z_2 are the location of the two detector rings (z_1 may equal to z_2).

SSRB is only accurate when the activity is concentrated near the axis of the scanner. In cases of extended activity distributions, such as whole-body FDG scans, SSRB will become less accurate and introduce distortions. A more accurate rebinning method called Fourier rebinning

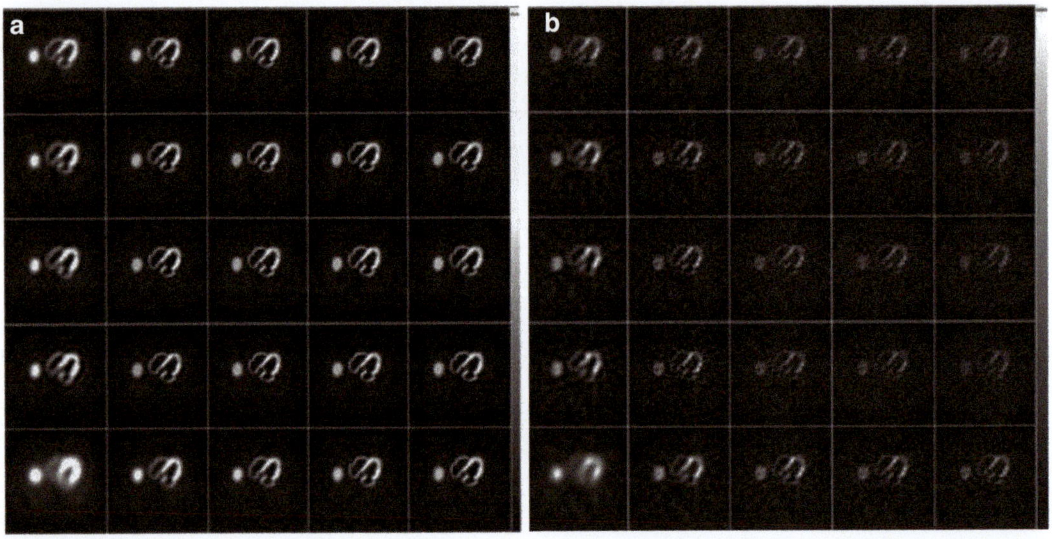

Fig. 11.4 Images reconstructed from simulated NCAT phantom (**a**) noiseless and (**b**) noisy data. *Top 4 rows* were reconstructed using Butterworth window with orders 2, 4, 8, and 32, respectively. *Bottom row* used Hann window. *Left to right*: cutoff frequencies of 0.1, 0.2, 0.3, 0.4, and 0.5 cycle/pixel, respectively (Reproduced from Tsui and Frey [6])

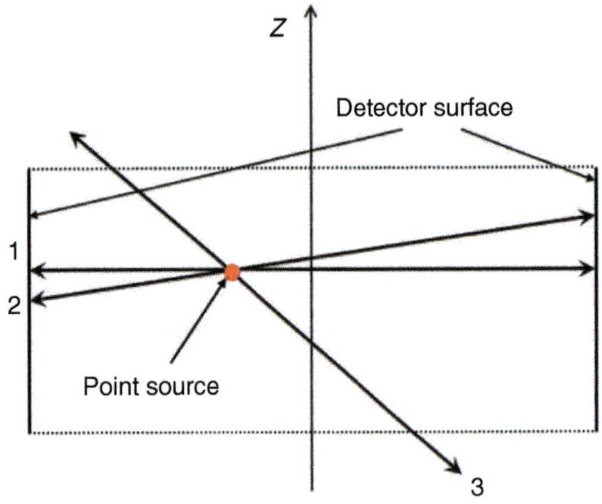

Fig. 11.5 Cross section of a PET scanner: events along LOR1 is acquired in 2D PET, LOR2 is acquired in 3D PET, while LOR3 is missing from the 3D PET data

(FORE) has been developed based on the relationship between the Fourier transforms of the 2D data and oblique data [10].

Following SSRB or FORE, a 2D reconstruction algorithm is applied to reconstruct each slice separately. The advantage of FORE is that it allows fast 2D reconstructions while retaining the SNR benefits from 3D data. Figure 11.6 shows a brain FDG scan data reconstructed using 3DRP and FORE+FBP. The image quality is comparable while the speed of FORE+FBP is more than ten times faster than 3DRP.

Although FORE has been widely used for clinical 3D PET image reconstruction, it is still based on the line integral geometric model and cannot model all the physical effects in PET data acquisition. In addition, FORE requires all the data corrections to be applied directly to the data (instead of being part of the system model), and therefore changes data noise properties which become difficult to model when a 2D iterative algorithm is used to reconstruct the rebinned dataset. As a result, fully 3D statistical reconstruction methods are preferable over FORE rebinning followed by 2D reconstruction methods.

11.3 Model-Based Statistical Reconstruction

Analytic image reconstruction methods inherently assume that noiseless line integrals of the image are available. In reality, data acquired in typical PET scanners are not exact line integrals, and there is significant statistical noise in almost all clinical datasets. Model-based statistical image

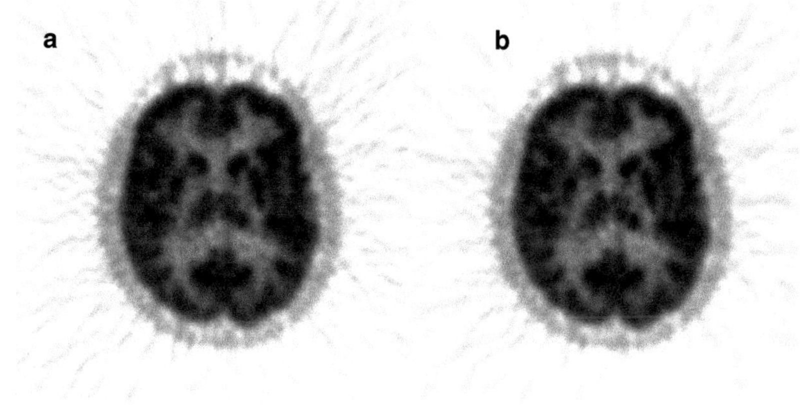

Fig. 11.6 A central transaxial slice of an FDG brain scan reconstructed using (**a**) 3DRP and (**b**) FORE+FBP [10]

reconstruction approaches are preferable due to their ability to model the physics and statistics of the imaging process and have become widely available in all commercial scanners. In this section, we first introduce statistical noise models for PET data and physical system models which describe the complex physics of data acquisition. We then review the methodology of maximum likelihood (ML) and maximum-a-posteriori (MAP) estimation and numerical optimization algorithms used to generate PET images. Due to the nonlinear, shift-varying and high-dimensional nature of statistical reconstruction algorithms, image resolution and noise analyses are complicated and are still an active research area. We will give a brief review on this topic in the end.

11.3.1 Noise Model

PET data is inherently noisy, and this fact has significant effects on reconstructed image quality. Statistical reconstruction algorithms model the noise in PET data explicitly and use iterative numerical optimization algorithms to solve the associated optimization problem. Over the last four decades, many model-based statistical image reconstruction algorithms have been proposed. Although the formulae of these methods are quite different, they are all designed to solve the following problem:

$$y = \bar{y}(x) + \text{noise} \tag{11.7}$$

where y is the measured data, $\bar{y}$ denotes the mean of the data, and x is the image of the unknown activity distribution. The number of events detected at a detector within a given time due to the radioactive decay inside the object can be accurately modeled by the Poisson distribution:

$$P(n \mid \lambda) = \frac{e^{-\lambda}\lambda^{n}}{n!} \tag{11.8}$$

where n is the number of decays and λ is the mean, which is equal to the variance.

If system dead time and detector pileup effects are ignored, then measured data can be modeled as independent Poisson random variables with joint distribution:

$$P(y \mid \bar{y}) = \prod_{i=1}^{M} \frac{e^{-\bar{y}_i}\bar{y}_i^{\,y_i}}{y_i!} \tag{11.9}$$

where y_i is the number of events detected in the ith LOR, $\bar{y}_i$ is the mean number of events in the ith LOR that can be calculated using the system model described in the next section, and M is the number of LORs.

While a Gaussian noise model may be used for low-noise data with acceptable accuracy, resulting in the weighted least square (WLS) approach for image reconstruction [11], most statistical approaches use the Poisson model.

In PET, a common practice is to subtract an estimate of the random events (e.g., using delayed window method) online to reduce the bandwidth needed for data transfer and storage space [12]. In that case, measured data at the ith LOR is given by

$$y_i = p_i - r_i \quad (11.10)$$

where p_i is the number of prompts and r_i is the number of delayed events for the ith LOR. While both p_i and r_i are independent Poisson random variables, the difference between the two is no longer Poisson. The distribution of y_i has a numerically intractable form. One can use Gaussian distribution as an approximation to the true distribution of the precorrected data. Yavuz and Fessler noticed that a simple but good approximation is to add $2\overline{r}_i$ to the data [13], where $\overline{r}_i$ is the mean of the delayed events estimated from the data and to model the resulting random variable as Poisson with mean and variance equal to $\overline{y}_i + 2\overline{r}_i$.

As we discussed previously, Fourier rebinning is commonly used to reduce the size of the dataset and reconstruction time. It has been shown that FORE rebinned data is no longer Poisson [14]. Similar to the approach for random precorrected data, Liu et al. used a simple scaling to match the mean and variance of the rebinned data [15]. Then a reconstruction algorithm based on the Poisson noise model can be used to reconstruct the resulting data.

11.3.2 System Model

The spatial resolution of PET is limited by several factors such as positron range, photon noncollinearity, and penetration and scattering of the photon in the detector. One critical limitation of analytic reconstruction methods is that these factors are neglected in the simple line integral model. With model-based statistical reconstruction, we use a system model to account for these resolution-deteriorating effects. Other factors may also be included in the system model such as the attenuation of the photons in the body, nonuniform efficiencies of the detectors, and random and scattered events.

In the absence of noise, we can model the data as a linear function of the image:

$$\overline{y}_i = \sum_{j=1}^{N} p_{ij} x_j + \overline{r}_i \quad (11.11)$$

or in matrix format $\overline{y} = Px + \overline{r}$

where $\overline{r}$ is the sum of mean of random and scattered events and P is the system matrix, which relates the image to the noiseless data, and can be expressed in factored form as [16]:

$$P = P_{\text{norm}} P_{\text{blur}} P_{\text{attn}} P_{\text{geom}} P_{\text{range}} \quad (11.12)$$

where P_{range} models the blurring due to positron range in image space [17, 18]; P_{geom} is the geometric projection matrix containing the geometric detection probabilities for each voxel and detector pair combination; P_{attn} is a diagonal matrix with attenuation factors; P_{blur} models the blurring in sinogram space due to photon pair noncollinearity, intercrystal penetration, and scattering; and P_{norm} is a diagonal matrix with normalization factors.

Matrix–vector multiplications with P and P^T (called forward and backprojection operations) are typically the most computationally intensive components of statistical reconstructions. Over the last decade, considerable amount of research has been done to speed up statistical reconstruction by reducing the time of forward and backprojections. Many algorithms have been developed that explore the symmetry of the scanner geometry [19] or use fast processors such as graphic processing units (GPUs) to achieve high performance at low cost [20].

It has been shown that the modeling of sinogram blurring is important for resolution recovery [16]. The central component of resolution recovery is the estimation of detector point spread functions (PSF). Such PSFs can be calculated analytically [21], estimated from Monte Carlo simulations [16], or measured from point source data [22, 23]. PSF kernels can either be estimated and stored nonparametrically [23], or the PSF measurements can be fit to a given model, such as asymmetric Gaussian functions [22], and the resulting model parameters can be stored. It has also been shown that for Fourier rebinned data, PSF kernels can be estimated from point source data [23, 24].

Another recent trend is to use an image-space PSF model to account for all resolution degrading effects in the imaging process:

$$P = P_{\text{norm}} P_{\text{attn}} P_{\text{geom}} P_{\text{psf}} \quad (11.13)$$

The image-space PSF P_{psf} can be estimated from an initial reconstruction of point sources without any resolution recovery and is easy to implement as an image-space blurring operation. Recently shift–variant PSFs have been designed to model the degradation of image resolution toward the edge of the field of view (FOV) [25].

Figure 11.7 shows a Hoffman brain phantom data reconstructed with and without PSF modeling. The PSF image shows better resolution and contrast.

One caveat of PSF modeling is that it can result in edge artifacts that have been shown to overestimate activity by up to 40 % in phantom studies [26]. Methods to mitigate edge artifacts include filtering [27] and under-modeling the PSF kernels [28]; however these approaches come at the expense of reduced resolution recovery.

11.3.3 Maximum Likelihood Estimation Methods

Once we have the noise model and system model, statistical methods can be used to estimate the image. Maximum likelihood (ML) is a widely used statistical estimation method and has been applied to PET image reconstruction.

The likelihood function of the data is the probability of observing the data given the image. Usually the logarithm of the likelihood function is used for easier calculation because the logarithm is a one-to-one monotonic function:

$$L(x) = \log\left(\text{Prob}(y \mid x)\right) \quad (11.14)$$

ML estimation seeks the image that maximizes the log-likelihood function:

$$x_{ML} = \arg\max_{x \geq 0} L(x) \quad (11.15)$$

The nonnegativity constraint is due to the fact that the concentration of radioactivity is not negative.

The log-likelihood function under the Poisson noise model is given by (omitting the $y_i!$ term which does not depend on x)

$$L(x) = \sum_{i=1}^{M} y_i \log \bar{y}_i(x) - \bar{y}_i(x) \quad (11.16)$$

ML estimation is a classic optimization problem, where the cost function (or objective function) is the log-likelihood function (Eq. 11.16). There are many numerical algorithms that can be used to find the ML estimate of the image, such as coordinate ascent or gradient-based methods. One of the earliest approaches used for ML PET image reconstruction is the expectation–maximization (EM) algorithm [29]. EM is a general framework to compute the ML solution through the use of "complete" but unobservable data and is composed of two steps. The first step, called the E-step, involves the calculation of the conditional expectation of the complete data, and the second step, called the M-step, maximizes this conditional expectation with respect to the image. In PET, a very common choice for complete data is the number of events detected by the *i*th LOR that are emitted from the *j*th voxel. Shepp and Vardi first applied EM to emission image reconstruction [30], and Lange and Carson extended the work to transmission image reconstruction [31].

The update equation of EM algorithm for emission image reconstruction is given by

$$x_j^{k+1} = \frac{x_j^k}{\sum_{i'} P_{i'j}} \sum_i P_{ij} \frac{y_i}{\sum_{j'} P_{ij'} x_{j'}^k} \quad (11.17)$$

where y_i is the number of events acquired in the *i*th LOR, P_{ij} is the element in the system matrix P described in the previous section, and x_j^k is the estimate of the *j*th image voxel at the *k*th iteration.

The EM algorithm is usually initialized using a uniform image. A new image is then calculated using Eq. 11.17. This process is repeated until a

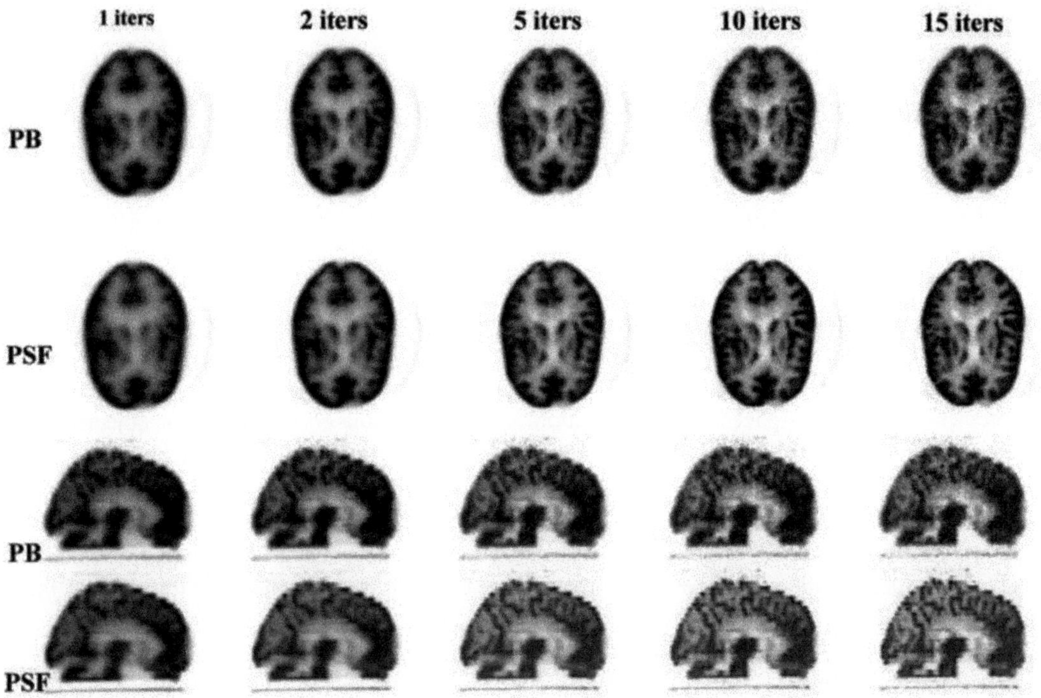

Fig. 11.7 Hoffman brain phantom reconstructions for various numbers of iterations. Upper images are transaxial views, and the lower images are sagittal views. *PB* parallel-beam, non-PSF [22]

certain number of iterations are reached. Typically a smoothing filter is applied afterward to reduce image noise.

It is interesting to note that the EM update equation can be derived in several ways. One approach is based on using the concavity of the Poisson log-likelihood function and Jensen's inequality [32]. In another work, Qi and Leahy showed that that EM algorithm is a functional substitution (FS) method [33]. FS is based on designing a surrogate function at each iteration which is easier to maximize than the original function. Under suitable conditions (equal function value and gradient with current estimated image, surrogate function always higher than the original function), it can be proven that the FS method converges to the maxima of the original function [34–36].

It has been shown that EM converges monotonically to the global maximum of the log-likelihood function and the image is guaranteed to be nonnegative if initialized with a nonnegative image [37]. These nice properties made EM a popular algorithm but unfortunately EM converges very slowly. Hundreds or thousands of iterations are usually necessary to ensure the convergence of EM. Hudson and Larkin observed that the convergence of EM algorithm could be significantly speeded up by dividing the projection data into nonoverlapping blocks, or subsets, and applying EM to each subset of the data [38] and named this method ordered subsets EM (OSEM).

OSEM can speed up the reconstruction almost linearly as a function of number of subsets in early iterations. As a result, it has been widely used in clinical PET and SPECT. The speedup of OSEM can be explained in part by viewing EM as a preconditioned gradient-ascent method:

$$x^{k+1} = x^k + D\left(x^k\right)\nabla L\left(x^k\right) \quad (11.18)$$

where $D(x^k)$ is a diagonal matrix with $D_{jj} = x_j^k / \sum_i p_{ij}$ and $\nabla L\left(x^k\right)$

denotes the gradient of the log-likelihood calculated at the kth iteration image. When the image is far away from the solution, the gradient computed from a subset of the data provides a satisfactory direction for increasing the log-likelihood function value [39].

Although OSEM is fast in the beginning, it is not guaranteed to converge to the ML solution, and the convergence depends on the selection of the subsets. In the original OSEM paper, subsets are chosen such that the detection probability of each voxel is equal for each subset, which is called subset balance. It has been proven that with consistent data and under the condition of subset balance, OSEM converges to the ML solution [38]. In practice subset balance is difficult to achieve due to differences in sensitivity and attenuation. A common practice is to choose the projections in each subset with maximum angular separation to avoid directional artifacts. Another OSEM algorithm convergent with consistent data is rescaled block-iterative EM (RBI-EM), in which the OSEM equation is written in gradient-ascent form and a voxel-independent scaling factor is used to avoid the requirement of subset balance [40].

In general PET data is not consistent due to noise, in which case OSEM usually enters a limit cycle [39]. One way to make OSEM converge with noisy data is to reduce the number of subsets: however convergence is then slowed down. Alternatively, we can use OSEM in the earlier iterations and switch to a convergent algorithm in later iterations [41].

Among other ML estimation approaches, Browne and De Pierro proposed a row-action maximum likelihood algorithm (RAMLA) [42], where the stepsize η_k at the kth iteration satisfies the following conditions:

$$\lim_{k\to 0}\eta_k = 0, \sum_{k=0}^{\infty}\eta_k = +\infty \qquad (11.19)$$

RAMLA converges to ML solution if the log-likelihood function is strictly concave [42]. However the convergence rate can be very slow.

Another way to achieve convergence is through the use of an augmented cost function [39], and an example of this method is the convergent OSEM algorithm (COSEM) [43].

Despite its convergence issues, OSEM is still by far the most popularly used iterative reconstruction algorithm in clinical nuclear medicine. Figure 11.8 shows OSEM images from a monkey brain phantom reconstructed using different numbers of iterations. It shows that image noise increases quickly as number of iterations is increased. As a result, clinical OSEM images are usually reconstructed using less than five iterations, and a smoothing filter is applied post-OSEM to reduce image noise.

In Fig. 11.8 we also show an image reconstructed using the maximum-a-posteriori (MAP) method. In MAP reconstruction regularization is used to ensure a stable solution is reached, as demonstrated by the MAP image after 25 iterations, which shows fine structures and low noise. We will introduce MAP reconstruction methods in the next section.

11.3.4 Maximum-a-Posteriori Estimation Methods

11.3.4.1 Prior Functions

It has been observed that with ML estimators such as EM or OSEM, iterating beyond a certain point will dramatically increase noise and decrease image quality [44]. The reason is the inherent ill-posedness of the PET inverse problem. The system matrix is ill-conditioned so that small differences in the data (which naturally occur due to photon counting noise) produce large changes in the ML solution. It can be shown that the variance of the estimator increases as voxel sizes are reduced [33]. The noise in the OSEM image can be controlled by stopping the algorithm before convergence [45] or post-smoothing the image after many iterations [46]. An alternative approach to dealing with the instability of the ML problem is to use regularization in image reconstruction. Here we take the Bayesian formulation and view the regularization function as the log of the prior function. Thus we have the following *maximum-a-posteriori* (MAP) estimator:

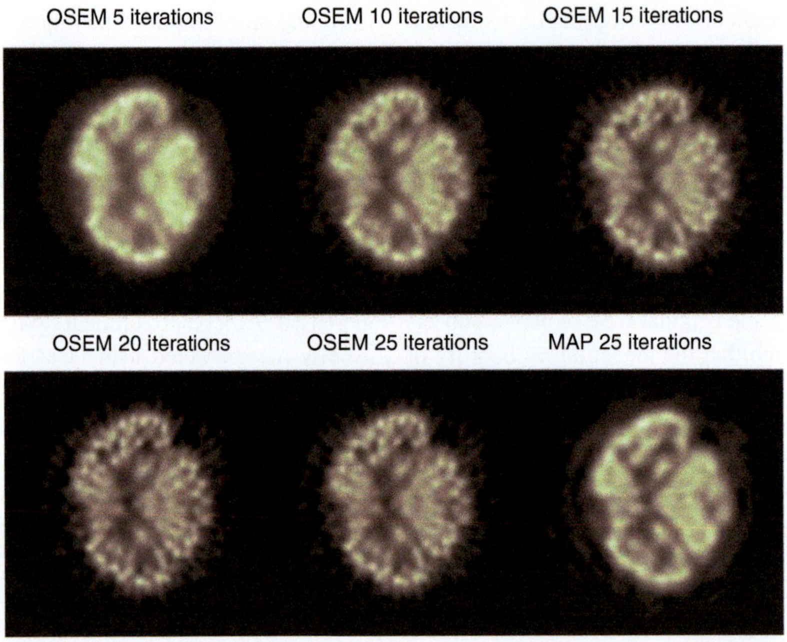

Fig. 11.8 Monkey brain phantom images reconstructed using OSEM with different number of iterations and MAP with 25 iterations

$$x_{MAP} = \arg\max_{x\geq 0} \Phi(x) = L(y \mid x) + p(x) \quad (11.20)$$

where $L(y|x)$ is the log-likelihood function and $p(x)$ is the log-prior (or penalty) function.

MAP estimation allows us to use other information about the image such as smoothness or anatomical information in the form of the prior function to improve image quality. The effect of the prior distribution is to choose among those images that have similar likelihood values the one that is most probable with respect to the prior.

There are many ways of designing the prior function for the image. One simple method is to ignore the statistical dependence of the pixels and treat each one separately. Independent Gaussian [21] and Gamma models [47] have been proposed. For these models, we need to estimate the mean image, which can be difficult and introduces significant bias. Several methods have been developed to estimate the mean image [48, 49]. The attraction of this model is that closed form update equations can be found in the generalized EM framework.

Independent voxel models are of limited value since the information we typically seek to capture in the prior is some degree of piecewise smoothness in the image. In order to model the local smoothness of the image, we can use Markov random field (MRF) models or Gibbs distributions [50]. The general form of a Gibbs distribution is given by

$$p(x \mid \beta) = \frac{1}{Z} e^{-\beta U(x)} \quad (11.21)$$

where Z is a normalization factor and $U(x)$ is the Gibbs energy function which is the sum of potentials. Each potential is defined on a subset of voxels called a "clique." The cliques are composed of neighboring voxels that are mutual neighbors [51]. β is a hyperparameter which controls the image smoothness.

The Gibbs distribution allows us to specify a prior in terms of local interactions since all MRFs have the property that the conditional probability of any voxel in the image depends only on the values of the voxels in a local neighborhood of that voxel. This not only allows us to model the desired local properties but also leads to computationally tractable MAP reconstruction algorithms.

To define a MRF prior, we need to specify the form of statistical interaction (or conditioning) between neighboring voxels. In image reconstruction, the potential functions are usually defined on pairwise voxels:

$$U(x)=\sum_{j=1}^{N}\sum_{k\in N_j,k>j}\phi(x_j-x_k) \quad (11.22)$$

with the constraint that $\phi(x_j-x_k)\geq 0$ and that the function is monotonically nondecreasing in $|x_j-x_k|$.

The function $\phi(x_i-x_j)$ determines the properties of the prior. The simplest one is the quadratic penalty: $\phi(x_i-x_j)=(x_i-x_j)^2$. When the image has the same value at each voxel, the potential functions and hence the energy function $U(x)$ are zero, and the probability density function $P(x)=1/Z\exp(-\beta U(x))$ is at its maximum value. As the difference between voxels increases, so does $U(x)$, with $P(x)$ decreasing correspondingly, indicating less likely images. The advantage of this weighting is that it tends to produce the most natural-looking images. However, quadratic prior functions are limited in their abilities to identify sharp changes in intensity. A large number of alternative functions have been explored that reduce the penalty for larger differences such as the generalized p-Gaussian model [52] and the Huber prior [16].

Recently total variation (TV) regularization has become increasingly popular in medical imaging, especially CT image reconstruction [53], but it can also be applied to PET and SPECT image reconstruction [54–56]. The TV prior is equivalent to the TV norm that is now commonly used in the context of sparse imaging [57].

11.3.4.2 Non-convex and Anatomical Priors

The above prior functions are convex. In order to further encourage sharp edges, non-convex functions have also been proposed [58]. Recently a relative distance prior has been proposed and used in clinical PET image reconstruction [59, 60]. The general goal of these functions is to assign lower probability to images that are not locally smooth but without over-penalizing occasional large changes that might correspond, for example, to organ boundaries.

When high-resolution anatomical information is available from co-registered MR or CT images, it is also possible to incorporate it into the prior function [61]. While anatomical and functional images clearly give very different views on the human body, it is also true that functional images, whether they represent metabolism, blood volume, or receptor binding, will exhibit a spatial morphology that reflects the underlying anatomy. It is reasonable to assume that most tracers exhibit distinct changes in activity across tissue boundaries, while inside each region the distribution is smooth, unless there is evidence to the contrary in the functional data itself. The important thing is that we do not force the abrupt change of activity across the boundaries but rather model changes in these locations as more likely. There are two main approaches to using anatomical information: In the first approach, edge or region information is used to penalize activity changes near the boundaries to a lesser degree. The other approach maximizes an information-based similarity measure between the anatomical and reconstructed functional image, such as the Kullback–Leibler (KL) distance, joint entropy (JE), or mutual information (MI) [61].

Figure 11.9 shows brain PET images reconstructed using FBP, MLEM, and MAP with JE prior. The MAP image has better resolution which clearly shows the fine structures in the brain.

Although there is improvement in quantitation and detection performance when the anatomical prior provides accurate information about the location of boundaries of lesions, these advantages are largely lost when the quality of the anatomical image deteriorates or when there is a mismatch between anatomical and functional boundaries. In addition, the resolution of images reconstructed using anatomical priors is anisotropic and spatially variant, making them more challenging to interpret. Anatomical priors have not been widely applied to clinical PET studies.

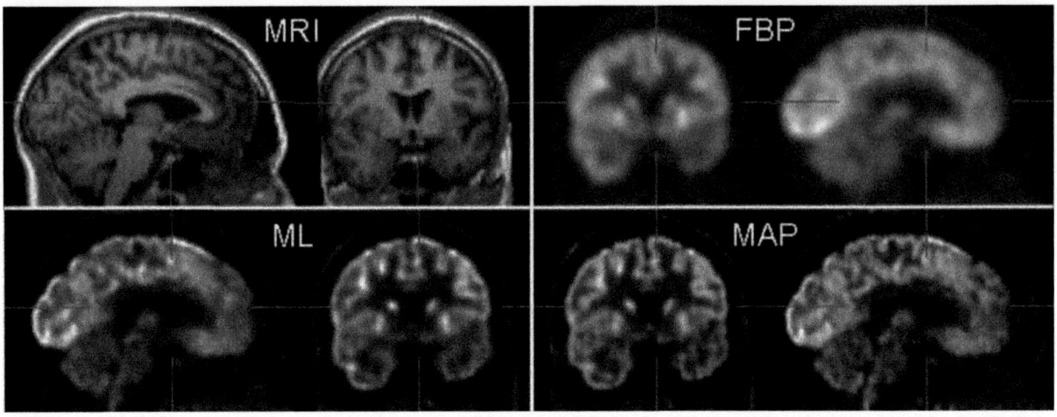

Fig. 11.9 Sagittal and coronal slices of MRI images and PET reconstruction with FBP, ML, and MAP (using JE prior) [62]

11.3.4.3 MAP Reconstruction Algorithms

Most of the optimization algorithms used for ML can be extended to MAP estimation. When EM is applied to MAP, the M-step has a closed form solution only when the prior function is spatially independent. For spatially coupled priors, an iterative method such as gradient or coordinate ascent can be applied in the M-step [63]. Green proposed the "one-step-late" (OSL) approach where the partial derivatives of the prior function are evaluated using the current estimate [64]. However the OSL method does not in general converge to the MAP solution, and the estimated image is not guaranteed to be nonnegative.

Another approach is to apply the FS methodology and design separable surrogate functions for the prior function [65]. In that case, a closed form solution can be found for the M-step.

Standard gradient-based methods can also be applied to the MAP estimation problem. For example, the preconditioned conjugate gradient algorithm has been used for PET image reconstruction [66]. The preconditioner is critical for the convergence of the algorithm. A simple diagonal preconditioner derived from the EM algorithm has been shown to be very effective [67]. Several methods have been proposed to approximate the ideal preconditioner (the inverse of the Hessian matrix), including using the inverse of the diagonal of the Hessian matrix [68], Fourier-based preconditioners [69], and matrix factorization [70].

Unlike the EM algorithm, the nonnegativity constraint in gradient-based methods needs to be handled explicitly. This can be achieved by several strategies, including restricting the step size [71], bent-line search followed by a second-line search [72], or using the active set [66]. Penalty functions [67] and interior point methods [68] have also been used.

MAP estimation problem is better conditioned than ML; thus reconstructed images are less noisy compared to ML. The convergence rate is also much faster, and good quality images can be reconstructed with tens of iterations instead of hundreds or thousands of iterations as in ML-EM. Another advantage of MAP estimators is that image quality can be controlled through carefully designed prior functions [33, 73]. We note that when the prior function contains data-dependent terms, the estimator is no longer truly a MAP estimator (these are typically referred to as penalized likelihood estimators since the second term is no longer a prior but a penalty that penalizes image roughness).

Figure 11.10 compares FBP with model-based statistical reconstruction of a monkey brain phantom data. The superior image quality resulting from the statistical algorithm is clear.

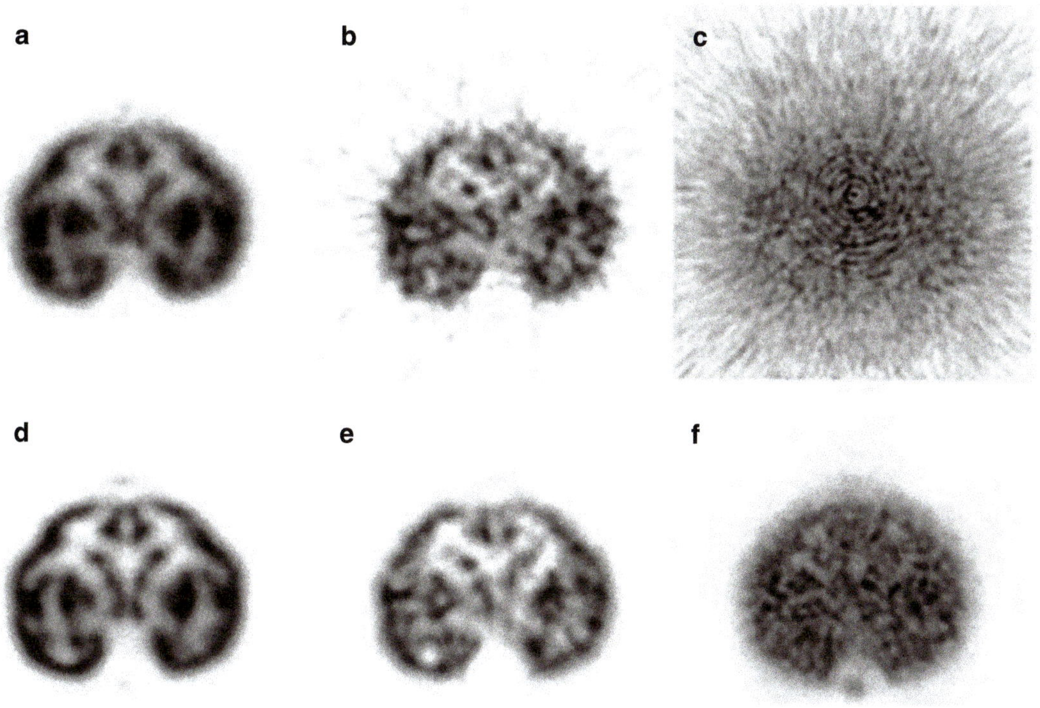

Fig. 11.10 Monkey brain phantom image from 60 scans. (**a–c**) FBP and (**d–f**) MAP. (**a**) Reconstructed from summed data. (**b**) From 1 scan. (**c**) Variance image [74]

11.3.5 Analysis of Image Properties

11.3.5.1 Image Resolution

Image properties of ML and MAP estimators are more difficult to analyze compared to analytic methods, because these methods are nonlinear and have large image and sinogram dimensions. For statistical image reconstruction, the system response is shift variant, especially for 3D systems. One way to quantify image resolution is by using the local impulse response (LIR) [75, 76]:

$$l^j(x) = \lim_{\delta \to 0} \frac{\mu(x + \delta e^j) - \mu(x)}{\delta} \quad (11.23)$$

where $\mu(x)$ is the mean of the estimated image when the true image is x. e^j denotes the unit vector where the jth voxel is 1 and all other voxels are 0. A good approximation to the mean of the estimated image can be obtained from the estimation of the noiseless data [76]. Analytic approximations of the LIR function for MAP estimators can also be derived [76]. The computation of the LIR involves the inversion of a large matrix composed of the Fisher information matrix (FIM) and the Hessian matrix of the prior function, an operation that is impractical for real data. Several Fourier transform-based approximations to the FIM have been proposed to make the inversion practical [77–79].

Interestingly, it has been shown that image resolution gets worse in regions with higher activity [76]. One can take the resolution analysis one step further and design spatially-variant weightings for the prior function to achieve desired image resolution, for example, to make the contrast recovery coefficient (CRC, defined as the peak of the LIR) spatially uniform [76, 77].

Not only is the resolution spatially variant for MAP, it is also non-isotropic. This results in distortion of the activity shape. Stayman and Fessler proposed to estimate the coefficients in the prior function to match a predefined target response function in shift-invariant imaging systems [73]. Later the method was generalized to more realistic, shift–variant PET and SPECT systems [80].

The above methods require iterative computation of the coefficients in the prior function. A simple, non-iterative method has been used in PET image reconstruction to achieve count-independent resolution [81]. The resulting image resolution is roughly data-independent, thus can be pre-calculated for different values of the hyperparameter β using phantom measurements or simulated data. In real patient or animal scans, the hyperparameter β can be selected for desired resolution [81]. Figure 11.11 shows the calibration result and measured resolution from a validation phantom scan. It shows that the predicted (ED) resolution is very close to the actual measured resolution. The slight mismatch is caused by the line-source location differences in calibration and validation scans.

11.3.5.2 Image Noise

Analytic expressions of image noise for MLEM have been derived and shown to be accurate for low-noise data [82]. Similar analyses have also been performed for MAP reconstructions [77, 83]. These methods can be used to characterize the reconstructed image and optimize imaging systems and reconstruction algorithms. In general, images with higher resolution also have higher noise; thus the image reconstruction approach needs to balance resolution and noise in order to achieve optimal image quality.

11.3.5.3 Image Property Measurements

In practice, phantom scans are frequently used to measure image resolution, contrast, and noise. For resolution measurements a point source or line source is typically scanned, and the full width at half maximum (FWHM) is measured from the reconstructed image profile through the source. However, when evaluating statistical reconstruction algorithms, the point source or line source needs to be surrounded by a warm background to avoid potential biases caused by the nonnegativity constraint. Figure 11.12 shows the resolution vs. noise plots measured from an 8.3 cm diameter cylindrical phantom on a microPET Focus220 scanner. Five needles were inserted into the phantom along a line with

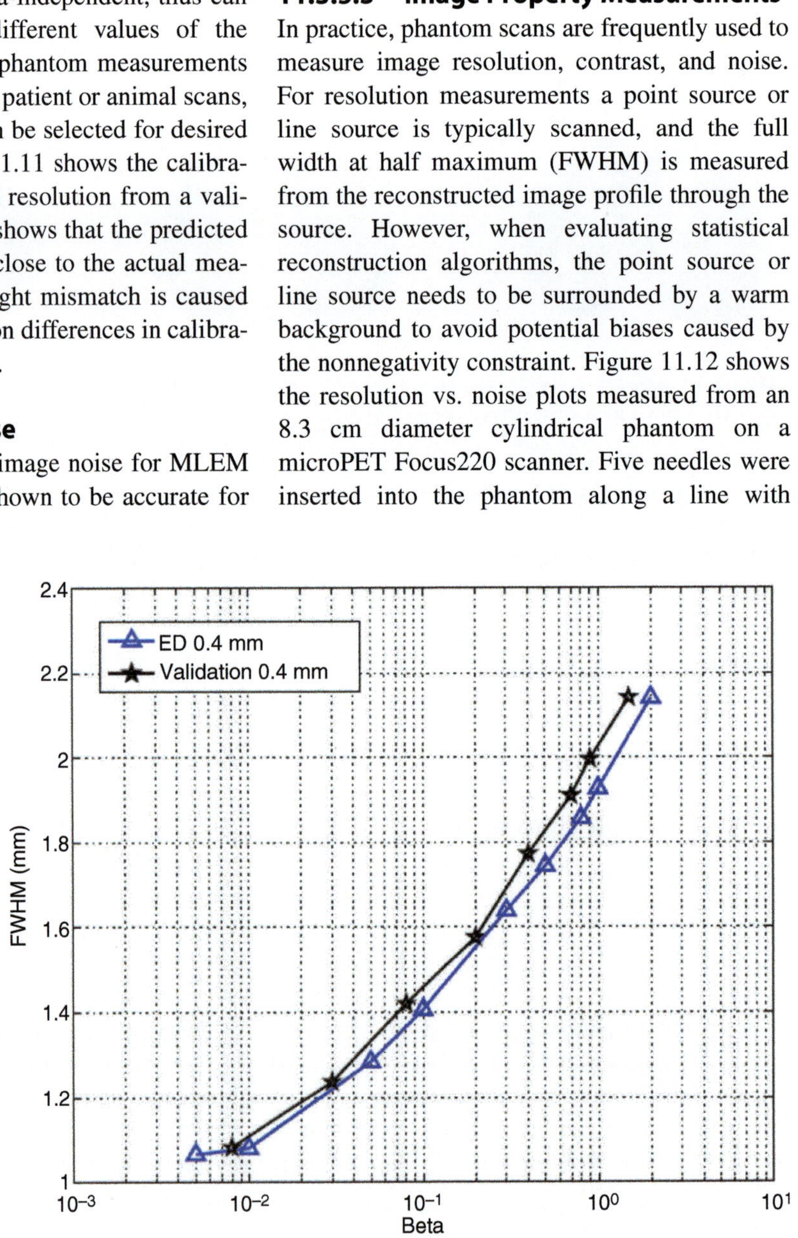

Fig. 11.11 Predicted and experimental resolution from phantom study. *ED* Experimentally generated table [81]

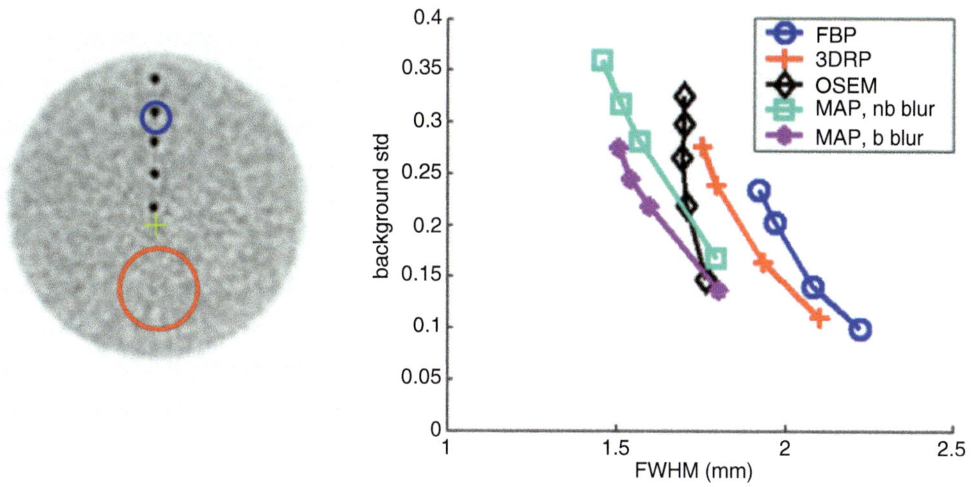

Fig. 11.12 Image resolution and noise measured using line sources in a cylindrical phantom. *Left*: central slice of the phantom. *Red circle* shows the background ROI; *blue circle* shows the ROI used to calculate resolution. *Right*: noise vs. resolution measurement

0.8 cm spacing in radial direction. One needle was placed at the center of the cylinder. The outer and inner diameters of the needles were 0.76 mm and 0.28 mm, respectively. The phantom was filled with a 69.8 MBq ^{18}F solution. The ratio between the concentrations of the activity in the needles and the background was 300:1. The phantom was placed at the center of the field of view and scanned for 15 min. Data were reconstructed using several algorithms including FBP, 3DRP, OSEM, and MAP with all the corrections. A large 3D region of interest (ROI) was selected in the background. The noise of the image is defined as the standard deviation of the 3D ROI normalized by the mean of the same ROI. Radial resolutions were calculated by selecting a small region around the line source 3 cm from the center in each image plane and fitting the profile through the peak to a Gaussian model. The FWHM of the 10 image planes at the axial center was averaged as the resolution of the image. For MAP reconstruction, four different smoothing parameters were used to achieve different resolution. System model using block and non-block blurring kernels was used for MAP reconstructions. The block blurring kernels model the PET scanner geometry more accurately. For OSEM a variety of number of iterations, ranging from 4 to 20, were used. FBP and 3DRP images were reconstructed with a ramp filter, followed by smoothing using Gaussian filters with different FWHM. The result shows that MAP with the block blurring kernels has the highest spatial resolution (smallest FWHM) at a given noise level, compared to other methods.

11.4 PET Image Quantitation

PET is a highly sensitive, quantitative molecular imaging technology, which is frequently used to measure the spatial and occasionally the temporal distribution of the radiotracers injected into the human or animal body. Accuracy of the PET measurement depends on many factors including patient physiology, scanner technology, and reconstruction method. Here we briefly describe the PET quantitation issues related to image reconstruction.

11.4.1 PET Data Corrections

The raw PET data is not only noisy but also distorted and corrupted during the acquisition process. Several corrections need to be applied in order to obtain quantitatively accurate and artifact-free PET images.

11.4.1.1 Normalization

In PET, the detector response varies due to the intrinsic properties of the detectors, geometry and changing count-rate [84]. Normalization is used to compensate for these variations. Accurate normalization is essential for reducing artifacts and for accurate quantitation in PET. Modern PET and PET/CT scanners usually use component-based approaches, where the normalization factors are decomposed into several factors, for example, detector efficiencies, geometric factors, and dead time factors [84–86]. To measure the components, a known source of activity is scanned, and then the normalization factors are estimated by comparing the ideal numbers of coincidences and those actually measured. Rotating rod sources, uniform plane sources, and uniform cylindrical sources have been used for normalization.

The normalization factors can be estimated sequentially. For example, the detector efficiencies can be estimated first, and then the data can be corrected using these estimated detector efficiencies before estimating the geometric factors [86]. Alternatively we can jointly estimate the count-rate-independent factors using statistical estimation methods, where the statistical noise can also be taken into account to significantly reduce the number of events needed for normalization scans [85]. Further discussion on detector normalization can be found in Chap. 10.

11.4.1.2 Attenuation Correction

Due to the interactions between photons and body tissues through Compton scattering and photoelectric absorption, a substantial fraction of the 511 keV photons resulting from positron–electron annihilation is attenuated in the body, and the number of counts along the directions in which the photons originally travel is reduced. It has been estimated that as much as 80 % of the photon pairs emitted from the center of the human brain are lost due to attenuation [87] and the number is even higher for body imaging.

On dedicated PET scanners, the attenuation correction factors are usually measured using an external source. Two scans are needed for this purpose: a blank scan in which the FOV is empty and a transmission scan, which is taken with the subject in the scanner. Correction factors can be computed as the ratio of blank to transmission data. The blank scan can be acquired for a long time to reduce the noise; however the transmission scan is usually short and the resulting data is therefore noisy. As a result, the calculated attenuation correction factors are quite noisy. To address this problem, the reconstruction–reprojection method has been proposed. In this method, an image of attenuation coefficients is computed, and attenuation correction factors are calculated from the projection of this image [88].

With the development of combined PET/CT and PET/MR scanners, it is possible to use the coregistered CT or MR image to calculate the attenuation correction factors. For CT it is relatively straightforward since the CT image is a measurement of the attenuation coefficient of the body, although with a lower, poly-energetic spectrum. It has been shown that a piecewise linear transform can be used to convert the CT Hounsfield units (HU) to the attenuation coefficients of 511 keV photons [89]. For MR the conversion is more difficult because of the lack of signal from the bone [90]. PET attenuation correction using MR image is still a very active research area. See Chap. 9.

11.4.1.3 Scattered and Random Events

The dominant interaction between 511 keV photons and the surrounding atoms is Compton scattering [91]. In 3D PET the portion of scattered coincidences in all detected events can be as high as 30–50 % compared to 10–15 % in the 2D case [92]. Scattered events are mispositioned in the recorded data, which introduce a smooth background in the reconstructed PET image.

The scatter distribution depends on the emission source distribution, the scattering medium, and the detector geometry. Deterministic algorithms for calculating scatter distributions have been proposed [93, 94]. With the computational power available today, it is also possible to estimate the scatter distribution using Monte Carlo simulations [95]. Since the distribution of scattered events is smooth, deterministic methods give reasonable results in most cases and are widely used, especially in commercial PET scanners [94].

A random event is recorded when two photons unrelated to each other are detected within the coincidence timing window. The fraction of random events depends on the amount of activity in the body and can be significant for studies using large amounts of radioactivity. Usually a "delayed window" method is used to estimate the amount of random events [12]. The measured "delayed events" are usually very noisy, and an iterative method has been proposed to estimate its mean [67].

Figure 11.13 shows a typical sequence of corrections applied to the data before it is input to a reconstruction algorithm. For analytic reconstruction methods, these corrections are applied to the data before the reconstruction. With statistical reconstruction methods, precorrection changes noise properties of the data, and the exact distribution of the corrected data is no longer Poisson and difficult to calculate. A better approach for statistical reconstruction methods is to incorporate the corrections in the system model, as previously presented.

11.4.2 PET Image Calibration

Value in the PET image represents the concentration of the radioisotope, usually in the units of Bq/ml or nCi/cc. For clinical PET/CT, a cross calibration procedure is usually performed. During cross calibration, a source (typically cylindrical ^{18}F or $^{68}Ge/^{68}Ga$ source) with known activity concentration is scanned in the scanner. A large ROI is drawn in the reconstructed image, and the mean of this ROI is measured to calculate the scaling factor that converts PET image values to standard units.

The decay of the radioactive nucleus and branching fraction also need to be considered when quantifying the PET image. PET scanner calibration and quality control procedures are reviewed in Chap. 10.

11.5 Recent Developments

11.5.1 Time of Flight PET

In time-of-flight (TOF) PET, the arrival times of the two 511 keV photons are measured. By calculating the difference between the arrival times, we can narrow down the location of the source to a portion of the LOR.

As with non-TOF-PET, both analytic and model-based statistical methods can be used to reconstruct TOF-PET data, with similar advantages and limitations. The additional TOF information can be used to improve image quality, especially for large patients.

All the model-based statistical reconstruction algorithms described in Section 3 can be extended directly to TOF data. The only changes are the

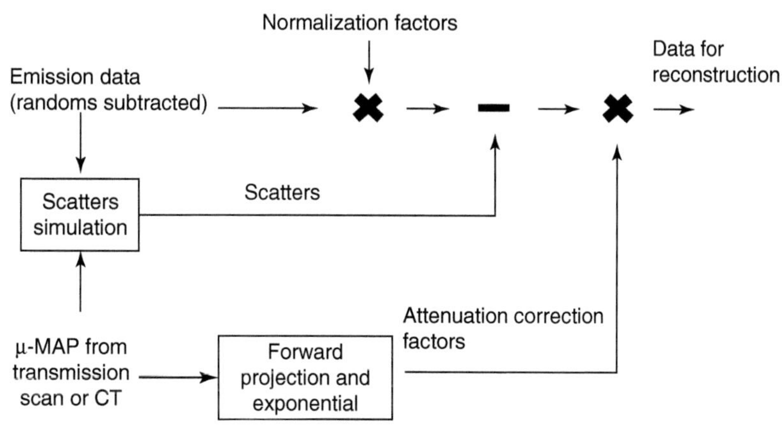

Fig. 11.13 Data corrections applied to PET data before reconstruction

following: (1) there is one more dimension of the data to represent TOF; (2) the system matrix needs to be modified to include TOF. For analytic reconstruction algorithms, TOF changes the reconstruction formula. The following discussion focuses on 2D case, and similar methods can also be derived for 3D TOF-PET.

2D TOF-PET data can be expressed as:

$$p(s,\phi,t) \approx \int_{-\infty}^{\infty} f(-s\sin\phi + l\cos\phi, s\cos\phi + l\sin\phi)h(t-l)\,dl \quad (11.24)$$

where t is the TOF variable. $h(\tau)$ is the TOF kernel, which is usually assumed to be a Gaussian function with FWHM determined by the system hardware and software.

It can be shown that the 2D Fourier transform of the 2D TOF sinogram in one projection is the FT of the image weighted by the 1D FT of the TOF kernel. FBP-type algorithms can be derived for TOF data. A general form of these methods in frequency domain is [96]

$$F(v) = \int_0^{\pi} \frac{W(\hat{u},v)P(\varphi,v)d\varphi}{\int_0^{\pi} W(\hat{u}',v)H(\hat{u}'\cdot v)d\varphi'} \quad (11.25)$$

where $F(v)$ is the 2D FT of the image, $P(\phi,v)$ is the 2D FT of the TOF projection at angle ϕ, $W(\hat{u},v)$ is a filter, which represents a weighting scheme of the projection data in frequency domain, $u = (-\sin\phi, \cos\phi)$ is the unit vector in the projection direction, and $H(\omega)$ is the 1D FT of the TOF kernel. Apparently the algorithm depends on the choice of the filter $W(\hat{u},v)$, which must satisfy the condition that

$$\int_0^{\pi} W(u,v)H(u\cdot v)d\phi \neq 0, \forall v \quad (11.26)$$

Due to the redundancy of the TOF data, FBP algorithm does not have a unique formula. In case of noiseless data, they give the same results. However, due to the noise of the data, the performance of the algorithms using different filters is not the same. A widely used method is confidence weighting, where the chosen filter is $W(u,v) = H(u\cdot v)$.

Given the current timing resolution of TOF-PET scanners (~500 pico-seconds, or 7.5 cm FWHM), the spatial resolution of TOF-PET images is essentially the same as non-TOF-PET. On the other hand, using the TOF information can improve the SNR of the image [96–98]. The improvement of SNR is approximately proportional to D/h, where D is the diameter of the object and h is the TOF spatial resolution. However TOF reconstruction is much slower due to the large dataset. Recently Cho et al. developed a generalized projection slice theorem and proposed a unified framework for mapping between different datasets, allowing us to explore and optimize the use of TOF and 3D PET information [99, 100]. Figure 11.14 displays the mappings between PET datasets.

Two Fourier rebinning algorithms of time-of-flight data (FORET) have been developed [100]. The 3D TOF data can be rebinned into 3D non-TOF data using FORET3D (or 2D non-TOF data using FORET2D), which is a weighted average of the TOF data in Fourier transform domain. The SNR of the data depends on the weighting scheme. Under reasonable assumptions, it can be proven that the best linear unbiased estimator of the 3D non-TOF data is achieved when using FORET3D to rebin 3D TOF data and the weight-

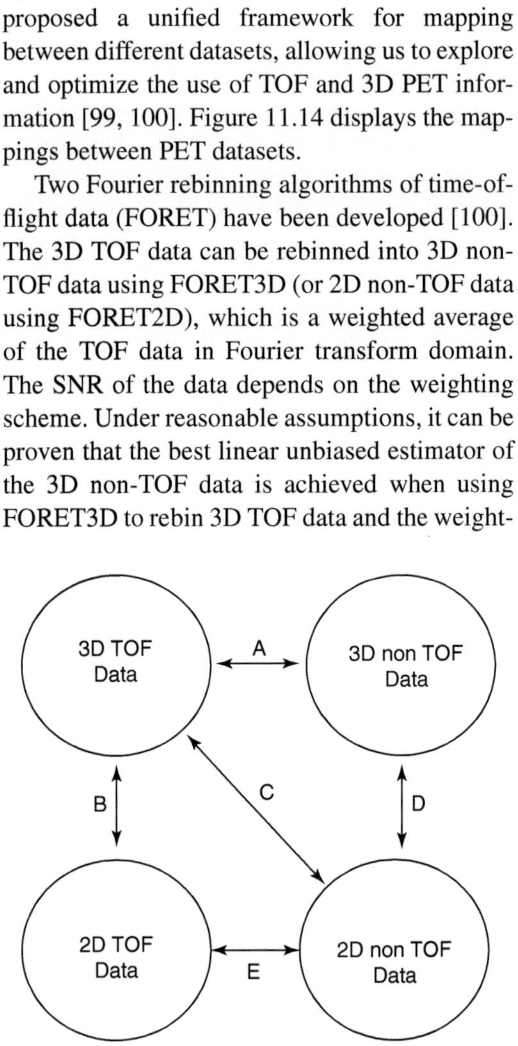

Fig. 11.14 Possible mappings between different PET data [100]

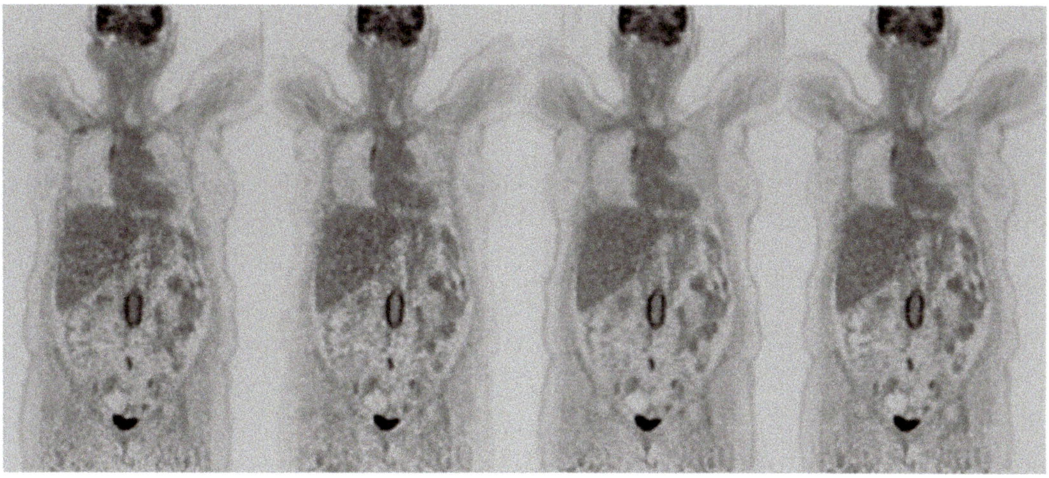

Fig. 11.15 FDG patient images. *Left to right*: non-TOF MAP, FORET2D+MAP, FORET3D+MAP, TOF MAP [24]

Table 11.1 Mean and noise measurements from the patient image in Fig. 11.15 [24]

Method	Mean	SD	%SD
TOF	0.577	0.109	18.9
FORET-3D	0.569	0.110	19.3
FORET-2D	0.617	0.151	24.5
Non-TOF	0.568	0.155	27.3

ing factors equal to the square of the Fourier transform of the TOF kernel [97]. The SNR gain is approximately a constant in this case. For FORET2D, which rebins 3D TOF data into 2D non-TOF data, it can be shown that the SNR gain is roughly constant for each 2D sinogram, which can be calculated very accurately [24]. Figure 11.15 shows a patient data reconstructed from non-TOF, FORET2D, FORET3D, and TOF data using a statistical algorithm. Table 11.1 shows the noise in the images measured from an ROI in the liver of the patient image in Fig. 11.15. The smoothing parameters were selected such that all the images have the same resolution (6 mm FWHM). These results show that the quality of FORET3D image is similar to TOF image, while FORET2D image is noisier than FORET3D, but still better than the non-TOF image. Since FORET uses FFT, the computation is very fast. The reconstruction speed of FORET3D is similar to non-TOF reconstruction, which is about five times faster than 3D TOF reconstruction. FORET2D can further increase the speed by a factor of 5, at the expense of more noise in the image.

11.5.2 Parametric Image Reconstruction

We focus on the reconstruction of static data in this chapter. PET is a dynamic modality where data can be acquired continuously for a period of time and useful kinetic parameters can be calculated from it [101]. A straightforward approach is to divide the data into many frames, reconstruct each frame, and then calculate the kinetic parameters (either voxel-wise or ROI-wise) from the time–activity curves extracted from these images. Another class of image reconstruction methods are designed to reconstruct kinetic parameters from the measurements directly [102–104]. Figure 11.16 shows a whole-body FDG patient study. The patient was stepped through the scanner twice and Patlak image calculated from the list-mode data. Static PET images were also calculated from the two passes. We note that although the visual difference between Patlak image and static images is subtle, the Patlak image is a voxel-wise quantitative image and the values are more informative. These direct and indirect parametric reconstruction methods require the estimation of the arterial input function which can either be measured during the scan by

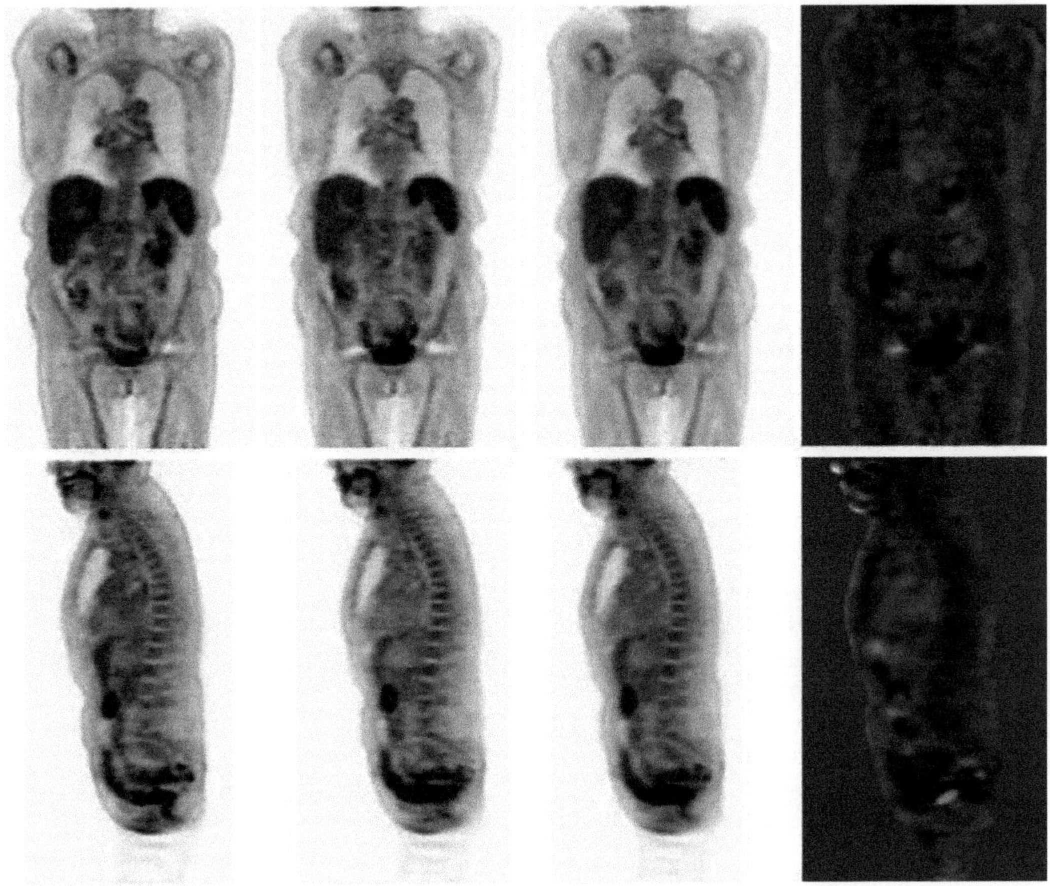

Fig. 11.16 Whole-body FDG patient images. From *left to right*: first frame, second frame, Patlak slope, %DSUV [102]

arterial blood sampling or from reconstructed multiframe images. In Fig. 11.16, the arterial input function was estimated using a hybrid approach which combines a population-based approach with a simplified exponential model [104].

Conclusions

The last two decades have seen tremendous progress in PET image reconstruction. Once considered slow and only used for research studies, model-based statistical reconstruction methods are now applied in nuclear medicine clinics every day for tumor detection and staging, assessment of therapy response, and other applications. By combining an appropriate noise model with an accurate system model, we are able to improve image resolution and noise properties, which increase the sensitivity and specificity of clinical studies. There has also been a lot of work in regularized reconstruction algorithms where we can effectively control image properties and optimize them for different tasks by designing appropriate regularization functions that might also include anatomical information. This is in contrast to the analytic methods, where the only control options are the ramp filter cutoff frequencies and any post-filters applied to the images. As a result, optimal results can be obtained for different imaging applications.

Coupled with the development of PET instrumentation, including the new detector material and data correction techniques, PET image quality and quantitative accuracy have improved significantly. Statistical PET image reconstruction is still an active research field, especially in TOF-PET, MR-PET, and parametric imaging.

References

1. Radon J. On determination of functions by their integral values along certain multiplicities. Ber Sachische Akad Wiss LeipzigGermany. 1917;69: 262–77.
2. Hounsfield GN. Computerized transverse axial scanning (tomography): part 1. Description of system. Br J Radiol. 1973;46(552):1016–22.
3. Natterer F. Computerized tomography. In: The mathematics of computerized tomography. New York: John Wiley and Sons Inc; 1986. p. 1–8.
4. Shepp LA, Logan B. The Fourier reconstruction of a head section. IEEE Trans Nucl Sci. 1974;21:21–33.
5. Farquhar TH, Chatziioannou A, Chinn G, Dahlbom M, Hoffman EJ. An investigation of filter choice for filtered back-projection reconstruction in PET. Presented at the Nuclear Science Symposium and Medical Imaging Conference, vol. 2; 1997. p. 1042–6.
6. Tsui B, Frey E. Analytic image reconstruction methods in emission computed tomography. In: Quantitative analysis in nuclear medicine imaging. New York: Springer; 2006. p. 82–106.
7. Colsher JG. Fully three-dimensional positron emission tomography. Phys Med Biol. 1980;25(1):103–15.
8. Kinahan PE, Rogers JG. Analytic 3D image reconstruction using all detected events. IEEE Trans Nucl Sci. 1989;36(1):964–8.
9. Daube-Witherspoon ME, Muehllehner G. Treatment of axial data in three-dimensional PET. J Nucl Med. 1987;28(11):1717–24.
10. Defrise M, Kinahan PE, Townsend DW, Michel C, Sibomana M, Newport DF. Exact and approximate rebinning algorithms for 3-D PET data. IEEE Trans Med Imaging. 1997;16(2):145–58.
11. Fessler JA. Penalized weighted least-squares image reconstruction for positron emission tomography. IEEE Trans Med Imaging. 1994;13(2):290–300.
12. Hoffman EJ, Huang S-C, Phelps ME, Kuhl DE. Quantitation in positron emission computed tomography: 4. Effect of accidental coincidences. J Comput Assist Tomogr. 1981;5(3):391–400.
13. Yavuz M, Fessler JA. Statistical image reconstruction methods for randoms-precorrected PET scans. Med Image Anal. 1998;2(4):369–78.
14. Comtat C, Kinahan PE, Defrise M, Michel C, Townsend DW. Fast reconstruction of 3D PET data with accurate statistical modeling. IEEE Trans Nucl Sci. 1998;45(3):1083–9.
15. Liu X, Comtat C, Michel C, Kinahan P, Defrise M, Townsend D. Comparison of 3-D reconstruction with 3D-OSEM and with FORE+OSEM for PET. IEEE Trans Med Imaging. 2001;20(8):804–14.
16. Qi J, Leahy RM, Cherry SR, Chatziioannou A, Farquhar TH. High-resolution 3D Bayesian image reconstruction using the microPET small-animal scanner. Phys Med Biol. 1998;43(4):1001–13.
17. Bai B, Ruangma A, Laforest R, Tai YC, Leahy RM. Positron range modeling for statistical PET image reconstruction. Presented at the Nuclear Science Symposium and Medical Imaging Conference Record, vol. 4; 2003. p. 2501–5.
18. Fu L, Qi J. A residual correction method for high-resolution PET reconstruction with application to on-the-fly Monte Carlo based model of positron range. Med Phys. 2010;37:704.
19. Hong I, Chung S, Kim H, Kim Y, Son Y, Cho Z. Ultra fast symmetry and SIMD-based projection-backprojection (SSP) algorithm for 3-D PET image reconstruction. IEEE Trans Med Imaging. 2007;26(6):789–803.
20. Pratx G, Chinn G, Olcott PD, Levin CS. Fast, accurate and shift-varying line projections for iterative reconstruction using the GPU. IEEE Trans Med Imaging. 2009;28(3):435–45.
21. Huesman RH, Klein GJ, Moses WW, Qi J, Reutter BW, Virador PR. List-mode maximum-likelihood reconstruction applied to positron emission mammography (PEM) with irregular sampling. IEEE Trans Med Imaging. 2000;19(5):532–7.
22. Panin VY, Kehren F, Michel C, Casey M. Fully 3-D PET reconstruction with system matrix derived from point source measurements. IEEE Trans Med Imaging. 2006;25(7):907–21.
23. Tohme MS, Qi J. Iterative image reconstruction for positron emission tomography based on a detector response function estimated from point source measurements. Phys Med Biol. 2009;54(12):3709.
24. Bai B, Lin Y, Zhu W, Ren R, Li Q, Dahlbom M, DiFilippo F, Leahy RM. MAP reconstruction for Fourier rebinned TOF-PET data. Phys Med Biol. 2014;59(4):925.
25. Rahmim A, Qi J, Sossi V. Resolution modeling in PET imaging: theory, practice, benefits, and pitfalls. Med Phys. 2013;40:064301.
26. Bai B, Esser PD. The effect of edge artifacts on quantification of Positron Emission Tomography. Presented at the Nuclear Science Symposium and Medical Imaging Conference Record (NSS/MIC); 2010. p. 2263–6.
27. Tong S, Alessio AM, Thielemans K, Stearns C, Ross S, Kinahan PE. Properties and mitigation of edge artifacts in PSF-based PET reconstruction. IEEE Trans Nucl Sci. 2011;58(5):2264–75.
28. Watson CC. Estimating effective model kernel widths for PSF reconstruction in PET. Presented at the Nuclear Science Symposium and Medical Imaging Conference (NSS/MIC); 2011. p. 2368–74.
29. Dempster AP, Laird NM, Rubin DB. Maximum likelihood from incomplete data via the EM algorithm. J R Stat Soc Ser B Methodol. 1977;39:1–38.
30. Shepp LA, Vardi Y. Maximum likelihood reconstruction for emission tomography. IEEE Trans Med Imaging. 1982;1(2):113–22.
31. Lange K, Carson R. EM reconstruction algorithms for emission and transmission tomography. J Comput Assist Tomogr. 1984;8(2):306–16.
32. De Pierro AR. On the relation between the ISRA and the EM algorithm for positron emission tomography. IEEE Trans Med Imaging. 1993;12(2):328–33.

33. Qi J, Leahy RM. Iterative reconstruction techniques in emission computed tomography. Phys Med Biol. 2006;51(15):R541–78.
34. Lange K, Fessler JA. Globally convergent algorithms for maximum a posteriori transmission tomography. IEEE Trans Image Process. 1995;4(10):1430–8.
35. Hunter DR, Lange K. A tutorial on MM algorithms. Am Stat. 2004;58(1):30–7.
36. Jacobson MW, Fessler JA. An expanded theoretical treatment of iteration-dependent majorize-minimize algorithms. IEEE Trans Image Process. 2007;16(10):2411–22.
37. Vardi Y, Shepp LA, Kaufman L. A statistical model for positron emission tomography. J Am Stat Assoc. 1985;80(389):8–20.
38. Hudson HM, Larkin RS. Accelerated image reconstruction using ordered subsets of projection data. IEEE Trans Med Imaging. 1994;13(4):601–9.
39. Ahn S, Fessler JA. Globally convergent image reconstruction for emission tomography using relaxed ordered subsets algorithms. IEEE Trans Med Imaging. 2003;22(5):613–26.
40. Byrne CL. Accelerating the EMML algorithm and related iterative algorithms by rescaled block-iterative methods. IEEE Trans Image Process. 1998;7(1):100–9.
41. Li Q, Ahn S, Leahy R. Fast hybrid algorithms for PET image reconstruction. Presented at the Nuclear Science Symposium and Medical Imaging Conference Record, vol. 4; 2005. p. 1851–5.
42. Browne J, De Pierro AB. A row-action alternative to the EM algorithm for maximizing likelihood in emission tomography. IEEE Trans Med Imaging. 1996;15(5):687–99.
43. Hsiao IT, Huang HM. An accelerated ordered subsets reconstruction algorithm using an accelerating power factor for emission tomography. Phys Med Biol. 2010;55(3):599–614.
44. Snyder DL, Miller MI, Thomas LJ, Politte DG. Noise and edge artifacts in maximum-likelihood reconstructions for emission tomography. IEEE Trans Med Imaging. 1987;6(3):228–38.
45. Veklerov E, Llacer J. Stopping rule for the MLE algorithm based on statistical hypothesis testing. IEEE Trans Med Imaging. 1987;6(4):313–9.
46. Llacer J, Veklerov E, Coakley KJ, Hoffman EJ, Nunez J. Statistical analysis of maximum likelihood estimator images of human brain FDG PET studies. IEEE Trans Med Imaging. 1993;12(2):215–31.
47. Lange K, Bahn M, Little R. A theoretical study of some maximum likelihood algorithms for emission and transmission tomography. IEEE Trans Med Imaging. 1987;6(2):106–14.
48. Alenius S, Ruotsalainen U. Bayesian image reconstruction for emission tomography based on median root prior. Eur J Nucl Med. 1997;24(3):258–65.
49. Hsiao T, Rangarajan A, Gindi G. A new convex edge-preserving median prior with applications to tomography. IEEE Trans Med Imaging. 2003;22(5):580–5.
50. Besag J. Spatial interaction and the statistical analysis of lattice systems. J R Stat Soc Ser B Methodol. 1974;36:192–236.
51. Geman S, Geman D. Stochastic relaxation, gibbs distributions, and the bayesian restoration of images. IEEE Trans Pattern Anal Mach Intell. 1984;6(6):721–41.
52. Bouman CA, Sauer K. A unified approach to statistical tomography using coordinate descent optimization. IEEE Trans Image Process. 1996;5(3):480–92.
53. Sidky EY, Pan X. Image reconstruction in circular cone-beam computed tomography by constrained, total-variation minimization. Phys Med Biol. 2008;53(17):4777.
54. Panin VY, Zeng GL, Gullberg GT. Total variation regulated EM algorithm [SPECT reconstruction]. IEEE Trans Nucl Sci. 1999;46(6):2202–10.
55. Bai B. An interior-point method for total variation regularized positron emission tomography image reconstruction; 2012. p. 83136B1–83136B6.
56. Wang G, Qi J. Edge-preserving PET image reconstruction using trust optimization transfer, Presented at the 12th International Meeting on fully three-dimensional image reconstruction in radiology and nuclear medicine; 2013. p. 70–3.
57. Candes EJ, Romberg J, Tao T. Robust uncertainty principles: exact signal reconstruction from highly incomplete frequency information. IEEE Trans Inf Theory. 2006;52(2):489–509.
58. Geman S, McClure D. Bayesian image analysis: an application to single photon emission tomography. Presented at the American Statistical Association; 1985. p. 12–8.
59. Ahn S, Ross SG, Asma E, Miao J, Jin X, Cheng L, Wollenweber SD, Manjeshwar RM. Quantitative comparison of OSEM and penalized likelihood image reconstruction using relative difference penalties for clinical PET. Phys Med Biol. 2015;60(15):5733.
60. Nuyts J, Bequé D, Dupont P, Mortelmans L. A concave prior penalizing relative differences for maximum-a-posteriori reconstruction in emission tomography. IEEE Trans Nucl Sci. 2002;49(1):56–60.
61. Bai B, Li Q, Leahy RM. Magnetic resonance-guided positron emission tomography image reconstruction. Presented at the Seminars in Nuclear Medicine, vol. 43;2013. p. 30–44.
62. Nuyts J. The use of mutual information and joint entropy for anatomical priors in emission tomography. Presented at the Nuclear Science Symposium Conference Record, 2007. NSS '07. IEEE, vol. 6; 2007. p. 4149–54.
63. Hebert T, Leahy R. A generalized EM algorithm for 3-D Bayesian reconstruction from Poisson data using Gibbs priors. IEEE Trans Med Imaging. 1989;8(2):194–202.

64. Green PJ. Bayesian reconstructions from emission tomography data using a modified EM algorithm. IEEE Trans Med Imaging. 1990;9(1):84–93.
65. De Pierro AR. A modified expectation maximization algorithm for penalized likelihood estimation in emission tomography. IEEE Trans Med Imaging. 1995;14(1):132–7.
66. √ú Mumcuoglu E, Leahy RM, Cherry SR. Bayesian reconstruction of PET images: methodology and performance analysis. Phys Med Biol. 1996;41(9):1777.
67. Mumcuoglu EU, Leahy R, Cherry SR, Zhou Z. Fast gradient-based methods for Bayesian reconstruction of transmission and emission PET images. IEEE Trans Med Imaging. 1994;13(4):687–701.
68. Johnson CA, Seidel J, Sofer A. Interior-point methodology for 3-D PET reconstruction. IEEE Trans Med Imaging. 2000;19(4):271–85.
69. Fessler JA, Booth SD. Conjugate-gradient preconditioning methods for shift-variant PET image reconstruction. IEEE Trans Image Process. 1999;8(5):688–99.
70. Chinn G, Huang S-C. A general class of preconditioners for statistical iterative reconstruction of emission computed tomography. IEEE Trans Med Imaging. 1997;16(1):1–10.
71. Kaufman L. Implementing and accelerating the EM algorithm for positron emission tomography. IEEE Trans Med Imaging. 1987;6(1):37–51.
72. Kaufman L. Maximum likelihood, least squares, and penalized least squares for PET. IEEE Trans Med Imaging. 1993;12(2):200–14.
73. Stayman JW, Fessler JA. Regularization for uniform spatial resolution properties in penalized-likelihood image reconstruction. IEEE Trans Med Imaging. 2000;19(6):601–15.
74. Chatziioannou A, Qi J, Moore A, Annala A, Nguyen K, Leahy R, Cherry SR. Comparison of 3-D maximum a posteriori and filtered backprojection algorithms for high-resolution animal imaging with microPET. IEEE Trans Med Imaging. 2000;19(5):507–12.
75. Wilson DW, Tsui BMW. Spacial resolution properties of FB and ML-EM reconstruction methods. Presented at the Nuclear Science Symposium and Medical Imaging Conference; 1993. p. 1189–93.
76. Fessler JA, Rogers WL. Spatial resolution properties of penalized-likelihood image reconstruction: space-invariant tomographs. IEEE Trans Image Process. 1996;5(9):1346–58.
77. Qi J, Leahy RM. Resolution and noise properties of MAP reconstruction for fully 3-D PET. IEEE Trans Med Imaging. 2000;19(5):493–506.
78. Fessler JA. Analytical approach to regularization design for isotropic spatial resolution. Presented at the Nuclear Science Symposium Conference Record, 2003 IEEE, vol. 3; 2003. p. 2022–6.
79. Vunckx K, Zhou L, Matej S, Defrise M, Nuyts J. Fisher information-based evaluation of image quality for time-of-flight PET. IEEE Trans Med Imaging. 2010;29(2):311–21.
80. Stayman JW, Fessler JA. Compensation for nonuniform resolution using penalized-likelihood reconstruction in space-variant imaging systems. IEEE Trans Med Imaging. 2004;23(3):269–84.
81. Li Q, Bai B, Cho S, Smith A, Leahy R. Count independent resolution and its calibration. Presented at the 10th International Meeting on fully three-dimensional image reconstruction in radiology and nuclear medicine; 2009. p. 223–6.
82. Barrett HH, Wilson DW, Tsui BM. Noise properties of the EM algorithm: I. Theory. Phys Med Biol. 1994;39(5):833–46.
83. Fessler JA. Mean and variance of implicitly defined biased estimators (such as penalized maximum likelihood): applications to tomography. IEEE Trans Image Process. 1996;5(3):493–506.
84. Badawi R, Marsden P. Developments in component-based normalization for 3D PET. Phys Med Biol. 1999;44(2):571.
85. Bai B, Li Q, Holdsworth CH, Asma E, Tai YC, Chatziioannou A, Leahy RM. Model-based normalization for iterative 3D PET image reconstruction. Phys Med Biol. 2002;47(15):2773–84.
86. Defrise M, Townsend DW, Bailey D, Geissbuhler A, Michel C, Jones T. A normalization technique for 3D PET data. Phys Med Biol. 1991;36(7):939–52.
87. Cherry SR, Phelps ME. Imaging brain function with positron emission tomography. In: Brain Mapping Methods. New York: Academic; 1996. p. 191–221.
88. Riederer SJ. Application of the noise power spectrum to positron emission CT self-absorption correction. Med Phys. 1981;8(2):220–4.
89. Carney J, Townsend DW, Rappoport V, Bendriem B. Method for transforming CT images for attenuation correction in PET/CT imaging. Med Phys. 2006;33(4):976–83.
90. Hofmann M, Pichler B, Schölkopf B, Beyer T. Towards quantitative PET/MRI: a review of MR-based attenuation correction techniques. Eur J Nucl Med Mol Imaging. 2009;36(1):93–104.
91. Cherry SR, Sorenson JA, Phelps ME. Physics in nuclear medicine. Philadelphia: Elsevier Health Sciences; 2012.
92. Watson CC, Newport D, Casey ME. A single scatter simulation technique for scatter correction in 3D PET. In: Three-dimensional image reconstruction in radiology and nuclear medicine. Boston: Kluwer Academic Publishers; 1996. p. 255–68.
93. Ollinger JM. Model-based scatter correction for fully 3D PET. Phys Med Biol. 1996;41(1):153.
94. Watson CC. New, faster, image-based scatter correction for 3D PET. IEEE Trans Nucl Sci. 2000;47(4):1587–94.
95. Holdsworth H, Levin C, Janecek M, Dahlbom M, Hoffman E. Performance analysis of an improved 3-D PET Monte Carlo simulation and scatter correction. IEEE Trans Nucl Sci. 2002;49(1):83–9.

96. Watson CC. An evaluation of image noise variance for time-of-flight PET. IEEE Trans Nucl Sci. 2007;54(5):1639–47.
97. Ahn S, Cho S, Li Q, Lin Y, Leahy RM. Optimal rebinning of time-of-flight PET data. IEEE Trans Med Imaging. 2011;30(10):1808–18.
98. Tomitani T. Image reconstruction and noise evaluation in photon time-of-flight assisted positron emission tomography. IEEE Trans Nucl Sci. 1981;28(6): 4581–9.
99. Cho S, Ahn S, Li Q, Leahy RM. Analytical properties of time-of-flight PET data. Phys Med Biol. 2008;53(11):2809–21.
100. Cho S, Ahn S, Li Q, Leahy RM. Exact and approximate Fourier rebinning of PET data from time-of-flight to non time-of-flight. Phys Med Biol. 2009;54(3):467–84.
101. Carson RE. Tracer kinetic modeling in PET. In: Positron emission tomography. London: Springer; 2005. p. 127–59.
102. Kamasak ME, Bouman CA, Morris ED, Sauer K. Direct reconstruction of kinetic parameter images from dynamic PET data. Med. Imaging IEEE Trans. 2005:636–50.
103. Karakatsanis NA, Lodge MA, Tahari AK, Zhou Y, Wahl RL, Rahmim A. Dynamic whole-body PET parametric imaging: I. Concept, acquisition protocol optimization and clinical application. Phys. Med. Biol. 2013;58:7391.
104. Zhu W, Bai B, Conti PS, Li Q, Leahy RM. Data correction methods for wholebody Patlak imaging from list-mode PET data. Presented at the 12th International Meeting on fully 3D image reconstruction in radiology and nuclear medicine, Lake Tahoe; 2013. p. 213–16.

Image Processing and Analysis of PET and Hybrid PET Imaging

12

Issam El Naqa

Contents

12.1	**Introduction**	286
12.2	**Image Features from PET**	286
12.2.1	Static PET Features	286
12.2.2	Dynamic PET Features	287
12.3	**Extension to PET/CT and PET/MR**	288
12.4	**Application of PET in Radiotherapy**	291
12.4.1	Biological Target Definition Using PET	291
12.4.2	PET Radiomics	293
12.5	**Current Issues and Future Directions**	294
12.5.1	PET Image Characteristics	294
12.5.2	Robustness and Stability of Extracted Image Features	295
12.5.3	Improved PET-Based Outcome Models	296
Conclusions		297
References		297

Abstract

PET imaging is a main diagnostic modality of different diseases including cancer. In the particular case of cancer, PET is widely used for staging of disease progression, identification of the treatment gross tumor volume, monitoring of disease, as well as prediction of outcomes and personalization of treatment regimens. Among the arsenal of different functional imaging modalities, PET has benefited from early adoption of quantitative image analysis starting from simple standard uptake value (SUV) normalization to more advanced extraction of complex imaging uptake patterns, thanks chiefly to the application of sophisticated image processing algorithms. In this chapter, we discuss the application of image processing techniques to PET imaging with special focus on the oncological radiotherapy domain starting from basic feature extraction to application in target definition using image segmentation/registration and more recent image-based outcome modeling in the radiomics field. We further extend the discussion into hybrid anatomical functional combinations of PET/CT and PET/MR multimodalities.

I. El Naqa, PhD, DABR
Department of Radiation Oncology, Physics Division, University of Michigan, 519 W. William St, Argus Bldg 1, Ann Arbor, MI 48103-4943, USA
e-mail: ielnaqa@med.umich.edu, https://sites.google.com/a/umich.edu/ielnaqa/

M.M. Khalil (ed.), *Basic Science of PET Imaging*, DOI 10.1007/978-3-319-40070-9_12

12.1 Introduction

Recent years have witnessed exponential growth in the use of imaging for diagnostic and therapeutic radiological purposes. In particular, positron emission tomography (PET) has been widely used in oncology for the purposes of diagnosis, grading, staging, and assessment of response. For instance, PET imaging with ^{18}F-FDG (fluoro-2-deoxy-d-glucose), a glucose metabolism analog, has been applied for diagnosis, staging, and treatment planning of lung cancer [1–10], head and neck cancer [11, 12], prostate cancer [13], cervical cancer [14, 15], colorectal cancer [16], lymphoma [17, 18], melanoma [19], and breast cancer [20–22]. Moreover, accumulating evidence supports that pretreatment or posttreatment FDG-PET uptake could be used as a prognostic factor for predicting outcomes [23–27]. For a review, see Chaps. 13 and 19.

Besides FDG-PET, other PET tracers have been also shown to be useful in interrogating tumor properties such as hypoxia by FMISO or Cu-ATSM and DNA synthesis and cell proliferation by FLT [28]. Interestingly, Denecke et al. compared CT, MRI, and FDG-PET in the prediction of outcomes to neoadjuvant radiochemotherapy in patients with locally advanced primary rectal cancer, demonstrating sensitivities of 100 % for FDG-PET, 54 % for CT, and 71 % for MRI and specificities of 60 % for FDG-PET, 80 % for CT, and 67 % for MRI [29]. Benz et al. showed that combined assessment of metabolic and volumetric changes predicts tumor response in patients with soft tissue sarcoma [30]. Similarly, Yang et al. showed that the combined evaluation of contrast-enhanced CT and FDG-PET/CT predicts the clinical outcomes in patients with aggressive non-Hodgkin's lymphoma [31]. Indeed, quantitative information from hybrid imaging modalities could be related to biological and clinical endpoints, a new emerging field referred to as "radiomics" [32, 33]. We were among the leading groups to demonstrate the potential of this new field to monitor and predict response to radiotherapy in head and neck [34], cervix [34, 35], and lung [36] cancers, in turn allowing for adapting and individualizing treatment regimens.

In this chapter, we discuss the application of advanced image processing techniques in PET imaging with specific focus on two major areas of better tumor target definition and image-based prediction of treatment outcomes.

12.2 Image Features from PET

A necessary prerequisite of image processing application in PET is the robust extraction of relevant imaging features, which could be used in varying applications. The features extracted from PET images could be divided into static (time-invariant) and dynamic (time-variant) features according to the acquisition protocol at the time of scanning and into pre- or intra-treatment features according to the scanning time point [37].

12.2.1 Static PET Features

(a) *Standard uptake value (SUV) descriptors*: SUV is a standard method in PET image quantitative analysis [38]. In this case, raw intensity values are converted into SUVs, and statistical descriptors such as maximum, minimum, mean, standard deviation (SD), and coefficient of variation (CV) are extracted.
(b) *Total lesion glycolysis (TLG)*: This is defined as the product of volume and mean SUV [5, 30, 39].
(c) *Intensity-volume histogram (IVH)*: This is analogous to the dose-volume histogram widely used in radiotherapy treatment planning in reducing complicated 3D data into a single easier to interpret curve. Each point on the IVH defines the absolute or relative volume of the structure that exceeds a variable intensity threshold as a percentage of the maximum intensity [34]. This method would allow for extracting several metrics from PET images for outcome analysis such as I_x (minimum intensity to $x\%$ highest intensity volume), V_x (percentage volume having at least x% intensity value), and descriptive statistics (mean, minimum, maximum, standard

deviation, etc.). We have reported the use of the IVH for predicting local control in lung cancer [36], where a combined metric from PET and CT image-based model provided a superior prediction power compared to commonly used dosimetric-based models of local treatment response.

(d) *Morphological features*: These are generally geometrical shape attributes such as eccentricity (a measure of non-circularity), which is useful for describing tumor growth directionality, and Euler number (the number of connected objects in a region minus the total number of holes in the objects) the solidity (this is a measurement of convexity), which may be a characteristic of benign lesions [40, 41]. An interesting demonstration of this principle is that a shape-based metric based on the deviation from an idealized ellipsoid structure (i.e., eccentricity) was found to have strong association with survival in patients with sarcoma [41, 42].

(e) *Texture features*: Texture in imaging refers to the relative distribution of intensity values within a given neighborhood. It integrates intensity with spatial information resulting in higher-order histograms when compared to common first-order intensity histograms. It should be emphasized that texture metrics are independent of tumor position, orientation, size, and brightness and take into account the local intensity spatial distribution [43, 44]. This is a crucial advantage over direct (first-order) histogram metrics (e.g., mean and standard deviation), which only measures intensity variability independent of the spatial distribution in the tumor microenvironment. Texture methods are broadly divided into three categories: statistical methods (e.g., high-order statistics, co-occurrence matrices, moment invariants), model-based methods (e.g., Markov random fields, Gabor filter, wavelet transform), and structural methods (e.g., topological descriptors, fractals) [45, 46]. Among these methods, statistical approaches based on the co-occurrence matrix and its variants such as the gray-level co-occurrence matrix (GLCM), neighborhood gray-tone difference matrix (NGTDM), run-length matrix (RLM), and gray-level size zone matrix (GLSZM) have been widely applied for characterizing FDG-PET heterogeneity [47].

Four commonly used features from the GLCM include energy, entropy, contrast, and homogeneity [44]. The NGTDM is thought to provide more humanlike perception of texture such as coarseness, contrast, busyness, and complexity. RLM and GLSZM emphasize regional effects. Textural map examples from multiple PET tracers are shown in Fig. 12.1.

These features were shown to predict response in cancers of the cervix [34], esophagus [48], head and neck [49], and lung cancer [50]. MaZda is a dedicated software for image feature analysis [51]. An example of PET different feature extraction from head and neck cancer is shown in Fig. 12.2.

12.2.2 Dynamic PET Features

These features are based on kinetic analysis using tissue compartment models and parameters related to transport and binding rates [52]. In the case of FDG, a three-compartment model could be used to depict the trapping of FDG-6-phosphate (FDG6P) in tumor [53, 54]. Using estimates from compartmental modeling, glucose metabolic uptake rate could be evaluated. The uptake rate and other compartment estimates themselves could form "parameter map" images, which previously described static features, and could be derived from as well (see Chap. 14).

Glucose metabolic rate was correlated with pathologic tumor control probability in lung cancer [55]. Thorwarth et al. published interesting data on the scatter of voxel-based measures of local perfusion and hypoxia in head and neck cancer [56, 57]. Tumors showing a wide spread in both showed less reoxygenation during a course of radiotherapy and had lower local control. A rather interesting approach to improve the robustness of such features is the use of advanced 4D iterative techniques; an example is given in Fig. 12.3. Further improvement could be achieved by utilizing multi-resolution transformations

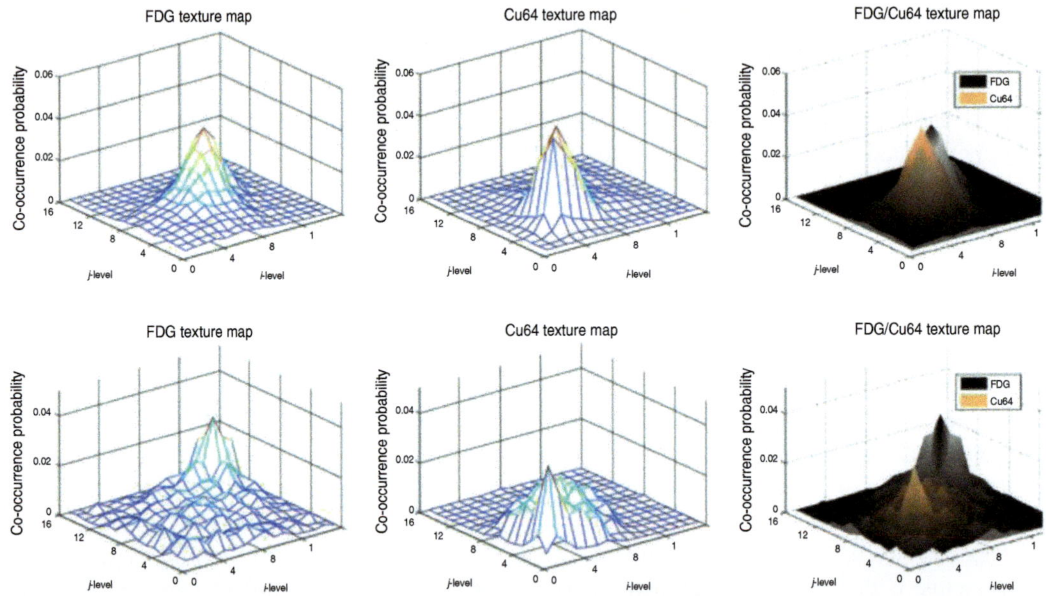

Fig. 12.1 The two rows, referring to an individual patient with primary cervical cancer, show texture maps for FDG (metabolic marker) and Cu-ATSM (hypoxia marker) alone and overlapping texture maps of the two markers [37]

(e.g., wavelet transform) to stabilize kinetic parameter estimates spatially [58].

12.3 Extension to PET/CT and PET/MR

Combining information from multiple modalities allows for better utilization of complementary features from different images. For instance, several studies have indicated that inter- and intra-observer variability of defining the tumor extent could be reduced by using PET/CT or PET/MR. Researchers in lung cancer reported reduced variability when using CT with PET for target definition [3, 10]. Furthermore, a study of fractionated stereotactic radiotherapy for meningioma patients demonstrated improved target definition by combining physiological information from PET, anatomical structure from CT, and soft tissue contrasts from MRI, resulting in alterations of the original contour definitions in 73 % of the cases [59]. However, this visual approach for integrating multimodality imaging information is prone to observer subjectivity and variations as contrasted to single image analysis as discussed later.

The PET imaging features presented as static metrics in Sect. 12.2.1 could be applied equally to PET/CT or PET/MR, where instead of SUV, Hounsfield units are used in the case of CT, and T1w or T2w images, for instance, could be used in the case of MRI, for instance, using its weighted relaxation times or proton density pixel intensities. In the case of dynamic MRI acquisitions, the corresponding pharmacokinetic models would be applied to extract the parametric maps such as extended Tofts model [60], which is also a three-compartment model, and extracted parameters include the transfer constant (K_{trans}), the extravascular-extracellular volume fraction (ve), and the blood volume (bv).

However, among the most challenging issues in multimodality imaging is the fusion of multiple imaging data from different scanners. This is typically carried out through a geometric transformation, i.e., image registration. This could be solved greatly using integrated hardware systems such as PET/CT scanners or PET/MRI scanners; otherwise, software solutions need to be deployed. These software solutions could be divided into rigid or deformable registration techniques [61]. In

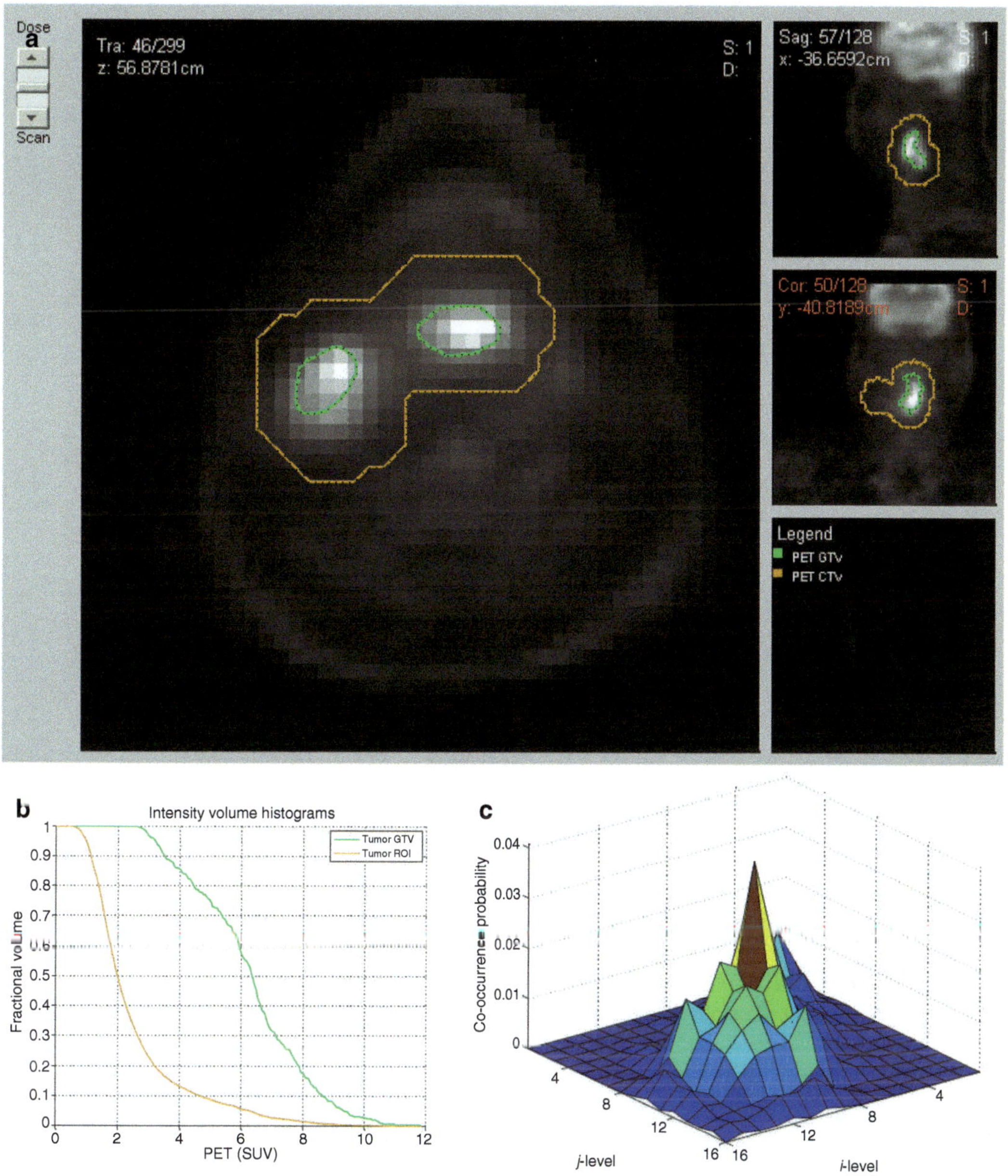

Fig. 12.2 A pretreatment PET scan of a head and neck cancer case of a patient who died from disease after radiotherapy treatment. (**a**) The head and neck tumor region of interest (*brown*) and the gross tumor volume (GTV) (*green*) were outlined by the physician. (**b**) An IVH plot, where I_x and V_x parameters are derived. (**c**) A texture map plot of the GTV heterogeneity through intensity spatial mapping

our previous work, we have developed several tools for this purpose such as MIASYS [62] and DIRART [63]. https://sites.google.com/a/umich.edu/ielnaqa/home/software-tools.

MIASYS is a dedicated open-source software tool developed in MATLAB for multimodality image analysis. The software tool aims to provide a comprehensive solution for 3D image segmentation by integrating automatic algorithms, manual contouring methods, image preprocessing filters, post-processing procedures, user-interactive features, and evaluation metrics.

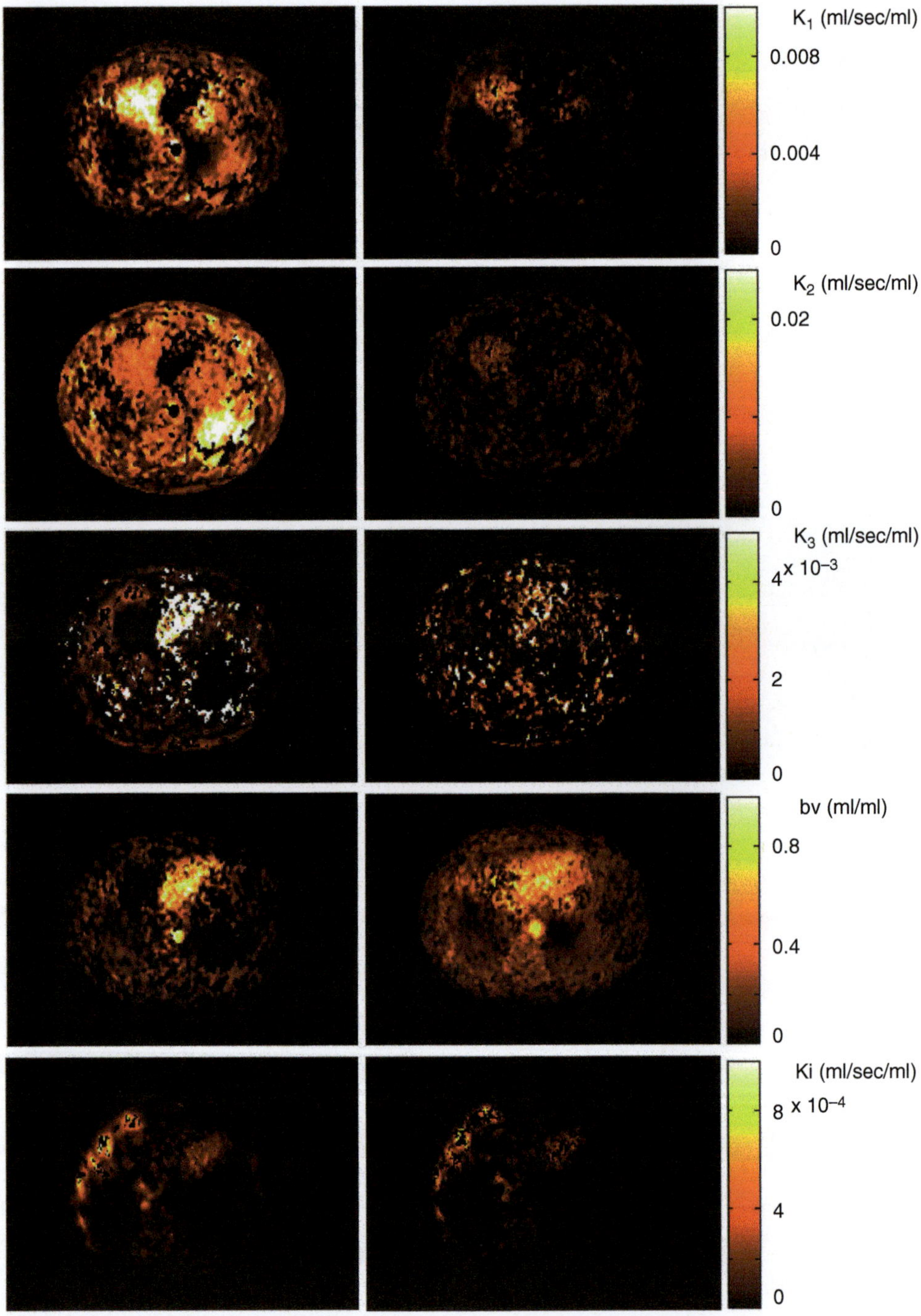

Fig. 12.3 An abdominal dynamic FDG-PET/CT kinetic analysis. The figure shows the three-compartment parameter map (K_1, k_2, k_3) model assuming irreversible kinetics ($k_4=0$), blood volume component ($bv=K_1/k_2$), and K_{FDG} net influx rate constant (*Ki*). In this case, the parameters were obtained using a 4D iterative technique (compared with simple differential methods) by estimation directly from the sinogram domain

The implemented methods include multiple image thresholding, clustering based on K-means and fuzzy C-means (FCM), and active contours based on snakes and level sets. Image registration is achieved via manual and automated rigid methods [62].

DIRART is also an open-source software implemented in MATLAB to support deformable image registration (DIR) for adaptive radiotherapy applications. Image registration in this regard computes voxel mapping between two image sets and is formulated as an optimization problem in which the solution is found by maximizing a similarity metric between the two images (e.g., mutual information). DIRART contains 20+ deformable image registration (DIR) algorithms including 12 different optical flow algorithms, different demon algorithms, and four level set algorithms. It also supports interface to ITK so that ITK DIR algorithms can be called from within DIRART. Currently five ITK DIR algorithms are supported, including demon algorithms and B-spline algorithms. In addition, the newer inverse consistency algorithms to provide consistent displacement vector field (DVF) in both forward and backward directions are implemented [63].

12.4 Application of PET in Radiotherapy

In the following, we discuss the application of PET to radiotherapy with focus on two cases, contouring of tumor/organs at risk in treatment planning and outcome prediction for clinical decision-making using radiomics.

12.4.1 Biological Target Definition Using PET

Medical image segmentation is a process to separate structures of interest in an image from its background or other neighboring structures. It is a necessary prerequisite step for many medical imaging applications in radiology and radiation therapy. These applications may include automatic organ delineation, quantitative tissue classification, surface extraction, visualization and image registration, etc. [64, 65]. For instance, Pham and coworkers divided segmentation algorithms into eight different categories: thresholding, region growing, classifiers, clustering, Markov random field models, artificial neural networks, deformable models, and atlas-guided approaches. In our work on PET-guided treatment planning in radiotherapy, we presented a comparative survey of the current methods applied for tumor segmentation [66, 67]; an example in head and neck cancer using different segmentation algorithms is presented in Fig. 12.4.

There are several commercial and academic software tools that support different segmentation algorithms. In general, commercial software packages have better implementations with a user-friendly interface for manual and semiautomatic segmentation methods, but often lag behind the latest development in the field. In contrast, academic software packages, such as ITK [68], BioImage Suite [69], MIPAV [70], ImageJ [71], and 3D slicer [72], may tend to be oriented toward single-modality applications and less friendly in handling multimodality images as proposed here.

Most automatic algorithms attempt to utilize image intensity variations or image gradient information. However, for low-contrast images, many of these algorithms tend to provide suboptimal solutions that are not clinically acceptable. For such cases, it has been demonstrated that if multiple images are available for the same object (the same image modality or different image modalities), all the available complementary information can be fed into the segmentation algorithms to define the so-called biophysical target [73]. Thus, the segmentation algorithms would benefit from the complementary information from different images, and consequently the accuracy of the final segmentation results could be improved. Similar approaches have been applied for detecting blood-wall interface of heart ventricles from CT, MRI, and ultrasound images using a snake deformable model [74], for classifying coronary artery plaque composition from multiple contrast MR images using K-means

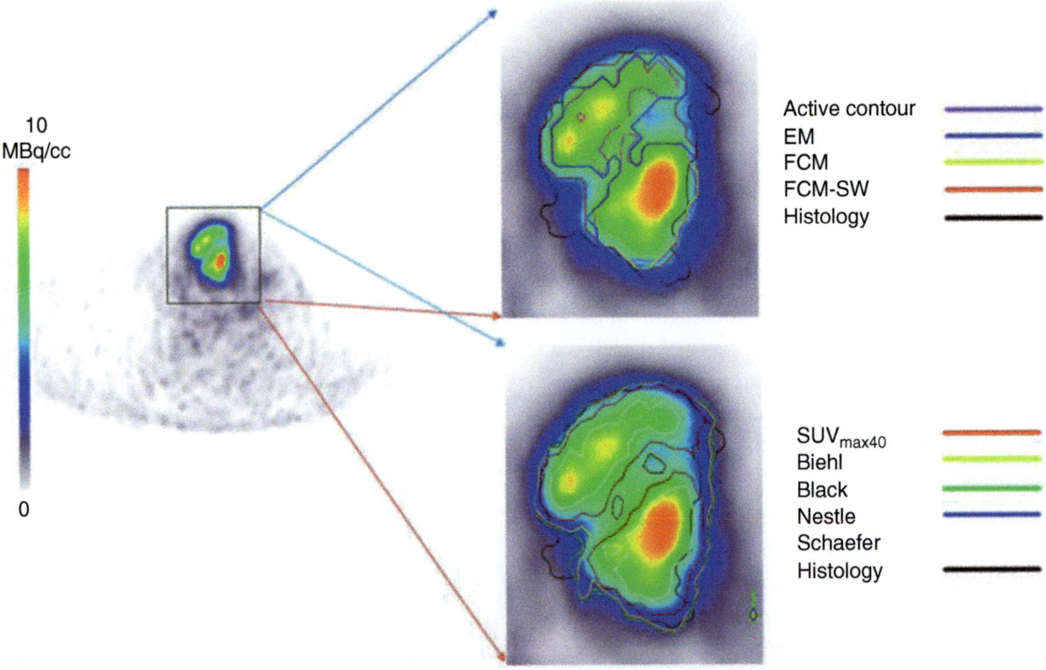

Fig. 12.4 Example of different PET segmentation methods of head and neck cancer. The methods include 40 % of SUV_{max} (SUV_{max40}) and the methods of Nestle, Black, Biehl, and Schaefer. This is in addition to the level set technique (active contour), the stochastic EM approach (EM), the FCM algorithm (FCM), and the FCM-SW variant of the FCM algorithm (FCM-SW). The 3D contour defined on the macroscopic tumor specimen is used as the reference for assessing the performance of the different segmentation techniques (From Zaidi et al. [66])

clustering algorithm [75], and for defining tumor target volumes using PET/CT/MR images for radiotherapy treatment planning by using a multivalued deformable level set approach as in our previous work. Mathematically, such an approach is a framework that could be thought of as a mapping from the imaging space to the "perception" space as identified by the radiologists [73]:

$$\text{Biophysical target} = f\left(\text{CT, PET, MRI, } \ldots, \lambda\right) \quad (12.1)$$

where $f(\cdot)$ is the mapping function from the different imaging modalities to the target space parameterized by λ, which represents users' defined set of parameters representing the prior knowledge. This framework is highlighted in Fig. 12.5.

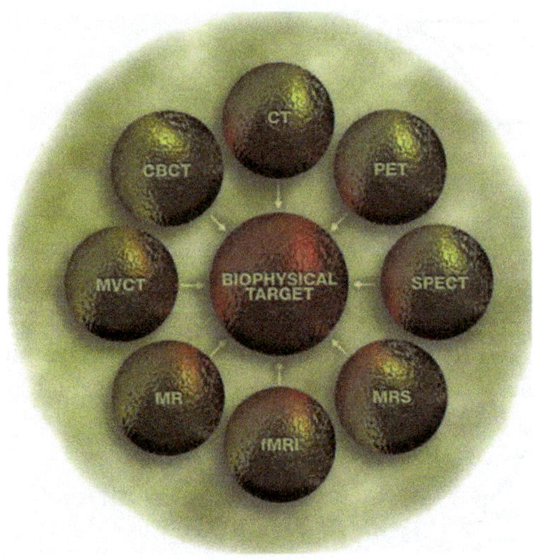

Fig. 12.5 Biophysical target as generated from multimodality imaging by combining anatomical and functional information

The robust image segmentations methods are based on deformable models, which are geometric representations of curves or surfaces that are defined explicitly or implicitly in the imaging domain. These models move under the influence of internal forces (contour curvature) and external forces (image boundary constraints) [76, 77]. The level set is a state-of-the-art variational method for shape recovery [76, 78–80]. They were originally developed in curve evolution theory to overcome the limitations encountered in parametric deformable models (e.g., snakes [81]) such as initialization requirement, generalization to 3D, and topological adaptation such as splitting or merging of model parts. Our generalization to multimodality imaging is based on redefining the concept of a boundary as a logical or "best" combination of multiple images by learning and incorporating expert's knowledge on subregional or even voxel levels. An example showing combination of PET/CT in lung cancer is shown in Fig. 12.6 using a multivalued level set algorithm [73].

In another example the PET/CT images were taken from patients with cervix cancer. The PET image was sharpened using a deconvolution approach [82]. The 40 % maximum SUV (standard uptake value) thresholding is adopted in many institutes to estimate gross tumor volume for cervix cancer patients due to the high target to background ratio of these tumors in PET and the difficulty to distinguish their boundary in CT. In Fig. 12.7, the active contour algorithm is initialized with a circle (in white) of 15.9 mm diameter around the PET lesion. The evolved contour took ten iterations (in blue) and the final estimated contours (in thick black) are shown. The algorithm converged in just 30 iterations. This fast convergence could be attributed in part to the almost spherical shape of the tumor and the sharpness of the gradient. It is noticed that the results of the algorithm match the PET ground truth (99 %) as delineated by an experienced nuclear medicine radiologist. Hence, the delineation results were explained mainly by PET in this case, although information from CT could still be used to steer the algorithm, if desired.

12.4.2 PET Radiomics

The extraction of quantitative information from imaging modalities and relating information to biological and clinical endpoints is a new emerging field referred to as "radiomics" [32, 33]. Traditionally, quantitative analysis of FDG-PET or other PET tracer uptake is conducted based on observed changes in the standard uptake value (SUV). For instance, decrease in SUV postirradiation has been associated with better outcomes in lung cancer [83, 84]. However, SUV measurements themselves are potentially pruned to errors due to the initial FDG uptake kinetics and radiotracer distribution, which are dependent on the initial dose and the elapsing time between injection and image acquisition. In addition, some commonly reported SUV measurements might be sensitive to changes in tumor volume definition (e.g., mean SUV). These factors and others might make such approach subject to significant intra- and inter-observer variability [25, 26, 34].

Radiomics consist of two main steps, extraction of static and dynamic features as discussed in Sect. 17.3 and outcome modeling as presented in the following. Outcomes in oncology and particularly in radiation oncology are characterized by tumor control probability (TCP) and the surrounding normal tissue complication probability (NTCP) [85, 86]. A detailed review of outcome modeling in radiotherapy is presented in our previous work [87]. DREES is a dedicated software tool for modeling of radiotherapy response [88]. In the context of image-based treatment outcome modeling, the observed outcome (e.g., TCP or NTCP) is considered to be adequately captured by extracted image features [34, 89]. We will highlight this approach using classical logistic regression.

Logistic modeling is a common tool for multimetric modeling. In our previous work [90, 91], a logit transformation was used:

$$f(\mathbf{x}_i) = \frac{e^{g(\mathbf{x}_i)}}{1+e^{g(\mathbf{x}_i)}}, \quad i = 1,\ldots,n, \qquad (12.2)$$

where n is the number of cases (patients) and $\mathbf{x}_i$ is a vector of the input variable values (i.e., image features) used to predict $f(\mathbf{x}_i)$ for outcome y_i (i.e., TCP or NTCP) of the i_{th} patient

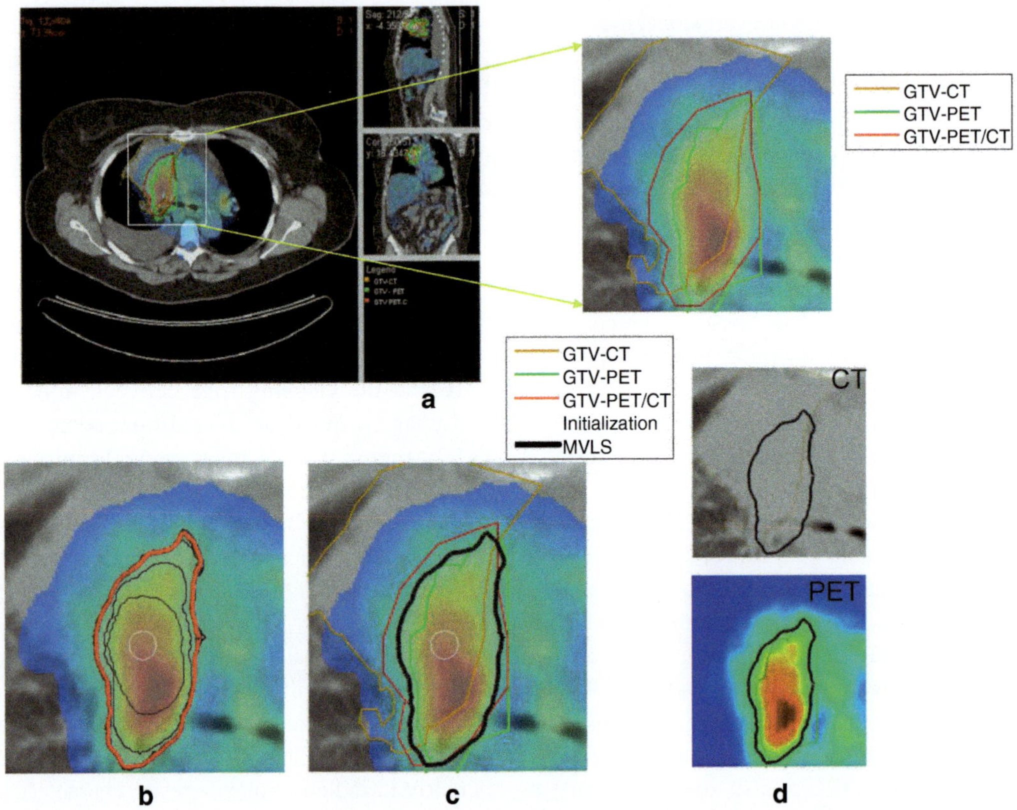

Fig. 12.6 Joint estimation of lung PET/CT target/disease volume. (**a**) A fused PET/CT displayed in CERR with manual contouring shown of the subject's right gross tumor volume. The contouring was performed separately for CT (*in orange*), PET (*in green*), and fused PET/CT (*in red*) images. (**b**) The MVLS algorithm was initialized with a circle (*in white*) of 9.8 mm diameter, an evolved contour in steps of ten iterations (*in black*), and the final estimated contour (*in thick red*). The algorithm converged in 120 iterations in few seconds. The PET/CT ratio weighting was selected as 1:1.65. (**c**) MVLS results are shown along with manual contour results on the fused PET/CT. Note the agreement of the fused PET/CT manual contour and MVLS (dice=0.87). (**d**) MVLS contour superimposed on CT (*top*) and PET (*bottom*) separately

$$g(\mathbf{x}_i) = \beta_o + \sum_{j=1}^{d} \beta_j x_{ij}, \quad i = 1,\ldots,n, \ j = 1,\ldots,d, \tag{12.3}$$

where d is the number of model variables and the βs are the set of model coefficients determined by maximizing the probability that the data gave rise to the observations. Resampling methods such as cross validation and bootstrapping methods could be used to determine optimal model order and parameter selection as shown in Fig. 12.8 for PET/CT modeling of lung cancer [36]. Interestingly, a model of two parameters from PET and CT based on intensity-volume histograms provided the best fit to local control.

12.5 Current Issues and Future Directions

12.5.1 PET Image Characteristics

Generally speaking, PET images have lower resolution than CT or MRI in the order of 3–5 mm, which is further worsened under cardiac or respiratory motion conditions due to longer acquisition periods. Moreover, PET images are susceptible to limited photon count noise. Advances in hardware such as crystal detector technologies [92] and software such as image reconstruction techniques [93] are poised to improve PET image quality and their subsequent use. See Chaps. 8 and 11.

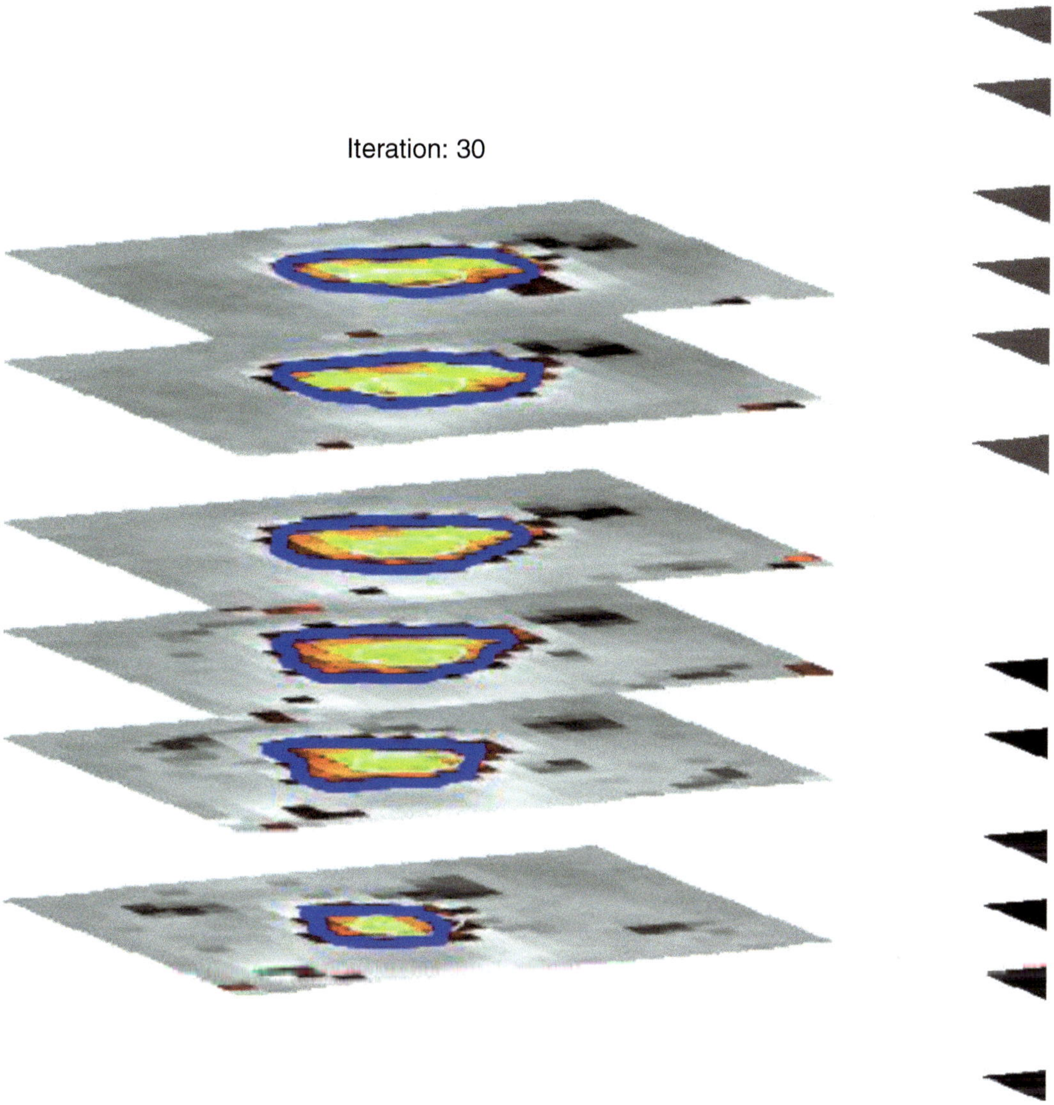

Fig. 12.7 A 3D generalization of multivalued level set (MVLS) algorithm in the case of PET/CT cervix. The MVLS algorithm is initialized with a sphere (*in white*) of 15.9 mm diameter, a curve evolution in steps of ten iterations (*in magenta*), and the final estimated contour (*in thick blue*). The algorithm converged in 30 iterations. MVLS estimated contour superimposed on CT. MVLS estimated contour superimposed on PET

12.5.2 Robustness and Stability of Extracted Image Features

It is well recognized that image acquisition protocols may impact the reproducibility of extracted features from PET images, which may consequently impact the robustness and stability of these features for image analysis. This includes static features such as SUV descriptors [94–96] and texture features [97, 98]. Interestingly, texture-based features were shown to have a reproducibility similar to or better than that of simple SUV descriptors [99]. Moreover, textural features from the GLCM seemed to exhibit lower variations than NGTDM features [97]. Other factors that may impact the stability of these features may include signal-to-noise ratio (SNR), partial volume effect, motion artifacts, parameter

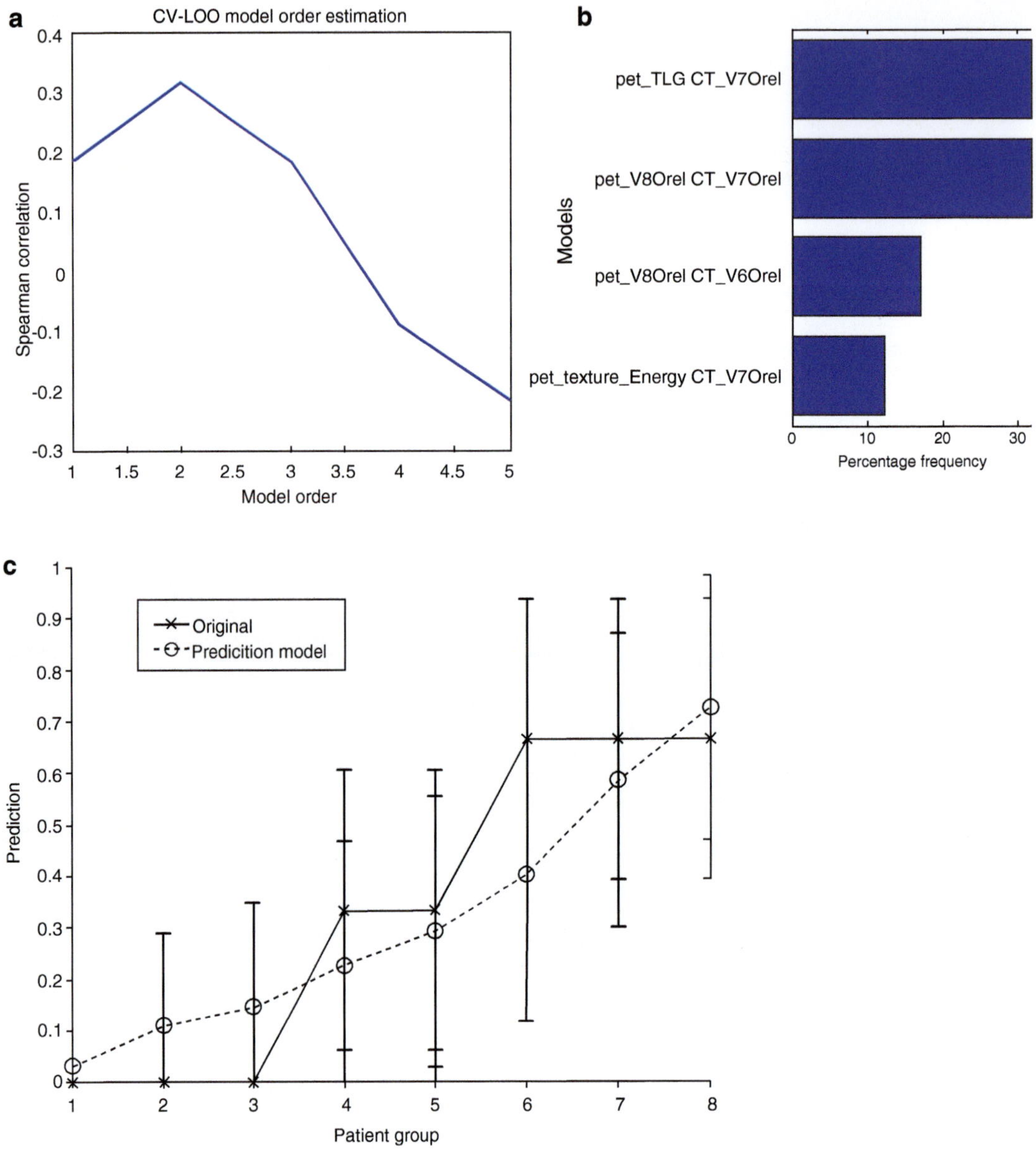

Fig. 12.8 Multi-metric modeling of local failure from PET/CT features. (**a**) Model-order selection using leave-one-out cross validation. (**b**) Most frequent model selection using bootstrap analysis where the *y*-axis represents the model selection frequency on resampled bootstrapped samples. (**c**) Plot of local failure probability as a function of patients binned into equal-size groups showing the model prediction of treatment failure risk and the original data (Reproduced with permission from Vaidya et al. [36])

settings, resampling size, and image quantization [34, 98]. Denoising methods for mitigation of noise in PET imaging follow their limited photon effects using traditional denoising filtering methods [66, 100] or more advanced methods based on combining wavelet and curvelet transform characteristics [101].

12.5.3 Improved PET-Based Outcome Models

In addition to using appropriate candidate image features for PET-based outcome modeling, "radiomics," a main weakness in using classical logistic regression formalism is that the model's capacity to follow details of the data trends is limited. In addition, Eq. (12.3) requires the user's feedback to determine whether interaction terms or higher-order terms should be added, making it a trial-and-error process. A solution to ameliorate this problem is offered by applying machine learning methods [102].

A class of machine learning methods that is particularly powerful, and which we propose to use for image-based outcome prediction, includes so-called kernel-based methods and their most prominent subtype, support vector machines (SVMs). These methods have been applied successfully in many diverse areas including outcome prediction [103–107]. Learning is defined in this context as estimating dependencies from data [108]. In the example of outcome prediction (i.e., discrimination between patients who are at low risk versus patients who are at high risk of local failure), the main function of the kernel-based technique would be to separate these two classes with "hyperplanes" that maximize the margin (separation) between the classes in the nonlinear feature space. The objective here is to minimize the bounds on the generalization error of a model on unseen data before rather than minimizing the mean-square error over the training dataset itself (data fitting). Note that the kernel in these cases acts as a similarity function between sample points in the feature space. Moreover, kernels enjoy closure properties, i.e., one can create admissible composite kernels by weighted addition and multiplication of elementary kernels. This flexibility allows for the construction of a neural network by using a combination of sigmoidal kernels. Alternatively, one could choose a logistic regression equivalent kernel by proper choice of the objective function itself.

Evaluation of radiomics in clinical trials is still in its infancy. According to the website clinicaltrials.gov, a registered trial for "Radiomics: A Study of Outcome in Lung Cancer" between the Maastro Clinic in the Netherlands, Moffitt Cancer Center and Research Institute from Florida, USA, and Gemelli Hospital from Rome, Italy, is reported. Another trial on "Radiomics Prediction of Long Term Survival and Local Failure After Stereotactic Radiotherapy for Brain Metastases" by the Maastro Clinic has been recently opened.

Conclusions

Image processing constitutes an indispensible set of tools for analyzing and extracting valuable information from PET images. We presented in this chapter an overview of different features that could be extracted from PET images for different applications including contouring and response prediction. We have shown that incorporation of different anatomical information from CT and MRI into PET is feasible and could yield better results. However, there are challenges still in the use of PET, some are related to inherited image quality, and others are related to standardization of image acquisition protocols and reconstruction algorithms. Nevertheless, advances in hardware and software technologies will further facilitate wider application of advanced image processing techniques to PET and hybrid imaging to achieve better clinical results. In particular, the synergy between image analysis and machine learning could provide powerful tools to strengthen and further the utilization of PET in clinical practice.

References

1. Verhagen AF, Bootsma GP, Tjan-Heijnen VC, van der Wilt GJ, Cox AL, Brouwer MH, et al. FDG-PET in staging lung cancer: how does it change the algorithm? Lung Cancer. 2004;44:175–81.
2. Bradley J, Thorstad WL, Mutic S, Miller TR, Dehdashti F, Siegel BA, et al. Impact of FDG-PET on radiation therapy volume delineation in non-small-cell lung cancer. Int J Radiat Oncol Biol Phys. 2004;59:78–86.
3. Bradley JD, Perez CA, Dehdashti F, Siegel BA. Implementing biologic target volumes in radiation treatment planning for non-small cell lung cancer. J Nucl Med. 2004;45 Suppl 1:96S–101.
4. Bradley J. Applications for FDG-PET in lung cancer; staging, targeting, and follow-up. Chicago: The Radiological Society of North America; 2004.
5. Erdi YE, Macapinlac H, Rosenzweig KE, Humm JL, Larson SM, Erdi AK, et al. Use of PET to monitor the response of lung cancer to radiation treatment. Eur J Nucl Med. 2000;27:861–6.

6. Mac Manus MP, Hicks RJ. PET scanning in lung cancer: current status and future directions. Semin Surg Oncol. 2003;21:149–55.
7. Mac Manus MP, Hicks RJ, Matthews JP, McKenzie A, Rischin D, Salminen EK, et al. Positron emission tomography is superior to computed tomography scanning for response-assessment after radical radiotherapy or chemoradiotherapy in patients with non-small-cell lung cancer. J Clin Oncol. 2003;21: 1285–92.
8. MacManus MR, Hicks R, Fisher R, Rischin D, Michael M, Wirth A, et al. FDG-PET-detected extracranial metastasis in patients with non-small cell lung cancer undergoing staging for surgery or radical radiotherapy – survival correlates with metastatic disease burden. Acta Oncol. 2003;42:48–54.
9. Pandit N, Gonen M, Krug L, Larson SM. Prognostic value of [18F]FDG-PET imaging in small cell lung cancer. Eur J Nucl Med Mol Imaging. 2003;30: 78–84.
10. Toloza EM, Harpole L, McCrory DC. Noninvasive staging of non-small cell lung cancer: a review of the current evidence. Chest. 2003;123:137S–46.
11. Schwartz DL, Ford E, Rajendran J, Yueh B, Coltrera MD, Virgin J, et al. FDG-PET/CT imaging for preradiotherapy staging of head-and-neck squamous cell carcinoma. Int J Radiat Oncol Biol Phys. 2005;61: 129–36.
12. Suarez Fernandez JP, Maldonado Suarez A, Dominguez Grande ML, Santos Ortega M, Rodriguez Villalba S, Garcia Camanaque L, et al. Positron emission tomography (PET) imaging in head and neck cancer. Acta Otorrinolaringol Esp. 2004;55:303–9.
13. Oyama N, Miller TR, Dehdashti F, Siegel BA, Fischer KC, Michalski JM, et al. 11C-acetate PET imaging of prostate cancer: detection of recurrent disease at PSA relapse. J Nucl Med. 2003;44: 549–55.
14. Mutic S, Malyapa RS, Grigsby PW, Dehdashti F, Miller TR, Zoberi I, et al. PET-guided IMRT for cervical carcinoma with positive para-aortic lymph nodes-a dose-escalation treatment planning study. Int J Radiat Oncol Biol Phys. 2003;55:28–35.
15. Miller TR, Grigsby PW. Measurement of tumor volume by PET to evaluate prognosis in patients with advanced cervical cancer treated by radiation therapy. Int J Radiat Oncol Biol Phys. 2002;53:353–9.
16. Ciernik IF. Radiotherapy of rectal cancer. Schweiz Rundsch Med Prax. 2004;93:1441–6.
17. Castellucci P, Zinzani P, Nanni C, Farsad M, Moretti A, Alinari L, et al. 18F-FDG PET early after radiotherapy in lymphoma patients. Cancer Biother Radiopharm. 2004;19:606–12.
18. Spaepen K, Stroobants S, Verhoef G, Mortelmans L. Positron emission tomography with [(18)F]FDG for therapy response monitoring in lymphoma patients. Eur J Nucl Med Mol Imaging. 2003;30 Suppl 1:S97–105.
19. Fogarty GB, Tartaglia CJ, Peters LJ. Primary melanoma of the oesophagus well palliated by radiotherapy. Br J Radiol. 2004;77:1050–2.
20. Biersack HJ, Bender H, Palmedo H. FDG-PET in monitoring therapy of breast cancer. Eur J Nucl Med Mol Imaging. 2004;31 Suppl 1:S112–7.
21. Lind P, Igerc I, Beyer T, Reinprecht P, Hausegger K. Advantages and limitations of FDG PET in the follow-up of breast cancer. Eur J Nucl Med Mol Imaging. 2004;31 Suppl 1:S125–34.
22. Zangheri B, Messa C, Picchio M, Gianolli L, Landoni C, Fazio F. PET/CT and breast cancer. Eur J Nucl Med Mol Imaging. 2004;31 Suppl 1:S135–42.
23. Brun E, Kjellen E, Tennvall J, Ohlsson T, Sandell A, Perfekt R, et al. FDG PET studies during treatment: prediction of therapy outcome in head and neck squamous cell carcinoma. Head Neck. 2002;24: 127–35.
24. Hope AJ, Saha P, Grigsby PW. FDG-PET in carcinoma of the uterine cervix with endometrial extension. Cancer. 2006;106:196–200.
25. Kalff V, Duong C, Drummond EG, Matthews JP, Hicks RJ. Findings on 18F-FDG PET scans after neoadjuvant chemoradiation provides prognostic stratification in patients with locally advanced rectal carcinoma subsequently treated by radical surgery. J Nucl Med. 2006;47:14–22.
26. Hicks RJ, Mac Manus MP, Matthews JP, Hogg A, Binns D, Rischin D, et al. Early FDG-PET imaging after radical radiotherapy for non-small-cell lung cancer: inflammatory changes in normal tissues correlate with tumor response and do not confound therapeutic response evaluation. Int J Radiat Oncol Biol Phys. 2004;60:412–8.
27. Grigsby PW, Siegel BA, Dehdashti F, Rader J, Zoberi I. Posttherapy [18F] fluorodeoxyglucose positron emission tomography in carcinoma of the cervix: response and outcome. J Clin Oncol. 2004;22:2167–71.
28. Shields AF. Positron emission tomography measurement of tumor metabolism and growth: its expanding role in oncology. Mol Imaging Biol. 2006;8:141–50.
29. Denecke T, Rau B, Hoffmann KT, Hildebrandt B, Ruf J, Gutberlet M, et al. Comparison of CT, MRI and FDG-PET in response prediction of patients with locally advanced rectal cancer after multimodal preoperative therapy: is there a benefit in using functional imaging? Eur Radiol. 2005;15:1658–66.
30. Benz MR, Allen-Auerbach MS, Eilber FC, Chen HJJ, Dry S, Phelps ME, et al. Combined assessment of metabolic and volumetric changes for assessment of tumor response in patients with soft-tissue sarcomas. J Nucl Med. 2008;49:1579–84. doi:10.2967/jnumed.108.053694.
31. Yang D-H, Min J-J, Jeong Y, Ahn J-S, Kim Y-K, Cho S-H, et al. The combined evaluation of interim contrast-enhanced computerized tomography (CT)

and FDG-PET/CT predicts the clinical outcomes and may impact on the therapeutic plans in patients with aggressive non-Hodgkin's lymphoma. Ann Hematol. 2009;88:425–32.
32. Lambin P, Rios-Velazquez E, Leijenaar R, Carvalho S, van Stiphout RG, Granton P, et al. Radiomics: extracting more information from medical images using advanced feature analysis. Eur J Cancer. 2012; 48:441–6.doi:10.1016/j.ejca.2011.11.036.doi:S0959-8049(11)00999-3 [pii].
33. Kumar V, Gu Y, Basu S, Berglund A, Eschrich SA, Schabath MB, et al. Radiomics: the process and the challenges. Magn Reson Imaging. 2012;30:1234–48. doi:10.1016/j.mri.2012.06.010. doi:S0730-725X(12)00220-2 [pii].
34. El Naqa I, Grigsby P, Apte A, Kidd E, Donnelly E, Khullar D, et al. Exploring feature-based approaches in PET images for predicting cancer treatment outcomes. Pattern Recognit. 2009;42:1162–71. doi:10.1016/j.patcog.2008.08.011.
35. Kidd EA, El Naqa I, Siegel BA, Dehdashti F, Grigsby PW. FDG-PET-based prognostic nomograms for locally advanced cervical cancer. Gynecol Oncol. 2012;127:136–40. doi:10.1016/j.ygyno.2012.06.027. doi:S0090-8258(12)00478-7 [pii].
36. Vaidya M, Creach KM, Frye J, Dehdashti F, Bradley JD, El Naqa I. Combined PET/CT image characteristics for radiotherapy tumor response in lung cancer. Radiother Oncol. 2012;102:239–45. doi:10.1016/j.radonc.2011.10.014. doi:S0167-8140(11)00626-8 [pii].
37. El Naqa I. The role of quantitative PET in predicting cancer treatment outcomes. Clin Transl Imaging. 2014;2:305–20. doi:10.1007/s40336-014-0063-1.
38. Strauss LG, Conti PS. The applications of PET in clinical oncology. J Nucl Med. 1991;32:623–48.
39. Larson SM, Erdi Y, Akhurst T, Mazumdar M, Macapinlac HA, Finn RD, et al. Tumor treatment response based on visual and quantitative changes in global tumor glycolysis using PET-FDG imaging. The visual response score and the change in total lesion glycolysis. Clin Positron Imaging. 1999;2: 159–71. doi:S1095039799000163 [pii].
40. Jain AK. Fundamentals of digital image processing. Englewood Cliffs: Prentice Hall; 1989.
41. O'Sullivan F, Roy S, O'Sullivan J, Vernon C, Eary J. Incorporation of tumor shape into an assessment of spatial heterogeneity for human sarcomas imaged with FDG-PET. Biostatistics. 2005;6:293–301. doi:10.1093/biostatistics/kxi010.
42. O'Sullivan F, Roy S, Eary J. A statistical measure of tissue heterogeneity with application to 3D PET sarcoma data. Biostatistics. 2003;4:433–48. doi:10.1093/biostatistics/4.3.433.
43. Castleman KR. Digital image processing. Englewood Cliffs: Prentice Hall; 1996.
44. Haralick R, Shanmugam K, Dinstein I. Texture features for image classification. IEEE Trans Sys Man Cyb SMC. 1973;3:610–21.
45. Zhang J, Tan T. Brief review of invariant texture analysis methods. Pattern Recognit. 2002;35:735–47. doi:http://dx.doi.org/10.1016/S0031-3203(01)00074-7.
46. Castellano G, Bonilha L, Li LM, Cendes F. Texture analysis of medical images. Clin Radiol. 2004;59: 1061–9. doi:http://dx.doi.org/10.1016/j.crad.2004.07.008.
47. Chicklore S, Goh V, Siddique M, Roy A, Marsden P, Cook GR. Quantifying tumour heterogeneity in 18F-FDG PET/CT imaging by texture analysis. Eur J Nucl Med Mol Imaging. 2013;40:133–40. doi:10.1007/s00259-012-2247-0.
48. Tixier F, Le Rest CC, Hatt M, Albarghach N, Pradier O, Metges J-P, et al. Intratumor heterogeneity characterized by textural features on baseline 18F-FDG PET images predicts response to concomitant radiochemotherapy in esophageal cancer. J Nucl Med. 2011;52:369–78. doi:10.2967/jnumed.110.082404.
49. Cheng N-M, Dean Fang Y-H, Tung-Chieh Chang J, Huang C-G, Tsan D-L, Ng S-H, et al. Textural features of pretreatment 18F-FDG PET/CT images: prognostic significance in patients with advanced T-stage oropharyngeal squamous cell carcinoma. J Nucl Med. 2013;54:1703–9. doi:10.2967/jnumed.112.119289.
50. Cook GJR, Yip C, Siddique M, Goh V, Chicklore S, Roy A, et al. Are pretreatment 18F-FDG PET tumor textural features in non–small cell lung cancer associated with response and survival after chemoradiotherapy? J Nucl Med. 2013;54:19–26. doi:10.2967/jnumed.112.107375.
51. Szczypinski PM, Strzelecki M, Materka A, Klepaczko A. MaZda – a software package for image texture analysis. Comput Methods Programs Biomed. 2009;94:66–76. doi:10.1016/j.cmpb.2008.08.005.
52. Watabe H, Ikoma Y, Kimura Y, Naganawa M, Shidahara M. PET kinetic analysis – compartmental model. Ann Nucl Med. 2006;20:583–8.
53. Graham MM, Peterson LM, Hayward RM. Comparison of simplified quantitative analyses of FDG uptake. Nucl Med Biol. 2000;27:647–55.
54. Patlak CS, Blasberg RG. Graphical evaluation of blood-to-brain transfer constants from multiple-time uptake data. Generalizations. J Cereb Blood Flow Metab. 1985;5:584–90.
55. Choi NC, Fischman AJ, Niemierko A, Ryu JS, Lynch T, Wain J, et al. Dose–response relationship between probability of pathologic tumor control and glucose metabolic rate measured with FDG PET after preoperative chemoradiotherapy in locally advanced non-small-cell lung cancer. Int J Radiat Oncol Biol Phys. 2002;54:1024–35. doi:S0360301602030389 [pii].
56. Thorwarth D, Eschmann S-M, Holzner F, Paulsen F, Alber M. Combined uptake of [18F]FDG and [18F]FMISO correlates with radiation therapy outcome in head-and-neck cancer patients. Radiother Oncol. 2006;80:151–6.

57. Thorwarth D, Eschmann S-M, Paulsen F, Alber M. A model of reoxygenation dynamics of head-and-neck tumors based on serial 18F-fluoromisonidazole positron emission tomography investigations. Int J Radiat Oncol Biol Phys. 2007;68:515–21.
58. Turkheimer FE, Aston JA, Asselin MC, Hinz R. Multi-resolution Bayesian regression in PET dynamic studies using wavelets. Neuroimage. 2006; 32:111–21. doi:10.1016/j.neuroimage.2006.03.002. doi:S1053-8119(06)00180-7 [pii].
59. Milker-Zabel S, Zabel-du Bois A, Henze M, Huber P, Schulz-Ertner D, Hoess A, et al. Improved target volume definition for fractionated stereotactic radiotherapy in patients with intracranial meningiomas by correlation of CT, MRI, and [68Ga]-DOTATOC-PET. Int J Radiat Oncol Biol Phys. 2006;65:222–7.
60. Tofts PS, Brix G, Buckley DL, Evelhoch JL, Henderson E, Knopp MV, et al. Estimating kinetic parameters from dynamic contrast-enhanced T(1)-weighted MRI of a diffusable tracer: standardized quantities and symbols. J Magn Reson Imaging. 1999;10:223–32. doi:10.1002/(SICI)1522-2586(199909)10:3<223::AID-JMRI2>3.0.CO;2-S [pii].
61. Hajnal JV, Hawkes DJ, Hill DLG. Medical image registration. Boca Raton: CRC Press; 2001.
62. Yang D, Zheng J, Nofal A, Wu Y, Deasy J, El Naqa I. Techniques and software tool for 3D multimodality medical image segmentation Journal of radiation oncology informatics. 2009:accepted.
63. Yang D, Brame S, El Naqa I, Aditya A, Wu Y, Goddu SM, et al. Technical note: DIRART – a software suite for deformable image registration and adaptive radiotherapy research. Med Phys. 2011;38: 67–77.
64. Pham DL, Xu C, Prince JL. Current methods in medical image segmentation. Annu Rev Biomed Eng. 2000;2:315–37.
65. Suri JS, Setarehdan SK, Singh S. Advanced algorithmic approaches to medical image segmentation: state-of-the-art applications in cardiology, neurology, mammography, and pathology. New York: Springer; 2002.
66. Zaidi H, Abdoli M, Fuentes CL, El Naqa IM. Comparative methods for PET image segmentation in pharyngolaryngeal squamous cell carcinoma. Eur J Nucl Med Mol Imaging. 2012;39(5):881–91. doi:10.1007/s00259-011-2053-0.
67. Zaidi H, El Naqa I. PET-guided delineation of radiation therapy treatment volumes: a survey of image segmentation techniques. Eur J Nucl Med Mol Imaging. 2010;37:2165–87. doi:10.1007/s00259-010-1423-3.
68. Yoo TS, Ackerman MJ, Lorensen WE, Schroeder W, Chalana V, Aylward S, et al. Engineering and algorithm design for an image processing API: a technical report on ITK – the insight toolkit. In: Proceedings of medicine meets virtual reality. 2002;586–92.
69. Papademetris X, Jackowski M, Rajeevan N, Constable RT, Staib L. BioImage suite: an integrated medical image analysis suite. Insight J. 2005; 2006:209.
70. McAuliffe MJ, Lalonde FM, McGarry D, Gandler W, Csaky K, Trus BL. Medical image processing, analysis & visualization in clinical research. In: Proceedings of the fourteenth IEEE symposium on computer-based medical systems. IEEE Computer Society. 2001.
71. Abramoff MD, Magelhaes PJ, Ram SJ. Image processing with imageJ. Biophotonics Int. 2004;11:36–42.
72. Fedorov A, Beichel R, Kalpathy-Cramer J, Finet J, Fillion-Robin JC, Pujol S, et al. 3D Slicer as an image computing platform for the quantitative imaging network. Magn Reson Imaging. 2012;30:1323–41. doi:10.1016/j.mri.2012.05.001.
73. El Naqa I, Yang D, Apte A, Khullar D, Mutic S, Zheng J, et al. Concurrent multimodality image segmentation by active contours for radiotherapy treatment planning. Med Phys. 2007;34:4738–49.
74. Sebbahi A, Herment A, de Cesare A, Mousseaux E. Multimodality cardiovascular image segmentation using a deformable contour model. Comput Med Imaging Graph. 1997;21:79–89.
75. Zheng J, Naqa IE, Rowold FE, Pilgram TK, Woodard PK, Saffitz JE, et al. Quantitative assessment of coronary artery plaque vulnerability by high-resolution magnetic resonance imaging and computational biomechanics: a pilot study ex vivo. Magn Reson Med. 2005;54:1360–8.
76. Sethian JA. Level set methods and fast marching methods: evolving interfaces in computational geometry, fluid mechanics, computer vision, and material science. 2nd ed. Cambridge: Cambridge University Press; 1999.
77. Xu C, Pham DL, Prince JL. Image segmentation using deformable models. In: Sonka M, Fitzpatrick JM, editors. Handbook of medical imaging: medical image processing and analysis. Bellingham: SPIE (The International Society for Optical Engineering) Press; 2002. p. 129–74.
78. Suri JS, Kecheng L, Singh S, Laxminarayan SN, Xiaolan Z, Reden L. Shape recovery algorithms using level sets in 2-D/3-D medical imagery: a state-of-the-art review. IEEE Trans Inf Technol Biomed. 2002;6:8–28.
79. Aubert G. Mathematical problems in image processing: partial differential equations and the calculus of variations. 2nd ed. New York: Springer; 2006.
80. Osher S, Fedkiw RP. Level set methods and dynamic implicit surfaces. New York: Springer; 2003.
81. Kass M, Witkin A, Terzopoulos. Snakes: active contour models. In: First international conference on computer vision, London. 1987;259–68.
82. El Naqa I, Low DA, Bradley JD, Vicic M, Deasy JO. Deblurring of breathing motion artifacts in thoracic PET images by deconvolution methods. Med Phys. 2006;33:3587–600.
83. Wong CY, Schmidt J, Bong JS, Chundru S, Kestin L, Yan D, et al. Correlating metabolic and anatomic

responses of primary lung cancers to radiotherapy by combined F-18 FDG PET-CT imaging. Radiat Oncol. 2007;2:18. doi:10.1186/1748-717X-2-18. doi:1748-717X-2-18 [pii].
84. Coon D, Gokhale AS, Burton SA, Heron DE, Ozhasoglu C, Christie N. Fractionated stereotactic body radiation therapy in the treatment of primary, recurrent, and metastatic lung tumors: the role of positron emission tomography/computed tomography-based treatment planning. Clin Lung Cancer. 2008;9:217–21. doi:10.3816/CLC.2008.n.032. doi:935437162W233526 [pii].
85. Steel GG. Basic clinical radiobiology. 3rd ed. London/New York/Arnold: Oxford University Press; 2002.
86. Webb S. The physics of three-dimensional radiation therapy: conformal radiotherapy, radiosurgery, and treatment planning. Bristol/Philadelphia: Institute of Physics Pub; 2001.
87. El Naqa I. Outcomes modeling. In: Starkschall G, Siochi C, editors. Informatics in radiation oncology. Boca Raton: CRC Press/Taylor and Francis; 2013. p. 257–75.
88. El Naqa I, Suneja G, Lindsay PE, Hope AJ, Alaly JR, Vicic M, et al. Dose response explorer: an integrated open-source tool for exploring and modelling radiotherapy dose-volume outcome relationships. Phys Med Biol. 2006;51:5719–35.
89. El-Naqa I, Yang Y, Galatsanos NP, Nishikawa RM, Wernick MN. A similarity learning approach to content-based image retrieval: application to digital mammography. IEEE Trans Med Imaging. 2004;23:1233–44. doi:10.1109/TMI.2004.834601.
90. Deasy JO, El Naqa I. Image-based modeling of normal tissue complication probability for radiation therapy. In: Mehta M, Bentzen S, editors. Radiation oncology advances. New York: Springer; 2007.
91. El Naqa I, Bradley JD, Lindsay PE, Blanco AI, Vicic M, Hope AJ, et al. Multi-variable modeling of radiotherapy outcomes including dose-volume and clinical factors. Int J Radiat Oncol Biol Phys. 2006;64:1275–86.
92. Moses WW. Fundamental limits of spatial resolution in PET. Nucl Instrum Meth Phys Res A Accelerators Spectrometers Detectors Assoc Equipment. 2011;648 Suppl 1:S236–40. doi:10.1016/j.nima.2010.11.092.
93. Tong S, Alessio AM, Kinahan PE. Image reconstruction for PET/CT scanners: past achievements and future challenges. Imaging Med. 2010;2:529–45. doi:10.2217/iim.10.49.
94. Nahmias C, Wahl LM. Reproducibility of standardized uptake value measurements determined by 18F-FDG PET in malignant tumors. J Nucl Med. 2008;49:1804–8. doi:10.2967/jnumed.108.054239.
95. Kinahan PE, Fletcher JW. Positron emission tomography-computed tomography standardized uptake values in clinical practice and assessing response to therapy. Semi Ultrasound CT MRI. 2010;31:496–505. doi:http://dx.doi.org/10.1053/j.sult.2010.10.001.
96. Hatt M, Cheze-Le Rest C, Aboagye EO, Kenny LM, Rosso L, Turkheimer FE, et al. Reproducibility of 18F-FDG and 3′-deoxy-3′-18F-fluorothymidine PET tumor volume measurements. J Nucl Med. 2010;51:1368–76. doi:10.2967/jnumed.110.078501.
97. Galavis PE, Hollensen C, Jallow N, Paliwal B, Jeraj R. Variability of textural features in FDG PET images due to different acquisition modes and reconstruction parameters. Acta Oncol. 2010;49:1012–6. doi:10.3109/0284186X.2010.498437.
98. Cheng NM, Fang YH, Yen TC. The promise and limits of PET texture analysis. Ann Nucl Med. 2013;27:867–9. doi:10.1007/s12149-013-0759-8.
99. Tixier F, Hatt M, Le Rest CC, Le Pogam A, Corcos L, Visvikis D. Reproducibility of tumor uptake heterogeneity characterization through textural feature analysis in 18F-FDG PET. J Nucl Med. 2012;53:693–700. doi:10.2967/jnumed.111.099127.
100. El Naqa I, Kawrakow I, Fippel M, Siebers JV, Lindsay PE, Wickerhauser MV, et al. A comparison of Monte Carlo dose calculation denoising techniques. Phys Med Biol. 2005;50:909–22. doi:10.1088/0031-9155/50/5/014. doi:S0031-9155(05)86128-7 [pii].
101. Le Pogam A, Hanzouli H, Hatt M, Cheze Le Rest C, Visvikis D. Denoising of PET images by combining wavelets and curvelets for improved preservation of resolution and quantitation. Med Image Anal. 2013;17:877–91. doi:10.1016/j.media.2013.05.005.
102. El Naqa I, Li R, Murphy MJ, editors. Machine learning in radiation oncology: theory and application. 1st ed. Cham: Springer International Publishing; 2015.
103. El Naqa I, Bradley J, Deasy J. Machine learning methods for radiobiological outcome modeling. In: Mehta M, Paliwal B, Bentzen S, editors. Physical, chemical, and biological targeting in radiation oncology. Madison: Medical Physics Publishing; 2005.
104. El-Naqa I, Yang Y, Galatsanos NP, Nishikawa RM, Wernick MN. A similarity learning approach to content-based image retrieval: application to digital mammography. IEEE Trans Med Imaging. 2004;23:1233–44.
105. El-Naqa I, Yang Y, Wernick MN, Galatsanos NP, Nishikawa RM. A support vector machine approach for detection of microcalcifications. IEEE Trans Med Imaging. 2002;21:1552–63.
106. Schèolkopf B, Tsuda K, Vert J-P. Kernel methods in computational biology. Cambridge, MA: MIT Press; 2004.
107. Shawe-Taylor J, Cristianini N. Kernel methods for pattern analysis. Cambridge/New York: Cambridge University Press; 2004.
108. Hastie T, Tibshirani R, Friedman JH. The elements of statistical learning: data mining, inference, and prediction: with 200 full-color illustrations. New York: Springer; 2001.

Basics and Advances of Quantitative PET Imaging

13

Magdy M. Khalil

Contents

13.1 **Introduction** 304

13.2 **PET Quantitation** 304
13.2.1 Spectrum of PET Quantitation 305
13.2.2 Static PET Imaging 305
13.2.3 Dynamic PET Imaging 306
13.2.4 Static Versus Dynamic PET 309

13.3 **Standardized Uptake Value (SUV)** 310
13.3.1 Drawbacks of SUV 311
13.3.2 SUV Variants 311

13.4 **Total Disease Burden** 312

13.5 **Factors Affecting Quantitative Measurements** 313
13.5.1 Biological Factors 314
13.5.2 Blood Glucose Level 314

13.6 **Response to Therapy** 315

13.7 **Tumor Texture Analysis** 317

Conclusion 318

References 318

Abstract

Positron emission tomography (PET) has been enjoying outstanding quantitative features since its inception in diagnostic clinical imaging. These capabilities have served the evolution and diagnostic performance of PET in many circumstances including research and development as well as clinical routines. However, this has been made with extensive efforts exerted on technical, physical, and instrumental levels. Quantitative PET can be very simple but also sometimes need to be very complicated and cumbersome. This depends heavily on the purpose of the imaging task. Static and dynamic PET are the two different modes of data acquisition from which the relevant type of information is extracted and physiologically interpreted. The most commonly used form of data quantitation in PET is the standardized uptake value (SUV) that may take several forms. This later quantitative index, despite being simple to calculate showing effectiveness in a number of malignancies, is prone to many technical and biological errors if not properly adjusted. All of the above have been reviewed in this chapter along with other new emerging volumetric and disease burden quantitative metrics.

M.M. Khalil, PhD
Medical Biophysics, Department of Physics,
Faculty of Science, Helwan University, Cairo, Egypt
e-mail: magdy_khalil@hotmail.com

M.M. Khalil (ed.), *Basic Science of PET Imaging*, DOI 10.1007/978-3-319-40070-9_13

13.1 Introduction

Positron emission tomography (PET) is a well-established and standard diagnostic imaging modality in clinical practice. The major role has become very evident in oncology with useful diagnostic capabilities in other areas of medicine that include neurology, cardiology, infection, and inflammation. In 2007, the Society of Nuclear Medicine and Molecular Imaging defined molecular imaging as "the visualization, characterization, and measurement of biological processes at the molecular and cellular levels in humans and other living systems." PET imaging using F18-flurodeoxyglucose has a high sensitivity in detecting glucose avid malignant tumors. This phenomenon was originally initiated by Warburg in 1930s [1, 2]. In contrast to normal differentiated cells, which rely primarily on mitochondrial oxidative phosphorylation to generate the energy needed for cellular processes, most cancer cells instead rely on the non-efficient aerobic glycolysis [3]. During this process, glucose uptake is enhanced by upregulation of glucose transporters (GLUT), increased levels of hexokinase, and decreased levels of glucose-6-phosphatase [4].

PET imaging has a unique molecular sensitivity as it can use very small amount of radiotracer in the range of nano- to picomolar concentration in detection of functional disorders within human body without disturbing the normal biochemistry or pharmacokinetics of the target tissue. This detection capability is a central point in characterizing PET systems over other imaging modalities. Therefore, there is a continuous interest to improve overall system performance in terms of spatial resolution, sensitivity, count rate performance, timing, and energy resolution in connection to developing new advanced correction and reconstruction algorithms. These developments have several consequences on image quality and quantitative accuracy of PET examinations.

PET is a multidisciplinary functional and molecular diagnostic tool with enhanced morphological features when combined with structural imaging modalities such as x-ray computed tomography (CT) and magnetic resonance imaging (MRI). These relatively new hybrid imaging modalities bring to reading physicians a significant amount of information not only on qualitative (i.e., visual assessment) level but also have a substantial influence on quantitative and semi-quantitative measurements.

PET/CT has gained a wide acceptance among nuclear medicine practitioners and scientific community owing to the fact of improved diagnostic performance and guiding clinicians toward better patient management. Applications of PET/CT in oncology are of particular importance and include initial diagnosis, staging, restaging, recurrence detection, monitoring response to treatment, as well as patient stratification and prognostication.

The multimodality hybrid imaging approach has proved its clinical significance in more than one aspect. Together with time reduction, speed of diagnosis, incremental diagnostic information, and advising on proper treatment strategy, hybrid imaging will play a very essential tool in future of modern medicine or more specifically on practice of what is recently called personalized or precision medicine [5].

13.2 PET Quantitation

Despite the fact that visual interpretation is the conventional method of reading PET imaging data, it has been shown that quantitative analysis allows an objective complement in supporting diagnostic and decision-making process [6]. The term "quantitation" has several interpretations among PET imaging practitioners, and range from simple detection and determination of tracer concentrations may be in units of kBq/ml, μCi/ml to more sophisticated mathematical algorithms that indicate rate of tracer transportation or exchange among different biochemical species or tissue space [7, 8]. What determines the level of complexity of quantitation is the target biological question and objective of the PET study which might be a development of new PET radiopharmaceutical and examining tracer biodistribution, diagnostic workup and staging, response to treatment, or investigating efficacy of new therapeutic drugs as can be seen and performed in clinical trials [9].

We may classify quantitative approaches in PET imaging into three major types, namely, qualitative methods using visual assessment, semiquantitative methods using standardized uptake value (SUV) and its variants, and absolute measurements of tracer pharmacokinetics using kinetic modeling analysis. Two major types of data acquisition are available in PET that permits one to perform the required type of image quantitation; these are static and dynamic imaging. Static images are normally acquired when the tracer is injected and an adequate time is given for tracer clearance from plasma and accumulation into the tissue to improve target-to-nontarget ratio. However, dynamic imaging as the name implies does capture the metabolic information on a real time fashion enabling one to derive valuable physiologic quantitative parameters as will be discussed later.

13.2.1 Spectrum of PET Quantitation

Interpretations of FDG PET scan depend in large part on well understanding of the normal physiologic uptake and associated normal variants in addition to imaging pitfalls. This supports the reading physician to come up with clear idea about abnormal finding whether it is a true pathology or normal physiologic uptake. However, this process is subject to a significant inter-reader variability and less quantitative base.

A reliable and reproducible measure of tracer uptake within different pathologic lesions of cancer as well as other disease pathologies has several advantages and benefits. Elimination of inter-reader variability is the first outcome of these quantitative or semiquantitative metrics in PET image interpretation. Another aim of having this type of measurement is the possibility of comparison among different patient studies typically in monitoring and assessment of response to treatment. A robust, reliable, and distinctive cutoff value of the response is ideally desirable to support the decision-making process for a given treatment line [10]. It would also be very helpful in predicting the success of a chosen therapy over others especially at early cycles of selected therapeutic regimen. On the other side, such a metric could provide a more insight into the spectrum and biological heterogeneity of a specific disease and particularly in inter-patient comparisons. The development of novel targeted tracers imposes the use of a suitable or optimal quantitative method as conventional quantitative metrics may not always be adapted for extracting relevant information [11].

A standardized imaging protocol and quantification strategy would also permit an easy comparison among different PET clinics to build up a knowledge base with minimal observer variability and methodological preferences. This can take place if the method is well defined and sources of technical errors and imaging pitfalls are recognized and eliminated [12]. Therefore, standardized quantification facilitates multicenter trials, allows comparison among different PET clinics, and supports the way toward personalized therapy [13]. These properties are not limited only to oncology applications, but there is a growing interest to use PET quantitative indices in infection and inflammatory disorders in addition to the existing interest in neurology and cardiology [14].

13.2.2 Static PET Imaging

After the advent of PET/CT more than a decade ago, there was a paradigm shift in the practice of PET imaging in terms of its impact on management of cancer patients and hence on clinical oncology [15]. The standard PET/CT imaging protocol in oncology is normally a whole-body scanning procedure that extends from skull base to mid-thigh. Most imaging procedures start around 60 min post-activity administration, and patient is allowed to relax in a room of moderate light intensity after intravenous injection. Patients should fast for 4–6 h to minimize the effect of endogenous glucose and avoid its competition with the injected glucose analogue F18-FDG during the uptake period. The CT examination often starts before the multiple bed positions used for acquiring the PET. The former is launched by acquiring a scout view that is then used by the user to delimit the whole-body segment required for CT and PET scan length. Contrast-enhanced CT might be performed after PET acquisition to avoid the possibility of image

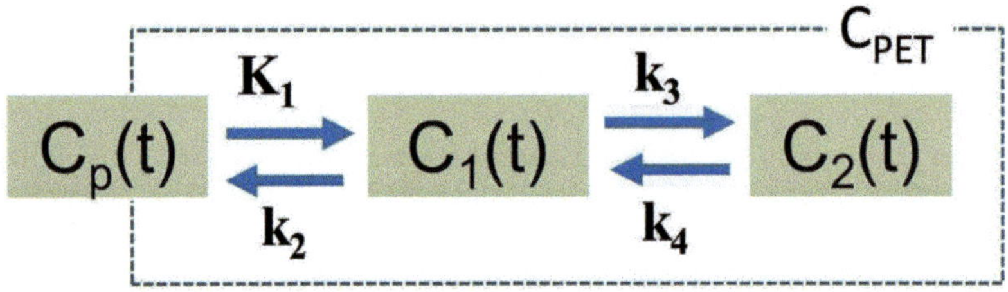

Fig. 13.1 The figure shows the structure of three-compartment model to quantitatively assess the transportation rate constants related to FDG metabolism, where C_p, C_1, and C_2 are the compartments for plasma, free, and metabolized tracer, respectively. C_{PET} represents what the scanner measures in a voxel or in a region of interest (ROI). The rate constants K_1–k_4 regulate the tracer transportation through the different compartments which could be a transfer from chemical species to another or from physical space to another physical space. Note that K_1 is the perfusion and has units in ml/g/min, while k_2–k_4 have units in 1/min. The measured PET signal is contaminated by a fraction of tracer concentration in plasma, and this question is addressed by including a portion of the input function in the kinetic model equation (Adapted from Bentourkia [7])

artifacts due to contrast deposition in some regions of the body [16, 17].

Image reconstruction using iterative techniques (reviewed in Chap. 11) has become widely available due to many reasons including improved noise characteristics, contrast and spatial resolution, and ultimately quantitative accuracy and image quality. As mentioned, the PET data are acquired using sequential multiple bed scanning approach applying 2–5 min for each bed position. This heavily depends on the adopted imaging protocol that is affected by PET system performance and the employed F18-FDG dosing and uptake period. The most common form of image quantitation is the use of the standardized uptake value (SUV) as an adjunct in image interpretation.

13.2.3 Dynamic PET Imaging

Apart from static whole-body PET examinations, dynamic imaging reveals several important physiologic and metabolic information of tracer pharmacokinetic behavior in tissues and has been extensively used in a number of potential applications in neurology, cardiology, and oncology [11, 18, 19]. It can be acquired with predetermined number of frames and the duration of each or group of frame(s). List mode data acquisition, however, is one tool that can be used to record events based on their specific attributes such as time and energy but at the cost of high storage demands. This type of acquisition provides opportunity to reframe acquired data at any arbitrary time frame.

Dynamic PET provides the possibility of absolute data quantitation based on compartmental or non-compartmental methods and quantitative estimation of tracer kinetics relying on region or voxel of interest analysis. The approach of using individual voxel as separate input to the pharmacokinetic model is termed parametric data analysis and provides more insights into spatial distribution of the radiotracer kinetics. However, it suffers from image noise and requires more computational resources [20]. Kinetic modeling does assist in deriving biologically relevant parameters, such as vascular transport and cellular metabolism, and asks for determination of the blood activity concentration of the native tracer over time as an input function to the model [21]. A compartment model of glucose metabolism is illustrated in Fig. 13.1. Mathematical bases of kinetic modeling are reviewed in Chap. 14.

In PET cardiac imaging, determination of myocardial blood flow and flow reserve can be measured using dynamic scanning of the heart region using some radiotracers such as O15-water, ammonia (N13), Rubidium-82 (Rb82), and other tracers that exhibit blood flow characteristics. Quantitation of myocardial blood flow using dynamic PET is reviewed in Chap. 19.

In neurology, dynamic PET has been a very useful tool in determination of important physiologic measures that reflect tracer receptor density, distribution volume, drug occupancy, and

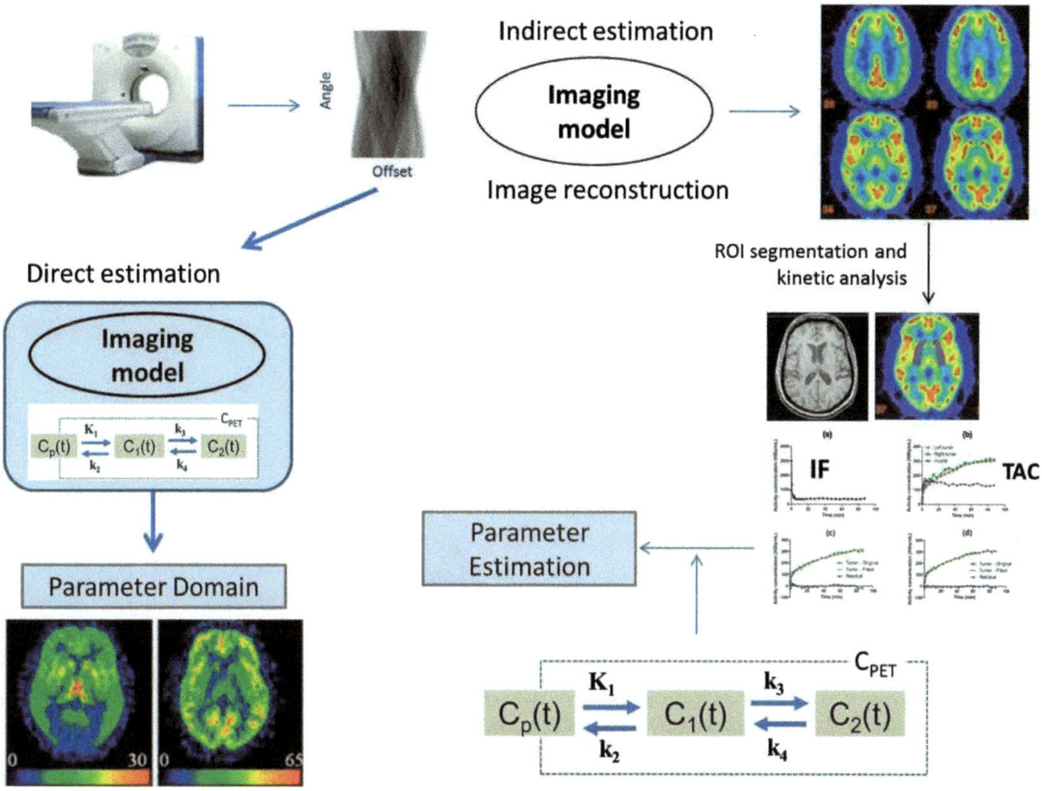

Fig. 13.2 Dynamic PET is used to determine valuable metabolic and functional parameters. The standard protocol relies on delineating regions of interest (ROIs) on a summed PET image reconstructed using the system model or a co-registered anatomical image. Time-activity curves (TACs) from the ROIs with collected information about tracer concentration in plasma (i.e., input function, IF) are used in the kinetic model to derive the physiologic tracer parameters. The other way around is to calculate rate parameters directly from sinogram data with less noisy estimates (Modified from Muzi et al. [21])

very instrumental tool in drug development [22]. In oncology, pharmacokinetic modeling provides valuable opportunities for measurements of receptor density of potential therapeutic targeting, determination of tumor blood flow, as well as measuring the efficacy of anticancer drugs [23].

Dynamic PET imaging-derived kinetic parameters, particularly transport (flow) and overall metabolic rate, have provided imaging endpoints for clinical trials at single-center institutions for years. However, dynamic imaging poses many challenges for multicenter clinical trial implementations from cross-center calibration to the inadequacy of a common informatics infrastructure [21]. Figure 13.2 illustrates the imaging workflow of static and dynamic PET image acquisition and data analysis. One recent study revealed that the influx rate constant K_i determined by Patlak graphical method in simulation and patient data has better contrast-to-noise ratio (a measure related to more reliable tumor detection), and this has remarkable advantage in lesions of high uptake surrounded by elevated but constant background levels such as liver lesions. Meanwhile, SUV performance was relatively poor [24]. Another study have used different methods for quantification of tumor activity (in a group of 40 patients with colon cancer metastatic to the liver) including SUV, Patlak graphical analysis, simplified kinetic model, and metabolic rate of glycolysis (MRGlu). Overall, Patlak was the best predictor of outcome and best discriminator between normal tissue and tumor results [25].

Several attempts have been devised to correlate the kinetically derived tracer influx rate constant K_i to SUV measurements by either making

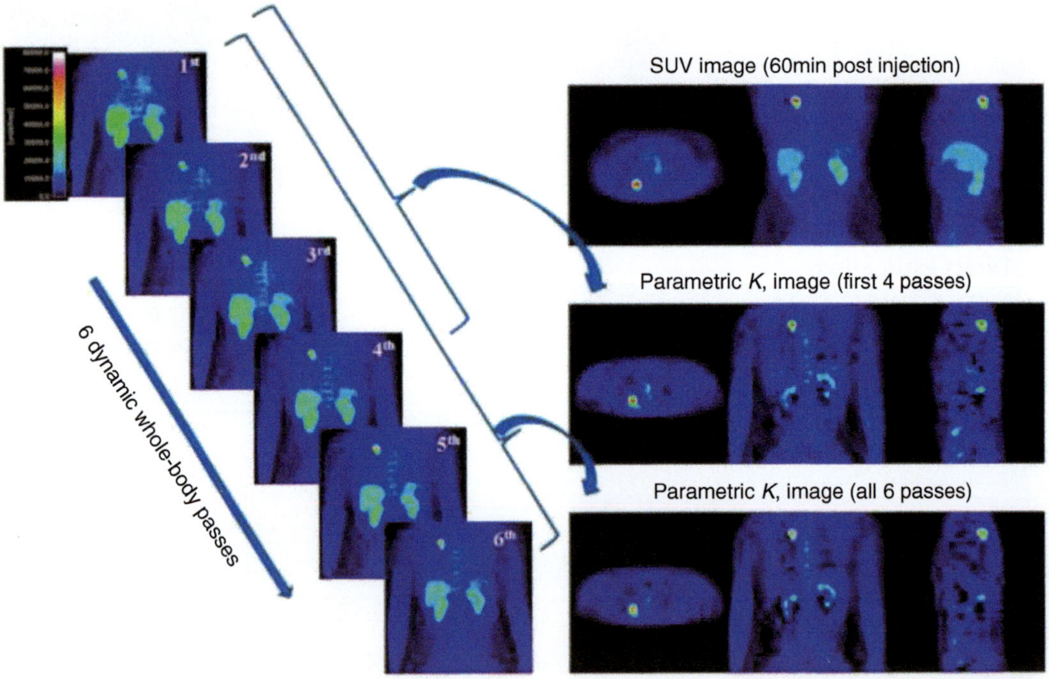

Fig. 13.3 Patlak analysis using six sequential whole-body PET scans. The last six whole-body dynamic frames are shown on the left side. On the right side: the SUV image, the K_i parametric image derived from all six last frames, and the K_i image after omitting the last two frames (Reprinted with permission from Karakatsanis et al. [24] and thanks to Dr Nicolas Karakatsanis for providing some clarification on the figure)

strong assumptions that could be violated in practice or still function of the imaging time point [26, 27]. The measuring time point is very crucial in estimating the metabolic activity, and wide variation could be found in different malignancies and in individual patients; therefore, quantitative image interpretation should be cautiously undertaken. Benign and inflammatory lesion uptake time could be within 30–60 min, while malignant tissues exhibit wide variation across patients that may reach plateau after 4 h [28]. Thus, recommendations are often taken to be within 50–70 min and not much longer to minimize the effect of tracer decay [29–31].

For example, dynamic F18-FDG PET imaging was found to accurately differentiate malignant from benign pulmonary lesions in patients with suspected malignant pulmonary lesions. SUV and visual assessment were outperformed by dynamic imaging data analysis in differentiating benign and malignant lesions [32]. However, whole-body dynamic PET imaging is not feasible at the moment due to limited axial field of view of most commercial PET scanners.

In a recent work, researchers proposed a new solution where dynamic whole-body imaging can be made feasible using the current PET/CT generation systems [24, 33]. It consists of a 6 min initial scan over the heart to extract the input function through image-based method to get rid of the cumbersome work associated with arterial catheterization. This action is followed by six passes of dynamic whole-body scanning including subsequent passes over the heart. Standard Patlak linear graphical analysis modeling is then applied at the voxel level to derive parametric images of K_i that reflects net tracer uptake [33]. The method looks interesting and combines between feasibility and advantages of dynamic quantitative features, but further work is needed to explore its potential in routine practice of patient diagnosis and therapeutic applications.

In Fig. 13.3 and in the SUV image, the patient was scanned with arms in the up position, according to the conventional whole-body PET protocol recommendations to limit the attenuation from the arms. However, for the whole-body dynamic protocol, the patient had to be scanned for approximately 45 min with arms down due to the lengthy period of the scan. It was observed that the additional attenuation that may be caused because of that position does not affect the quality of the data [24].

13.2.4 Static Versus Dynamic PET

As described, the net FDG influx rate constant K_i (mL blood/mL tissue/min) is a valuable quantitative measure that reflects the hexokinase and enzymatic capacity of the tumor cells. This measure was found to correlate with SUV measurements taking two conditions into account as outlined by Kotasidis et al. [26]:

1. The time integral of plasma FDG concentration is proportional to the injected dose divided by body weight (BW), lean body mass (LBM), or body surface area (BSA) as defined in the SUV formula. However, this assumption is not always valid due to, for example, treatment intervention that might interfere or influence dynamics of FDG in plasma, and a simple correlation with injected dose and BW, BSA, or LBM would not be effective.
2. Non-phosphorylated FDG that includes vascular and extravascular FDG should be negligible when compared to the phosphorylated FDG. This assumption can also be violated in FDG non-avid tumors where the vascular concentration and/or intracellular non-phosphorylated FDG are increased and the standard imaging time wouldn't be appropriate. In post-therapy conditions, there is also a chance to find an elevated background activity that impacts the SUV uptake profile taken over time [26].

From the above described points, one should be very careful in using the SUV in assessing response to treatment or using the SUV as a surrogate biomarker in clinical trials. The assumption that SUV is correlated with the metabolic rate of glycolysis (MRglu) and thus can be used as surrogate biomarker specially in clinical trials requires validation studies as some new drugs modify the FDG differential uptake due to, for example, increased inflammatory processes in other areas away from the tumor site(s) [27]. In some situations, it has been reported that up to 40% of FDG uptake occurs in non-tumor tissue in post-therapeutic evaluation [34].

Dual or multiple time point SUV measurement is an intermediate approach between static-based acquisitions and dynamic imaging. It considers the tumor uptake in timely spaced points instead of recording tumor uptake over a certain acquisition period while static because it doesn't look at tracer kinetics during data acquisition. It provides a good means for characterizing a given pathology whether inflammatory (or benign lesion) versus malignant lesions as the former generally shows a pattern of constant or tracer washout, while the malignant tissue often has a persistent or even accumulating uptake pattern (see Fig. 13.4).

Dual time point can serve to improve test sensitivity by improving lesion contrast and test specificity by excluding patients with abnormal or suspected findings. Its utility has been

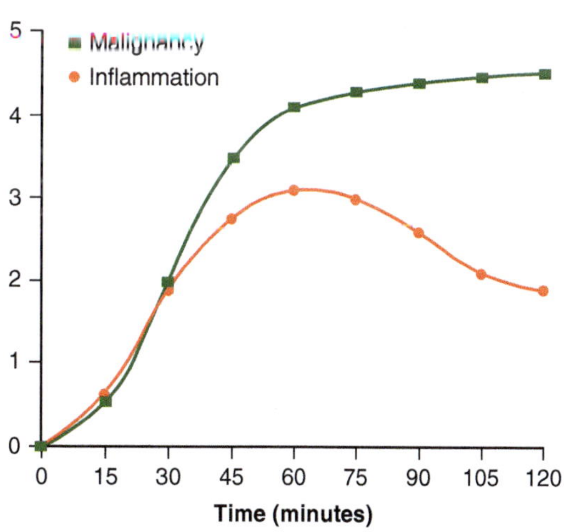

Fig. 13.4 General pattern of F18-FDG uptake in inflammatory and malignant lesions. Inflammatory cells exhibit a sort of transient retention and tracer washout, while cancer cells show a continuous tracer uptake over time (From Hess et al. [13] with permission from Springer Science+Business Media)

demonstrated in a number of malignancies including bone, head and neck, lung, breast, and colorectal cancers and infection or inflammatory disorders [35–38]. However, further efforts need to be exercised along with elaborate guidelines emphasizing the specifics of dual or multiple time points in routine clinical practice [39].

13.3 Standardized Uptake Value (SUV)

SUV is the most commonly used quantitative index in clinical PET imaging. SUV formula is very simple and this form is widely acceptable.

$$\text{SUV} = \frac{\text{Activity Concentration}\left(\text{Voxel or VOI}\right)}{\text{Normalized injected Activity}_{(\text{bw, lbm, or bsa})}}$$

Activity concentration is a quantity derived from a region of interest or voxel taken at a certain single region where the metabolic activity is of considerable clinical value. It can be kBq/ml or μCi/ml or any other equivalent unit.

Normalized injected activity is the administered PET tracer (i.e., injected dose) normalized to patient body weight (BW), body surface area (BSA), or lean body mass (LBM), and decay corrected to the PET acquisition start time. Note that the injected activity (e.g., MBq or mCi) should have the same unit like the one measured from the image 2D ROI, voxel or volume of interest (VOI).

Advantages of SUV are more than onefold. It is easy to calculate, available, and implemented as a built-in tool in viewing or processing workstations of all modern PET/CT scanners. It doesn't also require arterial blood sampling like other methods that rely on dynamic imaging and kinetic modeling as outlined earlier. It can principally be calculated at any single time point after tracer administration. There are several approaches devised to look for what is the most appropriate or representative voxel or group of voxels that accurately and reliably express metabolic activity within a given pathology. Therefore, there are a number of SUV variants that have been proposed in practice and will be discussed later.

Lesion contouring methods are also broad and range from very simple manual delineation to very sophisticated high-order automatic lesion segmentation. There are, however, some variables that need to be highlighted when attempts are made to work on PET data such as image noise, spatial resolution, image filtering, voxel size, degree of heterogeneity in the tumor, and uptake gradient within and outside the tumor relative to the background level [40]. Methods that can model or account for these variables while able to provide accurate and reproducible lesion segmentation can be the most preferable one for clinical adoption and standardization.

Substantial efforts have been carried out to address the problem of manual delineation that is prone to inter-subject and intra-subject variability. Several methods were developed for lesion segmentation task with different statistical or mathematical principles that may include thresholding; edge detection; watersheds; region growing; classifiers; clustering; gradient-based, fuzzy C-means or fuzzy locally adaptive Bayesian, Markov random field models; artificial neutral networks; deformable models; atlas-based methods; and others [41, 42]. Some studies were also conducted to address inherent differences and highlight the relative accuracies of those approaches [43]. However, there is no single optimal solution or consensus acceptable for all clinical problems in terms of accuracy, precision, and efficiency. This is particularly important in multicenter oncology studies where uniform delineation methods are required [44].

Investigators recognize that there is a substantial growing interest in applying fully automatic approaches that are clinically more feasible on efficiency and user-input levels [41]. Image segmentation in research could vary significantly based on the intended application and the adopted method together with the textural or morphological appearance of the oncologic lesions. Therefore, producing a benchmark database for validation and comparison of methods will be very beneficial for PET imaging detection tasks and image processing applications [41].

13.3.1 Drawbacks of SUV

Although the SUV has several quantitative and clinical implications, it has some potential drawbacks. It is simply a temporal and spatial oversimplification of the metabolic and biochemical process in question and doesn't provide a detailed description of tracer kinetics within different tissue compartments [28, 45]. The injected tracer undergoes a number of biochemical interactions that are not accounted for using SUV measurements and through which it may be converted from one chemical species to another or from vascular space to interstitial space or vice versa. Meanwhile, the SUV picks up only the total signal coming from the area of interest where all or some of these processes are taking place [46]. The biodistribution of tracer in a given lesion might include delivery, uptake, retention, and clearance, and these processes can't be separated by a single SUV metric. It is also impossible to separate the various components that contribute to the total signal such as specific binding, nonspecific binding, and free tracer in tissue [27].

Another quantitative shortcoming of SUV comes when using different radiotracers of tumor uptake that is not significantly different from healthy tissues. This situation stimulated researchers to look for alternative quantitative measures that potentially able to discriminate between pathologic lesion kinetics and other type of non-pathologic processes as demonstrated in 3′-[18 F]fluoro-3′-deoxythymidine (18 F-FLT) PET studies [11, 21].

13.3.2 SUV Variants

Quantitative PET and SUV metric has several levels of measurements based on the complexity of computation and the employed analytical methods [40]. The most commonly used SUV metrics are SUV_{mean}, SUV_{max}, and SUV_{peak}. The former is defined using the abovementioned formula for SUV calculations where the numerator is taken as the mean FDG or PET tracer concentration within the region or volume of interest. Measurements of SUV_{max} consider the maximal pixel concentration within the selected lesion. The SUV_{mean} is operator dependant and underestimates the true value especially in small lesions due to partial volume effect. On the other side, SUV_{max} is sensitive to noise as it increases positive bias as noise increases and a subject of debate in response to treatment monitoring [47, 48]. It has also some wrong implications and less representation in heterogenous tumor mass as more than SUV_{max} may exist within the same volume.

One study reported that the variability of SUV_{max} that can be attributed to image noise accounts for half of the overall variability [47]. They also reported that percentage change in $SUV_{max} < 30\,\%$ is still within the uncertainty of repeated measurement, and a positive bias of SUV_{max} can be as high as 30 % for short acquisition time (high noise level), evaluated as 1 min per bed position [47]. SUV_{mean} is much more variable due to operator-dependent factors including size and shape of mask delineation and location within or around a lesion, as well as the presence of tumor heterogeneity and variable level of background 18 F-FDG activity.

SUV_{peak} is the average SUV within a small, fixed-size region of interest (ROI peak) centered on a high-uptake part of the tumor. PET Response Criteria in Solid Tumors (PERCISTs) recommend SUV_{peak} taken for the lean body mass (i.e., SUL) as an index for tumor response [49]. It has several technical definitions as what are the most relevant ROI shape, size, and dimension. The shape can be square or cuboidal of side length of 7–15 mm. In terms of ROI geometries, it can be cylindrical, spherical, or even circular in diameters ranging from 9 to 17 mm [50]. For a given lesion, there might be more than one SUV_{peak}.

In a recent work, a number of 24 SUV_{peak} were used to look for the most appropriate variant in quantification of different tumor response using FLT as biomarker. ROI size was the most influential factor in SUV_{peak} variation when compared to ROI shape or location. In addition and generally, the intra-tumor SUV_{peak} tended to decrease, but its variation tended to increase as the size of ROI_{peak} increased [50]. Therefore, the SUV_{peak}

ROI candidate should be optimally chosen based on well-defined specific criterion in favor of accurate assessment of patient response for individual tumor. One report revealed that SUV_{peak} was the most robust method when using varying reconstruction methods, especially in small lesions when compared to SUV_{mean} and SUV_{max} [51]. In the same report, the latter two showed an increased variability in small lesions <5 ml, while SUV_{peak} remained more stable.

A robust and reliable estimate of SUV should be carried out based on standardized protocol and long-term observation on patient outcome. SUV measures are still "surrogate" biomarker and the accurate determinant, and reference gold standard is patient survival-based treatment response strategy [52]. In most cases, a number of lesion samples are taken to be quantified with less interest to cover all lesions and their metabolic volume or global metabolic activity leading to a relative sampling and assessment error based on the particular region selected. Nevertheless, a growing interest is currently being taken toward evaluating patients based on overall disease burden as follows in the next section.

13.4 Total Disease Burden

Total lesion glycolysis (TLG) is another metric that is used in quantifying total tumor burden. It is simply calculated by multiplying the SUV_{mean} by the lesion volume. This is for a single lesion, but when considering the whole-body tumor burden, then the values of all lesions TLG are summed up. Total metabolic tumor volume (TMTV) on the other hand reflects the total volume of all lesions within the whole body. These measures look at the overall or gross metabolic activity of cancer cells and eventually could be a potential measure of disease status and better candidates for monitoring response to treatment in comparison to uptake measures such as SUV and its variants [53–55].

It was first proposed in patients with Alzheimer to assess disease burden in an age-matched comparison along with partial volume correction [56]. The MR segmented brain structures were multiplied with the mean cerebral glycolytic activity, and end results showed that partial volume-corrected metabolic rates per unit weight of the brain were not significantly different in these cohorts, but that total brain metabolism was significantly lower in patients with Alzheimer. In addition, their efficacy and predictive power in correlation with recurrence-free survival or overall survival have then been investigated in the field of oncology. In cardiology, combining the FDG PET data and CT morphologic imaging of the chest covering the aortic region was proposed in calculating the atherosclerotic burden for each segment of the aorta by multiplying SUV with wall volume [57]. The arterial wall volume was calculated with the help of the CT contrast data delineating the inner and outer area of the aortic segment that appeared on each axial CT slice then subtracting to get the net volume.

In small-cell lung cancer, high TMTV and TLG were associated with poor survival outcomes, and both were reported to be significant independent prognostic factor, whereas SV_{mean} and SUV_{max} were poor measures and showed non-statistical significance in survival [58]. This was true especially in patients with limited disease rather than extended disease. However, finding a proper and reliable but may be combined prognostic indices could help physicians in taking risk-adapted therapeutic decision and better follow-up treatment strategy. For instance, SUV_{max} and MTV measured on pretreatment ^{18}F-FDG PET/CT in patients with oropharyngeal squamous cell carcinoma have shown to be independent variables in predicting clinical outcomes such as overall survival and disease-free survival [59].

In the context of head and neck cancer in response to chemoradiotherapy, multivariate analysis showed that high MTV (defined as tumor volume with SUV over 2.5) >25.0 mL and high TLG >144.8 g remained as independent significant predictors of incomplete response compared with low MTV and low TLG, respectively. However, predictive efficacy of pretreatment F18-FDG PET/CT varies with different primary sites and chosen parameters. Local response of laryngohypopharyngeal cancer was highly predictable by PET-/CT-based volume measurements [60].

Abgral et al. showed that the retention index (measured as percentage variation of SUV_{max}) and MTV measured for a cohort of head and neck squamous cell carcinoma patients using dual-phase (early-delay) technique were independently correlated with recurrence-free survival [61]. Global disease assessment will likely have great importance for improved pretreatment planning, patient selection for clinical trials, patient stratification, prediction of treatment response, and response assessment. Nevertheless, it was pointed out that the use of a whole-body metric involving TLG could be highly dependent on the severity of partial volume effect, and ignoring this pitfall in small lesions can greatly underestimate the total TLG compromising its potential prognostic value. However, this needs to be evaluated more thoroughly on an individual tumor basis [62].

Combining metabolic information and structural changes from PET and CT, respectively, was also an approach taken to monitor disease response to treatment. While a reduction in tumor volume using multi-detector row CT during chemotherapy for esophageal cancer was found a good predictor of histopathologic response [63], Larson et al. combined anatomic and functional information and monitoring changes using TLG derived from multiplying the tumor volume on CT with the FDG uptake on PET [64].

It should be noted that the new era of molecular-anatomical imaging has witnessed an emergence and advances not only from image co-registration and extracting invaluable diagnostic information but also on the way the data are quantified. Similarly, combining the powerful multiparametric concept in patient diagnosis to interrogate characteristic information of tumor biology within individual patients, despite expensive and technically demanding, can provide a wealth of information that guide physician to more accurate diagnosis and proper treatment.

13.5 Factors Affecting Quantitative Measurements

The quantitative approach implemented in SUV measurements has several sources of error and may lead to great under- or overestimation of the net results. It is not only related to biological factors or physiological conditions but also associated with quite large number of methodological and technical variables [65–67]. There are also some points that need to be addressed that influence SUV during patient preparation and radioactivity injection. Infiltrated or extravasated radioactivity during patient injection serves to underestimate the injected dose described in the SUV formula and hence compromise the SUV measurements [68].

Physical and technical or instrumental factors are also important variables and extend to include image acquisition and data reconstruction, uptake time, count density, reconstruction algorithm, examination time, scanner cross calibration with dose calibrator, and other corrections that include data normalization, dead time, random corrections, scatter and attenuation correction, and partial volume effect (PVE) (details can be found in Chap. 15). Reconstruction algorithm and selection of reconstruction parameters play an important role in the speed and rate of convergence and also to the final spatial resolution of the reconstructed image and might result in increased partial volume effects by making SUV more dependent on surrounding activity distributions [39, 51]. Other factors such as size, shape, and location of ROI/VOI used together with patient weight normalization factor are interplaying to determine the accuracy and reproducibility of SUV. In addition, application of contrast agents and the presence of metallic artifacts in CT images overestimate the attenuation factors and cause a significant elevation of SUV [69]. Patient stress and uncomfortable long waiting or exposure to cold conditions can cause increased uptake in muscle and brown fat affecting SUV measurements [70, 71].

Motion artifact is also one of the major issues in thoracic and abdominal PET imaging due to the blurring effect caused by organ motion during data acquisition. This is particularly important as it can reduce signal-to-noise ratio compromising delineation of lesion borders and corrupting SUV measurements together with less confidence in image interpretation. Several and extensive research works have been carried out to address this potential artifact and rectify the results of the SUV measurements. This topic was discussed in details in Chap. 16. Consequently, SUV should be carefully interpreted in body regions where motion exists, and thus special emphasis should be placed on longitudinal and follow-up studies [72].

13.5.1 Biological Factors

Accumulation and uptake of FDG within cells and tissues vary considerably, and a better understanding of the time activity profile of the tracer in a region of interest has important implications in data quantification. In the definition of SUV, the tracer concentration is the only variable for a given patient, and injected dose and hence an appropriate time point must be carefully selected to reflect clinically relevant information. This is also particularly important if the tracer accumulation and clearance occur at a relatively fast rate.

A number of studies have been conducted to look at the F18-FDG concentration over time to understand its kinetic parameters and biodistribution profile over body organs. This can potentially provide a baseline information to be used as guidelines for multiple point imaging sessions, using particular regions as reference for other pathologic lesions, or in delayed imaging protocol [73]. While FDG is taking up avidly by tumor cells of high glycolytic activity, its uptake value is less in some other types of tumor cells such as well-differentiated prostate adenocarcinoma and renal cell carcinoma [74, 75]. Furthermore, in poorly differentiated hepatocellular tumors, the degree of FDG uptake is relatively high when compared to well-differentiated tumors. An increased level of background activity can also be seen as concentration of dephosphorylating enzymatic activity (i.e., phosphatases) increases leading to FDG un-trapping and reuptake by normal liver cells. On the therapeutic level, high uptake by infiltrating immune cells can mask the decreased uptake by the dying tumor cells [76]. All the above scenarios have a confounding influence on the quantitative accuracy of PET data and should be placed into proper technical and clinical perspectives.

13.5.2 Blood Glucose Level

As mentioned earlier, the FDG molecule is taken avidly by tumor cells of high glycolytic activity. This interferes with the endogenous glucose to the extent that it may suppress the FDG uptake in the tumor or target cells especially at increased levels of blood glucose levels (e.g., diabetes). However, this was shown to have little effect in inflammatory cells [77]. FDG is a glucose analogue and competes with the plasma glucose through the transmembrane transporters (GLUTs) and intracellular enzymatic activity to enter into the cellular domain. Therefore, increased levels of blood glucose, as in hyperglycemia, play an important role in altering the relative uptake of FDG within different healthy tissues and unhealthy tumor cells. It can significantly reduce the retention of FDG in tumor cells underestimating the SUV measurements. Because of these shortcomings, guidelines have some recommendations of glucose levels for those referred for FDG PET scanning. The European Association of Nuclear Medicine (EANM) recommends that scanning be avoided above 11.1 mmol/L (about 200 mg/dL as an upper threshold limit), and for research the recommended upper plasma glucose levels may range between 7 and 8.3 mmol/L (126 and 150 mg/dL). Similarly, the Society of Nuclear Medicine and Molecular Imaging (SNMMI) recommends rescheduling the patient if the blood glucose level is greater than 150–200 mg/dL [78].

The use of insulin intervention to reduce glucose to normal levels has some characteristics that need to be understood. Insulin regulates glucose uptake into cells by recruiting membrane vesicles containing the GLUT glucose transporters from the interior of cells to the cell surface, where it allows glucose to enter cells by facultative diffusion. Increased levels of insulin in the blood therefore play a molecular role in eliciting the translocation of the GLUT protein transporter, and this phenomenon is significantly apparent in skeletal and cardiac muscles as well as adipose tissues [79].

While some recent optimized protocols for intravenous injection of insulin in diabetic patients were shown to lessen or avoid any abnormal FDG distribution, there are some other reports that show insulin may lead to unacceptable distribution of 25 % of diabetic cancer patients manifested by increased muscle uptake and decreased liver uptake [80]. It appears that insulin injection has some critical precautions that need to be placed into proper perspectives. The method of injection, the dose of insulin, the time between injection and imaging procedure, and the degree of hyperglycemia versus patient tolerance and response all seems to play a relative role in proper management of diabetic cancer patients [81].

In this context, it is important to mention that some drugs do alter the FDG uptake and significant change in SUV measurements can be observed. It has been shown that metformin, for example, significantly increases F18-FDG uptake in the colon and, to a lesser extent, in the small intestine, but lesion quantification might need further evaluation [82]. Stopping metformin has therefore been recommended so that lesion obliteration can be prevented [83]. For a review, see [84].

Attempts made to correct the SUV measurements for blood glucose level were reported to increase variability in test-retest studies when evaluating reproducibility in cancer-free population [85]. In obese patients, the fat contribution to the body composition is relatively large, and the FDG uptake is significantly low. This factor plays a role to overestimate the SUV measurements. This phenomenon is mitigated by using lean body mass or body surface area in SUV calculations [86, 87].

13.6 Response to Therapy

Evaluating patients after or during treatment of cancer represents one of the major challenges that physicians encounter in patient management. PET imaging continues to be a valuable tool to assess and manage cancer patients. A notable advantage of using FDG PET/CT in response monitoring is that metabolic changes often precede anatomical alterations [88]. Furthermore, newly developed targeted therapies may not even result in tumor shrinkage despite having a beneficial effect on patient outcome. FDG PET/CT has also been shown to have the potential to change in diagnosis and/or staging and/or treatment plan in more than one-third of patients with suspected or known malignant disease [89]. In addition, it has been demonstrated that it can detect therapeutic changes that permit physicians to revise or modify treatment protocol at early stages of therapeutic regimen. This has several implications in patient prognosis and survival rates.

The lack of metabolic response on FDG PET indicates primary resistance to the drug and may help identify patients who would benefit from another therapy, while re-emergence of metabolic activity within tumor sites following a period of therapeutic response indicates secondary resistance to the drug [90]. The importance of quantitative PET lies in inter-scan evaluation by providing valuable information about treatment efficacy as well as serving as objective measure of the clinical outcome. FDG uptake during treatment is different from uptake after treatment completion, and hence quantification comes into play [88]. It is not only F18-FDG which is used in drug evaluation and assessment of response to therapy, but also there are some other tracers such as F18-FLT that has been utilized in looking at proliferative capacity of the tumor cells. It has some early response capabilities in treatment monitoring and insensitivity to inflammatory lesions especially after radiotherapy and hence better characterization than FDG in this respect [91].

Some malignancies such as lymphoma can be qualitatively assessed for treatment response, whereas other tumors with less response success rate need a proper quantitative evaluation versus a particular therapy line. This is important to address partial metabolic response versus stable response or disease with further metabolic progression. Another valuable feature is obtained when successive measurements of treatment response would provide more insight into downstream outcomes such as survival [92].

A number of different treatment response criteria have been conducted to provide an objective and standardized assessment of therapy outcome and patient monitoring. Traditionally, the anatomically based tumor response criteria used were World Health Organization (WHO) and Response Evaluation Criteria in Solid Tumors (RECIST 1.0 and RECIST 1.1) which was introduced by the National Cancer Institute (NCI) [93–95]. The former defines the response as a decrease in the product of two perpendicular diameters of the tumor by 50 %, while RECIST defines partial response as a 30 % decrease in the sum of the diameters of target lesions [95].

In 1981, the WHO first published tumor response criteria, mainly for the use in trials where tumor response was the primary endpoint [96]. The criteria introduced the concept of an overall assessment of tumor burden by summing the products of the two longest perpendicular diameters of the measurable lesions and determined response to therapy by evaluation of change from baseline while on treatment. It is based on 2D lesion measurements, no specific requirements on the number of lesions or the smallest measurable lesion size, and therefore tends to be more subjective and time consuming.

On the other hand, key features of the original RECIST included definitions of minimum size of measurable lesions, instructions on how many lesions to follow (up to ten, a maximum five per organ site), and the use of one-dimensional rather than bidimensional measures for overall evaluation of tumor burden. These criteria have subsequently been widely adopted by several academic and nonacademic institutions as well as industry for trials where the primary endpoints are objective response or progression. There was also an interest from regulatory authorities in accepting RECIST as an appropriate guideline for these assessments [94].

There are two common criteria proposed when using metabolic imaging to evaluate tumor treatment response, namely, the European Organization for Research and Treatment of Cancer (EORTC) and PET Response Criteria in Solid Tumors (PERCISTs), and both have quite different approaches in lesion selection, ROI definition, body habitus normalization (body surface area versus lean body mass), and objective rank of disease status that includes progression or regression [49, 97]. Patients are then classified into different response categories based on the relative change in SUV. These categories include complete metabolic response, partial metabolic response, stable metabolic disease, and progressive metabolic disease.

The EORTC criteria were first published in 1999 and are based on baseline-chosen, lesion-specific regions of interest (ROIs) that are followed on each subsequent scan. The chosen lesions should be the most FDG avid. For SUV calculations, EORTC recommends that SUV should be normalized to body surface area [97]. However, the number of lesions to be measured and minimum measurable metabolic lesion was not specified leading to an increased inter-reader variability.

PERCIST was published in 2009, and some of the above shortcomings were circumvented such as determination of number of lesions, the minimum measurable lesion activity and background level, and the features that must exist in comparing between two scanning procedures [49]. This can improve interobserver variability and provide more reproducible data results. The target lesion is defined as the hottest single tumor lesion (SUL) of "maximal 1.2-cm diameter volume ROI in tumor" or SUL peak. PERCIST only evaluates the SUL peak of the hottest tumor. This is a possible limitation of the approach, and further work is warranted to determine how many lesions are needed for assessment [49].

This region is also selected on the basis of cancer stem cell theory regarded as an indicator of the patient's disease status at the given time point and no need to be located in the same lesion at every instance of evaluation. Conditions applied are such that the SUL peak is at least 1.5-fold greater than liver SUL mean + 2 SDs (in 3-cm spherical ROI in normal right lobe of the liver). If the liver is abnormal, primary tumor should have uptake greater than 2.0 x SUL mean of blood pool in 1-cm diameter ROI in descending thoracic aorta extended over 2-cm z-axis [49].

EORTC criteria was the first to provide a classification scheme based on patient treatment response: progressive or stable metabolic disease and partial or complete metabolic response that could be compared to traditional clinical trial endpoints such as overall survival. Its limitation might be ascribed to that fact that estimation parameters are outlined more as guidelines with options rather than clear definitions. This implies that the observer defines what the ROI size is, whether maximum or mean values should be chosen, how many and which target lesions should be registered, whether the SUVs should be summed or response should be calculated per tumor, and whether there should be a minimum SUV limit that a tumor should exceed in order to qualify as a target lesion [98]. Nevertheless, the EORTC criteria cover quantification of both metabolism and size of the tumor burden, whereas in PERCIST, disease status is determined by the most metabolically active portion of the tumor region.

13.7 Tumor Texture Analysis

Tumor heterogeneity is one of characteristics that can explain the underlying interplaying molecular and genetic factors for a given malignancy and possibly a given stage of disease development. At the time of clinical diagnosis, the majority of human tumors display remarkable heterogeneity in many morphological and physiological features, such as expression of cell surface receptors, and proliferative and angiogenic potential. This heterogeneity might be attributed substantially to morphological and epigenetic plasticity, but there is also strong evidence for the coexistence of genetically divergent tumor cell clones within tumors [99]. It is not generally easy to address this issue by just observing the different color or gray levels during image interpretation, and more objective descriptor can be a surrogate tool providing numerical evidence of tumor heterogeneity.

The process of identification, characterization, understanding, and possibly treatment of tumor heterogeneity is key challenges in oncology and can be an important aid in designing effective cancer therapeutics and monitoring strategies [100]. PET imaging is a promising candidate for determination of tumor heterogeneity within a given tumor mass due to its inherent molecular targeting and capabilities of image quantitation. Other methods have also been reported and of relative strength and weaknesses such as MRI, CT, ultrasonography, and also the use of pathological specimens in lesion characterization [101].

A standard image acquisition, reconstruction, and segmentation protocols are not only prerequisites for uniform data analysis among patients but also for other potential tasks such as establishing a criterion for tumor response assessment as well as in drug development process and clinical trials. Standards are needed to ensure that prospective studies that incorporate textural features are properly designed to measure true effects that may impact clinical outcomes as demonstrated by some investigators [102]. They also found complex trends in variability as a function of textural feature, lesion size, patient size, and reconstruction parameters. The sensitivity of PET textural features to normal stochastic image variation and imaging parameters was found large and is feature dependent.

To investigate the utility of texture analysis in real practice, several studies have been designed to address its clinical value in a number of malignancies. In patients presented with esophageal cancer and treated with combined radiochemotherapy, receiver-operating characteristic (ROC) curve analysis showed that tumor textural analysis was able to identify nonresponder, partial-responder, and complete-responder patients with higher sensitivity (76–92%) than any SUV measurement providing a stratification mechanism of esophageal carcinoma patients in the context of therapy-response prediction [103].

Pyka et al. and others demonstrated that evidences are growing to indicate that tumor heterogeneity as described by FDG PET texture is associated with response to radiation therapy in non-small cell lung cancer [104]. The results may be helpful into identifying patients who might profit from an intensified treatment regime. In another study from the same group, determination of tumor heterogeneity in pre-therapeutic 18 F-fluoroethyl-L-tyrosine (FET)-PET using textural features was beneficial for the subgrading of high-grade glioma as well as prediction of tumor progression and patient survival. It also showed improved performance compared to standard parameters such as tumor-background ratio and tumor volume [105]. Those two studies need further verification in a prospective patient cohort before being incorporated into routine clinical practice [104, 105].

Another report has shown that each subtype of non-small cell lung cancer, namely, adenocarcinoma and squamous cell carcinoma, has different metabolic heterogeneity supporting the use of textural parameters in FDG PET as an imaging biomarker [106]. There were 15 texture features that had significant different values between the two different tumor subtypes, and there was no high correlation between SUV_{max} and texture parameters ($|r| \leq 0.62$). Cheng et al. reported that uniformity extracted from the normalized gray-level co-occurrence matrix represents an independent prognostic predictor in patients with advanced T-stage oropharyngeal squamous cell carcinoma [107].

As described earlier, MTV is one of the potential prognostic indices, and correlation with tumor heterogeneity could provide complementary information in the same context. Volume and heterogeneity were found independent prognostic factors ($P = 0.0053$ and 0.0093, respectively) along with stage ($P = 0.002$) in non-small cell lung cancer, but in the esophageal tumors, volume and heterogeneity had less complementary value because of smaller overall volumes [108].

Conclusion

Image quantitation in PET examinations is one of the features that place PET in a unique position in morphological and molecular imaging matrix. Static imaging and dynamic imaging are the two common mode of data acquisition that can be used to derive the required sort of information. The former is the conventional type that used routinely in whole-body PET/CT during clinical practice, whereas dynamic imaging is limited to research activities but able to address "absolute" physiologic information of tracer pharmacokinetics. Due to technical limitation of current designs of PET systems, whole-body dynamic imaging can't be realized, but some trials are being done to overcome such limitation that could make it feasible in the clinic using modified acquisition protocols.

It has become evident that SUV measurements and its intrinsic characteristics of normalization to body weight, lean body mass, or surface body area could have an important implication on the accuracy and reproducibility of tracer quantitation. SUV measurements have several sources of error that could substantially impact its reliability, and thus careful measures need to be undertaken for successful adoption in the clinic.

Quantitative parameters derived from PET imaging data have valuable but differential diagnostic and predictive power in patient prognosis. Several challenges are facing nuclear medicine practitioners to standardize image acquisition, reconstruction, and data analysis so that any interinstitutional variability and systematic errors can be eliminated. This would help in correlating values among different clinics, building up large-scale database and providing more statistical power in data analysis. Now there are many quantitative measures that can be used in patient stratification, prognosis, and predicting tumor response to therapy; however, a universal guidance or general consensus from international societies should be in place to support and optimize the efforts toward finding the best approach for each malignancy.

References

1. Warburg O. On the origin of cancer cells. Science. 1956;123:309–14.
2. Warburg O, Posener K, Negelein E. Über den Stoffwechsel der Carcinomzelle. Biochem Z. 1924; 152:309–44.
3. Vander Heiden MG, Cantley LC, Thompson CB. Understanding the Warburg effect: the metabolic requirements of cell proliferation. Science. 2009; 324:1029–33.
4. Pauwels EK, Ribeiro MJ, Stoot JH, et al. FDG accumulation and tumor biology. Nucl Med Biol. 1998;25:317–22.
5. Hricak H. Oncologic imaging: a guiding hand of personalized cancer care. Radiology. 2011;259:633–40.
6. Vriens D, Visser EP, de Geus-Oei LF, Oyen WJ. Methodological considerations in quantification of

oncological FDG PET studies. Eur J Nucl Med Mol Imaging. 2009;37:1408–25.
7. Bentourkia M. Tracer kinetic modeling: methodology and applications. In: Khalil MM, editor. Basic sciences of nuclear medicine. Berlin/Heidelberg: Springer; 2011.
8. Kjell E. Tracer kinetic modeling: basics and concepts. In: Khalil MM, editor. Basic sciences of nuclear medicine. Berlin/Heidelberg: Springer; 2011.
9. Kostakoglu L, Gallamini A. Interim 18F-FDG PET in Hodgkin lymphoma: would PET-adapted clinical trials lead to a paradigm shift? J Nucl Med. 2013;54:1082–93.
10. Cistaro A, Quartuccio N, Mojtahedi A, et al. Prediction of 2 years-survival in patients with stage I and II non-small cell lung cancer utilizing (18) F-FDG PET/CT SUV quantification. Radiol Oncol. 2013;47:219–23.
11. Tomasi G, Turkheimer F, Aboagye E. Importance of quantification for the analysis of PET data in oncology: review of current methods and trends for the future. Mol Imaging Biol. 2011;14:131–46.
12. Boellaard R. Standards for PET image acquisition and quantitative data analysis. J Nucl Med. 2009;50 Suppl 1:11S–20.
13. Hess S, Blomberg B, Rakheja R, et al. A brief overview of novel approaches to FDG PET imaging and quantification. Clini Transl Imag. 2014;2:187–98.
14. Gholami S, Salavati A, Houshmand S, Werner TJ, Alavi A. Assessment of atherosclerosis in large vessel walls: a comprehensive review of FDG-PET/CT image acquisition protocols and methods for uptake quantification. J Nucl Cardiol. 2015;22:468–79.
15. von Schulthess GK, Steinert HC, Hany TF. Integrated PET/CT: current applications and future directions. Radiology. 2006;238:405–22.
16. Antoch G, Freudenberg LS, Egelhof T, et al. Focal tracer uptake: a potential artifact in contrast-enhanced dual-modality PET/CT scans. J Nucl Med. 2002;43:1339–42.
17. Brechtel K, Klein M, Vogel M, et al. Optimized contrast-enhanced CT protocols for diagnostic whole-body 18F-FDG PET/CT: technical aspects of single-phase versus multiphase CT imaging. J Nucl Med. 2006;47:470–6.
18. Varnas K, Varrone A, Farde L. Modeling of PET data in CNS drug discovery and development. J Pharmacokinet Pharmacodyn. 2013;40:267–79.
19. Klein R, Beanlands RS, deKemp RA. Quantification of myocardial blood flow and flow reserve: technical aspects. J Nucl Cardiol. 2010;17:555–70.
20. Dimitrakopoulou-Strauss A, Pan L, Strauss LG. Parametric imaging: a promising approach for the evaluation of dynamic PET-18F-FDG studies – the DKFZ experience. Hell J Nucl Med. 2010;13:18–22.
21. Muzi M, O'Sullivan F, Mankoff DA, et al. Quantitative assessment of dynamic PET imaging data in cancer imaging. Magn Reson Imaging. 2012;30:1203–15.
22. Jones T, Rabiner EA. The development, past achievements, and future directions of brain PET. J Cereb Blood Flow Metab. 2012;32:1426–54.
23. Watabe H, Ikoma Y, Kimura Y, Naganawa M, Shidahara M. PET kinetic analysis – compartmental model. Ann Nucl Med. 2006;20:583–8.
24. Karakatsanis NA, Lodge MA, Tahari AK, et al. Dynamic whole-body PET parametric imaging: I. Concept, acquisition protocol optimization and clinical application. Phys Med Biol. 2013;58:7391–418.
25. Graham MM, Peterson LM, Hayward RM. Comparison of simplified quantitative analyses of FDG uptake. Nucl Med Biol. 2000;27:647–55.
26. Kotasidis F, Tsoumpas C, Rahmim A. Advanced kinetic modelling strategies: towards adoption in clinical PET imaging. Clini Trans Imag. 2014;2:219–37.
27. Lammertsma A, Boellaard R. The need for quantitative PET in multicentre studies. Clini Transl Imag. 2014;2:277–80.
28. Hamberg LM, Hunter GJ, Alpert NM, et al. The dose uptake ratio as an index of glucose metabolism: useful parameter or oversimplification? J Nucl Med. 1994;35:1308–12.
29. Boellaard R, Delgado-Bolton R, Oyen WJ, et al. FDG PET/CT: EANM procedure guidelines for tumour imaging: version 2.0. Eur J Nucl Med Mol Imaging. 2015;42:328–54.
30. Boellaard R, O'Doherty MJ, Weber WA, et al. FDG PET and PET/CT: EANM procedure guidelines for tumour PET imaging: version 1.0. Eur J Nucl Med Mol Imaging. 2010;37:181–200.
31. Fukukita H, Suzuki K, Matsumoto K, et al. Japanese guideline for the oncology FDG-PET/CT data acquisition protocol: synopsis of Version 2.0. Ann Nucl Med. 2014;28:693–705.
32. Gupta N, Gill H, Graeber G, et al. Dynamic positron emission tomography with F 18 fluorodeoxyglucose imaging in differentiation of benign from malignant lung/mediastinal lesions. Chest. 1998;114:1105–11.
33. Karakatsanis NA, Lodge MA, Zhou Y, Wahl RL, Rahmim A. Dynamic whole-body PET parametric imaging: II. Task-oriented statistical estimation. Phys Med Biol. 2013;58:7419–45.
34. Kazama T, Faria SC, Varavithya V, et al. FDG PET in the evaluation of treatment for lymphoma: clinical usefulness and pitfalls. Radiographics. 2005;25:191–207.
35. Hustinx R, Smith RJ, Benard F, et al. Dual time point fluorine-18 fluorodeoxyglucose positron emission tomography: a potential method to differentiate malignancy from inflammation and normal tissue in the head and neck. Eur J Nucl Med. 1999;26:1345–8.
36. Sahlmann CO, Siefker U, Lehmann K, Meller J. Dual time point 2-[18F]fluoro-2′-deoxyglucose positron emission tomography in chronic bacterial osteomyelitis. Nucl Med Commun. 2004;25:819–23.
37. Tian R, Su M, Tian Y, et al. Dual-time point PET/CT with F-18 FDG for the differentiation of malignant and benign bone lesions. Skeletal Radiol. 2009;38:451–8.

38. Shimizu K, Okita R, Saisho S, et al. Clinical significance of dual-time-point 18F-FDG PET imaging in resectable non-small cell lung cancer. Ann Nucl Med. 2015;29:854–60.
39. Houshmand S, Salavati A, Hess S, et al. An update on novel quantitative techniques in the context of evolving whole-body PET imaging. PET Clini. 2015;10:45–58.
40. Carlier T, Bailly C. State-of-the-art and recent advances in quantification for therapeutic follow-up in oncology using PET. Front Med (Lausanne). 2015;2:18.
41. Foster B, Bagci U, Mansoor A, Xu Z, Mollura DJ. A review on segmentation of positron emission tomography images. Comput Biol Med. 2014;50:76–96.
42. Zaidi H, El Naqa I. PET-guided delineation of radiation therapy treatment volumes: a survey of image segmentation techniques. Eur J Nucl Med Mol Imaging. 2010;37:2165–87.
43. Tylski P, Stute S, Grotus N, et al. Comparative assessment of methods for estimating tumor volume and standardized uptake value in (18)F-FDG PET. J Nucl Med. 2010;51:268–76.
44. Boellaard R, Oyen WJ, Hoekstra CJ, et al. The Netherlands protocol for standardisation and quantification of FDG whole body PET studies in multicentre trials. Eur J Nucl Med Mol Imaging. 2008;35:2320–33.
45. Keyes Jr JW. SUV: standard uptake or silly useless value? J Nucl Med. 1995;36:1836–9.
46. Huang SC. Anatomy of SUV. Standardized uptake value. Nucl Med Biol. 2000;27:643–6.
47. Lodge MA, Chaudhry MA, Wahl RL. Noise considerations for PET quantification using maximum and peak standardized uptake value. J Nucl Med. 2012;53:1041–7.
48. Boellaard R, Krak NC, Hoekstra OS, Lammertsma AA. Effects of noise, image resolution, and ROI definition on the accuracy of standard uptake values: a simulation study. J Nucl Med. 2004;45:1519–27.
49. Wahl RL, Jacene H, Kasamon Y, Lodge MA. From RECIST to PERCIST: evolving considerations for PET response criteria in solid tumors. J Nucl Med. 2009;50 Suppl 1:122S–50.
50. Vanderhoek M, Perlman SB, Jeraj R. Impact of the definition of peak standardized uptake value on quantification of treatment response. J Nucl Med. 2012;53:4–11.
51. Brendle C, Kupferschlager J, Nikolaou K, et al. Is the standard uptake value (SUV) appropriate for quantification in clinical PET imaging? – variability induced by different SUV measurements and varying reconstruction methods. Eur J Radiol. 2014;84:158–62.
52. Weber WA. Assessing tumor response to therapy. J Nucl Med. 2009;50 Suppl 1:1S–0.
53. Manohar K, Mittal BR, Bhattacharya A, Malhotra P, Varma S. Prognostic value of quantitative parameters derived on initial staging 18F-fluorodeoxyglucose positron emission tomography/computed tomography in patients with high-grade non-Hodgkin's lymphoma. Nucl Med Commun. 2012;33:974–81.
54. Chung HH, Kwon HW, Kang KW, et al. Prognostic value of preoperative metabolic tumor volume and total lesion glycolysis in patients with epithelial ovarian cancer. Ann Surg Oncol. 2011;19:1966–72.
55. Liao S, Penney BC, Wroblewski K, et al. Prognostic value of metabolic tumor burden on 18F-FDG PET in nonsurgical patients with non-small cell lung cancer. Eur J Nucl Med Mol Imaging. 2012;39:27–38.
56. Alavi A, Newberg AB, Souder E, Berlin JA. Quantitative analysis of PET and MRI data in normal aging and Alzheimer's disease: atrophy weighted total brain metabolism and absolute whole brain metabolism as reliable discriminators. J Nucl Med. 1993;34:1681–7.
57. Bural GG, Torigian DA, Chamroonrat W, et al. Quantitative assessment of the atherosclerotic burden of the aorta by combined FDG-PET and CT image analysis: a new concept. Nucl Med Biol. 2006;33:1037–43.
58. Park SB, Choi JY, Moon SH, et al. Prognostic value of volumetric metabolic parameters measured by [18F] fluorodeoxyglucose-positron emission tomography/computed tomography in patients with small cell lung cancer. Cancer Imaging. 2014;14:2.
59. Kim JW, Oh JS, Roh JL, et al. Prognostic significance of standardized uptake value and metabolic tumour volume on (1)(8)F-FDG PET/CT in oropharyngeal squamous cell carcinoma. Eur J Nucl Med Mol Imaging. 2015;42:1353–61.
60. Hanamoto A, Tatsumi M, Takenaka Y, et al. Volumetric PET/CT parameters predict local response of head and neck squamous cell carcinoma to chemoradiotherapy. Cancer Med. 2014;3:1368–76.
61. Abgral R, Valette G, Robin P, et al. Prognostic evaluation of percentage variation of metabolic tumor burden calculated by dual-phase FDG PET-CT imaging in patients with head and neck cancer. Head Neck. 2016;38 Suppl 1:E600–6.
62. Hatt M, Le Pogam A, Visvikis D, Pradier O, Cheze Le Rest C. Impact of partial-volume effect correction on the predictive and prognostic value of baseline 18F-FDG PET images in esophageal cancer. J Nucl Med. 2012;53:12–20.
63. Beer AJ, Wieder HA, Lordick F, et al. Adenocarcinomas of esophagogastric junction: multi-detector row CT to evaluate early response to neoadjuvant chemotherapy. Radiology. 2006;239:472–80.
64. Larson SM, Erdi Y, Akhurst T, et al. Tumor treatment response based on visual and quantitative changes in global tumor glycolysis using PET-FDG imaging. The visual response score and the change in total lesion glycolysis. Clini Positron Imag. 1999;2:159–71.
65. Cook GJ, Wegner EA, Fogelman I. Pitfalls and artifacts in 18FDG PET and PET/CT oncologic imaging. Semin Nucl Med. 2004;34:122–33.
66. Gorospe L, Raman S, Echeveste J, et al. Whole-body PET/CT: spectrum of physiological variants, artifacts

and interpretative pitfalls in cancer patients. Nucl Med Commun. 2005;26:671–87.
67. Mawlawi O, Pan T, Macapinlac HA. PET/CT imaging techniques, considerations, and artifacts. J Thorac Imaging. 2006;21:99–110.
68. Silva-Rodriguez J, Aguiar P, Sanchez M, et al. Correction for FDG PET dose extravasations: Monte Carlo validation and quantitative evaluation of patient studies. Med Phys. 2014;41:052502.
69. Ahmadian A, Ay MR, Bidgoli JH, Sarkar S, Zaidi H. Correction of oral contrast artifacts in CT-based attenuation correction of PET images using an automated segmentation algorithm. Eur J Nucl Med Mol Imaging. 2008;35:1812–23.
70. Hao R, Yuan L, Zhang N, Li C, Yang J. Brown adipose tissue: distribution and influencing factors on FDG PET/CT scan. J Pediatr Endocrinol Metab. 2012;25:233–7.
71. Pace L, Nicolai E, D'Amico D, et al. Determinants of physiologic 18F-FDG uptake in brown adipose tissue in sequential PET/CT examinations. Mol Imaging Biol. 2010;13:1029–35.
72. Nehmeh SA, Erdi YE. Respiratory motion in positron emission tomography/computed tomography: a review. Semin Nucl Med. 2008;38:167–76.
73. Cheng G, Alavi A, Lim E, et al. Dynamic changes of FDG uptake and clearance in normal tissues. Mol Imaging Biol. 2013;15:345–52.
74. Delgado Bolton RC, Mucientes Rasilla J, Perez Castejon MJ, Carreras Delgado JL. Positron emission tomography (PET) and PET-CT in renal, bladder and prostate cancer: update. Actas Urol Esp. 2009;33:11–23.
75. Schoder H, Larson SM. Positron emission tomography for prostate, bladder, and renal cancer. Semin Nucl Med. 2004;34:274–92.
76. Merchant S, Witney T, Aboagye E. Imaging as a pharmacodynamic and response biomarker in cancer. Clini Trans Imag. 2014;2:13–31.
77. Zhao S, Kuge Y, Tsukamoto E, et al. Fluorodeoxyglucose uptake and glucose transporter expression in experimental inflammatory lesions and malignant tumours: effects of insulin and glucose loading. Nucl Med Commun. 2002;23:545–50.
78. Delbeke D, Coleman RE, Guiberteau MJ, et al. Procedure guideline for tumor imaging with 18F-FDG PET/CT 1.0. J Nucl Med. 2006;47:885–95.
79. Young LH, Coven DL, Russell 3rd RR. Cellular and molecular regulation of cardiac glucose transport. J Nucl Cardiol. 2000;7:267–76.
80. Roy FN, Beaulieu S, Boucher L, Bourdeau I, Cohade C. Impact of intravenous insulin on 18F-FDG PET in diabetic cancer patients. J Nucl Med. 2009;50:178–83.
81. Martin J, Saleem N. 18F-FDG PET-CT scanning and diabetic patients: what to do? Nucl Med Commun. 2014;35:1197–203.
82. Gontier E, Fourme E, Wartski M, et al. High and typical 18F-FDG bowel uptake in patients treated with metformin. Eur J Nucl Med Mol Imaging. 2008;35:95–9.
83. Ozulker T, Ozulker F, Mert M, Ozpacaci T. Clearance of the high intestinal (18)F-FDG uptake associated with metformin after stopping the drug. Eur J Nucl Med Mol Imaging. 2010;37:1011–7.
84. Surasi DS, Bhambhvani P, Baldwin JA, Almodovar SE, O'Malley JP. (1)(8)F-FDG PET and PET/CT patient preparation: a review of the literature. J Nucl Med Technol. 2014;42:5–13.
85. Paquet N, Albert A, Foidart J, Hustinx R. Within-patient variability of (18)F-FDG: standardized uptake values in normal tissues. J Nucl Med. 2004;45:784–8.
86. Kim CK, Gupta NC, Chandramouli B, Alavi A. Standardized uptake values of FDG: body surface area correction is preferable to body weight correction. J Nucl Med. 1994;35:164–7.
87. Kim CK, Gupta NC. Dependency of standardized uptake values of fluorine-18 fluorodeoxyglucose on body size: comparison of body surface area correction and lean body mass correction. Nucl Med Commun. 1996;17:890–4.
88. Allen-Auerbach M, Weber WA. Measuring response with FDG-PET: methodological aspects. Oncologist. 2009;14:369–77.
89. Hoilund-Carlsen PF, Gerke O, Vilstrup MH, et al. PET/CT without capacity limitations: a Danish experience from a European perspective. Eur Radiol. 2011;21:1277–85.
90. Van den Abbeele AD. The lessons of GIST – PET and PET/CT: a new paradigm for imaging. Oncologist. 2008;13 Suppl 2:8–13.
91. Bollineni VR, Kramer GM, Jansma EP, Liu Y, Oyen WJ. A systematic review on [F]FLT-PET uptake as a measure of treatment response in cancer patients. Eur J Cancer. 2016;55:81–97.
92. Doot RK, McDonald ES, Mankoff DA. Role of PET quantitation in the monitoring of cancer response to treatment: review of approaches and human clinical trials. Clini Transl Imag. 2014;2:295–303.
93. World, Health, Organization. WHO handbook of reporting results of cancer treatment. Geneva: World Health Organization; 1979.
94. Therasse P, Arbuck SG, Eisenhauer EA, et al. New guidelines to evaluate the response to treatment in solid tumors. European Organization for Research and Treatment of Cancer, National Cancer Institute of the United States, National Cancer Institute of Canada. J Natl Cancer Inst. 2000;92:205–16.
95. Eisenhauer EA, Therasse P, Bogaerts J, et al. New response evaluation criteria in solid tumours: revised RECIST guideline (version 1.1). Eur J Cancer. 2009;45:228–47.
96. Miller AB, Hoogstraten B, Staquet M, Winkler A. Reporting results of cancer treatment. Cancer. 1981;47:207–14.
97. Young H, Baum R, Cremerius U, et al. Measurement of clinical and subclinical tumour response using [18F]-fluorodeoxyglucose and positron emission

tomography: review and 1999 EORTC recommendations. European Organization for Research and Treatment of Cancer (EORTC) PET Study Group. Eur J Cancer. 1999;35:1773–82.
98. Skougaard K, Nielsen D, Jensen BV, Hendel HW. Comparison of EORTC criteria and PERCIST for PET/CT response evaluation of patients with metastatic colorectal cancer treated with irinotecan and cetuximab. J Nucl Med. 2013;54:1026–31.
99. Marusyk A, Polyak K. Tumor heterogeneity: causes and consequences. Biochim Biophys Acta. 1805; 2009:105–17.
100. Buvat I, Orhlac F, Soussan M. Tumor texture analysis in PET: where do we stand? J Nucl Med. 2015;56(11):1642–4.
101. Lubner MG, Stabo N, Lubner SJ, et al. CT textural analysis of hepatic metastatic colorectal cancer: pretreatment tumor heterogeneity correlates with pathology and clinical outcomes. Abdom Imaging. 2015;40:2331–7.
102. Nyflot MJ, Yang F, Byrd D, et al. Quantitative radiomics: impact of stochastic effects on textural feature analysis implies the need for standards. J Med Imag (Bellingham). 2015;2:041002.
103. Tixier F, Le Rest CC, Hatt M, et al. Intratumor heterogeneity characterized by textural features on baseline 18F-FDG PET images predicts response to concomitant radiochemotherapy in esophageal cancer. J Nucl Med. 2011;52:369–78.
104. Pyka T, Bundschuh RA, Andratschke N, et al. Textural features in pre-treatment [F18]-FDG-PET/CT are correlated with risk of local recurrence and disease-specific survival in early stage NSCLC patients receiving primary stereotactic radiation therapy. Radiat Oncol. 2015;10:100.
105. Pyka T, Gempt J, Hiob D, et al. Textural analysis of pre-therapeutic [18F]-FET-PET and its correlation with tumor grade and patient survival in high-grade gliomas. Eur J Nucl Med Mol Imaging. 2016;43:133–41.
106. Ha S, Choi H, Cheon GJ, et al. Autoclustering of non-small cell lung carcinoma subtypes on (18) F-FDG PET using texture analysis: a preliminary result. Nucl Med Mol Imag. 2015;48:278–86.
107. Cheng NM, Fang YH, Chang JT, et al. Textural features of pretreatment 18F-FDG PET/CT images: prognostic significance in patients with advanced T-stage oropharyngeal squamous cell carcinoma. J Nucl Med. 2013;54:1703–9.
108. Hatt M, Majdoub M, Vallieres M, et al. 18F-FDG PET uptake characterization through texture analysis: investigating the complementary nature of heterogeneity and functional tumor volume in a multi-cancer site patient cohort. J Nucl Med. 2015;56: 38–44.

14 Compartmental Modeling in PET Kinetics

Hiroshi Watabe

Contents

14.1	**Introduction**	323
14.2	**Basic Concepts for PET Data Analysis**	324
14.3	**Compartmental Model**	325
14.3.1	Definition and Assumptions of a Compartmental Model	325
14.3.2	Solutions of Compartmental Models	326
14.3.3	Parameter Estimation of Compartmental Model for PET Data	329
14.3.4	Linearization	333
14.4	**Physiological and Biological Basis of Compartmental Model**	338
14.4.1	Blood Flow and Oxygen Consumption	339
14.4.2	Partition Coefficient and Distribution Volume	340
14.4.3	In Vitro Receptor Binding Experiment and Binding Potential	340
14.5	**TAC and Input Function**	343
14.5.1	Acquisition of TAC	343
14.5.2	Acquisition of Input Function	344
Conclusions		349
References		349

H. Watabe, PhD
Division of Radiation Protection and Safety Control, Cyclotron and Radioisotope Center, Tohoku University, 6-3 Aoba, Aramaki, Aoba, Sendai 980-8578, Japan
e-mail: hwatabe@m.tohoku.ac.jp

Abstract

In this chapter, we explain how positron emission tomography (PET) data are analyzed to estimate behavior of radiotracer injected. For this purpose, compartmental model and its kinetic parameters are introduced, and concept, mathematical basis, and biological interpretation of the compartmental model and the kinetic parameters are described. General form of the compartmental model is brought for comprehensive understanding of the model. Several approaches for fast estimation of the kinetic parameters are introduced based on general compartmental model. The input function for the compartmental model is important for quantitative analysis of PET data, and the reference region model is one approach to avoid acquisition of the input function.

14.1 Introduction

Positron emission tomography (PET) enables us to quantitatively detect radiopharmaceuticals injected into a patient with very high sensitivity. The most widely used application for PET is the study with ^{18}F-fluorodeoxyglucose (^{18}F-FDG) for detecting tumor and monitoring cancer therapy. It uses the property of ^{18}F-FDG to accumulate cells in high energy demand. Usually in the ^{18}F-FDG

M.M. Khalil (ed.), *Basic Science of PET Imaging*, DOI 10.1007/978-3-319-40070-9_14

studies, only one static scan is performed at the certain time point after the administration of ^{18}F-FDG, and the medical doctor visually interprets the ^{18}F-FDG image whether the region of high uptake of ^{18}F-FDG exists or not, which is subjective and uses minimal advantages of PET. In this chapter, we describe several quantitative techniques for PET, which maximize potentials of PET. Especially basic idea and some applications for "compartmental modeling" will be discussed.

14.2 Basic Concepts for PET Data Analysis

For PET data analysis, it is important to understand the concept of "radiotracer" or, in short, "tracer." The "tracer" represents radiopharmaceutical used in general. PET study is initiated after injection of the tracer. If we consider the radiopharmaceutical as "tracer," we assume the amount of the tracer injected must be small enough, and it does not influence physiological processes and molecular interactions in the living body. Recently, PET microdosing studies have been introduced as a powerful tool of drug development [1]. In the microdosing studies, the pharmacokinetics of a new drug in the tissue targeted can be determined using PET with less than 1/100th of the dose of a test substance to yield a pharmacological effect or a maximum dose of ≤100 μg. To realize how small amount we inject, let's see the case of ^{18}F-FDG. The weight of ^{18}F-FDG is 181 g/mol, and if we inject 100 MBq of ^{18}F-FDG, the injected mole of ^{18}F-FDG is $100 \times 10^6/(\lambda \cdot N_A) = 1.58 \times 10^{-12}$ [mol] where λ is the decay constant of ^{18}F (1.05×10^{-4} [s^{-1}]) and N_A is the Avogadro constant (6.02×10^{23} [mol^{-1}]).[1] Therefore, the injected dose of ^{18}F-FDG corresponds to $181 \times 1.58 \times 10^{-12} = 0.286$ [ng], which is far below 100 μg of maximum microdosing dose. Another aspect of "tracer" is that the tracer's behavior represents behavior of the substance itself. Although the dose linearity in the microdosing studies is still an issue [1], we generally accept this assumption, and the quantitative outcomes from the tracer will represent the properties of the substance itself. However, the assumption may be invalid for brain receptor study. The specific activity (SA) is defined as the radioactivity per unit of substance (unit often used is GBq/nmol). In receptor study, if the tracer injected has very low SA, there are many nonradioactive molecules (carrier), and the carrier binds to the receptor, which consequently produces no signal from the tracer.

The standard uptake value (SUV) is the simplest and the most frequently used quantitative outcome of PET data analysis. The SUV is defined as the tissue concentration (Bq/kg) of tracer measured by PET scanner divided by the injected radioactivity (Bq) divided by body weight (kg) and unitless [2]. The SUV represents how much the tracer uptake exceeds under assumption of uniform distribution. Although the SUV is sometimes useful for diagnosis, the user of the SUV must pay caution to the meaning of SUV value. The SUV is actually referred to as semiquantitative parameter because there are many sources of variability such as subject's size, tracer concentration in blood, and time to be measured.

In principle, PET scanner detects 511 keV γ-rays emitted from the positron emitters and determines amounts and positions of the γ-ray sources, but it cannot distinguish physical and chemical properties of positron sources, and its signal in a voxel of PET image is composed of mixture of several photons from various sources such as the tracer binding to certain proteins, nonbinding tracer in plasma, and metabolized tracer which is altered in chemical form. In order to extract useful outcome from the mixed signal in a voxel, we must use temporal information of the tracers. To get the temporal information, dynamic data acquisition of PET must be performed, which results in time-activity curve (TAC) representing time course of radioactivity concentration of the tracer (Fig. 14.1. See Sect. 14.5 how to obtain TAC from PET image).

[1] We can also calculate the molar mass if we know the specific activity [GBq/nmol] of the tracer at the injection time.

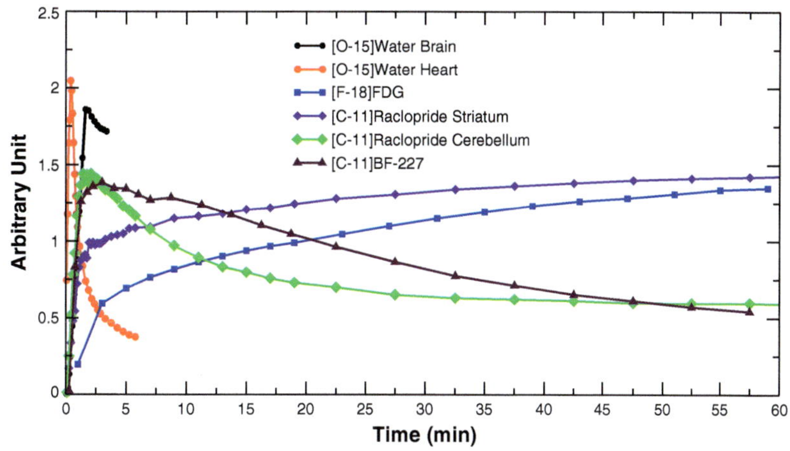

Fig. 14.1 Examples of TACs (time-activity curves) from several radiotracers

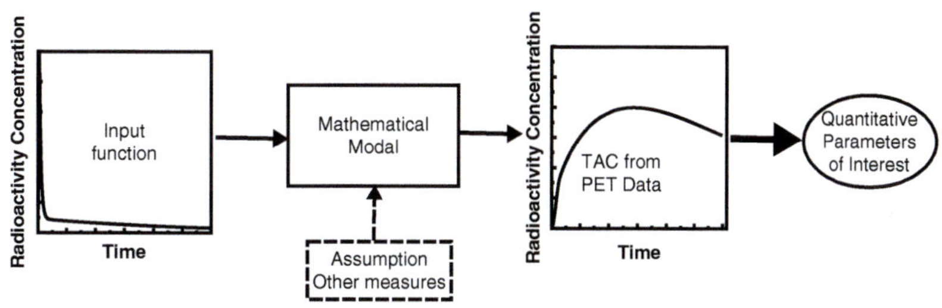

Fig. 14.2 Schematic diagram for analysis of tracer kinetics in PET data

Figure 14.2 shows scheme of PET data analysis. TAC of PET data is considered to be generated by input function under a mathematical model. The input function is the time course of radioactivity concentration of injected tracer in blood or plasma after the administration of the tracer and must be separately measured. The mathematical model consists of some parameters associated with certain physiological or biochemical information, and these parameters will be estimated by fitting the model to the observed TAC. It is important to choose the proper mathematical model to obtain meaningful results. The following section describes the most commonly used mathematical model, "compartmental model," [3] in detail.

14.3 Compartmental Model

This section describes compartmental model in mathematical point of view. Nomenclature and units in the text are tried to be consistent with recent consensus nomenclature [4].

14.3.1 Definition and Assumptions of a Compartmental Model

Figure 14.3 shows schematic drawings of three important compartmental models, namely, one-tissue compartmental model (1TC model), two-tissue compartmental model (2TC model), and three-tissue compartmental model (3TC model). As shown in this figure, several boxes are assumed to describe tracer's behavior inside the living organism. Each box is called "compartment" and represents a pool of homogeneous tracer substance. A tracer is transferred between compartments with a first-order rate constant (K_1, k_2, k_3, k_4, k_5, k_6 in Fig. 14.3) which is proportional to the concentration of the tracer in the compartment. The "compartment" is fairly conceptual and could be a spatial region or a chemical state.

$A(t)$ [Bq/mL] in Fig. 14.3 is time course (a function of time t [min]) of radioactivity concentration of the tracer, which delivers the tracer in the system and is called *input function*. The input function $A(t)$ is usually referred to the radioactivity concentration in blood or plasma

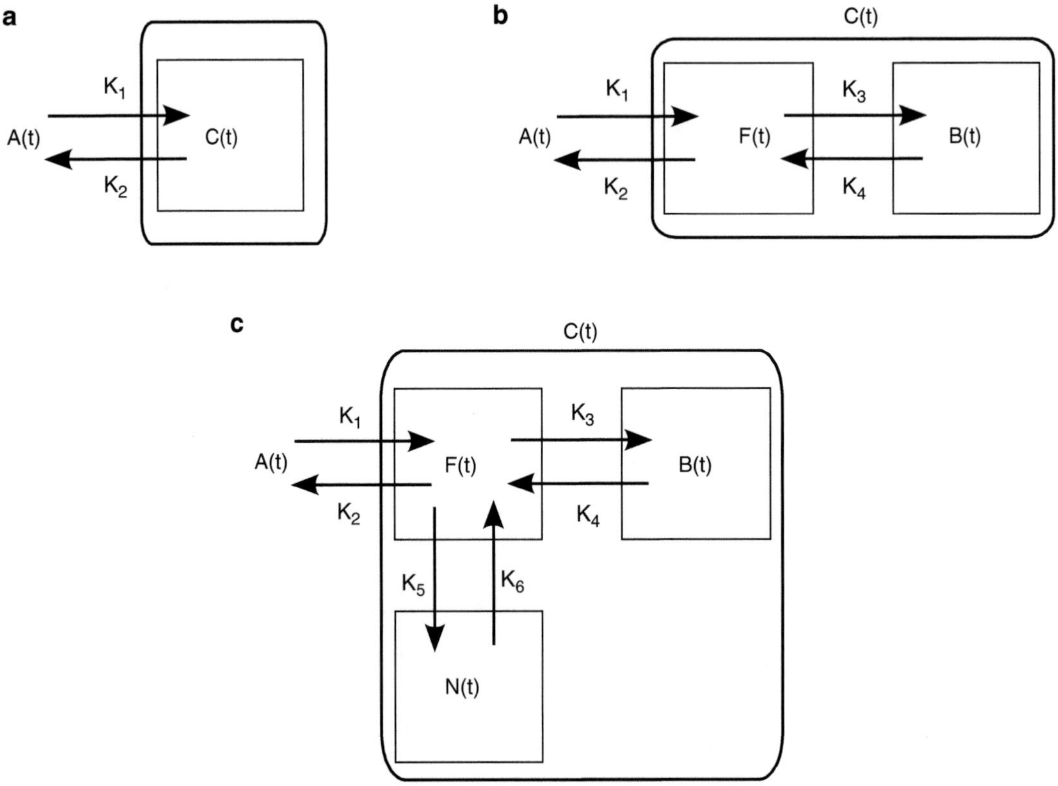

Fig. 14.3 Examples of compartmental models. (**a**) 1TC model, (**b**) 2TC model, and (**c**) 3TC model. *A*(*t*) input function, *F*(*t*) TAC in free (nondisplaceable) compartment, *B*(*t*) TAC in specific binding compartment, *N*(*t*) TAC in nonspecific binding compartment

and measured by frequent sampling of blood after administration of the radiotracer. The magnitude and shape of the input function are highly influenced by the manner of injection of the radiotracer. $C(t)$ [Bq/mL] in Fig. 14.3 is time course (a function of time t [min]) of the radiotracer in tissue measured by PET. Even though there are several compartments in tissue such as 2TC model and 3TC model in Fig. 14.3, PET can only measure total radioactivity concentrations of multiple compartments. We could refer $C(t)$ as a response of the system for the input function $A(t)$ (Fig. 14.2). The pharmacokinetics of most PET tracer can be expressed by either 1TC, 2TC, or 3TC model. Before analyzing PET data, we must choose the most proper model for the tracer of interest. It will be discussed how we select the proper model in the following sections.

14.3.2 Solutions of Compartmental Models

14.3.2.1 1TC Model

In 1TC model (Fig. 14.3a), the following differential equation is written between $A(t)$ [Bq/mL] and $C(t)$ [Bq/mL]:

$$\frac{dC(t)}{dt} = K_1 A(t) - k_2 C(t) \tag{14.1}$$

where rate constant from blood to tissue is K_1 [mL/cm^3/min] and rate constant from tissue to blood is k_2 [1/min]. Note that K in K_1 is capitalized to distinguish other rate constants which have unit of [1/min]. K_1 is unit of volume of blood (or plasma) (mL) per volume of tissue (cm^3) per minute. To solve differential equation with linear first-order parameters such as Eq. 14.1, Laplace transform can be utilized to solve the differential equation (Eq. 14.1) under the condition of $C(0)=0$ as follows:

$$C(t) = K_1 A(t) \otimes e^{-k_2 t} \tag{14.2}$$

where e is exponential function and $\otimes$ represents the convolution operation and is equivalent to

$$C(t) = K_1 \int_0^t e^{-k_2(t-\tau)} A(\tau)\, d\tau \tag{14.3}$$

Figure 14.4a shows an example of generated $C(t)$ from observed input function $A(t)$ by 1TC model (Eq. 14.2 or 14.3) with $K_1=0.5$ [mL/cm³/min] and $k_2=0.2$ [1/min]. For intuitively interpreting convolution operation, the above equation can be written as

$$\begin{aligned} C(t) &= \int_0^t K_1 e^{-k_2(t-\tau)} A(\tau)\, d\tau \\ &\simeq K_1 \sum_{\tau=0}^{\tau=t} e^{-k_2(t-\tau)} A(\tau) \Delta\tau \\ &\simeq K_1 \begin{pmatrix} e^{-k_2 t} A(0) + e^{-k_2(t-1)} A(1) + e^{-k_2(t-2)} \\ A(2) \cdots + A(t) \end{pmatrix} \end{aligned} \tag{14.4}$$

which indicates the $C(t)$ at time t is influenced by $A(t)$ in the past, i.e., $A(0)$ and $A(1)$ in Eq. 14.4. Figure 14.4b shows situation of Eq. 14.4 at time $t=10$ [min]. It is also noticed K_1 is scaling the input function and determinant of the magnitude of $C(t)$.

14.3.2.2 2TC Model

As shown in Fig. 14.3b, 2TC model has two compartments, and we often refer the first compartment as *free compartment* or *nondisplaceable compartment* (see detail in Sect. 14.4.2) and the second compartment as *binding compartment*, and their TACs are denoted $F(t)$ [Bq/mL] and $B(t)$ [Bq/mL], respectively. In 2TC model, two differential equations are derived with four parameters, K_1 [mL/cm³/min], k_2 [1/min], k_3 [1/min], and k_4 [1/min] as follows:

$$\frac{dF(t)}{dt} = K_1 A(t) - (k_2 + k_3) F(t) + k_4 B(t) \tag{14.5}$$

$$\frac{dB(t)}{dt} = k_3 F(t) - k_4 B(t) \tag{14.6}$$

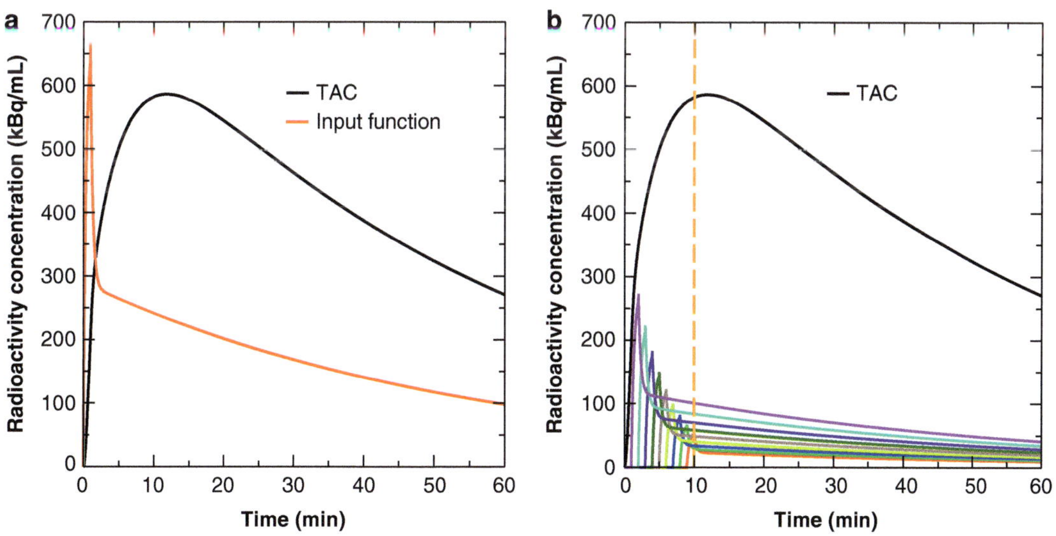

Fig. 14.4 (**a**) Input function (*red curve*) and generated TAC (*black curve*) by 1TC model (Eq. 14.2) with $K_1=0.5$ [mL/cm³/min] and $k_2=0.2$ [1/min] and (**b**) the input curve is scaled and shifted according to Eq. 14.4. Summed input curves at time 10 [min] generate TAC at time 10 [min]

PET cannot distinguish between $F(t)$ and $B(t)$ and can only detect summation of two compartments $C(t)$ expressed as

$$C(t) = F(t) + B(t) \tag{14.7}$$

Using Laplace transform and combining Eqs. 14.5, 14.6, and 14.7, $C(t)$ can be solved as follows:

$$C(t) = \frac{K_1}{\beta_2 - \beta_1}\left[(k_3 + k_4 - \beta_1)e^{-\beta_1 t} + (\beta_2 - k_3 - k_4)e^{-\beta_2 t}\right] \otimes A(t) \tag{14.8}$$

where β_1 and β_2 are defined as

$$\beta_{1,2} = \frac{1}{2}\left[(k_2 + k_3 + k_4) \mp \sqrt{(k_2 + k_3 + k_4)^2 - 4k_2k_4}\right] \tag{14.9}$$

There is a special case when k_4 is zero, which is often used for ^{18}F-FDG, and we call it *irreversible model* because the tracer will be trapped in one compartment (see Fig. 14.7c) (in contrary, the tracer which is not trapped in the compartment is called *reversible tracer*). For the irreversible model, Eq. 14.8 becomes by setting $k_4 = 0$

$$C(t) = \frac{K_1}{k_2 + k_3}\left[k_3 + k_2 e^{-(k_2 + k_3)t}\right] \otimes A(t) \tag{14.10}$$

14.3.2.3 3TC Model

As shown in Fig. 14.3c, 3TC model has three compartments in the tissue. TACs in the three compartments are often referred to as $F(t)$ [Bq/mL] for *free compartment*, $B(t)$ [Bq/mL] for *specific binding compartment*, and $N(t)$ [Bq/mL] for *nonspecific binding compartment*. The following three differential equations are given:

$$\begin{aligned}
\frac{dF(t)}{dt} &= K_1 A(t) - (k_2 + k_3 + k_5)F(t) + k_4 B(t) + k_6 N(t) \\
\frac{dB(t)}{dt} &= k_3 F(t) - k_4 B(t) \\
\frac{dN(t)}{dt} &= k_5 F(t) - k_6 N(t)
\end{aligned} \tag{14.11}$$

and the tissue TAC $C(t)$ [Bq/mL] observed by PET is the summation of three compartments as follows:

$$C(t) = F(t) + B(t) + N(t) \tag{14.12}$$

By using Laplace transform, the relationship between $A(t)$ and $C(t)$ can be expressed as

$$C(t) = K_1\left[\alpha_1 e^{-\beta_1 t} + \alpha_2 e^{-\beta_2 t} + \alpha_3 e^{-\beta_3 t}\right] \otimes A(t) \tag{14.13}$$

where β_1, β_2, and β_3 are three solutions of the cubic function below:

$$\begin{aligned}
&x^3 + (k_2 + k_3 + k_4 + k_5 + k_6)x^2 \\
&+ \left[k_4(k_2 + k_5 + k_6) + k_6(k_2 + k_3)\right]x \\
&+ k_2k_4k_6 = 0
\end{aligned} \tag{14.14}$$

Several methods have been proposed for solving the cubic function, such as Cardano's method. The α_1, α_2, and α_3 are defined as

$$\begin{aligned}
\alpha_1 &= \frac{\beta_1^2 + (k_3 + k_4 + k_5 + k_6)\beta_1 + k_4k_6 + k_3k_6 + k_4k_5}{(\beta_1 - \beta_2)(\beta_1 - \beta_3)} \\
\alpha_2 &= \frac{\beta_2^2 + (k_3 + k_4 + k_5 + k_6)\beta_2 + k_4k_6 + k_3k_6 + k_4k_5}{(\beta_2 - \beta_1)(\beta_2 - \beta_3)} \\
\alpha_3 &= \frac{\beta_3^2 + (k_3 + k_4 + k_5 + k_6)\beta_3 + k_4k_6 + k_3k_6 + k_4k_5}{(\beta_3 - \beta_1)(\beta_3 - \beta_2)}
\end{aligned} \tag{14.15}$$

3TC model with six parameters can be theoretically solved; however, in practical, it is too complicated to apply 3TC model for the actual PET data that the reduction of parameters and some assumptions to constrain parameters are required [5].

14.3.2.4 General Solution for Compartmental Model

Generally if there are n compartments in tissue, relationship between input function as $A(t)$ and TAC as $C(t)$ can be expressed as follows [6]:

$$C(t) = A(t) \otimes \sum_{i=1}^{n} \alpha_i e^{-\beta_i t} \tag{14.16}$$

The input function $A(t)$ is impulse or Dirac delta function, which is an infinite height at time 0 with an integral of one. If we define $R(t)$ as follows

$$R(t) = \sum_{i=1}^{n} \alpha_i e^{-\beta_i t} \tag{14.17}$$

Equation 14.16 can be rewritten as

$$C(t) = A(t) \otimes R(t) \tag{14.18}$$

We call the function $R(t)$ impulse response function (IRF) which is a system response against impulse input function. The α_i and β_i in $R(t)$ are combinations of several rate constants as shown in Eqs. 14.8 and 14.9 for 2TC model and Eqs. 14.14 and 14.15 for 3TC model. IRF describes the behavior of the compartmental model which reflects properties of the injected tracer and the tissue of interest (see Fig. 14.5 for two examples of IRF). On the other hand, the shape of the input function is highly dependent on how the radiotracer is injected. As shown in Fig. 14.6, two input functions (Fig. 14.6a) produce very different TACs from a unique IRF. It is also worth to note that there are many possibilities of compartmental models to produce the same IRF. Figure 14.7a, c shows conventional 2TC models (one is reversible and the other is irreversible) and Fig. 14.7b, d models of two independent compartments inside. Their biological contexts are very different, but they share equivalent IRF in mathematical sense. The rate constants such as K_1, k_2, k_3, and k_4 are called

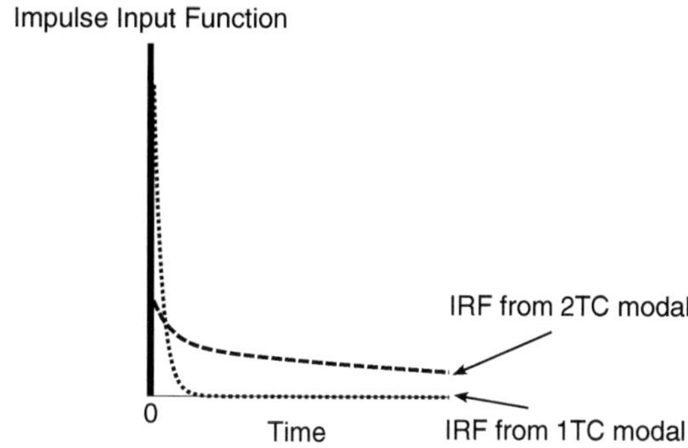

Fig. 14.5 Impulse input function and two response functions. *Dotted line* is generated from 1TC model and *dashed line* is generated from 2TC model

micro-parameters and sometimes difficult to estimate with high precision due to noise in PET data, and only *macro-parameters* which are α_i, β_i, or combinations of α_i and β_i are available. For example, one of the most frequently used macro-parameters, *total distribution volume* V_T [mL/cm^3], is defined as below using Eq. 14.17 (see Sect. 14.4.2 for physiological definition of V_T):

$$V_T = \int_0^{\infty} R(t)\,dt - \sum_{i=1}^{i=n} \frac{\alpha_i}{\beta_i} \tag{14.19}$$

14.3.3 Parameter Estimation of Compartmental Model for PET Data

We will estimate rate constants or macro-parameters which explain the time course of the measured PET data. Generally, from input function $A(t)$ and n data of TAC $C_{PET}(t_i)$ ($i = 1, \ldots, n$) measured by PET, the parameters will be estimated by minimizing χ^2 in equation below:

$$\chi^2 = \sum_{i=0}^{n} \omega_i \left(C_{PET}(t_i) - C(t_i)\right)^2 \tag{14.20}$$

where $C(t_i)$ is the estimated TAC at time t_i calculated by Eq. 14.18 and ω_i is the weighting factor at time t_i and is inversely proportional to the variance of measured data $C(t_i)$ (discussed below). Figure 14.8a shows examples of observed TAC and estimated TACs by 1TC model and 2TC

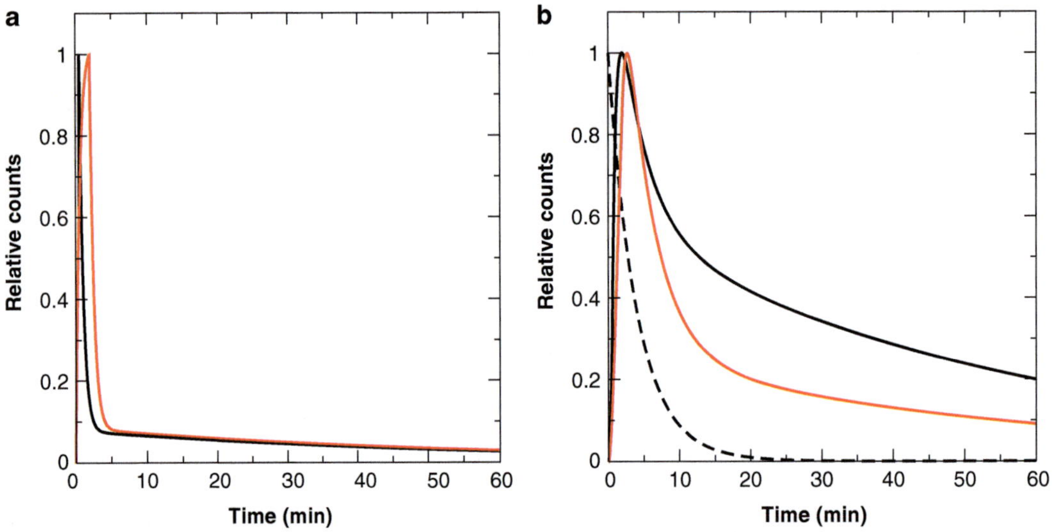

Fig. 14.6 (**a**) Two input functions, (**b**) IRF (*dashed line*), and two TACs generated from the two input functions (*black and red lines*)

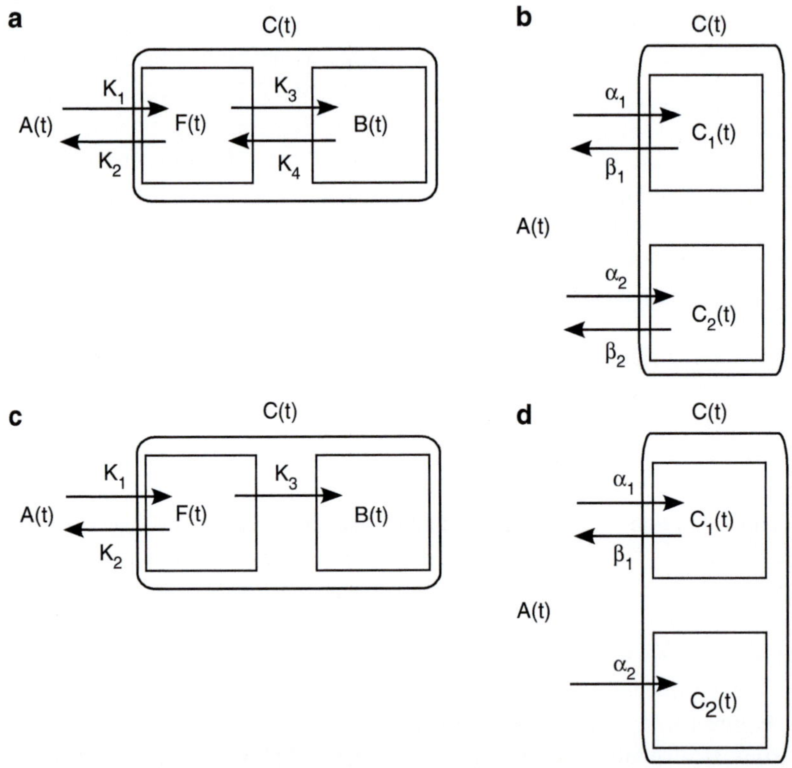

Fig. 14.7 Examples of compartmental models which have two compartments in tissue. (**a**) Conventional 2TC model, (**b**) model with two independent compartments, (**c**) conventional irreversible model for ^{18}F-FDG, and (**d**) model with two independent compartments: one is reversible and the other is irreversible compartment

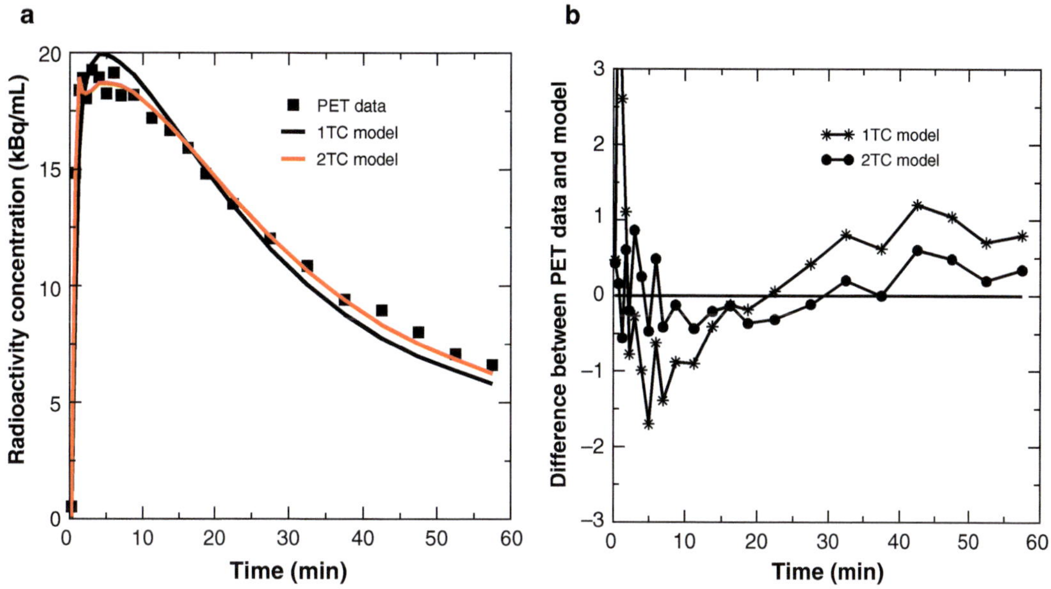

Fig. 14.8 Examples of fitting PET data by 1TC model or 2TC model. (**a**) Observed TAC data $C_{PET}(t_i)$ (*filled square*) and estimated TAC $C(t_i)$ by 1TC model (*black line*) and 2TC model (*red line*). (**b**) Differences between $C(t_i)$ and $C_{PET}(t_i)$

model. Figure 14.8b shows plots of $(C_{PET}(t_i) - C(t_i))$. So the minimum χ^2 in Eq. 14.20 has the smallest offset from zero line in Fig. 14.8b.

The problem to minimize χ^2 is called the weighted least squares problem. Especially, in the case of Eq. 14.18, $\partial R/\partial \beta_i$ in Eq. 14.17 is not independent to β_i, and we must deal with *nonlinear least squares problem* or *nonlinear fitting problem*. In general, to solve the nonlinear fitting problem, we must give the initial guesses of estimated parameters and iteratively calculate Eq. 14.20 until no further improvement is achieved. There are several techniques to update estimated parameters at each iteration. One major approach is to go to the steepest descent direction for each parameter by computing gradient of the parameter against Eq. 14.20. Another major approach known as the Gauss-Newton approach is to use the first-order Taylor series expansion which results in a linear function and can be solved by linear regression technique. The Marquardt-Levenberg algorithm is a composition of the steepest descent approach and Gauss-Newton approach [7]. The techniques mentioned above require calculation of derivatives, which sometimes introduces source of error since there is no analytic solution for the derivatives and numerical computation of derivatives must be carried out. Another approach, the downhill simplex method [8], requires no derivative calculation although the method itself is very slow.

The ω_i in Eq. 14.20 must be set before the parameter estimation. The variance of PET data is related to many factors, including events of random coincidence and scattered photon inside the field of view (FOV), reconstruction algorithm, size of region, time duration of data acquisition, and time passed after the injection of radiotracer. Therefore, ω_i must be set under assumption. The uniform weighting factor is often used, but this assumption must be used with caution especially for radiotracer with short half-lives such as ^{15}O (about 2 min of half-life) and ^{11}C (about 20 min of half-life), which have lower count rate at later time frames due to radioactive decay. By accounting for radioactive decay and frame duration, the weighting factor can be approximated as follows [9]:

$$\omega_i \propto \frac{\Delta t_i \cdot e^{-\lambda t_i}}{C_{PET}(t_i)} \tag{14.21}$$

where Δt_i [min] is the frame duration of PET data at time t_i and λ is the decay constant (0.340 [min^{-1}] for ^{15}O, 0.0340 [min^{-1}] for ^{11}C, and 0.00631 [min^{-1}] for ^{18}F). Alternatively, the inverse of noise equivalent counts (NEC) as a good guess of variance in PET data is employed for approximation of ω_i [10].

In contrast to the linear regression which has a unique solution without iterations, the nonlinear fitting does not guarantee to have one unique solution. Figure 14.9 shows schematic drawings to represent to search the solution in the nonlinear fitting. If the squared sum computed by given parameters looks like Fig. 14.9a, the solution is only one at the bottom of the valley. In the case of Fig. 14.9b, the sum of squares has many valleys (local minima), and estimated results are highly dependent on the starting point. In the case of Fig. 14.9c, there is only one valley of the squared sum, but many solutions are possible (Fig. 14.9).

In Fig. 14.8a, b, it is apparent the 2TC model is better than the 1TC model for fitting the PET data. Generally a model with more parameters (four parameters for 2TC model versus two parameters for 1TC model) gives better fitting results. However, it is not always implying a model with more parameters can describe more precisely

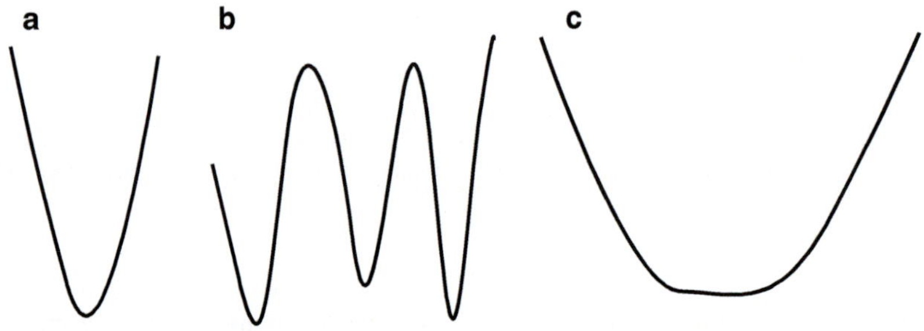

Fig. 14.9 Schematic drawings of solutions of nonlinear fitting. (**a**) Only one solution exists, (**b**) multiple local minima exist, and (**c**) many solutions are possible

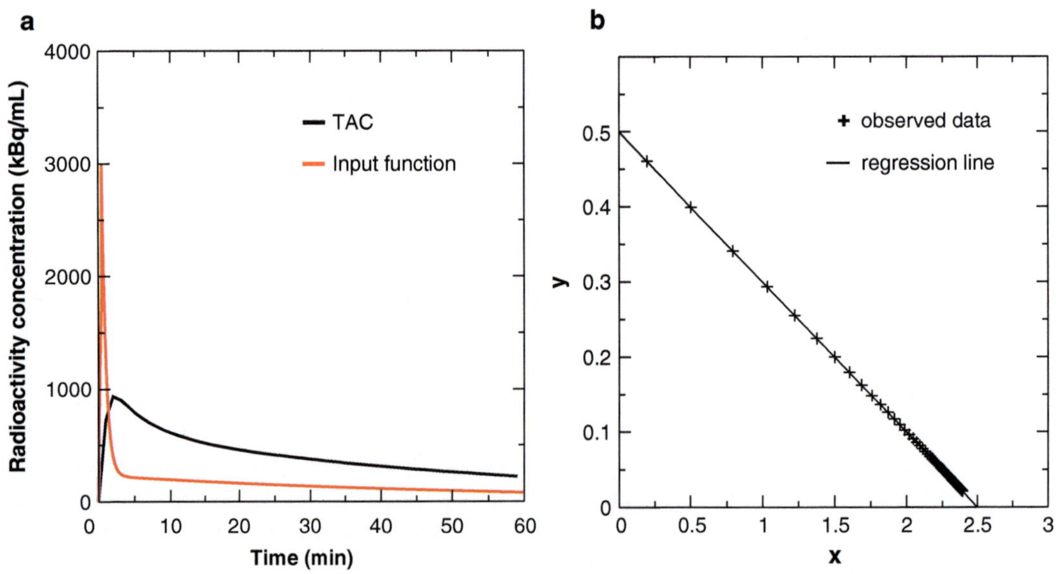

Fig. 14.10 (**a**) TAC (*black curve*) and input function (*red curve*). TAC is generated by 1TC model with $K_1 = 0.5$[mL/cm^3/min] and $k_2 = 0.2$[1/min]. (**b**) Plot of Eq. 14.24 and a regression line. Intercept of y-axis is 0.5[mL/cm^3/min] as K_1 and x-axis is 2.5 as K_1/k_2

physiological or biological properties than simpler model. There are several statistical tests that have been proposed to compare between the models such as the AIC (Akaike information criterion), SC (Schwarz criterion, also called Bayesian information criterion (BIC)), or F-test [11]. Impulse response fraction [12] can be employed to predict the reliability of the model with more than one compartments over the 1TC model. The impulse response fraction for 2TC model is defined as

$$f = \frac{\alpha_2\left[1-e^{-\beta_2 T}\right]/\beta_2}{\alpha_1\left[1-e^{-\beta_1 T}\right]/\beta_1+\alpha_2\left[1-e^{-\beta_2 T}\right]/\beta_2} \quad (14.22)$$

where α_1, α_2, β_1, and β_2 are from Eq. 14.16 under condition of $\beta_1<\beta_2$ and T is the duration of data acquisition. This equation implies the relative contribution of the second compartment against the first compartment. If this fraction is close to 0, it is difficult to distinguish two compartments separately. It is also important to be aware of the identifiability of each micro-parameter. If the cross correlation between two parameters is high and these parameters are not independently identified, only macro-parameters must be utilized with confidence, or the simpler model is recommended to be used. It often happened that the 1TC model must be employed for analysis even though 2TC and 3TC models are a biochemically proper choice [5].

14.3.4 Linearization

As described above, nonlinear fitting to estimate parameters has several drawbacks including computational burden, large parameter variation, and poor parameter identification due to local minima. To overcome these problems, "linearization" techniques have been proposed, in which linear least fitting procedure is performed instead of the nonlinear fitting.

14.3.4.1 1TC Model

Equation of 1TC model is relatively easy to linearize due to simplicity of the model. Integration of Eq. 14.1 from time zero to time t yields

$$C(t) = K_1\int_0^t A(\tau)d\tau - k_2\int_0^t C(\tau)d\tau \quad (14.23)$$

It is purposeful to use integration operation because PET scanner does not have enough temporal resolution to measure $C(t)$ instantaneously, and the scanner actually measures the integration of $C(t)$ over time. From the above equation, K_1 and k_2 can be solved by multiple linear regression technique between the dependent variable $C(t)$ and two regressors, $\int_0^t A(\tau)d\tau$ and $\int_0^t C(\tau)d\tau$. Furthermore, dividing both sides by $\int_0^t A(\tau)d\tau$, Eq. 14.23 can be rewritten [13]:

$$\frac{C(t)}{\int_0^t A(\tau)d\tau} = K_1 - k_2\frac{\int_0^t C(\tau)d\tau}{\int_0^t A(\tau)d\tau} \quad (14.24)$$

If we plot $\frac{\int_0^t C(\tau)d\tau}{\int_0^t A(\tau)d\tau}$ as x and $\frac{C(t)}{\int_0^t A(\tau)d\tau}$ as y and a regression line is computed, intercepts of y-axis and x-axis are K_1 and $V_T = K_1/k_2$, respectively.

Another popular linearization technique for 1TC model is an autoradiographic technique [14]. This technique is often used for measuring blood flow with $^{15}O\text{-}H_2O$. Here, we assume the ratio of tissue concentration C to concentration of input function A at equilibrium is constant. $p = C/A$ [mL/cm^3] at equilibrium is called *partition coefficient* and p can be expressed as K_1/k_2 for 1TC model. If p is constant and known, integration of Eq. 14.2 from time t_1 to t_2 becomes

$$\int_{t_1}^{t_2} C(\tau)d\tau = K_1\int_{t_1}^{t_2} A(\tau)\otimes e^{-\frac{K_1}{p}\tau}d\tau \quad (14.25)$$

The right side of Eq. 14.25 is precomputed within reasonable range of K_1 using measured input function $A(t)$ and fixed p value. By using this table (look-up table) and measured $\int_{t_1}^{t_2} C(\tau)d\tau$, K_1 is uniquely determined (Fig. 14.11).

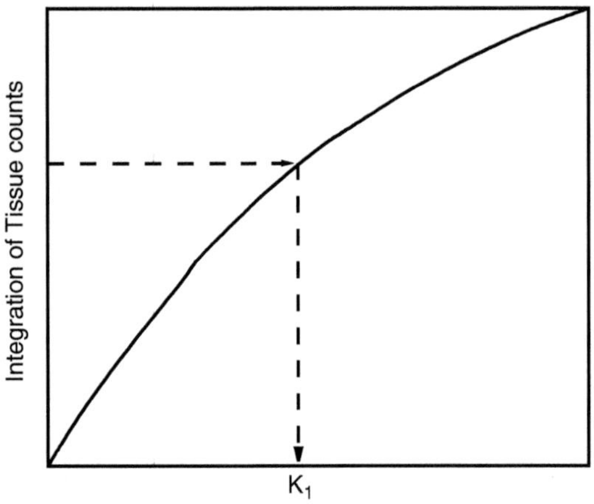

Fig. 14.11 Look-up table for autoradiographic technique. $\int_{t_1}^{t_2} C(\tau)d\tau$ (y-axis) for different K_1 values are precomputed, and from PET data, K_1 is uniquely determined

14.3.4.2 Logan Plot

The most frequently employed linearization for reversible tracer is so-called Logan plot [15]. The Logan plot is a model-free approach since it does not require any assumption about the number of compartments. In this section, the formula of the Logan plot is derived from model with two independent compartments (Fig. 14.7b), but it is easily extendable for general model expressed in Eq. 14.16. For each compartment, the following differential equation can be written as similar as 1TC model:

$$\begin{aligned} \frac{dC_1(t)}{dt} &= \alpha_1 A(t) - \beta_1 C_1(t) \\ \frac{dC_2(t)}{dt} &= \alpha_2 A(t) - \beta_2 C_2(t) \end{aligned} \tag{14.26}$$

As same as Eq. 14.23, integration of both sides from 0 to time t yields

$$\begin{aligned} C_1(t) &= \alpha_1 \int_0^t A(\tau)d\tau - \beta_1 \int_0^t C_1(\tau)d\tau \\ C_2(t) &= \alpha_2 \int_0^t A(\tau)d\tau - \beta_2 \int_0^t C_2(\tau)d\tau \end{aligned} \tag{14.27}$$

By arranging the above two equations and considering $C(t) = C_1(t) + C_2(t)$, we will get the following equation:

$$\int_0^t C(\tau)d\tau = \left(\frac{\alpha_1}{\beta_1} + \frac{\alpha_2}{\beta_2}\right)\int_0^t A(\tau)d\tau - \frac{\beta_2 C_1(t) + \beta_1 C_2(t)}{\beta_1\beta_2} \tag{14.28}$$

Both sides of the above equation is divided by $C(t)$, and the equation becomes

$$\begin{aligned} \frac{\int_0^t C(\tau)d\tau}{C(t)} &= \left(\frac{\alpha_1}{\beta_1} + \frac{\alpha_2}{\beta_2}\right)\frac{\int_0^t A(\tau)d\tau}{C(t)} - \frac{\beta_2 C_1(t) + \beta_1 C_2(t)}{\beta_1\beta_2 C(t)} \\ &= V_T \frac{\int_0^t A(\tau)d\tau}{C(t)} - \left[\frac{1}{\beta_1} + \frac{\beta_1 - \beta_2}{\beta_1\beta_2}\frac{C_2(t)}{C(t)}\right] \end{aligned} \tag{14.29}$$

where V_T is called the total distribution volume as defined by Eq. 14.19. If the Logan plot is the plot of $\frac{\int_0^t A(\tau)d\tau}{C(t)}$ as x and $\frac{\int_0^t C(\tau)d\tau}{C(t)}$ as y as shown in Fig. 14.12b), d, the plot is fitted well to straight line, and the slope of the line represents V_T. Equation 14.29 indicates two particular cases dependent on the second term on the left side of the equation. If β_2 has a similar range to β_1 and is relatively large (*fast kinetics* Fig. 14.12a, b), $C_2(t)/C(t)$ in the third term of Eq. 14.29 becomes constant. In this case, the Logan plot shows linearity from the beginning of the point (Fig. 14.12b). On the other hand, if β_2 is small and the tracer has *slow kinetics* (see TAC of $C_2(t)$

in Fig. 14.12c), only later points of the Logan plot become linear as shown in Fig. 14.12d. The time beyond which the Logan plot becomes linear is called t^*. The t^* must be carefully determined. The wrong t^* results in the underestimation of V_T [16]. Another pitfall of the Logan plot is the problem of noise in the data [17]. The $C(t)$ is in the denominators of both sides of Eq. 14.29, which introduces noise not only in the dependent variable (y) but also in the independent variable (x). To overcome these pitfalls, some attempts have been applied such as "multilinear analysis [16]" and "principle component analysis (PCA) [18]."

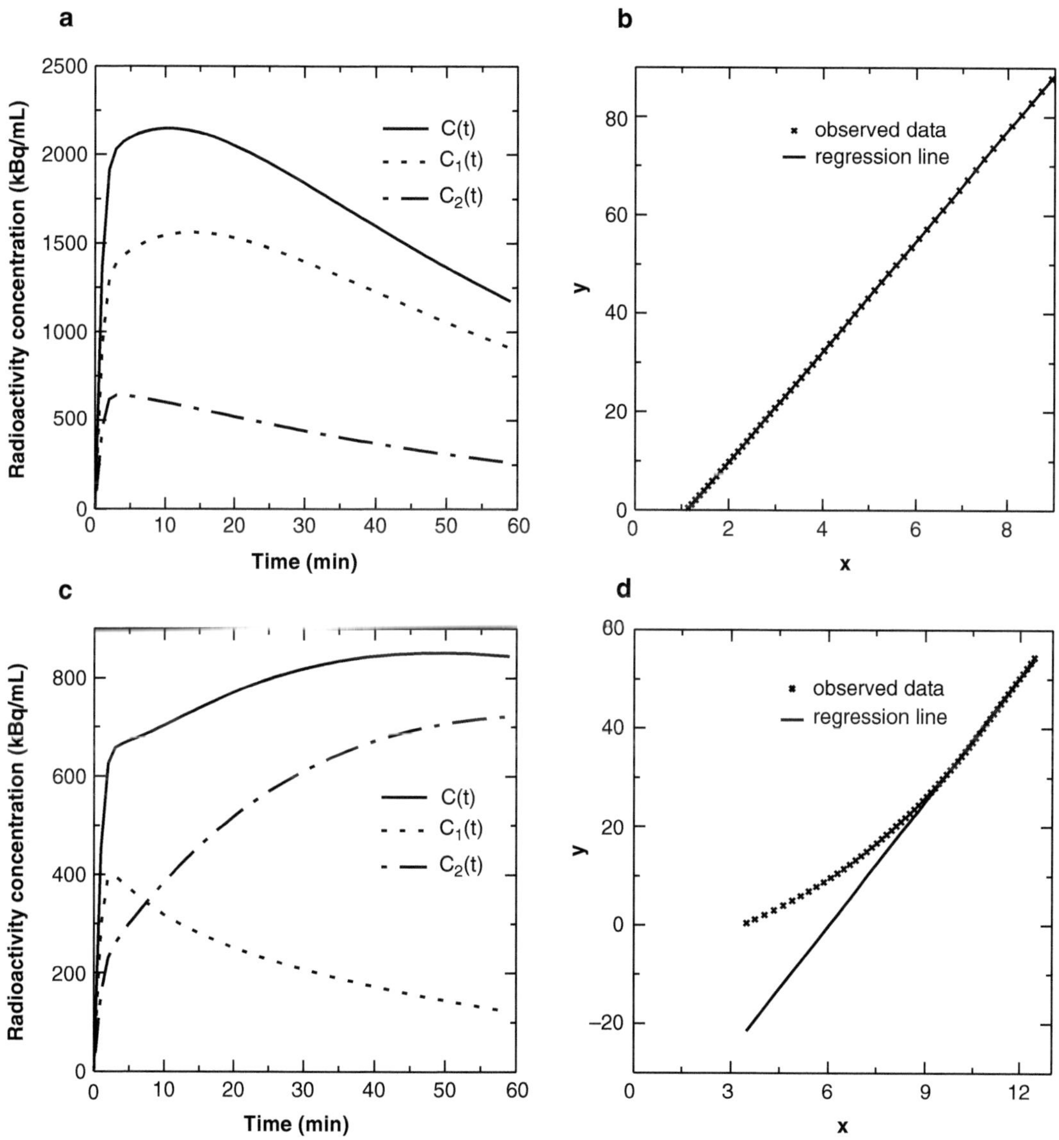

Fig. 14.12 Two cases (fast and slow kinetics) of TACs (**a**, **c**) and Logan plots (**b**, **d**). For fast kinetics, TACs of $C_1(t)$, $C_2(t)$, and $C(t)$ were generated with parameters of $\alpha_1=0.6$, $\alpha_2=0.3$, $\beta_1=0.07$, $\beta_2=0.11$, and for slow kinetics, TACs of $C_1(t)$, $C_2(t)$, and $C(t)$ were generated with parameters of $\alpha_1=0.2$, $\alpha_2=0.1$, $\beta_1=0.15$, $\beta_2=0.01$

14.3.4.3 Patlak Plot

The Patlak plot[2] is another important linearization approach for irreversible tracer [19, 20]. As same as the Logan plot, the Patlak plot is a model-free approach, but here we use model with two individual compartments for derivation of formula of the Patlak plot (Fig. 14.7d). Differential equations for the model are as follows:

$$\begin{aligned}\frac{dC_1(t)}{dt} &= \alpha_1 A(t) - \beta_1 C_1(t)\\ \frac{dC_2(t)}{dt} &= \alpha_2 A(t)\end{aligned} \quad (14.30)$$

Integration from time 0 to t for the above equations yields

$$\begin{aligned}C_1(t) &= \alpha_1 \int_0^t A(\tau)d\tau - \beta_1 \int_0^t C_1(\tau)d\tau\\ C_2(t) &= \alpha_2 \int_0^t A(\tau)d\tau\end{aligned} \quad (14.31)$$

The above equations are divided by $A(t)$:

$$\begin{aligned}\frac{C_1(t)}{A(t)} &= \alpha_1 \frac{\int_0^t A(\tau)d\tau}{A(t)} - \beta_1 \frac{\int_0^t C_1(\tau)d\tau}{A(t)}\\ \frac{C_2(t)}{A(t)} &= \alpha_2 \frac{\int_0^t A(\tau)d\tau}{A(t)}\end{aligned} \quad (14.32)$$

Combination of the above two equations with $C(t) = C_1(t) + C_2(t)$ makes the following equation:

$$\begin{aligned}\frac{C(t)}{A(t)} &= (\alpha_1+\alpha_2)\frac{\int_0^t A(\tau)d\tau}{A(t)} - \beta_1 \frac{\int_0^t C_1(\tau)d\tau}{A(t)}\\ &= \alpha_2 \frac{\int_0^t A(\tau)d\tau}{A(t)} + \frac{\alpha_1 \int_0^t A(\tau)d\tau - \beta_1 \int_0^t C_1(\tau)d\tau}{A(t)}\\ &= \alpha_2 \frac{\int_0^t A(\tau)d\tau}{A(t)} + \frac{C_1(t)}{A(t)}\end{aligned} \quad (14.33)$$

If time passes and $\frac{C_1(t)}{A(t)}$ becomes constant (expected constant value is α_1/β_1), Eq. 14.33 will be linear between $\frac{\int_0^t A(\tau)d\tau}{A(t)}$ and $\frac{C(t)}{A(t)}$. If we can consider the tracer's kinetics follows 2TC model, α_2 corresponds to $\frac{K_1 k_3}{k_2 + k_3}$ in Eq. 14.10, and it is often denoted as K_i and called metabolic rate.

[2] It is sometimes called *Gjedde-Patlak plot* named after two authors describing this approach.

Figure 14.13 shows two examples of Patlak plots (large k_3 and small k_3). K_i can be written as $K_i = \frac{K_1}{1+\frac{k_2}{k_3}}$; therefore, if the system has large k_3 (high affinity), K_i becomes highly dependent on K_1 (blood flow or transport of tracer from blood) and less sensitive against change of k_3. In the case of small k_3 (Fig. 14.13c, d), K_i value increased to 83 % when k_3 is changed from 0.01 to 0.02 [1/min]. And in the case of large k_3 (Fig. 14.13a, b), K_i value increased to only 33 % when k_3 is changed from 0.1 to 0.2 [1/min]. These phenomena are called "delivery/flow limitation effect."

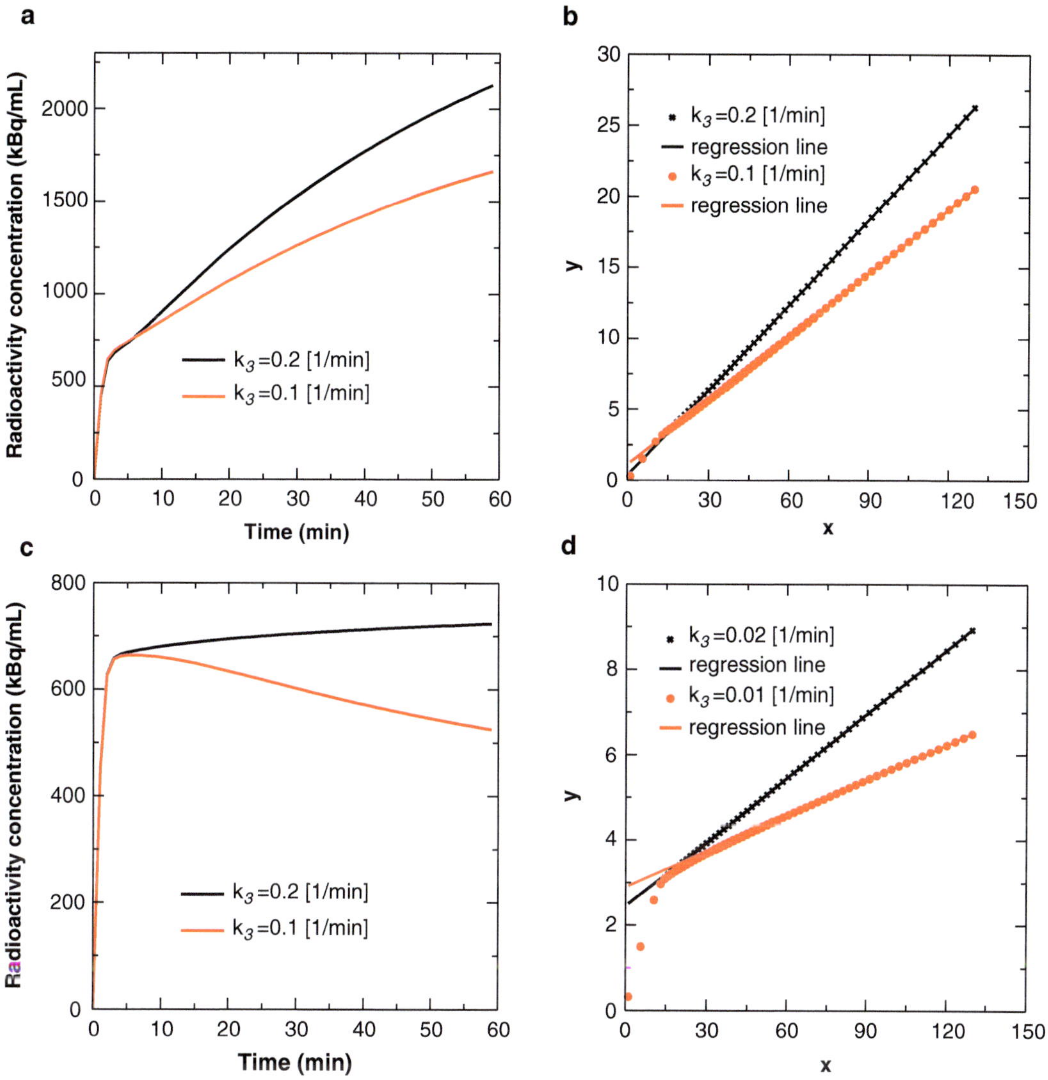

Fig. 14.13 Two cases (large k_3 and small k_3 kinetics) of TACs (**a**, **c**) and Patlak plots (**b**, **d**). In both cases, TACs are generated with $K_1 = 0.3$ and $k_2 = 0.1$

14.3.4.4 Spectral Analysis

Spectral analysis is a model-free method and even one can estimate how many compartments the system has by the spectral analysis [21, 22]. General compartmental model can be written according to Eq. 14.16:

$$C(t) = \sum_{i=1}^{n} \alpha_i e^{-\beta_i t} \otimes A(t) = \sum_{i=1}^{n} \alpha_i B_i(t)$$
$$B_i(t) = e^{-\beta_i t} \otimes A(t) \tag{14.34}$$

$B_i(t)$ is called *basis function*, and if $B_i(t)$ is predefined with N sets of discrete β_i values, the estimation of α_i becomes a linear equation. Strictly, α_i must not be negative, and nonnegative least squares (NNLS) algorithm and simplex algorithm are employed for estimation of α_i. Usually, a discrete set of β_i is chosen in physically and physiologically available range from physical decay constant (e.g., 0.000105 [s^{-1}] for ^{18}F) to 1 [s^{-1}]. Due to a large range of β_i, the range is

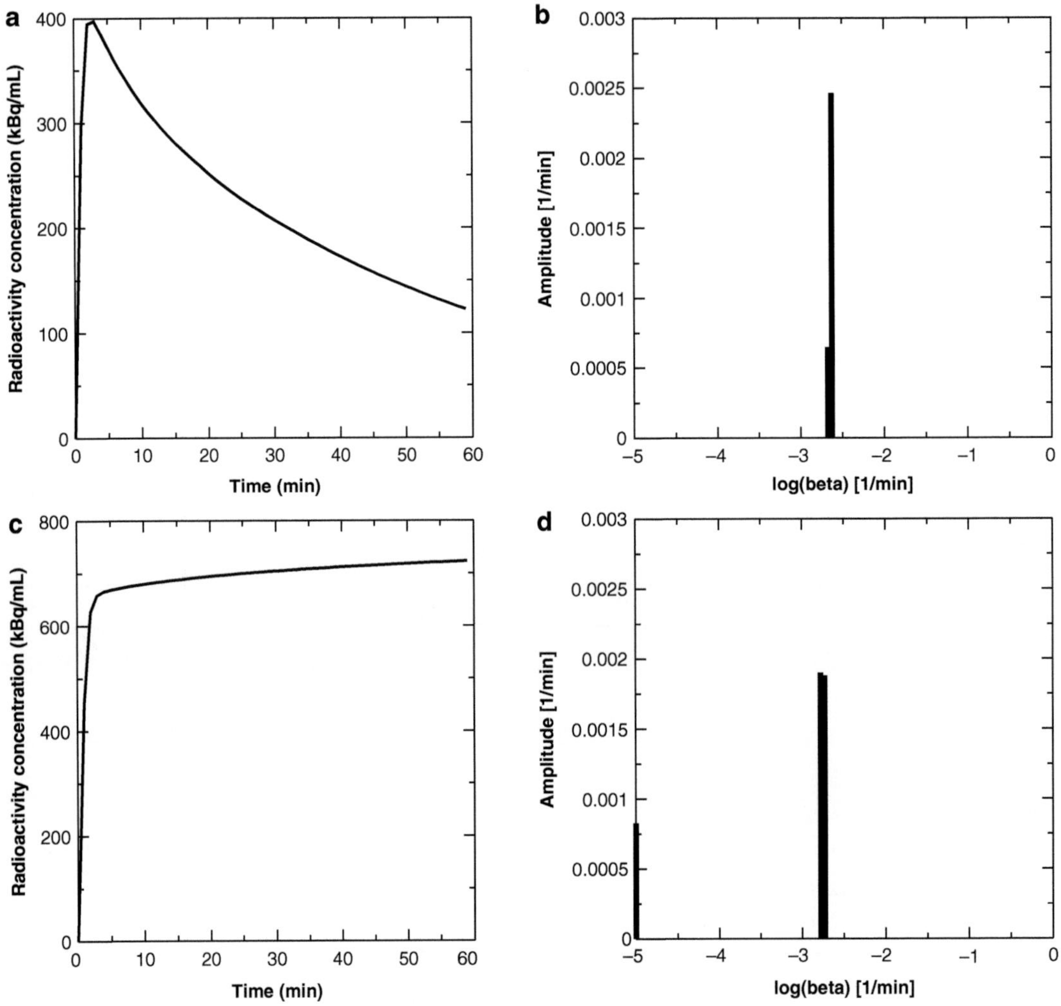

Fig. 14.14 Examples of spectral analysis. TAC of 1TC model (**a**) and its spectrum (**b**). TAC of irreversible 2TC model (**c**) and its spectrum (**d**)

logarithmically divided. The estimated α_i for each β_i is plotted as a spectrum (Fig. 14.14b, d). The number of peaks in the spectrum corresponds to the number of compartments in the system. The peak at the far left in Fig. 14.14d is trapped compartment. Although the spectral analysis has no ability to estimate micro-parameters of each compartment, the IRF $R(t)$ and V_T of the system can be calculated from results of the spectral analysis using Eqs. 14.17 and 14.19, respectively. Although the spectral analysis is a very powerful tool to estimate the number of compartments without any prior knowledge, the user must carefully interpret the spectrum because the spectral analysis is sensitive to the noise on the PET data, and the noise causes many peaks in the spectrum.

14.4 Physiological and Biological Basis of Compartmental Model

In this section, some physiological and biological concepts behind the compartmental model are discussed.

14.4.1 Blood Flow and Oxygen Consumption

Delivery of radiotracer into tissue is the first step for PET measurement. The transport of the radiotracer from blood to tissue is represented as K_1 in the compartmental model. K_1 is actually the product of blood flow or perfusion F [mL/min/cm^3] and first-pass extraction fraction E.

$$K_1 = F \cdot E \qquad (14.35)$$

F is the volume of blood passing through unit tissue volume per unit time, and E can be expressed according to Renkin-Crone capillary model [23, 24], which considers the capillary as a cylindrical tube (Fig. 14.15a) as follows:

$$E = 1 - e^{-\frac{P \cdot S}{F}} \qquad (14.36)$$

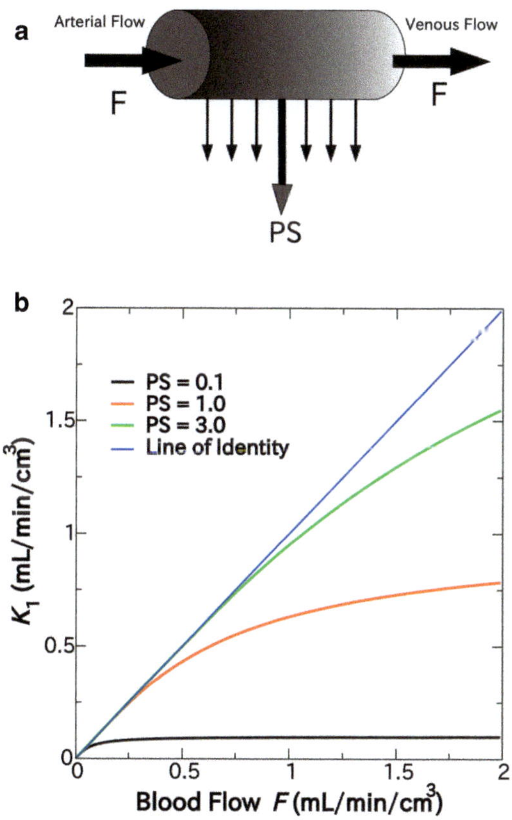

Fig. 14.15 (**a**) The Renkin-Crone capillary model. (**b**) Relationship between blood flow F and K_1 according to the Renkin-Crone model

where P is the permeability of the tracer across the capillary membrane and S is the capillary surface area per unit tissue volume. As shown in Eq. 14.36, E is a function of F and influenced by F (Fig. 14.15b). According to Eq. 14.36, when $P \cdot S$ is large relative to F, E reaches to one and $K_1 \simeq F$. The typical high E tracer is ^{15}O-water and often utilized for blood flow measurement. On the other hand, if $P \cdot S$ is small relative to F, the E becomes $P \cdot S/F$ and $K_1 \simeq P \cdot S$. The example of the low $P \cdot S$ is ^{18}F-FDOPA [25].

Consumption of molecular oxygen in tissue can be described as shown in Fig. 14.16 [26]. The left side of Fig. 14.16 corresponds to the intravascular space, and it is assumed when oxygen enters the tissue, oxygen is immediately metabolized to water and no oxygen in the extravascular tissue (Fig. 14.16 right). If the arterial and venous concentrations of oxygen (A_{O_2} and V_{O_2}, respectively) and blood flow are measured, metabolic rate of oxygen, MRO$_2$, can be calculated [27] as

$$\mathrm{MRO}_2 = F \cdot \left(A_{O_2} - V_{O_2}\right) \qquad (14.37)$$

Measurements of the arterial and venous concentrations of oxygen are invasive, and in order to measure MRO$_2$ by PET, not only ^{15}O-oxygen but also concentrations of ^{15}O-water (or ^{15}O-CO$_2$) and ^{15}O-CO are required to quantify metabolite of oxygen and vascular space, respectively [28].

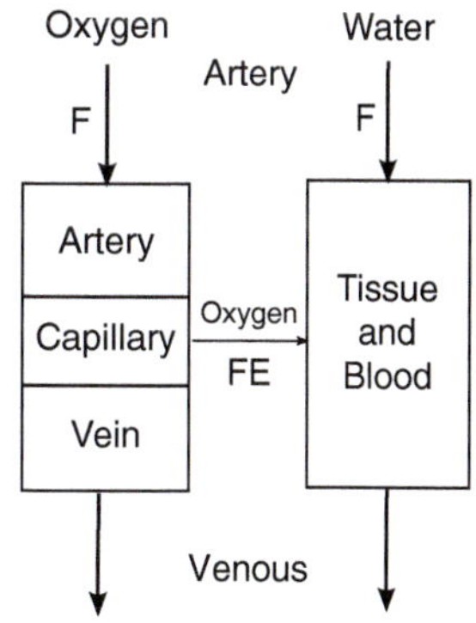

Fig. 14.16 Model to describe behavior of oxygen and water of metabolism

14.4.2 Partition Coefficient and Distribution Volume

The partition coefficient p is defined as the ratio of concentrations of two compartments at equilibrium condition. The *distribution volume* V [mL/cm^3] is numerically identical to p and one of the most frequently used macro-parameters. V implies the volume of blood that contains the same activity as unit volume of tissue. Especially, the ratio between radiotracer in tissue and radiotracer in blood at equilibrium condition is called "total distribution volume" V_T and can be expressed as $V_T = \frac{C}{A}$ at equilibrium condition. The relationship between micro-parameters and V_T depends on the compartmental model. For the 1TC model, V_T is equal to K_1/k_2. For the 2TC model, after becoming equilibrium condition, exchanges of substance between compartments are balanced, and we will see $K_1A = k_2F$ and $k_3F = k_4B$ (see Fig. 14.3b). Therefore, V_T for 2TC model is written as

$$V_T = \frac{C}{A} = \frac{F+B}{A} = \frac{K_1}{k_2}\left(1 + \frac{k_3}{k_4}\right) \quad (14.38)$$

Similarly, V_T for 3TC model is expressed as

$$V_T = \frac{K_1}{k_2}\left(1 + \frac{k_3}{k_4} + \frac{k_5}{k_6}\right) \quad (14.39)$$

The distribution volume for each compartment is also written as follows:

$$V_S = \frac{B}{A} = \frac{F}{A} \cdot \frac{B}{F} = \frac{K_1}{k_2} \cdot \frac{k_3}{k_4} \quad (14.40)$$

$$V_{NS} = \frac{N}{A} = \frac{F}{A} \cdot \frac{N}{F} = \frac{K_1}{k_2} \cdot \frac{k_5}{k_6} \quad (14.41)$$

$$V_{ND} = \frac{F+N}{A} = \frac{F}{A} + \frac{N}{A} = \frac{K_1}{k_2}\left(1 + \frac{k_5}{k_6}\right) \quad (14.42)$$

where summation of free (F) and nonspecific bound (N) compartments is called *nondisplaceable* and is denoted as suffix ND because, unlike ND compartment, binding compartment B is saturable and displaceable by nonradioactive molecules of same chemical form. As mentioned in Sect. 14.3.2.3, 3TC model is impractical for actual PET data, and compartments F and N are not distinguishable in most cases. For this reason, free compartment F in 2TC model is often referred to as nondisplaceable compartment ND. The fraction of free component in ND at equilibrium is defined as $f_{ND} = \frac{F}{F+N}$.

14.4.3 In Vitro Receptor Binding Experiment and Binding Potential

It is worth to review in vitro receptor binding experiment and its concept to understand PET neuro-receptor studies. Usual procedures for in vitro receptor binding experiments involve homogenizing and centrifuging tissue, adding radiotracer, and incubating to observe the ligand-receptor interaction. In in vitro binding assay, "the law of mass action" is used to describe reaction between ligand and receptor. This law states that the rate of reaction between unbound ligand and unbound receptor (association) is dependent on the concentrations of the ligand [L] (nM) and the receptor [R] (nM), and the rate of dissociation of the ligand-receptor complex is proportional to the concentration of ligand-receptor complex [LR] (nM):

$$L + R \underset{k_{on}}{\overset{k_{off}}{\Leftrightarrow}} LR \quad (14.43)$$

The rate constants for association and dissociation are k_{on} (nM$^{-1}\cdot$min^{-1}) and k_{off} (min^{-1}), respectively. By the "the law of mass action," the association and the dissociation rates are defined as k_{on} [L] [R] and k_{off} [LR], respectively. Initially when the ligand is added to the receptor pool, the association rate is greater than the dissociation rate because [LR] is zero and gradually [L] and [R] decrease and association rate decreases as well. After some time, the association and dissociation rates are equal, which we call "equilibrium state." Actually, this state is a dynamic equilibrium because the association and dissociation rates are not zero and the ligand still binds to the receptor and unbinds from the receptor.

During the equilibrium state, the following relation is obtained:

$$k_{on}[R][L] = k_{off}[LR]$$
$$\frac{[R][L]}{[LR]} = \frac{k_{off}}{k_{on}} = K_D \quad (14.44)$$

where K_D is called the equilibrium dissociation constant and the unit of K_D is nM. As the equation implies, K_D is inversely related to the affinity of the ligand for the receptor, and a high K_D value corresponds to low affinity to the receptor, and a low K_D value corresponds to high affinity to the receptor.

Here, we introduce other nomenclatures to connect between in vitro experiments and PET neuro-receptor studies. B_{max} is the total receptor concentration (bound to ligand and unbound to ligand) and defined as $B_{max} \equiv [R] + [LR]$. F is free ligand as $[L]$ and B is bound ligand as $[LR]$. By substituting these symbols in Eq. 14.44, the equation becomes as follows:

$$K_D = \frac{F(B_{max} - B)}{B} \quad (14.45)$$

which is rearranged for B as follows:

$$B = \frac{B_{max}F}{K_D + F} \quad (14.46)$$

The above equation is called Michaelis-Menten equation which originally states the relationship between reactions of enzyme and substrate. As shown in Fig. 14.17a, when B is plotted as a function of F, the curve is hyperbolic with an asymptote at B_{max}. This curve tells if enough amount of ligand is supplied, the ligand finally saturates all receptors and B will equal to the maximum concentration of receptor B_{max}. The amount of free ligand for saturation is dependent on K_D value as shown in this figure (see $K_D = 10$ (nM) for black line and $K_D = 3$ (nM) for red line). If $B = \frac{1}{2}B_{max}$ is substituted in Eq. 14.48, the equation becomes $F = K_D$, which means K_D corresponds to the concentration of free ligand required to saturate half of receptors. In the the case of Fig. 14.17a, 3 (nM) of free ligand is required to occupy 50 % of receptors for $K_D = 3$ (nM) (red line), and 10 (nM) of free ligand is required to occupy 50 % of receptors for $K_D = 10$ (nM) (black line). Thus, the case of $K_D = 3$ (nM) has more affinity than the case of $K_D = 10$ (nM).

Equation 14.45 is also rewritten as follows:

$$B = \left(\frac{B_{max}}{K_D} - \frac{B}{K_D}\right)F \quad (14.47)$$

which implies that at low concentration of F and B, initial slope (dashed lines in Fig. 14.17a) will be $\frac{B_{max}}{K_D}$. As shown in this figure, the ligand with higher affinity ($K_D = 3$ (nM) (red dashed line)) has larger slope than the ligand with lower affinity ($K_D = 10$ (nM) (black dashed line)). Finally Eq. 14.47 becomes

$$\frac{B}{F} = \frac{B_{max}}{K_D} - \frac{1}{K_D}B \quad (14.48)$$

As shown in Fig. 14.17b, if bound/free ligand (B/F) is plotted as a function of B, the plot becomes a straight line with a slope of ($1/K_D$) and an intercept of (B_{max}/K_D), which is called Scatchard plot. The intercept of y-axis for the black line in Fig. 14.17(b) corresponds to $B_{max}/K_D = 100/10$, and the intercept of y-axis for the red line in Fig. 14.17b corresponds to $B_{max}/K_D = 100/3$. The intercepts of x-axis for both plots are equal to $B_{max} = 100$ (nM). If we obtain at least two data points by receptor binding experiments, we will be able to estimate B_{max} and K_D separately using the Scatchard plot.

As mentioned above, the slope (B/F) at low F and B corresponds to the ratio of B_{max} and K_D. Most PET neuro-receptor studies are performed at the portion in which there is linear relationship between F and B. Thus, B/F is constant, and if F becomes doubled, B is also doubled. The constant B/F is regarded as product of B_{max} and affinity ($1/K_D$), and in PET neuro-receptor study, we call the constant "binding potential" (BP), and it is considered as one of the most important parameters in PET neuro-receptor study. Actually, since concentrations of free ligands and bounding ligands in PET neuro-receptor study are very low, we will not solely estimate B_{max} value by PET

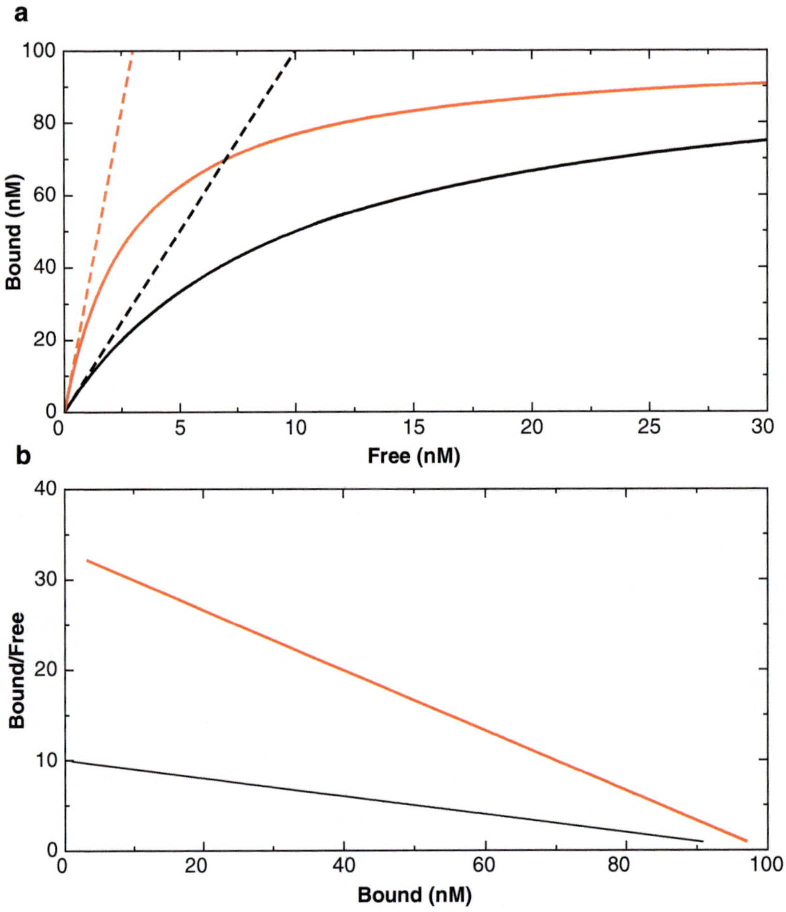

Fig. 14.17 (**a**) The relationship between free and bound ligand concentration as expressed in the Michaelis-Menten equation with two situations of $B_{max}=100$ (nM) and $K_D=10$ (nM) (*black line*) and $B_{max}=100$ (nM) and $K_D=3$ (nM) (*red line*). The dashed lines are initial slopes of two curves which correspond to $\frac{B_{max}}{K_D}$ (**b**) Scatchard plot. The Michaelis-Menten equation (Eq. 14.46) is linearized as Eq. 14.48

data (see Fig. 14.17a) but only estimate BP value. Because BP value is a product of B_{max} and $1/K_D$, the one with a high BP value implies either high B_{max} value or low K_D value.

The discussion above is for in vitro experiment, and in order to interpret in vivo PET data, some conversions are required. Only subset of receptors is available in PET study due to occupation of receptors by endogenous transmitter and it is called B_{avail} instead of B_{max}. Also regarding to the input function A, only free radiotracer in the plasma must be considered, and fraction between free and protein binding radiotracers is called "plasma free fraction" f_p. Analogy to the in vitro experiment, BP observed by PET under assumption of 3TC model is

$$\mathrm{BP_F} = \frac{B_{avail}}{K_D} = \frac{B}{F} \tag{14.49}$$

However, we usually observe PET data as 2TC model, and the following relationships are derived with definitions of BP_F (binding potential against free tracer), $\mathrm{BP_{ND}}$ (binding potential against nondisplaceable tracer), and BP_p (binding potential against plasma arterial input function):

$$\mathrm{BP_F} = \frac{B}{F} = \frac{B}{f_{\mathrm{ND}} \cdot ND} = \frac{1}{f_{\mathrm{ND}}} \mathrm{BP_{ND}} = \frac{B}{f_\mathrm{p} \cdot A} = \frac{1}{f_\mathrm{p}} \mathrm{BP_p} \tag{14.50}$$

where we assume $f_{\mathrm{ND}} \cdot ND = f_\mathrm{p} \cdot A$, which implies the free radiotracer in plasma equals to free radiotracer in tissue after reaching equilibrium. We rather employ the f_p because the f_{ND} is commonly not detectable from PET data, but f_p is measurable from sampled blood. Moreover, normally we will not achieve equilibrium condition during PET study, and BP must be determined from estimated micro-parameters. If the micro-parameters of 2TC model are estimated, the following equations are obtained (see Eqs. 14.40, 14.41, and 14.42):

$$\mathrm{BP}_F = \frac{K_1 k_3}{f_\mathrm{p} k_2 k_4},\ \mathrm{BP}_p = \frac{K_1 k_3}{k_2 k_4},\ \mathrm{BP_{ND}} = \frac{k_3}{k_4} \tag{14.51}$$

If only the macro-parameters V_T and V_{ND} are available, we also estimate BP from Eqs. 14.39 and 14.42 as

$$\mathrm{BP}_F = \frac{V_\mathrm{T} - V_{\mathrm{ND}}}{f_\mathrm{p}},\ \mathrm{BP_p} = V_\mathrm{T} - V_{\mathrm{ND}},\ \mathrm{BP_{ND}} = \frac{V_\mathrm{T} - V_{\mathrm{ND}}}{V_{\mathrm{ND}}} \tag{14.52}$$

14.5 TAC and Input Function

14.5.1 Acquisition of TAC

TAC $C(t_i)$. One common method to obtain TAC is getting averaged value inside a priori defined region of interest (ROI)[3] (ROI-based method) (Fig. 14.18). Alternatively, TAC can be generated for each pixel (voxel), which results in so-called parametric image (voxel-based method). The TAC by the ROI-based method has less noise than the voxel-based method, and estimated parameters by the ROI-based method have less variance. The ROI-based method is, however, a time-consuming task to manually delineate many ROIs and there is large interoperator variability. There have be several attempts to do automatic delineation of ROIs especially in brain image [29], in which standardized ROIs are employed after normalizing PET image to anatomical standard template from magnetic resonance image. In heart study, the PET image is often reoriented to short-axis image (slices perpendicular to the line from the apex to the mitral valve), and automatically segmented cardiac ROIs (for instance, 17 segmented ROIs proposed by the American Heart Association, AHA) are generated. By the voxel-based method, we will get an image of function, which makes easy for researchers to visually interpret the results, and it is further possible to perform voxel-by-voxel statistical test by using software package such as SPM (statistical parametric mapping, http://www.fil.ion.ucl.ac.uk/spm/). However, compared to the ROI-based method, the voxel-based method requests more computational burden, and the TAC by the voxel-based method has large noise, and it is difficult to reliably estimate micro-parameters. Therefore, in order to apply the voxel-based method, we must use simpler model, reduce parameters, or utilize acceleration techniques such as linearization (Sect. 14.3.4). Either while applying the ROI-based method or voxel-based method, we assume homogeneous distribution of radiotracer inside the region or voxel of interest; however, in reality, even one voxel contains many cells with different functions, and voxel counts are influenced by neighbor voxels due to limited spatial resolution of PET scanner (we call this phenomena partial volume effect, PVE). Although many techniques have been proposed to correct PVE [30], bias due to inhomogeneous region of interest should be acknowledged.

It is sometimes important to consider blood component in voxels of PET image. If C_B is the radioactivity concentration of the whole blood and V_B ($0 \le V_\mathrm{B} \le 1$) is fraction of blood component in the ROI, the measured total radioactivity concentration $ROI(t)$ in the ROI is

[3] If the region is in three-dimensional volume, it is called volume of interest (VOI).

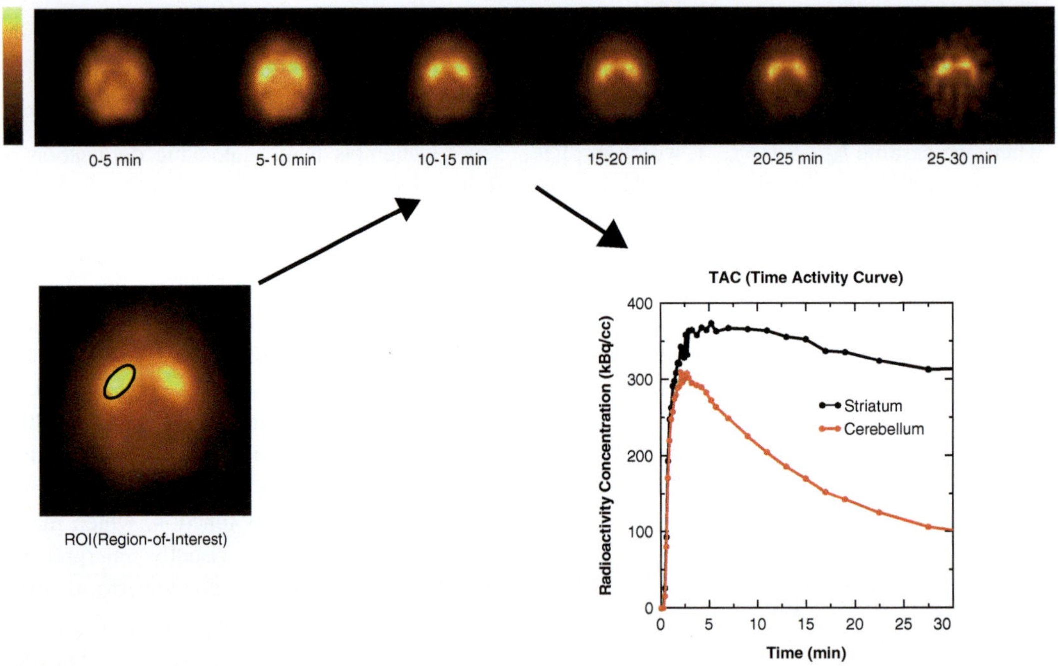

Fig. 14.18 Schematic drawings to obtain TAC from region of interest (ROI)

$$\mathrm{ROI}(t) = (1 - V_{\mathrm{B}})C(t) + V_{\mathrm{B}}C_{\mathrm{B}}(t) \tag{14.53}$$

It is possible to include V_{B} as one of estimated parameters during the fitting procedure. In brain study, the V_{B} is about 5 % and the influence of the blood component is not serious, and sometimes fixed value is used especially in the voxel-based method. However, if the target region has large contribution from blood component such as the heart, kidney, and liver [31], the consideration of the blood volume is required. Note that $C_{\mathrm{B}}(t)$ is radioactivity concentration in whole blood, and it is not necessary to match to the input function $A(t)$ (see further discussion of $A(t)$ in the next section).

14.5.2 Acquisition of Input Function

As already mentioned, the accurate input function is essential for the success of PET tracer analysis. In order to measure the input function, arterial blood must be frequently sampled after injection of radiotracer. If it is required to get radioactivity concentration in plasma, the sampled blood must be cetrifugated to separate plasma from whole blood. Moreover, in case that radioactive metabolites in the blood must be considered, the fraction of metabolites in the plasma must be measured usually by high-pressure liquid chromatography (HPLC). Because the data from the manual sampling are often sparse and discrete, the input function may be determined by being fitted to a mathematical form such as [32]

$$A(t) = (A_1 t - A_2 - A_3)e^{\lambda_1 t} + A_2 e^{\lambda_2 t} + A_3 e^{\lambda_3 t} \tag{14.54}$$

where A_1, A_2, A_3, λ_1, λ_2, and λ_3 are parameters to be estimated.

Manual sampling of blood (usually from the radial artery) is labor intensive, and automatic sampling technique is sometimes preferable although this technique only obtains radioactivity in whole blood, and if needed, another blood samples for separation of plasma and metabolites must be performed. In this technique, after the catheter is inserted into the artery, the arterial blood is continuously withdrawn through tube by pump during PET study, and the concentration of the radioactivity in the arterial blood is monitored by means of radiation detector [33, 34]. Some calibration

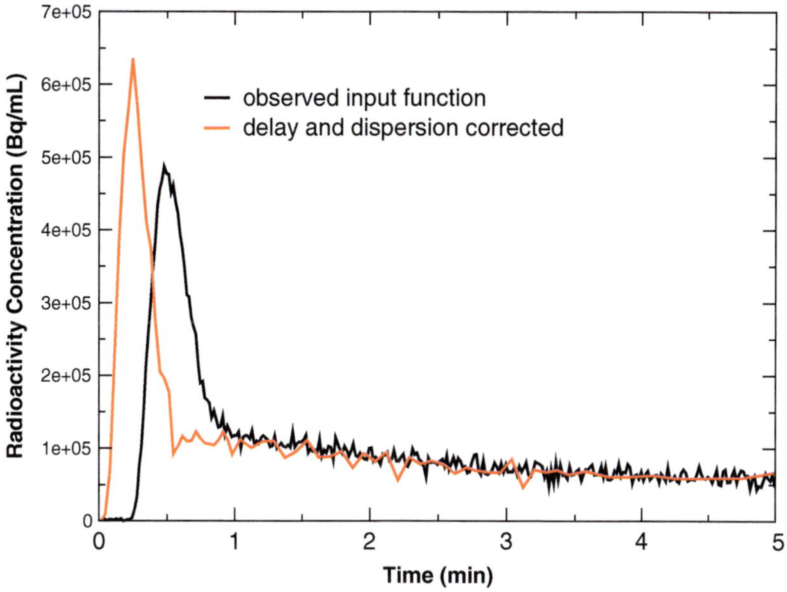

Fig. 14.19 Observed input function by the radiation detector and true input function. There is time shift between two curves (delay), and the observed input curve is dispersed compared to the true input curve

procedures are essential for this approach. The cross calibration between radioactivity concentration measured by PET scanner and the radiation detector for the blood sampling must be performed routinely. The difference between arrival time of tracer at the target organ and time of detection by the radiation detector (delay time) must be corrected. Especially the correction of the delay time is important for ^{15}O tracer due to its short physical half-life of 2 min. Moreover, the dispersion of shape of input curve is observed for the time passing through tube (see Fig. 14.19), and the dispersion correction must be applied. Often used dispersion function [35] is defined as

$$A_o(t) = A(t) \otimes \left(\frac{1}{\tau} e^{-\frac{t}{\tau}} \right) \quad (14.55)$$

where $A_0(t)$ is the observed input curve and τ [s] is the dispersion time constant. The deconvolution operation is required to solve the above equation, which introduces noise on the input function. Alternatively, parameters of the delay and dispersion are included in the model; both parameters are simultaneously estimated with other kinetic parameters [36]. This approach is attractive; however, more parameters to be solved result in large variance in the estimated parameters, and the careful attention to the obtained results must be paid.

There have been several attempts to extract input function from PET images. By this methodology, blood sampling is not required (or only one point blood sample is enough for scaling the input function), and error due to delay and dispersion could be minimized. If the left ventricle (LV) is in the field of view (FOV) of the PET scanner, the input function can be directly estimated from VOI on the LV of PET images [37]. The image of the descent aorta is also used to extract the input function because the descent aorta is a relatively isolated region and expected to have minimum influence from surrounding tissue [38]. But, generally, due to limited spatial resolution of PET scanner, PVE must be corrected in some extent. In brain study, carotid artery is often a target region for the extraction of input function [39]. Image segmentation algorithms such as principle component analysis, factor analysis, and independent component analysis are applied to separate signal of blood from tissue [40–43]. As same as the automatic sampling technique, image-based input function can only represent radioactivity from whole blood, and if one requires separation of plasma and whole blood or non-metabolite fraction in blood, additional blood sampling is necessary. Another attempt to estimate the input function is the compartmental model with PVE correction. In myocardium blood flow (MBF) study with ^{15}O-water, the following model equation of 1TC model is employed with MBF f [44, 45]:

$$C(t) = \alpha f A(t) \otimes \exp\left(-\frac{f}{p}t\right) + V_a A(t) \quad (14.56)$$

where α is the so-called perfusable tissue fraction which implies fraction of available tissue in the ROI and V_a is the fraction of vascular component in the ROI. The p is the partition coefficient with fixed value. Three unknown parameters α, f, and V_a will be estimated by means of the nonlinear least squares technique. The true f value is underestimated due to PVE and only apparent K_1 (αf) value is only observed. But under assumption that washout of water can be observed without influence of PVE by washout rate of $\frac{f}{p}$, the MBF f without PVE can be determined.

An alternative approach to get the input function invasively is to use population-based input function [46, 47]. In this approach, blood samples were carried out previously for certain numbers of patients or normal volunteers, and averaged input function is computed as the population-based input function. The population-based input function must be used in caution if the group participated for the PET study is different from the group in which the blood sampling was carried out.

14.5.2.1 Continuous Infusion

Compartmental model generally consists of series of differential equations such as Eq. 14.1, and if the TAC along time becomes constant, the left side of the differential equation is equal to zero, and solving the compartmental model will be easier. If the input function is constant, only one blood sample is enough to determine the input function. The so-called steady-state technique, the continuous administration of ^{15}O labeled gasses of CO_2, O_2, and CO, is one of the classical applications of PET to measure cerebral blood flow (CBF), oxygen extraction fraction (OEF), cerebral metabolic rate of oxygen ($CMRO_2$), and cerebral blood volume (CBV) [28, 48]. For example, by the steady-state technique according to Eq. 14.1, CBF(f) can be computed by a blood sample A_C and PET count C_C as follows ($A(t)$ and $C(t)$ are not decay corrected):

$$\frac{dC(t)}{dt}(=0) = fA(t) - \left(\frac{f}{p} + \lambda\right)C(t)$$
$$f\left(A - \frac{C}{p}\right) = \lambda C \quad (14.57)$$
$$f = \frac{p\lambda}{p\frac{A_C}{C_C} - 1}$$

where λ and p are fixed value as the physical decay constant of ^{15}O and the partition coefficient of water, respectively.

In neuro-receptor study, as described at Sect. 14.4.3, several physiological parameters including BP and V_T can be obtained at equilibrium condition. The "bolus + infusion" (B/I) approach was developed to make the equilibrium condition during PET study. In order to rapidly make equilibrium condition, the radiotracer is first delivered as a bolus followed by a continuous infusion [49]. In order to determine how the radiotracer is infused during PET study, first we will carry out PET study with bolus injection in order to obtain the IRF $R_i(t)$ ($i = 1 \ldots M$) of regions of interest (ROI) or input function (M is numbers of regions of interest). Infusion protocol $H(t)$ of the radiotracer for B/I approach can be defined as a combination of bolus plus continuous infusion over time T and written as

$$H(t) = \frac{K_{bol}\delta(t) + \theta(t) - \theta(t - T)}{K_{bol} + T} \quad (14.58)$$

where $\delta(t)$ is the Dirac delta function representing bolus injection and $\theta(t)$ is a step function (0 for $t < 0$, 1 for $t > 0$) representing infusion phase. K_{bol} is the magnitude of the bolus component with unit of time and implies that bolus dose corresponds to K_{bol} minutes of infusion. The $C_i(t_j)$ ($j = 1..N$), N numbers of points of TAC by B/I protocol, can be written as similar to Eq. 14.18

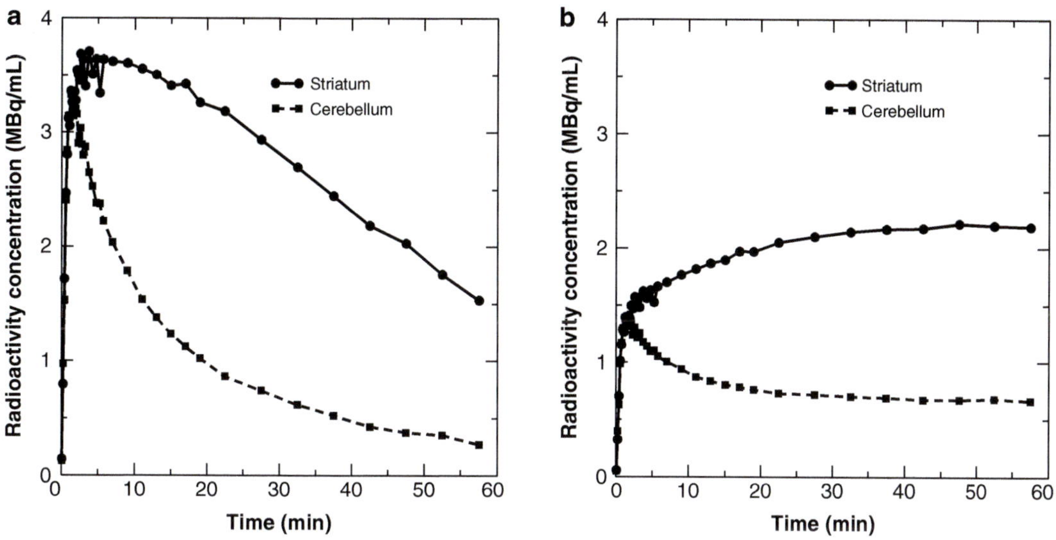

Fig. 14.20 Bolus + infusion approach (**a**) observed TACs after bolus injection of ^{11}C-raclopride and (**b**) expected TACs after B/I protocol with optimal K_{bol} obtained using Eq. 14.60

$$C_i(t) = H(t) \otimes R_i(t) \frac{K_{bol} R_i(t) + \int_0^t R_i(\tau)\, d\tau}{K_{bol} + T} \quad (14.59)$$

Optimized K_{bol} is guessed by minimizing Φ in the following equations by means of the least squares fitting approach:

$$\Phi = \sum_{i=1}^{M} \sum_{j=1}^{N} \left[\frac{C_i(t_j)}{C_i(T)} - 1 \right]^2 \quad (14.60)$$

Examples of TAC after B/I protocol are shown in Fig. 14.20. The B/I approach is easily extended to neurotransmitter-change experiment by perturbing the endogenous neurotransmitter after reaching the equilibrium condition [50].

14.5.2.2 Reference Region Model

To avoid arterial blood sampling, there are several approaches which have been already discussed in the above section such as employment of the image-based input function. The reference region (tissue) model approach described in this section is an approach to eliminate component of the input function by assuming two regions (target region which has specific binding of the tracer and reference region which has no specific binding of the tracer) share the same input function. Although the "full reference region model" is referred to as 2TC model for the target region and 1TC model for the reference region [51], there are many variations of the reference region model by how we define the compartmental model for the target region and the reference region (Fig. 14.21). The simplified reference region model (often called simplified reference tissue model, SRTM) [52, 53] is the most popular reference region model which uses 1TC models for both the target and the reference regions (Fig. 14.21c). Let's derive the operation equation for the SRTM. We start as we did in the section of Logan plot (Sect. 14.3.4.2):

$$\begin{aligned} \frac{dC(t)}{dt} &= K_1 A(t) - k_2 C(t) \\ \frac{dC'(t)}{dt} &= K_1' A(t) - k_2' C'(t) \end{aligned} \quad (14.61)$$

From the above equations, common term $A(t)$ can be eliminated:

$$\frac{\frac{dC(t)}{dt} + k_2 C(t)}{K_1} = \frac{\frac{dC'(t)}{dt} + k_2' C'(t)}{K_1'} \quad (14.62)$$

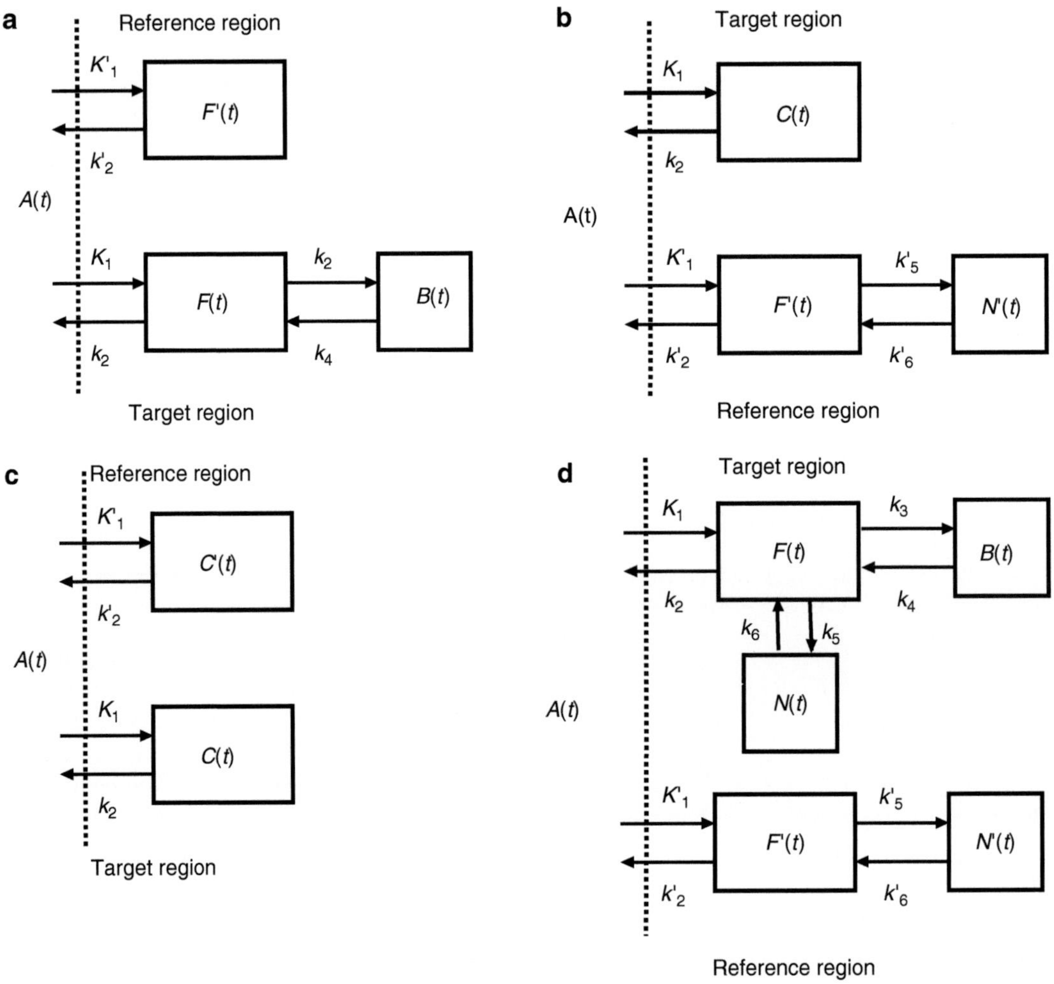

Fig. 14.21 Variety of the reference region models. (**a**) 2TC model for the target region and 1TC model for the reference region, (**b**) 1TC model for the target region and 2TC model for the reference region, (**c**) 1TC models for both target and reference regions, (**d**) 3TC model for the target region and 2TC model for the reference region

If we define $R_1 = K_1/K'_1$ and Laplace transform is employed to solve the differential equation above

$$\begin{aligned}(s+k_2)C(s) &= R_1\left[(s+k_2')C'(s)\right]\\ C(s) &= R_1\left[\frac{s+k_2'}{s+k_2}C'(s)\right]\\ &= R_1\left[C'(s)+\frac{k_2'-k_2}{s+k_2}C'(s)\right]\\ C(t) &= R_1C'(t)+R_1(k_2'-k_2)C'(t)\otimes e^{-k_2t}\end{aligned} \qquad (14.63)$$

Total distribution volumes for the target region (V_T) and the reference region (V'_T) can be written as

$$V_T = \frac{K_1}{k_2} = V_{ND}(1+BP_{ND}) \qquad (14.64)$$

$$V_T' = \frac{K_1'}{k_2'} = V_{ND} \qquad (14.65)$$

where BP_{ND} and V_{ND} are binding potential and distribution volume for nondisplaceable compartment defined in Sect. 14.4.3. If we assume the target region and reference region have same V_{ND}, from the above equations, BP_{ND} is derived as

$$BP_{ND} = \frac{R_1k_2'}{k_2} - 1 \qquad (14.66)$$

Three parameters of R_1, k_2, and k'_2 can be estimated using Eq. 14.63 by means of nonlinear least squares fitting. For voxel-by-voxel computation, basis function method (BFM) [54] as similar manner as the spectral analysis (Sect. 14.3.4.4) is often employed, in which the convolution term in Eq. 14.63 is once calculated within available range of k_2, and other parameters are rapidly solved by the linear least squares fitting.

Alternatively, the SRTM can be solved by integration as same as we did in Sect. 14.3.4.2. Integration over time is applied for both equations in Eq. 14.61 as follows:

$$\begin{aligned} C(t) &= K_1\int_0^t A(\tau)d\tau - k_2\int_0^\tau C(\tau)d\tau \\ C'(t) &= K'_1\int_0^t A(\tau)d\tau - k'_2\int_0^\tau C'(\tau)d\tau \end{aligned} \quad (14.67)$$

Eliminating common term $\int_0^t A(\tau)d\tau$ from the above equations results in

$$\begin{aligned} &\frac{C(t)+k_2\int_0^\tau C(\tau)d\tau}{K_1} = \frac{C'(t)+k'_2\int_0^\tau C'(\tau)d\tau}{K'_1} \\ &C(t)+k_2\int_0^\tau C(\tau)d\tau = R_1\left[C'(t)+k'_2\int_0^\tau C'(\tau)d\tau\right] \\ &C(t) = R_1C'(t)+R_1k'_2\int_0^\tau C'(\tau)d\tau - k_2\int_0^\tau C(\tau)d\tau \end{aligned} \quad (14.68)$$

Equation 14.68 is a multiple linear form and R_1, k_2, and k'_2 can be directly derived by multilinear regression technique. The technique is utilized for neuro-receptor study [55] but is also applicable for CBF estimation [56]. Equation 14.68 can be rearranged as

$$\frac{\int_0^\tau C(\tau)d\tau}{C(t)} = \frac{R_1k'_2}{k_2}\frac{\int_0^\tau C'(\tau)d\tau + C'(t)/k'_2}{C(t)} - \frac{R_1k'_2}{k_2} \quad (14.69)$$

which is another popular noninvasive approach called "Logan reference tissue model" [57] and $\frac{R_1k'_2}{k_2} = \frac{V_T}{V'_T}$ is called "distribution volume ratio" (DVR). Here k'_2 is a tracer clearance rate constant from the reference region and must be determined prior to the Logan analysis.

The reference region approach is very attractive since no blood sampling and metabolite correction are required, and if the reference region is available, the reference region analysis is nowadays the first choice in clinical study. However, due to the discrepancy between real data and assumption of the reference region model, the biases of estimated parameters are often observed and the model must be employed with caution [58].

Conclusions

In this chapter, we have explained how PET data are analyzed to estimate behavior of radiotracer injected. The PET data only represent distribution of positron emitter, and the SUV is not enough parameter to properly interpret PET data. The compartmental model is introduced to explain behavior of the radiotracer. Mathematical basis and biological meaning of the compartmental models including 1TC, 2TC, and 3TC models have been described. Several methodologies such as Logan plot, Patlak plot, B/I approach, spectral analysis, and reference region approach have been explained in this chapter, and we have seen that the root of methodologies to analyze PET data is common among many radiotracers and can be understandable by concept of general compartmental model with combination of IRF and input function. For the selection of the compartmental model and analyzed approach, we need not only biological and physiological background of the tracer but also basic concept and limitation of the compartmental model.

References

1. Wagner CC, Langer O. Approaches using molecular imaging technology use of PET in clinical microdose studies. Adv Drug Deliv Rev. 2011;63:539–46.
2. Keyes JW. SUV: standard uptake or silly useless value? J Nucl Med. 1995;36:1836–9.
3. Watabe H, Ikoma Y, Kimura Y, Naganawa M, Shidahara M. Pet kinetic analysis–compartmental model. Ann Nucl Med. 2006;20:583–9.
4. Innis RB, Cunningham VJ, Delforge J, Fujita M, Gjedde A, Gunn RN, Holden J, Houle S, Huang

SC, Ichise M, Iida H, Ito H, Kimura Y, Koeppe RA, Knudsen GM, Knuuti J, Lammertsma AA, Laruelle M, Logan J, Maguire RP, Mintun MA, Morris ED, Parsey R, Price JC, Slifstein M, Sossi V, Suhara T, Votaw JR, Wong DF, Carson RE. Consensus nomenclature for in vivo imaging of reversibly binding radioligands. J Cereb Blood Flow Metab. 2007;27:1533–9.
5. Watabe H, Channing M, Der M, Adams H, Jagoda E, Herscovitch P, Eckelman W, Carson R. Kinetic analysis of the 5-HT2A ligand [11C]MDL 100,907. J Cereb Blood Flow Metab. 2000;20:899–909.
6. Gunn R, Gunn S, Cunningham V. Positron emission tomography compartmental models. J Cereb Blood Flow Metab. 2001;21:635–52.
7. Marquardt DW. An algorithm for least-squares estimation of nonlinear parameters. J Soc Indust Appl Math. 1963;11:431–41.
8. Nelder JA, Mead R. A simplex method for function minimization. Comput J. 1965;7:308–13.
9. Logan J, Fowler J, Volkow N, Ding Y, Wang G, Alexoff D. A strategy for removing the bias in the graphical analysis method. J Cereb Blood Flow Metab. 2001;21:307–20.
10. Watabe H, Endres C, Breier A, Schmall B, Eckelman W, Carson R. Measurement of dopamine release with continuous infusion of [11C]raclopride: optimization and signal-to-noise considerations. J Nucl Med. 2000;41:522–30.
11. Landaw EM, DiStefano JJ. Multiexponential, multicompartmental, and noncompartmental modeling. II data analysis and statistical considerations. Am J Physiol. 1984;246:R665–77.
12. Carson R, Kiesewetter D, Jagoda E, Der M, Herscovitch P, Eckelman W. Muscarinic cholinergic receptor measurements with [18f]fp-tztp: control and competition studies. J Cereb Blood Flow Metab. 1998;18:1130–42.
13. Jvd H, Burchert W, Müller-Schauenburg W, Meyer G, Hundeshagen H. Accurate local blood flow measurements with dynamic PET: fast determination of input function delay and dispersion by multilinear minimization. J Nucl Med. 1993;34:1770–7.
14. Raichle ME, Martin WR, Herscovitch P, Mintun MA, Markham J. Brain blood flow measured with intravenous H2(15)O. II. implementation and validation. J Nucl Med : Off Publ, Soc Nucl Med. 1983;24:790–8.
15. Logan J, Fowler J, Volkow N, Wolf A, Dewey S, Schlyer D, MacGregor R, Hitzemann R, Bendriem B, Gatley S. Graphical analysis of reversible radioligand binding from time-activity measurements applied to [N-11C-methyl]-(−)-cocaine PET studies in human subjects. J Cereb Blood Flow Metab. 1990;10:740–7.
16. Ichise M, Toyama H, Innis R, Carson R. Strategies to improve neuroreceptor parameter estimation by linear regression analysis. J Cereb Blood Flow Metab. 2002;22:1271–81.
17. Kimura Y, Naganawa M, Shidahara M, Ikoma Y, Watabe H. PET kinetic analysis pitfalls and a solution for the logan plot. Ann Nucl Med. 2007;21:1–8.
18. Varga J, Szabo Z. Modified regression model for the Logan plot. J Cereb Blood Flow Metab. 2002;22:240–4.
19. Gjedde A. Calculation of cerebral glucose phosphorylation from brain uptake of glucose analogs in vivo: a re-examination. Brain Res. 1982;257:237–74.
20. Patlak C, Blasberg R, Fenstermacher J. Graphical evaluation of blood-to-brain transfer constants from multiple-time uptake data. J Cereb Blood Flow Metab. 1983;3:1–7.
21. Cunningham V, Jones T. Spectral analysis of dynamic PET studies. J Cereb Blood Flow Metab. 1993;13:15–23.
22. Turkheimer F, Sokoloff L, Bertoldo A, Lucignani G, Reivich M, Jaggi JL, Schmidt K. Estimation of component and parameter distributions in spectral analysis. J Cereb Blood Flow Metab. 1998;18:1211–22.
23. Renkin EM. Transport of potassium-42 from blood to tissue in isolated mammalian skeletal muscles. Am J Physiol. 1959;197:1205–10.
24. Crone C. The permeability of capillaries in various organs as determined by use of the 'indicator diffusion' method. Acta Physiol Scand. 1963;58:292–305.
25. Matsubara K, Watabe H, Kumakura Y, Hayashi T, Endres CJ, Minato K, Iida H. Sensitivity of kinetic macro-parameters to changes in dopamine synthesis, storage and metabolism: a simulation study for [(18) F]FDOPA PET by a model with detailed dopamine pathway. Synapse. 2011;65:751–62.
26. Mintun M, Raichle M, Martin W, Herscovitch P. Brain oxygen utilization measured with O-15 radiotracers and positron emission tomography. J Nucl Med. 1984;25:177–87.
27. Kudomi N, Hayashi T, Watabe H, Teramoto N, Piao R, Ose T, Koshino K, Ohta Y, Iida H. A physiological model for recirculation water correction in CMRO2 assessment with 15O2 inhalation PET. J Cereb Blood Flow Metab. 2009;29:355–64.
28. Frackowiak RS, Lenzi GL, Jones T, Heather JD. Quantitative measurement of regional cerebral blood flow and oxygen metabolism in man using 15O and positron emission tomography: theory, procedure, and normal values. J Comput Assist Tomogr. 1980;4:727–36.
29. Schain M, Varnäs K, Cselényi Z, Halldin C, Farde L, Varrone A. Evaluation of two automated methods for PET region of interest analysis. Neuroinformatics. 2014;12:551–62.
30. Erlandsson K, Buvat I, Pretorius PH, Thomas BA, Hutton BF. A review of partial volume correction techniques for emission tomography and their applications in neurology, cardiology and oncology. Phys Med Biol. 2012;57:R119–59.

31. Kudomi N, Slimani L, Järvisalo M, Kiss J, Lautamäki R, Naum G, Savunen T, Knuuti J, Iida H, Nuutila P, Iozzo P. Non-invasive estimation of hepatic blood perfusion from H(2)(15)O PET images using tissue-derived arterial and portal input functions. Eur J Nucl Med Mol Imaging. 2008;35:1899–911.
32. Feng D, Wong KP, Wu CM, Siu WC. A technique for extracting physiological parameters and the required input function simultaneously from pet image measurements: theory and simulation study. IEEE Trans Inf Technol Biomed. 1997;1:243–54.
33. Kanno I, Iida H, Miura S, Murakami M, Takahashi K, Sasaki H, Inugami A, Shishido F, Uemura K. A system for cerebral blood flow measurement using an H215O autoradiographic method and positron emission tomography. J Cereb Blood Flow Metab. 1987;7:143–53.
34. Kudomi N, Choi E, Yamamoto S, Watabe H, Kim K, Shidahara M, Ogawa M, Teramoto N, Sakamoto E, Iida H. Development of a GSO detector assembly for a continuous blood sampling system. IEEE Trans Nucl Sci. 2003;50:70–3.
35. Iida H, Kanno I, Miura S, Murakami M, Takahashi K, Uemura K. Error analysis of a quantitative cerebral blood flow measurement using H2(15)O autoradiography and positron emission tomography, with respect to the dispersion of the input function. J Cereb Blood Flow Metab. 1986;6:536–45.
36. Meyer E. Simultaneous correction for tracer arrival delay and dispersion in CBF measurements by the H215O autoradiographic method and dynamic PET. J Nucl Med. 1989;30:1069–78.
37. Weinberg IN, Huang SC, Hoffman EJ, Araujo L, Nienaber C, Grover-McKay M, Dahlbom M, Schelbert H. Validation of PET-acquired input functions for cardiac studies. J Nucl Med. 1988;29:241–7.
38. Watabe H, Channing M, Riddell C, Jousse F, Libutti S, Carrasquillo J, Bacharach S, Carson R. Noninvasive estimation of the aorta input function for measurement of tumor blood flow with [15o]water. IEEE Trans Med Imaging. 2001;20:164–74.
39. Lyoo CH, Zanotti-Fregonara P, Zoghbi SS, Liow JS, Xu R, Pike VW, Zarate CA, Fujita M, Innis RB. Image-derived input function derived from a supervised clustering algorithm: methodology and validation in a clinical protocol using [11C](R)-rolipram. PLoS One. 2014;9:e89101.
40. Ahn J, Lee D, Lee J, Kim S, Cheon G, Yeo J, Shin S, Chung J, Lee M. Quantification of regional myocardial blood flow using dynamic H2(15)O pet and factor analysis. J Nucl Med. 2001;42:782–7.
41. Lee J, Lee D, Ahn J, Cheon G, Kim S, Yeo J, Seo K, Park K, Chung J, Lee M. Blind separation of cardiac components and extraction of input function from h(2)(15)o dynamic myocardial pet using independent component analysis. J Nucl Med. 2001;42:938–43.
42. Naganawa M, Kimura Y, Ishii K, Oda K, Ishiwata K, Matani A. Extraction of a plasma time-activity curve from dynamic brain PET images based on independent component analysis. IEEE Trans Biomed Eng. 2005;52:201–10.
43. Suk H, Lee JS, Li JH, Yang YW, Liu RS, Chen JC. Partial volume correction of the microPET blood input function using ensemble learning independent component analysis. Phys Med Biol. 2009;54: 1823–46.
44. Iida H, Rhodes C, Rd S, Araujo L, Bloomfield P, Lammertsma A, Jones T. Use of the left ventricular time-activity curve as a noninvasive input function in dynamic oxygen-15-water positron emission tomography. J Nucl Med. 1992;33:1669–77.
45. Watabe H, Jino H, Kawachi N, Teramoto N, Hayashi T, Ohta Y, Iida H. Parametric imaging of myocardial blood flow with 15O-water and PET using the basis function method. J Nucl Med. 2005;46:1219–24.
46. Eberl S, Anayat A, Fulton R, Hooper P, Fulham M. Evaluation of two population-based input functions for quantitative neurological FDG PET studies. Eur J Nucl Med. 1997;24:299–304.
47. Zanotti-Fregonara P, Hines CS, Zoghbi SS, Liow JS, Zhang Y, Pike VW, Drevets WC, Mallinger AG, Zarate CA, Fujita M, Innis RB. Population-based input function and image-derived input function for [11C](R)-rolipram PET imaging: methodology, validation and application to the study of major depressive disorder. Neuroimage. 2012;63:1532–41.
48. Watabe T, Shimosegawa E, Watabe H, Kanai Y, Hanaoka K, Ueguchi T, Isohashi K, Kato H, Tatsumi M, Hatazawa J. Quantitative evaluation of cerebral blood flow and oxygen metabolism in normal anesthetized rats: 15O-labeled gas inhalation PET with MRI fusion. J Nucl Med. 2013;54:283–90.
49. Carson R, Channing M, Blasberg R, Dunn B, Cohen R, Rice K, Herscovitch P. Comparison of bolus and infusion methods for receptor quantitation: application to [18F]cyclofoxy and positron emission tomography. J Cereb Blood Flow Metab. 1993;13:24–42.
50. Endres C, Kolachana B, Saunders R, Su T, Weinberger D, Breier A, Eckelman W, Carson R. Kinetic modeling of [11C]raclopride: combined PET-microdialysis studies. J Cereb Blood Flow Metab. 1997;17:932–42.
51. Lammertsma A, Bench C, Hume S, Osman S, Gunn K, Brooks D, Frackowiak R. Comparison of methods for analysis of clinical [11C]raclopride studies. J Cereb Blood Flow Metab. 1996;16:42–52.
52. Lammertsma A, Hume S. Simplified reference tissue model for pet receptor studies. Neuroimage. 1996;4:153–8.
53. Wu Y, Carson RE. Noise reduction in the simplified reference tissue model for neuroreceptor functional imaging. J Cereb Blood Flow Metab. 2002;22: 1440–52.

54. Gunn R, Lammertsma A, Hume S, Cunningham V. Parametric imaging of ligand-receptor binding in PET using a simplified reference region model. Neuroimage. 1997;6:279–87.
55. Ichise M, Liow JS, Lu JQ, Takano A, Model K, Toyama H, Suhara T, Suzuki K, Innis RB, Carson RE. Linearized reference tissue parametric imaging methods: application to [11C]DASB positron emission tomography studies of the serotonin transporter in human brain. J Cereb Blood Flow Metab. 2003;23:1096–112.
56. Watabe H, Itoh M, Cunningham V, Lammertsma A, Bloomfield P, Mejia M, Fujiwara T, Jones A, Jones T, Nakamura T. Noninvasive quantification of rcbf using positron emission tomography. J Cereb Blood Flow Metab. 1996;16:311–9.
57. Logan J, Fowler J, Volkow N, Wang G, Ding Y, Alexoff D. Distribution volume ratios without blood sampling from graphical analysis of PET data. J Cereb Blood Flow Metab. 1996;16:834–40.
58. Folkersma H, Boellaard R, Vandertop WP, Kloet RW, Lubberink M, Lammertsma AA, Berckel BNM. Reference tissue models and blood–brain barrier disruption: lessons from (R)-[11C]PK11195 in traumatic brain injury. J Nucl Med Off Publ Soc Nucl Med. 2009;50:1975–9.

Part V

PET Imaging Artifacts and Correction Techniques

Partial Volume Correction in PET Imaging

15

Kjell Erlandsson

Contents

15.1 **Introduction** 356
15.1.1 Background 356
15.1.2 The Partial Volume Effect 356
15.1.3 The Point Spread Function 358
15.1.4 The Tissue Fraction Effect 358
15.1.5 Clinical Implications 359
15.1.6 Partial Volume Correction 359

15.2 **Theory** 360
15.2.1 Deconvolution 360
15.2.2 Motion 361
15.2.3 Region-Based PVC 361
15.2.4 Voxel-Based PVC 362
15.2.5 Combined PVC Methods 363

15.3 **PVC Examples** 363
15.3.1 Data Generation 363
15.3.2 Example 1: Oncology 364
15.3.3 Example 2: Cardiology 364
15.3.4 Example 3: Neurology 366

15.4 **Practical Considerations** 366
15.4.1 Accuracy 366
15.4.2 Resolution 366
15.4.3 Co-registration 369
15.4.4 Segmentation 369
15.4.5 Sampling 370

15.5 **Advanced Topics** 370
15.5.1 Alternative Correction Approaches 370
15.5.2 Alternative Correction Methods 370
15.5.3 Alternative Classification Methods 370

15.6 **Clinical Applications** 371
15.6.1 Cardiology 371
15.6.2 Neurology 372
15.6.3 Oncology 372

15.7 **Summary** 373

15.8 **Appendix: PVC Methods** 373

References 375

Abstract

Spill over of data between different regions in a PET image is known as the "partial volume effect" (PVE) and leads to errors in the quantification of local tracer concentration. PVE can be a confounding factor in clinical studies if the effect changes over time or between subjects, and it is then important to correct for PVE. Such a correction procedure is known as "partial volume correction" (PVC). Since the PVE depends on the spatial resolution of the PET images, some degree of compensation can be

K. Erlandsson
Institute of Nuclear Medicine,
University College London, London, UK
e-mail: k.erlandsson@ucl.ac.uk

M.M. Khalil (ed.), *Basic Science of PET Imaging*, DOI 10.1007/978-3-319-40070-9_15

obtained using resolution recovery or deconvolution algorithms. However, these algorithms should not be considered as PVC algorithms, as they simply provide alternative bias vs. noise trade-off solutions from the same measured data. More accurate correction methods can be implemented by utilising high-resolution anatomical information from co-registered MRI or CT images, which would typically first be segmented into a number of regions. Different PVC methods have been developed, which are based on different assumptions. The corrected values should therefore be regarded as approximations of the true values. Also, the results are sensitive to errors in co-registration and segmentation of the anatomical images, as well as in the estimation of the system point spread function. Despite these limitations, the importance of PVC has been demonstrated in a number of clinical neurology, oncology and cardiology studies.

15.1 Introduction

15.1.1 Background

"Unclear medicine" – This is a term sometimes used jokingly when referring to nuclear medicine. The basis for the joke is the blurry appearance of PET and SPECT images when compared to CT or MRI images due to the relatively poor spatial resolution. The consequence of this qualitative blurry appearance, from a quantitative point of view, is known as the "partial volume effect" (PVE). This effect results in spill over of data between different image regions. With respect to a particular region, two separate PVEs can be distinguished: spill-in and spill-out (see Fig. 15.1). However these are not separate effects, as spill-in to one region is spill-out from another region or regions. This chapter will discuss methods to correct for PVEs, which are known as partial volume correction (PVC) methods.

In order to obtain accurate quantitative values from PET data, it is necessary to correct for a number of physical effects, including random coincidences, electronic dead time, detector efficiency variations, photon attenuation, Compton scattering, patient motion and PVE. Most of these effects are well understood, and correction methods have been developed and are being used routinely. Also PVE is a well-understood effect and a number of correction methods have been developed over the years. However, these are not generally being used routinely. There are several reasons for this: additional data are required, complex image processing is involved, and the result is sensitive to small errors at various stages of processing.

The PVE can be described using the point spread function (PSF) of the system, which essentially corresponds to the image of a point source. The PSF is often characterised mathematically by a Gaussian function, and the amount of blurring is determined by the full width at half maximum (FWHM) of this function. If every point in the actual distribution is blurred by the same amount, then the measured image is described as a convolution between the true image and the PSF. Convolution is a mathematical integral operation between two functions (see, e.g. [1]).

15.1.2 The Partial Volume Effect

Figure 15.2 shows an illustration of the PVE in 3D. The true object was a cylindrical phantom (20 cm in diameter) containing six spherical inserts (diameters 6, 9, 12, 15, 18 and 24 mm) with a sphere-to-background contrast[1] of 4. The phantom was blurred with a 3D Gaussian PSF with a 6-mm FWHM (typical for the resolution of current PET systems). The figure includes cross sections of the original and blurred phantoms, as

[1] Contrast is defined as $C=(T-B)/B$, where T and B are the target and background values, respectively.

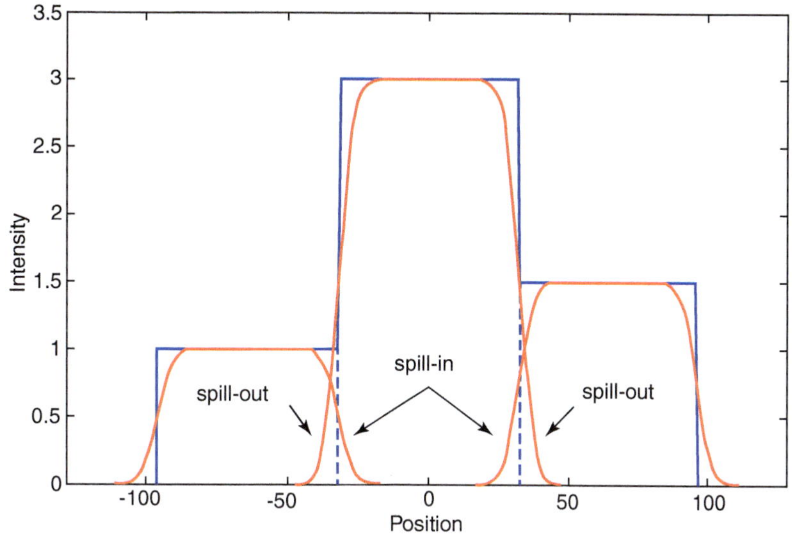

Fig. 15.1 1D illustration of the spill-in and spill-out effects. The *solid blue line* represents the true distribution, the *dashed blue lines* indicate the edges of the target region, and the *red line* represents the blurred contributions from the target and background regions separately

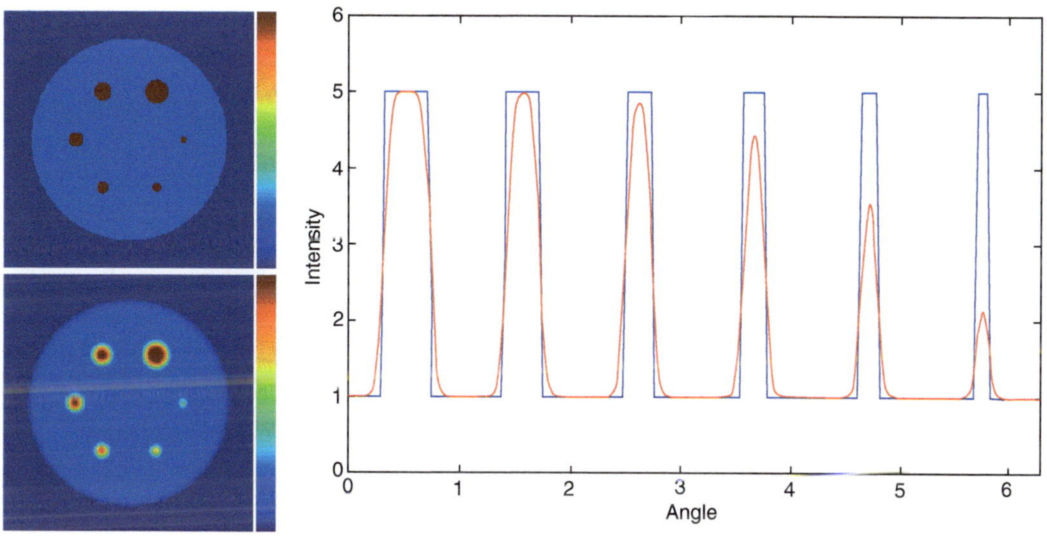

Fig. 15.2 Illustration of 3D PVE. The images on the left hand side show transaxial sections of the original phantom (*top*) and the blurred image (*bottom*) (intensity scale, 0–5). The graph on the right hand side shows a circular profile through the spheres. The *blue line* represents the true data and the *red line* represents the blurred data

well as a circular profile through the spheres. In the largest spheres, there is a section where the measured values coincide with the true values. In the smaller spheres, on the other hand, the maximum measured value is reduced in comparison to the true value. There is therefore a limit in terms of object size, above which the measured max value can be used as an estimation of the true mean value (under the assumption that the object is homogeneous and noise-free). In fact, to use the maximum value in a region is one way to mitigate the effect of PVE. This is a simple method that may work for relatively large, uniform objects, although it is very sensitive to noise. The max and mean values in each sphere are shown in Fig. 15.3 as a function of sphere diameter. It can be seen that the point at which the max value starts to drop below the true value is ~3·FWHM. The mean

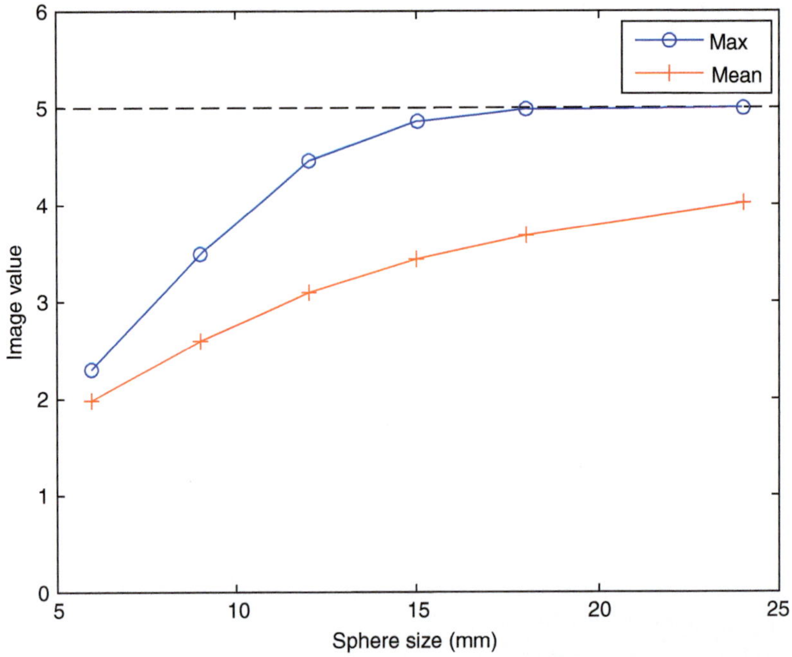

Fig. 15.3 Mean and maximum values in the spheres in Fig. 15.2 as a function of sphere diameter

value always underestimates the true mean value, but it is less noise sensitive than the max value, and the amount of underestimation can be predicted.

15.1.3 The Point Spread Function

In PET, the PSF can often be modelled as a Gaussian function, and the FWHM is sometimes assumed to be constant over the field of view (FOV). In general, the PSF actually varies over the FOV due to the geometry of the detector system. The resolution is determined by the "tubes of response", defined by two opposing detectors. The scintillation crystals used in PET scanners typically have a small cross section in order to give high resolution, but are quite long in the radial direction for high sensitivity. This means that, as you move away from the centre of the scanner, the photons can hit the crystals at an oblique angle, leading to what is known as the "parallax effect" and resulting in broadening of the tubes of response and degradation of the spatial resolution (Fig. 15.4a).

In SPECT, the PSF also varies over the FOV, but for a different reason. The resolution is defined mainly by the geometry of the collimator, resulting in a "cone of response" for a given detector position. This means that the resolution becomes worse with increasing distance from the detector, as the cone becomes wider (Fig. 15.4b). In SPECT, it is easier to model the resolution during forward and back projection, and it can therefore be advantageous to perform PVC during the reconstruction process (see, e.g. [2]). If the image space PSF can be accurately estimated, then post-reconstruction PVC can also be performed in SPECT, using the same methods as in PET.

15.1.4 The Tissue Fraction Effect

PVEs are also said to occur in MRI and CT images. However, in this context, the term does not refer to the effect of the limited spatial resolution of the system, but to the effect of the finite size of the image voxels. Those voxels which are on the boundaries between different organs or tissues would in principle correspond to a mixture of tissue types. We will refer to this sub-voxel effect as the "tissue fraction effect" (TFE). PET images would also be affected by

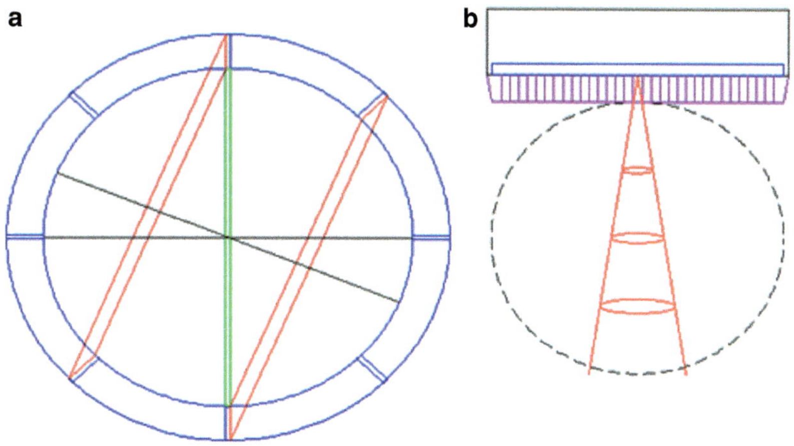

Fig. 15.4 PSF variation in (**a**) PET with a scanner, consisting of a ring of detectors (only a small number are shown), and (**b**) SPECT using a rotating scintillation camera (The effects have been exaggerated for illustration purposes)

this, but the main cause of PVE in PET is the system PSF. The TFE can usually be addressed to some extent by simply using smaller voxels (although it is arguably always present).

15.1.5 Clinical Implications

In clinical studies, if no correction for PVEs is performed, an implicit assumption is made that the PVE is either negligible or constant in space or in time or across subjects.

In neurological studies, most PET tracers used are primarily taken up in grey matter (GM). The GM layer in the cerebral cortex is only a few mm thick, resulting in a significant amount of PVE. In elderly patients suffering from dementia, there is often a certain degree of atrophy, which further reduces the cortical thickness. In this situation, it is not possible to determine whether a reduction in image intensity is due to reduced tracer concentration in GM or is a result of increased PVE due to reduced cortical thickness.

In cardiac studies, various tracers are used that are taken up in the myocardium. The myocardial wall has a thickness of ~10 mm, but it changes over the cardiac cycle, the wall being thicker at end systole as compared to end diastole. This leads to a change in PVE and, consequently, in image intensity. This "systolic brightening" can actually be clinically useful, as it provides indirect information about the myocardial wall thickening.

In oncology, PET studies are often acquired before and after therapy, in order to monitor the effect of the therapy on the tumour. The follow-up study would typically be done a few weeks after the baseline study, during which time the tumour size may have changed and therefore also the PVE. The change in image intensity will be a combination of both the change in tracer uptake and in tumour size. Reduction in tracer uptake or in tumour size both results in reduced image intensity and is an indication of a positive therapy outcome. Therefore, it is not always considered necessary to correct for PVE in this type of study. On the other hand, it may be more useful to obtain the information about tumour size and tracer uptake separately, rather than as a combined outcome measure, as the change in tumour volume may conceal preserved or incremented activity concentration in a small sub-volume that may merit further treatment.

15.1.6 Partial Volume Correction

Methods to correct for PVE are known as "partial volume correction" (PVC) method, although sometimes the term "partial volume effect correction" has been used. The basic principle behind PVC is to utilise the high-resolution anatomical structural information from CT or MRI data to improve the quality of the PET images, with the assumption that the tracer uptake is controlled by the anatomical boundaries. The anatomical image has to be aligned with the PET image, and it usually also needs to be segmented/parcellated into anatomical regions that can be assumed to be relatively uniform in terms of tracer uptake. PVC methods can be divided into region-based and voxel-based methods, depending on whether they provide only corrected regional mean values or a corrected image. In both cases, anatomical regions need to be defined. A number of PVC methods have been proposed over the years, but we will not attempt to cover all of them in this chapter. Instead, we will primarily focus on the most commonly used methods, but we also will describe some of the more advanced techniques that may have future appeal. A recent review of PVC methods can be found in [3].

15.2 Theory

15.2.1 Deconvolution

As mentioned above, PVEs are caused by convolution of the true object distribution with the system PSF. Therefore, it would seem reasonable to believe that PVC could be performed by an inverse convolution, or deconvolution, procedure. Such a procedure can be implemented either during or after the image reconstruction and can provide a certain degree of resolution recovery, resulting in a reduction of PVEs. However, a full correction cannot be achieved with these methods, partly due to information that is lost and cannot be recovered and partly due to an increased noise level and image artefacts.

Convolution of the true image by the PSF results in an attenuation of mid-range frequency information and a loss of high-frequency information. The former can be restored by various types of deconvolution of inverse-filtering techniques, but the latter can never be recovered from the blurred data. At higher frequencies, the data is usually dominated by noise, and any attempt to restore the high-frequency components will result in noise amplification. Sharp boundaries in images are represented using high-frequency components. If these are lost from the image, any algorithm attempting to restore the sharp boundaries will attempt to do so using components from lower frequencies, resulting in oscillations, with over- and undershoots on both sides of the boundaries. This is the so-called Gibb's effect.

Since no new information is introduced, deconvolution algorithms can only provide alternative solutions with different resolution vs. noise trade-offs, based on the original data. The procedure is therefore analogous (but with opposite effect) to smoothing with a low-pass filter. These algorithms should be regarded as optional steps in the image reconstruction process and not as PVC algorithms. Here we will use the term "PVC algorithm" only for those algorithms that utilise structural anatomical information from CT or MRI images (sometimes known as "anatomically guided PVC algorithms"). The role of the anatomical data is to provide local high-frequency information, corresponding to anatomical boundaries.

Figure 15.5 shows the effect of applying an iterative deconvolution algorithm [4] to the blurred image from Fig. 15.2. It can be seen that this algorithm results in ring artefacts in the larger spheres, overcorrection at the centre of the medium-size spheres and under-correction in the smallest sphere. For comparison, the image obtained by using the anatomically guided PVC algorithm region-based voxel-wise correction (RBV) [5] is also shown. This image is identical to the original phantom, which shows how powerful PVC, based on anatomical information, can be. It should also be said that iterative deconvolution algorithms can be improved by incorporating so-called edge-preserving smoothness constraints. This corresponds to utilising a priori information about the expected image, assuming that it should be piecewise constant. The information about the location of the edges must, however, be extracted from the PET data itself.

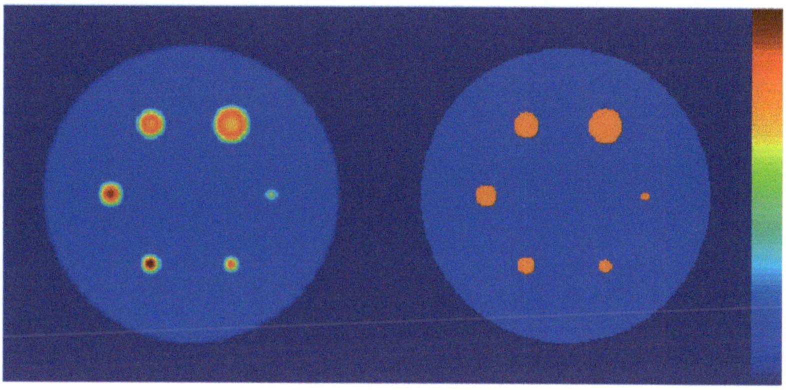

Fig. 15.5 Restoration of the blurred image in Fig. 15.2 using an iterative deconvolution algorithm (*left*) and an anatomically guided PVC algorithm (*right*) (intensity scale, 0–6.5)

15.2.2 Motion

Blurring in PET images can also be caused by motion, such as respiratory, cardiac or patient body motion. However, this is a different effect to the blurring caused by the system PSF and should be treated differently. The blurring caused by motion cannot, in most cases, be described by a simple Gaussian function and cannot be assumed to be uniform. There is no way to avoid the PSF blurring, but motion blurring, on the other hand, can be reduced or even eliminated completely by simply using shorter time frames. It then becomes a motion correction problem (see Chap. 16). The two effects are independent and can be treated separately; motion correction should be applied first and then PVC.

15.2.3 Region-Based PVC

We will now describe a series of PVC methods to correct for the system PSF only. (A more detailed mathematical description can be found in the appendix.) Figure 15.6 shows a scheme representing the early developments of PVC methods, including some still commonly used ones. In 1979, Hoffman et al. introduced the term PVE and proposed a method for correcting the mean value in a volume of interest (VOI), assuming a uniform distribution within the VOI and no background activity [6]. The true mean value is obtained by simply dividing the measured mean value within the VOI by a recovery coefficient (RC), precalculated based on the shape and size of the VOI and the system PSF. This method is therefore corrected for spill-out but not for spill-in. Later, Kessler et al. calculated RC values for cases with a non-zero background activity [7]. In this way, correction could be done for both spill-in and spill-out at the same time, but it was necessary to know the true target-to-background contrast in order to select the correct RC values.

A different approach was chosen by Henze et al. for cardiac studies [8] (see also [9]). They developed a method to correct for the crosstalk between two different VOIs, corresponding to the myocardium of the left ventricle (LV) and the blood pool inside the LV. The contributions from each VOI to the other one and to itself were calculated based on the system PSF. A system of two linear equations was then set up, which could easily be solved by matrix inversion, resulting in the true mean values in the two VOIs.

The same principle was later used by Rousset et al. for neurological studies [10]. In this case, the brain was parcellated into multiple VOIs, based on MRI data. This method can in principle handle any number of VOIs, although the matrix inversion operation can become numerically unstable with too many VOIs. The authors called the crosstalk matrix the "geometric transfer matrix" (GTM), and the method became known as the GTM method. Another method, proposed by Labbé et al., was based on a slightly different formulation with a much larger crosstalk matrix [11]. In the original paper, the authors used an algorithm based on singular value decomposition to calculate the matrix inverse; however, a more practical solu-

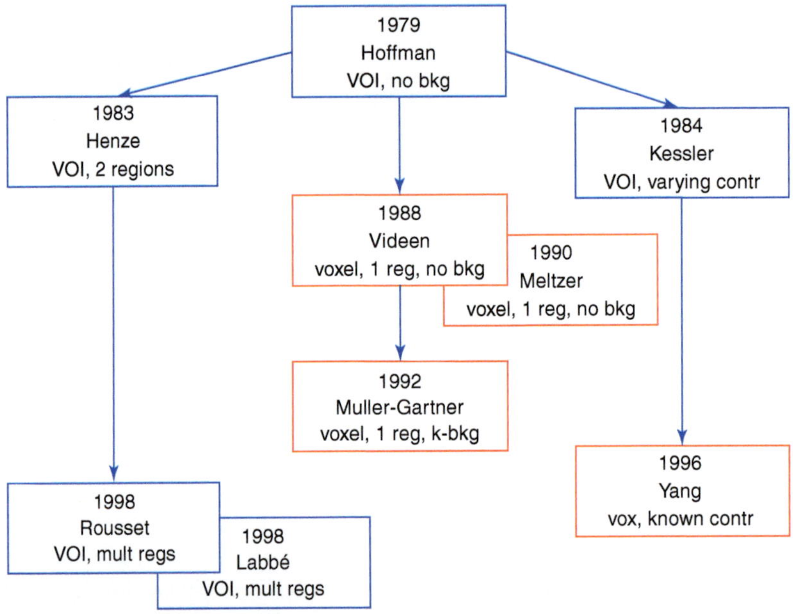

Fig. 15.6 Development of traditional PVC techniques

tion is obtained by using the Moore-Penrose pseudo-inverse instead. The method then becomes very similar to the GTM method. In both cases, the image is parcellated into a number of VOIs. In the GTM method, the image is then sampled using the original VOIs, while in the Labbé method, the VOIs are first blurred by the system PSF. This leads to a different cross-talk matrix, but the output from both methods will be the corrected mean values in the original VOIs. The theoretical difference between these two methods is that the Labbé method in principle utilises all the data corresponding to each VOI in the estimation of their mean values, resulting in a slightly different accuracy vs. precision trade-off.

A simple region-based PVC method was developed by Hofheinz et al. for oncology [12]. It is based on the definition of three regions (VOIs) for each tumour: a target region, corresponding to the actual tumour; a "spill-out" region, surrounding the target region; and a background region, surrounding the spill-out region. First a background term is estimated using the background region and subtracted from the spill-out region. The true activity concentration in the target region is then determined as the total activity in the target and spill-out regions divided by the volume of the target region. The advantage with this method is that it is not very sensitive to an accurate estimation of the PSF.

15.2.4 Voxel-Based PVC

In the methods described above, the image was divided into a number of regions (or VOIs), and the goal of the PVC was to estimate the true mean value within these regions. For voxel-based PVC, it is still (in general) necessary to divide the image into regions, but the correction is then applied to each voxel within these regions separately, thereby producing a new, corrected image. The basic idea is to correct for the spill over from one region to another, but the correction is different for each voxel, as the spill over is not uniformly distributed.

The first voxel-based PVC method was presented by Videen et al. [13]. It was essentially an extension of the Hoffman method. One target VOI was defined and RC values were calculated for each voxel within this VOI, correcting for spill-out but not spill-in. The method was intended for neurological studies and was based on a CT image, segmented into brain and non-brain regions. The brain region included both grey matter (GM) and white matter (WM). This method was later implemented by Meltzer et al. [14], using MRI instead of CT data, and is often cited through this reference.

Later, Müller-Gärtner et al. improved the method by incorporating spill-in correction [15]. In this case, the brain was segmented into three regions: GM, WM and cerebrospinal fluid (CSF). The target region was GM, while WM was considered as a background region. The activity concentration in CSF was assumed to be zero, but it was necessary to know the true value in WM for the spill-in correction. This could be estimated from a WM region, less likely to be affected by PVE. The spill-in from WM to GM was calculated and subtracted, before using the voxel-based RCs to correct for spill-out. This is an additive-multiplicative method, in which PVC is applied to the target region (GM) only.

An alternative approach was used by Yang et al. in their voxel-based PVC method [16]. This method can be seen as an extension of the Kessler method. Multiplicative correction factors are generated for each voxel in the whole image, correcting for both spill-in and spill out simultaneously. This method requires prior knowledge of the contrast between the different regions. In Yang et al. [16] the method was implemented for brain studies with a 3-class segmentation into GM, WM and CSF, assuming relative activity concentrations of 4, 1 and 0, respectively.

15.2.5 Combined PVC Methods

The PVC methods mentioned above have certain advantages and disadvantages: the region-based methods can only provide mean regional values, while the voxel-based ones require various types of prior information. However, by combining the two approaches, you can get the best of both worlds. Figure 15.7 shows a schematic illustration for how this can be done. The procedure consists of the following four steps:

1. The anatomical image is segmented/parcellated into a number of VOIs.
2. Region-based PVC is applied to obtain the mean values in each VOI.
3. A piecewise constant pseudo-image is generated, where all voxels in each region contain the corresponding mean value.
4. The pseudo-image is finally used to perform a voxel-based PVC.

In step 2, either the GTM method or the Labbé method can be used. In step 4, either a Müller-Gärtner-type or a Yang-type correction can be used. Two such algorithms have been proposed: the "multi-target correction" (MTC) method [17] and the "region-based voxel-wise correction" (RBV) method [5]. Another alternative is a method known as "iterative Yang" (iY), proposed in [3], in which the regional mean values are estimated in an iterative procedure with a Yang-type correction, avoiding the GTM step.

Recently a new PVC method was introduced, called "single target correction" (STC) [18]. This method only requires segmentation of the region to be corrected and does not need any a priori information regarding the activity distribution. It operates using region-based spill-out correction and voxel-based spill-in correction, which are applied to both target and background regions.

15.3 PVC Examples

15.3.1 Data Generation

We simulated PET data corresponding to various digital phantoms using the following procedure: (1) the true activity distribution was blurred in the image domain with a 3D Gaussian function with a FWHM of 6 mm, representing the system PSF; (2) the resulting image was forward projected into 180 angles over 180° and multiplied by a forward projected attenuation map; (3) a uniform background was added, representing randoms and scattered events, corresponding to 33 % of

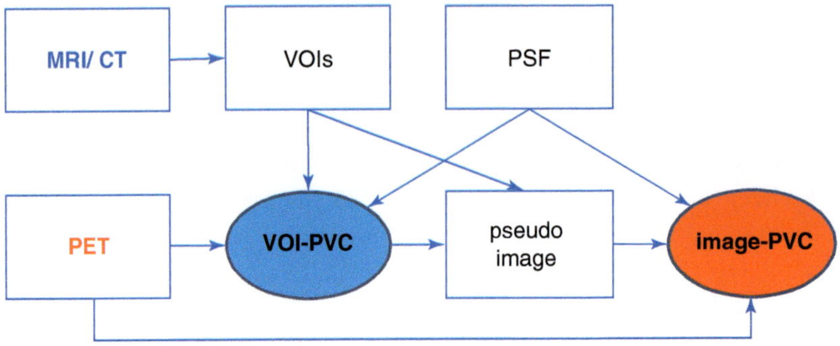

Fig. 15.7 Schematic illustration of the combination of region- and voxel-based PVC. Region-based PVC is performed first, using VOIs defined in the MRI or CT image and the system PSF. Voxel-based PVC can then be performed, using a piecewise constant pseudo-image, generated based on the corrected VOI mean values, resulting in a corrected image (See text for step-by-step description)

the data; (4) the projection data were scaled so as to obtain a realistic total number of counts, and Poisson distributed data were generated using a random number generator; (5) images were reconstructed using FBP, after background and attenuation correction; and (6) the reconstructed images were smoothed with a 3D Gaussian with a FWHM of ~5.3 mm for noise-reduction purposes. For each phantom, the simulations were repeated with 30 different noise realisations.

15.3.2 Example 1: Oncology

We simulated data corresponding to an oncology study using the NCAT torso phantom [19], including respiratory and cardiac motion with periods of 5 s and 1 s, respectively. Data was generated for 40 frames (gates) over one respiratory period. Two spherical tumours (20 mm diameter) were added to the phantom, one in the lung and one in the liver. After reconstructing each frame independently, motion correction (MC) was applied, using an estimated motion pattern. PVC was then applied to each tumour using STC [18].

Figure 15.8 shows a coronal section of the true distribution as well as the reconstructed image without correction, after MC only and after both MC and PVC. Profiles through the tumours are shown in Fig. 15.9, and the mean values in the tumours are presented in Table 15.1, including results obtained with the Hofheinz method [12].

In the uncorrected image, the tumours are elongated due to motion blurring. MC restores their round shape and increases the intensity. PVC improves the uniformity in the tumours and further increases the intensity. Quantitatively, the correction is not perfect. This could be due approximations in the motion pattern or in the PSF. The Hofheinz method seems to give slightly higher accuracy than STC in the liver tumour. This could be because it is less dependent on the PSF. However, it relies on a uniform background and does not produce a new image.

15.3.3 Example 2: Cardiology

The same phantom was used as in the previous example, but without tumours. MC was applied and the image frames were merged into eight cardiac gates. PVC was applied to the myocardium using STC [18]. The heart was reoriented into standard short- and long-axis sections.

Images with and without correction are shown in Fig. 15.10 for the end systole (ES) and end diastole (ED) phases of the cardiac cycle, and quantitative results are presented in Table 15.2.

In the uncorrected images, there is underestimation of the myocardial image intensity, and there is a difference between ES and ED. After MC, the intensity is increased and the ES-ED difference is reduced. After MC+PVC, there is further increase in intensity, and the difference is reduced to <1 %.

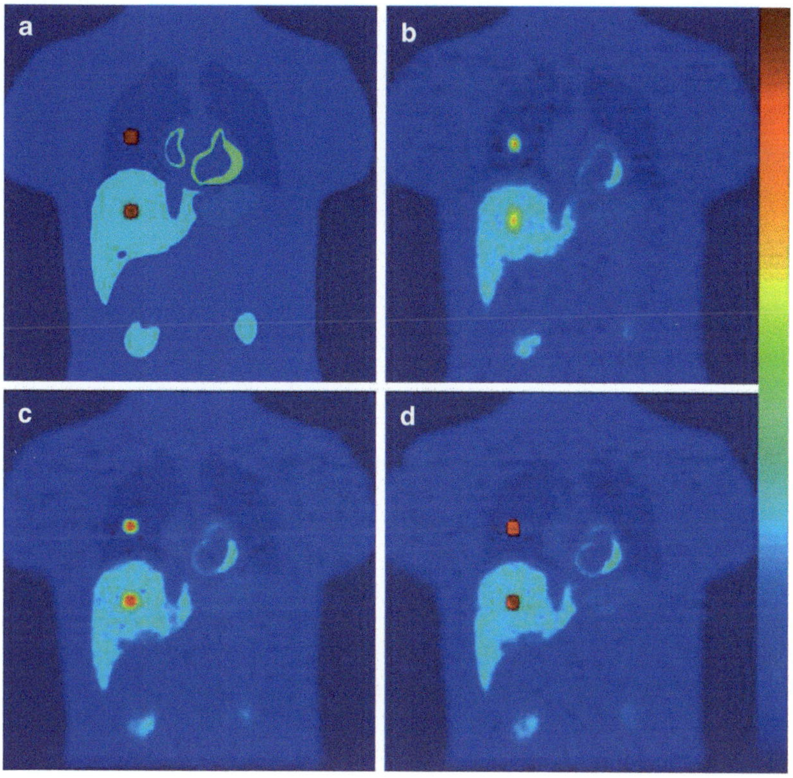

Fig. 15.8 Simulated oncology study. (**a**) Original phantom (single frame), (**b**) simulated PET image including motion blurring and PVE, (**c**) image after MC, (**d**) image after MC and PVC (STC)

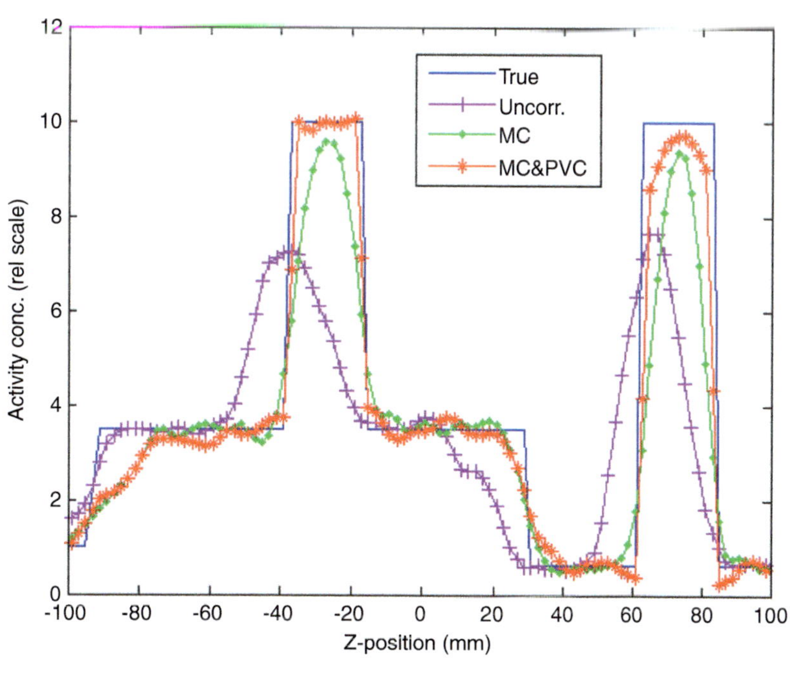

Fig. 15.9 Vertical profiles through the images in Fig. 15.8a–d, passing through the two tumours

Table 15.1 Quantitative results of the oncology simulation experiment (%, mean ± SD)

	Method	Lung tumour	Liver tumour
Corrections		Mean ± SD	Mean ± SD
Uncorrected		46.97 ± 0.34	58.49 ± 0.36
MC		57.22 ± 0.28	71.11 ± 0.37
MC + PVC	Hofheinz	89.75 ± 0.76	96.49 ± 1.15
	STC	89.79 ± 0.50	93.69 ± 0.70

15.3.4 Example 3: Neurology

We used a brain phantom [20] for testing several of the PVC methods developed for neurology studies. The phantom contained a number of cortical and subcortical regions (Fig. 15.11). The matrix size was 256 × 256 × 128 and the voxel size 1.1 × 1.1 × 1.4 mm. From the original phantom, we generated a segmented version, containing regions for grey matter (GM), white matter (WM) and cerebrospinal fluid (CSF) (Fig. 15.11), and also an activity distribution, with values of 0.8–1.2 in the GM regions, 0.25 in WM and 0.01 in CSF. A sinusoidal pattern was added to the image, in order to introduce some intra-regional variation (Fig. 15.12). We applied five different PVC methods to the reconstructed image: (1) Videen/Meltzer (V/M) [13, 14], (2) Müller-Gärtner (MG) [15], (3) GTM [10], (4) MTC [17] and (5) RBV [5].

The resulting images are shown in Fig. 15.12 and some quantitative results in Fig. 15.13. The V/M method gives a very limited correction, as it does not separate between GM and WM (no image shown). The GTM method produces only regional mean values, so all intra-regional variation is lost. The MG method performs a voxel-wise correction and therefore retains some of the original intra-regional variation, but only within the GM region. (It assumes the true WM mean value can be estimated separately.) Also, it only corrects for spill over between GM and WM, not between different GM regions. Therefore, the quantitative accuracy is limited (see, e.g. the insula region). The MTC and RBV methods both perform voxel-wise correction of the entire image, retaining some intra-regional variation (see, e.g. the putamen region). Both methods also give accurate regional mean values, but the RBV results are less noisy.

15.4 Practical Considerations

15.4.1 Accuracy

The PVC procedure consists of a number of separate steps, and many things can go wrong along the way. As mentioned previously, the final result of PVC is sensitive to small errors in various steps of the process. The key steps are (1) estimation of the system PSF, (2) co-registration of the PET and anatomical images and (3) segmentation and/or parcellation of the anatomical image into different tissue types and anatomical regions.

One way to deal with the possibility of misregistration is to use blurred anatomical labels instead of the original ones, to reflect the uncertainty in the co-registration [21, 22]. This would reduce any potential artefacts, but also the accuracy of the correction. Various groups have investigated the robustness of different PVC methods [23–25]. Validation of PVC methods is usually performed with simulated data, as it requires knowledge of ground truth in terms of activity concentration. It can, however, be difficult to simulate data that are clinically realistic and also independent of the PVC methods used.

15.4.2 Resolution

The PSF of the system depends on several factors: the range of the positrons before annihilation, the non-colinearity of the annihilation photons, the geometry and intrinsic resolution of the detector system and the image reconstruction algorithm.

The magnitude of the positron range depends on the radionuclide used. It is not very large for ^{18}F, but becomes a more important factor for other radionuclides, such as ^{82}Rb. The range also depends on the tissue density, being longer in the lung and air and shorter in the soft tissue and bone. Johnson et al. looked at the difference in

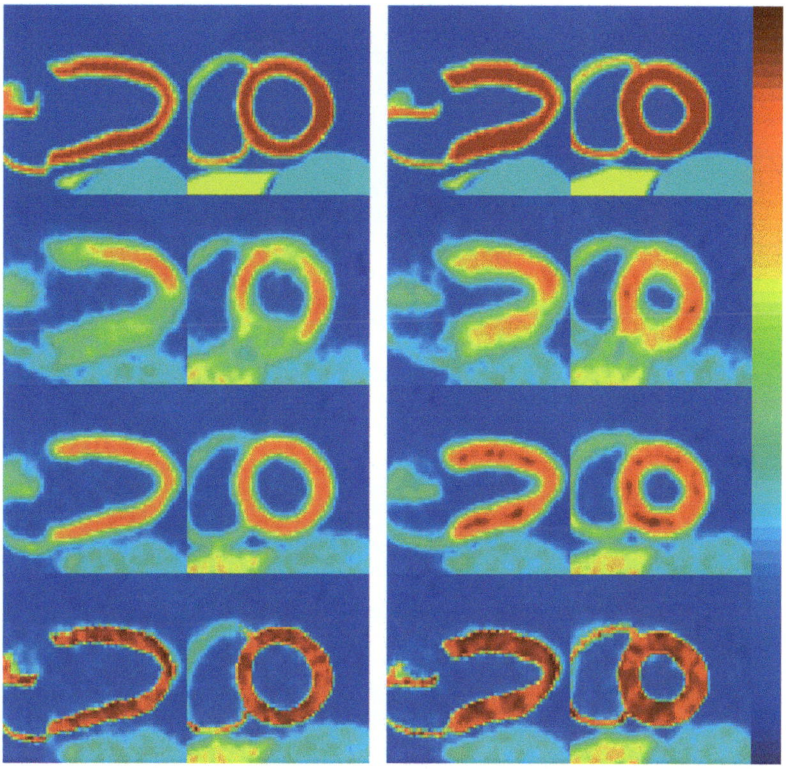

Fig. 15.10 Cardiac phantom for end diastole (*left panel*) and end systole (*right panel*) gates, including vertical long-axis (*first column*) and short-axis (*second column*) sections. The *top row* shows true activity distribution with MC; the *second row*, uncorrected images; the *third row*, images after MC only; and the *bottom row* images obtained after MC and PVC (STC)

PVC factors in cardiac studies between ^{18}F and ^{82}Rb [26]. They found an average whole heart cycle PVC factor of 1.23 for ^{82}Rb, as compared to 1.14 for ^{18}F.

In most PET scanners, the resolution is spatially variant, i.e. it depends on the position in the field of view (FOV). This is due to the parallax effect, which results in a PSF that becomes more and more elongated in the radial direction, as you move further away from the central axis of the scanner. For brain studies, it may be adequate to assume a spatially invariant PSF (for simplicity), although higher accuracy is achieved by taking this variability into account [27].

If the PET scanner has a very good spatial resolution, then the PVE will be small and PVC may not even be necessary. For example, Uchida et al. found that serotonin-2A receptor binding, measured with the HRRT PET scanner, decreased with age, consistent before and after PVC, suggesting that PVC may not be necessary with the HRRT scanner, which has a resolution of ~2.8 mm [28].

Table 15.2 Quantitative results from the cardiac phantom simulation experiment

	End diastole	End systole	Difference (%)
True values	100	100	0
Uncorrected	65.0	70.0	7.53
MC	75.5	78.5	3.88
MC and PVC	93.2	94.0	0.84

The PSF also depends on the reconstruction algorithm used: whether it is analytical or iterative; whether or not any low-pass filter was used before, after or during reconstruction; and whether resolution recovery was included or not. Analytical reconstruction algorithms (such as FBP) are linear, and the PSF can be accurately estimated using point source measurements. Iterative algorithms (such as ML-EM, OS-EM or MAP-EM), on the other hand, are nonlinear, and the PSF in the reconstructed image will depend not only on the number of iterations and number of subsets used but also on the activity distribution in the object being imaged. The speed of

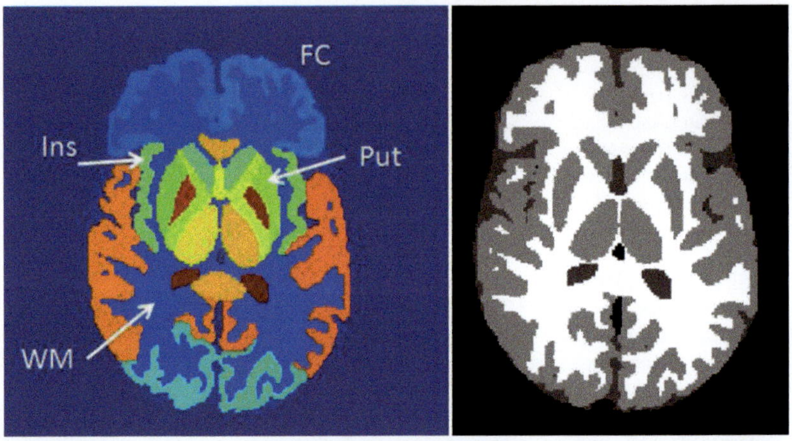

Fig. 15.11 *Left*: mask of the brain phantom with different colours for different regions, including the frontal cortex (*FC*), putamen (*Put*), insula (*Ins*) and white matter (*WM*). *Right*: segmentation of the brain phantom into CSF (*dark grey*), GM (*light grey*) and WM (*white*)

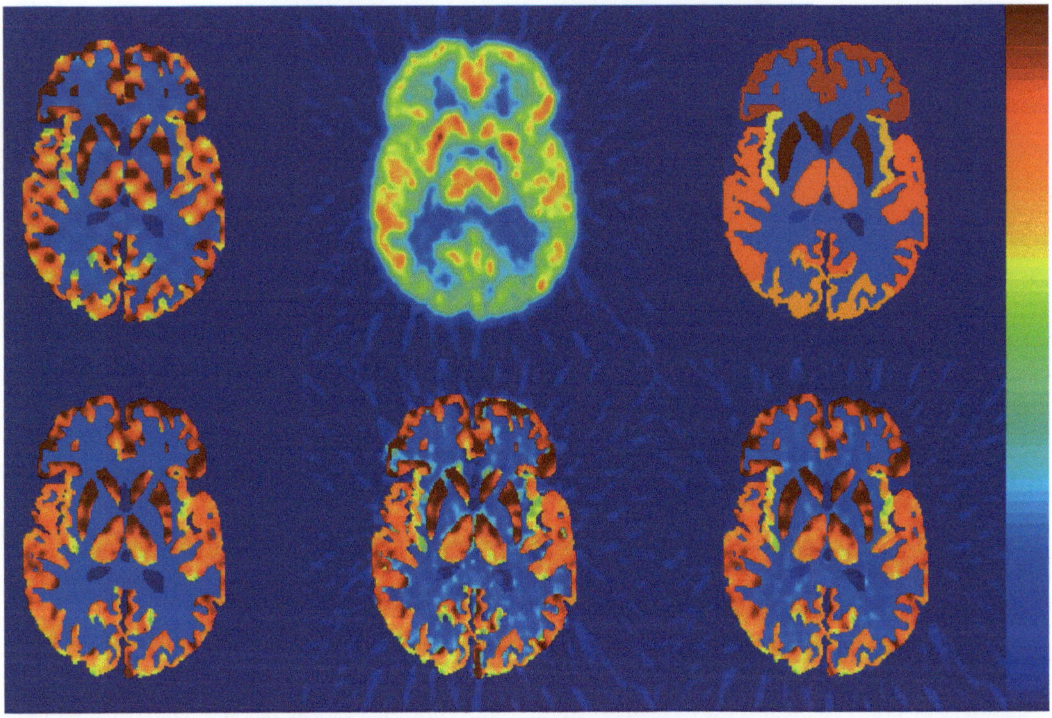

Fig. 15.12 Results of the brain phantom experiment, from *left to right* and *top to bottom*: the true activity distribution, the uncorrected image and images corrected using the GTM, MG, MTC and RBV methods

convergence of the algorithm will also be object dependent. *Further details on image reconstruction can be found in* Chap. 11.

In the case of iterative reconstruction, the PSF can be estimated using the perturbation technique [29], which can be described as follows: a point source with a very low intensity (a perturbation) is added to an image, which is then forward projected, and a new image is reconstructed. By subtracting the image reconstructed without the perturbation, an image of the point source is obtained, which should represent the PSF corresponding to the original image at a specific location, for a particular reconstruction procedure. A similar approach has been described for directly estimating regional crosstalk coefficients [30].

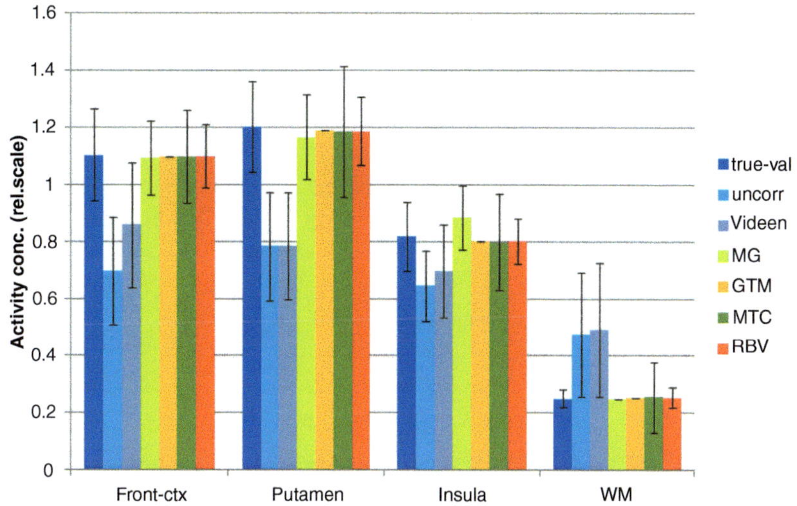

Fig. 15.13 Quantitative analysis of brain PVC methods. The *error bars* represent SD across voxels within each region

15.4.3 Co-registration

A fundamental step for the correction is to co-register the PET and anatomical images. This typically involves maximising a measure of similarity (cost-function) between a transformed image and a fixed image. There are a number of choices that have to be made: which should be the transformed and which should be the fixed image? Should a rigid, affine or nonlinear transformation be used? What cost-function and interpolation method should be used? In general, the best procedure to follow will depend on the type of data involved. You need to consider that, if a transformation is applied to the PET image, the interpolation will introduce some extra blurring, causing more PVE. For brain studies, a rigid transformation would in principle be sufficient. However, it could be necessary to use an affine transformation, e.g. to take into account possible MRI distortions. For non-brain studies, a nonlinear transformation is usually required. With regard to the cost-function, when co-registering images from different modalities, the best choice would be to use either mutual information (MI) [31] or normalised MI [32].

With dual-modality scanners such as PET/CT or PET/MRI, you might think that no co-registration would be needed, as the two images should be automatically registered. However, even if the patient does not leave the bed, there can still be some patient motion between the acquisitions of the two data sets, and even a small misregistration can cause significant errors in the PVC. Also, the FOV can be different for the two modalities, and PVC will only be possible in the region where there is an overlap. For further information on image registration, see one of the following reviews [33–37].

15.4.4 Segmentation

In cardiac studies, the anatomical image needs to be segmented into the myocardium and blood pool, which are of primary interest for PVC, and also neighbouring structures such as the lungs and liver, for background activity [38]. It may also be important to segment severe uptake defects as independent regions [39]. If a CT image is used, it will be necessary to use contrast enhancement in order to distinguish the myocardium and the blood pool [39, 40], but this is not needed with MRI [41]. There is therefore an advantage in hybrid PET/MR over PET/CT for quantitative cardiac imaging. To reduce motion blur in cardiac studies, ECG and respiratory gating can be used.

In neurological studies, the MRI image, first of all, has to be segmented into different tissue types: GM, WM and CSF. This type of segmentation can be done based on the voxel intensities in the MRI image and is sufficient for some PVC methods. Other methods require further subdivision into various cortical and subcortical anatomical brain structures. This is known as parcellation, and it cannot be done using intensity information only. However, automatic methods have been developed using probabilistic atlases, based on manual labelling [42–44].

Zaidi et al. and Gutierrez et al. performed a comparative evaluation of various algorithms for segmentation of brain MRI images for PVC using simulated and clinical data [45, 46]. They found substantial differences between algorithms and concluded that a careful choice of the segmentation algorithm for PVC is needed.

15.4.5 Sampling

The sampling rate required in a digital image depends on the highest frequency present in the data. According to the Nyquist sampling theorem, the sampling rate should be $1/d = 2 \cdot \nu_{max}$, where d is the distance between samples (voxels) and ν_{max} is the highest frequency [1]. As CT and MRI images have better spatial resolution than PET images, they need smaller voxel sizes. Due to the difference in the voxel size, it will be necessary to resample either the PET or the anatomical image for the purpose of PVC. Usually, the anatomical image is down-sampled, and the PVC is applied with the original PET voxel size. In this case, it is possible to utilise the higher original sampling of the anatomical image to produce a "fuzzy" segmentation [38]. This means that voxels at the edge between two regions have a certain probability, p ($0 \leq p \leq 1$), to belong to one of the regions and a probability ($1-p$) to belong to the other. (There could also be more than two regions involved.) On the other hand, if you consider that the fundamental purpose of PVC is to improve the spatial resolution in the PET image (at least locally), it should make more sense to use a smaller voxel size for the corrected image. From this point of view, it would be better to up-sample the PET images to the voxel size of the anatomical image. This also allows for the use of a binary rather than a fuzzy segmentation, which simplifies the correction procedure. The downside is that it will be slower and require more space for data storage. It will also be necessary to consider which interpolation method to use for resampling the PET image. Due to the usually noisy nature of PET images, the safest choice would typically be trilinear interpolation.

15.5 Advanced Topics

15.5.1 Alternative Correction Approaches

We have so far only considered PVC methods that are applied to the reconstructed PET image, i.e. post-reconstruction methods. An alternative approach is to incorporate the anatomical data as prior information in the reconstruction process (see Ref. [47] for a review). This approach can produce better results than post-reconstruction algorithms, but is more complex and requires access to the raw projection data. (See also Chap. 11.)

15.5.2 Alternative Correction Methods

The fundamental objective of PVC can be described as transfer of high-frequency information from a high-resolution anatomical image to a lower-resolution PET image. All voxel-based PVC methods mentioned above do this. An alternative way to achieve the same objective has been proposed, based on the multiresolution property of the wavelet transform [48, 49]. In this method, high-resolution components of the PET image are replaced, in part, with those of the anatomical image after appropriate scaling.

15.5.3 Alternative Classification Methods

For PVC we need to subdivide an image into different image components or tissue classes. Previously we have assumed that this is achieved by segmentation of an anatomical image. However, there are other ways in which this can be done.

If one of the components is blood, it is possible to obtain an image of the blood distribution by doing a separate PET scan with a tracer that stays in the intravascular space, such as $C^{15}O$ [50].

With dynamic data, it is also possible to separate between different components or tissue types by the shape of the corresponding time-activity curves. In this case, the crosstalk coefficients can be incorporated into a kinetic model and estimated together with the standard kinetic parameters. This has been utilised to distinguish blood and myocardium in cardiac studies [51] and between GM and WM in brain studies [52].

If, on the other hand, a standard PVC method is applied to dynamic PET data, it is important to take into account the fact that since the activity distribution in the object changes with time, so does the PVE. This means that the PVC must be performed before the kinetic modelling, rather than being applied to a parametric image [27].

Several methods have been proposed for performing resolution recovery combined with anatomically guided smoothing procedures, which do not require segmentation or parcellation of the anatomical data. These methods use a neighbourhood defined around each image voxel. Ardekani et al. proposed a method based on smoothing kernel with weights determined based on the difference in the MRI image values [53]. Bowsher et al. proposed a method, in which voxels are chosen within the neighbourhood, such that the difference between the anatomical image values is minimised [54]. Yan et al. proposed another method, in which a linear relationship is assumed to exist between the anatomical image values and the PET values within the neighbourhood [55]. The first two methods are reconstruction based, while the third one is a post-reconstruction method.

15.6 Clinical Applications

Below is a summary of some of the studies, in which the clinical usefulness of PVC has been investigated. Most of the clinical studies with PVC have been in neurology, and in most of these, the MG method [15] was used. PVC has also been used in a number of oncological studies, mostly using a RC method, with or without the background being taken into account. In cardiology, there have only been a few clinical studies, using a range of different PVC methods. In most cases, PVC was found to be clinically useful, but not always. Sometimes PVC improved the diagnostic accuracy of a method, and sometimes it changed a clinical finding.

15.6.1 Cardiology

Herrero et al. applied the Henze PVC method [8] to dynamic $H_2{}^{15}O$ PET data from dog studies to obtain quantitative estimations of myocardial blood flow [9]. They used data from a study with $C^{15}0$ (which labels only red blood cells) to estimate the dimensions of the ventricular cavity and an average literature value for the myocardial wall thickness. Their results correlated closely with flow values obtained with a standard technique using radiolabeled microspheres.

Iida et al. compared two different methods of correcting for PVE in cardiac PET studies, based on the measurement of tissue fraction and extravascular density, respectively [50]. The tissue fraction was determined from dynamic $H_2{}^{15}O$ PET studies, by assuming it was directly proportional to the volume of distribution of water. The extravascular tissue density was obtained by subtraction of a blood volume image, derived from the $C^{15}0$ PET scan, from a tissue density image, obtained from a transmission scan [56]. They found that the tissue fraction was ~10 % larger than the extravascular density in normal tissue regions, but that this ratio was reduced in regions of infarction, and concluded that the combined use of these two techniques may aid in the differentiation between perfusable and non-perfusable tissue in the infarcted myocardium.

Johnson et al. demonstrated the importance of PVC in quantitative myocardial perfusion studies, using clinical data from ECG-gated ^{82}Rb PET studies [26]. First, diastolic PVC was performed relative to systole, based on the systolic/diastolic activity ratio, and then systolic PVC was performed, based on phantom data combined with the systolic left ventricular wall thicknesses. They determined a whole heart cycle PVC factor for ungated images of 1.23.

15.6.2 Neurology

Meltzer et al. found a mild but significant inverse correlation between age and cortical CBF in the uncorrected data but not in the data corrected for PVE using an MRI-based method [57]. The authors concluded that the decline seen in the uncorrected data was caused by increased PVE due to age-related cerebral atrophy rather than a real decrease in CBF.

Giovacchini et al. evaluated the effect of healthy ageing on brain incorporation of ^{11}C-arachidonic acid [58]. They found reduction in tracer uptake in the frontal lobe in old subjects as compared to young ones, which were significant before but not after PVC.

Bencherif et al. studied the influence of PVC on analysis of age effects on μ-opioid receptor (μ-OR) binding using ^{11}C-carfentanil PET in healthy subjects [59]. Without PVC, they found no significant relationship with age. However, after PVC, they found that μ-OR binding in the left temporal cortex increased with age, which is consistent with the results from autoradiographic studies.

Yanase et al. investigate the effects of atrophy correction on ^{18}F-FDG PET studies in the context of normal ageing [60]. They found that significant negative correlations between age and relative FDG activity, observed before PVC, were largely resolved after PVC.

Curiati et al. performed a study in order to test whether there is regional cerebral age-related hypometabolism in later stages of life, using ^{18}F-FDG PET studies in cognitively healthy elderly subjects [61]. Their study revealed significant sex-specific age-related metabolic decrease in various brain regions before PVC, which did not remained significant after PVC. They concluded that age-related functional brain variability is largely secondary to regional brain atrophy.

Samuraki et al. investigated the effects of PVC on ^{18}F-FDG PET studies in patients with mild Alzheimer's disease (AD) [62]. They found that FDG uptake in the posterior cingulate gyri and parietotemporal lobes was reduced in AD regardless of whether or not PVC was applied, supporting the notion that the reduced FDG uptake in these areas was not the result of atrophy. In this study, PVC also revealed that FDG uptake in medial temporal lobe, including hippocampal areas, was relatively preserved, despite grey matter loss, as revealed by voxel-based morphometry.

15.6.3 Oncology

Vesselle et al. examined the relationship between ^{18}F-FDG uptake and surgical stage in non-small cell lung cancer (NSCLC) [63]. Tracer uptake was quantified by maximum standardised uptake value (SUV_{max}) in the tumour. PVC was performed using recovery coefficients (RC), with background correction. The RC values were dependent on lesion size, which was estimated from CT images. They found an association between tumour stage and FDG uptake before, but not after PVC.

Vesselle et al. compared primary NSCLC ^{18}F-FDG uptake in PET with tumour Ki-67 proliferation index [64]. There was a significant positive correlation between FDG uptake and Ki-67 scores. Partial volume correction increased the strength of this correlation while also diminishing the positive correlation between FDG uptake and tumour size.

Tsujikawa et al. investigated the relationship between ^{18}F-FDG uptake in PET and the clinical aggressiveness of non-Hodgkin's lymphoma [65]. FDG uptake was quantified by SUV_{max} values, and PVC was performed using RC values. They found that the diagnostic accuracy was higher without than with PVC. The authors assumed this was because the uncorrected values contain information about lesion size as well as FDG uptake. These two quantities would have similar effects on the image values: a reduced lesion size leads to increased PVE and hence reduced image values and vice versa. On the other hand, after PVC, the image values depend only on ^{18}F-FDG uptake. (The lesion size information would still have been available separately, of course, but this was not considered.)

Sakaguchi et al. investigated the diagnostic ability of ^{18}F-FDG PET for lymph node metastasis [66]. FDG uptake was quantified by SUV_{max} and PVC was performed using RC values dependent on lesion size, as measured from CT images, as well as lesion-to-background ratio. They found that the difference in SUV_{max} between malignant and benign lymph nodes became more prominent after correction, so that PVC improved the diagnostic accuracy.

Maruoka et al. evaluate the clinical usefulness of PVC in ^{18}F-FDG PET/CT studies for predicting accumulation of ^{131}I in metastatic lymph nodes during ^{131}I-therapy [67]. Uptake of FDG was quantified by SUV_{max} and PVC was performed using RC values. They found that the accuracy in predictability for ^{131}I accumulation was significantly better with than without PVC.

15.7 Summary

PVC is important when absolute quantification of activity concentration is required. It is also important in situations in which there is a change in PVE between two studies. This could happen if the dimensions of organ or tissue of interest changes due to, e.g. atrophy, muscular contraction or disease progression, or if the activity distribution changes due to tracer kinetics. In these situations, the PVE could be a confounding factor, resulting in misinterpretation of the data.

Resolution-recovery or deconvolution algorithms can reduce the PVE, but a more accurate correction can be obtained when high-resolution anatomical information from CT or MRI is available. A number of PVC methods that utilise anatomical information have been proposed over the years, based on different assumptions and data requirements (see Erlandsson et al. [3] for review).

In this chapter, various PVC methods for PET have been described, but we have largely ignored all the work that has been done on PVC for SPECT. The reason for this was to avoid having to introduce extra complexities, as there are several technical issues related to PVC in SPECT, which are not relevant for PET.

The PVC procedure is sensitive to errors in various data processing steps, such as PSF estimation, anatomical segmentation and parcellation and image co-registration. It is therefore worthwhile putting some care into each of these steps. It should also be remembered that, due to some of the assumptions involve (e.g. regional uniformity), PVC is in general just an approximate correction.

Different methods tend to be used for different type of studies, e.g. the MG method or the GTM method is often used in neurology, while in oncological studies, various RC techniques are typically applied (see Soret et al. [68]). These methods all have limitations, and it could be advantageous to use a method such as RBV [5], which provides a voxel-based correction of the whole image.

Comparison of different PVC methods is not trivial, as assumptions made when generating the test data may favour one method over another one [69]. In order to facilitate this type of comparison, Thomas et al. propose a methodology for simulation of PET and MR images, based on real patient data [70]. This methodology attempts to avoid assumptions about the activity distribution, so as to allow a fair comparison between methods.

The availability of PET/MRI greatly improves the logistics of acquiring well-registered PET and MRI data in individuals and so should encourage routine PV correction in the future.

Acknowledgements The author wishes to thank Prof. Brian Hutton, INM, UCL, UK, for revising the text and providing useful comments and suggestions.

15.8 Appendix: PVC Methods

A PET image, $g(\cdot)$, can be described by a convolution operation between the true image, $f(\cdot)$, and the system PSF, $h(\cdot)$:

$$g(x) = \int f(x')h(x - x')dx' \triangleq \{f \otimes h\}(x)$$

where $\boldsymbol{x}$ and $\boldsymbol{x}'$ are coordinates in 3D space.

In the Hoffman PVC method [6], the mean value, m_V, in a region, V, in the uncorrected image is first calculated:

$$m_V = \overline{g(\boldsymbol{x})}\Big|_{\boldsymbol{x}\in V}$$

Next, a region-specific recovery coefficient, C_V, is calculated:

$$C_V = \overline{J_V(\boldsymbol{x})}\Big|_{\boldsymbol{x}\in V}$$

where $J_V(\cdot)$ is a blurred version of the indicator function, $I_V(\cdot)$, for region V:

$$J_V(\boldsymbol{x}) = \{I_V \otimes h\}(\boldsymbol{x})$$

$$I_V(\boldsymbol{x}) = \begin{cases} 1; \boldsymbol{x}\in V \\ 0; \boldsymbol{x}\notin V \end{cases}$$

The correct mean value, $\hat{\mu}_V$, can then be estimated as

$$\hat{\mu}_V = \frac{1}{C_V} m_V$$

The Henze method [8] corrects for crosstalk between two regions, V_1 and V_2, by solving a system of linear equations:

$$\begin{cases} m_1 = c_{11}\mu_1 + c_{12}\mu_2 \\ m_2 = c_{21}\mu_1 + c_{22}\mu_2 \end{cases}$$

where

$$c_{ij} = \overline{J_{V_j}(\boldsymbol{x})}\Big|_{\boldsymbol{x}\in V_i}$$

The solution is obtained by matrix inversion:

$$\begin{pmatrix} \hat{\mu}_1 \\ \hat{\mu}_2 \end{pmatrix} = \boldsymbol{C}^{-1} \begin{pmatrix} m_1 \\ m_2 \end{pmatrix}$$

where C is a 2×2 matrix with elements c_{ij}.

The Kessler method [7] is an extension of the Hoffman method with a non-zero background. The recovery coefficient can then be calculated as

$$C_{V_1} = c_{11} + \left(\frac{\mu_2}{\mu_1}\right) c_{12}$$

where V_1 is the target region and V_2 the background region. It is necessary to know the true target-to-background ratio, μ_1/μ_2.

The Videen method [13] is a voxel-by-voxel implementation of the Hoffman method and can be described as

$$\hat{f}(\boldsymbol{x}) = \frac{g(\boldsymbol{x})}{J_V(\boldsymbol{x})}; \boldsymbol{x}\in V$$

This correction is only valid for voxels inside V, and it corrects for spill-out only.

The Müller-Gärtner method [15] is an extension of this method that incorporates spill-in correction and can be described as follows:

$$\hat{f}(\boldsymbol{x}) = \frac{g(\boldsymbol{x}) - b(\boldsymbol{x})}{J_1(\boldsymbol{x})}; \boldsymbol{x}\in V_1$$

$$b(\boldsymbol{x}) = \mu_2 J_2(\boldsymbol{x})$$

The correction is valid for voxels inside region V_1, and the spill-in correction is performed as a background subtraction due to activity in the background region V_2. It is necessary to know the true background mean value, μ_2.

The Yang method [16] starts with the generation of a pseudo-image, $\psi(\cdot)$:

$$\psi(\boldsymbol{x}) = \sum_{i=1}^{N} \tilde{\mu}_i I_i(\boldsymbol{x})$$

And the correction can then be described as

$$\hat{f}(\boldsymbol{x}) = g(\boldsymbol{x}) \frac{\psi(\boldsymbol{x})}{\{\psi \otimes h\}(\boldsymbol{x})}$$

This method corrects for both spill-out and spill-in and is valid in the entire image, but it is necessary to know the relative mean values, $\tilde{\mu}_i$, in the N different regions.

The GTM method [10] is similar to the Henze method described above, but with a larger number of regions. An alternative description is given below. The original image is first sampled, based on N different regions:

$$s_i = \int g(\boldsymbol{x}) I_i(\boldsymbol{x}) d\boldsymbol{x};\ i = 1,\ldots N$$

Next, a system of linear equations is set up:

$$\left\{ s_i = \sum_{j=1}^{N} a_{ij} m_j \right\};\ i = 1,\ldots N$$

where

$$a_{ij} = \int J_j(\boldsymbol{x}) I_i(\boldsymbol{x}) d\boldsymbol{x}$$

The solution can then be obtained as

$$\left(\hat{\mu}_1,\ldots\hat{\mu}_N\right)^T = \boldsymbol{A}^{-1}\left(s_1,\ldots s_N\right)^T$$

where $\boldsymbol{A}$ is an $N \times N$ matrix with elements a_{ij}.

The Labbé method [11] is very similar to the GTM method. The difference is that the sampling of the original image is done using the blurred regions instead of the original ones:

$$t_i = \int g(\boldsymbol{x}) J_i(\boldsymbol{x}) d\boldsymbol{x};\ i = 1,\ldots N$$

And the solution is given by

$$\left(\hat{\mu}_1,\ldots\hat{\mu}_N\right)^T = \boldsymbol{B}^{-1}\left(t_1,\ldots t_N\right)^T$$

where $\boldsymbol{B}$ is an NxN matrix with elements b_{ij}:

$$b_{ij} = \int J_j(\boldsymbol{x}) J_i(\boldsymbol{x}) d\boldsymbol{x}$$

The MTC method [17] is an extension of the Müller-Gärtner method, which allows correction of the entire image using a large number of regions. It starts by using the GTM method to obtain an estimate of the true mean values, μ_i, in each region. It then applies the Müller-Gärtner correction to each region, one at a time, while treating all other regions as background regions:

$$\hat{f}(\boldsymbol{x}) = \sum_{i=1}^{N} I_i(\boldsymbol{x}) \frac{g(\boldsymbol{x}) - b_i(\boldsymbol{x})}{J_i(\boldsymbol{x})}$$

$$b_i(\boldsymbol{x}) = \sum_{j \neq i} \hat{\mu}_j J_j(\boldsymbol{x})$$

The RBV method [5] is an alternative to MTC, which also starts with the GTM method, but then applies the Yang method to obtain a corrected image. The iterative Yang method [3] is similar, but avoids the use of GTM by estimating the mean values from the current image within an iterative loop, in which the Yang correction is applied repeatedly with increasingly more accurate mean values. Typically, 5–10 iterations are sufficient.

Finally, the novel STC method can be described as follows:

$$\hat{f}^{k+1}(\boldsymbol{x}) = \sum_{i=1}^{2} I_i(\boldsymbol{x}) \frac{g(\boldsymbol{x}) - b_i^k(\boldsymbol{x})}{J_i(\boldsymbol{x})}$$

Where

$$b_i^k(\boldsymbol{x}) = \left[\hat{f}^k(\boldsymbol{x})\left(1 - I_i(\boldsymbol{x})\right)\right] \otimes h(\boldsymbol{x})$$

$\hat{f}^k(\cdot)$ is the corrected image after k iterations, and $i = 1/2$ refers to the target and background regions, respectively.

References

1. Brigham EO. The fast Fourier transform. Englewood Cliffs: Prentice-Hall, Inc.; 1974.
2. Erlandsson K, Thomas BA, Dickson J, Hutton BF. Partial volume correction in SPECT reconstruction with OSEM. Nucl Instr Meth A. 2011;648:S85–8.
3. Erlandsson K, Buvat I, Pretorius PH, Thomas BA, Hutton BF. A review of partial volume correction techniques for emission tomography and their applications in neurology, cardiology and oncology. Phys Med Biol. 2012;57:R119–59.
4. Tohka J, Reilhac A. Deconvolution-based partial volume correction in raclopride-PET and Monte Carlo comparison to MR-based method. Neuroimage. 2008;39:1570–84.
5. Thomas BA, Erlandsson K, Modat M, Thurfjell L, Vandenberghe R, Ourselin S, et al. The importance of appropriate partial volume correction for PET quantification in Alzheimer's disease. Eur J Nucl Med Mol Imaging. 2011;38:1104–19.
6. Hoffman EJ, Huang SC, Phelps ME. Quantitation in positron emission computed tomography: 1. Effect of object size. J Comput Assist Tomogr. 1979;3:299–308.
7. Kessler RM, Ellis Jr JR, Eden M. Analysis of emission tomographic scan data: limitations imposed by resolution and background. J Comput Assist Tomogr. 1984;8:514–22.
8. Henze E, Huang SC, Ratib O, Hoffman E, Phelps ME, Schelbert HR. Measurements of regional tissue and blood-pool radiotracer concentrations from serial

tomographic images of the heart. J Nucl Med. 1983;24:987–96.

9. Herrero P, Markham J, Myears DW, Weinheimer CJ, Bergmann SR. Measurement of myocardial blood flow with positron emission tomography: correction for count spillover and partial volume effects. Math Comput Modelling. 1988;11:807–12.
10. Rousset OG, Ma Y, Evans AC. Correction for partial volume effects in PET: principle and validation. J Nucl Med. 1998;39:904–11.
11. Labbé C, Koepp MJ, Ashburner J, Spinks T, Richardson M, Duncan J, et al. Absolute PET quantification with correction for partial volume effects within cerebral structures. In: Carson RE D-WM, Herscovitch P, editors. Quantitative functional brain imaging with positron emission tomography. San Diego: Academic; 1998. p. 59–66.
12. Hofheinz F, Langner J, Petr J, Beuthien-Baumann B, Oehme L, Steinbach J, et al. A method for model-free partial volume correction in oncological PET. EJNMMI Res. 2012;2:16.
13. Videen TO, Perlmutter JS, Mintun MA, Raichle ME. Regional correction of positron emission tomography data for the effects of cerebral atrophy. J Cereb Blood Flow Metab. 1988;8:662–70.
14. Meltzer CC, Leal JP, Mayberg HS, Wagner Jr HN, Frost JJ. Correction of PET data for partial volume effects in human cerebral cortex by MR imaging. J Comput Assist Tomogr. 1990;14:561–70.
15. Müller-Gartner HW, Links JM, Prince JL, Bryan RN, McVeigh E, Leal JP, et al. Measurement of radiotracer concentration in brain gray matter using positron emission tomography: MRI-based correction for partial volume effects. J Cereb Blood Flow Metab. 1992;12:571–83.
16. Yang J, Huang SC, Mega M, Lin KP, Toga AW, Small GW, et al. Investigation of partial volume correction methods for brain FDG PET studies. IEEE Trans Nucl Sci. 1996;43:3322–7.
17. Erlandsson K, Wong AT, van Heertum R, Mann JJ, Parsey RV. An improved method for voxel-based partial volume correction in PET and SPECT. Neuroimage. 2006;31:T84.
18. Erlandson K, Hutton BF. A novel voxel-based partial volume correction method for single regions of interest. J Nucl Med. 2014;55:2123.
19. Segars WP, Tsui BMW. Study of the efficacy of respiratory gating in myocardial SPECT using the New 4-D NCAT phantom. IEEE Trans Nucl Sci. 2002;49:675–9.
20. Zubal IG, Harrell CR, Smith EO, Rattner Z, Gindi G, Hoffer PB. Computerized three-dimensional segmented human anatomy. Med Phys. 1994;21:299–302.
21. Fessler JA, Clinthorne NH, Rogers WL. Regularized emission image reconstruction using imperfect side information. IEEE Trans Nucl Sci. 1992;39:1464–71.
22. Comtat C, Kinahan PE, Fessler JA, Beyer T, Townsend DW, Defrise M, et al. Clinically feasible reconstruction of 3D whole-body PET/CT data using blurred anatomical labels. Phys Med Biol. 2002;47:1–20.
23. Strul D, Bendriem B. Robustness of anatomically guided pixel-by-pixel algorithms for partial volume effect correction in positron emission tomography. J Cereb Blood Flow Metab. 1999;19:547–59.
24. Frouin V, Comtat C, Reilhac A, Gregoire MC. Correction of partial-volume effect for PET striatal imaging: fast implementation and study of robustness. J Nucl Med. 2002;43:1715–26.
25. Quarantelli M, Berkouk K, Prinster A, Landeau B, Svarer C, Balkay L, et al. Integrated software for the analysis of brain PET/SPECT studies with partial-volume-effect correction. J Nucl Med. 2004;45:192–201.
26. Johnson NP, Sdringola S, Gould KL. Partial volume correction incorporating Rb-82 positron range for quantitative myocardial perfusion PET based on systolic-diastolic activity ratios and phantom measurements. J Nucl Cardiol. 2011;18:247–58.
27. Bowen SL, Byars LG, Michel CJ, Chonde DB, Catana C. Influence of the partial volume correction method on (18)F-fluorodeoxyglucose brain kinetic modelling from dynamic PET images reconstructed with resolution model based OSEM. Phys Med Biol. 2013;58:7081–106.
28. Uchida H, Chow TW, Mamo DC, Kapur S, Mulsant BH, Houle S, et al. Effects of aging on 5-HT(2A) R binding: a HRRT PET study with and without partial volume corrections. Int J Geriatr Psychiatry. 2011;26:1300–8.
29. Stamos JA, Rogers WL, Clinthorne NH, Koral KF. Object dependent performance comparison of two iterative reconstruction algorithms. IEEE Trans Nucl Sci. 1988;35:611–4.
30. Du Y, Tsui BM, Frey EC. Partial volume effect compensation for quantitative brain SPECT imaging. IEEE Trans Med Imaging. 2005;24:969–76.
31. Maes F, Collignon A, Vandermeulen D, Marchal G, Suetens P. Multimodality image registration by maximization of mutual information. IEEE Trans Med Imaging. 1997;16:187–98.
32. Studholme C, Hill DLG, Hawkes DJ. An overlap invariant entropy measure of 3D medical image alignment, pattern recognition. Pattern Recogn. 1999;32:71–86.
33. Hutton BF, Braun M. Software for image registration: algorithms, accuracy, efficacy. Semin Nucl Med. 2003;33:180–92.
34. Hutton BF, Braun M, Slomka P. Image registration techniques in nuclear medicine imaging. In: Zaidi H, editor. Quantitative analysis in nuclear medicine imaging. New York: Springer; 2006. p. 272–307.
35. Slomka PJ, Baum RP. Multimodality image registration with software: state-of-the-art. Eur J Nucl Med Mol Imaging. 2009;36 Suppl 1:S44–55.
36. Klein A, Andersson J, Ardekani BA, Ashburner J, Avants B, Chiang MC, et al. Evaluation of 14 nonlinear deformation algorithms applied to human brain MRI registration. Neuroimage. 2009;46:786–802.
37. Oliveira FP, Tavares JM. Medical image registration: a review. Comput Methods Biomech Biomed Engin. 2014;17(2):73–93.

38. Pretorius PH, King MA. Diminishing the impact of the partial volume effect in cardiac SPECT perfusion imaging. Med Phys. 2009;36:105–15.
39. Du Y, Madar I, Stumpf MJ, Rong X, Fung GS, Frey EC. Compensation for spill-in and spill-out partial volume effects in cardiac PET imaging. J Nucl Cardiol. 2013;20:84–98.
40. Pretorius PH, Pan TS, Narayanan MV, King MA. A study of the influence of local variations in myocardial thickness on SPECT perfusion imaging. IEEE Trans Nucl Sci. 2002;49:2304–8.
41. Petitjean C, Dacher JN. A review of segmentation methods in short axis cardiac MR images. Med Image Anal. 2011;15:169–84.
42. Fischl B, Salat DH, Busa E, Albert M, Dieterich M, Haselgrove C, et al. Whole brain segmentation: automated labeling of neuroanatomical structures in the human brain. Neuron. 2002;33:341–55.
43. Fischl B, van der Kouwe A, Destrieux C, Halgren E, Segonne F, Salat DH, et al. Automatically parcellating the human cerebral cortex. Cereb Cortex. 2004;14:11–22.
44. Cabezas M, Oliver A, Llado X, Freixenet J, Cuadra MB. A review of atlas-based segmentation for magnetic resonance brain images. Comput Methods Programs Biomed. 2011;104:e158–77.
45. Zaidi H, Ruest T, Schoenahl F, Montandon ML. Comparative assessment of statistical brain MR image segmentation algorithms and their impact on partial volume correction in PET. Neuroimage. 2006;32:1591–607.
46. Gutierrez D, Montandon ML, Assal F, Allaoua M, Ratib O, Lovblad KO, et al. Anatomically guided voxel-based partial volume effect correction in brain PET: impact of MRI segmentation. Comput Med Imaging Graph. 2012;36:610–9.
47. Bai B, Li Q, Leahy RM. Magnetic resonance-guided positron emission tomography image reconstruction. Semin Nucl Med. 2013;43:30–44.
48. Boussion N, Hatt M, Lamare F, Bizais Y, Turzo A, Cheze-Le Rest C, et al. A multiresolution image based approach for correction of partial volume effects in emission tomography. Phys Med Biol. 2006;51:1857–76.
49. Shidahara M, Tsoumpas C, Hammers A, Boussion N, Visvikis D, Suhara T, et al. Functional and structural synergy for resolution recovery and partial volume correction in brain PET. Neuroimage. 2009;44:340–8.
50. Iida H, Rhodes CG, de Silva R, Yamamoto Y, Araujo LI, Maseri A, et al. Myocardial tissue fraction--correction for partial volume effects and measure of tissue viability. J Nucl Med. 1991;32:2169–75.
51. Lin KP, Huang SC, Choi Y, Brunken RC, Schelbert HR, Phelps ME. Correction of spillover radioactivities for estimation of the blood time-activity curve from the imaged LV chamber in cardiac dynamic FDG PET studies. Phys Med Biol. 1995;40:629–42.
52. Iida H, Law I, Pakkenberg B, Krarup-Hansen A, Eberl S, Holm S, et al. Quantitation of regional cerebral blood flow corrected for partial volume effect using O-15 water and PET: I. Theory, error analysis, and stereologic comparison. J Cereb Blood Flow Metab. 2000;20:1237–51.
53. Ardekani BA, Braun M, Hutton BF, Kanno I, Iida H. Minimum cross-entropy reconstruction of PET images using prior anatomical information. Phys Med Biol. 1996;41:2497–517.
54. Bowsher JE, Yuan H, Hedlund LW, Turkington TG, Akabani G, Badea A, et al. Utilizing MRI information to estimate F18-FDG distributions in rat flank tumors," In: IEEE nuclear science symposium and medical imaging conference, Rome; 2004. p. 2488–92.
55. Yan J, Lim JC, Townsend DW. MRI-guided brain PET image filtering and partial volume correction. Phys Med Biol. 2015;60:961–76.
56. Rhodes CG, Wollmer P, Fazio F, Jones T. Quantitative measurement of regional extravascular lung density using positron emission and transmission tomography. J Comput Assist Tomogr. 1981;5:783–91.
57. Meltzer CC, Cantwell MN, Greer PJ, Ben-Eliezer D, Smith G, Frank G, et al. Does cerebral blood flow decline in healthy aging? A PET study with partial-volume correction. J Nucl Med. 2000;41:1842–8.
58. Giovacchini G, Lerner A, Toczek MT, Fraser C, Ma K, DeMar JC, et al. Brain incorporation of 11C-arachidonic acid, blood volume, and blood flow in healthy aging: a study with partial-volume correction. J Nucl Med. 2004;45:1471–9.
59. Bencherif B, Stumpf MJ, Links JM, Frost JJ. Application of MRI-based partial-volume correction to the analysis of PET images of mu-opioid receptors using statistical parametric mapping. J Nucl Med. 2004;45:402–8.
60. Yanase D, Matsunari I, Yajima K, Chen W, Fujikawa A, Nishimura S, et al. Brain FDG PET study of normal aging in Japanese: effect of atrophy correction. Eur J Nucl Med Mol Imaging. 2005;32:794–805.
61. Curiati PK, Tamashiro-Duran JH, Duran FL, Buchpiguel CA, Squarzoni P, Romano DC, et al. Age-related metabolic profiles in cognitively healthy elders: results from a voxel-based [18F]fluorodeoxy-glucose-positron-emission tomography study with partial volume effects correction. AJNR Am J Neuroradiol. 2011;32:560–5.
62. Samuraki M, Matsunari I, Chen WP, Yajima K, Yanase D, Fujikawa A, et al. Partial volume effect-corrected FDG PET and grey matter volume loss in patients with mild Alzheimer's disease. Eur J Nucl Med Mol Imaging. 2007;34:1658–69.
63. Vesselle H, Turcotte E, Wiens L, Schmidt R, Takasugi JE, Lalani T, et al. Relationship between non-small cell lung cancer fluorodeoxyglucose uptake at positron emission tomography and surgical stage with relevance to patient prognosis. Clin Cancer Res. 2004;10:4709–16.
64. Vesselle H, Salskov A, Turcotte E, Wiens L, Schmidt R, Jordan CD, et al. Relationship between non-small cell lung cancer FDG uptake at PET, tumor histology, and Ki-67 proliferation index. J Thorac Oncol. 2008;3:971–8.

65. Tsujikawa T, Otsuka H, Morita N, Saegusa H, Kobayashi M, Okazawa H, et al. Does partial volume corrected maximum SUV based on count recovery coefficient in 3D-PET/CT correlate with clinical aggressiveness of non-Hodgkin's lymphoma? Ann Nucl Med. 2008;22:23–30.
66. Sakaguchi Y, Mizoguchi N, Mitsumoto T, Mitsumoto K, Himuro K, Ohya N, et al. A simple table lookup method for PET/CT partial volume correction using a point-spread function in diagnosing lymph node metastasis. Ann Nucl Med. 2010;24:585–91.
67. Maruoka Y, Abe K, Baba S, Isoda T, Kitamura Y, Mizoguchi N, et al. Usefulness of partial volume effect-corrected F-18 FDG PET/CT for predicting I-131 accumulation in the metastatic lymph nodes of patients with thyroid carcinoma. Ann Nucl Med. 2013;27:873–9.
68. Soret M, Bacharach SL, Buvat I. Partial-volume effect in PET tumor imaging. J Nucl Med. 2007;48:932–45.
69. Hutton BF, Thomas BA, Erlandson K, Bousse A, Reilhac-Laborde A, Kazantsev D, et al. What approach to brain partial volume correction is best for PET/MRI? Nucl Instr Meth A. 2013;702:29–33.
70. Thomas BA, Erlandsson K, Drobnjak I, Pedemonte S, Vunckx K, Bousse A, et al. Framework for the construction of a Monte Carlo simulated brain PET–MR image database. Nucl Inst Methods Phys Res A. 2014;734:162–5.

Motion Artifacts and Correction Techniques in PET/CT

16

Tinsu Pan

Contents

16.1 **Introduction** 380
16.1.1 Causes of Artifacts from Respiratory Motion 380
16.1.2 Misregistration of Fast Helical CT and PET 383
16.1.3 Average CT (ACT) of Less Than 1 mSv to Reduce Misregistration 387
16.1.4 4D-PET 392
16.1.5 4D-PET/CT = 4D-PET + 4D-CT 393
16.2 **Summary** 394
References 394

Abstract

PET/CT is a very important imaging tool in the management of the oncology patients. PET/CT hardware registration between the sequential imaging of CT and PET with the same imaging table has significantly improved the registration between the anatomy in CT and the functional information in PET. However, registration between the CT and PET images remains an issue in the thorax and the abdomen, where the anatomy moves with the respiratory motion and the snapshot CT images may not register well with the average PET images. Respiratory gating has been proposed for CT and PET, but its adaption in the clinic can only be found with the respiratory-gated CT or 4D-CT in radiation therapy treatment planning. Majority of the PET/CT practices are not using any CT or PET gating duc to the complexity of gating and the challenge of finding the right patient for gating before PET/CT imaging. In this chapter, we will not only cover the more complex gated CT and gated PET techniques but also introduce the simple average CT technique of less than 1 mSv to improve the registration of CT and PET and to provide the important CT data for dose calculation and image guidance in radiation therapy.

T. Pan, PhD
Department of Imaging Physics – Unit 1352, M.D. Anderson Cancer Center, University of Texas, 1515 Holcome Blvd., Houston, TX 77030, USA
e-mail: tpan@mdanderson.org

M.M. Khalil (ed.), *Basic Science of PET Imaging*, DOI 10.1007/978-3-319-40070-9_16

16.1 Introduction

PET/CT was developed in 1998 [1]. The first commercial PET/CT scanner was available in 2001 [2]. Since 2005, stand-alone PET scanners have not been in production [3]. Today, PET and PET/CT are synonymous to each other. Prior to PET/CT, the CT and PET data were acquired in two different scanners and in two different sessions. Fusion of the PET and CT data was performed with software techniques [4]. Registration of the PET and CT data was more successful for brain studies with rigid translation but not very successful for the other regions of the body, in particular in the thorax or the abdomen, due to the difficulty in repositioning the patient in two separate sessions and the non-rigid nature of the organs. The advent of PET/CT scanners made it possible for the first time that a single imaging table transports the patient between PET and CT to hardware-fuse the PET and CT data without a repeat of patient setup. Hardware fusion is more accurate than software fusion, in particular in the area of tumor infiltration of adjacent structures that could not be conclusively assessed using the separate CT and PET data [5].

Application of PET/CT is over 90 % on oncology with ^{18}F-FDG [6–10] and less than 5 % on cardiology with ^{82}Rb or ^{13}NH3 for myocardial perfusion imaging [11]. PET/CT also plays an important role in image-guided radiation therapy [12] and treatment response assessment [13]. Integration of functional PET data with anatomical CT data is critical in radiation therapy [8]. However, it remains a challenge to quantify the improvement of simulation with PET/CT over CT in treatment planning for radiation treatment as conclusive clinical data are not yet available. Early studies have found PET/CT has advantages over CT in standardization of volume delineation [14, 15], in reduction of the risk for geometrical misses [16], and in minimization of radiation dose to the nontarget organs [7, 9, 17]. Utilization of PET/CT is expected to grow as more molecular-targeted imaging agents are being developed [18].

There are still some challenges in PET/CT imaging. PET needs CT data for tumor localization, attenuation correction, and quantification. Incorporation of CT for PET attenuation correction improves the throughput of PET/CT scan and patient comfort by replacing the long transmission scan time of rotating rod sources with the short scan time of CT. Application of PET/CT in diagnosis is a task of detection and quantitation based on standardized uptake value (SUV) [19, 20]. A physician can sometimes mentally reconstruct the suppose-to-be images in his/her brain even if the images were with artifacts. If the artifacts are not significant, they could simply be read through. Inconsistency between the CT and PET data in PET/CT may compromise localization and quantification of the PET data and may impact the diagnostic accuracy of a PET/CT scan. Patient motion between the CT and PET scans is another source of artifact because the scans are taken in a sequential order of mostly CT followed by PET. Registration with the rigid translation and/or rotation of the CT images to match with the PET images may be sufficient to fix the brain images such as the patient study in Fig. 16.1. An example of misregistration at the heart and the liver, corrected by two stages of registration, one for the heart and the other one for the liver, is in Fig. 16.2. This example indicated that a patient motion could cause different complexities of misregistration, and a simple rigid-body registration might not be able to fix the problem. We will focus this chapter on the attenuation correction strategies in PET/CT to mitigate the respiration-induced artifacts in PET/CT, which are more difficult to correct with post-processing registration software.

16.1.1 Causes of Artifacts from Respiratory Motion

CT is mostly a 2D whereas PET is a 3D imaging device. A CT scanner is composed of an X-ray source and a bank of detector modules arranged in fan beam, which needs to rotate at least 180° plus 60° fan angle to produce a tomographic image. The detector coverage along the cranio-caudal or table direction at the imaging center or isocenter is 2 cm for a 16-slice or 4 cm for a

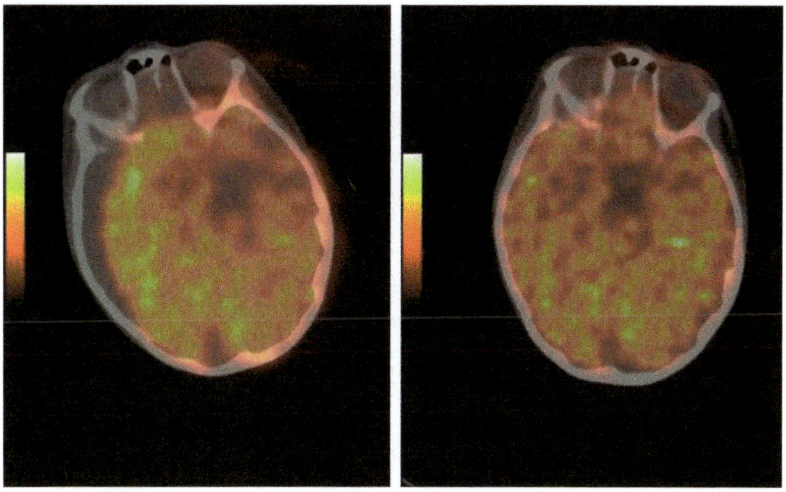

Fig. 16.1 Incorrect quantification of the ^{18}F-FDG activity in the brain due to the head motion causing misregistration between the CT and PET on the *left*. Software registration of the CT to the PET data improves the quantification (Reproduced from the Pan and Zaidi [61]; with permission)

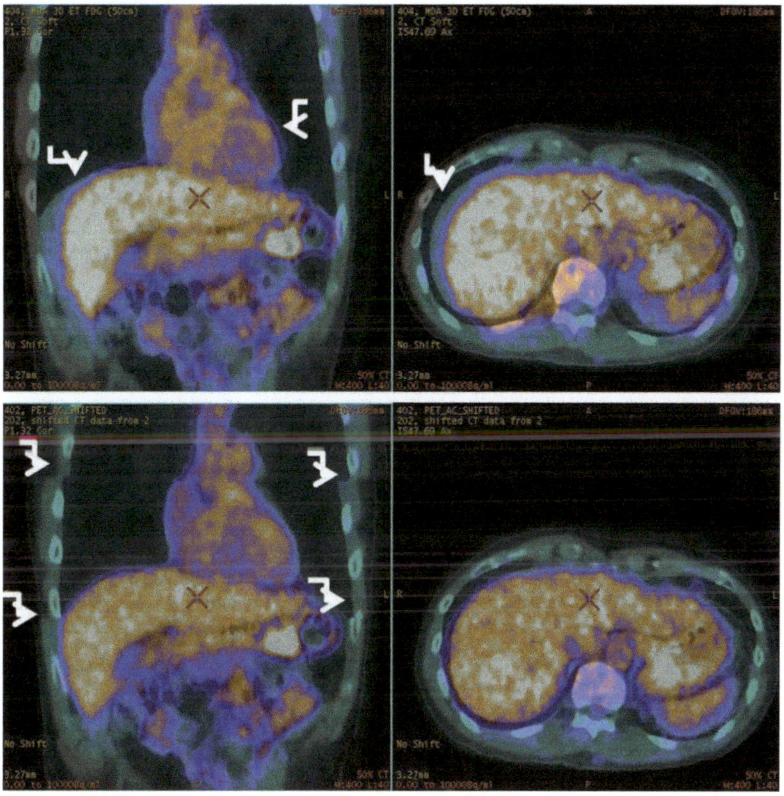

Fig. 16.2 *Top panel* shows the coronal and axial view of a patient study whose CT and PET data were not registered in the heart and the liver due to patient motion. *Bottom panel* shows the results of a two-stage registration: one for the heart and one for the liver. There were discontinuities marked by the *arrows* on the rib cage to indicate the improved registration for the heart and the liver at the expense of rib cage registration

64-slice GE CT scanner.[1] A helical CT scan of 100 cm from the orbit to the mid-thigh in a typical PET/CT scan can be performed in less than 20 s on a 16-slice or less than 10 s on a 64-slice PET/CT. The speed of helical CT is determined by the following three components: gantry rotation cycle time, width of X-ray collimation, and pitch factor defined as the ratio of table translation distance per rotation to the width of X-ray collimation. A faster CT scan can be accomplished with a fast gantry rotation cycle time of

[1]It is a 19.2-mm detector coverage on a 20-, 40-, or 64-slice Siemens mCT scanner.

0.5 s, the X-ray collimation of 2 cm for a 16-slice or 4 cm for a 64-slice CT, and a pitch factor of 1.375 for the scan speed of 5.5 and 11 cm/s for a 16-slice and 64-slice CT, respectively. On the other hand, combination of a slow gantry rotation cycle time of 1 s, a smaller X-ray collimation of 1 cm for a 16-slice or 2 cm for a 64-slice CT, and a pitch factor of 1 would make the scan speeds of 1 and 2 cm/s for a 16-slice and 64-slice CT, respectively. Note that the pitch factor closest to 1 on the GE CT scanner is 0.9375 (15/16 on a 16 slice), 0.96875 (31/32 on a 64 slice), or 0.984 (63/64 on a 64 slice).

The 3D volume of a CT scan is composed of a stack of 2D CT images acquired in the craniocaudal direction. Fast CT gantry rotation time of sub-second improves the temporal resolution of the CT image to sub-second, making the CT image almost free of respiratory motion artifacts. However, these 2D CT images, almost free of respiratory motion artifacts, cannot guarantee consistency of the 3D CT anatomy in the craniocaudal direction because each CT image is a snapshot of the anatomy at a particular phase of a respiratory cycle when the patient free-breathes during the CT data acquisition of a PET/CT scan. A phase is determined as a percentage in a breath cycle between two consecutive end-inspiration phases, which typically correspond to a local maximum in amplitude. On the other hand, end-expiration phases correspond to a local minimum in amplitude. End-inspiration phase is 0 % and end-expiration phase is around 40–60 %. The maximum and minimum amplitudes are by convention assigned to end-inspiration and end-expiration phases, respectively. An example of the inconsistence is illustrated in the sagittal view CT image of a patient in Fig. 16.3, where the respiratory and cardiac motion artifacts are highlighted.

Most of the PET acquisitions today are in the 3D acquisition mode without the septa to improve the sensitivity of detecting annihilation photons of 511 keV. The scan coverage of a GE PET detector module in the craniocaudal direction is 15.4 cm, much larger than the CT detector module of 2 cm for the 16 slice or 4 cm for the 64 slice. The PET detectors are arranged in a ring geometry without space or gap to improve also the sensitivity. The duration of a PET scan at each bed position is typically 2–3 min, and it can be shortened by utilizing a larger axial field of view such as the 21.6 cm detector on the Siemens mCT scanner to further improve the sensitivity of PET imaging. There is no guarantee that the CT images from a fast scan CT at the temporal resolution of sub-second would match temporally with the PET images of a slow PET scan. It is this mismatch in temporal resolution between the CT and PET data acquisitions that causes misregistration between the CT and PET images in PET/CT imaging of a patient at free breathing.

The current design of PET/CT only matches the spatial resolution of the CT and PET data by

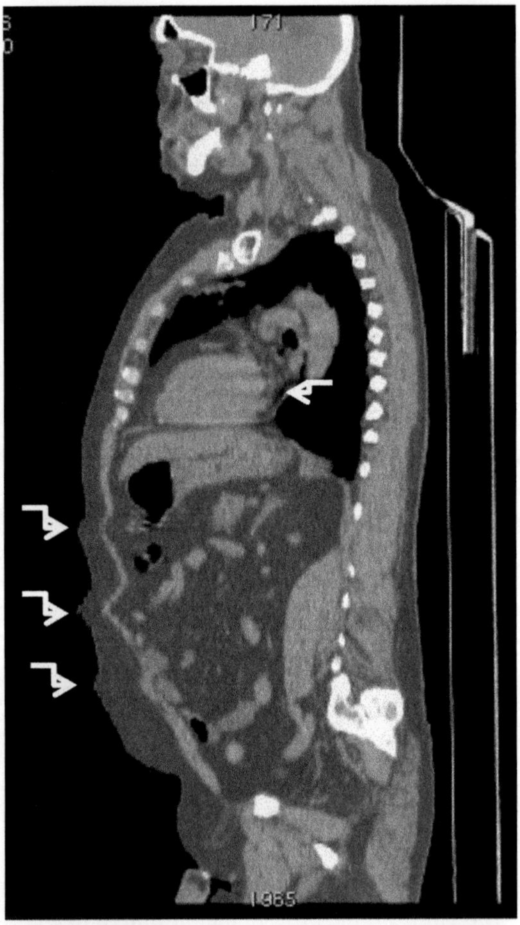

Fig. 16.3 A sagittal view of a CT scan in PET/CT with the helical CT protocol of 16×0.625 mm, 0.8 s gantry rotation, and pitch 1.375:1. There were three skinfold artifacts on the abdomen and some pulsating artifacts on the heart. The speed of CT scan in the table direction is 17.2 mm/s (Reproduced from Zaid and Pan [62]; with permission)

blurring the CT images so that the spatial resolution of the CT images matches with the spatial resolution of the PET images. There has been no attempt from manufacturers to match the temporal resolutions of CT and PET for a routine whole-body PET/CT scan. For any measure to match the temporal resolution of the PET and CT data, additional acquisition time cannot be too long and post-processing cannot be too cumbersome. It is because the patient normally is asked to position his/her arms over the head during data acquisition of the CT and PET data in order to improve the image quality of the thorax and abdomen. In this position, an average person can maintain stationary for about 15–20 min and not more than 30 min at maximum. Any scan over 30 min is susceptible to patient motion due to discomfort at a still location for a prolonged period of time.

16.1.2 Misregistration of Fast Helical CT and PET

Misregistration between the CT and the PET data is typically identified by a curvilinear white band or photopenic region near the diaphragm in the PET images (Fig. 16.4). Existence of a white band suggests a misregistration near the diaphragm. It is possible to have a combination of good or misregistration at the tumor location and good or misregistration at the diaphragm position. The combination depends on the tumor location, the CT scan speed (cm/s), and the time at which the tumor (at one phase of a breath cycle) was scanned by CT. A tumor may become smaller (or larger) than it really was if the CT scan is in the same (or opposite to the) direction of the tumor motion when the CT scans the tumor. In cardiac imaging, the heart is always nearby the diaphragm. The problem of misregistration can be more of an issue in cardiac PET than in oncological PET.

Since we tend to spend more time in expiration than in inspiration, the PET data averaged over several minutes is closer to end expiration than end inspiration. If the CT data is acquired near the end expiration, then the CT and PET data will have a better chance of registration with each other. On the other hand, if the CT data is acquired in or near end inspiration, the inflated lungs from inspiration of more air will be larger than the deflated lungs at expiration. The larger area of the inflated lungs in CT renders less attenuation correction in the reconstruction of the PET data near the diaphragm where the inflated lungs push the diaphragm lower toward the feet in CT than the average diaphragm position in PET. The result is a white band region identified as a misregistered region or a photopenic region.

It was reported that respiration-induced artifacts can be reduced in both magnitude and prominence for a free-breathing PET/CT scan by employing CT components of six or more detector rows [21]. The number of skinfolds shown in Fig. 16.3 can be reduced with a fast CT scan by spreading the skinfolds further apart with more CT detector rows. However, a fast helical CT scan of six or more detector rows cannot eliminate misregistration between the CT and the PET data.

Coaching the patient to hold breath at mid-expiration during the CT acquisition was suggested as an alternative to improve the registration between the CT and PET data [22]. However, the outcomes were mixed because coaching the patient to hold breath at a certain state during CT data acquisition is not very reliable from both the perspectives of the patient and the technologist operating the PET/CT scanner. In our study of 100 patients coached to hold breath at mid-expiration, 50 patient data sets exhibited a misregistration of more than 1 cm between the CT and PET data [23]. It was because interpretation of a mid-expiration position can vary from patient to patient. It may not be easy to train a patient or technologist that the breath-hold CT to best match with PET should be taken at the mid-expiration in light breathing not in deep breath in and deep breath out as shown in Fig. 16.5. Adding to the difficulty is that the technologist does not have any measure to ensure the patient follows his/her instructions. However, in a cardiac PET imaging session of only one bed position, it is possible to observe the patient's breathing pattern in light breathing and to ask the patient to breath-hold at mid- or near

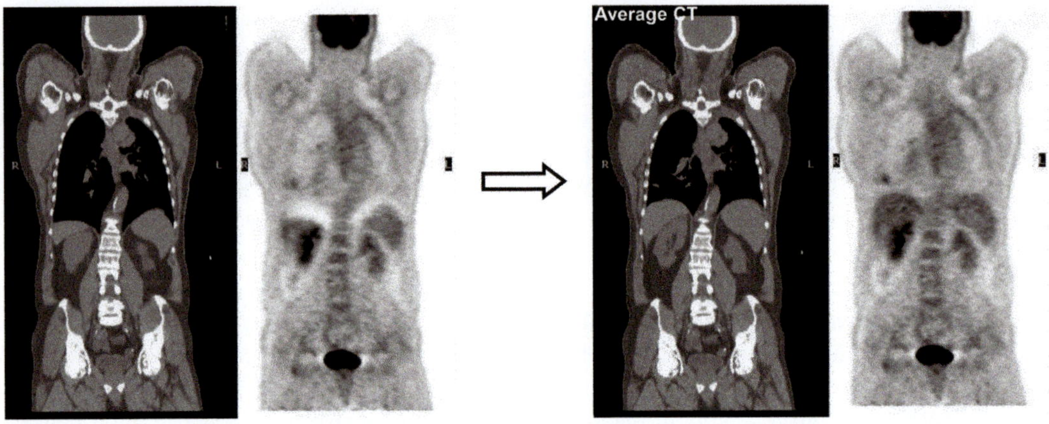

Fig. 16.4 (*Left panel*) A patient breath-held at mid-expiration when the CT data had a lower (inferior) diaphragm position than the PET average data of free breathing, resulting in a photopenic region with an underestimation of ^{18}F-FDG uptake. (*Right panel*) After correction with the average CT data, the photopenic region disappeared, and the SUV_{max} of the tumor (above the diaphragm) increased by 57% from 2.3 to 3.6 (Reproduced from Zaidi and Pan [62]; with permission)

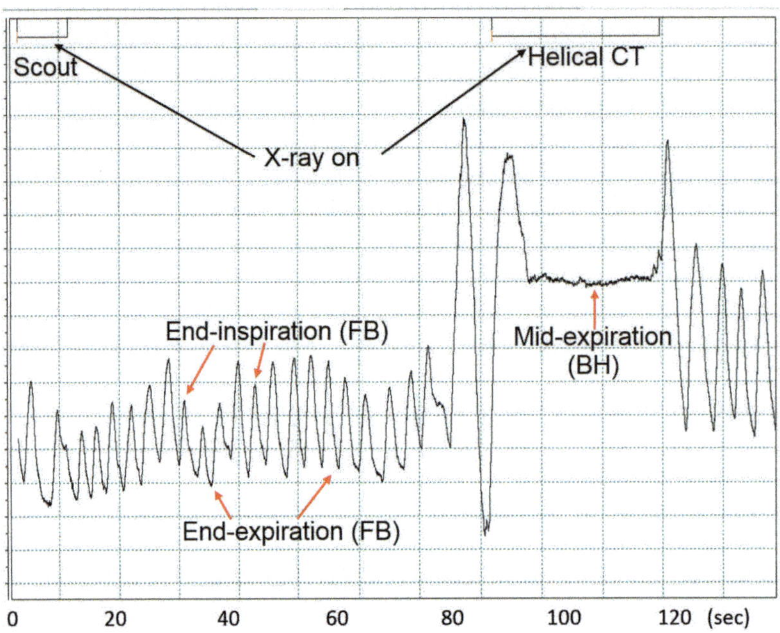

Fig. 16.5 A breathing trace of a patient exercising mid-expiration breath-hold during the helical CT scan. The duration of X-ray for both the scout and helical CT is shown at the top. The patient was free-breathing during the scout scan and remained so until a breathing instruction of "breath in, breath out, and hold your breath at mid-expiration" was given to the patient. Although the patient was holding at the mid-expiration in deep breath in and breath out, the mid-expiration state during the helical CT was at a very different breathing state from the average breathing state in free breathing where the patient's PET data was taken (Reproduced from Pan et al. [23]; with permission)

end expiration because the CT scan can be completed in 3 to 4 s to scan the single bed position of about 15.4 cm on the GE PET/CT scanner.

As long as the CT scan is conducted when the patient is free breathing, there is always a possibility that the CT and the PET data may be misaligned due to the fact that some CT slices are taken at inspiration and some at expiration, whereas the PET data is averaged over several minutes. The distance between two consecutive end-expiration phases can become longer (or shorter) with a faster (or slower) speed helical CT scan typically realized by more CT detector rows. Let us go back to the example in Fig. 16.3, which shows the CT images taken when the patient was free breathing during a CT scan at the speed of 1.72 cm/s. There were skinfold artifacts on the abdomen and cardiac pulsation artifacts on the heart. These artifacts may not be obvious in the review of each individual CT slice. By measuring the distance between the adjacent peaks of the respiratory (cardiac pulsation) artifacts and dividing the distance by the table translation speed of the CT scan, one can estimate the breathing cycle and the heart rate of the patient to be about 4.7 s and 50 beats per minute, respectively. These artifacts were due to the respiration and the heart beatings of the patient.

Three more clinical examples of misregistration in the lungs are shown in Figs. 16.6, 16.7, and 16.8. It was not always the case that the SUV_{max} will increase with correction of the misregistration artifact with average CT. The changes in SUV_{max} in Figs. 16.6 and 16.8 potentially indicated a partial response with the same PET data attenuation correction with the free-breathing helical CT and the free-breathing average CT. Figure 16.7 shows an improvement on localization of a lung tumor in both the average CT and the PET data.

16.1.2.1 Frequency of Misregistration and Its Impact

The rate of misregistration can be as high as 68 % [24] to 84 % [25] and may only impact 2 % of diagnosis in the whole-body ^{18}F-FDG PET/CT imaging [26]. However, in the cardiac PET/CT studies, since the heart is adjacent and superior to the diaphragm, it has been shown to cause a false-positive rate of up to 40 % without software registration of the CT and PET data [27]. In a whole-body PET/CT, the tumor(s) of interest may not be close to the diaphragm where most misregistrations occur, and the task of diagnosis may not be compromised by misregistration between the CT and PET data. Since the heart is right above the diaphragm and the diagnostic quality of the cardiac PET imaging is dependent on accurate quantification of the PET data, a more stringent requirement in registration is needed for the cardiac PET/CT than for the whole-body PET/CT.

Most of the modern PET/CT scanners provide a rigid-body registration software utility to help mitigate the problem of misregistration between the CT and PET data. An automatic registration tool has become commercially available to tackle the misregistration issue for the cardiac PET/CT studies [28]. It was found that automatic registration can perform just as well as manual registration and can save time for the

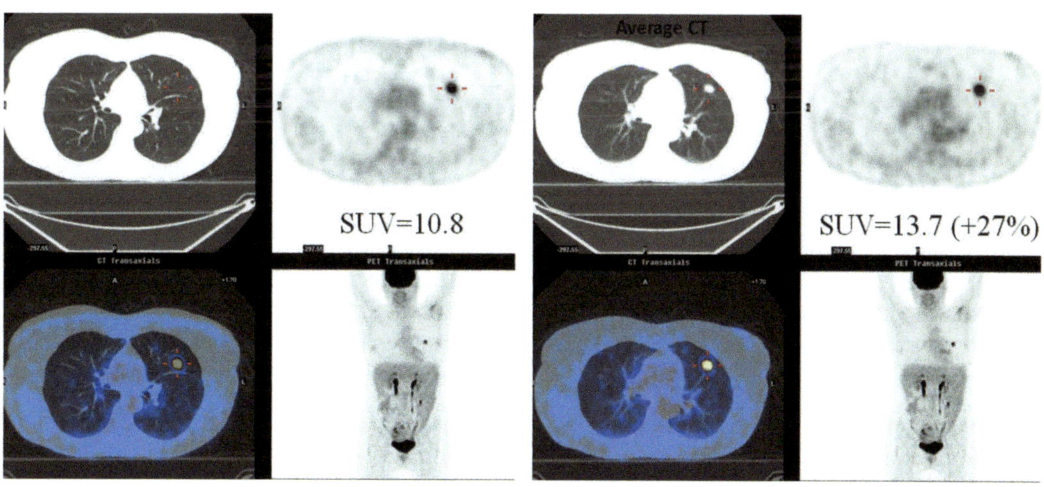

Fig. 16.6 (*Left panel*) The PET/CT data of a patient free-breathed during the helical CT. The panel shows the CT, PET, PET MIP, and fused PET/CT in clockwise. After correction with the average CT, the SUV_{max} of the tumor increased by 27 % from 10.8 to 13.7 in addition to a consistent registration of the tumor shown in both the CT and the PET images

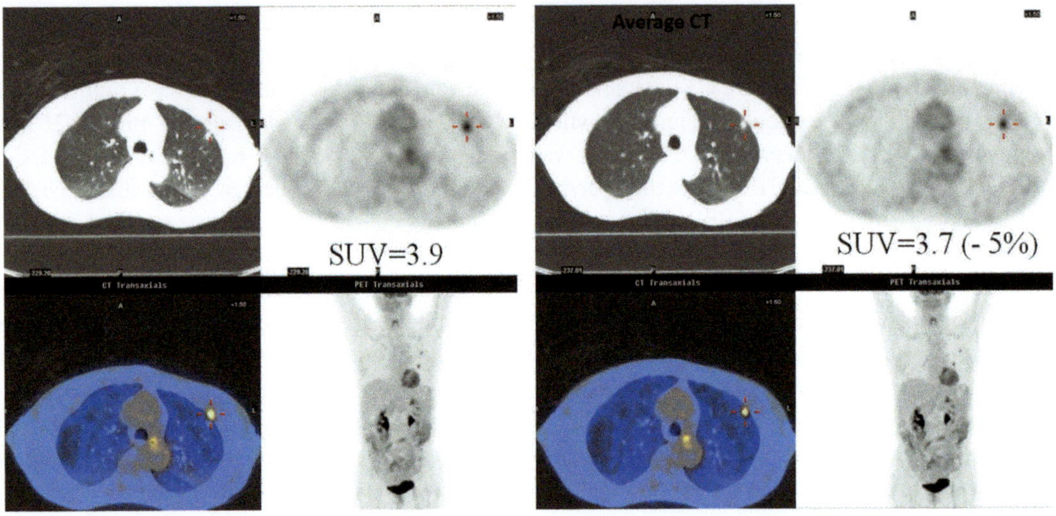

Fig. 16.7 (*Left panel*) The PET/CT data of a patient free-breathed during the helical CT. The panel shows the CT, PET, PET MIP, and fused PET/CT in clockwise. The CT shows the tumor in the lungs, whereas the PET shows the tumor in the chest walls. After correction with the average CT, the SUV_{max} of the tumor decreased by 5 % from 3.9 to 3.7. The CT and PET tumor locations were consistent in the lungs

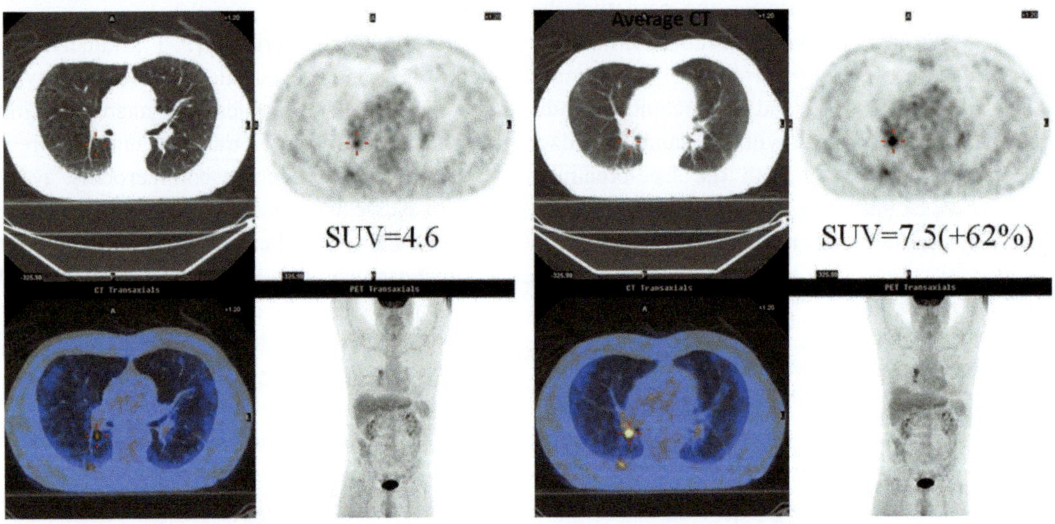

Fig. 16.8 (*Left panel*) The PET/CT data of a patient free-breathed during the helical CT. The panel shows the CT, PET, PET MIP, and fused PET/CT in clockwise. The CT shows an ^{18}F-FDG uptake in the low CT density region of the lung parenchyma and by the chest walls. After correction with average CT, the SUV_{max} of the tumor increased 62 % from 4.6 to 7.5. The uptake is now supported by the soft tissues not in the lung parenchyma, and the tumor against the chest walls was more elevated

technologist to register the CT and PET data. However, it was also noted that automatic registration should be performed only with supervision and when there was misregistration between the CT and PET data to avoid false-negative cases [28].

For radiation therapy, we have reported a study of 216 patients in quantification with SUV and gross target volume (GTV) delineation [24]. There were 68 % of the patients with at least one respiratory artifact, and 10 % of the misregistrations in PET/CT studies could cause an SUV change of over 25 %, which can be a threshold indicating a partial response to therapy [29]. The small tumors of <50 cm^3 in size near the diaphragm could have a shift of the centroid tumor location of 2.4 mm and a GTV change of over 154 % and an SUV change of 21 %. It is clear that many whole-body PET/CT exams are with misregistration between the CT and PET data, but only a small portion of the scans with small tumors near the diaphragm could be impacted by misregistration.

16.1.3 Average CT (ACT) of Less Than 1 mSv to Reduce Misregistration

One approach to improve registration between the CT and PET data is to bring the temporal resolution of the CT images to that of the PET data [23]. Recognizing that a PET image is averaged over many breath cycles, a CT image averaged over one breath cycle could approach the temporal resolution of the PET image and register better with the PET image. Figure 16.4 shows an example of misregistration between the CT and PET data and correction of the misregistration by the use of average CT. This concept of average CT is very similar to the one on a stand-alone PET scanner whereby two to three rotating transmission rod sources of ^{68}Ge were used to obtain the transmission map for attenuation correction of the PET data. The transmission map has been shown to register well with the emission PET data [30]. Since most PET/CT scanners are not equipped with transmission rod sources, average CT can serve as an alternative for the transmission rod sources. The advantages of average CT over transmission rod sources are (1) short acquisition time, 1 min for average CT and 10 min per bed position for transmission imaging, and (2) high photon flux and less noisy attenuation maps. The disadvantages are (1) radiation dose of <1 mSv from average CT than about 0.13 mSv from the transmission rod sources [30]. Average CT has been shown to be effective in attenuation correction of the PET data not only in oncological imaging with ^{18}F-FDG but also in cardiac imaging as we demonstrated in reference [31] and confirmed by others [32, 33].

Acquiring cine CT images for average CT can be accomplished by scanning at the same location with a fast gantry rotation of sub-second over a breath cycle of 3–5 s. It does not need to record the respiratory signal while acquiring this type of data on the GE scanner, but GE needs the user to purchase their 4D-CT in order to derive average CT. Other vendors do not even allow data acquisition of a low-pitch helical CT to mimic the cine CT scan mode on the GE CT scanner without 4D-CT. There are two key components in the implementation of the average CT: one is to scan at a fast gantry rotation to achieve high temporal resolution and to minimize motion artifacts in each CT image; the other one is to scan over one breath cycle of 3–5 s to produce sufficient samples of the CT images across the multiple phases of a respiratory cycle to achieve the averaging effect like PET (Fig. 16.9). There is no need to have a respiratory monitoring device in acquiring the cine CT data for average CT as we have demonstrated with an in-house software on the GE CT or PET/CT scanners [31]. Unfortunately, all manufacturers require the purchase of 4D-CT to enable average CT. The conventional approach of using a slow-scan CT of several seconds per gantry rotation to generate slow CT to mimic average CT is not effective and should be discouraged [31, 34]. The slow-scan CT acquires data over one CT gantry rotation of several seconds, typically 2 or 4 s on the GE CT scanner. This scan technique could cause severe reconstruction artifacts. Figure 16.10 shows a clinical example of a patient scanned with the slow-scan CT of 4 s per gantry rotation and the average CT by the cine CT of fast gantry rotation of 0.5 s for 4 s. There were severe reconstruction artifacts caused by the respiratory motion in the images of the slow 4-s gantry rotation because the projection data of the slow 4-s CT were not consistent over one revolution of the CT scan due to the breathing motion, in violation of the basic tomographic image reconstruction principle which requires the imaged object to be stationary during data acquisition. Except some blurring at

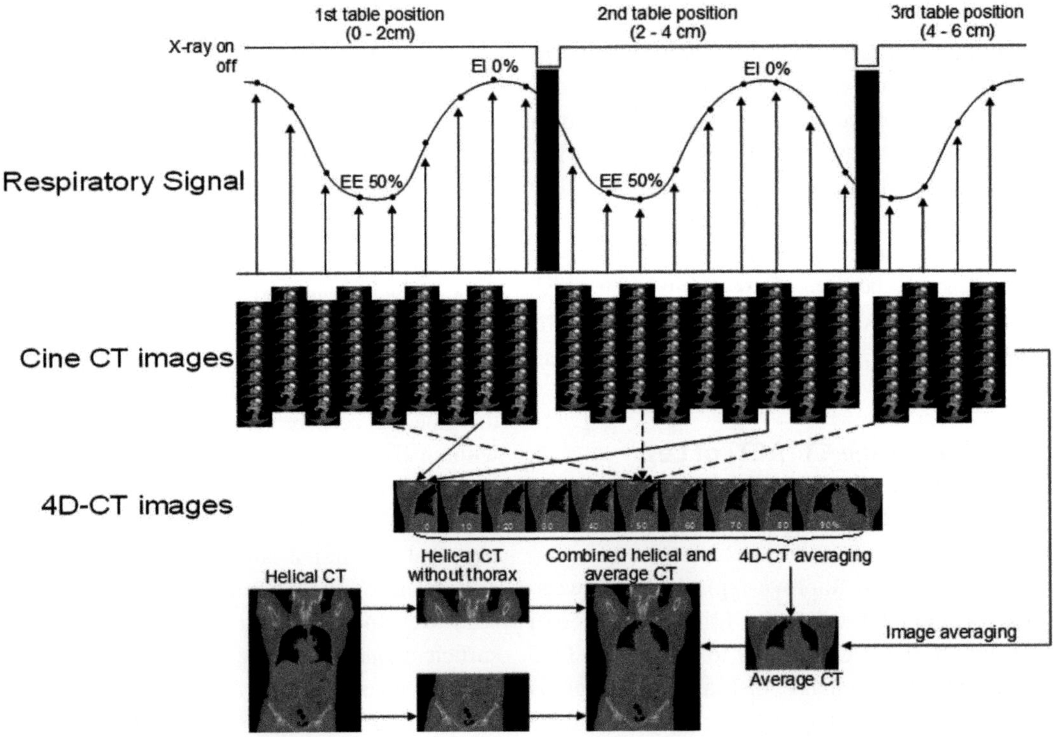

Fig. 16.9 Cine CT data acquisition of multiple table positions of 2 cm to generate many phases of a respiratory cycle for average CT. The thoracic region of misregistration was replaced with the average CT images for attenuation correction. The effective radiation dose for average CT is less than 0.87 mSv for 14 cm coverage, much less than the average lung screening CT dose of 1.4 mSv. The implementation does not need gating. However, GE requires 4D-CT which requires gating in order to generate average CT

the boundary of the liver, there were no artifacts in the average CT over a breath cycle of the CT images of high temporal resolution. The average CT and PET data are similar in temporal resolution and the average CT is without the artifacts in the slow CT.

Scan with either cine CT on the GE scanner or low-pitch helical CT (pitch <0.1) on the PET/CT scanners of the other manufacturers can be adopted to obtain average CT and has been available in 4D-CT imaging [35–37]. However, it is not clear whether the setup of 4D-CT imaging primarily for the assessment of tumor motion in radiation therapy with a respiratory monitoring device is ideal for obtaining the average CT when the majority of PET/CT scanners are in diagnostic imaging and are not equipped with 4D-CT with a respiratory monitoring device.

We have designed a practical approach to acquire average CT without a respiratory monitoring device and without 4D-CT to improve quantification of the PET data [31, 38] because the cine CT scan mode is available on any GE PET/CT scanner. We averaged the cine CT images for average CT and replace the portion of the helical CT data corresponding in location to the average CT data for attenuation correction of the PET data. The radiation exposure with average CT is about 4.4 mGy for the technique of 120 kV, 10 mA, 0.5 seconds gantry rotation, 8 × 2.5 mm collimation, and 5-s cine duration or 0.86 mSv for the coverage of 14 cm on the GE CT scanner (sufficient to cover the heart). In comparison, the low-dose lung screening CT has a higher effective dose of 1.4 mSv [39]. The scan time of the cine CT for average CT is less than 1 min. Software processing for average CT can be automated in the clinic. For example, once the cine CT scan is completed after a cardiac stress perfusion PET scan, the

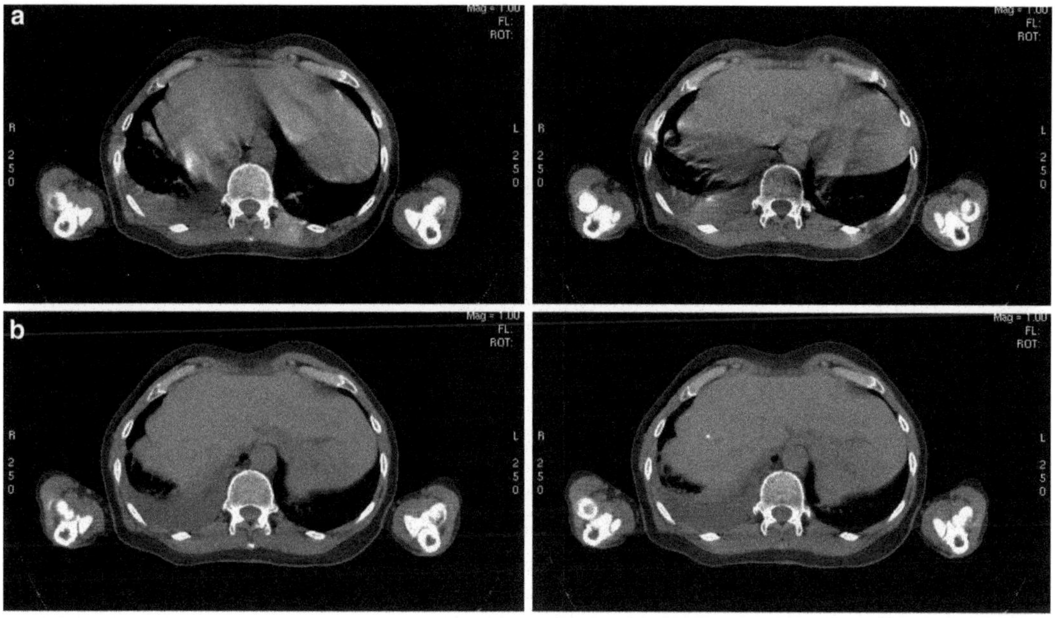

Fig. 16.10 The average CT and the slow-scan CT images of a patient with an average breath cycle of 4 s. The slow-scan CT images in (**a**) were taken with one single CT gantry rotation of 4 s, and the two images were 2.5 mm apart and 2.5 mm thick. The corresponding average CT images in (**b**), obtained by averaging the cine CT images, were averaged from 4 s of data collection over 8 gantry rotations. The average CT images were almost free of reconstruction artifacts, which were observed in the SSCT images (Reproduced from Pan et al. [31]; with permission)

technologist enters the scanner room to unload the patient from the imaging table. By the time the technologist is back to the scanner console in a couple of minutes, the task of computing for average CT is already finished, not impacting the overall scan time of a PET/CT procedure.

In a whole-body PET/CT scan, the CT images are typically acquired before PET. The technologist can determine if a cine or average CT scan is needed when the CT and PET images of the thorax and abdomen, which are more likely to be impacted by the mismatch of the CT and PET images, are available for review before completion of the PET scan. Therefore, not every patient data needs an average CT, and radiation dose can be further reduced or targeted to the patient data with misregistration. The coverage of 14 cm can be further reduced to save radiation dose if the target tumor area is small.

There was an approach of interpolated average CT to reduce radiation dose of average CT by only acquiring the end-inspiration and end-expiration phases and interpolating the between phases from the two acquired phases [40]. This interpolated average CT approach requires gating, patient coaching, and complex deformable image registration. Its application may be limited as the average CT from over one respiratory cycle does not require gating or patient coaching and has been utilized in cardiac PET for over 6,000 patients with automation since its clinical use in 2006 [27].

16.1.3.1 Benefits of Average CT for Radiation Therapy

Radiation therapy has embraced the use of average CT for dose calculation for conventional radiation therapy [41] and in particular for proton beam therapy [42] when the respiratory motion may alter the dose calculation. Average CT has also been shown to benefit the alignment with the cone-beam CT images taken right before radiation treatment in image-guided radiation therapy [43]. Average CT can be generated from the cine CT scan by averaging the cine CT images without a respiratory gating device [38, 44, 45], which means that it can be derived on all GE

PET/CT scanners for the purposes of attenuation correction of PET images, dose calculation for radiation therapy with photon and proton in particular, and alignment with cone-beam CT for image-guided radiation therapy. Unfortunately, most manufacturers only offer average CT in 4D-CT, i.e., average CT can only be generated in 4D-CT with the optical sensing device of the real-time position management (RPM) respiratory gating system (Varian Medical Systems, Palo Alto, CA), the pressure sensor device AZ-733V (Anzai Medical Corporation, Tokyo, Japan), or the air bellow combined with a pressure sensor (Philips Medical Systems, Andover, MA). Although we have developed in house the software for average CT, many PET/CT sites are limited by the availability of average CT only from 4D-CT.

From the same scan data for average CT, the maximum intensity projection (MIP) CT images can be derived by finding the maximum pixel value at each pixel location from all the images of cine CT or 4D-CT [36, 38]. It has been shown that MIP CT images are effective in depicting the extent of tumor motion [46, 47]. For peripheral lung tumors (surrounded by the lower density air in the lungs), MIP CT images can be used to assist the determination of the tumor target volume and to avoid ambiguity in using a threshold of SUV to determine the target volume in PET. Any ^{18}F-FDG uptake in the lungs should be supported by the soft tissues depicted in the MIP images. Any PET GTV determined with an SUV threshold should not exceed the soft-tissue boundary in the MIP images. Their application for treatment planning for stereotactic body radiation therapy has been demonstrated in [48]. The MIP CT images can help determine the tumor volume in the thorax. Figure 16.11 shows an example of determining the extent of PET GTV with MIP CT to avoid the uncertainty of thresholding a functional tumor with SUV. A similar concept has been attempted with the regular helical CT data for peripheral non-small cell lung cancer (NSCLC) by Biehl et al. [49], when the boarder of the tumor can be identified by the CT data.

Figure 16.12 shows an example of misregistration that caused a false-negative diagnosis and a change of the gross target volume for radiation therapy when the misregistration was removed with average CT. In the era of image-guided radiation therapy to deliver a very high dose of radiation at a great precision, it is very important to pay attention to any misregistration between the CT and the PET images during tumor delineation when PET/CT images are used in the treatment planning. At the MD Anderson Cancer Center, we routinely use 4D-CT data for treatment simulation with the fusion of the PET/CT data from patient diagnosis and staging in diagnostic imaging. The most ideal approach is to conduct PET/CT and 4D-CT in the same simulation session. However, insurance providers only pay for one

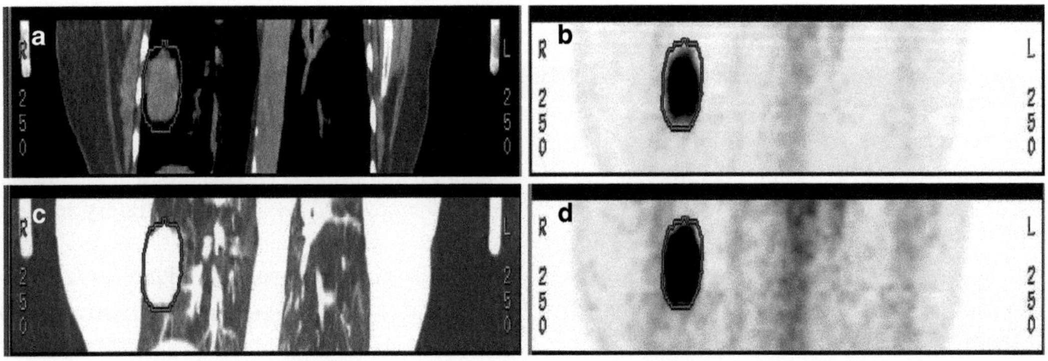

Fig. 16.11 The MIP CT and PET images of a patient. The MIP CT in (**a**) is displayed with (window, level) = (400, 40) and PET in (**b**) with a threshold of 40 % of the maximum SUV of the tumor. The images of (**a**) and (**b**) are displayed again with (1000,–700) in (**c**) and the threshold of 20 % in (**d**), respectively. The tumor contour in (**c**) is superimposed in (**a**, **b**), and (**d**) to demonstrate the effect on tumor size by display parameters

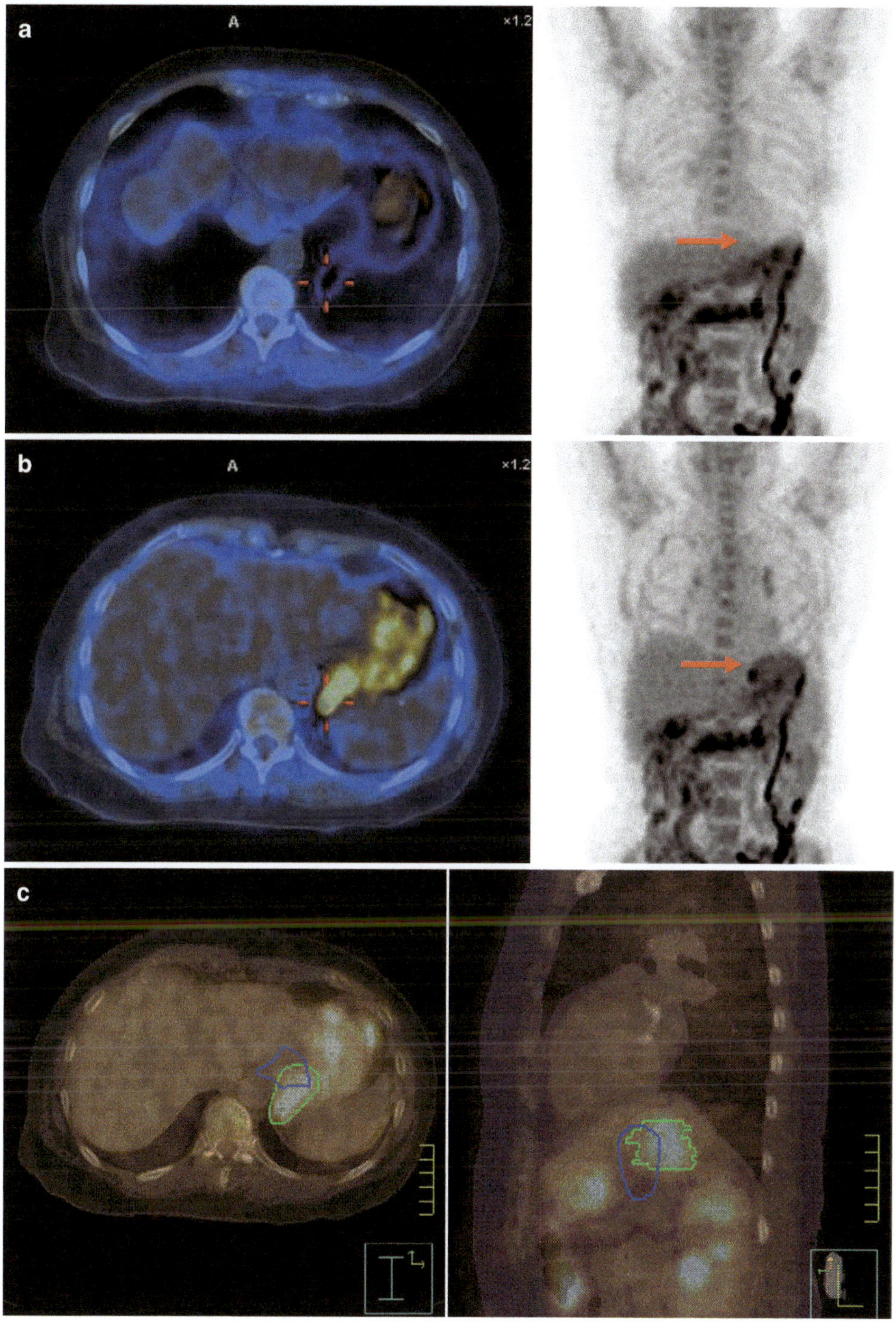

Fig. 16.12 The PET/CT images of a 69-year-old female patient with an esophageal tumor after an induction chemotherapy. (**a**) shows an axial slice of the fused clinical CT and PET image at the level of the esophageal tumor (*left*) and the PET image in coronal view (*right*). The radiology report indicated the patient had a positive response to the chemotherapy. After removal of misalignment by the average CT, the tumor reappeared in the same PET data set in (**b**). The *arrows* pointed to the tumor location. The gross target volumes drawn in the images of (**a**) and (**b**) are shown in blue and in green, respectively, in (**c**). The patient was treated with the tumor volume in green, and the radiology report was corrected by the average CT (Reproduced from Pan and Mawlawi [63]; with permission)

PET/CT before cancer treatment, and this issue has resulted in a decline of interest in application of PET/CT for radiation therapy simulation.

16.1.4 4D-PET

4D-PET was first developed for cardiac imaging to assess myocardial motion and to obtain ejection fraction [50]. 4D-PET was adopted for tumor imaging of the thorax [51–54] at about the same time when 4D-CT was developed [35–37, 55, 56]. Today, 4D-PET for cardiac imaging is routinely practiced, and 4D-CT is standard in CT simulation of the tumor motion for radiation therapy. 4D-PET for tumor imaging is still mainly a research tool because (1) its impact on diagnosis, staging, or treatment planning over the conventional PET/CT has not been established and (2) its workflow in setup for acquisition and data processing is relatively cumbersome. It could take several minutes to ensure (1) the scan field of view covering the target tumor, (2) the respiratory monitoring device on the patient producing triggers to the scanner, and (3) the gating parameters such as the number of bins for amplitude or phase binning properly set according to the patient's breathing pattern. A 4D-PET scan of an average duration of 10 min conducted after a whole-body PET/CT would lengthen the total time of a patient on the imaging table over 30–40 min. The setup of gating, binning, and post-processing can be intimidating to the technologist. As the patient is often instructed to hold his/her arms over the head to avoid attenuation by the arms for 30–40 min, patient motion or irregular respiratory cycles due to patient discomfort are likely to happen and could degrade the value of 4D-PET imaging.

In 4D-PET, the data are split into several exclusive bins. There can be 8 bins of 500 ms for an average respiratory cycle of 4 s. Because of insufficient photons per bin obtained in PET imaging of 2–3 min in each bed location, the duration of a 4D-PET scan has to be over 10 min to ensure sufficient counts recorded in each bin. It may be necessary to scan for two bed positions if a tumor is not at the center of the PET detector field of view to account for the high sensitivity at the center and low sensitivity at the edge of the PET detector in the 3D data acquisition without the septa.

Image reconstruction of 4D-PET is performed on the data of each bin, and the result is a set of 3D PET images over a respiratory cycle for assessment of tumor motion and quantification. Even though the number of photons in each bin can be small in 4D-PET, resulting in higher noise in the 4D-PET images, the 4D-PET images can potentially be used for accurate assessment of ^{18}F-FDG uptake [54].

Most modern PET/CT scanners are equipped with the list-mode data acquisition whereby events from each coincidence pair of 511 keV photons can be stored in a list stream for subsequent static, dynamic, or gated reconstruction (Fig. 16.11). List-mode data acquisition can be performed with either cardiac or respiratory triggering during a normal static image acquisition [57]. This functionality offers the capability of retrospectively mapping the coincidence events into multiple phases/bins for the reconstruction of 4D-PET images. The PET scanners can be configured to acquire the list-mode data which can produce prospectively static PET data as a standard data set and retrospectively 4D-PET data to freeze the tumor motion. Although it is still cumbersome to acquire 4D-PET data due to its prolonged acquisition time, it is expected that both large detector coverage and new digital photomultipliers may allow easy positioning of a tumor near the center of field of view and short acquisition time to make 4D-PET a clinically feasible solution to improving the quantification accuracy of a tumor or the heart in motion.

One important logistical issue with 4D-PET is that it is not clear which patients are going to benefit from 4D-PET. The tumors near the diaphragm such as some lung tumors, liver tumors (typically from the colorectal cancer), or esophageal tumors near the gastroesophageal junction may benefit from the 4D-PET imaging by reducing the impact of blurring on the PET images from the respiratory motion. However, as most PET/CT scans are conducted in a diagnostic setting of covering the orbit to the mid-thigh, we may not know the locations of the targeted tumors prior to the first PET/CT scan to determine the application of 4D-PET. The setup of a respiratory monitoring device for sending triggers in 4D-PET has to be read on the patient before the patient scan. This is a dilemma in the application of 4D-PET, which requires 10 more minutes in data acquisition and likely equal amount of time in locating a bed position to cover the tumor and setting up a 4D-PET acquisition. On the other hand, 4D-CT has become a standard clinical procedure for the treatment simulation of a lung or liver tumor because the physician needs the 4D-CT data to determine the envelope of tumor motion in treatment planning. The diagnosis has been made, and the targeted area is local for radiation therapy, which is different from whole-body PET/CT.

16.1.5 4D-PET/CT = 4D-PET + 4D-CT

4D-CT [35–37] may be needed for accurate quantification of 4D-PET data as each phase of PET data may need its own CT data for attenuation correction [54]. 4D-CT has found its acceptance in radiation therapy for providing the gated CT images of multiple phases over a respiratory cycle to assist contouring the envelope of tumor motion. 4D-CT takes less time in data acquisition than 4D-PET does. It normally takes less than 2 min to cover 35 cm in the craniocaudal direction on an 8- or 16-slice CT. The scan coverage of 4D-CT for radiation therapy is typically the whole lungs, whereas the coverage for average CT for diagnostic PET/CT should be limited to the tumor or the heart region. Radiation dose for 4D-CT is about 50 mGy and should be less than 5 mGy for average CT for diagnostic PET/CT.

Two data acquisition modes can be used in 4D-CT. One is cine CT and the other one is low-pitch helical CT. Both acquisitions need to scan a prescribed volume for over one breath cycle to produce the multiple phases of 4D-CT images over a respiratory cycle. Both require the respiratory monitoring devices. Cine 4D-CT uses less radiation and generates thinner slices than low-pitch helical 4D-CT. On the other hand, helical 4D-CT is faster than cine 4D-CT because it does not pause between two table positions as in the cine 4D-CT [58]. The cine 4D-CT is available on the GE 4-, 8-, 16-, or 64-slice CT scanners, and the helical 4D-CT is only available on newer 16- or 64-slice CT scanners. There has been no PET/CT scanner with more than 64 slice. The Siemens 128-slice PET/CT has only 64 slice, and its claim of 128 slice was from the flying focal spot, which simulates the effect of 128 slice. However, the 128-slice mode is typically used to obtain the high-resolution CT images of 0.3 mm and is not applicable for 4D-CT. Figure 16.13 illustrates an example of 4D-PET/CT in 6 bins over 13 min of data acquisition. Quantification of the tumor in SUV changed from 5 to 8.5 at the end-expiration phase in this example. Image reconstruction can also be applied on 4D-PET, based on the tumor motion from 4D-CT, to deform/register the multiple phases of PET data to a single "motion freeze" PET data set to reduce the noise in 4D-PET data and to improve tumor quantification [59]. There has been no clinical data to suggest this single freeze PET image can be accomplished in the clinical setting because it relies on the motion information either from 4D-CT or 4D-PET. As most 4D-PET is con-

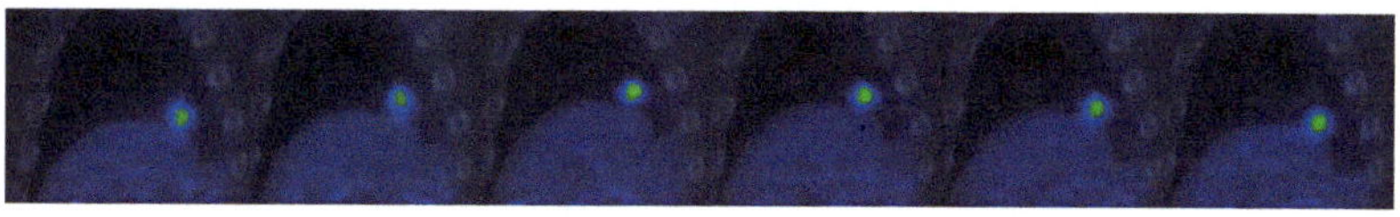

Fig. 16.13 A 4D-PET/CT patient study. The acquisition time for the 4D-PET was 13 min, and the PET data were gated into 6 phases. Attenuation of the 4D-PET data was corrected with the corresponding 4D-CT data. Quantification of the tumor in SUV went from 5.0 in the static PET without gating to 8.5 in the end-expiration phase of the 4D-PET (Reproduced from the Pan and Zaidi [61]; with permission)

ducted without 4D-CT, the reliability of motion information from 4D-PET is questionable.

16.2 Summary

In the early days of PET/CT, misregistration of the CT and PET data was recognized as a new artifact from the combined PET/CT scanner sharing the same imaging table [60]. Since it was not possible to slow down the CT gantry rotation (currently at 2 s and was at 4 s per revolution) to mimic the slow scanning with transmission rod sources like in a stand-alone PET scanner, other approaches to coach the patient to hold breath at the average PET position and to use a fast CT scanner of more than six detector rows have been proposed with limited success. The misregistration artifacts due to the respiration have been understood and can compromise tumor quantification. However, the artifacts can be effectively fixed by average CT or 4D-PET/CT.

Average CT is a viable solution without excessive radiation on the patient (less than 1 mSv) or without too much imaging time (less than 1 min) to match the temporal resolution of the CT data and the temporal resolution of the PET data without an elaborated gating scheme of 4D-PET or 4D-PET/CT. Average CT can be derived from the cine CT scan, available on all the GE PET/CT scanners, to help improve the registration of the CT and PET data and to help calculate the radiation dose in radiation therapy with photon and in particular with proton beam which requires a more stringent requirement to account for uncertainty. Average CT derived from averaging the CT images of high temporal resolution acquired over a respiratory cycle at sub-second gantry rotation has been shown to be effective in improving the registration of the CT and the PET data, resulting in improvement on quantification of the PET data both for tumor imaging and cardiac imaging. In addition, average CT can also be applied in dose calculation and image-guided radiation therapy. Its companion MIP images, derived from the same cine CT or 4D-CT data for average CT, play a very important role in tumor delineation of a moving lung tumor in treatment simulation and are likely the first image data set out of 4D-CT in tumor delineation by a radiation oncology physician. Radiation dose of average CT is <1 mSv, and application of average CT can be limited to only the patients whose PET data and CT data do not register. With the development of 4D-CT, the difficulties in imaging the tumor motion with CT in the thorax or the abdomen have been largely eliminated.

List-mode data acquisition, although not new, has been very useful to allow the post-processing of the 4D-PET data for static PET as a baseline data. 4D-PET and 4D-PET/CT are emerging as the next frontier for researchers and clinicians to put into the clinical use. The bottleneck in 4D-PET and 4D-PET/CT is the long acquisition time for acquiring the 4D-PET data. It is hoped that future instrumentation can significantly improve the sensitivity of PET imaging so that every whole-body PET imaging can become a 4D-PET imaging without a significant increase of the scan time.

References

1. Beyer T, et al. A combined PET/CT scanner for clinical oncology. J Nucl Med. 2000;41(8):1369–79.
2. Townsend DW, Beyer T. A combined PET/CT scanner: the path to true image fusion. Br J Radiol. 2002;75 Spec No:S24–30.
3. Blodgett TM, Meltzer CC, Townsend DW. PET/CT: form and function. Radiology. 2007;242(2):360–85.
4. Hutton BF, Braun M. Software for image registration: algorithms, accuracy, efficacy. Semin Nucl Med. 2003;33(3):180–92.
5. Reinartz P, et al. Side-by-side reading of PET and CT scans in oncology: which patients might profit from integrated PET/CT? Eur J Nucl Med Mol Imaging. 2004;31(11):1456–61.
6. Bradley J, et al. Impact of FDG-PET on radiation therapy volume delineation in non-small-cell lung cancer. Int J Radiat Oncol Biol Phys. 2004;59(1):78–86.
7. Ciernik IF, et al. Radiation treatment planning with an integrated positron emission and computer tomography (PET/CT): a feasibility study. Int J Radiat Oncol Biol Phys. 2003;57(3):853–63.
8. Mah K, et al. The impact of (18)FDG-PET on target and critical organs in CT-based treatment planning of patients with poorly defined non-small-cell lung

carcinoma: a prospective study. Int J Radiat Oncol Biol Phys. 2002;52(2):339–50.
9. van Baardwijk A, et al. The current status of FDG-PET in tumour volume definition in radiotherapy treatment planning. Cancer Treat Rev. 2006;32(4):245–60.
10. Messa C, et al. PET/CT and radiotherapy. Q J Nucl Med Mol Imaging. 2006;50(1):4–14.
11. Di Carli MF, et al. Clinical myocardial perfusion PET/CT. J Nucl Med. 2007;48(5):783–93.
12. Stewart RD, Li XA. BGRT: Biologically guided radiation therapy – the future is fast approaching. Med Phys. 2007;34(10):3739–51.
13. Gregory DL, et al. Effect of PET/CT on management of patients with non-small cell lung cancer: results of a prospective study with 5-year survival data. J Nucl Med. 2012;53(7):1007–15.
14. Steenbakkers RJ, et al. Reduction of observer variation using matched CT-PET for lung cancer delineation: a three-dimensional analysis. Int J Radiat Oncol Biol Phys. 2006;64(2):435–48.
15. Ashamalla H, et al. The contribution of integrated PET/CT to the evolving definition of treatment volumes in radiation treatment planning in lung cancer. Int J Radiat Oncol Biol Phys. 2005;63(4):1016–23.
16. Erdi YE, et al. Radiotherapy treatment planning for patients with non-small cell lung cancer using positron emission tomography (PET). Radiother Oncol. 2002;62(1):51–60.
17. Schwartz DL, et al. FDG-PET/CT-guided intensity modulated head and neck radiotherapy: a pilot investigation. Head Neck. 2005;27(6):478–87.
18. Chao KS, et al. A novel approach to overcome hypoxic tumor resistance: Cu-ATSM-guided intensity-modulated radiation therapy. Int J Radiat Oncol Biol Phys. 2001;49(4):1171–82.
19. Zasadny KR, Wahl RL. Standardized uptake values of normal tissues at PET with 2-[fluorine-18]-fluoro-2-deoxy-D-glucose: variations with body weight and a method for correction. Radiology. 1993;189(3):847–50.
20. Keyes Jr JW. SUV: standard uptake or silly useless value? J Nucl Med. 1995;36(10):1836–9.
21. Beyer T, et al. Respiration artifacts in whole-body (18)F-FDG PET/CT studies with combined PET/CT tomographs employing spiral CT technology with 1 to 16 detector rows. Eur J Nucl Med Mol Imaging. 2005;32(12):1429–39.
22. Goerres GW, et al. PET/CT of the abdomen: optimizing the patient breathing pattern. Eur Radiol. 2003;13(4):734–9.
23. Pan T, et al. Attenuation correction of PET images with respiration-averaged CT images in PET/CT. J Nucl Med. 2005;46(9):1481–7.
24. Chi PC, et al. Effects of respiration-averaged computed tomography on positron emission tomography/computed tomography quantification and its potential impact on gross tumor volume delineation. Int J Radiat Oncol Biol Phys. 2008;71(3):890–9.
25. Osman MM, et al. Respiratory motion artifacts on PET emission images obtained using CT attenuation correction on PET-CT. Eur J Nucl Med Mol Imaging. 2003;30(4):603–6.
26. Osman MM, et al. Clinically significant inaccurate localization of lesions with PET/CT: frequency in 300 patients. J Nucl Med. 2003;44(2):240–3.
27. Gould KL, et al. Frequent diagnostic errors in cardiac PET/CT due to misregistration of CT attenuation and emission PET images: a definitive analysis of causes, consequences, and corrections. J Nucl Med. 2007;48(7):1112–21.
28. Slomka PJ, et al. Automatic registration of misaligned CT attenuation correction maps in Rb-82 PET/CT improves detection of angiographically significant coronary artery disease. J Nucl Cardiol. 2015;22(6):1285–95.
29. Young H, et al. Measurement of clinical and subclinical tumour response using [18F]-fluorodeoxyglucose and positron emission tomography: review and 1999 EORTC recommendations. European Organization for Research and Treatment of Cancer (EORTC) PET Study Group. Eur J Cancer. 1999;35(13):1773–82.
30. Papathanassiou D, et al. Respiratory motion artefact in the liver dome on FDG PET/CT: comparison of attenuation correction with CT and a caesium external source. Eur J Nucl Med Mol Imaging. 2005;32(12):1422–8.
31. Pan T, et al. Attenuation correction of PET cardiac data with low-dose average CT in PET/CT. Med Phys. 2006;33(10):3931–8.
32. Cook RA, et al. Respiration-averaged CT for attenuation correction in canine cardiac PET/CT. J Nucl Med. 2007;48(5):811–8.
33. Alessio AM, et al. Cine CT for attenuation correction in cardiac PET/CT. J Nucl Med. 2007;48(5):794–801.
34. Keall PJ, et al. The management of respiratory motion in radiation oncology report of AAPM Task Group 76. Med Phys. 2006;33(10):3874–900.
35. Low DA, et al. A method for the reconstruction of four-dimensional synchronized CT scans acquired during free breathing. Med Phys. 2003;30(6):1254–63.
36. Pan T, et al. 4D-CT imaging of a volume influenced by respiratory motion on multi-slice CT. Med Phys. 2004;31(2):333–40.
37. Keall PJ, et al. Acquiring 4D thoracic CT scans using a multislice helical method. Phys Med Biol. 2004;49(10):2053–67.
38. Pan T, Sun X, Luo D. Improvement of the cine-CT based 4D-CT imaging. Med Phys. 2007;34(11):4499–503.
39. Larke FJ, et al. Estimated radiation dose associated with low-dose chest CT of average-size participants in the National Lung Screening Trial. AJR Am J Roentgenol. 2011;197(5):1165–9.
40. Sun T, et al. Low dose interpolated average CT for thoracic PET/CT attenuation correction using an active breathing controller. Med Phys. 2013;40(10):102507.
41. Riegel AC, et al. Dose calculation with respiration-averaged CT processed from cine CT without a respiratory surrogate. Med Phys. 2008;35(12):5738–47.
42. Cai J, et al. Estimation of error in maximal intensity projection-based internal target volume of lung

tumors: a simulation and comparison study using dynamic magnetic resonance imaging. Int J Radiat Oncol Biol Phys. 2007;69(3):895–902.
43. Shirai K, et al. Phantom and clinical study of differences in cone beam computed tomographic registration when aligned to maximum and average intensity projection. Int J Radiat Oncol Biol Phys. 2014;88(1):189–94.
44. Chi P-CM, et al. Effects of respiration-averaged computed tomography on positron emission tomography/computed tomography quantification and its potential impact on gross tumor volume delineation. Int J Radiat Oncol Biol Phys. 2008;71(3):890–9.
45. Riegel AC, et al. Cine computed tomography without respiratory surrogate in planning stereotactic radiotherapy for non-small-cell lung cancer. Int J Radiat Oncol Biol Phys. 2009;73(2):433–41.
46. Underberg RW, et al. Use of maximum intensity projections (MIP) for target volume generation in 4DCT scans for lung cancer. Int J Radiat Oncol Biol Phys. 2005;63(1):253–60.
47. Bradley JD, et al. Comparison of helical, maximum intensity projection (MIP), and averaged intensity (AI) 4D CT imaging for stereotactic body radiation therapy (SBRT) planning in lung cancer. Radiother Oncol. 2006;81(3):264–8.
48. Riegel AC, et al. Cine computed tomography without respiratory surrogate in planning stereotactic radiotherapy for non-small-cell lung cancer. Int J Radiat Oncol Biol Phys. 2009;73(2):433–41.
49. Biehl KJ, et al. 18F-FDG PET definition of gross tumor volume for radiotherapy of non-small cell lung cancer: is a single standardized uptake value threshold approach appropriate? J Nucl Med. 2006;47(11):1808–12.
50. Hoffman EJ, et al. Electrocardiographic gating in positron emission computed tomography. J Comput Assist Tomogr. 1979;3(6):733–9.
51. Nehmeh SA, et al. Effect of respiratory gating on quantifying PET images of lung cancer. J Nucl Med. 2002;43(7):876–81.
52. Nehmeh SA, et al. Effect of respiratory gating on reducing lung motion artifacts in PET imaging of lung cancer. Med Phys. 2002;29(3):366–71.
53. Nehmeh SA, et al. Reduction of respiratory motion artifacts in PET imaging of lung cancer by respiratory correlated dynamic PET: methodology and comparison with respiratory gated PET. J Nucl Med. 2003;44(10):1644–8.
54. Nehmeh SA, et al. Four-dimensional (4D) PET/CT imaging of the thorax. Med Phys. 2004;31(12):3179–86.
55. Vedam SS, et al. Acquiring a four-dimensional computed tomography dataset using an external respiratory signal. Phys Med Biol. 2003;48(1):45–62.
56. Mageras GS, et al. Measurement of lung tumor motion using respiration-correlated CT. Int J Radiat Oncol Biol Phys. 2004;60(3):933–41.
57. Kinahan PE, et al. Whole-body respiratory gated PET/CT. J Nucl Med. 2006;47(1):187P.
58. Pan T. Comparison of helical and cine acquisitions for 4D-CT imaging with multislice CT. Med Phys. 2005;32(2):627–34.
59. Li T, et al. Model-based image reconstruction for four-dimensional PET. Med Phys. 2006;33(5):1288–98.
60. Bacharach SL. PET/CT attenuation correction: breathing lessons. J Nucl Med. 2007;48(5):677–9.
61. Pan T, Zaidi H. Attenuation correction strategies for PET and 4D PET/CT. PET Clin. 2013;8:37–50.
62. Zaid H, Pan T. Recent advances in hybrid imaging for radiation therapy planning: the cutting edge. PET Clin. 2011;6:207–26.
63. Pan T, Mawlawi O. PET/CT in Radiation Oncology. Med Phys. 2008;35(11):4955–66.

Part VI

Scientific and Clinical Basis of PET Applications

Physiologic and Molecular Basis of PET in Cancer Imaging

17

Abhishek Mahajan and Gary Cook

Contents

17.1	**Introduction**	400
17.2	**Why PET/CT?**	401
17.3	**Underlying Tumour Biology and FDG**	401
17.4	**Beyond FDG**	404
17.4.1	PET Tracers for Imaging Tumour Amino-Acid Metabolism	404
17.4.2	Natural Amino Acids	404
17.4.3	Synthetic Amino Acids	404
17.5	**PET Tracers for Imaging Phospholipid Metabolism**	405
17.6	**PET Tracers for Imaging Tumour Angiogenesis**	406
17.7	**PET Tracers for Imaging Tumour Hypoxia**	408
17.8	**PET Tracers for Imaging Apoptosis**	410
17.9	**PET Tracers for Imaging Tumour Cell Proliferation**	411
17.10	**PET Tracers for Imaging Epidermal Growth Factor Receptors**	414
17.11	**PET Tracers for Imaging Somatostatin Receptors**	415
17.12	**PET Tracers for Imaging Bone Metabolism**	416
17.13	**PET Tracers for Imaging Agents Targeting Chemokine Receptor**	417
17.14	**PET Tracers for Imaging Multidrug Resistance in Cancer**	417
Conclusion		418
References		418

Abstract

Over the last 25 years, PET has seen the progress from a research tool mainly for neurological applications to becoming one of the major imaging methods for assessing cancer. Whilst FDG remains the most commonly used PET tracer to measure tumour glucose transport and glycolysis, there are a number of tumours that are not FDG avid and a number of important underlying biological events in the cancer cell that can be more directly reported with alternative tracers. Beyond tumour glycolysis, other underlying processes, including proliferation, amino-acid transport, cell membrane and phospholipid metabolism, apoptosis, angiogenesis and hypoxia, are all highly

A. Mahajan, MBBS, MD
Department of Radiodiagnosis, Tata Memorial Hospital, Mumbai 400012, India
e-mail: drabhishek.mahajan@yahoo.in

G. Cook, MB BS, MSc, MD, FRCR, FRCP (✉)
Division of Imaging Sciences and Biomedical Engineering, King's College London and the King's College London and Guys & St Thomas' PET Centre, St Thomas' Hospital, London, UK
e-mail: gary.cook@kcl.ac.uk

M.M. Khalil (ed.), *Basic Science of PET Imaging*, DOI 10.1007/978-3-319-40070-9_17

relevant aspects of tumour biology that can be imaged and quantified with PET. Many of these tracers are used primarily for research applications, but a number have been translated into clinical practice, either for tumours that are not FDG avid, e.g. choline tracers in prostate cancer and somatostatin receptor imaging in neuroendocrine tumours, or when a more specific biomarker is required to interrogate underlying changes in tumour biology.

In tandem with the development and translation of novel tracers, there is improvement in hardware, e.g. PET/CT and PET/MRI, and software, e.g. reconstruction algorithms, that have allowed PET to become one of the essential and leading imaging modalities in clinical and research cancer applications.

17.1 Introduction

Cancer is one of the leading causes of death worldwide [1]. Optimising the patient's therapeutic management needs accurate diagnosis, staging, therapeutic response assessment and restaging of the disease [2]. Imaging plays an indispensable role in the management of cancer patients [3]. Imaging modalities such as plain radiography, computed tomography (CT) and magnetic resonance imaging (MRI) provide anatomical detail that helps to detect and localise tumours. Of late, biochemical, molecular and functional imaging technologies such as positron emission tomography (PET) play a complementary role to the anatomical information gained from other imaging modalities such as CT and MRI and has significant impact on individualised cancer care and management [4, 5].

Biologically important small molecules such as glucose, amino acids and peptides, nucleic acids, water and receptor ligands labelled with positron-emitting radionuclides form the basis of PET imaging [6]. The radioactive decay resulting in a positron that interacts with an electron to produce subsequent annihilation radiation (two 511 KeV gamma ray photons), which are detected by a PET scanner, allows the spatial and temporal distribution of these compounds to be measured to create "physiological maps" of the functional and molecular processes relevant to the labelled biological target molecule [7].

There are numerous radioactive tracers used for PET imaging, but the most important, which is used for the majority of clinical oncological PET imaging, is the analogue of glucose, 18F-2-fluoro-2-deoxy-D-glucose (FDG) [8]. First made 75 years ago, FDG as a PET tracer images tumour glucose metabolic rate by taking advantage of malignant cells having higher rates of glucose transport and glycolysis than normal cells [9]. FDG was the first Food and Drug Administration (FDA)-approved PET radiopharmaceutical and is used in 90% of oncological studies [7, 10]. Though FDG is not a perfect oncology imaging tracer (some malignant lesions are not FDG avid and some benign lesions show FDG avidity), it still proves to be very useful in most malignant tumours of clinical importance [10–12]. Recently the FDA has approved 11C-choline for prostate cancer and Sodium Fluoride F18 for bone imaging [11–13].

FDG-PET/CT imaging is primarily applied for staging and restaging of tumours to guide clinical patient care. Other important applications include assessment of response to drug therapy, often possible before actual tumour size reduction occurs [14, 15]. In certain tumours, such as lymphoma, oesophageal cancer and non-small-cell lung cancer, FDG-PET/CT has become the primary imaging modality for clinical management decision making and shows significant correlation with clinical endpoints and survival [14, 15].

FDG-PET/CT is also particularly useful for detecting recurrence, especially in asymptomatic patients with rising tumour marker levels and those with negative or equivocal conventional imaging findings [15, 16]. Yet there are some limitations and areas of uncertainty, mainly regarding the lack of specificity of FDG uptake and the variable avidity of some cancers for this tracer [7]. This has led to the development of more tumour-specific non-FDG-PET tracers that have been extensively studied in understanding the tumourigenesis-related pathways such as tumour proliferation, metabolism, hypoxia, angiogenesis and apoptosis. These tracers have

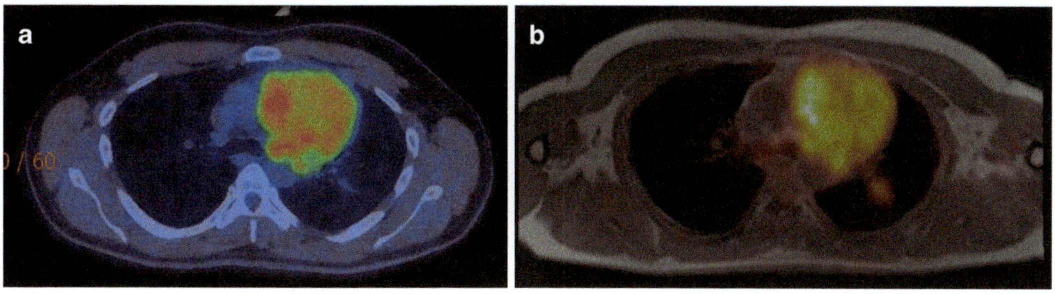

Fig. 17.1 A young male patient with a mediastinal germ cell tumour. 18F-FDG-PET/CT (**a**) and PET/MRI (**b**) trans-axial images through the upper thorax

been found to have a role in imaging tumours with low avidity for FDG [17, 18].

17.2 Why PET/CT?

To understand the role of biological imaging in cancer patient management in the present era, it is important to recognise the unmet diagnostic needs. These include accurate detection and staging, better understanding of tumour biology and phenotype, early and predictive therapeutic response assessment and personalised management of patients [19].

Over the last 20 years, CT has been the cornerstone of cancer imaging but is limited in its ability to delineate the critical differences in physiology and biology of tumours. Whilst progress with MRI allows whole-body imaging and the addition of functional information to anatomical data (e.g. diffusion-weighted imaging), PET imaging shows advantages, particularly its sensitivity in determining the physiology and metabolic activity of tumours, but lacks anatomical information [20, 21]. Integrated data sets from hybrid PET and CT or MRI offer the best of the available imaging modalities for oncologic imaging and significantly improve diagnostic accuracy [20–22]. For example, the diagnostic accuracy of detecting lymph node metastases is improved with the use of combined anatomical imaging by CT and increased glucose uptake on FDG-PET [23].

Before combined PET/CT scanners, the metabolic information was visually fused with the anatomical information by reviewing the separate PET and CT images and mentally synthesising the combined information [24, 25]. Fusion software helped to some extent, but the availability of combined hybrid PET/CT scanners has revolutionised the role of PET in oncologic imaging [26, 27]. More recently, hybrid PET/MRI scanners have become available allowing the combination of anatomical, functional and molecular imaging in a single acquisition. Whilst PET/CT has remained a sequential modality, PET/MRI scanners allow simultaneous data acquisition [13] (Fig. 17.1).

17.3 Underlying Tumour Biology and FDG

The progression from a few cancer cells to the formation of macroscopic solid tumours is a complex process of activation of specific metabolic pathways providing oxygen, glucose, other nutrients and growth factors which are critical for the growth of cancer cells [28]. Sokoloff et al. were the first to report FDG in their work on measuring regional cerebral glucose metabolism in animals using 14C-deoxyglucose autoradiography [29]. Subsequently FDG was developed for PET imaging which provided similar quantification of regional concentrations in humans. It was the Warburg observations in the 1930s, showing a high rate of glycolysis in cancer cells, which led to use of FDG as a tumour imaging agent. There is a complex process which regulates the multiple factors that influence the rate of glucose flux which can be measured by FDG-PET [30].

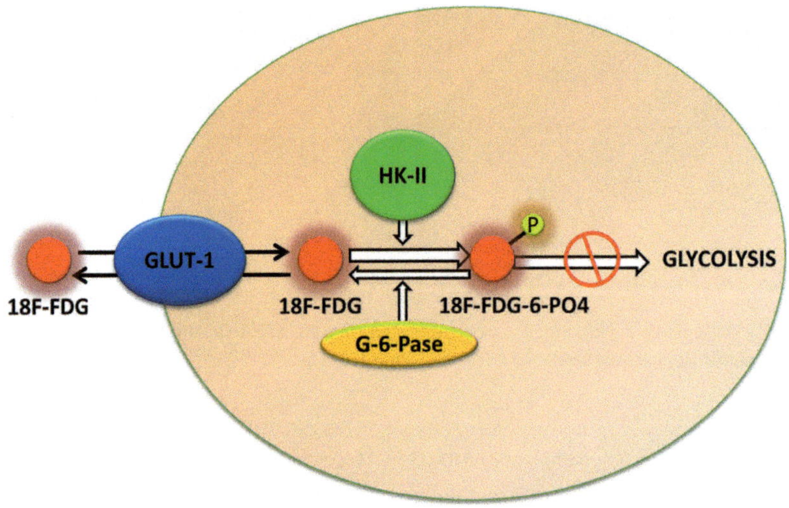

Fig. 17.2 Principles of 18F-FDG metabolism and signal amplification: like glucose, 18F-FDG is transported into the cells by the glucose transporter (*GLUT-1*); however, this happens at a much higher rate. This is then phosphorylated by hexokinase II (*HK-II*) to form 18F-FDG-6-PO4. Unlike glucose, further metabolism is arrested due to the presence of fluorine at the carbon-2 position of the ring instead of the hydroxyl group in glucose. 18F-FDG-6-PO4 does not enter the standard metabolism that glucose-6-PO4 does, and hence it remains trapped within the cell. This "metabolic trapping" of 18F-FDG-6-PO4 within the cell leads to signal amplification and forms the basis of the analysis of PET data

Membrane transporters for glucose are involved in the uptake of FDG by the cell. FDG is then phosphorylated by hexokinase to form FDG-6-phosphate in the cell. Unlike glucose-6-phosphate, FDG-6-phosphate is metabolically trapped and does not undergo further significant enzymatic reactions [31]. The primary exception to metabolic trapping of FDG is in the liver, where a large concentration of phosphatase enzymes results in dephosphorylation of FDG-6-phosphate and clearance of FDG from hepatocytes [32, 33]. Being a polar molecule, it cannot easily pass through the cell membrane to be redistributed out of the cell. With high levels of glucose-6-phosphatase, the phosphate group is cleaved off to regenerate FDG which can diffuse out of the cell and is redistributed elsewhere. Studies have shown FDG uptake for most tumours is mediated by (Fig. 17.2):

(a) Increased levels of membrane transporters for glucose (especially GLUT-1)
(b) Increased levels of hexokinases (HK-II)
(c) Stable or low levels of glucose-6-phosphatase (G-6-Pase) [34]

It has been shown that aberrant glycolysis decreases metabolic stress-induced apoptosis and leads to uncontrolled proliferation of cancer cells which is essential to the malignant tissue phenotype [35]. There is debate on the relative importance of glucose transporters versus the hexokinase activity in predicting the FDG uptake rate in cancer cells [36]. However, both in vitro and in vivo studies have shown that it is the phosphorylation status, and not the membrane transporters, that determine the rate of FDG uptake in most circumstances [37, 38].

As the tumour grows, hypoxia occurs and this is usually present 100–150 μm from the nearest blood supply. Hypoxia and rapid tumoural cell growth force the cells to be dependent on the anaerobic metabolism of glucose. This adaptive behaviour of tumour cells is one of the most crucial steps in tumour survival and progression [39]. There are various proposed molecular targets which are involved in tumourigenesis, and one such factor is hypoxia-inducible factor (HIF)-1, also known as pro-survival transcription factor. HIF-1 has two subunits, HIF-1α and HIF-1β, of which HIF-1α undergoes rapid degradation under normoxic conditions and the β subunit is the one which is constitutively expressed [40]. However, under hypoxic conditions, HIF-1α is stable and undergoes dimerisation with HIF-1β to form an active transcription factor. This dimer binds to the promoter of target genes, i.e. DNA sequence 5′-RCGTG-3′ (hypoxia response element, HRE), which leads to activation of angiogenic pathways, tumoural progression pathways and overexpression of glycolytic enzymes and vascular endothelial growth factor (VEGF) [39, 41]. Tumour hypoxia is one of the most important factors leading to an increased rate of FDG metabolism by anaerobic glycolysis [40]. The understanding of active molecular pathways involved in accelerated cellular proliferation such as mitogen-activated protein kinases and reduced apoptosis like AKT (alpha serine-/threonine-specific protein kinase) in carcinogenesis are shown to be responsible for rapid glucose uptake for glycolysis [42]. These pathways are well known to stimulate glycolysis. Studies have shown that as the AKT activity decreases, there is associated decline in the transcription of glycolytic enzymes, including GLUT transporter expression [43, 44].

There are other features which have led to widespread use of FDG in the clinical setting [8]. Unlike glucose, FDG is filtered and excreted by the kidneys leading to substantial clearance of FDG within 1 h of administration. Increased levels of the highly active hexokinase enzyme effectively trap FDG from the blood pool and are responsible for FDG retention in tumours in a short period after injection. This combined effect of increased tissue uptake and rapid blood pool clearance of FDG forms the basis of the resultant high-contrast images [45]. Most clinical oncology PET imaging protocols allow 60–90 min after the injection of FDG for tissue uptake and background and blood pool clearance before image acquisition [46].

Regional glucose metabolism can be quantified in detail using the dynamic PET imaging method which measures FDG accumulation in the tissue of interest for 60–90 min after injection to produce a tissue uptake curve [46]. This can be combined with direct arterial activity sampling or image-derived arterial activity (e.g. left ventricle or aorta) so that physiological rate constants can be estimated by applying compartmental modelling to these data sets [47, 48]. The metabolic rate of FDG can then be quantified in mmol/min/g [29, 33]. Dynamic imaging of FDG is time consuming and difficult for patients in clinical practice, and it is not possible to extend acquisitions over the whole body with current scanners field of view [46]. Whilst dynamic imaging and arterial sampling is valuable for research applications, the most commonly used clinical imaging method is a single image acquisition of FDG uptake after 60–90 min after injection over a number of consecutive bed positions to cover the required extent of the body [46]. This static uptake image gives an approximate indicator of glucose metabolism [29, 33]. The uptake can be measured semi-quantitatively as the standardised uptake value (SUV) which can be calculated as SUV = Ct/(i.d./wt), where Ct is the tissue FDG uptake from the image (kBq/mL or μCi/ml), i.d. is injected dose (e.g. MBq) and wt is the patient weight (kg). A uniform distribution of tracer is represented by an SUV of 1, and SUV > 1 is an indicator of specific accumulation of tracer [46, 48]. Tumours show variable uptake but most untreated lesions have SUVs of 3 or higher [49]. However, there is overlap between benign and malignant tumours and other non-malignant pathological processes including inflammation [49, 50]. The 110 min half-life of 18F allows regional distribution of FDG from a central cyclotron and radiochemistry facility. Keeping in mind all these attributes, FDG is the most commonly used clinical oncological imaging agent [51].

Currently the Centers for Medicare and Medicaid Services (CMS) recommends the clinical applications of FDG-PET in initial and subsequent treatment strategies of most common cancers such as colorectal, oesophagus, thyroid, head and neck, lymphoma and non-small-cell lung cancers. A few other cancers such as cervix, melanoma and breast are covered with exceptions and are reimbursable under CMS [10, 11].

17.4 Beyond FDG

Over decades FDG has played an indispensable role in clinical oncology. However, other PET tracers contribute to the molecular imaging abnormal tumour biology as there are known limitations of FDG [8]. Apart from imaging FDG-based energy metabolic changes related to tumour growth, there are various other biological pathways such as tissue repair, hypoxia, angiogenesis, apoptosis, cell invasion and migration which are not directly reflected with FDG-PET imaging [52]. The future of oncological therapy includes targeted therapies and individualised management which may need more specific PET radiopharmaceuticals that will help us guide personalised patient treatment by prediction and quantification of therapeutic response and identification of factors causing therapeutic resistance [53, 54]. Many more isotopes/molecules/markers and techniques are being constantly studied and are set to revolutionise personalised medicine. These have most potential in oncology, immunology and neurological disorders [19, 55].

17.4.1 PET Tracers for Imaging Tumour Amino-Acid Metabolism

Similar to increased glucose uptake and metabolism, tumour cells also have upregulation of protein synthesis and increased expression of the cell membrane transporters involved in transport of the amino acids [56]. Upregulated amino-acid metabolism forms the basis of amino-acid-based targeted PET imaging. The radiolabelled amino-acid tracers are metabolised and transported across the cellular membranes in a similar way to endogenous amino acids [57]. The major route providing amino-acid transport is the sodium-independent amino-acid transport system L, and studies have shown that tumour cells exhibit upregulation of L-type amino-acid transporter 1 (LAT1) expression. Increased LAT1 as a target has been used for PET tumour imaging [58]. PET imaging using amino acids includes natural and synthetic amino acids.

17.4.2 Natural Amino Acids

Of the various natural amino acids which are radiolabelled, the role of L-[methyl-11C] methionine (11C-Met) has been extensively evaluated in oncology [59]. 11C-Met was first developed by Comar et al. in 1976 [60]. Kubota et al. reported the first study which showed the potential role of 11C-Met in the diagnosis of lung cancer [61]. Following this, Sasaki et al. demonstrated the potential role of 11C-Met in differentiating various grades of astrocytomas. A recently published study from Koizumi et al. found that 11C-Met has a predictive role in recurrent rectal cancer treated with carbon ion radiotherapy (CIRT) [62]. 11C-Met-PET imaging has shown promising results in detection and delineation of viable tumour, especially in low-grade gliomas. Recent studies have shown that 11C-Met-PET imaging has a promising role in the clinical management of cerebral gliomas, not only for initial diagnosis, grading, prognostication and therapy planning but also for differentiation of tumour recurrence, biopsy planning, surgical resection, radiotherapy planning and assessment of response to therapy [63–65] (Fig. 17.3). Other clinical indications which are under evaluation include the differentiation of benign and malignant lesions in head and neck cancer, melanoma, ovarian cancer and other tumours [66, 67]. However, the short physical half-life of 11C-Met prevents its use in most nuclear medicine departments unless there is an on-site cyclotron [7].

17.4.3 Synthetic Amino Acids

Due to inherent limitations of labelled natural amino acids, synthetic labelled amino-acid analogues have been developed. These synthetic amino-acid tracers can be classified into two groups: aromatic amino acids and non-aromatic amino acids. These are non-metabolisable compounds which show limited or no efflux from the cellular compartment leading to high accumulation and better imaging properties [68, 69].

Radiolabelled aromatic amino-acid tracers are usually tyrosine or phenylalanine primarily system L substrates. These include L-3-18F-alpha-methyl

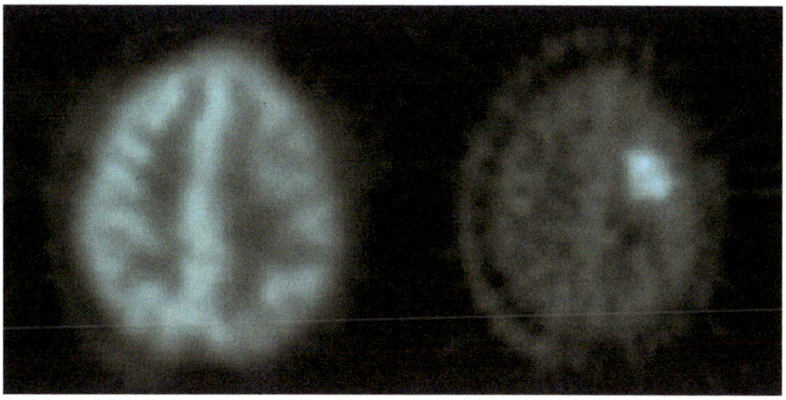

Fig. 17.3 A patient with a low-grade left frontal glioma. There is low 18F-FDG uptake (*left*) compared to normal brain cortex but a much greater tumour-to-background ratio with the 11C-methionine scan (*right*)

tyrosine (18F-FMT), 2-18F-fluoro-L-tyrosine (18F-TYR), O-(2-18F-Fluoroethyl)-l-tyrosine (18F-FET) and 6-18F-fluoro-L-3,4-dihydroxyphenylalanine (18F-FDOPA) [70]. 18F-FET and 18F-FDOPA have been extensively evaluated in humans. 18F-FET and 18F-FDOPA-PET/CT have demonstrated promise for assessing brain tumours, particularly low-grade gliomas where FDG shows limitations. 18F-FET-PET is found to be 92 % specific and 92 % sensitive for differentiating grade I and II recurrent gliomas from grade III and IV recurrent lesions [71]. 18F-FET-PET is also found to be a valuable prognostication marker in operated cases of glioblastoma multiforme [72].

Similarly, 18F-FDOPA-PET has shown utility in clinical brain tumour imaging and is found to have a sensitivity of 96 %, as opposed to 61 % for FDG for detection of primary and recurrent brain tumours [73, 74]. 18F-FDOPA has potential to differentiate low-grade from high-grade tumours and has been used to evaluate extracranial neuroendocrine tumours [75, 76].

Another category of synthetic amino-acid tracers includes alicyclic amino acids and 1-aminocycloalkane-1-carboxylic acids; they are neither metabolised nor readily incorporated into protein [77]. There are various alicyclic amino-acid tracers that have demonstrated value in human imaging including 1-amino-cyclobutane-1-carboxylic acid (ACBC) and its 3-fluoro analogue anti-1-amino-3-18F-fluorocyclobutane-1-carboxylic acid (anti-18F-FACBC) and 1-amino-cyclopentane-1-carboxylic acid (ACPC). Anti-18F-FACBC, a leucine analogue, has been studied in human glioblastoma multiforme lesions with promising results [77]. Due to its minimal renal excretion compared to FDG, it has also shown promise in genitourinary cancer imaging, including prostate cancer, renal cell carcinoma and pelvic malignancies [78, 79]. Increased uptake of anti-18F-FACBC in renal papillary cell carcinoma is shown to differentiate it from clear cell carcinoma [80]. There is growing evidence to support the potential utility of 18F-FACBC as it has shown superior ability to target prostate cancer when compared to ProstaScint and 11C-choline PET/CT [79, 81]. In detecting recurrent disease in prostate cancer, 18F-FACBC has shown improved sensitivity compared to 11C-choline PET/CT [79]. Anti-3-18F-FACBC is found to be 89 % sensitive (36 patients) for detecting tumours in the prostate bed and 100 % sensitive in detecting an extraprostatic recurrence (10 patients) [82]. Studies in animals have shown that 18F-FACBC-PET imaging is not only useful in detecting prostatic cancers but also in differentiation of tumoural lesions from inflammatory pathologies and benign prostatic hyperplasia [83].

17.5 PET Tracers for Imaging Phospholipid Metabolism

Choline is a precursor of phosphatidylcholine and uptake correlates with cell proliferation [84]. Choline is an essential component of cell membrane phospholipid synthesis. Tumours, including prostate cancer, have an increased requirement for cell membrane synthesis, and it has been shown that prostate cancer cells have an increased intracellular transport of choline, increased choline kinase expression and increased choline metabolism [85, 86]. This led to introduction of carbon-11 choline (11C-choline) as a promising PET tracer for evaluation of various malignancies such as brain tumours, lung cancer, gastrointestinal and genitourinary malignancies and particularly prostate cancer. 11C-choline overcomes some of the limitations of FDG which is excreted through the urinary system which leads to increased background activity in the pelvis [87]. At the same time, it matches FDG in differentiating benign from malignant pathologies. All these features make 11C-choline an important tracer for imaging prostate cancer [88, 89] (Fig. 17.4). Other applications include meningiomas, head and neck and primary hepatic malignancies [88, 90]. Another choline tracer is 18F-choline which has a longer half-life in comparison to that of C-11 and is extensively used to study patients with biochemical recurrence of prostate cancer and has potential to be used as a marker of therapeutic response in prostate cancer with bone metastases [91, 92].

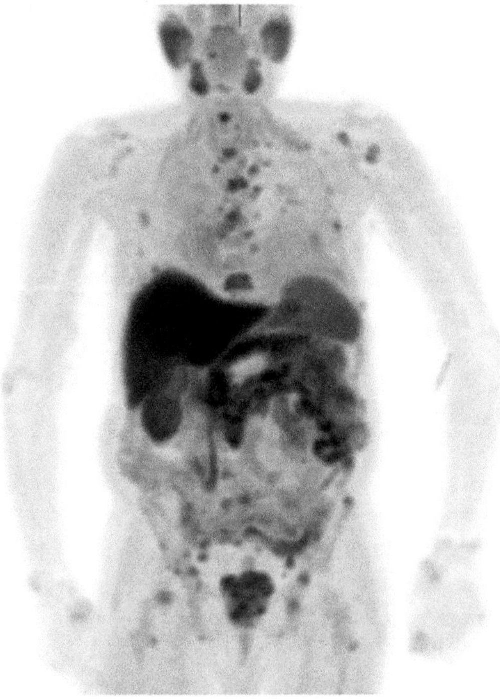

Fig. 17.4 11C-choline MIP image. A man with metastatic prostate cancer showing abnormal 11C-choline activity in a large primary prostate tumour with lymph node metastases in the pelvis and multiple bone metastases

17.6 PET Tracers for Imaging Tumour Angiogenesis

Angiogenesis which is pivotal for tumourigenesis is defined as the formation of new blood vessels from existing vascular structures [93]. The increased cellular proliferation in tumours needs an increased supply of metabolites and at the same time removal of metabolic waste products. Tumour hypoxia is the key factor which triggers neoangiogenesis and is found to be caused by proangiogenic growth factors [94]. The resultant neovasculature is disordered and usually does not meet the needs of the growing tumour leading to deoxyhaemoglobin and lactacidosis [93, 94].

Tumour angiogenesis is a complex multistep process which involves multiple growth factors which are involved in the activation of endothelial cells, degradation of basement membrane, migration of endothelial cells and angiogenic remodelling and vessel formation [95]. Some of the most important factors which are involved in neoangiogenesis are vascular endothelial growth factor (VEGF), epidermal growth factor receptor (EGFR), the acidic and basic fibroblast growth factors (aFGF and bFGF) and platelet-derived endothelial cell growth factor (PD-ECGF); these growth factors are secreted by tumour cells or by the fibroblast and endothelial cells in the peritumoural environment and extracellular matrix (ECM) [96]. Overexpression of the dimeric transmembrane integrin $\alpha v\beta 3$ by activated endothelial cells occurs with angiogenesis. This integrin regulates endothelial cell migration and the matrix metalloproteinase (MMPs) family in matrix degradation, facilitating cell invasion, and angiogenesis. These molecules form the basis for targeted imaging of angiogenesis and the development of tracers for tumour angiogenesis imaging [97].

Dynamic 15O-water PET has been used to study tumour blood flow in vivo, as a pharmacodynamic marker to study the mechanism of novel anticancer drugs such as endostatin and to monitor delivery of radiolabelled drugs to the target [98, 99]. 15O-water is the gold standard for assessment of blood flow/tissue perfusion and provides a physiological measure. 15O-water PET not only provides information regarding the pharmacokinetics but also assess whether single agent of combination therapies have different effects on tumour perfusion [100, 101]. Other molecules used for imaging tumour vascularity include 11C-carbon monoxide but has logistic issues and low signal-to-noise. 11C-carbon monoxide PET is reported to measure blood volume up to approximately 0.1–0.2 ml blood ml^{-1} tissue in renal cancer which is characterised by a high vascular phenotype [102]. Anderson and co-workers reported the rapid changes in blood volume following treatment with combretastatin A4 phosphate (CA4P) [103].

Integrins are a family of heterodimeric cell surface receptors (24 subtypes) composed of two non-covalently bound α- and β-subunits involved in cell-extracellular matrix and cell-cell interactions [104]. Integrins mediate these by transducing signals into the cells and out of the cells directly or indirectly regulating cellular functions such as cell survival, proliferation, adhesion, migration and invasion as well as angiogenesis, thrombosis, apoptosis and differentiation in various pathological processes [104, 105]. Many cancer cells have been found to overexpress the integrin αvβ3, which binds to arginine-glycine-aspartic acid (RGD)-containing components of the interstitial matrix such as vitronectin, fibronectin and thrombospondin [104]. Upregulation of these pathways has been shown in melanoma, ovarian cancer and late-stage glioblastomas. Based on these findings, linear as well as cyclic RGD peptides, which show very high binding affinity and selectivity for integrin αvβ3, have been labelled with positron-emitting radionuclides to serve as PET radiotracers [105, 106]. Initial studies revealed tumour-specific uptake but also significant hepatobiliary elimination leading to high background activity in the hepatic parenchyma and small bowel. To improve the pharmacokinetics of these radiohalogenated peptides, several modifications have been attempted, including labelling with sugar moieties, hydrophilic amino acids and polyethylene glycol (PEG) [107]. One such example is a glycopeptide based on cyclo (Arg-Gly-Asp-D-Phe-Lys). In an integrin-positive M21 melanoma xenograft model, 18F-galacto-RGD showed integrin αvβ3-specific tumour uptake. Initial safety studies of 18F-galacto-RGD in humans have been performed, and it is found to specifically delineate integrin-positive lesions, and its good tumour-to-background ratio suggests that it can be used as a surrogate marker of angiogenesis [108]. In various tumour studies, no obvious correlation was found between FDG and 18F-galacto-RGD, and it was shown that integrin αvβ3 expression and glucose metabolism were not closely correlated in tumour lesions. Hence, imaging based on these traces provides complementary information in cancer patients [109, 110]. Newer tracers such as 18F- and 64Cu-labelled RGD-containing peptides have shown better pharmacokinetics, tumour uptake and retention of the RGD peptides [111, 112]. For example, compared to a non-PEGylated ligand 64Cu-DOTA-RGD, PEGylated RGD peptide 64Cu-DOTA-PEG-3400-RGD is found to have low hepatic and small bowel uptake with no significant change in tumour-specific uptake and retention and hence was suitable for visualising lesions above the liver [113]. PEGylation using 18F-FB-PEG3400-RGD PEGylation showed significant and prolonged tracer retention in tumour without any comprise on the desired rapid clearance [113].

A series of multimetric RGD peptides labelled with 18F have been developed for PET imaging and have improved pharmacokinetics, tumour uptake and retention patterns. One such example is the dimeric RGD peptide-based tracer 18F-FB-E[c(RGDyK)]2 (18F-FRGD2) [114]. In small-animal imaging, it showed predominant renal excretion, and when compared with the monomeric tracer 18F-FB-c(RGDyK), it showed nearly twice as much tumour uptake. A comparison of monomeric and dimeric RGD analogues with tetrameric RGD peptide-based tracer, 18F-FB-E[E[c(RGDfK)]2]2 in xenograft-bearing mice revealed significantly higher receptor binding affinity and faster clearance from blood pool, better metabolic stability, predominant renal excretion and significant receptor-mediated tumour uptake providing better tumour contrast [115, 116].

Recent advances in radiolabelled nanoparticles, including inorganic and organic nanoparticles targeting integrin αvβ3, are a newer class of probes shown to have a potential role in research as well as clinical oncology [117]. Examples of these tracers include inorganic single-walled carbon nanotubes (SWNTs) coated non-covalently with PEG and with cyclic RGD peptides and DOTA for 64Cu chelation which have unique size, shape and physical properties [118, 119]. These properties of SWNTs make them a promising material that can be used for multimodality imaging, such as PET/CT, PET/MRI and PET/optical imaging [120].

Another important angiogenic process studied and used for imaging is the VEGF/VEGF receptor signalling pathway. The development of VEGF- or VEGFR-targeted PET imaging probes could serve as an important tool for understanding VEGF/VEGFR in angiogenesis-related tumourigenesis and drug delivery and assessing response to therapy with anti-angiogenic agents [121, 122]. Tracers such as 124I-labelled VG76e, which is an IgG1 monoclonal antibody against human VEGF, have been used in PET imaging of solid tumour xenograft models. However, this had the limitation of poor immune reactivity [123]. Another tracer, 124I-labelled HuMV833, has shown success in the phase I trials [124]. Recent development of bevacizumab labelled with 111In and 89Zr for SPECT and PET imaging, respectively, has led to better understanding of angiogenesis in human ovarian cancer xenograft models [125]. VEGF121 labelled with 64Cu has been used for VEGF receptor expression, and 1,4,7,10-tetraazacyclododecane-N,N′,N″,N‴-tetraacetic acid (DOTA)-VEGF121 has been used for receptor-specific imaging for VEGFR-2 [126]. Small-animal PET imaging using 64Cu-DOTA-VEGF121 has been validated in small U87MG tumours showing increased expression of VEGFR-2 [127]. Tracers such as15O-water and 13N-NH3 are used for dynamic PET blood flow imaging and have been applied in brain tumours to study anti-angiogenic therapy and grading of tumours [128–130].

17.7 PET Tracers for Imaging Tumour Hypoxia

The presence of hypoxic/anoxic regions is a characteristic feature of 50–60 % of locally advanced solid tumours and has been described in a wide range of human malignancies, including cancer of the breast, uterine cervix, vulva, head and neck, prostate, rectum and pancreas as well as in brain tumours, soft tissue sarcomas and malignant melanomas [131, 132]. Tumour hypoxia is orchestrated by the transcription factor hypoxia-inducible factor (HIF)-1, which has been verified as a master regulator of oxygen homeostasis under hypoxic conditions. The resulting adaptive changes in the proteome and genome of the tumour cells are believed to lead to more aggressive clones which are better adapted to survive in the compromised environment. Subsequent selection and clonal expansion of these cells lead to a more adapted and aggressive tumour cell population [133].

Hypoxia has also been shown to reduce chemotherapeutic and radiotherapeutic efficacy by causing cells within hypoxic regions to cycle more slowly and by providing a selection mechanism for cells with reduced susceptibility for apoptosis [134]. As therapeutically modifying hypoxia may have potential to change therapy outcome in patients, non-invasive PET imaging for identification and quantitation of tumour hypoxia status could play a key role in predicting and monitoring treatment response [135, 136].

Of the non-invasive imaging modalities to image hypoxia, radionuclide studies using PET tracers are the most extensively studied [137]. Parametric PET hypoxia imaging of tissue using inhalation of $15O_2$ by measuring regional oxygen extraction fraction and metabolic rate is shown to be more accurate than the invasive methods [137, 138]. $15O_2$ PET imaging is currently a "gold standard" for non-invasive imaging of tissue oxygen levels; however, because of logistics and technical issues such as very short half-life of

$15O_2$ (~2 min) and also being an expensive technique, it is not widely used in experimental or clinical settings [139]. Nitroimidazoles have shown very high selectivity in targeting hypoxic tissue and also have radiosensitising properties [140]. Nitroimidazole derivatives such as pimonidazole or 2-(2-nitro-1H-imidazol-1-yl)-N-(2,2,3,3,3-pentafluoropropyl) acetamide (EF5) can be analysed using invasive methods such as immunohistochemical analysis or cell-sorting techniques [141]. The first reported PET tracer used for hypoxia imaging focused on radiolabelled 2-nitroimidazole analogues. Intracellular reductases reduce these tracer analogues into reactive intermediary metabolites, accumulation of which shows an inverse correlation with the level of tissue oxygenation. The formed intermediary molecules form covalent bonds with thiol groups of the intracellular proteins and tend to accumulate in hypoxic cells. Many nitroimidazole compounds with varied properties have been developed and tested in imaging hypoxia [142, 143].

18F-labelled fluoromisonidazole (18F-FMISO) was the first hypoxia PET tracer which was found to have tumour specificity. It has been extensively used both in preclinical and clinical studies [144]. Preclinical studies in the 36B10 glioma rat xenograft model have evaluated the role of 18F-FMISO uptake in hypoxic tumours and assessment of hypoxic fraction. It was found that retention of the 18F-FMISO correlated with the degree of tissue hypoxia [145]. Another study performed in a rhabdomyosarcoma rat xenograft model correlated 18F-FMISO uptake with other markers of hypoxia such as pimonidazole and carbonic anhydrase IX (CA IX). 18F-FMISO-PET was found to be accurate in measuring hypoxia and correlated well with the hypoxic volumes derived from pimonidazole- and CA IX-stained tumour sections [146]. Clinical studies evaluating the role of 18F-FMISO and FDG in head and neck cancer patients found no correlation between pO_2 measurements and FDG uptake but good correlation with 18F-FMISO uptake. No correlation was found between FDG and 18F-FMISO uptake suggesting different tumour uptake mechanisms and characteristics [147, 148]. Another study in head and neck cancer showed the potential role of pre-therapy 18F-FMISO-PET imaging as an independent prognostic marker and that post-therapy changes in the uptake of 18F-FMISO-PET may predict disease free and overall survival [149]. Although 18F-FMISO has been studied extensively for imaging tumour hypoxia, its widespread application is limited by slow tumour-specific accumulation and nonspecific washout.

In an attempt to overcome the disadvantages of 18F-FMISO, second-generation 2-nitroimidazole tracers like 18F-fluoroazomycin arabinoside (18F-FAZA), 18F-fluoroerythronitroimidazole (18F-FETNIM) and 18F-tri-fluoroetanidazole (18F-FETA) were developed which showed better clearance and hydrophilicity characteristics. Preclinical studies have compared 18F-FMISO and 18F-FAZA in tumour xenograft models and found that 18F-FAZA has better pharmacokinetics than 18F-FMISO with higher tumour-to-background and tumour-to-muscle and tumour-to-blood ratios [150, 151]. Clinical studies evaluating the role of 18F-FAZA imaging in identifying tumour hypoxia in head and neck cancer have found it to have a potential role in dose painting for radiotherapy planning [152].

Third-generation hypoxia tracers such as 18F-flortanidazole (18F-HX4) have been developed with a 1,2,3-anti-triazole moiety that makes it more hydrophilic than 18F-FMISO [153]. It is found to have tumour-to-reference tissue values similar to 18F-FMISO at relatively early time points and hence a potential advantage of shorter acquisition times. It has also been evaluated in a preclinical rhabdomyosarcoma tumour model, and the uptake was confirmed to be dependent on tumour oxygenation status. Phase I clinical studies have demonstrated that hypoxia imaging using 18F-HX4 is feasible and nontoxic [154]. A recent comparative study in preclinical animal models showed a clear relationship between the immunohistochemical staining for perfusion, hypoxia and carbonic anhydrase IX and the level of uptake of 18F-FMISO, 18F-FAZA and 18F-HX4. It has been shown that both the 18F-FAZA- and 18F-FMISO-based PET tumour hypoxia uptake for patients in clinical studies have prognostic potential [155].

Other tracers for hypoxia imaging include 64Cu-bis(thiosemicarbazone) complexes (64Cu-ATSM and 64Cu-ATSE). Similarly 64Cu(II)-ATSM has shown promising results in studying tumour hypoxia. Being a neutral lipophilic molecule, it has high membrane permeability, and after cellular uptake, it is converted to [Cu(I)-ATSM] which is negatively charged in hypoxic cells and is trapped [156, 157]. Preclinical studies in R3230 mammary adenocarcinomas, fibrosarcomas and 9L gliomas have shown correlations of 64Cu-ATSM PET hypoxia imaging with other hypoxia markers such as EF5, pimonidazole and CA IX [158]. Preclinical and clinical studies comparing 64Cu-ATSM with 18F-FMISO have shown that regional distribution of 18F-FMISO at 2 h correlates well with the distribution of 64Cu-ATSM at 10 min or 24 h in 9L gliosarcoma tumours and 64Cu-ATSM has been shown to be a safe radiopharmaceutical for imaging tumour hypoxia in human cancers [159, 160].

17.8 PET Tracers for Imaging Apoptosis

Apoptosis or type I programmed cell death is a hallmark of cancer cells and has been extensively exploited to develop novel drug therapies [161]. The various steps in the process of programmed cell death are triggered by appropriate internal and/or external signals leading to preprogrammed cytoplasmic shrinkage and formation of membrane blebs. The process does not incite any inflammatory response [162]. Both radiation therapy and chemotherapy can induce apoptosis in tumour cells, and the rate and extent of apoptosis can be imaged by PET. This information is therefore of great potential interest in monitoring the efficacy of anticancer treatment [163]. Resistance to apoptosis or programmed cell death, a hallmark of cancer cells, has been exploited to develop novel drug therapies. Apoptosis is triggered by endogenous and exogenous stimuli leading to activation of intrinsic and extrinsic pathways of cell death, respectively. These pathways lead to activation of subsets of proteases such as caspase-3, 6 and 7 which target the intracellular proteins involved in DNA damage repair. These agents binding to cell surface proteases have been used to image apoptosis [164, 165]. Annexin-V is a protein that strongly binds phosphatidylserine residue that is externalised to the outer surface of apoptotic cells and is one of the most important probes used in optical and radionuclide imaging. Radiolabelled caspase tracers have also been recently developed [166].

The main methods for imaging apoptosis have been through targeting phosphatidylserine presentation or caspase activation. Recent advances for apoptosis imaging include radiolabelled caspase-3 substrates and inhibitors and monoclonal antibodies targeted to human annexin-V [167].

Agents binding to cell surface proteases that help dying cells to attract phagocytes have been used to image apoptosis. Annexin-V and its derivatives are extensively studied probes targeting apoptosis. 99mTc-labelled annexin-V was the first tracer used to detect cell death in the blood clots of patients who had atrial fibrillation [168]. The first reported use was in an experimental mouse lymphoma model treated with cyclophosphamide. Compared to the untreated mouse, the treated ones showed a 300 % increase in annexin-V uptake 20 h after chemotherapy. Other newer tracers include 99mTc-N2S2-rh annexin-V, used in the clinical setting of lung cancer and lymphomas. 99mTc-labelled annexin-V has also been applied to testing response to radiotherapy. 99mTc-labelled annexin-V scintigraphy [TAVS] was performed in 11 follicular lymphomas patients, and posttreatment TAVS findings matched with posttreatment cytology in 10 patients, confirming TAVS to be a noninvasive imaging modality to detect in vivo apoptosis following radiotherapy [169]. Another annexin-V-labelled tracer is 124I-annexin-V (124I-Anx5) which has been investigated for studying Fas-mediated hepatic cell death in BDF-1 mice using PET. An alternative to annexin-based probes for imaging apoptosis-targeting peptide-1 (ApoPep-1), a hexapeptide that binds to the histone H1 protein in the nucleus, was labelled with 131I to study the biodistribution in normal rats and labelled with 124I for the detection of apoptosis in A549 cell tumours in nude mice [170].

Another molecule which has been extensively studied for PET-based apoptosis imaging is caspase-3. One of the first caspase probes investigated for apoptosis imaging was 131I-labelled benzyloxycarbonyl-Val-Ala-DL-Asp(O-methyl)-fluoromethyl ketone (Z-VAD-fmk) which is a pan-caspase inhibitor. It was studied in Morris hepatoma cells (MH3924Atk8), which showed expression of the herpes simplex virus thymidine kinase (HSVtk) gene. Ganciclovir-induced apoptosis in these cells showed a twofold increase in 131I-Z-VAD-fmk uptake at the end of treatment [171, 172]. Other potential tracers are isatin sulfonamide analogue -based PET probes such as 18F-WC-II-89 and 18F-ICMT-11. 18F-WC-II-89 using micro-PET imaging has been used for studying caspase-3 inside the cell. Preclinical studies have evaluated the role of 18F-ICMT-11 as a caspase-3 specific PET imaging radiotracer and have shown its potential for the assessment of tumour apoptosis in anticancer drug development and the monitoring of early responses to therapy [171]. Though the isatin-based PET probes have shown promising results in imaging of apoptosis, the specificity of these tracers needs to be validated in in vivo models as most of the studies are in a preclinical setting and need validation in a clinical setting [173].

Other radiolabelled imaging targets which have tested in preclinical studies include 99mTc-labelled C2A for studying apoptosis induced by paclitaxel treatment in lung carcinoma and 18F-ML-10-targeted amphipathic apoptosis markers (ApoSense–targeting the cell membrane of apoptotic cells) have been used for clinical imaging and have progressed to phase I/II clinical trials [174, 175].

17.9 PET Tracers for Imaging Tumour Cell Proliferation

Upregulation of cellular proliferation is another hallmark of malignant transformation. PET imaging has played a significant role in imaging cellular proliferation and assessment of therapeutic interventions. One of the first PET radiotracers used for imaging cellular proliferation in tumours was 11C-thymidine [176]. Thymidine is a native nucleoside and is integrated into deoxyribonucleic acids to form DNA. It is taken up by the nucleoside transporters present in the cellular membranes. Once it enters the cell, the enzyme thymidine kinase 1 (TK1) phosphorylates it to thymidine monophosphate. Overexpression of the enzyme TK1 is commonly seen in proliferating tumours and forms the basis of thymidine-based radiolabelled imaging. However, the short 20 min half-life of 11C is the main limiting factor for use of 11C-thymidine in routine clinical practice. Hence, a variety of alternative radiolabelled thymidine tracers have been developed; these include 18F-labelled analogues, 3′-deoxy-3′-18F-fluorothymidine (18F-FLT) and 1-(2′-deoxy-2′-18F-fluoro-β-d-arabinofuranosyl) thymine (18F-FMAU) [177]. Once taken up by the cell, 18F-FLT is phosphorylated by TK1 to 18F-FLT monophosphate and further to 18F-FLT triphosphonate by nucleotide diphosphate kinase, which does not get assimilated into the growing DNA chain as the 3′-position is substituted by 18F and hence undergoes intracellular trapping. Intracellular 18F-FLT retention is quantified and used for measuring the cellular TK1 activity and is an indirect measure of the cellular proliferation rate [178]. It has been shown that the uptake of 18F-FLT increases with increasing TK1 activity in human tumour cell lines, and this uptake was validated with an independent measure of DNA synthesis in tissue. The protein Ki-67 which is a histopathological marker of cellular proliferation, identified by MIB-1 antibody staining, correlates with the level of 18F-FLT uptake measured by PET. This forms the basis of its use as a surrogate marker as an early quantitative measure of drug-induced changes in cellular proliferation [179, 180].

Several studies have shown the promise of 18F-FLT in in vivo imaging, one such example is non-invasive in vitro measurement of growth inhibition of tumour cells caused by a novel histone deacetylase inhibitor (LAQ824) in HCT-116 colon carcinoma xenografts [181]. Several studies concluded that 18F-FLT uptake correlated with histopathological Ki-67 expression and was identified to be an indirect measure of tumour proliferation in non-small-cell lung cancer [180]

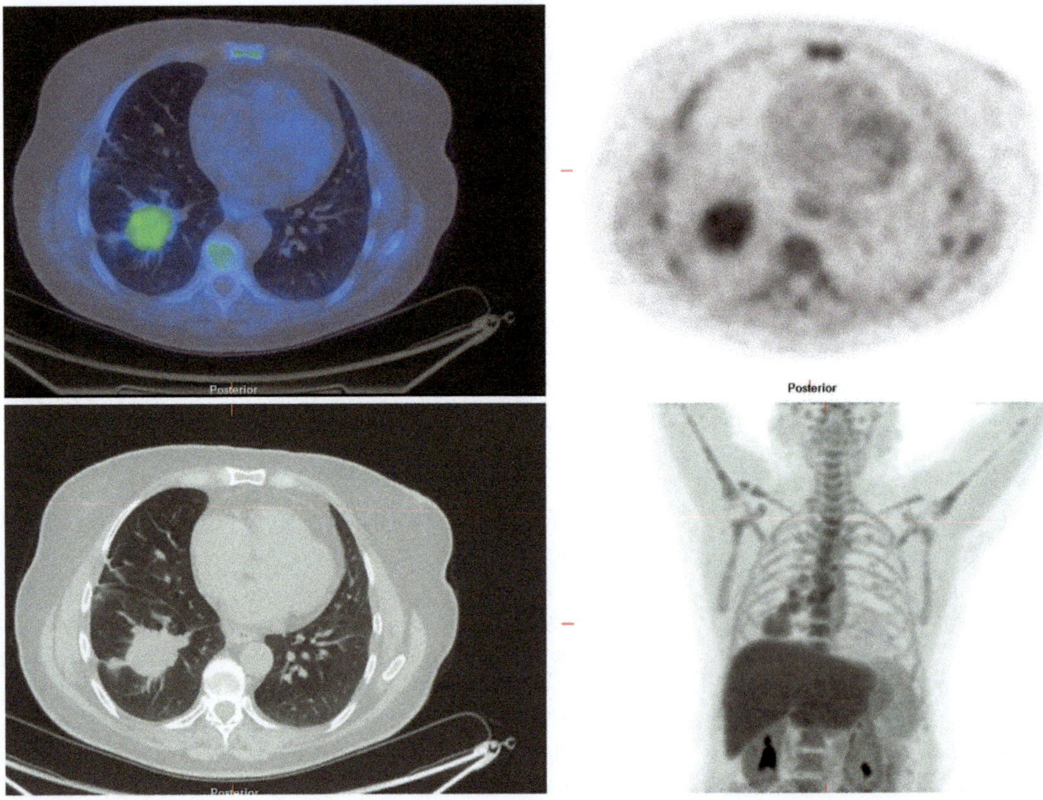

Fig. 17.5 18F-FLT-PET/CT scan of a patient with NSCLC showing increased uptake in the primary tumour as well as hilar and mediastinal lymph nodes (seen on the MIP image)

(Fig. 17.5). Similar results were seen in newly diagnosed/recurrent high-grade gliomas, and 18F-FLT was found to be more sensitive than FDG for detection of tumours in this setting. Also 18F-FLT correlated better with Ki-67 proliferation index and was found to be a better predictor of tumour progression and survival [182]. A clinical study in patients with primary/metastatic breast cancer treated with chemotherapy or hormonal therapy and imaged with 18F-FLT and FDG before, 2 weeks after therapy and at the end of treatment or after 1 year if the therapy was not terminated, revealed that the treatment-induced changes were consistent in both the tracer imaging studies. However, the changes in serum tumour markers correlated more strongly with 18F-FLT uptake than with FDG uptake, and 2-week 18F-FLT uptake correlated with long-term treatment efficacy [183]. Similar results were found in a study reported by Kenny et al. in stage II–IV breast cancer. They concluded that 18F-FLT-PET imaging can predict therapy response to 5-fluorouracil, epirubicin and cyclophosphamide 1 week after initiation of the therapy [184]. Results have been reproduced in several clinical studies in a variety of tumours treated with single or combination therapies. The uptake of 18F-FLT of tumours is dependent on the TK1 activity. Therapy-induced activation of salvage pathways and nucleoside transporter expression also determines the 18F-FLT uptake [185, 186]. Hence drugs such as cytostatic agents which cause cell cycle arrest in the S-phase may increase 18F-FLT uptake [187]. Similarly, agents blocking the endogenous pathway can lead to upregulation of the salvage pathway and increase tumour 18F-FLT uptake. Agents that block both the pathways lead to reduction in 18F-FLT uptake [188]. Despite the promising preclinical and clinical data, limitations are noted in 18F-FLT imag-

Table 17.1 Clinical experience with 18F-FLT

Tumour	Preclinical and clinical application of 18F-FLT	Comments
Breast cancer	Significant correlation with histopathology for assessment of proliferation with Ki67	Limited clinical studies with small population data
Gastrointestinal cancers	More specific than FDG for metastatic nodal assessment in oesophageal cancers Better gross tumour volume delineation for radiation treatment planning in oesophageal cancer	Physiological uptake in the liver, marrow and kidneys limits it widespread clinical use
Genitourinary cancers	Challenging in the urinary tract (route of excretion) Promising results in areas such as identifying malignancy in renal cysts	Potential clinical use in cystic renal, ovarian and testicular tumours
Head and neck cancers	Preclinical and clinical studies have shown its role in planning radiation treatment, and early follow-up may help with prediction of outcome	Large population studies needed in this area
Central nervous system cancers	Studies have shown promise in imaging recurrent high-grade tumours, and it is found to correlate better with Ki-67 values and is a more powerful predictor of tumour progression and survival	Limited experience and more studies needed in this area
Sarcomas	Studies have shown its role in differentiating low-grade from high-grade soft tissue sarcomas and have found that uptake of 18F-FLT correlates well with the proliferation rate. High 18F-FLT uptake – better response to treatment	Limited experience and more studies needed in this area

ing such as the complex metabolism of 18F-FLT, heterogeneous uptake in tumour tissue, reduced sensitivity in tumours having low expression of TK1 and high background activity in bone marrow and hepatic parenchyma making it more difficult to use in these regions. The clinical utilisation for imaging response of primary and metastatic tumour lesions to therapy therefore remains unclear [189–191] (Table 17.1).

Other cell proliferation imaging tracers include 18F-FMAU which is manufactured by labelling either the 5-methyl group of the pyrimidine base with 11C or at the 2′-fluoro position of the sugar with 18F. Preclinical data on the role of 18F-FMAU in tumour imaging has shown its uptake and retention in both tumour and non-tumour tissue reflecting that it gets incorporated into DNA [192]. It is highly resistant to in vivo catabolism, and maximum activity is seen within the first hour after injection [193, 194]. Compared to 18F-FLT, clinical studies of 11C- or 18F-FMAU have shown comparable tumour uptake with higher renal, hepatic and myocardium uptake yet relatively lower uptake in bone marrow and rate of urinary excretion. Studies have also shown rapid blood clearance of 11C- or 18F-FMAU and tumour uptake reaching a plateau by about 10 min after bolus injection of the radiotracer. These properties have been exploited for its clinical application in assessment of bone metastasis and in pelvic tumours [195, 196]. Overall, because 18F-FMAU can be incorporated into DNA, it appears to be a promising PET tracer to directly measure cell proliferation and a potential biomarker for evaluation of anticancer treatment response in both preclinical and clinical settings.

Another important cell proliferation biomarker for tumour detection and monitoring treatment is sigma-2 (σ2) receptors. Their expression is 10 times greater in tumour cells than in normal cells [197, 198]. The first radiolabelled σ2 receptor which showed tumour binding specificity was a benzamide radioligand with σ2 receptor [199]. Sigma-2 receptors imaging using *N*-(4-(6,7-dimethoxy-3,4-dihydroisoquinolin-2-1H-yl)butyl) and 2-(2-18F-fluoroethoxy)-5-methylbenzamide have shown potential for cell proliferation-based tumour imaging and assessment of targeted therapies [200, 201].

17.10 PET Tracers for Imaging Epidermal Growth Factor Receptors

Epidermal growth factor receptor (EGFR) is a well-known and extensively studied proto-oncogene associated with tumour progression [202]. It belongs to the structurally similar ErbB family of receptor tyrosine kinases and includes four receptors: HER1 (ErbB1), HER2 (ErbB2), HER3 (ErbB3) and HER4 (ErbB4) [203, 204]. Once activated, EGFR modulates many pathways in tumourigenesis, and its overexpression is found to be a prognostic indicator and predictive marker of poor survival. Recent studies have found that the monoclonal antibodies (mAbs) towards EGFR receptor that block the binding of EGF to its extracellular ligand-binding domain have potential both for targeted therapy and PET imaging [205].

Erbitux (cetuximab, ImClone LLC, New York, NY) was the first US Food and Drug Administration (FDA)-approved mAb targeted against EGFR used for treating EGFR-expressing metastatic colorectal carcinoma [206]. The 64Cu-labelled DOTA-cetuximab conjugate (64Cu-DOTA-cetuximab) is a novel radiolabelled tracer used for EGFR-based tumour imaging and has been studied in seven xenograft tumour mouse models [207]. Its uptake was compared in major organs and was tested in seven tumour models (U87MG human glioblastoma, PC-3 human prostate carcinoma, CT-26 murine colorectal carcinoma, HCT-8, HCT-116, SW620 human colorectal carcinoma and MDA-MB-435 human breast cancer). Good correlation was noted between tumour uptake and EGFR expression tested by the Western blot method. U87MG and PC-3 tumours showed the highest uptake (13.2 % ID/g and 12.8 % ID/g, respectively).

Panitumumab (ABX-EGF) is another important radiolabelled mAb targeted against EGFR [208–210]. Recently reported small-animal PET studies with 64Cu-labelled panitumumab in nude mice bearing human head and neck squamous cell carcinoma (HNSCC) from three cell lines with different levels of EGFR expression and antibody distribution confirmed by ex vivo immunostaining showed that UM-SCC-22B tumours with the lowest EGFR protein expression had the highest 64Cu-DOTA-panitumumab accumulation, whereas SQB20 tumours with the highest EGFR expression showed the lowest 64Cu-DOTA-panitumumab accumulation. The results from this study provide evidence for differential efficacy and rate of complications of anti-EGFR mAb therapy for HNSCC and other malignancies [208, 211].

In vitro studies have shown promising results for the recombinant human EGF DOTA conjugate (68Ga-DOTA-hEGF) PET imaging of HER1 and 68Ga-labelled F(ab′)2 fragment of herceptin (68Ga-DOTA-F(ab′)2-herceptin) PET imaging of HER2 [212]. 68Ga-DOTA-hEGF tracer has high binding affinity, rapid internalisation of radiotracer and good retention in EGFR-expressing cell lines such as U343 glioma and A431 cervical carcinoma. Biodistribution studies in tumour xenografts revealed a tumour-to-blood ratio at 30 min postinjection of 4.5 (2.7 % ID/g in tumour) with excellent tumour localisation. Similar results were seen in 68Ga-DOTA-F(ab′)2-herceptin-based HER2 imaging in BT474 breast tumour xenografts downregulated by heat shock protein (Hsp90) inhibitor [213]. PET imaging before and after treatment with the Hsp90 inhibitor 17-allylamino-17-demethoxygeldanamycin (17-AAG) revealed a significant reduction in expression of HER2 within 24 h, and it was noted that tumour uptake of FDG remained unchanged. The study concluded that the 68Ga-DOTA-F(ab′)2-herceptin-based HER2 PET imaging is superior to FDG imaging for evaluating tumour response to 17-AAG therapy.

Other novel PET probes such as 89Zr-trastuzumab can serve as an early biomarker for HSP90 inhibition in HER2-positive metastatic breast cancer patients and can potentially be used to provide whole-body insights into response of HER2-amplified breast cancer to NVP-AUY922 [214]. A further application of 89Zr-trastuzumab PET is in predefining areas within the tumour that may not respond to targeted treatment with HSP90 inhibitors such as NVP-AUY922 [215, 216].

17.11 PET Tracers for Imaging Somatostatin Receptors

Neuroendocrine tumours (NETs) have secretory granules which can produce biogenic amines and polypeptide hormones, and all of them share features of the neuroendocrine cell system [217]. NETs have particular characteristics that include low incidence, low proliferation rate as well as hypersecretion of biologically active substances. The commonest primary tumour sites are in the gastrointestinal and bronchopulmonary tracts. The clinical spectrum includes functioning and non-functioning tumours. The presence of peptide receptors and transporters at the cell membrane and the neuroamine uptake mechanisms of NETs is the principle behind clinical use of specific radiolabelled ligands for imaging and therapy [218, 219].

Somatostatin (SST) exists in two isoforms: a short peptide that has 14 amino acids and a second peptide that has 28 amino acids, both bind with high affinity to five receptor subtypes [220]. A majority of malignant tumours, such as neuroendocrine tumour (NET), small-cell lung cancer, breast cancer and malignant lymphoma, show overexpression of multiple somatostatin receptor subtypes. Of all the somatostatin receptor subtypes, the somatostatin receptor 2 (SST2) subtype is the commonest. Imaging of SST subtype 2 (SST2) NETs has been developed and has had extensive clinical applications for almost two decades [221]. Octreotide and octreotate are widely used as SST analogues and are radiolabelled with various radioisotopes for imaging of these tumours. Various studies have shown the impact of somatostatin receptors in the management of neuroendocrine tumours [222, 223]. Tumour grading is of pivotal importance in prognostic risk stratification and has been frequently utilised for treatment decision making [224]. In this regard, the Ki-67 labelling index (depicting Ki-67-positive tumour cells that represent the fraction that is in the proliferative phases of the cell cycle, i.e. G1, S, G2 and mitosis) or the MIB-1 labelling index, which has the advantage of being estimated on formalin-fixed, paraffin-embedded sections, are the common determinants [225, 226]. Both somatostatin receptor-targeted molecular imaging and FDG-PET/CT imaging have been utilised for the evaluation of NETs though the former is used for evaluating somatostatin receptor positivity and deciding upon the suitability of peptide receptor radionuclide therapy (PRRT) [227]. On the other hand, FDG-PET/CT gives assessment of glycolytic metabolism, and its higher uptake is associated with tumour aggressiveness. Dichotomous behaviour has been observed between both of these tracers in well-differentiated and poorly differentiated NETs [228].

68Ga is a generator-produced positron emitter and does not therefore depend on a cyclotron. The 68 min half-life is suitable for tumour imaging, and 68Ga-labelled SST analogues have great potential for PET imaging of NETs and their metastases. Studies have shown superiority of 68Ga-labelled peptides to 111In-DTPA-octreotide, and 68Ga-labelled SST is used as a tracer in the diagnosis, staging and restaging of patients with NETs. 68Ga-DOTA0-Tyr3-octreotide (68Ga DOTATOC), 68Ga-DOTA0,1NaI3-octreotide (68Ga-DOTANOC) and 68Ga-DOTA0-Tyr3-octreotate (68Ga-DOTATATE) are three 68Ga-labelled SST analogues widely utilised in NET imaging [229–231]. These tracers demonstrate slight differences in the affinity for the somatostatin receptor (SSTR) subtypes. 68Ga-DOTATATE has high affinity for the SSTR2 subtype with a 10-fold higher affinity for SSTR2 than that of 68Ga-DOTATOC which is selective for SSTR2 and SSTR5 subtypes. The sensitivity and specificity of labelled peptide PET or PET/CT have been reported to be 93 % and 91 %, respectively, in detecting thoracic and/or GEP-NETs [229]. The reported sensitivity and specificity of 68Ga-DOTATATE PET/CT in the diagnosis of primary or metastatic lesions in NETs range from 80 to 100 % and 82 to 90 %, respectively. Compared to 111In-DTPA-octreotide, MIBG scintigraphy and conventional imaging, 68Ga-DOTATATE PET/CT is reported to provide additional information which results in change in

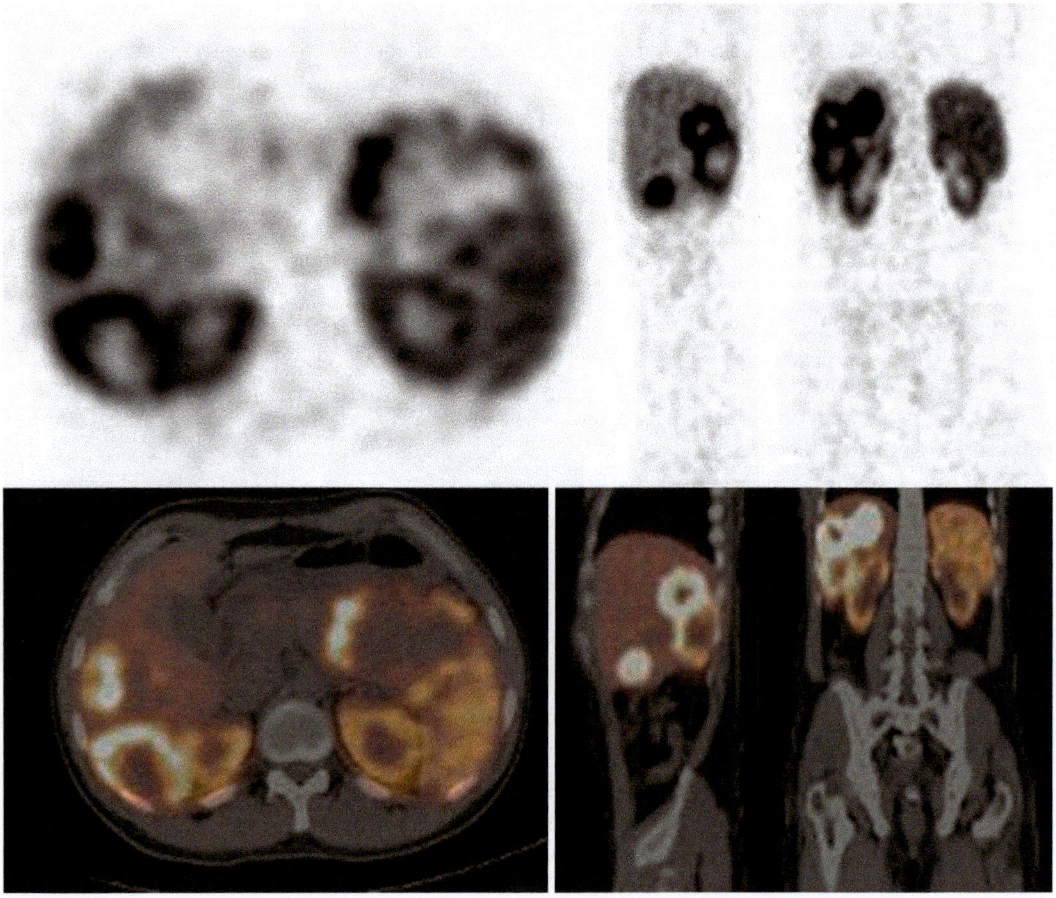

Fig. 17.6 A 35-year-old man presented with abdominal pain and vomiting and ultrasound and contrast-enhanced CT detected multiple large hepatic metastases from pancreatic NET (mass at body and tail). MIB-1 (or the Ki67) index less than 2 %. The patient was being evaluated for feasibility of PRRT. 68Ga-DOTATATE PET-CT (MIP and multiplanar images) demonstrating intense tracer uptake (signifying somatostatin receptor positivity) in the metastatic lesions with central necrosis

clinical management in 70.6–81 % of patients [230]. A significant impact has been seen in the following areas: a modified stage leading to a change in treatment plan, potential to prevent unnecessary intervention (surgery/PRRT) and potential to predict therapy response earlier in tumours [231]. Surgery is still the therapy of first choice when feasible but a majority of NETs still require further treatment with SST analogues and/or interferon [232]. The predominant expression of SST2 receptors in NETs is essential for the application of radiolabelled octapeptide SST analogues, as well as for PRRT using 90Y- and 177Lu-DOTATATE/DOTATOC [233]. SSTR PET positivity is an important criterion for selection of candidates for PRRT [234]. Decreased 68Ga-DOTATATE uptake after the first cycle of PRRT correlates with improvement of clinical symptoms and predicts time to progression in well-differentiated NET patients [235]. PRRT is a promising new method in the treatment of patients with inoperable or metastasised NETs because of fewer side effects, less toxicity and better therapeutic effect [236] (Fig. 17.6).

17.12 PET Tracers for Imaging Bone Metabolism

PET imaging of bone metabolism using 18F-fluoride (18F-NaF) may augment bone imaging in the future, particularly if the supply of

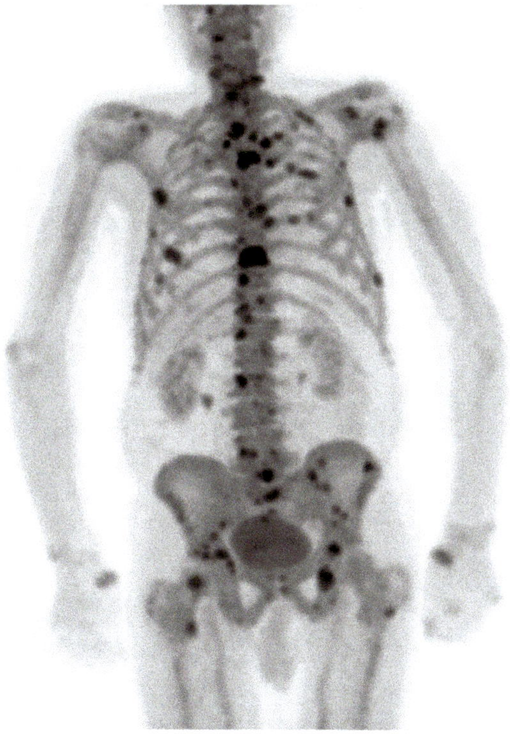

Fig. 17.7 18F-fluoride MIP image. A man with metastatic prostate cancer (same patient as Fig. 17.4) showing abnormal 18F-fluoride activity in multiple bone metastases

99m-technetium becomes more problematic [237]. 18F-NaF uptake shares similar mechanisms to 99mTc radiolabelled diphosphonates and correlates with osteoblastic metabolism and local bone turnover [238]. 18F-NaF imaging has a number of advantages over routine bone scintigraphy. High-contrast 18F-NaF images can be acquired as soon as 1 h after injection and show better image quality in view of the higher spatial resolution of PET compared to gamma camera imaging [239, 240].

Bone imaging using 18F-NaF has shown promise in staging various malignancies such as prostate cancer and lung and breast tumours and is found to have a very high diagnostic accuracy compared with bone scintigraphy, by reaching maximal rates (100 %) of sensitivity and specificity versus 92 % and 82 %, respectively, for 99mTc-MDP scintigraphy [241] (Fig. 17.7). It has shown high sensitivity for detecting both sclerotic and lytic bone lesions. However, 18F-fluoride for clinical oncological imaging lacks specificity for differentiating benign from malignant lesions although this is largely overcome by the use of combined morphological and functional imaging, as in hybrid PET/CT systems that may help to overcome potential false-positive findings [242, 243].

17.13 PET Tracers for Imaging Agents Targeting Chemokine Receptor

Chemokine receptor CXCR4 and its ligand CXCL12 mediated tumour cell migration, and hence metastasis is a key pathway in tumourigenesis [244, 245]. They are responsible for leukocyte trafficking and homing, and studies have shown that CXCR4 expression is responsible for metastatic progression in breast and head and neck cancers [246, 247]. CXCR4 imaging is a potential biomarker for studying metastases in distant organs. These chemokine receptors have been radiolabelled with various molecules such as peptides, mAbs, CXCL12 and anti-CXCR4 [248]. Because of low stability and slow blood clearance of peptides and antibodies in in vivo studies, they have not yet shown as much promise in clinical use. The recently developed bicyclam CXCR4 compound, AMD3100, is the only clinical agent to target CXCR4, which can be efficiently radiolabelled with metals, such as Cu-64, through cyclam chelation. However, its sensitivity and pharmacokinetics to effectively detect small metastatic foci is still under investigation [249, 250]. Another novel F-18-labelled small non-cyclam CXCR4 PET tracer (18F-M508F) has a faster clearance from blood and better sensitivity and is convenient for patients with a shorter waiting period between injection of radiotracer and image acquisition [251].

17.14 PET Tracers for Imaging Multidrug Resistance in Cancer

Multidrug Resistance (MDR) is defined as resistance of tumour cells to structurally unrelated drugs including taxanes and anthracyclines amongst others [252]. There are many mechanisms which are involved in MDR for chemotherapeutic drugs including drug efflux pumps, P-glycoprotein (Pgp) and multidrug resistance-associated protein (MRP) [253]. Functional imaging of MDR in cancer using SPECT or PET helps to identify clinically unfavourable prognoses and patients who will be more susceptible to develop drug toxicities and resistance. Radiolabelled metallic complexes and small organic molecular targets have been used to noninvasively study the Pgp transport substrates by PET or SPECT [254]. 99mTc-sestamibi and 99mTc-tetrofosmin have been used to study the Pgp-mediated transporter activity in vivo in humans [255]. Other novel tracers include gallium (III)-(bis(3-ethoxy-2-hydroxy-benzylidene)-N, N′-bis(2,2-dimethyl-3-amino-propyl) ethylenediamine) (Ga-[3-ethoxy-ENBDMPI])(+) for SPECT (67Ga) and generator-produced 68Ga for PET imaging. Some other radiolabelled agents such as 11C-colchicine and 11C-verapamil for PET imaging can be used to quantify Pgp-mediated transport in vivo [256, 257]. Other studied MDR proteins which are being evaluated include multidrug resistance protein 1 (MRP1, gene symbol ABCC1), MRP2 (gene symbol ABCC2) and breast cancer resistance protein (BCRP, gene symbol ABCG2) [253, 254]. 99mTc-sestamibi is a lipophilic cationic radiotracer commonly used for studying MDR proteins in cancer and has been used in in vivo studies for breast, head and neck, hepatobiliary, gastric and lung cancers [258]. In a study of lung cancer patients, it has shown sensitivity, specificity and accuracy of 94, 90 and 92 %, for predicting response to chemotherapy [259].

Conclusion

In the modern era of cancer imaging, molecular and functional imaging by PET has an increasingly important role and evidence continues to accumulate. Utility includes clinical applications ranging from cancer staging to response evaluation and personalised medicine. Though FDG as a PET tracer has shown great success in oncological imaging, it has some limitations that make non-FDG-PET tracers important in a number of clinical settings. Various non-FDG-PET tracers have been developed based on other features of tumour biology, tumour metabolism and the tumour microenvironment such as proliferation, hypoxia, angiogenesis and apoptosis. Better understanding of tumourigenesis and the discovery and validation of these novel PET tracers for imaging biomarkers will lead us nearer to the development of personalised patient care.

References

1. DeSantis CE, Lin CC, Mariotto AB, Siegel RL, et al. Cancer treatment and survivorship statistics, 2014. CA Cancer J Clin. 2014;64(4):252–71.
2. Yang DJ, Pham L, Liao MH, Kong FL, Uemura H, Shih YY. Advances in molecular pathway-directed cancer systems imaging and therapy. Biomed Res Int. 2014;2014:639475. doi:10.1155/2014/639475. Epub 2014 Dec 21.
3. Fass L. Imaging and cancer: a review. Mol Oncol. 2008;2:115–52.
4. Desar IM, van Herpen CM, van Laarhoven HW, Barentsz JO, Oyen WJ, van der Graaf WT. Beyond RECIST: molecular and functional imaging techniques for evaluation of response to targeted therapy. Cancer Treat Rev. 2009;35:309–21.
5. Puttick S, Bell C, Dowson N, Rose S, Fay M. PET, MRI, and simultaneous PET/MRI in the development of diagnostic and therapeutic strategies for glioma. Drug Discov Today. 2015;20(3):306–17. pii: S1359-6446(14)00421-8.
6. Griffeth LK. Use of PET/CT scanning in cancer patients: technical and practical considerations. Proc (Bayl Univ Med Cent). 2005;18(4):321–30.
7. Zhu A, Lee D, Shim H. Metabolic PET imaging in cancer detection and therapy response. Semin Oncol. 2011;38(1):55–69.
8. Kelloff GJ, Hoffman JM, Johnson B, et al. Progress and promise of FDG-PET imaging for cancer patient management and oncologic drug development. Clin Cancer Res. 2005;11:2785–808.
9. Warburg O. In: Dickens F, editor. The metabolism of tumors. London: Constable; 1930. p. 129–69.
10. http://www.cms.gov/Regulations-and-Guidance/Guidance/Transmittals/downloads/R168NCD.pdf.
11. http://www.cms.gov/Regulations-and-Guidance/Guidance/Transmittals/downloads/R119NCD.pdf.
12. http://www.fda.gov/Drugs/DevelopmentApprovalProcess/Manufacturing/ucm085783.htm.
13. Peller P, et al. editors. PET-CT and PET-MRI in oncology, medical radiology. Diagnostic Imaging. Berlin/Heidelberg:Springer;2012.doi:10.1007/174_2012_703.
14. Fletcher JW, Djulbegovic B, Soares HP, Siegel BA, Lowe VJ, Lyman GH, Coleman RE, Wahl R, Paschold

JC, Avril N, Einhorn LH, Suh WW, Samson D, Delbeke D, Gorman M, Shields AF. Recommendations on the use of 18F-FDG PET in oncology. J Nucl Med. 2008;49(3):480–508.
15. Hillner BE, Siegel BA, Shields AF, Liu D, Gareen IF, Hanna L, Stine SH, Coleman RE. The impact of positron emission tomography (PET) on expected management during cancer treatment: findings of the National Oncologic PET Registry. Cancer. 2009; 115(2):410–8.
16. Mahajan A, Goh V, Basu S, Vaish R, Weeks AJ, Thakur MH, Cook GJ. Bench to bedside molecular functional imaging in translational cancer medicine: to image or to imagine? Clin Radiol. 2015;70(10): 1060–82.
17. Wester HJ. Nuclear imaging probes: from bench to bedside. Clin Cancer Res. 2007;13:3476–81.
18. Kelloff GJ, Krohn KA, Larson SM, et al. The progress and promise of molecular imaging probes in oncologic drug development. Clin Cancer Res. 2005;11:7967–85.
19. Blasburg R. Imaging update: new windows, new views. Clin Cancer Res. 2007;13:3444–8.
20. Padhani AR, Koh DM, Collins DJ. Whole-body diffusion-weighted MR imaging in cancer: current status and research directions. Radiology. 2011; 261(3):700–18.
21. Mera Iglesias M, AramburuNúñez D, Del Olmo Claudio JL, et al. Multimodality functional imaging in radiation therapy planning: relationships between dynamic contrast-enhanced MRI, diffusion-weighted MRI, and 18F-FDG PET. Comput Math Methods Med. 2015;2015:103843. doi:10.1155/2015/103843. Epub 2015 Feb 19.
22. Beyer T, Townsend DW, Brun T, Kinahan PE, Charron M, Roddy R, Jerin J, Young J, Byars L, Nutt R. A combined PET/CT scanner for clinical oncology. J Nucl Med. 2000;41:1369–79.
23. Eubank WB, Mankoff DA, Schmiedl UP, et al. Imaging of oncologic patients: benefit of combined CT and FDG PET in the diagnosis of malignancy. AJR Am J Roentgenol. 1998;171:1103–10.
24. Blodgett TM, Meltzer CC, Townsend DW. PET/CT: form and function. Radiology. 2007;242(2):360–85.
25. Wahl RL, Wagner Jr HN, editors. Principles and practice of PET and PET/CT. 2nd ed. Philadelphia: Lippincott Williams & Wilkins; 2008.
26. Cohade C, Osman M, Marshall LT, Wahl RL. PET-CT: accuracy of PET and CT spatial registration of lung lesions. Eur J Nucl Med Mol Imaging. 2003;30:721–6.
27. von Schulthess GK, Steinert HC, Hany TF. Integrated PET/CT: current applications and future directions. Radiology. 2006;238:405–22.
28. Mankoff DA, Krohn KA. PET imaging of response and resistance to cancer therapy. In: Teicher B, editor. Drug resistance in cancer. Totowa: Humana Press; 2006. p. 105–22.
29. Sokoloff L, Reivich M, Kennedy C, et al. The [14C] deoxyglucose method for the measurement of local cerebral glucose utilization: theory, procedure, and normal values in the conscious and anesthetized albino rat. J Neurochem. 1977;28:897–916.
30. Warburg O. The metabolism of tumors. New York: Richard R. Smith; 1931.
31. Som P, Atkins HL, Bandoypadhyay D, et al. A fluorinated glucose analog, 2-fluoro-2-deoxy-D-glucose (F-18): nontoxic tracer for rapid tumor detection. J Nucl Med. 1980;21(7):670–5.
32. Phelps M, Huang S, Hoffman E. Tomographic measurement of local cerebral glucose metabolic rate in humans with (18F)2-fluoro-2-deoxy-D-glucose: validation of method. Ann Neurol. 1979;6:371.
33. Krohn KA, Mankoff DA, Muzi M, Link JM, Spence AM. True tracers: comparing FDG with glucose and FLT with thymidine. Nucl Med Biol. 2005;32:663–71.
34. Mamede M, Higashi T, Kitaichi M, Ishizu K, Ishimori T, Nakamoto Y, Yanagihara K, Li M, Tanaka F, Wada H, Manabe T, Saga T. [18F]FDG uptake and PCNA, Glut-1, and Hexokinase-II expressions in cancers and inflammatory lesions of the lung. Neoplasia. 2005; 7:369–79.
35. Gatenby RA, Gillies RJ. Why do cancers have high aerobic glycolysis? Nat Rev Cancer. 2004;4:891–9.
36. Aloj L, Caraco C, Jagoda E, Eckelman WC, Neumann RD. Glut-1 and hexokinase expression: relationship with 2-fluoro-2-deoxy-D-glucose uptake in A31 and T47D cells in culture. Cancer Res. 1999;59:4709–14.
37. Mathapala S, Rempel A, Pederson P. Aberrant glycolytic metabolism of cancer cells: a remarkable coordination of genetic, transcriptional, post-translational, and mutational events that lead to a critical role for type II hexokinase. J Bioenerg Biomembr. 1997;29:339–43.
38. Tseng J, Dunnwald LK, Schubert EK, et al. 18F-FDG kinetics in locally advanced breast cancer: correlation with tumour blood flow and changes in response to neoadjuvant chemotherapy. J Nucl Med. 2004;45:1829–37.
39. Semenza GL, Jiang BH, Leung SW, et al. Hypoxia response elements in the aldolase A, enolase 1, and lactate dehydrogenase A gene promoters contain essential binding sites for hypoxia-inducible factor 1. J Biol Chem. 1996;271(51):32529–37.
40. Clavo AC, Brown RS, Wahl RL. Fluorodeoxyglucose uptake in human cancer cell lines is increased by hypoxia. J Nucl Med. 1995;36:1625–32.
41. Semenza GL, Roth PH, Fang HM, Wang GL. Transcriptional regulation of genes encoding glycolytic enzymes by hypoxia-inducible factor 1. J Biol Chem. 1994;269(38):23757–63.
42. Sebolt-Leopold JS, Herrera R. Targeting the mitogen-activated protein kinase cascade to treat cancer. Nat Rev Cancer. 2004;4:937–47.
43. Thompson JE, Thompson CB. Putting the rap on Akt. J Clin Oncol. 2004;22:4217–26.
44. Majumder PK, Febbo PG, Bikoff R, et al. mTOR inhibition reverses Akt-dependent prostate intraepithelial neoplasia through regulation of apoptotic and HIF-1-dependent pathways. Nat Med. 2004;10:594–601.

45. Mankoff DA, Eary JF, Link JM, Muzi M, Rajendran JG, Spence AM, Krohn KA. Tumor-specific positron emission tomography imaging in patients: [18F] fluorodeoxyglucose and beyond. Clin Cancer Res. 2007;13(12):3460–9.
46. Shankar LK, Hoffman JM, Bacharach S, et al. Consensus recommendations for the use of 18F-FDG PET as an indicator of therapeutic response in patients in National Cancer Institute Trials. J Nucl Med. 2006;47:1059–66.
47. Mankoff DA, Dunnwald LK, Gralow JR, et al. Changes in blood flow and metabolism in locally advanced breast cancer treated with neoadjuvant chemotherapy. J Nucl Med. 2003;44:1806–14.
48. Huang S-C. Anatomy of SUV. Nucl Med Biol. 2000;27:643–6.
49. Zasadny KR, Wahl RL. Standardized uptake values of normal tissues at PET with 2-[fluorine-18]-fluoro-2-deoxy-D-glucose: variations with body weight and a method for correction. Radiology. 1993;189:847–50.
50. Zhuang H, Pourdehnad M, Lambright ES, et al. Dual time point 18F-FDG PET imaging for differentiating malignant from inflammatory processes. J Nucl Med. 2001;42:1412–7.
51. Gambhir SS, Czernin J, Schwimmer J, et al. A tabulated summary of the FDG PET literature. J Nucl Med. 2001;42:1S–93.
52. Krohn KA, Mankoff DA, Eary JF. Imaging cellular proliferation as a measure of response to therapy. J Clin Pharmacol. 2001;41:96S–103.
53. Kim CK, Beheshti M. PET tracers beyond FDG: normal variations and benign findings. PET Clin. 2014;9(3):xi–xii.
54. Antunovic L, Rodari M, Rossi P, Chiti A. Standardization and quantification in PET/CT imaging: tracers beyond FDG. PET Clin. 2014;9(3):259–66.
55. Saga T, Koizumi M, Furukawa T, Yoshikawa K, Fujibayashi Y. Molecular imaging of cancer: evaluating characters of individual cancer by PET/SPECT imaging. Cancer Sci. 2009;100(3):375–81.
56. Kaira K, Oriuchi N, Imai H, et al. l-type amino acid transporter 1 and CD98 expression in primary and metastatic sites of human neoplasms. Cancer Sci. 2008;99(12):2380–6.
57. Christensen HN. Role of amino acid transport and countertransport in nutrition and metabolism. Physiol Rev. 1990;70(1):43–77.
58. Yanagida O, Kanai Y, Chairoungdua A, et al. Human L-type amino acid transporter 1 (LAT1): characterization of function and expression in tumor cell lines. Biochim Biophys Acta. 2001;1514(2):291–302.
59. Singhal T, Narayanan TK, Jain V, Mukherjee J, Mantil J. 11C-L-methionine positron emission tomography in the clinical management of cerebral gliomas. Mol Imaging Biol. 2008;10(1):1–18.
60. Comar D, Cartron J, Maziere M, et al. Labeling and metabolism of methioninemethyl-11C. Eur J Nucl Med. 1976;1:11–4.
61. Kubota K, Matsuzawa T, Ito M, Ito K, Fujiwara T, Abe Y, Yoshioka S, Fukuda H, Hatazawa J, Iwata R, et al. Lung tumor imaging by positron emission tomography using C-11 L-methionine. J Nucl Med. 1985;26(1):37–42.
62. Koizumi M, Saga T, Yoshikawa K, Suzuki K, Yamada S, Hasebe M, Ohashi S, Abd-Elrazek S, Ishikawa H, Sagou K, Tamura K, Hara R, Kato H, Yasuda S, Yanagi T, Tsujii H. 11C-methionine-PET for evaluation of carbon ion radiotherapy in patients with pelvic recurrence of rectal cancer. Mol Imaging Biol. 2008;10:374–80.
63. Becherer A, Karanikas G, Szabo M, et al. Brain tumour imaging with PET: a comparison between [18F]fluorodopa and [11C]methionine. Eur J Nucl Med Mol Imaging. 2003;30(11):1561–7.
64. Shinozaki N, Uchino Y, Yoshikawa K, Matsutani T, Hasegawa A, Saeki N, Iwadate Y. Discrimination between low-grade oligodendrogliomas and diffuse astrocytoma with the aid of 11C-methionine positron emission tomography. J Neurosurg. 2011;114:1640–7.
65. Coope DJ, Cízek J, Eggers C, Vollmar S, Heiss WD, Herholz K. Evaluation of primary brain tumors using 11C-methionine PET with reference to a normal methionine uptake map. J Nucl Med. 2007;48:1971–80.
66. Inoue T, Kim EE, Wong FC, et al. Comparison of fluorine-18-fluorodeoxyglucose and carbon-11-methionine PET in detection of malignant tumors. J Nucl Med. 1996;37(9):1472–6.
67. Isohashi K, Shimosegawa E, Kato H, Kanai Y, Naka S, Fujino K, Watabe H, Hatazawa J. Optimization of [11C]methionine PET study: appropriate scan timing and effect of plasma amino acid concentrations on the SUV. EJNMMI Res. 2013;3(1):27.
68. Couturier O, Luxen A, Chatal JF, Vuillez JP, Rigo P, Hustinx R. Fluorinated tracers for imaging cancer with positron emission tomography. Eur J Nucl Med Mol Imaging. 2004;31(8):1182–206.
69. Laverman P, Boerman OC, Corstens FH, Oyen WJ. Fluorinated amino acids for tumour imaging with positron emission tomography. Eur J Nucl Med Mol Imaging. 2002;29(5):681–90.
70. McConathy J, Goodman MM. Non-natural amino acids for tumor imaging using positron emission tomography and single photon emission computed tomography. Cancer Metastasis Rev. 2008;27(4):555–73.
71. Popperl G, Kreth FW, Herms J, et al. Analysis of 18F-FET PET for grading of recurrent gliomas: is evaluation of uptake kinetics superior to standard methods? J Nucl Med. 2006;47(3):393–403.
72. Thiele F, Ehmer J, Piroth MD, et al. The quantification of dynamic FET PET imaging and correlation with the clinical outcome in patients with glioblastoma. Phys Med Biol. 2009;54(18):5525–39.
73. Tripathi M, Sharma R, D'Souza M, et al. Comparative evaluation of F-18 FDOPA, F-18 FDG, and F-18 FLT-PET/CT for metabolic imaging of low grade gliomas. Clin Nucl Med. 2009;34(12):878–83.
74. Chen W, Silverman DH, Delaloye S, et al. 18F-FDOPA PET imaging of brain tumors: comparison study with 18F-FDG PET and evaluation of diagnostic accuracy. J Nucl Med. 2006;47(6):904–11.

75. Schiepers C, Chen W, Cloughesy T, Dahlbom M, Huang SC. 18F-FDOPA kinetics in brain tumors. J Nucl Med. 2007;48(10):1651–61.
76. Koopmans KP, de Vries EG, Kema IP, et al. Staging of carcinoid tumours with 18F-DOPA PET: a prospective, diagnostic accuracy study. Lancet Oncol. 2006;7(9):728–34.
77. Shoup TM, Olson J, Hoffman JM, et al. Synthesis and evaluation of [18F]1-amino-3-fluorocyclobutane-1-carboxylic acid to image brain tumors. J Nucl Med. 1999;40(2):331–8.
78. Schuster DM, Votaw JR, Nieh PT, et al. Initial experience with the radiotracer anti-1-amino-3-18F--fluorocyclobutane-1-carboxylic acid with PET/CT in prostate carcinoma. J Nucl Med. 2007;48(1): 56–63.
79. Nanni C, Schiavina R, Boschi S, et al. Comparison of 18F-FACBC and 11C-choline PET/CT in patients with radically treated prostate cancer and biochemical relapse: preliminary results. Eur J Nucl Med Mol Imaging. 2013;40:S11–7.
80. Schuster DM, Nye JA, Nieh PT, et al. Initial experience with the radiotracer anti-1-amino-3-[18F] Fluorocyclobutane-1-carboxylic acid (anti-[18F] FACBC) with PET in renal carcinoma. Mol Imaging Biol. 2009;11(6):434–8.
81. Kairemo K, Rasulova N, Partanen K, Joensuu T. Preliminary clinical experience of trans-1-amino-3-(18) F-fluorocyclobutanecarboxylic acid (anti-(18)F-FACBC) PET/CT imaging in prostate cancer patients. BioMed Res Int. 2014;2014:305182.
82. Schuster DM, Savir-Baruch B, Nieh PT, et al. Detection of recurrent prostate carcinoma with anti-1-amino-3-18F-fluorocyclobutane-1-carboxylic acid PET/CT and 111In–capromab pendetide SPECT/CT. Radiology. 2011;259(3):852–61.
83. Oka S, Hattori R, Kurosaki F, et al. A preliminary study of anti-1-amino-3-18f-fluorocyclobutyl-1-carboxylic acid for the detection of prostate cancer. J Nucl Med. 2007;48(1):46–55.
84. Yoshimoto M, Waki A, Obata A, Furukawa T, Yonekura Y, Fujibayashi Y. Radiolabeled choline as a proliferation marker: comparison with radiolabeled acetate. Nucl Med Biol. 2004;31(7): 859–65.
85. McCarthy M, Siew T, Campbell A, et al. [18] F-Fluoromethylcholine (FCH) PET imaging in patients with castration-resistant prostate cancer: prospective comparison with standard imaging. Eur J Nucl Med Mol Imaging. 2011;38:14–22.
86. Kurhanewicz J, Vigneron DB, Hricak H, Narayan P, Carroll P, Nelson SJ. Three-dimensional H-1 MR spectroscopic imaging of the in situ human prostate with high (0.23-0.7 cm3) spatial resolution. Radiology. 1996;198:795–805.
87. Hara T, Kosaka N, Kishi H. Development of 18F-fluoroethylcholine for cancer imaging with PET: synthesis, biochemistry, and prostate cancer imaging. J Nucl Med. 2002;43(2):187–99.
88. Tian M, Zhang H, Oriuchi N, Higuchi T, Endo K. Comparison of 11C-choline PET and FDG PET for the differential diagnosis of malignant tumors. Eur J Nucl Med Mol Imaging. 2004;31(8):1064–72.
89. Umbehr MH, Müntener M, Hany T, Sulser T, Bachmann LM. The role of 11C-choline and 18F-fluorocholine positron emission tomography (PET) and PET/CT in prostate cancer: a systematic review and meta-analysis. Eur Urol. 2013;64(1): 106–17.
90. Khan N, Oriuchi N, Ninomiya H, Higuchi T, Kamada H, Endo K. Positron emission tomographic imaging with 11C-choline in differential diagnosis of head and neck tumors: comparison with 18F-FDG PET. Ann Nucl Med. 2004;18(5):409–17.
91. Bouchelouche K, Tagawa ST, Goldsmith SJ, Turkbey B, Capala J, Choyke P. PET/CT imaging and radioimmunotherapy of prostate cancer. Semin Nucl Med. 2011;41(1):29–44.
92. Kitajima K, Murphy RC, Nathan MA. Choline PET/CT for imaging prostate cancer: an update. Ann Nucl Med. 2013;27(7):581–91.
93. Carmeliet P. Angiogenesis in health and disease. Nat Med. 2003;9:653–60.
94. Bergers G, Benjamin LE. Tumorigenesis and the angiogenic switch. Nat Rev Cancer. 2003;3:401–10.
95. Ellis LM, Liu W, Ahmad SA, et al. Overview of angiogenesis: biologic implications for antiangiogenic therapy. Semin Oncol. 2001;28:94–104.
96. Carmeliet P, Jain RK. Angiogenesis in cancer and other diseases. Nature. 2000;407:249–57.
97. Eliceiri BP, Cheresh DA. The role of alphav integrins during angiogenesis. Mol Med. 1998;4:741–50.
98. Aboagye EO, Gilbert FJ, Fleming IN, Beer AJ, Cunningham VJ, Marsden PK, Visvikis D, Gee AD, Groves AM, Kenny LM, Cook GJ, Kinahan PE, Myers M, Clarke L; Experimental Cancer Medicine Centre 13 Imaging Network Group. Recommendations for measurement of tumour vascularity with positron emission tomography in early phase clinical trials. EurRadiol. 2012;22(7):1465–78.
99. Kötz B, West C, Saleem A, Jones T, Price P. Blood flow and Vd (water): both biomarkers required for interpreting the effects of vascular targeting agents on tumor and normal tissue. Mol Cancer Ther. 2009;8(2):303–9.
100. Saleem A, Yap J, Osman S, et al. Modulation of fluorouracil tissue pharmacokinetics by eniluracil: in-vivo imaging of drug action. Lancet. 2000;355(9221): 2125–31.
101. Gupta N, Saleem A, Kötz B, et al. Carbogen and nicotinamide increase blood flow and 5-fluorouracil delivery but not 5-fluorouracil retention in colorectal cancer metastases in patients. Clin Cancer Res. 2006;12(10):3115–23.
102. Kurdziel KA, Figg WD, Carrasquillo JA, et al. Using positron emission tomography 2-deoxy-2-[18F] fluoro-D-glucose, 11CO, and 15O-water for monitoring androgen independent prostate cancer. Mol Imaging Biol. 2003;5(2):86–93.
103. Anderson HL, Yap JT, Miller MP, Robbins A, Jones T, Price PM. Assessment of pharmacodynamic

vascular response in a phase I trial of combretastatin A4 phosphate. J Clin Oncol. 2003;21(15):2823–30.
104. Xiong JP, Stehle T, Zhang R, et al. Crystal structure of the extracellular segment of integrin αvβ3 in complex with an Arg-Gly-Asp ligand. Science. 2002;296: 151–5.
105. Haubner R, Weber WA, Beer AJ, et al. Noninvasive visualization of the activated alphavbeta3 integrin in cancer patients by positron emission tomography and [18F]Galacto-RGD. PLoS Med. 2005;2(3):e70. Epub 2005 Mar 29.
106. Cai W, Gambhir SS, Chen X. Multimodality tumor imaging targeting integrin αvβ3. Biotechniques. 2005;39(suppl):S6–17.
107. Zhang X, Xiong Z, Wu Y, et al. Quantitative PET imaging of tumor integrin αvβ3 expression with 18F-FRGD2. J Nucl Med. 2006;47:113–21.
108. Haubner R. αvβ3-Integrin imaging: a new approach to characterise angiogenesis? Eur J Nucl Med Mol Imaging. 2006;33 suppl 13:54–63.
109. Dumont RA, Deininger F, Haubner R, Maecke HR, Weber WA, Fani M. Novel (64)Cu- and (68) Ga-labeled RGD conjugates show improved PET imaging of α(ν)β(3) integrin expression and facile radiosynthesis. J Nucl Med. 2011;52(8):1276–84.
110. Beer AJ, Lorenzen S, Metz S, et al. Comparison of integrin alphaVbeta3 expression and glucose metabolism in primary and metastatic lesions in cancer patients: a PET study using 18F-galacto-RGD and18F-FDG. J Nucl Med. 2008;49:22–9.
111. Haubner R, Decristoforo C. Radiolabelled RGD peptides and peptidomimetics for tumour targeting. Front Biosci. 2009;14:872–86.
112. Chen X, Hou Y, Tohme M, et al. Pegylated Arg-Gly-Asp peptide: 64Cu labeling and PET imaging of brain tumor alphavbeta3-integrin expression. J Nucl Med. 2004;45:1776–83.
113. Chen X, Park R, Hou Y, Khankaldyyan V, et al. MicroPET imaging of brain tumor angiogenesis with 18F-labeled PEGylated RGD peptide. Eur J Nucl Med Mol Imaging. 2004;31(8):1081–9. Epub 2004 Apr 29.
114. Chen X, Tohme M, Park R, Hou Y, Bading JR, Conti PS. Micro-PET imaging of alphavbeta3-integrin expression with 18F-labeled dimeric RGD peptide. Mol Imaging. 2004;3:96–104.
115. Wu Z, Li ZB, Chen K, Cai W, He L, Chin FT, et al. microPET of tumor integrin alphavbeta3 expression using 18F-labeled PEGylated tetrameric RGD peptide (18F-FPRGD4). J Nucl Med. 2007;48:1536–44.
116. Haubner R, Maschauer S, Prante O. PET radiopharmaceuticals for imaging integrin expression: tracers in clinical studies and recent developments. BioMed Res Int. 2014;2014:871609.
117. De la Zerda A, Zavaleta C, Keren S, et al. Carbon nanotubes as photoacoustic molecular imaging agents in living mice. Nat Nanotechnol. 2008;3(9): 557–62.
118. Liu Z, Cai W, He L, et al. In vivo biodistribution and highly efficient tumour targeting of carbon nanotubes in mice. Nat Nanotechnol. 2007;2:47–52.
119. Almutairi A, Rossin R, Shokeen M, et al. Biodegradable dendritic positron-emitting nanoprobes for the noninvasive imaging of angiogenesis. Proc Natl Acad Sci U S A. 2009;106:685–90.
120. Hong H, Gao T, Cai W. Molecular imaging with single-walled carbon nanotubes. Nano Today. 2009; 4:252–61.
121. Rüegg C, Alghisi GC. Vascular integrins: therapeutic and imaging targets of tumor angiogenesis. Recent Results Cancer Res. 2010;180:83–101.
122. Reichardt W, Hu-Lowe D, Torres D, Weissleder R, Bogdanov Jr A. Imaging of VEGF receptor kinase inhibitor-induced antiangiogenic effects in drug-resistant human adenocarcinoma model. Neoplasia. 2005;7(9):847–53.
123. Li S, Peck-Radosavljevic M, Koller E, et al. Characterization of (123)I-vascular endothelial growth factor-binding sites expressed on human tumour cells: possible implication for tumour scintigraphy. Int J Cancer. 2001;91:789–96.
124. Jayson GC, Zweit J, Jackson A, et al. Molecular imaging and biological evaluation of HuMV833 anti-VEGF antibody: implications for trial design of antiangiogenic antibodies. J Natl Cancer Inst. 2002; 94:1484–93.
125. Deri MA, Zeglis BM, Francesconi LC, Lewis JS. PET imaging with 89Zr: from radiochemistry to the clinic. Nucl Med Biol. 2013;40(1):3–14.
126. Cai W, Chen X. Multimodality molecular imaging of tumor angiogenesis. J Nucl Med. 2008;49 Suppl 2:113S–28.
127. Cai W, Chen K, Mohamedali KA, et al. PET of vascular endothelial growth factor receptor expression. J Nucl Med. 2006;47:2048–56.
128. Xiangsong Z, Xinjian W, Yong Z, Weian C. 13N-NH3: a selective contrast-enhancing tracer for brain tumor. Nucl Med Commun. 2008;29: 1052–8.
129. de Langen AJ, van den Boogaart VE, Marcus JT, Lubberink M. Use of H2(15)O-PET and DCE-MRI to measure tumor blood flow. Oncologist. 2008;13: 631–44.
130. Verwer EE, Boellaard R, van der Veldt AA. Positron emission tomography to assess hypoxia and perfusion in lung cancer. World J Clin Oncol. 2014;5(5): 824–44.
131. Vaupel P, Harrison L. Tumor hypoxia: causative factors, compensatory mechanisms, and cellular response. Oncologist. 2004;9 Suppl 5:4–9.
132. Hockel M, Vaupel P. Tumor hypoxia: definitions and current clinical, biologic, and molecular aspects. J Natl Cancer Inst. 2001;93:266–76.
133. Vaupel P, Mayer A. Hypoxia in cancer: significance and impact on clinical outcome. Cancer Metastasis Rev. 2007;26:225–39.

134. Fyles AW, Milosevic M, Wong R, et al. Oxygenation predicts radiation response and survival in patients with cervix cancer. Radiother Oncol. 1998;48:149–56.
135. Krohn KA, Link JM, Mason RP. Molecular imaging of hypoxia. J Nucl Med. 2008;49 Suppl 2:129S–48.
136. Zheng X, Wang X, Mao H, Wu W, Liu B, Jiang X. Hypoxia-specific ultrasensitive detection of tumours and cancer cells in vivo. Nat Commun. 2015;6:5834.
137. Chia K, Fleming IN, Blower PJ. Hypoxia imaging with PET: which tracers and why? Nucl Med Commun. 2012;33(3):217–22.
138. Carlin S, Humm JL. PET of hypoxia: current and future perspectives. J Nucl Med. 2012;53(8):1171–4.
139. Serganova I, Humm J, Ling C, Blasberg R. Tumor hypoxia imaging. Clin Cancer Res. 2006;12(18):5260–4.
140. Peeters SG, Zegers CM, Yaromina A, van Elmpt W, Dubois L, Lambin P. Current pre-clinical and clinical applications of hypoxia PET imaging using 2-nitroimidazoles. Q J Nucl Med Mol Imaging. 2015;59(1):39–57.
141. Chitneni SK, Palmer GM, Zalutsky MR, Dewhirst MW. Molecular imaging of hypoxia. J Nucl Med. 2011;52(2):165–8.
142. Sun X, Niu G, Chan N, Shen B, Chen X. Tumor hypoxia imaging. Mol Imaging Biol. 2011;13:399–410.
143. Jiang L, Tu Y, Shi H, Cheng Z. PET probes beyond (18)F-FDG. J Biomed Res. 2014;28(6):435–46.
144. Mees G, Dierckx R, Vangestel C, Van de Wiele C. Molecular imaging of hypoxia with radiolabelled agents. Eur J Nucl Med Mol Imaging. 2009;36:1674–86.
145. Rasey JS, Casciari JJ, Hofstrand PD, Muzi M, Graham MM, Chin LK. Determining hypoxic fraction in a rat glioma by uptake of radiolabeled fluoromisonidazole. Radiat Res. 2000;153:84–92.
146. Dubois L, Landuyt W, Haustermans K, Dupont P, Bormans G, Vermaelen P, et al. Evaluation of hypoxia in an experimental rat tumour model by [(18)F]fluoromisonidazole PET and immunohistochemistry. Br J Cancer. 2004;91:1947–54.
147. Zimny M, Gagel B, DiMartino E, et al. FDG—a marker of tumour hypoxia? A comparison with [18F]fluoromisonidazole and pO2-polarography in metastatic head and neck cancer. Eur J Nucl Med Mol Imaging. 2006;33:1426–31.
148. Gagel B, Piroth M, Pinkawa M, et al. pO polarography, contrast enhanced color duplex sonography (CDS), [18F] fluoromisonidazole and [18F] fluorodeoxyglucose positron emission tomography: validated methods for the evaluation of therapy-relevant tumor oxygenation or only bricks in the puzzle of tumor hypoxia?? BMC Cancer. 2007;7:113.
149. Rajendran JG, Schwartz DL, O'Sullivan J, et al. Tumor hypoxia imaging with [F-18] fluoromisonidazole positron emission tomography in head and neck cancer. Clin Cancer Res. 2006;12:5435–41.
150. Piert M, Machulla HJ, Picchio M, et al. Hypoxia-specific tumor imaging with 18F-fluoroazomycin arabinoside. J Nucl Med. 2005;46:106–13.
151. Reischl G, Dorow DS, Cullinane C, et al. Imaging of tumor hypoxia with [124I]IAZA in comparison with [18F]FMISO and [18F]FAZA—first small animal PET results. J Pharm Pharm Sci. 2007;10:203–11.
152. Grosu AL, Souvatzoglou M, Roper B, et al. Hypoxia imaging with FAZA-PET and theoretical considerations with regard to dose painting for individualization of radiotherapy in patients with head and neck cancer. Int J Radiat Oncol Biol Phys. 2007;69:541–51.
153. Dubois LJ, Lieuwes NG, Janssen MH, et al. Preclinical evaluation and validation of [18f]hx4, a promising hypoxia marker for pet imaging. Proc Natl Acad Sci U S A. 2011;108:14620–5.
154. van Loon J, Janssen MH, Ollers M, et al. Pet imaging of hypoxia using [18f]hx4: a phase i trial. Eur J Nucl Med Mol Imaging. 2010;37:1663–8.
155. Carlin S, Zhang H, Reese M, et al. A comparison of the imaging characteristics and microregional distribution of 4 hypoxia PET tracers. J Nucl Med. 2014;55:515–21.
156. Fujibayashi Y, Taniuchi H, Yonekura Y, Ohtani H, Konishi J, Yokoyama A. Copper-62-ATSM: a new hypoxia imaging agent with high membrane permeability and low redox potential. J Nucl Med. 1997;38:1155–60.
157. Maurer RI, Blower PJ, Dilworth JR, Reynolds CA, Zheng Y, Mullen GE. Studies on the mechanism of hypoxic selectivity in copper bis(thiosemicarbazone) radiopharmaceuticals. J Med Chem. 2002;45:1420–31.
158. Yuan H, Schroeder T, Bowsher JE, Hedlund LW, Wong T, Dewhirst MW. Intertumoral differences in hypoxia selectivity of the PET imaging agent 64Cu(II)-diacetyl-bis(N4-methylthiosemicarbazone). J Nucl Med. 2006;47:989–98.
159. Dence CS, Ponde DE, Welch MJ, Lewis JS. Autoradiographic and small-animal PET comparisons between (18)F-FMISO, (18)F-FDG, (18)F-FLT and the hypoxic selective (64)Cu-ATSM in a rodent model of cancer. Nucl Med Biol. 2008;35:713–20.
160. Lewis JS, Laforest R, Dehdashti F, Grigsby PW, Welch MJ, Siegel BA. An imaging comparison of64Cu-ATSM and 60Cu-ATSM in cancer of the uterine cervix. J Nucl Med. 2008;49:1177–82.
161. Cotter TG. Apoptosis and cancer: the genesis of a research field. Nat Rev Cancer. 2009;9:501–7.
162. De Saint-Hubert M, Prinsen K, Mortelmans L, Verbruggen A, Mottaghy FM. Molecular imaging of cell death. Methods. 2009;48:178–87.
163. Haberkorn U, Markert A, Mier W, Askoxylakis V, Altmann A. Molecular imaging of tumor metabolism and apoptosis. Oncogene. 2011;30(40):4141–51.
164. Blankenberg FG. In vivo imaging of apoptosis. Cancer Biol Ther. 2008;7:1525–32.

165. Hengartner MO. The biochemistry of apoptosis. Nature. 2000;407:770–6.
166. Blankenberg FG. Recent advances in the imaging of programmed cell death. Curr Pharm Des. 2004;10: 1457–67.
167. Boersma HH, Kietselaer BL, Stolk LM, et al. Past, present, and future of annexin A5: from protein discovery to clinical applications. J Nucl Med. 2005;46: 2035–50.
168. Tait JF. Imaging of apoptosis. J Nucl Med. 2008; 49:1573–6.
169. Haas RL, de Jong D, Valdes Olmos RA, Hoefnagel CA, Van Den Heuvel I, Zerp SF, et al. In vivo imaging of radiation-induced apoptosis in follicular lymphoma patients. Int J Radiat Oncol Biol Phys. 2004;59:782–7.
170. Chopra A. 124/131I-Labeled apoptosis-targeting peptide-1 (ApoPep-1) 2011 Nov 8 [Updated 1 Dec 2011]. In: Molecular imaging and contrast agent database (MICAD) [Internet]. Bethesda: National Center for Biotechnology Information (US); 2004–2013. Available from: http://www.ncbi.nlm.nih.gov/books/NBK82381/.
171. Niu G, Chen X. Apoptosis imaging: beyond annexin V. J Nucl Med. 2010;51:1659–62.
172. Wang F, Fang W, Zhao M, et al. Imaging paclitaxel (chemotherapy)-induced tumor apoptosis with 99mTc C2A, a domain of synaptotagmin I: a preliminary study. Nucl Med Biol. 2008;35(3):359–64.
173. Nguyen QD, Smith G, Glaser M, Perumal M, Arstad E, Aboagye EO. Positron emission tomography imaging of drug-induced tumor apoptosis with a caspase-3/7 specific [18F]-labeled isatin sulfonamide. Proc Natl Acad Sci U S A. 2009;106:16375–80.
174. Vangestel C, Peeters M, Mees G, et al. In vivo imaging of apoptosis in oncology: an update. Mol Imaging. 2011;10(5):340–58.
175. Oborski MJ, Laymon CM, Lieberman FS, Drappatz J, Hamilton RL, Mountz JM. First use of (18)F-labeled ML-10 PET to assess apoptosis change in a newly diagnosed glioblastoma multiforme patient before and early after therapy. Brain Behav. 2014;4(2):312–5.
176. Wells P, Gunn RN, Alison M, et al. Assessment of proliferation in vivo using 2-[(11)C]thymidine positron emission tomography in advanced intra-abdominal malignancies. Cancer Res. 2002;62:5698–702.
177. Shields AF. Positron emission tomography measurement of tumor metabolism and growth: its expanding role in oncology. Mol Imaging Biol. 2006;8:141–50.
178. Shields AF, Grierson JR, Dohmen BM, et al. Imaging proliferation in vivo with [F-18]FLT and positron emission tomography. Nat Med. 1998;4:1334–6.
179. Chalkidou A, Landau DB, Odell EW, Cornelius VR, O'Doherty MJ, Marsden PK. Correlation between Ki-67 immunohistochemistry and 18F-fluorothymidine uptake in patients with cancer: a systematic review and meta-analysis. Eur J Cancer. 2012;48(18):3499–513.
180. Yamamoto Y, Nishiyama Y, Ishikawa S, et al. Correlation of 18F-FLT and 18F-FDG uptake on PET with Ki-67 immunohistochemistry in non-small cell lung cancer. Eur J Nucl Med Mol Imaging. 2007;34(10):1610–6.
181. Leyton J, Alao JP, Da Costa M, et al. In vivo biological activity of the histone deacetylase inhibitor LAQ824 is detectable with 3′-deoxy-3′-[18F]fluorothymidine positron emission tomography. Cancer Res. 2006;66:7621–9.
182. Yamamoto Y, Ono Y, Aga F, Kawai N, Kudomi N, Nishiyama Y. Correlation of 18F-FLT uptake with tumor grade and Ki-67 immunohistochemistry in patients with newly diagnosed and recurrent gliomas. J Nucl Med. 2012;53(12):1911–5.
183. Pio BS, Park CK, Pietras R, et al. Usefulness of 3′-[F-18]fluoro-3′-deoxythymidine with positron emission tomography in predicting breast cancer response to therapy. Mol Imaging Biol. 2006;8: 36–42.
184. Kenny L, Coombes RC, Vigushin DM, Al-Nahhas A, Shousha S, Aboagye EO. Imaging early changes in proliferation at 1 week post chemotherapy: a pilot study in breast cancer patients with 3′-deoxy-3′-[18F]fluorothymidine positron emission tomography. Eur J Nucl Med Mol Imaging. 2007;34:1339–47.
185. Dittmann H, Dohmen BM, Kehlbach R, Bartusek G, Pritzkow M, Sarbia M, et al. Early changes in [18F] FLT uptake after chemotherapy: an experimental study. Eur J Nucl Med Mol Imaging. 2002;29: 1462–9.
186. Schwartz JL, Tamura Y, Jordan R, Grierson JR, Krohn KA. Monitoring tumor cell proliferation by targeting DNA synthetic processes with thymidine and thymidine analogs. J Nucl Med. 2003;44:2027–32.
187. Barwick T, Bencherif B, Mountz JM, Avril N. Molecular PET and PET/CT imaging of tumour cell proliferation using F-18 fluoro-L-thymidine: a comprehensive evaluation. Nucl Med Commun. 2009;30(12):908–17.
188. Bading JR, Shields AF. Imaging of cell proliferation: status and prospects. J Nucl Med. 2008;49 Suppl 2:64S–80.
189. Been LB, Suurmeijer AJ, Cobben DC, Jager PL, Hoekstra HJ, Elsinga PH. [18F]FLT-PET in oncology: current status and opportunities. Eur J Nucl Med Mol Imaging. 2004;31:1659–72.
190. Reske SN, Deisenhofer S. Is 3-deoxy-3-(18) F-fluorothymidine a better marker for tumour response than (18)F-fluorodeoxyglucose? Eur J Nucl Med Mol Imaging. 2006;33 Suppl 13:38–43.
191. Kenny LM, Vigushin DM, Al-Nahhas A, et al. Quantification of cellular proliferation in tumor and normal tissues of patients with breast cancer by [18F]fluorothymidine-positron emission tomography imaging: evaluation of analytical methods. Cancer Res. 2005;65:10104–12.
192. Conti PS, Alauddin MM, Fissekis JR, Schmall B, Watanabe KA. Synthesis of 2′-fluoro-5-[11C]-methyl-1-beta-D-arabinofuranosyluracil ([11C]-FMAU): a potential nucleoside analog for in vivo study of cellular proliferation with PET. Nucl Med Biol. 1995;22:783–9.

193. Bading JR, Shahinian AH, Vail A, et al. Pharmacokinetics of the thymidine analog 2′-fluoro-5-methyl-1-beta-D-arabinofuranosyluracil (FMAU) in tumor-bearing rats. Nucl Med Biol. 2004;31:407–18.
194. Sun H, Mangner TJ, Collins JM, Muzik O, Douglas K, Shields AF. Imaging DNA synthesis in vivo with 18F-FMAU and PET. J Nucl Med. 2005;46:292–6.
195. Sun H, Sloan A, Mangner TJ, et al. Imaging DNA synthesis with [18F]FMAU and positron emission tomography in patients with cancer. Eur J Nucl Med Mol Imaging. 2005;32:15–22.
196. Muzi M, Spence AM, O'Sullivan F, et al. Kinetic analysis of 3′-deoxy-3′-18F-fluorothymidine in patients with gliomas. J Nucl Med. 2006;47:1612–21.
197. Wheeler KT, Wang LM, Wallen CA, Childers SR, Cline JM, Keng PC, et al. Sigma-2 receptors as a biomarker of proliferation in solid tumours. Br J Cancer. 2000;82:1223–32.
198. Hashimoto K, Ishiwata K. Sigma receptor ligands: possible application as therapeutic drugs and as radiopharmaceuticals. Curr Pharm Des. 2006;12:3857–76.
199. Al-Nabulsi I, Mach RH, Wang LM, Wallen CA, Keng PC, Sten K, et al. Effect of ploidy, recruitment, environmental factors, and tamoxifen treatment on the expression of sigma-2 receptors in proliferating and quiescent tumour cells. Br J Cancer. 1999;81:925–33.
200. Tu Z, Xu J, Jones LA, Li S, Dumstorff C, Vangveravong S, et al. Fluorine-18-labeled benzamide analogues for imaging the sigma2 receptor status of solid tumors with positron emission tomography. J Med Chem. 2007;50:3194–204.
201. Tu Z, Xu J, Jones LA, Li S, Zeng D, Kung MP, et al. Radiosynthesis and biological evaluation of a promising sigma(2)-receptor ligand radiolabeled with fluorine-18 or iodine-125 as a PET/SPECT probe for imaging breast cancer. Appl Radiat Isot. 2010;68:2268–73.
202. Salomon DS, Brandt R, Ciardiello F, Normanno N. Epidermal growth factor-related peptides and their receptors in human malignancies. Crit Rev Oncol Hematol. 1995;19:183–232.
203. Laskin JJ, Sandler AB. Epidermal growth factor receptor: a promising target in solid tumours. Cancer Treat Rev. 2004;30:1–17.
204. Hynes NE, Lane HA. ERBB receptors and cancer: the complexity of targeted inhibitors. Nat Rev Cancer. 2005;5:341–54.
205. Niesen J, Stein C, Brehm H, Hehmann-Titt G, Fendel R, Melmer G, Fischer R, Barth S. Novel EGFR-specific immunotoxins based on panitumumab and cetuximab show in vitro and ex vivo activity against different tumor entities. J Cancer Res Clin Oncol. 2015;141(6):1049–61.
206. Fan Z, Masui H, Altas I, Mendelsohn J. Blockade of epidermal growth factor receptor function by bivalent and monovalent fragments of 225 anti-epidermal growth factor receptor monoclonal antibodies. Cancer Res. 1993;53:4322–8.
207. Cai W, Chen K, He L, Cao Q, Koong A, Chen X. Quantitative PET of EGFR expression in xenograft-bearing mice using 64Cu-labeled cetuximab, a chimeric anti-EGFR monoclonal antibody. Eur J Nucl Med Mol Imaging. 2007;34:850–8.
208. Niu G, Li Z, Xie J, Le QT, Chen X. PET of EGFR antibody distribution in head and neck squamous cell carcinoma models. J Nucl Med. 2009;50:1116–23.
209. Mortimer JE, Bading JR, Colcher DM, Conti PS, Frankel PH, Carroll MI, Tong S, Poku E, Miles JK, Shively JE, Raubitschek AA. Functional imaging of human epidermal growth factor receptor 2-positive metastatic breast cancer using (64)Cu-DOTA-trastuzumab PET. J Nucl Med. 2014;55(1):23–9.
210. Liu Z, Liu Y, Jia B, et al. Epidermal growth factor receptor–targeted radioimmunotherapy of human head and neck cancer xenografts using 90Y-labeled fully human antibody panitumumab. Mol Cancer Ther. 2010;9(8):2297–308.
211. Niu G, Cai W, Chen X. Molecular imaging of human epidermal growth factor receptor 2 (HER-2) expression. Front Biosci. 2008;13:790–805.
212. Velikyan I, Sundberg AL, Lindhe O, et al. Preparation and evaluation of (68)Ga-DOTA-hEGF for visualization of EGFR expression in malignant tumors. J Nucl Med. 2005;46:1881–8.
213. Smith-Jones PM, Solit D, Afroze F, Rosen N, Larson SM. Early tumor response to Hsp90 therapy using HER2 PET: comparison with 18F-FDG PET. J Nucl Med. 2006;47:793–6.
214. Dijkers EC, Oude Munnink TH, Kosterink JG, Brouwers AH, Jager PL, de Jong JR, van Dongen GA, Schröder CP, Lub-de Hooge MN, de Vries EG. Biodistribution of 89Zr-trastuzumab and PET imaging of HER2-positive lesions in patients with metastatic breast cancer. Clin Pharmacol Ther. 2010;87(5):586–92.
215. Oude Munnink TH, Korte MA, Nagengast WB, Timmer-Bosscha H, Schröder CP, Jong JR, Dongen GA, Jensen MR, Quadt C, Hooge MN, Vries EG. (89)Zr-trastuzumab PET visualises HER2 downregulation by the HSP90 inhibitor NVP-AUY922 in a human tumour xenograft. Eur J Cancer. 2010;46(3):678–84.
216. van de Watering FC, Rijpkema M, Perk L, Brinkmann U, Oyen WJ, Boerman OC. Zirconium-89 labeled antibodies: a new tool for molecular imaging in cancer patients. Biomed Res Int. 2014;2014:203601. doi:10.1155/2014/203601. Epub 2014 May 28.
217. Bodei L, Paganelli G, Mariani G. Receptor radionuclide therapy of tumors: a road from basic research to clinical applications. J Nucl Med. 2006;47:375–7.
218. Reubi JC, Maecke HR. Peptide-based probes for cancer imaging. J Nucl Med. 2008;49(11):1735–8.
219. Reubi JC, Waser B. Concomitant expression of several peptide receptors in neuroendocrine tumours:

molecular basis for in vivo multireceptor tumour targeting. Eur J Nucl Med Mol Imaging. 2003;30: 781–93.
220. Scarpignato C, Pelosini I. Somatostatin analogs for cancer treatment and diagnosis: an overview. Chemotherapy. 2001;47 Suppl 2:1–29.
221. Forrer F, Valkema R, Kwekkeboom DJ, de Jong M, Krenning EP. Neuroendocrine tumors. Peptide receptor radionuclide therapy. Best Pract Res Clin Endocrinol Metab. 2007;21:111–29.
222. Rindi G, Klöppel G, Couvelard A, Komminoth P, Körner M, Lopes JM, McNicol AM, Nilsson O, Perren A, Scarpa A, Scoazec JY, Wiedenmann B. TNM staging of midgut and hindgut (neuro) endocrine tumors: a consensus proposal including a grading system. Virchows Arch. 2007;451(4):757–62.
223. Wang L, Tang K, Zhang Q, Li H, Wen Z, Zhang H, Zhang H. Somatostatin receptor-based molecular imaging and therapy for neuroendocrine tumors. Biomed Res Int. 2013;2013:102819.
224. Seregni E, Chiti A, Bombardieri E. Radionuclide imaging of neuroendocrine tumours: biological basis and diagnostic results. Eur J Nucl Med. 1998;25(6): 639–58. Review.
225. Klimstra DS, Modlin IR, Coppola D, Lloyd RV, Suster S. The pathologic classification of neuroendocrine tumors: a review of nomenclature, grading, and staging systems. Pancreas. 2010;39:707–12.
226. Koopmans KP, Neels ON, Kema IP, Elsinga PH, Links TP, de Vries EG, Jager PL. Molecular imaging in neuroendocrine tumors: molecular uptake mechanisms and clinical results. Crit Rev Oncol Hematol. 2009;71(3):199–213.
227. Kwekkeboom DJ, de Herder WW, van Eijck CHJ, et al. Peptide receptor radionuclide therapy in patients with gastroenteropancreatic neuroendocrine tumors. Semin Nucl Med. 2010;40(2):78–88.
228. Xu C, Zhang H. Somatostatin receptor based imaging and radionuclide therapy. Biomed Res Int. 2015;2015:917968. Epub 2015 Mar 24.
229. Ambrosini V, Campana D, Tomassetti P, Fanti S. 68Ga-labelled peptides for diagnosis of gastroenteropancreatic NET. Eur J Nucl Med Mol Imaging. 2012;39 Suppl 1:S52–60.
230. Mojtahedi A, Thamake S, Tworowska I, Ranganathan D, Delpassand ES. The value of 68Ga-DOTATATE PET/CT in diagnosis and management of neuroendocrine tumors compared to current FDA approved imaging modalities: a review of literature. Am J Nucl Med Mol Imaging. 2014;4(5):426–34.
231. Bison SM, Konijnenberg MW, Melis M, et al. Peptide receptor radionuclide therapy using radiolabeled somatostatin analogs: focus on future developments. Clin Transl Imaging. 2014;2(1):55–66.
232. Teunissen JJ, Kwekkeboom DJ, Valkema R, Krenning EP. Nuclear medicine techniques for the imaging and treatment of neuroendocrine tumours. Endocr Relat Cancer. 2011;18 Suppl 1:S27–51.
233. Koukouraki S, Strauss LG, Georgoulias V, Eisenhut M, Haberkorn U, Dimitrakopoulou-Strauss A. Comparison of the pharmacokinetics of 68Ga-DOTATOC and [18F] FDG in patients with metastatic neuroendocrine tumours scheduled for 90Y-DOTATOC therapy. Eur J Nucl Med Mol Imaging. 2006;33(10):1115–22.
234. Haug AR, Auernhammer CJ, Wängler B, Schmidt GP, Uebleis C, Göke B, Cumming P, Bartenstein P, Tiling R, Hacker M. 68Ga-DOTATATE PET/CT for the early prediction of response to somatostatin receptor-mediated radionuclide therapy in patients with well-differentiated neuroendocrine tumors. J Nucl Med. 2010;51(9):1349–56.
235. Koukouraki S, Strauss LG, Georgoulias V, et al. Evaluation of the pharmacokinetics of 68Ga-DOTATOC in patients with metastatic neuroendocrine tumours scheduled for 90Y-DOTATOC therapy. Eur J Nucl Med Mol Imaging. 2006;33(4):460–6.
236. Poeppel TD, Binse I, Petersenn S, et al. 68Ga-DOTATOC versus 68Ga-DOTATATE PET/CT in functional imaging of neuroendocrine tumors. J Nucl Med. 2011;52(12):1864–70.
237. Blau M, Nagler W, Bender MA. A new isotope for bone scanning. J Nucl Med. 1962;3:332–4.
238. Fischer DR, Maquieira GJ, Espinosa N, et al. Therapeutic impact of [(18)F]fluoride positron-emission tomography/computed tomography on patients with unclear foot pain. Skeletal Radiol. 2010;39(10):987–97.
239. Vallabhajosula S. 18F-labeled positron emission tomographic radiopharmaceuticals in oncology: an overview of radiochemistry and mechanisms of tumor localization. Semin Nucl Med. 2007;37:400–19.
240. Hetzel M, Arslandemir C, Konig HH, et al. F-18 NaF PET for detection of bone metastases in lung cancer: accuracy, cost-effectiveness, and impact on patient management. J Bone Miner Res. 2003;18:2206–14.
241. Groves AM, Win T, Ben Haim S, et al. Non-[18F] FDG PET in clinical oncology. Lancet Oncol. 2007;8:822–30.
242. Even-Sapir E, Metser U, Flusser G, et al. Assessment of malignant skeletal disease with 18F-fluoride PET/CT. J Nucl Med. 2004;45:272–8.
243. Iagaru A, Mittra E, Yaghoubi SS, et al. Novel strategy for cocktail 18F-flouride and 18F-FDG PET/CT scan for evaluation of malignancy: results of a pilot-phase study. J Nucl Med. 2009;50:501–5.
244. Megalizzi V, Le Mercier M, Decaestecker C. Sigma receptors and their ligands in cancer biology: overview and new perspectives for cancer therapy. Med Res Rev. 2012;32(2):410–27.
245. Balkwill F. The significance of cancer cell expression of the chemokine receptor CXCR4. Semin Cancer Biol. 2004;14:171–9.
246. Jacobson O, Weiss ID, Kiesewetter DO, Farber JM, Chen X. PET of tumor CXCR4 expression with 4-18F-T140. J Nucl Med. 2010;51:1796–804.
247. Shim H, Oishi S, Fujii N. Chemokine receptor CXCR4 as a therapeutic target for neuroectodermal tumors. Semin Cancer Biol. 2009;19:123–34.
248. Misra P, Lebeche D, Ly H, Schwarzkopf M, Diaz G, Hajjar RJ, et al. Quantitation of CXCR4 expression

in myocardial infarction using 99mTc-labeled SDF-1alpha. J Nucl Med. 2008;49:963–9.
249. Jacobson O, Weiss ID, Szajek L, Farber JM, Kiesewetter DO. 64Cu-AMD3100–a novel imaging agent for targeting chemokine receptor CXCR4. Bioorg Med Chem. 2009;17:1486–93.
250. Nimmagadda S, Pullambhatla M, Stone K, Green G, Bhujwalla ZM, Pomper MG. Molecular imaging of CXCR4 receptor expression in human cancer xenografts with [64Cu]AMD3100 positron emission tomography. Cancer Res. 2010;70:3935–44.
251. Shim H, Zhu A, Yoon Y, Liang Z, Voll R, Goodman MM. Development of novel small molecule F-18 labeled CXCR4 PET tracer for head and neck cancer. RSNA 2010. ID 9012133, Chicago.
252. Szakács G, Paterson JK, Ludwig JA, Booth-Genthe C, Gottesman MM. Targeting multidrug resistance in cancer. Nat Rev Drug Discov. 2006; 5:219–34.
253. Ling V. Multidrug resistance: molecular mechanisms and clinical relevance. Cancer Chemother Pharmacol. 1997;40(Suppl):S3–8.
254. Dizdarevic S, Peters AM. Imaging of multidrug resistance in cancer. Cancer Imaging. 2011;11:1–8.
255. Kyle SD, Law WP, Miles KA. Predicting tumour response. Cancer Imaging. 2013;13(3):381–90.
256. Nagengast WB, Oude Munnink TH, Dijkers EC, et al. Multidrug resistance in oncology and beyond: from imaging of drug efflux pumps to cellular drug targets. Methods Mol Biol. 2010; 596:15–31.
257. Sharma V, Prior JL, Belinsky MG, Kruh GD, Piwnica-Worms D. Characterization of a 67Ga/68Ga radiopharmaceutical for SPECT and PET of MDR1 P-glycoprotein transport activity in vivo: validation in multidrug-resistant tumors and at the blood–brain barrier. J Nucl Med. 2005;46:354–64.
258. Kannan P, John C, Zoghbi SS, Halldin C, Gottesman MM, Innis RB, Hall MD. Imaging the function of P-glycoprotein with radiotracers: pharmacokinetics and in vivo applications. Clin Pharmacol Ther. 2009;86(4):368–77.
259. Mohan HK, Miles KA. Cost-effectiveness of 99mTc-sestamibi in predicting response to chemotherapy in patients with lung cancer: systematic review and meta-analysis. J Nucl Med. 2009; 50(3):376–81.

18 Clinical Applications of PET/CT in Oncology

Abhishek Mahajan and Gary Cook

Contents

18.1 **Introduction** 430

18.2 **FDG-PET for Tumour Detection and Monitoring Tumour Response** 430

18.3 **Lung Cancer** 431

18.4 **Lymphoma** 432

18.5 **Breast Cancer** 435

18.6 **Malignant Melanoma** 437

18.7 **Head and Neck Cancer** 437

18.8 **Thyroid Cancer** 438

18.9 **Oesophageal Cancer** 438

18.10 **Colorectal Cancer** 439

18.11 **Gynaecological Cancers** 441
18.11.1 Cervical Cancer 441
18.11.2 Ovarian Cancer 441

18.12 **Pitfalls** 443

18.13 **PET in Clinical Trials** 443

18.14 **The Future** 443

Conclusion 443

References 444

Abstract

FDG-PET, and more recently PET/CT, has become an established clinical tool for aiding cancer management. Despite a number of new tracers that have specific clinical and research applications, FDG remains the most commonly used radiopharmaceutical for tumour characterisation, staging, response assessment and surveillance. FDG-PET/CT is now a routine investigation in many common cancers, including lung, lymphoma, oesophageal and colorectal cancers, affecting management decisions at a number of points in the treatment pathway.

In addition, FDG-PET/CT, as a downstream marker of drug effect, is now more commonly adopted into clinical trials as an imaging biomarker to determine early therapeutic response to novel cancer therapeutics with the development of quantitative and semiquantitative methods for objective measurements and response categorisation.

A. Mahajan, MBBS, MD
Department of Radiodiagnosis, Tata Memorial Hospital, Mumbai 400012, India
e-mail: drabhishek.mahajan@yahoo.in

G. Cook, MB BS, MSc, MD, FRCR, FRCP (✉)
Division of Imaging Sciences and Biomedical Engineering, King's College London and the King's College London and Guys & St Thomas' PET Centre, St Thomas' Hospital, London, UK
e-mail: gary.cook@kcl.ac.uk

M.M. Khalil (ed.), *Basic Science of PET Imaging*, DOI 10.1007/978-3-319-40070-9_18

With continued improvements in scanner design, reconstruction and analysis software, as well as the introduction of hybrid PET/MRI, it is highly likely that FDG-PET will remain an important clinical cancer imaging tool for years to come.

18.1 Introduction

In the previous chapter, we illustrated that non-FDG-PET tracer imaging using positron-emitting radioisotopes coupled to specific ligands is emerging as a sensitive molecular imaging technique. A wide range of biological pathways and molecular aberrations can be imaged with these radiolabelled ligands. However FDG-PET/CT still remains the bedrock imaging modality that provides combined anatomic and functional information and plays an intricate role in oncological imaging. With the extensive clinical experience with FDG for varied applications in oncology, FDG is an important agent in the assessment of tumour biology and therapy response assessment. We will highlight the main applications, advantages and limitations of FDG-PET/CT in oncology that will provide guidance for medical/radiation/surgical oncologists and other imaging and oncological specialists on the use of FDG-PET/CT in oncology.

18.2 FDG-PET for Tumour Detection and Monitoring Tumour Response

FDG-PET/CT has a wide application in clinical oncology ranging from tumour detection to staging of disease and diagnosis of residual or recurrent cancer [1]. The most common cancers imaged include lymphoma, lung, oesophagus, breast, colorectal, melanoma, head and neck, cervical and thyroid [2–4]. Tumours such as melanoma, high-grade lymphomas and most lung cancers show high FDG avidity [2, 3, 5]. In contrast tumours such as well-differentiated hepatocellular carcinoma and prostate cancers generally show low uptake making FDG-PET imaging of limited clinical utility in the detection and staging of these tumours [6, 7]. Some other tumours such as breast and thyroid cancers and sarcomas have variable FDG uptake, which, in addition to differences in underlying histological subtype and level of differentiation, is dependent on a number of biological factors which are not all completely understood [8–11].

For example, differentiated thyroid cancer that retains iodine avidity and androgen-sensitive differentiated prostate cancer tend to have low FDG uptake. In contrast, their dedifferentiated types, i.e. iodine negative thyroid cancers and androgen refractory prostate cancers, are typically FDG avid and easily detected by FDG-PET imaging [12, 13]. As the increased rate of metabolism is not specific to malignant cells, many non-malignant tissues may show avid FDG uptake causing potential false-positive diagnoses [14, 15]. Examples include inflammation, activated brown fat and active skeletal muscles. Though combined PET and CT fused images enhance specificity in sites unrelated to malignant tissue, substantial expertise is needed to accurately interpret FDG-PET/CT data. Low sensitivity and moderate specificity for detecting early-stage tumours, in general, limit the use of FDG-PET imaging for cancer screening. However, the judicial use of FDG in the appropriate clinical setting makes FDG-PET/CT a valuable clinical imaging tool [16].

Evidence for the utilisation of FDG-PET imaging to monitor response to therapy was delayed in comparison to its use for pretherapy staging [1]. One of the earliest reported studies which evaluated the role of FDG-PET in response assessment evaluated the role of FDG-PET to assess response to chemotherapy in advanced breast cancer and correlated it with response on histopathology [17, 18]. Currently in the United States, the use of FDG-PET is approved only for initial antitumour treatment strategy evaluation for breast cancer [1].

Following this, many studies have supported the role of FDG-PET in response assessment in a variety of malignancies treated with various single or combination therapies. In a number of studies, it showed correlation with outcome, such as progression-free, disease-free and overall survival [1, 19–23]. FDG-PET is found to have the ability to discern post cytotoxic chemotherapy response after a single cycle of chemotherapy in some cancers such as lymphomas, breast cancers and gastrointestinal cancers [17, 19, 20, 24–26].

The biology behind regression of FDG uptake after chemotherapy is not completely understood. However, a reduction in the number of viable tumour cells and the rate at which glucose is consumed per cell has shown correlation with reduction in FDG uptake [25]. Early data using C11-thymidine PET in small-cell lung cancer and high-grade sarcoma have revealed that tumour proliferation declines prior to changes seen in glycolysis. Recent studies on the mechanism of alteration in FDG uptake after imatinib therapy for gastrointestinal stromal tumours which inhibits the c-kit pathway revealed that regression in glycolysis and hence FDG uptake takes place within 1–2 days after initiation of therapy [27–30]. In this case, changes in FDG uptake were found to precede changes in tumour proliferation and tumour cell death. These mechanisms are not completely understood; recent studies have implicated a rapid decline of glucose transporter expression for it [31]. However, further studies are needed to elucidate the precise mechanisms underlying changes in FDG PET and its role in evaluating early response to this class of drugs [31, 32].

Rather than a decrease in FDG uptake, some studies have shown a flare of FDG uptake after therapy which predicts a response to therapy. Mortimer et al. evaluated the role of FDG-PET in biopsy-proven advanced ER-positive {ER(+)} breast cancer treated with tamoxifen and found increased uptake of FDG uptake 1–2 weeks after commencing therapy. This increased FDG uptake indicated early agonist or "flare" associated with tamoxifen therapy [33]. Similar findings are noted in assessing response to radiotherapy where FDG uptake may increase early after radiotherapy [34]. The mechanism underlying this finding was found to be associated with a different and more prolonged period of cell viability and attempted repair before cell death for radiotherapy versus chemotherapy in addition to an inflammatory response to radiotherapy with associated white cell FDG activity [16, 35]. An increase in FDG uptake following radiotherapy is seen to be a predictive marker of better outcome in high-grade gliomas [35]. An increase in FDG metabolic rate from pre- to post-RT in adults with malignant gliomas having longer survival was postulated to be due to one or more of the following reasons: (a) apoptosis of tumour cells in response to RT requires energy; (b) decreased tumour cell density by the RT leaves normal cells with higher metabolism; or (c) inflammatory cells infiltrate and take up glucose or FDG where tumour cells are dying [35].

Interpreting response data from FDG-PET needs caution, as most of the data is from smaller trials that have compared the findings with standard size-based response criteria. Some studies did have relevant end points, correlating the post-therapy FDG-PET findings to time to progression, disease-free survival and overall survival [7, 19, 20, 36–38]. For response, FDG-PET is most commonly used in lymphoma and breast cancer, where it has approval for Medicare payment for response evaluation. Multicentre trials are being undertaken to evaluate the predictive role of serial FDG-PET imaging in head and neck cancer, sarcoma, lung cancer and other tumours [34].

18.3 Lung Cancer

Lung cancer is the leading cause of cancer-related death in both men and women. Nearly 80% of lung cancers are non-small-cell lung cancer (NSCLC). Otherwise difficult to treat with significant morbidity and mortality, early-stage NSCLC has the potential to be radically cured by surgery. The role of FDG-PET has been extensively evaluated in lung cancers, and it has been found to be of value in not only diagnosing and staging early disease (e.g. solitary pulmonary nodule characterisation, nodal and distant metastasis detection) but has a very high overall sensitivity, specificity and accuracy in detecting residual and recurrent lung cancer [39–42]. The use of FDG-PET for initial and subsequent treatment strategies of NSCLC is covered under CMS. The clinical indication of FDG-PET/CT indeterminate solitary pulmonary nodules (SPNs) is reserved for cases where CT-guided fine-needle biopsy either is technically difficult or has been non-diagnostic [43]. The sensitivity of FDG-PET is comparable to CT. However, FDG-PET has shown higher specificity for depicting malignancy in SPNs, the reported values ranging from 81 % to 100 % and from 63 % to 100 %, respectively [44–46].

FDG-PET/CT imaging is shown to be the most accurate imaging modality for staging NSCLC, with accuracies for tumour (T), nodal (N) and metastases (M) staging of 70–97 %, 78–93 % and 83–96 %, respectively [47, 48]. In a systematic review, the pooled sensitivity and specificity of FDG-PET for differentiating benign from malignant pulmonary nodules in over 1200 patients were found to be 96 % and 80 %, respectively, and for nodal staging it was 88 % and 92 % [49]. The PET in Lung Cancer Staging (PLUS) study showed that FDG-PET is more accurate than conventional imaging for staging workup and significantly improved the management of the patients with unresectable disease. Compared to patients staged by conventional imaging, the overall healthcare costs and morbidity were reduced by preventing futile thoracotomies in patients with locally advanced disease or metastatic disease staged by using FDG-PET [50]. For predicting mediastinal nodal disease, FDG-PET was reported to have a sensitivity and specificity of 67–92 % and 82–99 %, respectively, which was significantly higher than that for CT alone (25–71 % and 66–98 %, respectively). Overall, correct staging by FDG-PET was documented in 85–96 % and was seen to be 58–59 % by conventional CT alone [51–53]. FDG-PET had a negative predictive value of 97 % for mediastinal nodal disease, and this high NPV of FDG-PET/CT is the basis of the current recommendations to omit mediastinoscopy in patients with FDG-PET/CT-negative mediastinal nodes [54–57]. However, central tumours have a higher incidence of occult N2 disease and this needs consideration while staging with FDG-PET/CT [58, 59]. Another study evaluating the role of FDG-PET for monitoring therapy response and prediction of patient outcome after neoadjuvant radiochemotherapy in 70 patients with NSCLC showed sensitivity, specificity and overall accuracy of 95 %, 80 % and 91 %, respectively, for the detection of viable residual primary tumour and 77 %, 68 % and 73 %, respectively, for detecting lymph node metastases [60]. As it allows more accurate initial staging, FDG-PET is strongly recommended for guiding radiation therapy planning. This potentially reduces the elective radiation to the uninvolved nodal stations and allows inclusion of otherwise occult nodal disease as well as changing management in patients who have occult distant metastases [61–63]. See Chap. 22 for further details.

FDG-PET also has a role in the detection of recurrence and restaging of lung cancers after therapy. Studies on the use of FDG-PET in differentiation of recurrent or small residual tumours from post-therapy changes, which may appear identical on conventional CT imaging, have revealed very high overall sensitivity, specificity and accuracy. Combined FDG-PET/CT has significantly improved the detection of extrathoracic metastatic disease involving the liver, bones and adrenal glands [64, 65] (Fig. 18.1).

FDG-PET has also shown promise in early assessment of targeted therapies [66, 67]. Post-therapy residual FDG uptake in the tumour is a poor prognostic marker [68]. Irrespective of the cell type or neoadjuvant treatment, regression of baseline SUVmax by 80 % is a predictive marker of complete pathological response and with a sensitivity, specificity and accuracy of 90 %, 100 % and 96 % [69].

18.4 Lymphoma

Lymphomas are the most common and most curable form of primary haematological cancer. Surgery has a limited role in management of these patients and the mainstay of treatment is chemotherapy and radiotherapy. With overall survival rates as high as 90 %, early detection and accurate staging are crucial for appropriate treatment planning, and FDG-PET/CT

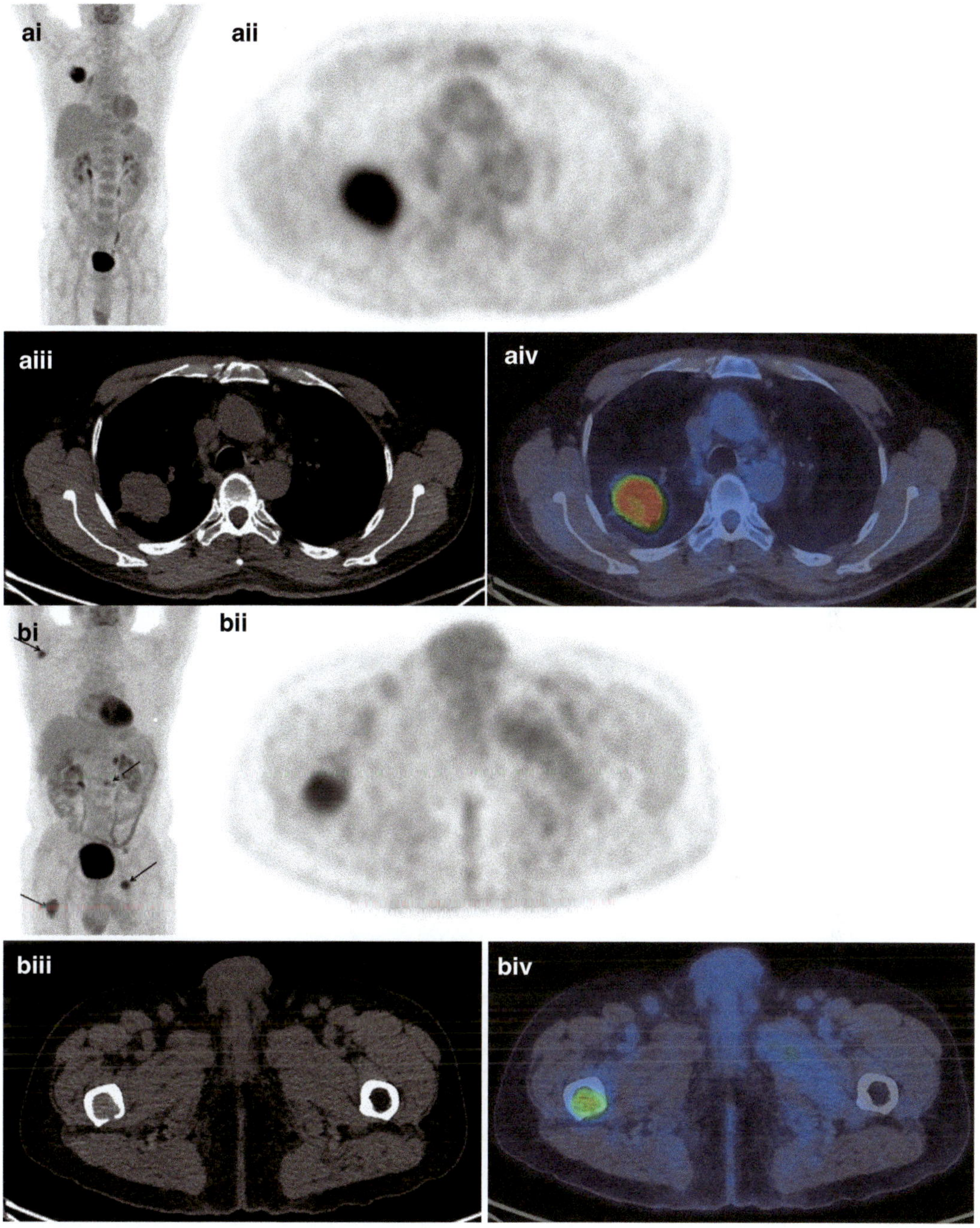

Fig. 18.1 A 67-year-old man had a right upper lobe NSCLC resected. (**a**) FDG-PET/CT scan (i) MIP, (ii) PET, (iii) CT and (iv) fused PET/CT axial images through the thorax demonstrating an active right upper lobe carcinoma with ipsilateral hilar nodal involvement. One year later he complained of bone pain and a follow-up FDG-PET/CT scan (**b**) (i) MIP, (ii) PET, (iii) CT and (iv) fused PET/CT axial images through the right femur showed bone (*right* femur, *left* pelvis, *right* scapula, L2; *arrows*) and left adrenal gland metastases

is recommended for initial staging, assessing response to therapy and post-therapy staging of patients with Hodgkin's disease and high-grade non-Hodgkin lymphomas [70, 71] (Fig. 18.2).

Overall sensitivity and specificity for staging and restaging of Hodgkin's lymphoma are 86 % and 96 %, respectively, which is significantly higher than that by conventional CT imaging (81 % and 41 %, respectively) [72]. Nodal and organ involvement can be predicted with a sensitivity and specificity of 94 % and 100 % with FDG-PET compared to 88 % and 100 % with CT, respectively [73]. FDG-PET/CT is routinely used in diffuse large B-cell lymphoma staging and helps in detecting nodal and extranodal disease sites such as the skeleton, liver and lung [74–76]. In a retrospective review conducted on 130 diffuse large B-cell lymphoma (DLBCL) patients, compared to bone marrow trephine biopsy, FDG-PET/CT was found to have higher overall accuracy in detecting bone and bone marrow (B/BM) involvement by lymphoma, with a sensitivity and specificity of 40 % and 100 % and 94 % and 100 %, respectively. The negative and positive predictive values were 98 % and 100 %, respectively [74]. Low-grade lymphomas, e.g. MALT (mucosa-associated lymphoid tissue) and low-grade follicular lymphoma, are not highly FDG avid and may show higher false-negative rates than in high-grade lymphomas [77, 78].

FDG-PET is useful in differentiating residual tumour from posttreatment fibrosis within residual radiographic masses [79]. Such lesions are seen in up to 50 % of non-Hodgkin's lymphoma and 66 % of Hodgkin's disease, and of

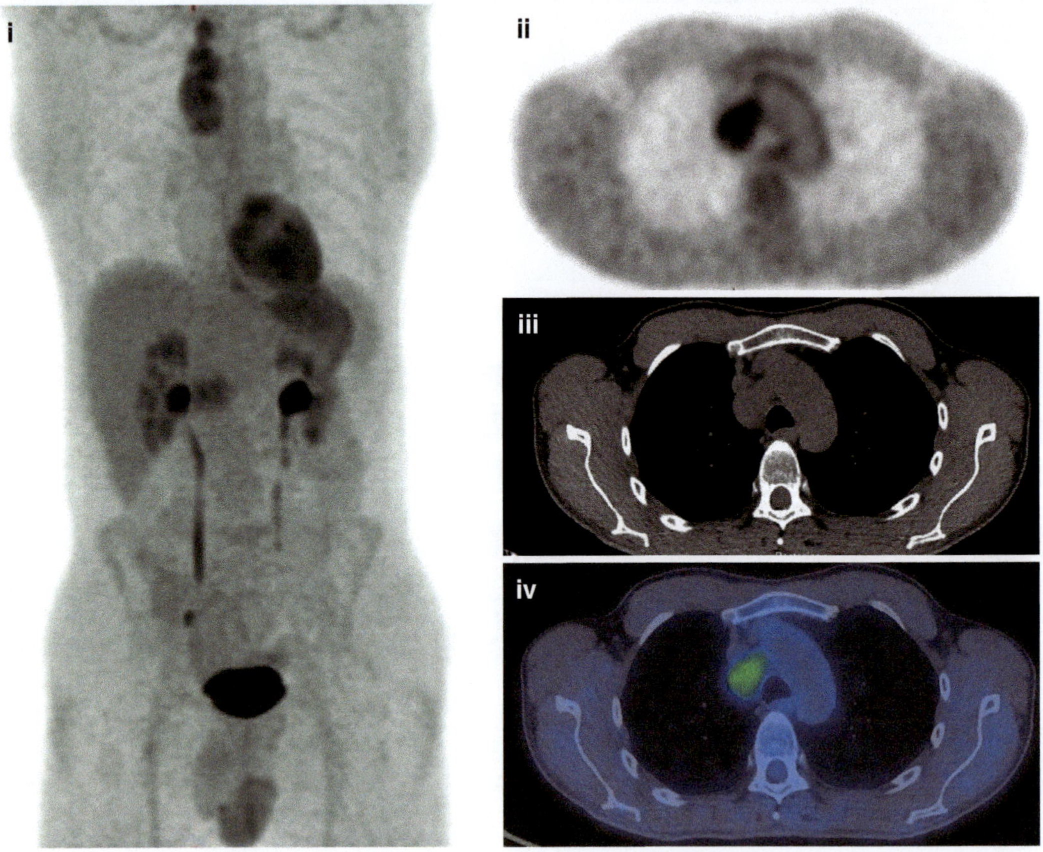

Fig. 18.2 A 27-year-old male with a new diagnosis of Hodgkin's lymphoma showing FDG-avid nodal disease in the mediastinum with no evidence of extranodal disease. FDG-PET/CT scan (i) MIP, (ii) PET, (iii) CT and (iv) fused PET/CT axial images through the mediastinum

these only up to 25 % of non-Hodgkin's lymphoma and 30 % of Hodgkin's disease patients eventually relapse [80, 81]. A prospective study of 58 patients of which 43 were Hodgkin's disease with posttreatment residual disease monitored using FDG-PET showed that SUV ≤3 predicts lack of recurrence ($P = 0.004$) and longer progression-free survival (PFS) ($P < 0.00001$) [82]. Studies have shown that response assessed on mid-treatment FDG-PET is a prognostic indicator for disease-free and overall survival in HL and aggressive NHL, as early as after one to three cycles of chemotherapy. Residual post-therapy disease is seen up to 85 % of cases of HL and up to 40 % of the cases of NHL. Early interim imaging after 2–4 cycles using FDG-PET/CT is found to correlate well with event-free survival in HL and high-grade NHL [83, 84]. FDG-PET imaging is used to tailor therapies by categorising patients with a worse prognosis into subgroups who will benefit from different types of treatment, such as additional radiotherapy to areas of bulky disease or myeloablative chemotherapy followed by stem cell transplantation [79, 85, 86].

18.5 Breast Cancer

Breast cancer is the commonest malignancy in females and is the second leading cause of death. The 5-year survival for localised cancers is approximately 96 % which decreases significantly with regional and distant metastases. FDG-PET is mostly used in the evaluation of recurrent or advanced breast cancer. Other potential clinical applications include staging of axillary lymph nodes and monitoring of response to chemotherapy [87, 88].

Studies have shown no proven role in detecting small and non-invasive primary carcinomas; the overall sensitivity is shown to be only 68 % for tumours of size <2 cm [88, 89]. Dense glandular tissue has relatively high uptake of FDG when compared to adipose tissue within the breast, and hence the tumour contrast is less reliable in dense breast parenchyma [90, 91]. Clinical utility has been shown in the detection of primary invasive breast cancers, mainly infiltrating ductal carcinomas, and in the detection of internal mammary and mediastinal metastases [92]. Further studies reported that the sensitivity of FDG-PET/CT for primary lesions <5 mm was 53 % and 92 % for lesions >20 mm [92]. In large primary cancers with a mean tumour size of 4.3 ± 1.4 cm, the reported sensitivity and specificity of FDG-PET/CT was 77 % and 80 %, respectively [87]. Nodal status is a prognostic and predictive marker of survival in patients with breast cancer. Many clinical studies have evaluated the accuracy of PET imaging in axillary nodal staging of operable breast cancer [93–95]. A systematic review and meta-analysis in 2,460 breast cancer patients revealed that FDG-PET has a wide range of sensitivity ranging from 20 to 100 % and specificity ranging from 65 to 100 % for detecting axillary node metastases [96]. Variable sensitivity (79–94 %) and specificity (86–92 %), and hence insufficient predictive accuracy for axillary nodal staging, preclude the use of FDG-PET as a modality for routine use [97].

For detection of relapse, FDG-PET/CT is found to be more sensitive than the serum tumour marker CA 15-3. It has shown high overall sensitivity, specificity and accuracy for the detection of locoregional recurrence (89 %, 84 % and 87 %, respectively) and distant metastases (100 %, 97 % and 98 %, respectively) [98] (Fig. 18.3). Despite limitations in identifying micrometastases, FDG-PET has an important role in the assessment of breast cancer response to chemotherapy as well as other treatments such as hormonal therapy and radiation [99, 100]. FDG-PET has been used to evaluate response to chemotherapy, and studies have demonstrated that responding tumours have a 40 % or more regression of SUVmax, whereas nonresponding tumours may show increased, stable or a slight decline of SUVmax which is not more than 24 %. The prognosis also correlates in a similar pattern, and patients who show more than a 40 % decrease in SUVmax are found to have a better prognosis [24, 87, 98, 101]. Reduction in FDG activity in cases of bone metastases with associated sclerosis in the CT component of FDG-PET/CT is a sign of response and bone healing [102, 103].

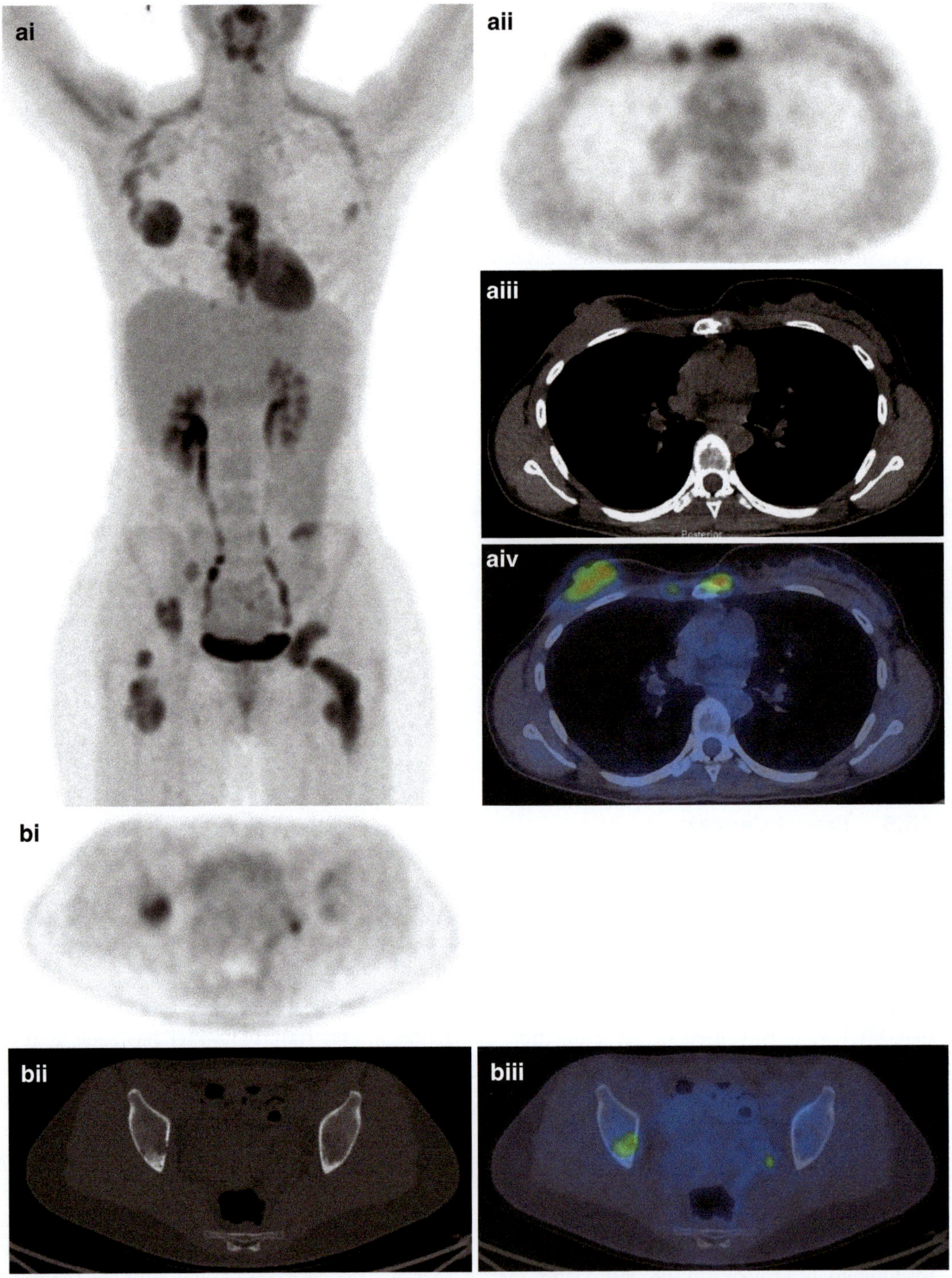

Fig. 18.3 A 39-year-old female with a 3-year history of breast cancer and known relapse referred for restaging. The FDG-PET/CT scan (i) MIP, (ii) PET, (iii) CT and (iv) fused PET/CT axial images through the right breast (**a**) and right pelvis (**b**) shows right breast recurrence with several bone metastases including the sternum, pelvis and femora. There is some physiological brown fat activity but also some right axillary nodal recurrence (ai)

Another important PET tracer is 18 F-fluoroestradiol (FES) which is found to correlate with oestrogen receptor (ER) expression has been used to localise ER-expressing tumours. It has been shown to predict response to salvage hormonal treatment in heavily pretreated metastatic breast cancer patients [104]. In a study of 47 patients with recurrent or metastatic breast cancer with ER-positive tumours, the treatment selection-based quantitative FES-PET showed that the response rate increased from 23 to 34 % overall and from 29 to 46 % in patients lacking HER2/neu overexpression suggesting that quantitative FES-PET can be used for guiding treatment selection [105].

18.6 Malignant Melanoma

Malignant melanomas are known to metastasise extensively anywhere in the body including unusual sites such as meninges, the gastrointestinal tract and myocardium [106, 107]. As these tumours show high FDG uptake, FDG-PET is a sensitive modality for staging patients with high-risk melanomas [108–110]. The reported sensitivity of FDG-PET for detecting visceral and abdominal nodal metastases is as high as 100 % with an accuracy of 100 % for superficial lymph node metastases. However, it has a lower sensitivity for pulmonary metastases, and the CT component of a combined FDG-PET/CT scan allows better evaluation of small pulmonary metastases [111]. A known limitation is in detecting metastases in the brain where normal parenchyma has a high background activity. As compared to CT imaging alone and PET alone, the overall diagnostic accuracy for M staging is significantly higher for FDG-PET/CT (84 %, 93 % vs. 98 %, respectively) (Fig. 18.4). Similarly for N staging, the diagnostic accuracy of CT alone is reported to be 86 %, whereas for FDG-PET/CT, it is 98 %. Baseline PET/CT staging in stage I–IV patients may change treatment in 48.4 % of patients [108, 111–113].

18.7 Head and Neck Cancer

PET imaging using FDG has a significant role in both newly diagnosed as well as treated patients with head and neck cancers [114]. Compared to CT imaging alone, FDG-PET/CT changes the initial clinical stage and TNM category of tumours in 14–57 % of patients with a diagnostic accuracy of approximately 90 % compared with 86 % for conventional CT [115–118]. For lymph node metastases, the per-patient sensitivity and specificity of FDG-PET/CT are reported as 94 % and 84 %, respectively, in comparison to 78 and 84 % for CT alone [119]. FDG-PET/CT imaging has been reported to change the initial management in 18–37 % of patients. It may detect synchronous lesions in 8.1 %, the site of unknown primaries in 73 % and distant metastatic lesions in 15.4 % of patients with head and neck cancer [117, 120]. It also has implications in radiotherapy planning and may influence changes due to the gross tumour volume (GTV) planned by FDG-PET/CT in 57 % of patients leading to a change in the planning radiotherapy field in approximately 29 % of patients [121, 122]. The sensitivity, specificity and accuracy of FDG-PET/CT in restaging patients with head and neck cancer have been reported to be 88 %, 78 % and 86 %, respectively [123].

The pretreatment SUV of the tumour on FDG-PET may have prognostic potential. Machtay et al. found that patients whose lesions showed maximum SUV <9 had 72 % disease-free survival compared to 37 % in patients with lesions having SUV >9. FDG-PET is found to have a very high negative predictive value for the detection of post-therapy recurrence [124]. However, in this setting FDG-PET has a low predictive value in detecting occult nodal metastases with a low positive predictive value due to false-positive lesions related to infective and inflammatory lesions or posttreatment effects. This limitation is partially overcome by FDG-PET/CT, as the posttreatment changes, inflammatory lesions and physiological structures such as brown fat are easily distinguishable from abnormalities on

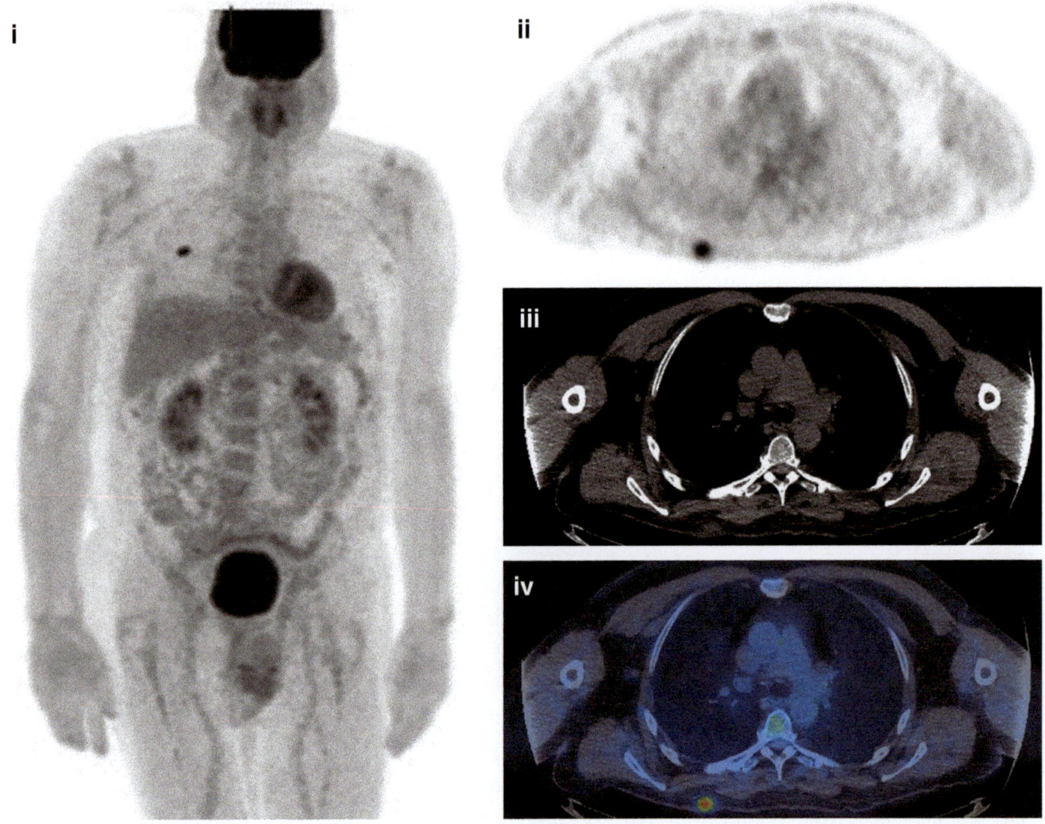

Fig. 18.4 A 30-year-old male with a previous history of a back melanoma referred for routine follow-up imaging. The FDG-PET/CT scan, (i) MIP, (ii) PET, (iii) CT and (iv) fused PET/CT axial images through the thorax, shows a small recurrent skin lesion on the back

FDG-PET/CT images, yet are more challenging to differentiate by PET or CT alone [125–127]. For the detection of primary site residual/recurrent disease and nodal recurrence, FDG-PET/CT is found to have higher sensitivity (88–100 %) and specificity (75–100 %) than CT alone (sensitivity, 38–90 %; specificity, 38–85 %) [128].

18.8 Thyroid Cancer

Approximately 90 % of thyroid malignancies are papillary and follicular carcinomas with well-differentiated morphology [129]. As the tumours become dedifferentiated, they tend to lose sodium iodide symporter expression; this causes inability of the cells to concentrate radioiodine. Similar features are seen in recurrent thyroid cancers and metastatic tumours [130]. In a multicentre trial in patients with increased levels of thyroglobulin and negative whole-body 131-iodine scans, FDG-PET/CT has shown a sensitivity of 85 % and it changed clinical management in 23–51 % of patients [131]. In iodine-refractory thyroid cancer, FDG-PET is found to be a predictive marker for tumour aggressiveness [132–135] (Fig. 18.5).

18.9 Oesophageal Cancer

FDG-PET/CT is recommended for initial M staging of oesophageal cancer and detects unexpected metastatic foci which are present in up to 30 % of patients [136–138]. Synchronous primary oesophageal tumours are detected in 5.5 % of patients which otherwise were not identified on conventional imaging [139–141]. It results in downstaging of disease in 5–7 % and upstaging in 15–20 %.

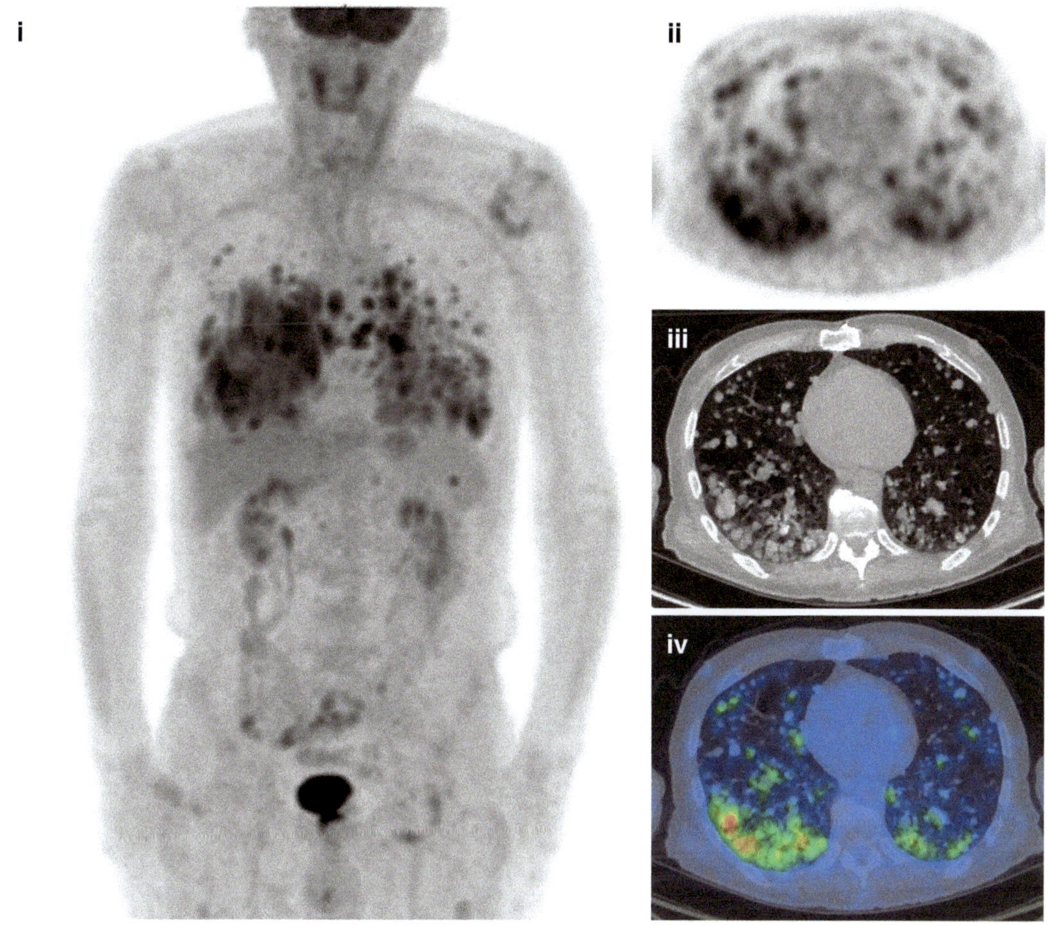

Fig. 18.5 A 62-year-old male with undifferentiated thyroid cancer demonstrating many FDG-avid pulmonary metastases. 131 iodine scans were negative. (i) MIP, (ii) PET, (iii) CT and (iv) fused PET/CT axial images through the thorax

For the detection of distant metastases, FDG-PET/CT has an overall sensitivity, specificity and accuracy of 43–78 %, 93–99 % and 62–86 %, respectively, which is better than CT and endoscopic ultrasound (EUS) [142, 143] (Fig. 18.6). FDG-PET has a diagnostic accuracy of 85 % in assessment of therapeutic response to neoadjuvant chemotherapy and is found to be an important prognostic factor [144, 145]. Thirty percent or more regression in the SUVmax is found to be a predictive marker of response to the chemotherapy, and 50 % or more decrease in SUVmax correlates with long-term disease-free survival and overall survival [146, 147]. For inoperable cases FDG-PET has been found to help in radiotherapy planning and has shown 56 % modification of gross tumour volume leading to alteration of treating volume in 53 % patients [148]. FDG-PET is highly sensitive in detecting regional and distant recurrent lesions with a reported sensitivity, specificity and accuracy of 94 %, 82 % and 87 %, respectively, in comparison to 81 %, 82 % and 81 % for conventional imaging [149].

18.10 Colorectal Cancer

FDG-PET/CT has a role in therapy assessment, imaging of recurrent disease, localisation of recurrent disease in unexplained raised serum carcinoembryonic antigen (CEA) levels and staging before surgical resection of local recurrence and distant metastatic disease in colorectal malignancy [150–152]. Routine use of FDG-PET/CT in the initial staging is not usually justified and is reserved as a problem solving tool for evaluation of high-risk patients such as CEA levels >10 ng/ml with locally advanced disease or equivocal findings on conventional imaging [153–155]. FDG-PET/CT not only detects unsuspected metastatic disease but also helps determine the nature of indeterminate lesions, and in turn it is found to change management in 18–24 % of these high-risk category patients [156–158]. In patients with raised CEA and negative or equivocal conventional imaging, FDG-PET/CT has shown a sensitivity of 88 %, specificity of 94 % and accuracy of 92 % for the detection of extrahepatic intra-abdominal colorectal recurrence and 95 %, 100 % and 99 %, respectively, for extra-abdominal and/or hepatic recurrences (Fig. 18.7). The overall sensitivity, specificity and accuracy for diagnosing recurrent colorectal disease are 89 %, 92 % and 90 %, respectively [159].

Furthermore FDG-PET/CT is a potentially valuable technique in radiotherapy planning and

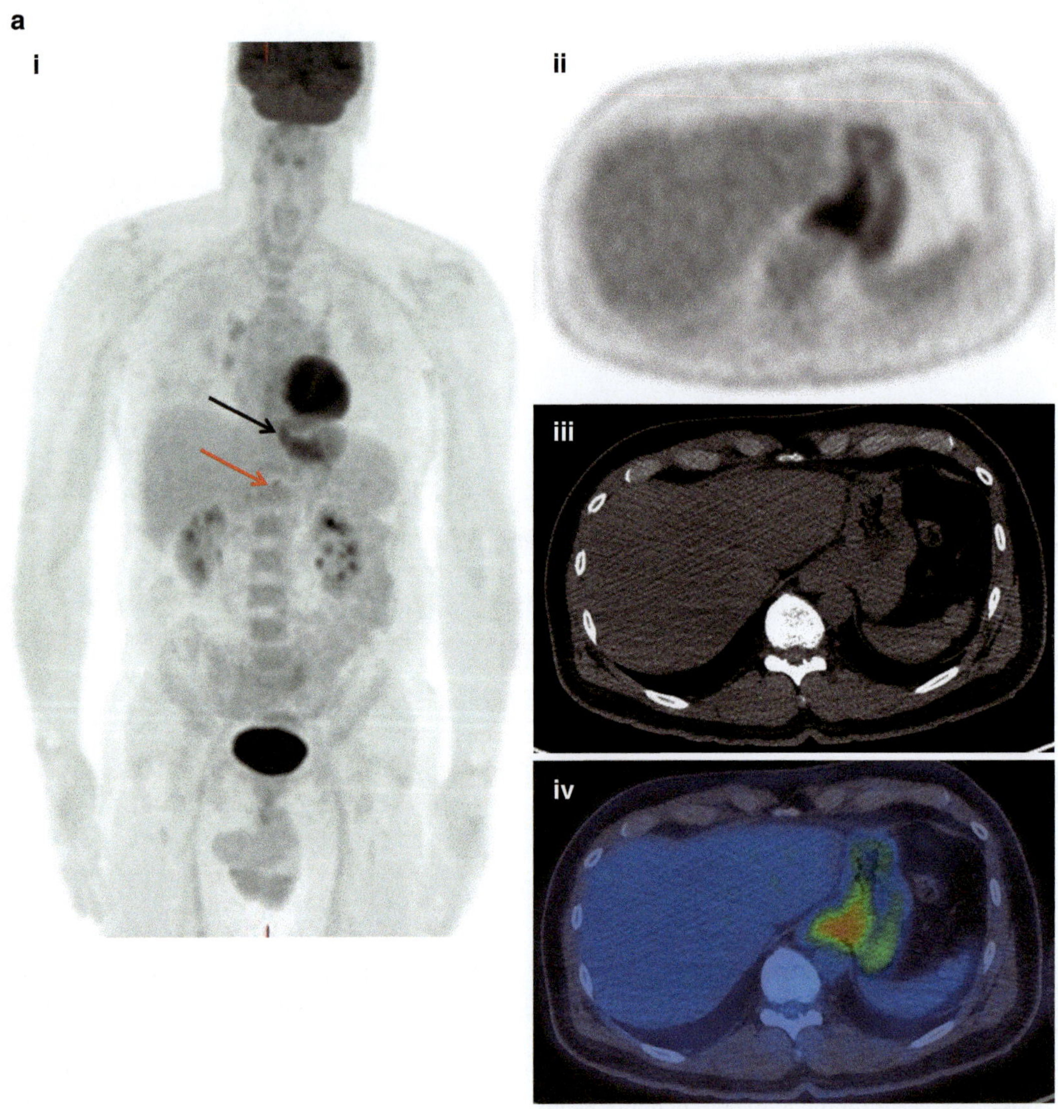

Fig. 18.6 A 74-year-old male with carcinoma of the gastro-oesophageal junction. FDG-PET/CT shows increased activity in the primary tumour (*black arrow*) (**a**) as well as an involved coeliac lymph node (*red arrow*) (**b**). (i) MIP, (ii) PET, (iii) CT and (iv) fused PET/CT axial images through the primary tumour (**a**) and upper abdomen (**b**)

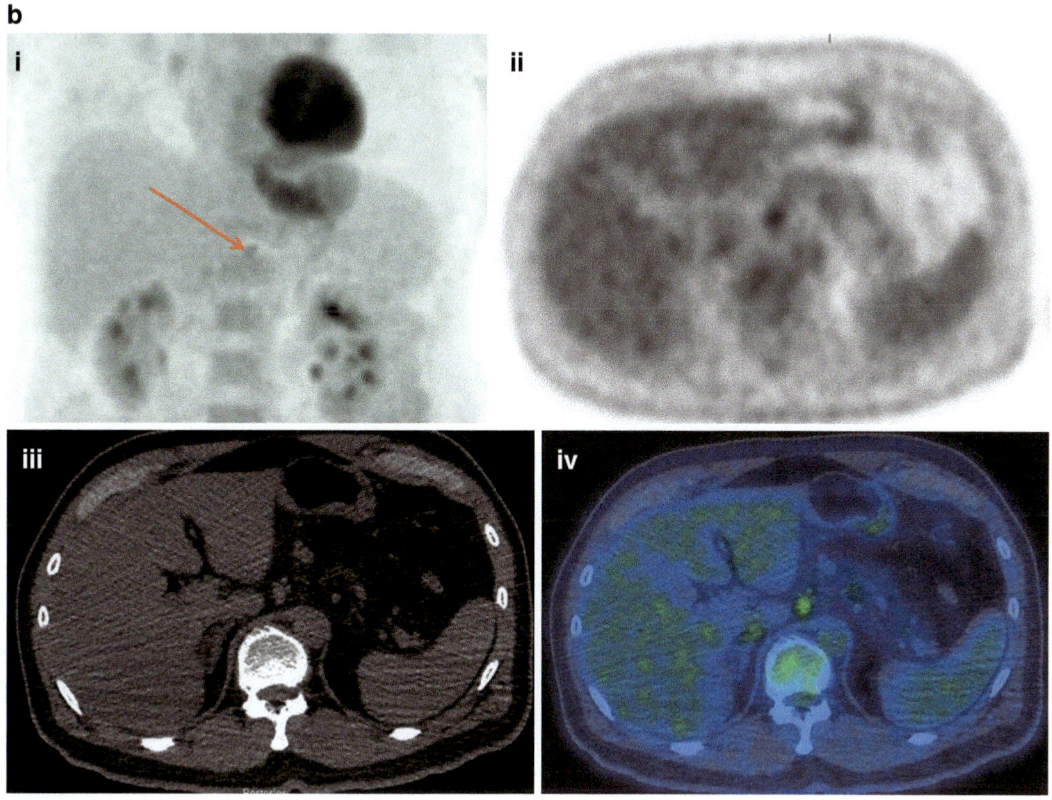

Fig. 18.6 (continued)

increases the gross tumour volume estimation in 25 % patients and clinical target volume in 4 % patients. It is also useful in the prediction and evaluation of response to radiotherapy [160, 161].

18.11 Gynaecological Cancers

18.11.1 Cervical Cancer

In advanced cervical cancer, FDG-PET/CT has an established role in preoperative staging and post-therapy restaging [162, 163]. For the detection of para-aortic nodal disease in advanced cervical cancer with negative conventional CT imaging, FDG-PET has shown a sensitivity, specificity and accuracy of 86 %, 94 % and 92 %, respectively. Preoperative FDG-PET imaging has been found to influence patient management in 18 % of patients [164]. For the detection of recurrent disease, FDG-PET imaging has an overall sensitivity and specificity of 86–94 % and 76–100 %, respectively. Post-therapy absence of FDG uptake is found to correlate with 2-year progression-free survival (86 % compared to 40 % in patients who showed persistent residual FDG uptake) [165, 166].

18.11.2 Ovarian Cancer

FDG-PET/CT is not routinely used for the detection of ovarian cancer [167, 168]. Studies have reported a sensitivity of 87 % and specificity of 100 % for differentiating benign from malignant ovarian cancer. However, it has a low diagnostic value in differentiating between borderline and benign tumours. Lesions up to 5 mm can be diagnosed [169]. Though it has a high specificity, its sensitivity is much lower than that of sonography [170, 171]. FDG-PET/CT is useful in evaluating distant metastatic disease. Pretreatment staging accuracy of FDG-PET/CT

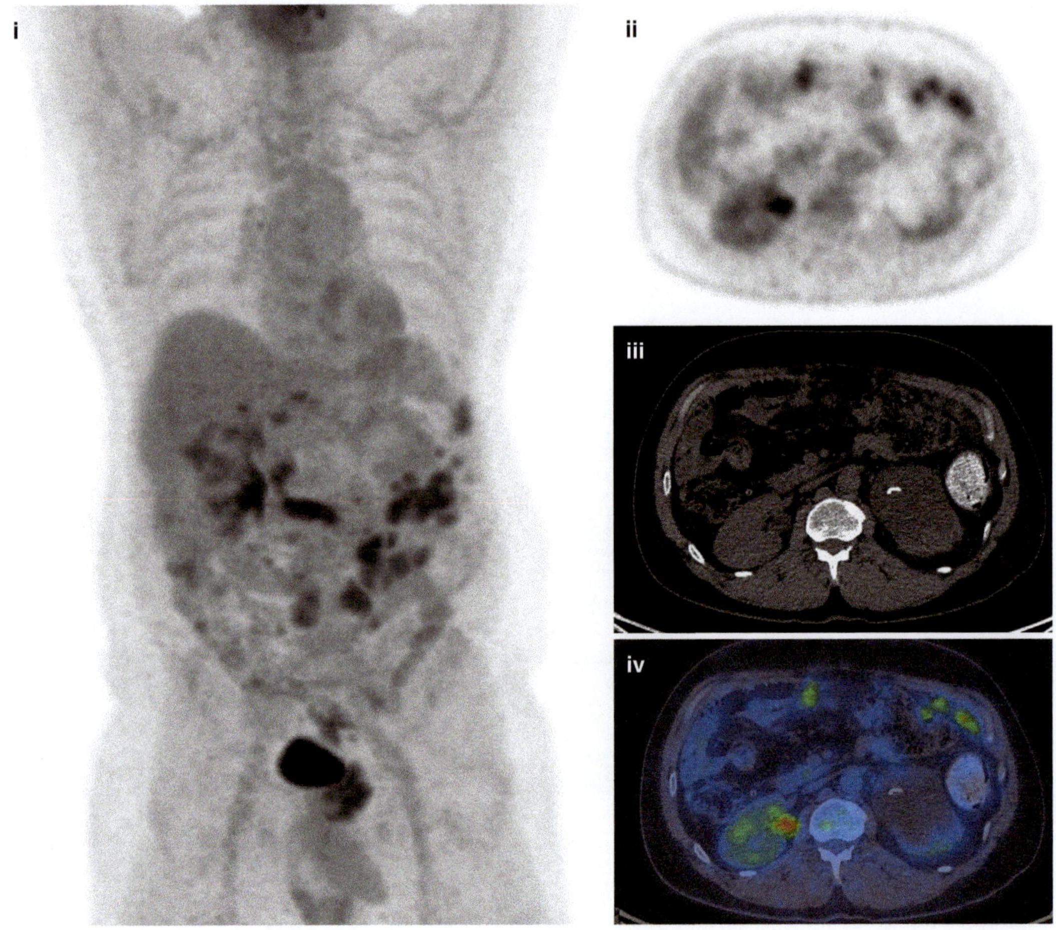

Fig. 18.7 A 58-year-old male with a history of rectal cancer with a rising CEA during follow-up. FDG-PET/CT scan shows active peritoneal metastases. (i) MIP, (ii) PET, (iii) CT and (iv) fused PET/CT axial images through the upper abdomen. A left ureteric stent is present as the patient had presented with hydronephrosis

is found to be 69–75 %, compared with 53–55 % with CT alone [172, 173]. High sensitivity has been reported for identifying peritoneal deposits larger than 1 cm and lymph nodes larger than 7 mm [174]. FDG-PET/CT identifies patients who are not suitable candidates for optimal debulking and would need preoperative chemotherapy. Early diagnosis of recurrence and exact anatomic localisation of metastatic disease are crucial for determination of the best treatment strategy [175–177]. There are limited data available regarding the role of FDG-PET or FDG-PET/CT to monitor therapy response in ovarian cancer. In one study sequential FDG-PET/CT used to predict patient outcome showed a significant correlation between changes in tumour FDG uptake after the first and third cycles of neoadjuvant chemotherapy in advanced-stage (International Federation of Gynecology and Obstetrics stages IIIC and IV) ovarian cancer, but not with conventional clinical or CA-125 response criteria [178, 179]. High rates of complete tumour resection were achieved in cases which showed more than 20 % regression in SUV from baseline after the first cycle and 50 % after the third cycle than in nonresponders. Also the rate of macroscopic tumour-free surgical resection was 33 % in metabolic responders vs. only 13 % in nonresponders [179]. In recurrent ovarian cancers with raised serum CA-125 and negative conventional imaging, FDG-PET/CT has a reported sensitivity and PPV of 83.3 % and

93.8 %, respectively, for the detection of recurrent disease at least 1 cm in size [180].

18.12 Pitfalls

Important pitfalls of FDG-PET/CT imaging can be seen during interpretation of scans. The factors which have been proved to cause variation in the detection of tumour include tumour size, tumour metabolic activity, background activity of surrounding tissue and serum glucose levels. False-negatives are commonly found in smaller lesions (<7 mm), tumours having low metabolic rate, interference from cytostatic treatments which cause a decrease in the tumour FDG uptake in the presence of viable tumour and suboptimal patient preparation, especially in patients with glucose intolerance or diabetes leading to a decrease in FDG uptake in tumours owing to competitive inhibition with glucose. Other known limitations are high background physiological FDG activity such as in the brain parenchyma and the genitourinary tract which may mask malignant pathologies and hence reduce lesion detection. Benign pathologies such as infections, inflammatory processes and postoperative and post-radiation changes may lead to increased FDG uptake and false-positive results.

18.13 PET in Clinical Trials

There is increasing interest in using functional imaging biomarkers in clinical trials as surrogate end points of drug effect. This has frequently been an exploratory objective in clinical trial design, but with greater confidence and more data to support functional imaging end points, PET is being considered more frequently. There has been development of quantitative response measures for FDG-PET from the relatively straightforward EORTC criteria [181] to the more recent introduction of PERCIST criteria [182]. Lymphoma trials have developed alternative Deauville criteria which are straightforward, semiquantitative and reproducible [183]. Key to multicentre trials is standardisation of image acquisition and quality as well as subsequent analysis. This has been pioneered in the United Kingdom by the National Cancer Research Institute PET core lab [184] and in the United States by the American College of Radiology Imaging Network. There are early examples of trials where FDG-PET has been used for response-adapted therapy in lymphoma [185, 186], 18F-fluoride for response assessment of bone metastases in prostate cancer [187] and 18F-FLT PET for assessment of primary brain tumours [188].

18.14 The Future

Possible future directions include exploring the use of FDG-PET/CT in predicting early response to therapy with hard end points, such as time to progression or overall survival. Well-designed large clinical studies are likely to answer this question and will lead to formulation of guidelines for more widespread approved clinical indications in this context. At the same time with the changing demands of clinical practice, there is a need to evaluate other areas of tumour biology such as tumour angiogenesis, hypoxia, cell proliferation and tumour receptors and incorporation of targeted tracers into clinical trials that will lead to greater clinical acceptance with time. Other future directions include development of higher-resolution PET scanners, the introduction of PET/MRI scanners as well as organ-specific scanners (such as breast PET scanners) and improvement in the speed of acquisition of studies, which will improve patient comfort and scanner throughput.

Conclusion

Over the past decade, combined FDG-PET/CT has become the cornerstone and standard of imaging care for many oncology indications. It not only has improved the localisation of tumours with greater confidence but has also impacted the staging and follow-up of the disease. Moving from its primary indication in tumour staging and restaging, FDG-PET/CT has proved to be a seminal tool for disease prognostication and compass for tailoring treatment in clinical oncology. However, the current challenges in its role as a unit for measuring tumour burden and quantification of disease load have led to foundation of new frontiers in the field of molecular imaging research.

References

1. Kelloff GJ, Hoffman JM, Johnson B, et al. Progress and promise of FDG-PET imaging for cancer patient management and oncologic drug development. Clin Cancer Res. 2005;11:2785–808.
2. Vansteenkiste JF. PET scan in the staging of non-small cell lung cancer. Lung Cancer. 2003;42 Suppl 1:S27–37.
3. Weber WA, Petersen V, Schmidt B, et al. Positron emission tomography in non-small-cell lung cancer: prediction of response to chemotherapy by quantitative assessment of glucose use. J Clin Oncol. 2003;21:2651–7.
4. Eubank W, Mankoff D. Current and future uses of PET in breast cancer imaging. Semin Nucl Med. 2004;34:224–40.
5. Macapinlac HA. FDG PET, and PET/CT imaging in lymphoma and melanoma. Cancer J. 2004;10: 262–70.
6. Khan MA, Combs CS, Brunt EM, et al. Positron emission tomography scanning in the evaluation of hepatocellular carcinoma. J Hepatol. 2000;32: 792–7.
7. Hoh CK, Seltzer MA, Franklin J, et al. Positron emission tomography in urological oncology. J Urol. 1998;159:347–56.
8. Avril N, Menzel M, Dose J, et al. Glucose metabolism of breast cancer assessed by 18F-FDG PET: histologic and immunohistochemical tissue analysis. J Nucl Med. 2001;42:9–16.
9. Bos R, van Der Hoeven JJ, van Der Wall E, et al. Biologic correlates of (18) fluorodeoxyglucose uptake in human breast cancer measured by positron emission tomography. J Clin Oncol. 2002;20:3 79–87.
10. Eary JF, O'Sullivan F, Powitan Y, et al. Sarcoma tumor FDG uptake measured by PET and patient outcome: a retrospective analysis. Eur J Nucl Med Mol Imaging. 2002;29:1149–54.
11. Wang W, Larson SM, Fazzari M, et al. Prognostic value of [18F] fluorodeoxyglucose positron emission tomographic scanning in patients with thyroid cancer. J Clin Endocrinol Metab. 2000;85:1107–13.
12. Morris MJ, Akhurst T, Osman I, et al. Fluorinated deoxyglucose positron emission tomography imaging in progressive metastatic prostate cancer. Urology. 2002;59:913–8.
13. Wang W, Larson SM, Tuttle RM, et al. Resistance of [18F]-fluorodeoxyglucose-avid metastatic thyroid cancer lesions to treatment with high-dose radioactive iodine. Thyroid. 2001;11:1169–75.
14. Mankoff D, Bellon J. PET imaging of cancer: FDG and beyond. Semin Radiat Oncol. 2001;11:16–27.
15. Rohren EM, Turkington TG, Coleman RE. Clinical applications of PET in oncology. Radiology. 2004; 231:305–32.
16. Mankoff DA, Eary JF, Link JM, et al. Tumor-specific positron emission tomography imaging in patients: [18F] fluorodeoxyglucose and beyond. Clin Cancer Res. 2007;13(12):3460–9.
17. Wahl RL, Zasadny K, Helvie M, et al. Metabolic monitoring of breast cancer chemohormonotherapy using positron emission tomography: initial evaluation. J Clin Oncol. 1993;11:2101–11.
18. Minn H, Soini I. [18F]fluorodeoxyglucose scintigraphy in diagnosis and follow up of treatment in advanced breast cancer. Eur J Nucl Med. 1989;15:61–6.
19. Ott K, Weber WA, Lordick F, et al. Metabolic imaging predicts response, survival, and recurrence in adenocarcinomas of the esophagogastric junction. J Clin Oncol. 2006;24:4692–8.
20. Romer W, Hanauske AR, Ziegler S, et al. Positron emission tomography in non-Hodgkin's lymphoma: assessment of chemotherapy with fluorodeoxyglucose. Blood. 1998;91:4464–71.
21. Mac Manus MP, Hicks RJ, Matthews JP, et al. Positron emission tomography is superior to computed tomography scanning for response-assessment after radical radiotherapy or chemoradiotherapy in patients with non-small-cell lung cancer. J Clin Oncol. 2003;21:1285–92.
22. Mankoff DA, Dunnwald LK, Gralow JR, et al. Changes in blood flow and metabolism in locally advanced breast cancer treated with neoadjuvant chemotherapy. J Nucl Med. 2003;44:1806–14.
23. Pfannenberg AC, Aschoff P, Brechtel K, et al. Low dose non-enhanced CT versus standard dose contrast-enhanced CT in combined PET/CT protocols for staging and therapy planning in non-small cell lung cancer. Eur J Nucl Med Mol Imaging. 2007;34:36–44.
24. Schelling M, Avril N, Nahrig J, et al. Positron emission tomography using [18F] fluorodeoxyglucose for monitoring primary chemotherapy in breast cancer. J Clin Oncol. 2000;18:1689–95.
25. Shields AF, Mankoff DA, Link JM, et al. Carbon-11-thymidine and FDG to measure therapy response. J Nucl Med. 1998;39:1757–62.
26. Smith I, Welch A, Hutcheon A, et al. Positron emission tomography using [18F]-fluorodeoxy-D-glucose to predict the pathologic response of breast cancer to primary chemotherapy. J Clin Oncol. 2000;18: 1676–88.
27. Demetri GD, von Mehren M, Blanke CD, et al. Efficacy and safety of imatinibmesylate in advanced gastrointestinal stromal tumors. N Engl J Med. 2002;347:472–80.

28. Gayed I, Vu T, Iyer R, et al. The role of [18F]-FDG PET in staging and early prediction of response to therapy of recurrent gastrointestinal stromal tumors. J Nucl Med. 2004;45:17–21.
29. Stroobants S, Goeminne J, Seegers M, et al. 18FDG-positron emission tomography for the early prediction of response in advanced soft tissue sarcoma treated with imatinibmesylate (Glivec). Eur J Cancer. 2003;39:2012–20.
30. Van den Abbeele AD, Group ftGCPS. [F-18]-FDG in PET provides early evidence of biological response to ST1571 in patients with malignant gastrointestinal stromal tumors (GIST). Proc Am Soc Clin Oncol. 2001;20:362a.
31. Su H, Bodenstein C, Dumont RA, et al. Monitoring tumor glucose utilization by positron emission tomography for the prediction of treatment response to epidermal growth factor receptor kinase inhibitors. Clin Cancer Res. 2006;12:5659–67.
32. Linden HM, Krohn KA, Livingston RB, Mankoff DA. Monitoring targeted therapy: is fluorodeoxyglucose uptake a marker of early response? Clin Cancer Res. 2006;12:5608–10.
33. Mortimer JE, Dehdashti F, Siegel BA, et al. Metabolic flare: indicator of hormone responsiveness in advanced breast cancer. J Clin Oncol. 2001;19:2797–803.
34. Hicks RJ. The role of PET in monitoring therapy. Cancer Imaging. 2005;5:51–7.
35. Spence AM, Muzi M, Graham MM, et al. 2-[(18)F] Fluoro-2-deoxyglucose and glucose uptake in malignant gliomas before and after radiotherapy: correlation with outcome. Clin Cancer Res. 2002;8:971–9.
36. Cachin F, Prince HM, Hogg A, Ware RE, Hicks RJ. Powerful prognostic stratification by [18F]fluorodeoxyglucose positron emission tomography in patients with metastatic breast cancer treated with high-dose chemotherapy. J Clin Oncol. 2006;24:3026–31.
37. Hawkins DS, Schuetze SM, Butrynski JE, et al. [18F]Fluorodeoxyglucose positron emission tomography predicts outcome for Ewing sarcoma family of tumors. J Clin Oncol. 2005;23:8828–34.
38. Fletcher JW, Djulbegovic B, Soares HP, et al. Recommendations on the use of 18F-FDG PET in oncology. J Nucl Med. 2008;49(3):480–508.
39. Oyen WJ, Bussink J, Verhagen AF, Corstens FH, Bootsma GP. Role of FDG-PET in the diagnosis and management of lung cancer. Expert Rev Anticancer Ther. 2004;4(4):561–7.
40. Schmid RA, Hautmann H, Poellinger B, et al. Staging of recurrent and advanced lung cancer with 18F-FDG PET in a coincidence technique (hybrid PET). Nucl Med Commun. 2003;24(1):37–45.
41. Hicks RJ, Kalff V, MacManus MP, et al. The utility of 18F-FDG PET for suspected recurrent non-small cell lung cancer after potentially curative therapy: impact on management and prognostic stratification. J Nucl Med. 2001;42(11):1605–13.
42. Hicks RJ. Role of 18F-FDG PET in assessment of response in non-small cell lung cancer. J Nucl Med. 2009;50(1):31S–42.
43. Joshi SC, Pant I, Hamzah F, Kumar G, Shukla AN. Integrated positron emission tomography/computed tomography fusion imaging: an emerging gold standard in lung cancer. Indian J Cancer. 2008;45:137–41.
44. Lowe V, Naunheim K. Positron emission tomography in lung cancer. Ann Thorac Surg. 1998;65:1821–9.
45. Behzadi A, Ung Y, Lowe V, Deschamps C. The role of positron emission tomography in the management of non-small cell lung cancer. Can J Surg. 2009;52:235–42.
46. Fletcher JW, Kymes SM, Gould M, et al. A comparison of the diagnostic accuracy of 18F-FDG PET and CT in the characterization of solitary pulmonary nodules. J Nucl Med. 2008;49:179–85.
47. Lardinois D, Weder W, Hany T, et al. Staging of non-small cell lung cancer with integrated positron-emission tomography. J Nucl Med. 2003;348:2500–7.
48. Sachelarie I, Kerr K, Ghesani M, et al. Integrated PET-CT: evidence-based review of oncology indications. Oncology (Williston Park). 2005;19:481–90.
49. Reske SN, Kotzerke J. FDG-PET for clinical use. Results of the 3rd German Interdisciplinary Consensus Conference, "Onko-PET III", 21 July and 19 September 2000. Eur J Nucl Med. 2001;28(11):1707–23.
50. Verboom P, van Tinteren H, Hoekstra OS, et al. Cost-effectiveness of FDG-PET in staging non-small cell lung cancer: the PLUS study. Eur J Nucl Med Mol Imaging. 2003;30(11):1444–9.
51. Steinert HC, Hauser M, Allemann F, et al. Non-small cell lung cancer: nodal staging with FDG PET versus CT with correlative lymph node mapping and sampling. Radiology. 1997;202:441–6.
52. Marom EM, McAdams HP, Erasmus JJ, et al. Staging non-small cell lung cancer with whole-body PET. Radiology. 1999;212:803–9.
53. Gould MK, Kuschner WG, Rydzak CE, et al. Test performance of positron emission tomography and computed tomography for mediastinal staging in patients with non-small-cell lung cancer: a meta-analysis. Ann Intern Med. 2003;139:879–92.
54. Pieterman RM, van Putten JW, Meuzelaar JJ, et al. Preoperative staging of non-small-cell lung cancer with positron-emission tomography. N Engl J Med. 2000;343:254–61.
55. Verhagen AF, Bootsma GP, Tjan-Heijnen VC, et al. FDG-PET in staging lung cancer: how does it change the algorithm? Lung Cancer. 2004;44:175–81.
56. Jett JR. How to optimize staging in early non-small cell lung cancer. Lung Cancer. 2002;38:S13–6.
57. Kramer H, Groen HJ. Current concepts in the mediastinal lymph node staging of nonsmall cell lung cancer. Ann Surg. 2003;238:180–8.
58. Al-Sarraf N, Aziz R, Gately K, et al. Pattern and predictors of occult mediastinal lymph node involvement in non-small cell lung cancer patients with negative mediastinal uptake on positron emission tomography. Eur J Cardiothorac Surg. 2008;33:104–9.

59. Silvestri GA, Tanoue LT, Margolis ML, Barker J, Detterbeck F. The noninvasive staging of non-small cell lung cancer: the guidelines. Chest. 2003;123: 147S–56.
60. Eschmann SM, Friedel G, Paulsen F, et al. 18F-FDG PET for assessment of therapy response and preoperative re-evaluation after neoadjuvant radio-chemotherapy in stage III non-small cell lung cancer. Eur J Nucl Med Mol Imaging. 2007;34(4):463–71.
61. De Ruysscher D, Wanders S, van Haren E, et al. Selective mediastinal node irradiation based on FDG-PET scan data in patients with non-small-cell lung cancer: a prospective clinical study. Int J Radiat Oncol Biol Phys. 2005;62:988–94.
62. Bradley J, Thorstad WL, Mutic S, et al. Impact of FDG-PET on radiation therapy volume delineation in non-small-cell lung cancer. Int J Radiat Oncol Biol Phys. 2004;59:78–86.
63. van Loon J, Offermann C, Bosmans G, et al. 18FDG-PET based radiation planning of mediastinal lymph nodes in limited disease small cell lung cancer changes radiotherapy fields: a planning study. Radiother Oncol. 2008;87:49–54.
64. Tulchinsky M, Coquia S, Wagner H. Small bowel metastasis from lung cancer detected on FDG PET/CT. Clin Nucl Med. 2009;34(7):446–8.
65. Liu N, Ma L, Zhou W, et al. Bone metastasis in patients with non-small cell lung cancer: the diagnostic role of F-18 FDG PET/CT. Eur J Radiol. 2010;74(1):231–5.
66. Yamamoto Y, Kameyama R, Murota M, et al. Early assessment of therapeutic response using FDG PET in small cell lung cancer. Mol Imaging Biol. 2009; 11(6):467–72.
67. Sunaga N, Oriuchi N, Kaira K, et al. Usefulness of FDG-PET for early prediction of the response to gefitinib in non-small cell lung cancer. Lung Cancer. 2008;59(2):203–10.
68. Rohren EM, Lowe VJ. Update in PET imaging of nonsmall cell lung cancer. Semin Nucl Med. 2004;34:134–53.
69. Cerfolio RJ, Bryant AS, Winokur TS, Ohja B, Bartolucci AA. Repeat FDG-PET after neoadjuvant therapy is a predictor of pathologic response in patients with non-small cell lung cancer. Ann Thorac Surg. 2004;78:1903–9.
70. Dhanapathi H, Kumar R. F-18 FDG PET/PET-CT in the management of lymphoma. Indian J Med Pediatr Oncol. 2007;28:17–23.
71. Elstrom R, Guan L, Baker G, et al. Utility of FDG-PET scanning in lymphoma by WHO classification. Blood. 2003;101:3875–6.
72. Stumpe KD, Urbinelli M, Steinert HC, et al. Whole-body positron emission tomography using fluorodeoxyglucose for staging of lymphoma: effectiveness and comparison with computed tomography. Eur J Nucl Med. 1998;25:721–8.
73. Schaefer NG, Hany TF, Taverna C, et al. Non-Hodgkin lymphoma and Hodgkin disease: coregistered FDG PET and CT at staging and restaging: do we need contrast-enhanced CT? Radiology. 2004;232:823–89.
74. Elstrom RL, Leonard JP, Coleman M, Brown RK. Combined PET and low-dose, noncontrast CT scanning obviates the need for additional diagnostic contrast-enhanced CT scans in patients undergoing staging or restaging for lymphoma. Ann Oncol. 2008;19:1770–3.
75. Khan AB, Barrington SF, Mikhaeel NG, et al. PET-CT staging of DLBCL accurately identifies and provides new insight into the clinical significance of bone marrow involvement. Blood. 2013;122:61–7.
76. Avigdor A. Staging DLBCL: bone marrow biopsy or PET-CT? Blood. 2013;122:4–5.
77. Hoffmann M, Kletter K, Diemling M, et al. Positron emission tomography with fluorine-18-2-fluoro-2-deoxy-D-glucose (F18-FDG) does not visualize extranodal B-cell lymphoma of the mucosa-associated lymphoid tissue (MALT)-type. Ann Oncol. 1999;10:1185–9.
78. Schöder H, Noy A, Gönen M, et al. Intensity of 18fluorodeoxyglucose uptake in positron emission tomography distinguishes between indolent and aggressive non-Hodgkin's lymphoma. J Clin Oncol. 2005;23:4643–51.
79. Spaepen K, Stroobants S, Dupont P, et al. Prognostic value of positron emission tomography (PET) with fluorine-18 fluorodeoxyglucose ([18F]FDG) after first-line chemotherapy in non-Hodgkin's lymphoma: is [18F]FDG-PET a valid alternative to conventional diagnostic methods? J Clin Oncol. 2001;19:414–9.
80. de Wit M, Bumann D, Beyer W, et al. Whole-body positron emission tomography (PET) for diagnosis of residual mass in patients with lymphoma. Ann Oncol. 1997;8:57–60.
81. Reske SN. PET and restaging of malignant lymphoma including residual masses and relapse. Eur J Nucl Med Mol Imaging. 2003;30:S89–96.
82. Naumann R, Vaic A, Beuthien-Baumann B, et al. Prognostic value of positron emission tomography in the evaluation of post-treatment residual mass in patients with Hodgkin's disease and non-Hodgkin's lymphoma. Br J Haematol. 2001;115:793–800.
83. Cremerius U, Fabry U, Neuerburg J, Zimny M, Osieka R, Buell U. Positron emission tomography with 18F-FDG to detect residual disease after therapy for malignant lymphoma. Nucl Med Commun. 1998;19:1055–63.
84. Talbot JN, Haioun C, Rain JD, et al. [18F]-FDG positron imaging in clinical management of lymphoma patients. Crit Rev Oncol Hematol. 2001; 38:193–221.
85. Jerusalem G, Beguin Y, Fassotte MF, et al. Whole-body positron emission tomography using 18F-fluorodeoxyglucose for posttreatment evaluation in Hodgkin's disease and non-Hodgkin's lymphoma has higher diagnostic and prognostic value than classical computed tomography scan imaging. Blood. 1999;94:429–33.

86. Foo SS, Mitchell PL, Berlangieri SU, et al. Positron emission tomography scanning in the assessment of patients with lymphoma. Intern Med J. 2004;34: 388–97.
87. Duch J, Fuster D, Munoz M, et al. 18F-FDG PET/CT for early prediction of response to neoadjuvant chemotherapy in breast cancer. Eur J Nucl Med Mol Imaging. 2009;36(10):1551–7.
88. Yang SK, Cho N, Moon WK. The role of PET/CT for evaluating breast cancer. Korean J Radiol. 2007;8:429–37.
89. Avril N, Rosé CA, Schelling M, et al. Breast imaging with positron emission tomography and fluorine-18 fluorodeoxyglucose: use and limitations. J Clin Oncol. 2000;18:3495–502.
90. Cermik TF, Mavi A, Basu S, Alavi A. Impact of FDG PET on the preoperative staging of newly diagnosed breast cancer. Eur J Nucl Med Mol Imaging. 2008;35(3):475–83.
91. Belohlavek O. What is the role of FDG-PET in the initial staging of breast cancer? Eur J Nucl Med Mol Imaging. 2008;35(3):472–4.
92. Eubank WB, Mankoff DA. Evolving role of positron emission tomography in breast cancer imaging. Semin Nucl Med. 2005;35:84–99.
93. Crippa F, Gerali A, Alessi A, Agresti R, Bombardieri E. FDG-PET for axillary lymph node staging in primary breast cancer. Eur J Nucl Med Mol Imaging. 2004;31(1):S97–102.
94. Sloka JS, Hollett PD, Mathews M. A quantitative review of the use of FDG-PET in the axillary staging of breast cancer. Med Sci Monit. 2007;13(3): RA37–46.
95. Ueda S, Tsuda H, Asakawa H, et al. Utility of 18F-fluorodeoxyglucose emission tomography/computed tomography fusion imaging (18F-FDG PET/CT) in combination with ultrasonography for axillary staging in primary breast cancer. BMC Cancer. 2008;8:165.
96. Peare R, Staff RT, Heys SD. The use of FDG-PET in assessing axillary lymph node status in breast cancer: a systematic review and meta-analysis of the literature. Breast Cancer Res Treat. 2010;123(1): 281–90.
97. Straver ME, Aukema TS, Olmos RAV, et al. Feasibility of FDG PET/CT to monitor the response of axillary lymph node metastases to neoadjuvant chemotherapy in breast cancer patients. Eur J Nucl Med Mol Imaging. 2010;37(6):1069–76. doi:10.1007/s00259-009-1343-2.
98. Kamel EM, Wyss MT, Fehr MK, von Schulthess GK, Goerres GW. [18F]-Fluorodeoxyglucose positron emission tomography in patients with suspected recurrence of breast cancer. J Cancer Res Clin Oncol. 2003;129:147–53.
99. Kumar A, Kumar R, Seenu V, et al. The role of 18F-FDG PET/CT in evaluation of early response to neoadjuvant chemotherapy in patients with locally advanced breast cancer. Eur Radiol. 2009;19(6): 1347–57.
100. Momiyama N, Ishikawa T, Ichikawa Y, et al. Early prediction of response to primary chemotherapy by sequential FDG -PET in patients with advanced breast cancer. Nippon Rinsho. 2007;65(6):385–8.
101. Dose Schwarz J, Bader M, Jenicke L, et al. Early prediction of response to chemotherapy in metastatic breast cancer using sequential 18F-FDG PET. J Nucl Med. 2005;46:1144–50.
102. Long NM, Smith CS. Causes and imaging features of false positives and false negatives on 18F-PET/CT in oncologic imaging. Insights Imaging. 2011;2(6): 679–98. doi:10.1007/s13244-010-0062-3.
103. Cook GJ, Houston S, Rubens R, et al. Detection of bone metastases in breast cancer by 18FDG PET: differing metabolic activity in osteoblastic and osteolytic lesions. J Clin Oncol. 1998;16:3375–9.
104. vanKruchten M, de Vries EG, Brown M, et al. PET imaging of oestrogen receptors in patients with breast cancer. Lancet Oncol. 2013;14(11):e465–75.
105. Linden HM, Stekhova SA, Link JM, et al. Quantitative fluoroestradiol positron emission tomography imaging predicts response to endocrine treatment in breast cancer. J Clin Oncol. 2006;24(18):2793–9. Epub 2006 May 8.
106. Eigtved A, Andersson AP, Dahlstrom K, et al. Use of fluorine-18-fluorodeoxyglucose positron emission tomography in the detection of silent metastases from malignant melanoma. Eur J Nucl Med. 2000;27:70–5.
107. Tyler DS, Onaitis M, Kherani A, et al. Positron emission tomography scanning in malignant melanoma: clinical utility in patients with stage III disease. Cancer. 2000;89:1019–25.
108. Strobel K, Dummer R, Husarik DB, et al. High-risk melanoma: accuracy of FDG PET/CT with added CT morphologic information for detection of metastases. Radiology. 2007;244(2):566–74.
109. Mansour 3rd AA, Kelley MC, Hatmaker AR, Holt GE, Schwartz HS. Verification of Musculoskeletal FDG-PET-CT findings performed for melanoma staging. Ann Surg Oncol. 2009;36(10):1551–7.
110. Jimenez-Requena F, Delgado-Bolton RC, Fernandez-Perez C, et al. Meta-analysis of the performance of 18F-FDG PET in cutaneous melanoma. Eur J Nucl Med Mol Imaging. 2010;37(2): 284–300.
111. Havenga K, Cobben DC, Oyen WJ, et al. Fluorodeoxyglucose-positron emission tomography and sentinel lymph node biopsy in staging primary cutaneous melanoma. Eur J Surg Oncol. 2003; 29:662–4.
112. Reinhardt MJ, Joe AY, Jaeger U, et al. Diagnostic performance of whole-body 18FDG PET/CT imaging for N- and M-staging of malignant melanoma: experience with 250 consecutive patients. J Clin Oncol. 2006;24:1178–87.
113. Bastiaannet E, Oyen WJ, Meijer S, et al. Impact of [18F]fluorodeoxyglucose positron emission tomography on surgical management of melanoma patients. Br J Surg. 2006;93:243–9.

114. Fleming Jr AJ, Johansen ME. The clinician's expectations from the use of positron emission tomography/computed tomography scanning in untreated and treated head and neck cancer patients. Curr Opin Otolaryngol Head Neck Surg. 2008;16:127–34.
115. Koshy M, Paulino AC, Howell R, et al. F-18 FDG PET-CT fusion in radiotherapy treatment planning for head and neck cancer. Head Neck. 2005;27: 494–502.
116. Wang D, Schultz CJ, Jursinic PA, et al. Initial experience of FDG-PET/CT guided IMRT of head-and-neck carcinoma. Int J Radiat Oncol Biol Phys. 2006;65:143–51.
117. Fleming Jr AJ, Smith Jr SP, Paul CM, et al. Impact of [18F]-2-fluorodeoxyglucose-positron emission tomography/computed tomography on previously untreated head and neck cancer patients. Laryngoscope. 2007;117:1173–9.
118. Gordin A, Golz A, Keidar Z, et al. The role of FDG-PET/CT imaging in head and neck malignant conditions: impact on diagnostic accuracy and patient care. Otolaryngol Head Neck Surg. 2007;137: 130–7.
119. Yamamoto Y, Wong T, Turkington T, Hawk T, Coleman R. Head and neck cancer: dedicated FDG PET/CT protocol for detection – phantom and initial clinical studies. Radiology. 2007;244:263–72.
120. Zanation AM, Sutton DK, Couch ME, et al. Use, accuracy, and implications for patient management of [18F]-2-fluorodeoxyglucose-positron emission/computerized tomography for head and neck tumors. Laryngoscope. 2005;115:1186–90.
121. Deantonio L, Beldì D, Gambaro G, et al. FDG-PET/CT imaging for staging and radiotherapy treatment planning of head and neck carcinoma. Radiat Oncol. 2008;3:29.
122. Schwartz DL, Ford E, Rajendran J, et al. FDG-PET/CT imaging for preradiotherapy staging of head-and-neck squamous cell carcinoma. Int J Radiat Oncol Biol Phys. 2005;61:129–36.
123. Halpern BS, Yeom K, Fueger BJ, Lufkin RB, Czernin J, Allen-Auerbach M. Evaluation of suspected local recurrence in head and neck cancer: a comparison between PET and PET/CT for biopsy proven lesions. Eur J Radiol. 2007;62:199–204.
124. Machtay M, Natwa M, Andrel J, et al. Pretreatment FDG-PET standardized uptake value as a prognostic factor for outcome in head and neck cancer. Head Neck. 2009;31(2):195–201.
125. Branstetter 4th BF, Blodgett TM, Zimmer LA, et al. Head and neck malignancy: is PET/CT more accurate than PET or CT alone? Radiology. 2005;235(2):580–6.
126. Fukui MB, Blodgett TM, Meltzer CC. PET/CT imaging in recurrent head and neck cancer. Semin Ultrasound CT MR. 2003;24(3):157–63.
127. Nguyen BD, Ram PC, Roarke MC. Endotracheal metastasis from squamous cell cancer of the head and neck: PET/CT imaging. Clin Nucl Med. 2008;33(5):340–1.
128. Zhu A, Lee D, Shim H. Metabolic PET imaging in cancer detection and therapy response. Semin Oncol. 2011;38(1):55–69.
129. Sherman SI. Thyroid carcinoma. Lancet. 2003;361: 501–11.
130. Min JJ, Chung JK, Lee YJ, et al. Relationship between expression of the sodium/iodide symporter and 131I uptake in recurrent lesions of differentiated thyroid carcinoma. Eur J Nucl Med. 2001;28:639–45.
131. Horn J, Lock-Andersen J, Sjostrand H, Loft A. Routine use of FDG-PET scans in melanoma patients with positive sentinel node biopsy. Eur J Nucl Med Mol Imaging. 2006;33:887–92.
132. Grünwald F, Kälicke T, Feine U, et al. Fluorine-18 fluorodeoxyglucose positron emission tomography in thyroid cancer: results of a multicentre study. Eur J Nucl Med. 1999;26:1547–52.
133. Nahas Z, Goldenberg D, Fakhry C, et al. The role of positron emission tomography/computed tomography in the management of recurrent papillary thyroid carcinoma. Laryngoscope. 2005;115:237–43.
134. Iagaru A, Kalinyak JE, McDougall IR. F-18 FDG PET/CT in the management of thyroid cancer. Clin Nucl Med. 2007;32:690–5.
135. Shammas A, Degirmenci B, Mountz JM, et al. 18F-FDG PET/CT in patients with suspected recurrent or metastatic well-differentiated thyroid cancer. J Nucl Med. 2007;48:221–6.
136. Kato H, Miyazaki T, Nakajima M, et al. The incremental effect of positron emission tomography on diagnostic accuracy in the initial staging of esophageal carcinoma. Cancer. 2005;103:148–56.
137. Choi JY, Lee KH, Shim YM, et al. Improved detection of individual nodal involvement in squamous cell carcinoma of the esophagus by FDG PET. J Nucl Med. 2000;41:808–15.
138. Barber TW, Duong CP, Leong T, et al. 18F-FDG PET/CT has a high impact on patient management and provides powerful prognostic stratification in the primary staging of esophageal cancer: a prospective study with mature survival data. J Nucl Med. 2012; 53(6):864–71.
139. Heeren PA, Jager PL, Bongaerts F, et al. Detection of distant metastases in esophageal cancer with (18) F-FDG PET. J Nucl Med. 2004;45:980–7.
140. Flamen P, Lerut A, Van Cutsem E, et al. Utility of positron emission tomography for the staging of patients with potentially operable esophageal carcinoma. J Clin Oncol. 2000;18:3202–10.
141. van Westreenen HL, Westerterp M, Jager PL, et al. Synchronous primary neoplasms detected on 18F-FDG PET in staging of patients with esophageal cancer. J Nucl Med. 2005;46:1321–5.
142. Yoon YC, Lee KS, Shim YM, et al. Metastasis to regional lymph nodes in patients with esophageal squamous cell carcinoma: CT versus FDG PET for presurgical detection prospective study. Radiology. 2003;227:764–70.
143. Luketich JD, Friedman DM, Weigel TL, et al. Evaluation of distant metastases in esophageal can-

cer: 100 consecutive positron emission tomography scans. Ann Thorac Surg. 1999;68:1133–6.
144. Brücher BL, Weber W, Bauer M, et al. Neoadjuvant therapy of esophageal squamous cell carcinoma: response evaluation by positron emission tomography. Ann Surg. 2001;233:300–9.
145. Westerterp M, van Westreenen HL, Reitsma JB, et al. Esophageal cancer: CT, endoscopic US, and FDG PET for assessment of response to neoadjuvant therapy–systematic review. Radiology. 2005;326:841–51.
146. Klaeser B, Nitzsche E, Schuller JC, et al. Limited predictive value of FDG-PET for response assessment in the preoperative treatment of esophageal cancer: results of a prospective multi-center trial (SAKK 75/02). Onkologie. 2009;32(12):724–30.
147. Isa T, Kaneshiro T, Yamamoto H, et al. Case of esophageal cancer successfully performed in early response evaluation for preoperative chemotherapy by FDG-PET. Nihon Shokakibyo Gakkai Zasshi. 2008;105(8):1193–9.
148. Krause BJ, Herrmann K, Wieder H, zumBuschenfelde CM. 18F-FDG PET and 18F-FDG PET/CT for assessing response to therapy in esophageal cancer. J Nucl Med. 2009;50 Suppl 1:89S–96.
149. Flamen P, Lerut A, Van Cutsem E, et al. The utility of positron emission tomography for the diagnosis and staging of recurrent esophageal cancer. J Thorac Cardiovasc Surg. 2000;120:1085–92.
150. De Geus-Oei LF, Ruers TJ, Punt CJ, et al. FDG-PET in colorectal cancer. Cancer Imaging. 2006;6:S71–81.
151. Chessin DB, Kiran RP, Akhurst T, Guillem JG. The emerging role of 18F fluorodeoxyglucose positron emission tomography in the management of primary and recurrent rectal cancer. J Am Coll Surg. 2005; 201:948–56.
152. Ogunbiyi OA, Flanagan FL, Dehdashti F, et al. Detection of recurrent and metastatic colorectal cancer: comparison of positron emission tomography and computed tomography. Ann Surg Oncol. 1997; 4:613–20.
153. Petersen RK, Hess S, Alavi A, Høilund-Carlsen PF. Clinical impact of FDG-PET/CT on colorectal cancer staging and treatment strategy. Am J Nucl Med Mol Imaging. 2014;4(5):471–82.
154. Delbeke D, Martin WH. FDG PET and PET/CT for colorectal cancer. Methods Mol Biol. 2011;727: 77–103.
155. Flamen P, Hoekstra OS, Homans F, et al. Unexplained rising carcinoembryonic antigen (CEA) in the postoperative surveillance of colorectal cancer: the utility of positron emission tomography (PET). Eur J Cancer. 2001;37:862–9.
156. Agarwal A, Marcus C, Xiao J, et al. FDG PET/CT in the management of colorectal and anal cancers. AJR Am J Roentgenol. 2014;203(5):1109–19.
157. Imdahl A, Reinhardt MJ, Nitzsche EU, et al. Impact of 18F-FDG-positron emission tomography for decision making in colorectal cancer recurrences. Langenbecks Arch Surg. 2000;385:129–34.
158. Huebner RH, Park KC, Shepherd JE, et al. A meta-analysis of the literature for whole-body FDG PET detection of recurrent colorectal cancer. J Nucl Med. 2000;41:1177–89.
159. Votrubova J, Belohlavek O, Jaruskova M, et al. The role of FDG-PET/CT in the detection of recurrent colorectal cancer. Eur J Nucl Med Mol Imaging. 2006;33:779–84.
160. Ciernik IF, Dizendorf E, Baumert BG, et al. Radiation treatment planning with an integrated positron emission and computer tomography (PET/CT): a feasibility study. Int J Radiat Oncol Biol Phys. 2003;57:853–63.
161. Bassi MC, Turri L, Sacchetti G, et al. FDG-PET/CT imaging for staging and target volume delineation in preoperative conformal radiotherapy of rectal cancer. Int J Radiat Oncol Biol Phys. 2008;70:1423–6.
162. Tsakiris P, De la Rosette J. Imaging in genitourinary cancer from the urologists' perspective. Cancer Imaging. 2007;7:84–92.
163. Nakamoto Y, Saga T, Fujii S. Positron emission tomography application for gynecologic tumors. Int J Gynecol Cancer. 2005;15:701–9.
164. Basu S, Li G, Alavi A. PET and PET-CT imaging of gynecological malignancies: present role and future promise. Expert Rev Anticancer Ther. 2009;9: 75–96.
165. Lin WC, Hung YC, Yeh LS, et al. Usefulness of (18) F-fluorodeoxyglucose positron emission tomography to detect para-aortic lymph nodal metastasis in advanced cervical cancer with negative computed tomography findings. Gynecol Oncol. 2003;89: 73–6.
166. Belhocine T, Thille A, Fridman V, et al. Contribution of whole-body 18FDG PET imaging in the management of cervical cancer. Gynecol Oncol. 2002;87:90–7.
167. Havrilesky LJ, Kulasingam SL, Matchar DB, Myers ER. FDG-PET for management of cervical and ovarian cancer. Gynecol Oncol. 2005;97:183–91.
168. Zimny M, Siggelkow W. Positron emission tomography scanning in gynecologic and breast cancers. Curr Opin Obstet Gynecol. 2003;15:69–75.
169. De Iaco P, Musto A, Orazi L, et al. FDG-PET/CT in advanced ovarian cancer staging: value and pitfalls in detecting lesions in different abdominal and pelvic quadrants compared with laparoscopy. Eur J Radiol. 2011;80:e98–103.
170. Castellucci P, Perrone AM, Picchio M. Diagnostic accuracy of 18F-FDG PET/CT in characterizing ovarian lesions and staging ovarian cancer: correlation with transvaginal ultrasonography, computed tomography, and histology. Nucl Med Commun. 2007;28:589–95.
171. Prakash P, Cronin CG, Blake MA. Role of PET/CT in ovarian cancer. AJR Am J Roentgenol. 2010; 194(6):W464–70.
172. Liu Y. Benign ovarian and endometrial uptake on FDG PET-CT: patterns and pitfalls. Ann Nucl Med. 2009;23:107–12.

173. Hynninen J, Auranen A, Carpen O, et al. FDG PET/CT in staging of advanced epithelial ovarian cancer: frequency of supradiaphragmatic lymph node metastasis challenges the traditional pattern of disease spread. Gynecol Oncol. 2012;126:64–8.
174. Kitajima K, Murakami K, Yamasaki E. Diagnostic accuracy of integrated FDG-PET/contrast-enhanced CT in staging ovarian cancer: comparison with enhanced CT. Eur J Nucl Med Mol Imaging. 2008;35:1912–20.
175. Sironi S, Messa C, Mangili G, et al. Integrated FDG PET/CT in patients with persistent ovarian cancer: correlation with histological findings. Radiology. 2004;233:433–40.
176. Chung HH, Kang WJ, Kim JW, et al. Role of [18F] FDG PET/CT in the assessment of suspected recurrent ovarian cancer: correlation with clinical or histological findings. Eur J Nucl Med Mol Imaging. 2007;34:480–6.
177. Sebastian S, Lee SI, Horowitz NS, et al. PET-CT vs CT alone in ovarian cancer recurrence. Abdom Imaging. 2008;33:112–8.
178. Rustin GJ, Nelstrop AE, Tuxen MK, Lambert HE. Defining progression of ovarian carcinoma during follow-up according to CA 125: a North Thames Ovary Group study. Ann Oncol. 1996;7:361–4.
179. Avril N, Sassen S, Schmalfeldt B, et al. Prediction of response to neoadjuvant chemotherapy by sequential F-18-fluorodeoxyglucose positron emission tomography in patients with advanced-stage ovarian cancer. J Clin Oncol. 2005;23(30):7445–53. Epub 2005 Sep 12. Erratum in: J ClinOncol. 2005 Dec 20; 23(36):9445.
180. Grigsby PW, Siegel BA, Dehdashti F, Mutch DG. Posttherapy surveillance monitoring of cervical cancer by FDG-PET. Int J Radiat Oncol Biol Phys. 2003;55:907–13.
181. Young H, Baum R, Cremerius U, et al. Measurement of clinical and subclinical tumour response using [18F]-fluorodeoxyglucose and positron emission tomography: review and 1999 EORTC recommendations. European Organization for Research and Treatment of Cancer (EORTC) PET Study Group. Eur J Cancer. 1999;35(13):1773–82.
182. Wahl RL, Jacene H, Kasamon Y, Lodge MA. From RECIST to PERCIST: evolving considerations for PET response criteria in solid tumors. J Nucl Med. 2009;50 Suppl 1:122S–50.
183. Barrington SF, Mikhaeel NG, Kostakoglu L, et al. Role of imaging in the staging and response assessment of lymphoma: consensus of the International Conference on Malignant Lymphomas Imaging Working Group. J Clin Oncol. 2014;32(27):3048–58.
184. Barrington SF, Mackewn JE, Schleyer P, et al. Establishment of a UK-wide network to facilitate the acquisition of quality assured FDG-PET data for clinical trials in lymphoma. Ann Oncol. 2011; 22(3):739–45.
185. Radford J, Illidge T, Counsell N, Hancock B, et al. Results of a trial of PET-directed therapy for early-stage Hodgkin's lymphoma. N Engl J Med. 2015;372(17):1598–607.
186. Swinnen LJ, Li H, Quon A, et al. Response-adapted therapy for aggressive non-Hodgkin's lymphomas based on early [18F] FDG-PET scanning: ECOG-ACRIN Cancer Research Group study (E3404). Br J Haematol. 2015;170(1):56–65.
187. Yu EY, Duan F, Muzi M, et al. Castration-resistant prostate cancer bone metastasis response measured by 18F-fluoride PET after treatment with dasatinib and correlation with progression-free survival: results https://www.acrin.org/TabID/638/Default.aspx from American College of Radiology Imaging Network 6687. J Nucl Med. 2015;56(3):354–60.
188. Ferdová E, Ferda J, Baxa J, Tupý R, Mraček J, Topolčan O, Hes O. Assessment of grading in newly-diagnosed glioma using 18F-fluorothymidine PET/CT. Anticancer Res. 2015;35(2):955–9.

Cardiac PET Imaging: Principles and New Developments

19

Ran Klein and Robert A. deKemp

Contents

19.1	**Background**	451
19.2	**Instrumentation**	453
19.3	**Cardiac PET Tracers**	454
19.4	**Perfusion**	454
19.4.1	Myocardial Perfusion Imaging	454
19.4.2	Stress Protocols	456
19.4.3	ECG-Gated Imaging	464
19.4.4	MPI Tracers	464
19.5	**Metabolic Imaging**	467
19.5.1	Carbohydrate Metabolism	467
19.5.2	Fatty Acid Metabolism	468
19.5.3	Oxidative Metabolism	469
19.5.4	Viability Imaging	469
19.5.5	Metabolic Alteration Studies	471
19.5.6	Quantification of Metabolism	471
19.6	**Myocardial Inflammation**	472
19.7	**Vascular Inflammation**	472
19.8	**Cell Signaling**	473
19.8.1	Neurocrine (ANS, RAAS) and Endocrine (Adrenalin, Angiotensin)	473
19.8.2	Paracrine (e.g., Nitric Oxide) and Autocrine (Immune)	477
19.9	**Cardiac PET in Clinical Trials**	478
19.10	**Future Directions**	479
	References	479

R. Klein, PhD (✉)
Department of Nuclear Medicine,
The Ottawa Hospital, 1053 Carling Ave.,
Ottawa, ON, K1Y 4E9, Canada
e-mail: rklein@toh.on.ca

R.A. deKemp, PhD, PEng, PPhys
National Cardiac PET Centre, Cardiac Imaging,
The University of Ottawa Heart Institute,
40 Ruskin St., Ottawa, ON, K1Y 4W7, Canada
e-mail: radekemp@ottawaheart.ca

Abstract

A growing interest in cardiac physiology, disease, and treatment has fuelled the development of cardiac PET applications both for research and clinical use. Imaging of the heart poses unique challenges, including the presence of cardiac, respiratory, and organ motions and complex anatomy. As with other organs, common challenges include physiologic interactions from the systematic level down to the molecular level and a broad range of diseases. Since cardiology includes mechanical, electrical, blood flow, metabolic, neurohormonal, immunological, and genetic aspects, cardiac imaging is a broad field with a wide range of tracers and applications designed to probe all of these mechanisms. This chapter provides an overview of existing applications and recent developments of cardiac PET imaging.

19.1 Background

Cardiac imaging has typically been a distinct subfield of radiology or nuclear medicine, and PET is no exception. Imaging of the heart poses

M.M. Khalil (ed.), *Basic Science of PET Imaging*, DOI 10.1007/978-3-319-40070-9_19

unique challenges due to its anatomy, physiology, and function. At the macroscopic level, the heart is a large, highly-perfused muscle that contracts around large blood pools in order to pump blood to the body tissues and lungs. The heart is encased in a thin layer of pericardial fluid that is contained within the pericardial sac. The heart is mostly surrounded by aerated lung tissue with the anterior region pressed against the sternum and the inferior region resting against the diaphragm and in close proximity to the liver, upper stomach, or spleen, which can all be potential sources of PET signal contamination due to partial volume averaging and spillover effects. Likewise tracer activity in the blood, including the right and left ventricles and atrial blood pools, as well as the arterial blood perfusing the myocardial tissue, may impact accurate quantification of tracer concentrations in the myocardium.

The left ventricle (LV) myocardium is the largest structure in the heart and has a wall thickness of approximately 1 cm at end diastole, which is on the order of the spatial resolution of PET. The right ventricle (RV) wall is approximately one-third to one-half the LV thickness and feature in cardiac PET images, but with more substantial partial volume loss. The atrial walls are thinner still (1–2 mm) and have therefore not been amenable to PET imaging until the most recent PET technologies, with improved spatial resolution and lower image noise. Therefore, the LV has been of major interest in cardiac PET, but imaging of the RV and the atria is of increasing interest.

A key challenge in cardiac imaging is motion. The human heart contracts roughly one to three times per second at rest or peak stress, resulting in cardiac motion blurring in PET images which are acquired over several seconds to several minutes. A secondary source of motion in cardiac PET is associated with respiratory motion of the heart, as the diaphragm pushes against the inferior wall of the LV myocardium. Heart creep may also be present as the heart settles in the thorax as a result of soft tissue compliance to the force of gravity after the patient has transitioned from upright to a supine position, as the patient relaxes during the imaging procedure, or as they recover from deep breathing following treadmill exercise stress. A final source of motion, as with all PET imaging, is voluntary and involuntary patient body motion (e.g., coughing, fidgeting, and repositioning due to discomfort).

Because all PET projection data is acquired simultaneously (as opposed to single-photon emission computed tomography – SPECT), motion is manifested as incremental blurring in the reconstructed images, and the associated partial volume effects adversely impact quantification of tracer concentrations. Furthermore, motion can result in partial misregistration between the emission and transmission images used for attenuation correction. Misregistration artifacts are especially noticeable in regions with sharp attenuation changes such as the interface between the heart and the lungs (e.g., lateral wall of the LV). While PET data are acquired over all phases of the cardiac and respiratory cycles, x-ray CT data for attenuation correction is captured mid-breath and even mid-cardiac stroke, and therefore perfect alignment is uncommon. However, during regular breathing, more time is spent in the end-expiration phase, which has become the standard target for PET-CT attenuation correction. Attenuation misregistration artifacts may manifest as either an over- or underestimation of tracer concentration depending on the direction of misalignment, and therefore quality assurance prior to reconstruction is essential. A large amount of research is devoted to reducing motion artifacts, but current guidelines recommend acquisition of attenuation CT without ECG triggering, at mid-to-end exhalation, low current, and high pitch in order to freeze the effects of respiratory motion and reduce patient dose [1]. Motion artifacts and correction techniques are discussed in Chap. 16.

On a smaller scale, the heart structure appears less uniform, with the coronary vasculature arguably producing the most significant effects in the context of cardiac PET. The heart muscle is perfused by a large amount of blood (up to 15 % of the cardiac output) through a fractal network of arteries originating at the root of the aorta and branching out on the epicardial surface of the

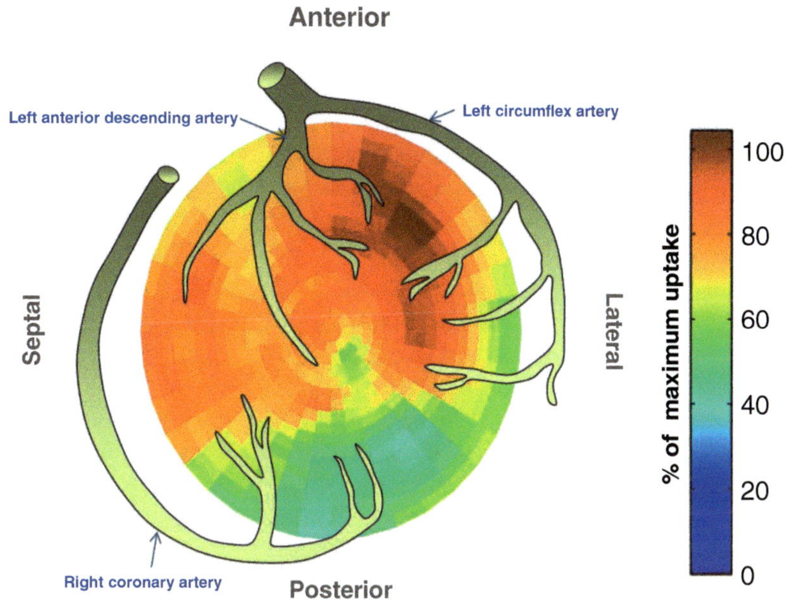

Fig. 19.1 Typical coronary anatomy. The LAD, LCx, and RCA are the three main coronary arteries that perfuse the LV myocardium. The colored polar map is an example image of relative tracer uptake (% of maximum) in the LV

ventricles. Distal branches penetrate the surface of the muscle delivering blood to the tissue via a fine mesh of capillaries. While a typical pattern is demonstrated in Fig. 19.1, a wide spectrum of anatomies can exist. Imaging all individual vessels is not possible with PET; however, their net effect on tracer distribution to territories supplied by these vessels is the basis of cardiac PET perfusion imaging for the diagnosis of coronary artery disease (CAD).

While cardiac SPECT is the workhorse of nuclear cardiology with an estimated 20,000 procedures per day in the USA alone being performed, cardiac PET is firmly established for state-of-the-art research applications and is exponentially expanding into clinical use. With the expected increases in SPECT radiopharmaceuticals costs, it is expected that the clinical use of cardiac PET will continue to grow in the coming decade [2]. Other imaging modalities (i.e., MRI, x-ray CT, and ultrasound) for cardiac applications are inherently different in their ability to image anatomy and tissue characterization, but less so for imaging molecular function, and therefore complement PET, hence the continued interest in hybrid imaging solutions such as PET-CT and PET-MR in cardiology.

19.2 Instrumentation

While most PET instrumentation has been designed with oncology application in mind, several adaptations have been crucial to enable cardiac PET. In the early 2000s, recognizing the increasing prevalence of obese patients, PET design shifted toward larger gantries with >60 cm diameter openings and beds capable of supporting upward of 200 kg patients. Faster, multislice diagnostic CT scanners became available as part of hybrid systems enabling coronary CT angiography and PET in a single imaging session – however, the routine clinical application remains rare.

ECG gating was introduced as a means to bin data into several (e.g., 8–24) phases of the cardiac cycle. Each coincidence event is placed in a bin corresponding to its cardiac contractile phase, and each bin is reconstructed individually producing a cine image of the beating heart. By viewing a single cardiac phase, a motion-free image is produced, offering greater spatial resolution. The greater the number of bins however, the fewer counts are available in each bin resulting in noisier images. In research applications, visualization of the mid-to-end diastolic (e.g., 70–80 % of the R–R interval) phase has been utilized as a relatively simple method to maximize image spatial resolution as the heart is nearly dilated (highest feature separation) and least moving (reduced motion blur).

The adoption of 3D PET acquisition highly benefited cardiac applications due to the two- to fivefold increase in camera sensitivity overall and as much as an order of magnitude increase in the central planes, which enables improved image quality especially with ECG-gated imaging [3]. Dynamic imaging with short imaging time frames also benefited from the improved count statistics of 3D PET. In static imaging, the increased camera sensitivity could be leveraged for shorter imaging times, radiation dose reductions, and/or reduced image noise. The addition of iterative statistical reconstruction and time-of-flight technologies has complemented 3D PET acquisition to further improve the effective sensitivity of cardiac PET.

With the exponential increase in data storage capacity, list-mode data acquisition has become a clinical reality and is offered by all vendors. In cardiac PET list-mode acquisitions were instrumental in enabling simultaneous acquisition of static, gated, and dynamic image series, primarily benefiting myocardial perfusion imaging (MPI) tests which is the most widely used application of cardiac PET [4]. A routine MPI exam consists of static and ECG-gated imaging of the tracer uptake for evaluating perfusion and cardiac function, respectively. An increasing number of centers also acquire a dynamic image sequence from the start of tracer administration to the end of initial distribution which is used to quantify myocardial blood flow (MBF), requiring early start of the image acquisition to measure the first-pass transit of tracer through the heart.

With the recent introduction of PET-MR hybrid scanners, new cardiac applications are being explored. One clinically relevant application of these hybrid systems is simultaneous PET and MR acquisition to reduce patient body and organ motion [5]. The MR images can be used to detect and characterize the motion, which is then incorporated into the PET image reconstruction to produce motion-free images. Furthermore, integration of PET acquisition with sophisticated cardiac MR protocols promises simultaneous acquisition of physiologic function from PET and high-quality anatomical and tissue characterization information from MR [6].

On the small animal imaging front, cameras have evolved to become extremely sensitive using longer bores and tightly packed detectors, enabling the use of lower tracer activities, even in the context of mice and rat imaging, keeping PET at the forefront of molecular imaging. Meanwhile, with continued improvements in imaging hardware and reconstruction algorithm, submillimeter imaging resolution is possible, but remains limited by the range of positrons leaving the atomic nucleus before combining with a free electron to produce the annihilation photons for PET imaging.

19.3 Cardiac PET Tracers

Cardiac PET applications are entirely dependent on the range of available molecules that can be imaged in vivo and therefore remains an active research field [7]. A unique advantage of PET over other noninvasive imaging modalities is the ability to image and quantify tracer concentrations in miniscule amounts due to the specific signal of the tracer and the very high sensitivity of PET instrumentation [8]. The molecular amount of radiolabeled molecule required for routine imaging is therefore in the pico- to femtomolar range, which is crucial to achieving trace quantities that do not invoke a physiologic response from the patient, organs, or cells [9, 10]. This property of PET is especially advantageous when probing mechanisms with limited binding capacity such as receptor signaling. Table 19.1 lists some of the more commonly used cardiac PET tracers, their characteristics, and their applications.

19.4 Perfusion

19.4.1 Myocardial Perfusion Imaging

Myocardial perfusion imaging (MPI) with SPECT is widely used to diagnose epicardial coronary artery disease (CAD), to prognosticate for risk stratification, and to guide therapy [11]. PET has been shown to be cost-effective

Table 19.1 Common cardiac tracers and their indicators

Tracer	Radioactive half-life (min)	Mean positron range in water (mm)	Production	Indications	Comments
^{82}Rb-rubidium chloride	1.27	2.60	Generator (^{82}Sr) eluate	Myocardial perfusion and blood flow quantification	Reasonable uptake-to-flow relationship Requires direct injection system Suitable for rapid serial imaging
^{13}N-ammonia	10.0	0.57	Cyclotron – purified	Myocardial perfusion and blood flow quantification	Excellent uptake-to-flow relationship
^{15}O-water	2.05	1.02	Cyclotron – synthesized	Myocardial blood flow quantification	Requires direct injection from bedside synthesis unit Ideal uptake-to-flow relationship MPI not possible
^{18}F-flurpiridaz	109.8	0.23	Cyclotron – synthesized	Myocardial perfusion and blood flow quantification	Excellent uptake-to-flow relationship
^{62}Cu-pyruvaldehyde bis(N-methyl-thiosemicarbazone) (PTSM)	9.67	4.39	Generator (^{62}Zn) eluate	Myocardial perfusion and blood flow quantification	Short parent isotope half-life has limited application
^{18}F-fluorodeoxyglucose (FDG)	109.8	0.23	Cyclotron – synthesized	Myocardial viability Inflammation (e.g., cardiac sarcoidosis, vulnerable plaque, device infection) Glucose uptake	Nonspecific cell target – explored for many biomarkers
^{11}C-glucose	20.3	0.42	Cyclotron – synthesized	Myocardial viability Glucose metabolism	Radiolabeled metabolites complicate quantification
^{18}F-fluorodeoxymannose (FDM)	109.8	0.23	Cyclotron – synthesized	Macrophage activity Glucose metabolism	Early studies for inflammation and oncology applications
^{11}C-acetate	20.3	0.42	Cyclotron – synthesized	Oxygen consumption myocardial perfusion and blood flow quantification	Indirect oxidative metabolism
^{18}F-fluorothia-6-heptadecanoic acid (FTHA)	109.8	0.23	Cyclotron – synthesized	Fatty acid uptake	

(continued)

Table 19.1 (continued)

Tracer	Radioactive half-life (min)	Mean positron range in water (mm)	Production	Indications	Comments
16-[^{18}F] fluoro-4-thia-palmitate (FTP)	109.8	0.23	Cyclotron – synthesized	Fatty acid uptake and metabolism	Hypoxia-dependent tissue uptake
Trans-9(RS)-18F-fluoro-3,4(RS,RS)-methyleneheptadecanoic acid (FCPHA)	109.8	0.23	Cyclotron – synthesized	Fatty acid uptake	High cardiac tissue uptake and retention
^{11}C-palmitate	20.3	0.42	Cyclotron – synthesized	Fatty acid metabolism	Difficult kinetics due to metabolites
^{11}C-lactate	20.3	0.42	Cyclotron – synthesized	Lactate metabolism	
$^{15}O_2$	2.05	1.02	Cyclotron – purified	Oxygen consumption	
^{11}C-carbon monoxide	20.3	0.42	Cyclotron – synthesized	Blood volume imaging	
^{15}O-carbon monoxide	2.05	1.02	Cyclotron	Blood volume imaging	Requires direct inhalation from bedside synthesis unit Often used in conjunction with ^{15}O-water perfusion scans
^{11}C-hydroxyephedrine (HED)	20.3	0.42	Cyclotron – synthesized	Sympathetic innervation	

compared to alternative imaging modalities [12]. Patients are imaged at rest and following either exercise or pharmacologic stress. The reconstructed images are evaluated in conjunction to evaluate rest perfusion, stress perfusion, stress-rest reversibility (ischemia), and stress-rest flow reserve (the capacity to increase perfusion). MPI with PET has been shown to have improved diagnostic accuracy [13] and prognostic value [14, 15], largely due to improved image quality and robust attenuation correction. A recent meta-analysis of the current literature concluded that ^{82}Rb-PET was superior to ^{99m}Tc-SPECT for detection of obstructive CAD (as defined by invasive coronary angiography) with 90 % vs. 85 % sensitivity and 88 % vs. 85 % specificity [16]. Consequently the use of PET to guide CAD patient management has been demonstrated to result in up to 50 % fewer invasive procedures, 30 % cost savings, and favorable outcomes when compared to SPECT [17]. However, due to the higher cost of PET, it has not been widely applied for MPI. The increasing availability of lower-cost PET cameras, the adoption of generator-produced ^{82}Rb in high-throughput clinics, and the increasing costs of ^{99m}Tc isotope for SPECT tracers are fuelling the growth of the cardiac PET MPI market. Currently, ^{82}Rb, ^{13}N-ammonia, and ^{15}O-water are approved for myocardial perfusion indications in some jurisdictions, with new tracers in various stages of regulatory review.

19.4.2 Stress Protocols

In general, exercise stress (e.g., treadmill) is preferred clinically, unless contraindicated, as it most accurately simulates real-life exertion and patient symptoms [18]. However, due to the short half-life of PET tracers, pharmacologic stress is routinely used for MPI studies. A variety of pharmacologic agents are available for inducing hyperemic flow during imaging, as listed in Table 19.2. Pharmacologic stress PET is advantageous for

Table 19.2 Commonly use cardiac stress agents in clinical MPI and MBF quantification

Agent	Response	Mechanism	Dose	Half-life	Remarks	Specific contraindications
Adenosine	Vasodilation	Coronary A_{2a} smooth vessel agonist	0.14 mg/kg/min	30 s	Caffeine has similar structure and also is an agonist of A_1,A_{2B},A_3 receptors	Asthma >Second-degree AV block or sinus node dysfunction (without artificial pacemaker) Bradycardia SBP <90 mmHg Unstable acute MI or coronary syndrome
Dipyridamole (Persantine)	Vasodilation	Inhibit adenosine reuptake and increases the intramyocardial concentration	0.14 mg/kg/min	40 min	Aminophylline used as antidote	
Regadenoson	Vasodilation	Coronary smooth vessel agonist on A_{2a}	0.4 mg	2–3 min	No need to stop β-blockers. No need for IV line (bolus injection)	>Second-degree AV block or sinus node dysfunction (without artificial pacemaker) SBP <90 mmHg
Dobutamine	Chronotropic and inotropic	Strong β_1, moderate β_2, and mild α_1 adrenergic receptor agonist	10–40 μg/kg/min	Very short	Could be combined with atropine	Recent MI Unstable angina Severe LV outflow obstruction History or risk of LV tachycardia Uncontrolled hypertension Aortic dissection or aneurysm Use of β-blockers

Common contraindications: recent use of dipyridamole <48 h prior, recent use of methyl xanthenes <24 h prior, caffeine consumption <12 h prior, and known hypersensitivity imaging at peak stress, as opposed to post-stress imaging which is performed with treadmill exercise and SPECT imaging. Some agents are designed to stimulate the sympathetic nervous system both directly and indirectly, and others induce vasodilation of coronary vessels, resulting in increased cardiac output to maintain arterial blood pressure. Since caffeine is a competing vasodilation agonist, absence of caffeine intake for >12 h is recommended to achieve maximum response between rest and stress [19].

Combined use of different stress agents can be used to evaluate individual contributing mechanisms to myocardial flow reserve. A common example is the use of the cold pressor test (CPT), in which a limb is submerged into ice-cold water, invoking a systemic vascular response which is dependent on endothelial function through adrenergic stimulation. The endothelium-mediated vasodilation represents a fraction of the total maximal flow obtained from stress agents above [20]. CPT and rest flow measurement have been used to demonstrate endothelial dysfunction in smokers compared to nonsmokers and that endothelial function may be rapidly restored with smoking cessation [21]. CPT can be unpleasant and difficult to endure, and alternative agonists of the sympathetic system such as induced hypercapnia [22] or salbutamol [23] are under investigation.

19.4.2.1 MPI Interpretation

Regional myocardial perfusion is evaluated visually by comparing tracer uptake in different regions of the myocardium against a reference region of maximum uptake, which is assumed to be normally perfused. Regions with homogeneous uptake at rest and stress are interpreted as normal. Regions with relatively reduced tracer uptake at stress that normalize at rest are interpreted as ischemic, while regions with relatively reduced uptake at both rest and stress are interpreted as myocardial scar [18]. The rest and stress images are reoriented to a standard orientation that can be viewed as a series of short-axis (SA) slices transecting the LV from apex to base as demonstrated in the top rows of Fig. 19.2. Orthogonal slices may be displayed to generate horizontal and vertical long axis (HLA and VLA, respectively) views of the heart (middle and bottom row on images). A more concise presentation of the LV is using polar maps (right bottom) which sample the mid myocardium contour. The apex is presented at the center of the polar map with the base at the radial extreme; the septum and anterior, lateral, and posterior walls are on the left, top, right, and bottom, respectively, as illustrated in Fig. 19.1.

LV polar maps can be segmented into regions which are each scored individually to generate a semiquantitative score of defect severity. Most commonly a 17-segment model is used with scores ranging from 0 to 4 corresponding to normal perfusion, mild reduction, moderate reduction, severe reduction, and an absence of tracer uptake [24]. Summation of the segment scores produces summed stress and rest scores (SSS and SRS) which are global metrics of defect extent and severity. The summed difference score (SDS) is a global indicator of reversible ischemia. SSS >3 is a commonly used threshold for the presence of disease with SRS >3 and SDS >1 indicating the presence of nonreversible scar. A limitation of these scores is the dependence on segment alignment and visual assessment (including overriding of automatically generated scores) which reduces their reproducibility [25]. The total perfusion deficit (TPD) is a quantitative alternative which does not rely on polar map segmentation [26] and is therefore increasing in popularity.

Relative uptake image interpretation, however, is susceptible to misdiagnosing or underdiagnosing CAD in patient with uniform reduction in perfusion such as in balanced disease in multiple coronary vessels and in distributed disease of the microvasculature (e.g., associated with diabetes mellitus). Furthermore, since the most commonly used PET MPI tracer (^{82}Rb) is extracted nonlinearly with blood flow, mild perfusion deficits may be difficult to detect. Absolute quantification of myocardial blood flow helps to address these limitations of relative-scale MPI.

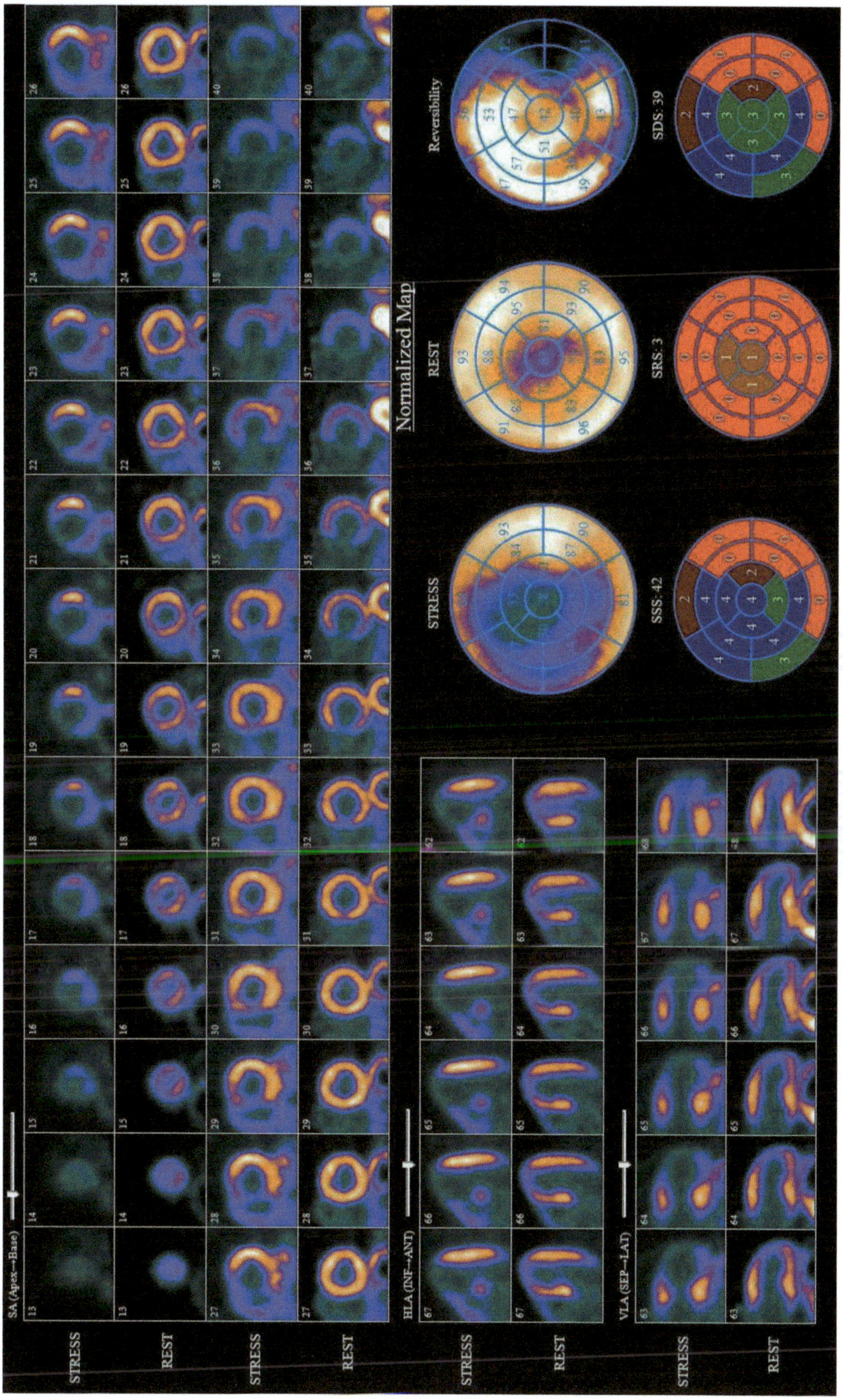

Fig. 19.2 Example of myocardial perfusion (MPI) report for a 54-year-old male patient using ^{82}Rb PET. A large uptake deficit in the septal, anterior, posterior, and apical regions at stress that is resolved at rest as indicated by the reversibility polar map

19.4.2.2 Myocardial Blood Flow (MBF) and Flow Reserve (MFR) Quantification

With dynamic PET imaging, absolute myocardial blood flow (MBF) can be quantified at peak stress and at rest in units of mL/min per g of tissue (mL/min/g) (Fig. 19.4). The ratio of the two is termed the myocardial flow reserve (MFR) and indicates the capacity to increase blood flow to the heart in order to meet demand with exercise [4]. Flow difference (delta), the difference between MBF at stress and rest, may also be used to describe reserve in absolute terms (mL/min/g). MFR has been shown to increase sensitivity for detection of balanced multivessel disease, where the relative perfusion is normalized to the area of highest perfusion which is itself underperfused and therefore would appear normal on standard relative MPI. MBF and MFR in this region would be low, thereby unmasking ischemia [27–29]. In addition MFR has been shown to detect diffuse disease of the microvasculature as well as endothelial dysfunction which are markers of incipient epicardial CAD [30]. As a result, MFR has demonstrated prognostic value incremental to relative MPI for prediction of both mortality and major adverse coronary events [29]. Normal human populations have been used to define thresholds for abnormal MBF and MFR values. Typically MFR values >2.5 are associated with normal myocardial perfusion and blood flow. Conversely, an MFR <2 is associated with CAD and/or microvascular disease [31–33].

Stress MBF and MFR have been proposed as potential differentiators between functionally significant and benign coronary lesions. MBF at maximum hyperemia decreases progressively once the stenosis is greater than 40–50 % of the vessel diameter, while resting MBF remains normal until there is a diameter stenosis of 80–90 % [34], leading to the use of invasive assessment of fractional flow reserve (FFR) to guide invasive interventions with better specificity and outcomes [35]. MBF can be increased with revascularization [34], but in diabetics with focal narrowing, revascularization leads to only mildly improved blood flow [36]. These findings confirm that MFR is determined by a combination of epicardial vessel flow, functional microvasculature, and cell integrity [34]. While it has been demonstrated that spatial patterns of MPI along with other information can result in better patient outcomes when used to guide therapy [14], the same has not yet been demonstrated for absolute MBF and MFR quantification.

Quantification of MBF requires dynamic imaging from the time of tracer administration until distribution is achieved (typically 5–10 min). The acquisition is binned into predefined time frames ranging from several seconds long in the early time frames, where rapid dynamics are occurring, to a few minutes in length in the late time frames, where the dynamics are slow and count rates are relatively low. The dynamic image sequence is then processed using specialized software that models the tracer kinetics in the myocardial tissue and the arterial blood that perfuses it. In most cases myocardial regions of interest (ROI) are automatically, semi-automatically, or manually defined using an uptake image in which the myocardium is clearly visible. Likewise an arterial ROI is defined in the left ventricle, left atrium, or aorta. The ROIs are then used to sample the dynamic sequence to measure time-activity curves (TAC) of the blood (input) and myocardium (output). A parameterized kinetic model is used to describe the relationship between the blood and myocardium TACs. The model parameters are fit to the measured TACs. Typically a two-compartment (blood and tissue) model is sufficient [37], of which the blood-to-myocardium uptake parameter (*K1*) is related to MBF [4, 38]. A tissue washout parameter (*k2*) may be associated with tissue integrity, viability, or perfusion, depending on the tracer. *K1* values must be corrected for flow-dependent extraction as discussed in the MPI tracer section in order to estimate MBF. See Chap. 14.

Special considerations must be given to tracer administration with dynamic PET imaging especially with short-lived isotopes such as ^{82}Rb. Early in the imaging process, the tracer activity is concentrated in a relatively small blood volume, but is then distributed throughout the entire body and undergoes radioactive decay. Thus, early time frames may experience count rates of 3–4

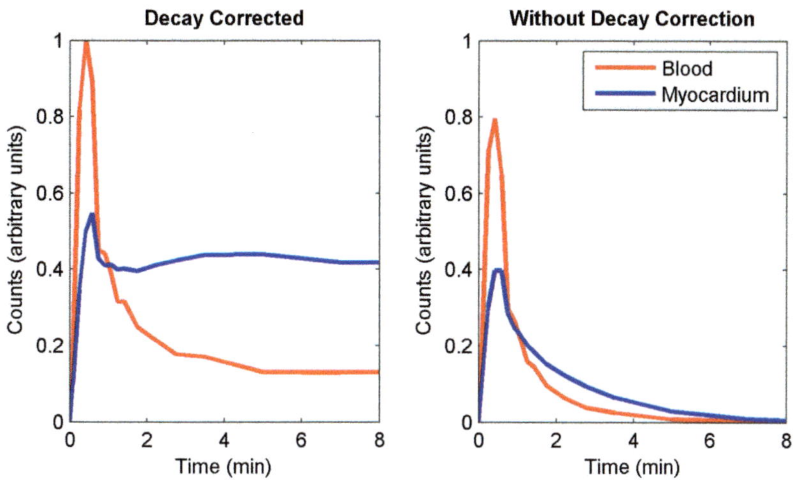

Fig. 19.3 Blood and myocardial time-activity curves of a ^{82}Rb stress scan with and without isotope decay correction. While for kinetic modeling decay correction is required, in practice the PET camera measures the activity without decay correction, which varies over several orders of magnitude during the scan due to tracer distribution and radioactive decay

orders of magnitude greater than those at late time frames as demonstrated in Fig. 19.3.

MBF and MFR analysis of the same patient as in Figs. 19.2 and 19.4 is shown in Fig. 19.5. While the MPI interpretation suggests ischemia in much of the LV territory that is resolved at rest, MBF and MFR paint a more severe picture of abnormally low MBF at stress in almost the entire LV and uniformly low rest MBF as well. Abnormal MFR (<2) and delta (<1 mL/min/g) are indicated in a larger territory (58 % of the myocardium) than with MPI, suggesting involvement of more tissue than indicated by MPI. Finally, cardiac steal (lower flow at stress than at rest) is indicated in 26 % of the LV also demonstrating severe obstruction of the blood supply in the territory of LAD artery.

Using automated classification rules [32], the territories associated with the left anterior descending (LAD) and mid to distal left circumflex (LCx) and right coronary arteries (RCA) were suspected to have obstructive stenoses. These findings were confirmed using invasive angiography as shown in Fig. 19.6 which indicated 100 % obstruction of the mid-LAD artery, 90 % stenosis in the first diagonal, >70 % stenoses in the proximal LCx and its branches, and >80 % stenoses in the distal RCA branches.

In MPI imaging, patient, organ and respiratory motions is manifested as a blur in the direction of motion which can lead to artifactual uptake deficits in opposing cardiac walls [39]. In MBF quantification these same motions can further result in inconsistent ROI sampling and attenuation misalignment artifacts that propagate to inaccurate TACs and MBF measurement errors. Quality assurance at each processing step can often expose the presence to motion clewing the reader to potentially unreliable MBF estimates. Robust motion detection and correction algorithms are an active area of research, but are complicated by rapid changes of the tracer distribution in the early time frames of the dynamic image sequence.

The effects of cardiac motion on MBF quantification are assumed to be small due to partial volume correction and due to improved normal-to-defect wall contrast as a result of tracer extraction correction. However in MPI, cardiac motion can produce regionally varying partial volume effects that can mask defects. For example, a hypokinetic wall region with mild uptake deficit may appear as bright as a normally perfused region with preserved wall motion and partial volume loses. For this and other reasons, MPI images should be interpreted in conjunction with ECG-gated imaging.

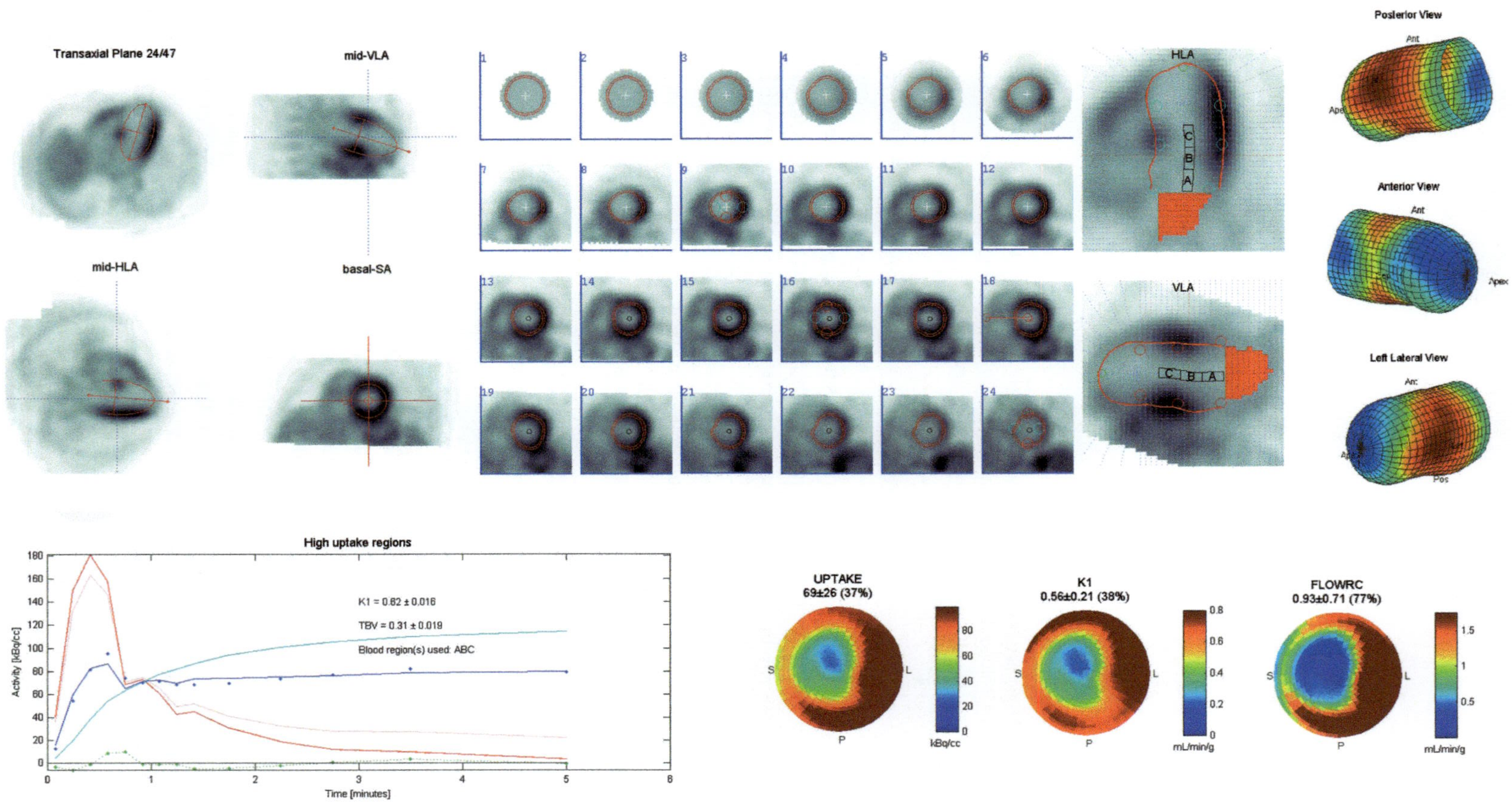

Fig. 19.4 Myocardial blood flow quantification using a dynamic ^{82}Rb scan (same stress scan in Fig. 19.2). An uptake image is generated using the late time frames and is reoriented (*top left*) to generate standard SA, HLA, and VLA views (*top center*) on which LV myocardium contours are defined (*red lines*) along with blood pool regions (*A*, *B*, and *C* regions). 3D meshes (*top right*) are displayed corresponding to the uptake polar map (*bottom center*). A one-tissue compartment model can be fit to myocardial (*blue*) and blood (*red*) time-activity curves (*bottom left*) to generate *K1* and extraction corrected flow polar maps (*bottom right*) in units of mL/min/g

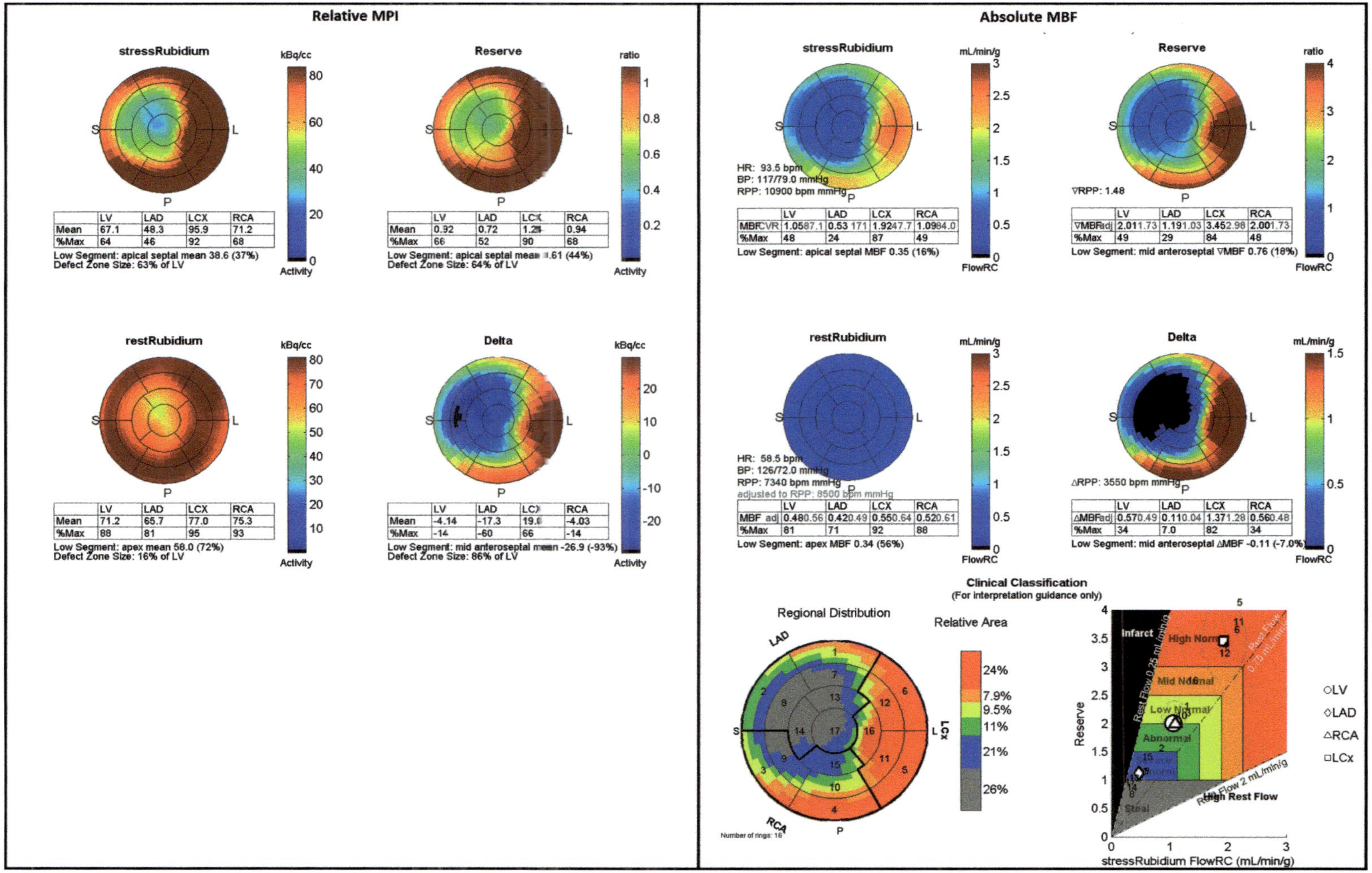

Fig. 19.5 Flow reserve using relative MPI (*left*) and absolute MBF (*right*) for the same patient as in Figs. 19.2 and 19.4. Similar stress deficit patterns are observed with both MPI and MBF, with more contrast and broader extent using MBF. Rest flow is uniform in both cases indicating stress-induced ischemia. The reserve and delta polar maps tell a similar story; however, MBF indicates a much more severe deficit than MPI, as indicated by cardiac steal (lower stress than rest flows) in 26 % of the LV territories using the clinical classification rules

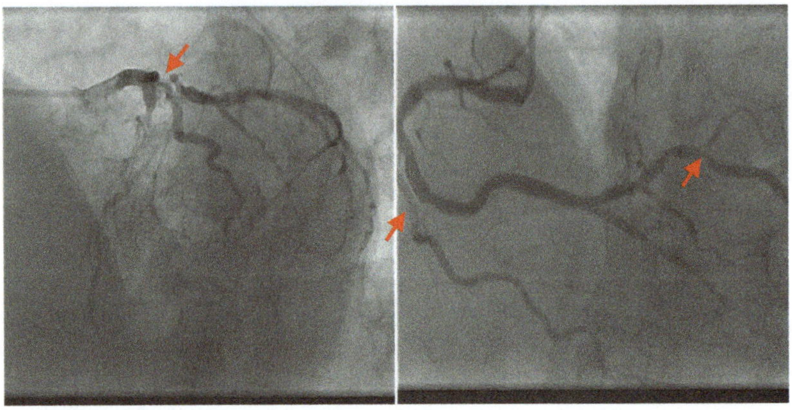

Fig. 19.6 Angiography for the same case as in Figs. 19.2, 19.4, and 19.5, indicating severe 100 % obstruction of the mid-LAD artery, 90 % stenosis in the first diagonal, >70 % stenoses in the proximal LCx and its branches (*left*), and >80 % stenoses in the distal RCA branches (*right*). Location of stenoses are indicated by *red arrows*

19.4.3 ECG-Gated Imaging

Whenever possible, ventricular function with gated imaging should be interpreted as part of MPI, as wall motion and wall thickening can be used to differentiate between ischemia and residual attenuation artifacts in regions with reduced tracer uptake [13]. Hypoperfused regions associated with wall motion abnormalities often signify scarred, stunned, or hibernating myocardium. However, if wall motion is preserved, apparent perfusion defects may be artifacts (e.g., attenuation misregistration, motion). Areas of normal perfusion with hypokinesis may be markers of myocardial stunning after an acute ischemic insult [11] or markers of mild perfusion deficit that are masked by lower regional partial volume losses (associated with reduced motion) compared to normal reference regions.

All current PET scanners offer the possibility of ECG gating and list-mode acquisition and therefore are able to reconstruct cine-gated images, dynamic images, and static (ungated) uptake MPI from a single injection and acquisition. An important advantage of physiologic stressing and image acquisition at peak stress is that wall motion abnormalities can be observed at peak stress, making PET more sensitive than conventional SPECT practice to detect regional and global wall motion abnormalities, which may otherwise resolve with post-stress imaging [13]. For the example case in Figs. 19.4, 19.5, and 19.6, the gated stress image indicated hypokinesis of the septal wall and dyskinesis of the apex, consistent with the findings of severe ischemia and steal from the MPI and MBF interpretations (Fig. 19.7).

19.4.4 MPI Tracers

As Table 19.2 demonstrates, several PET perfusion tracers are available, of which ^{82}Rb is the most widely used. ^{82}Rb is generator produced, and therefore does not require an on-site cyclotron compared to ^{13}N-ammonia, ^{11}C-acetate, or ^{15}O-water. Flurpiridaz, as with other ^{18}F-based MPI tracers, has a 2-h physical half-life and therefore may be distributed over large distances as is common with FDG and thus may become a clinically relevant alternative in the future.

The short half-life of ^{82}Rb implies low radiation dose to the patient [40] and staff, but can contribute to low count statistics in late uptake images. Furthermore ^{82}Rb has a relatively high positron range which can degrade the image spatial resolution slightly. ^{82}Rb is extracted from the blood into perfused tissue both through diffusion and active ion transport, as it is a potassium analogue. Consequently, tracer extraction from the blood into the tissue space is limited (Table 19.3) and decreases nonlinearly with flow as demonstrated in Fig. 19.8. This effect must be accounted for in MBF quantification using an extraction correction function [4, 33, 41–43]. Thus *K1* estimation error is amplified during conversion to MBF, especially at high stress flow values. As demonstrated in Fig. 19.8, several extraction

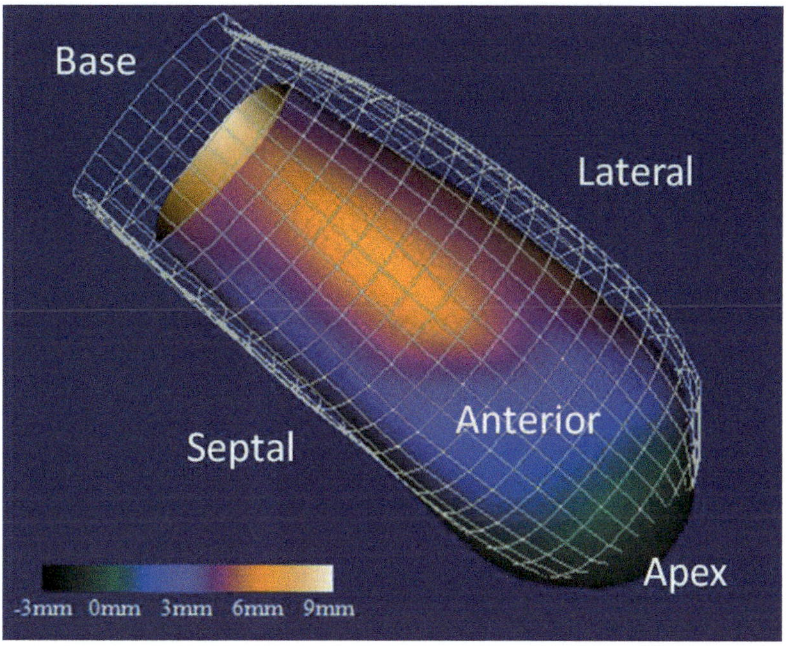

Fig. 19.7 Cardiac wall motion at peak stress for the same patient example as in Figs. 19.2, 19.4, 19.5, and 19.6. The *white mesh* indicates LV cavity contours at end diastole and the color surface at end systole. The *surface color* indicates the extent of cardiac wall motion of the respective territory. The septal wall is hypokinetic, and the apex is dyskinetic corresponding to the MPI and MBF findings

correction functions have been reported in the literature; their differences likely demonstrate the use of different imaging equipment, analysis software, experimental approaches, and patient cohorts, and therefore the extraction function can also be interpreted as a calibration function of *K1* to MBF (Fig. 19.8-right). Nevertheless, equivalent results have been demonstrated across commercially available software packages when using the one-tissue compartment model and the Lortie extraction function [44, 45]. The move to 3D PET imaging with higher count-rate capabilities is expected to improve the precision and accuracy of MBF using ^{82}Rb in particular.

^{15}O-water PET is regarded widely as the gold standard for noninvasive MBF quantification. Water is freely diffusible through the capillary cellular membranes and therefore has 100% extraction, eliminating the need for extraction correction. Likewise, water freely diffuses out of the cellular space, and therefore a simple one-tissue kinetic model with proportional *K1* and *k2* parameters can be resolved robustly to quantify MBF. Since the tracer is not trapped in the myocardium, however, late uptake images have no contrast between blood and tissue, so standard MPI interpretation is not possible. Likewise gated images of the beating heart are not readily available to assess cardiac function. Compounded by the need for an on-site cyclotron with direct line to the patient, water PET has mostly been applied in research settings.

^{13}N-ammonia is avidly extracted and retained in the myocardium making for an excellent perfusion agent; however, it too requires an on-site cyclotron making it less than ideal for widespread use. Ammonia is taken up by the liver (and to a lesser extent by the lungs), and images often result in difficult interpretation of the inferior wall of the heart due to inadequate spatial resolution or separation. Finally, ammonia metabolites accumulate in the blood which can have a small effect on blood-to-myocardium contrast and need to be corrected for accurate MBF quantification. ^{13}N-ammonia also has a reported normal variant reduction of tracer retention in the lateral wall that complicates the interpretation of disease in the LCX artery [46].

^{18}F-flurpiridaz is a relatively new tracer, developed specifically for PET MPI and MBF. It has almost ideal imaging properties including high extraction and retention, low positron energy, and slow radioactive decay. However, due to the long radioactive and biological life of

Table 19.3 Commonly use PET MPI and MBF tracer properties

Tracer	First-pass extraction	Image spatial resolution	Extracardiac interference	Injected activity with 3D PET (approximate)	Effective dose	Comments
^{82}Rb-rubidium chloride	40–100 % dependent on flow	8–12 mm	Stomach wall	1000 MBq	0.8 mSv/GBq	Fast serial imaging ^{82}Sr/^{82}Rb generator with 1–2 month supply Exercise stress not practical
^{13}N-ammonia	>95 %	6–10 mm	Liver, lung, and blood metabolites	500 MBq	4.1 mSv/GBq	Requires on-site cyclotron High lung uptake in smokers and heart failure patients Normal variant lateral wall defect
^{15}O-water	100 %	6–10 mm	Blood, liver, diaphragm, stomach, spleen	1110 MBq	2.2 mSv/GBq	Requires on-site cyclotron MPI not possible Cardiac function difficult
^{18}F-flurpiridaz	~96 %	6–10 mm	Liver and blood binding	Rest: 111 MBq Stress: 409 MBq	66 mSv/GBq 15–19 mSv/GBq	In phase 3 clinical trials Binds to albumin complicating MBF quantification
^{62}Cu-PTSM	45 %	9–13 mm	Liver	500 MBq	3 mSv/GBq	In phase 3 clinical trials ^{62}Zn/^{62}Cu generator with 1 day supply Lower spatial resolution due to high positron range (>4 mm)

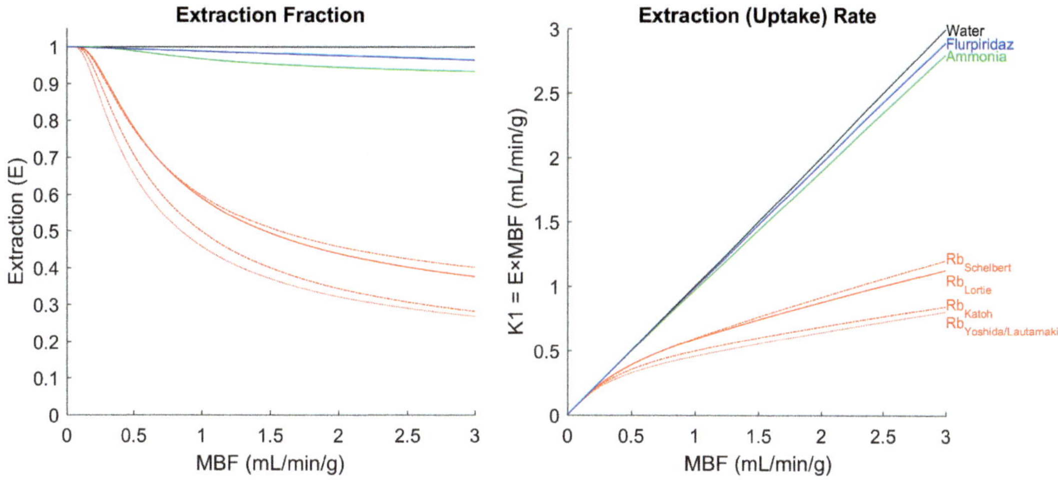

Fig. 19.8 Tracer extraction by myocardial tissue versus myocardial blood flow (*MBF*) and resulting rate of uptake (*K1*)

the tracer, rest-stress imaging must be performed either on separate days or with correction of the second image for residual activity from the first image or by overdosing the second injection. As expected, the radiation dose is relatively high compared to other PET perfusion tracers, but remains well below that of current SPECT tracers [47]. Other ^{18}F-based perfusion tracers (e.g., (4-[^{18}F]fluorophenyl) triphenyl phosphonium (^{18}F-FTPP) and ^{18}F-fluorobenzyl triphenyl phosphonium (^{18}F-FBnTP)) have shown similar promise, but are in less advanced stages of clinical validation.

^{62}Cu-PTSM has favorable kinetic properties including high first-pass extraction, rapid blood clearance, and long myocardial retention. However, the short half-life of the parent isotope ^{62}Zn ($t_{1/2}$=9.1 h) required daily supply of generators, which has limited widespread adoption.

Image intensity in MPI is dependent on tracer retention in the cardiac tissue. Since retention depends on both uptake (measured by *K1*) and washout (*k2*) rates, tracer retention fractions are always lower than *K1*. For this reason, *K1* uptake polar maps produce higher normal-to-defect region contrast than MPI uptake polar maps. The nonlinear extraction correction of *K1* to estimate MBF further increases this contrast, making defect severity and extent more pronounced with MBF quantification compared to MPI, as demonstrated in the polar maps of Fig. 19.4.

19.5 Metabolic Imaging

Cardiac myocytes can utilize a number of substrates for their energy needs including fatty acids, carbohydrates, lactate, and ketones [48]. To elucidate metabolic pathways, evaluate metabolic rates, and interrogate metabolic alterations with disease and therapies, a wide variety of tracers have been developed as demonstrated in Fig. 19.9. Diet and hormones (e.g., insulin) can be controlled to condition the patient's metabolic state to achieve a wide range of imaging applications, using even a subset of the available tracers.

19.5.1 Carbohydrate Metabolism

FDG as a glucose analogue is taken up into metabolically active cells using active glucose transporters (of which GLUT4 is the primary variety in myocytes) and mediated by insulin. Upon phosphorylation, however, FDG-6-phosphate cannot be further metabolized, unlike native glucose, and the radiolabeled FDG-P

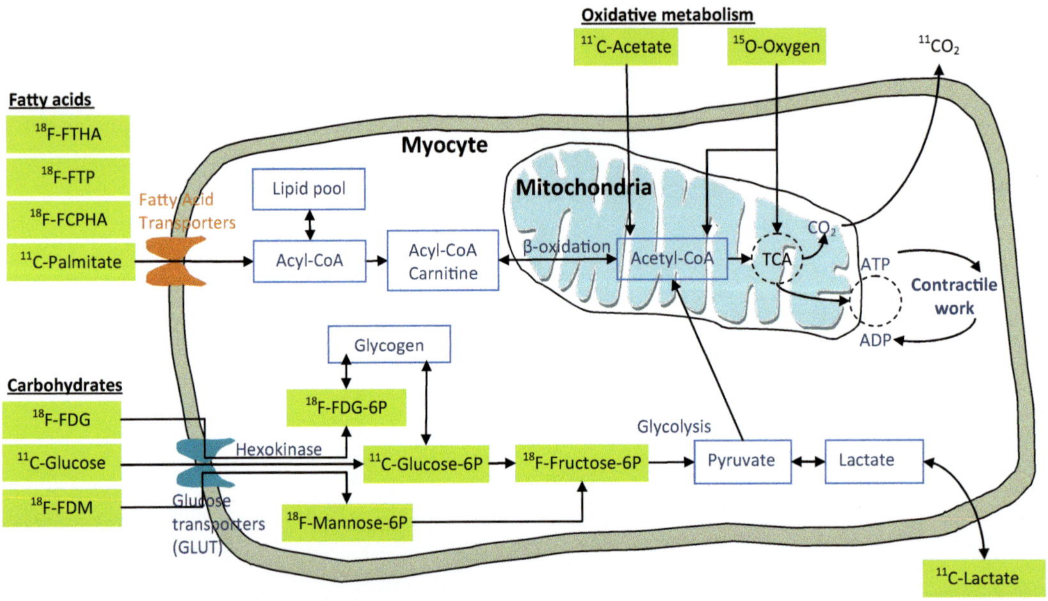

Fig. 19.9 Cardiomyocyte metabolism diagram demonstrating fatty acid and glucose energy substrates and related PET tracers for probing metabolic activity. *Yellow*-labeled molecules are positron emitting tracers of relevance to metabolic imaging

becomes trapped in the cell. Therefore, FDG is an excellent marker of glucose uptake, and it is convenient to use due to its widespread availability. Alternatives to FDG include ^{11}C-glucose which is metabolized like the non-radiolabeled molecule and is therefore considered to be the most accurate marker of glucose utilization. However, its kinetic modeling is complicated by the production of radioactive metabolites (e.g., $^{11}CO_2$, ^{11}C-pyruvate, ^{11}C-lactate) that propagate the metabolic pathways including washout of wastes, making quantification challenging. ^{18}F-mannose is an isomer of glucose and has been gaining interest as an alternative to FDG imaging since its affinity may be more specific than that of FDG to certain cell types such as inflammatory macrophages [49], and it is less sensitive to plasma glucose levels [50]. The feasibility of PET imaging of ^{11}C-lactate, a carbohydrate energy source for the heart, has also been demonstrated under a range of metabolic alterations [51]. FDG is by far the most commonly used tracer for glucose metabolic imaging.

19.5.2 Fatty Acid Metabolism

Free fatty acids (FFA) are the preferred source of energy by myocytes (60–90 % at fasting state), so long as sufficient oxygen is available to support β-oxidization in the mitochondria. FFAs, such as palmitate, are extracted from the blood and therefore can be labeled for metabolic imaging. ^{11}C-palmitate is metabolized rapidly and fully producing radiolabeled metabolites that complicate quantification of FA utilization. ^{18}F-FTHA (^{18}F-fluorothia-6-heptadecanoic acid) is the most commonly used PET tracer to measure FA uptake. It is not ideal, as retention levels have been shown to be insensitive to hypoxia [52]. FTP (16-[^{18}F] fluoro-4-thia-palmitate) was developed as a hypoxia-sensitive alternative and has been shown to be an accurate indicator of fatty acid oxidation [53]. ^{18}F-FCPHA (trans-9(RS)-^{18}F-fluoro-3,4(RS,RS)-methyleneheptadecanoic acid) is another fatty acid analogue that undergoes rapid cardiac uptake and clearance from the blood, but does not readily oxidize, resulting in high myocardial to blood contrast [54]. Fatty acid imaging has been performed for over three decades using ^{123}I-BMIPP SPECT, and clinical results have demonstrated its ability to detect ischemia and predict adverse cardiac events; it is reasonable to expect that PET imaging will have similar benefits with the added benefit of accurate quantification and improved image quality.

19.5.3 Oxidative Metabolism

FFA metabolism requires oxygen, which is replenished by the perfusing blood, and produces waste CO_2 which is carried away by the blood. Myocardial oxygen consumption (MVO_2) can be measured directly using $^{15}O_2$ or indirectly using ^{11}C-acetate [55] to interrogate the metabolic state of cardiac tissue.

19.5.4 Viability Imaging

Viability imaging is used to predict cardiac function recovery and patient outcome benefit after revascularization. When considering viability, the clinician is most concerned with identifying myocardium that has potential for recovery. Resting myocardial dysfunction may be attributed to ischemic or non-ischemic causes. Ischemic causes can be due to ongoing ischemia (hibernating), resolved ischemia (stunning), or previous ischemic injury (scar). Hibernation is a state of metabolic downregulation due to repeated episodes of ischemia but is potentially reversible with adequate revascularization [56].

FDG is taken up avidly by hibernating myocardium in which the myocytes favor anaerobic glucose utilization over oxygen-dependent FFA metabolism. FDG-PET is performed in conjunction with a rest perfusion scan (using ^{82}Rb or ^{13}N-ammonia) and is recognized as the most sensitive means of identifying hibernating myocardium, the amount of which has been shown to be the best predictor of outcome benefit from revascularization [57]. FDG-PET is typically performed with either oral glucose loading or euglycemic insulin clamp (especially in diabetics) to induce a metabolic state favoring glucose use as a primary energy source and increasing the sensitivity of the test. Regions of normal perfusion are presumed viable. Regions with reduced resting perfusion and *matched* reduced metabolic activity (uptake) are presumed to be fibrotic scar that will not recover function, while regions with *mismatch* (hibernating) metabolic uptake are viable and hypoperfused. Regions with preserved perfusion and *reverse-mismatched* reduced metabolic activity may be seen after an acute ischemic event or in the case of left bundle branch block and is of uncertain clinical significance [1]. Figure 19.10 demonstrates interpretation of a perfusion-viability mismatch study.

Observational studies have shown that FDG-PET can successfully identify patients that may benefit from revascularization [58–61]. The PARR-2 study was a prospective randomized trial where patients being considered for revascularization due to ischemic cardiomyopathy were assigned to undergo an FDG-PET scan or not (standard care). A trend toward better outcomes (cardiac death and major adverse cardiac outcomes) in the PET cohort was noted, but did not reach statistical significance in the original multicenter analysis [62]. However, a follow-up analysis of only the patients who adhered to the recommendations of the PET scan for intervention showed a significant reduction in adverse cardiac events versus those that did not undergo FDG-PET [63].

Various FDG imaging protocols have been developed; all with the common goal of switching the metabolic state to favor glucose utilization prior to FDG administration. In general the patient is fasted for >6 h and a baseline blood glucose measurement is used to guide glucose loading. For simplicity, oral glucose loading (25–100 g) to drive endogenous production of insulin is most commonly used clinically, but IV glucose (dextrose) infusion enables more accurate control of blood glucose levels. In diabetics glucose loading is more challenging due to low levels of endogenous insulin or cellular insensitivity to insulin. In most cases administration of insulin with glucose results in good image quality, but euglycemic

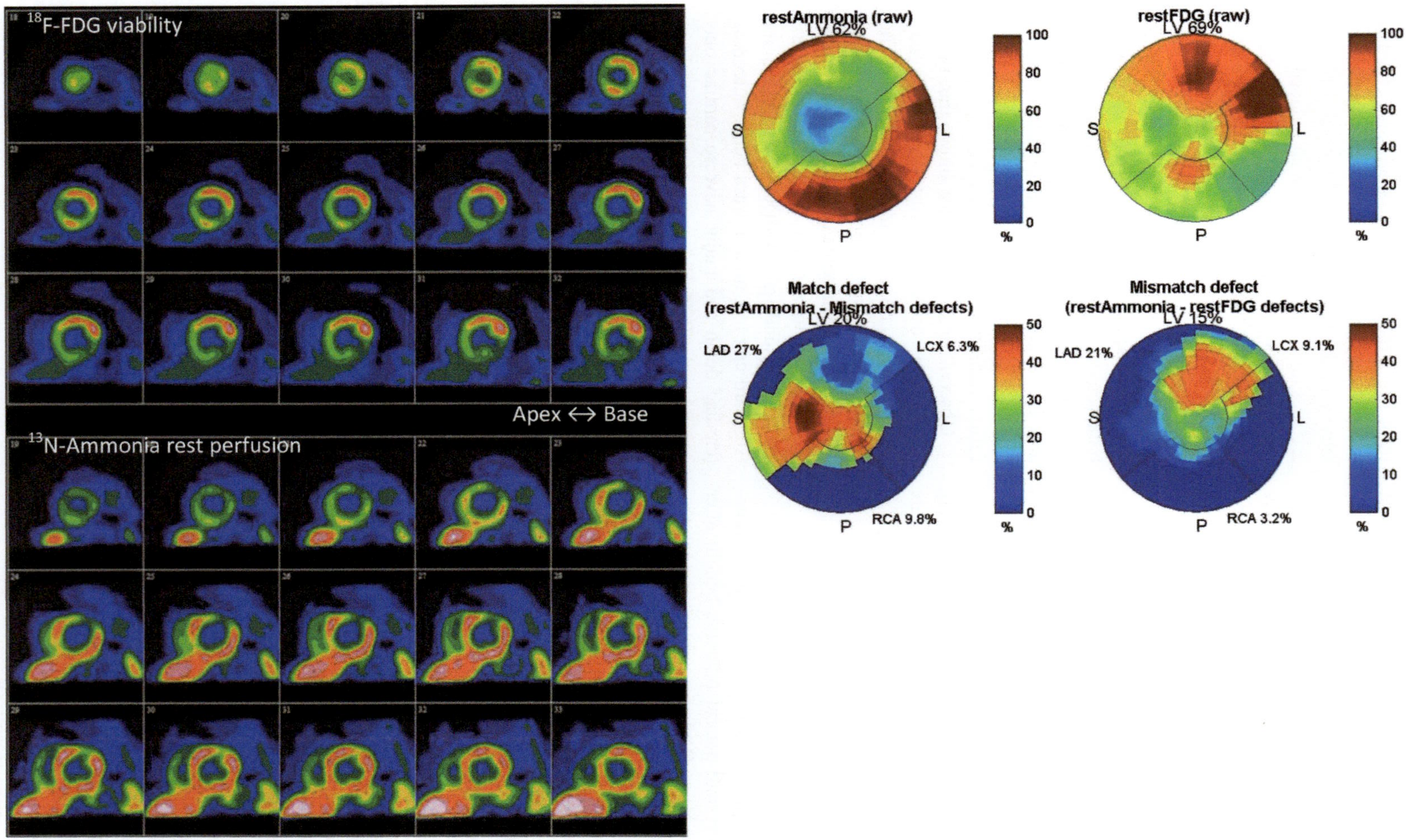

Fig. 19.10 Viability and perfusion images (*left*) and polar map analysis (*right*) of a 72-year-old woman assessed for bypass surgery. She had a 2-year history heart failure (class III) with paroxysmal nocturnal dyspnea (PND) and orthopnea, no history of myocardial infarction (MI), and recent complaints of increase of shortness of breath. She was found to have triple-vessel disease with PET, severe ischemic cardiomyopathy with a MRI ejection fraction of about 13–15 %, and no major valvular dysfunction with echocardiography. Her angiogram showed that she had narrowing of the right coronary 100 %, a lesion in the LAD, and disease of her circumflex, and therefore she was thought to be a bypass candidate. The PET viability exam showed about 20 % scar, and about 15 % of the left ventricle was hibernating myocardium and the rest was viable. Therefore, she was recommended for surgery

hyperinsulinemic clamp enables more precise control to achieve superior imaging quality. A detailed protocol is available in [1].

Multimodal imaging including metabolic cardiac PET is instrumental for elucidating mechanistic and adaptive changes in new diseases such as heart failure, right ventricular hypertrophy, and pulmonary artery hypertension both in human populations and in animal models.

19.5.5 Metabolic Alteration Studies

Complete metabolism of FA substrates requires oxidation and therefore is almost immediately downregulated under conditions of ischemia, while anaerobic glucose and lactate utilization is upregulated. This metabolic shift leads to less efficient production of ATP and can lead to reduced contractile function of the myocytes. FA utilization may be restored with reperfusion of ischemic tissue, but the phenomenon of "ischemic memory" has been well observed in which stunned myocardial tissue continues to operate in an anaerobic state favoring glucose utilization even after reperfusion [64]. FA imaging has therefore been shown to correlate well with perfusion imaging, but with higher prognostic power in acute myocardial ischemia [65]. With prolonged ischemia, little FA utilization recovery is to be expected. Thus, cardiac applications have thus leveraged radiolabeled metabolic substrates to differentiate ischemic and stunned myocardium and thus identify viable myocardium that is characterized by the presence of FDG uptake and reduced FTHA uptake, from normal myocardium having both FTHA and FDG uptake [48].

Metabolic shifts from FA metabolism to glycolysis (e.g., Randall cycle) have been associated with diabetes, obesity, non-ischemic dilated cardiomyopathy, and chronic kidney disease. While FA metabolism may be reduced with downregulation of β-oxidation (e.g., diabetes, dilated cardiomyopathy), circulating FA may remain high leading to elevated FA uptake and lipid storage within the myocytes and production of toxic, non-oxidized FA intermediates. FA imaging in conjunction with oxidative imaging (^{11}C-acetate) can differentiate between FA metabolism and storage (increased and reduced uptake, respectively).

19.5.6 Quantification of Metabolism

As with perfusion imaging, one of the key advantages of PET over competing modalities is the ability to quantify biochemical rates. Quantification of metabolic rates is instrumental to detect metabolic changes with disease progression, response to therapy, and differentiation between cohorts and to quantify the ratios between substrate utilizations. Commonly, a two-tissue compartment model (Fig. 19.11) is utilized to model blood plasma to tissue extraction (*K1*) and washout back into the plasma (*k2*). The parameter *k3* may represent the rate at which the tracer is metabolized or trapped. The *k4* parameter may represent back conversion of the trapped tracer or set to 0 if the conversion is known to be unidirectional. The interpretation of these parameters must be performed within the context of the tracer and its assumed metabolic mechanism. Tracer uptake (*K1*) is dependent on myocardial blood flow and the initial (first-pass) extraction fraction. More complex kinetic models may be required to fully model a tracer that is metabolized in cascade [66].

Since tissue TACs are contaminated by blood signal, due to actual perfusion and partial volume effects, tissue partial volume must be accounted for.

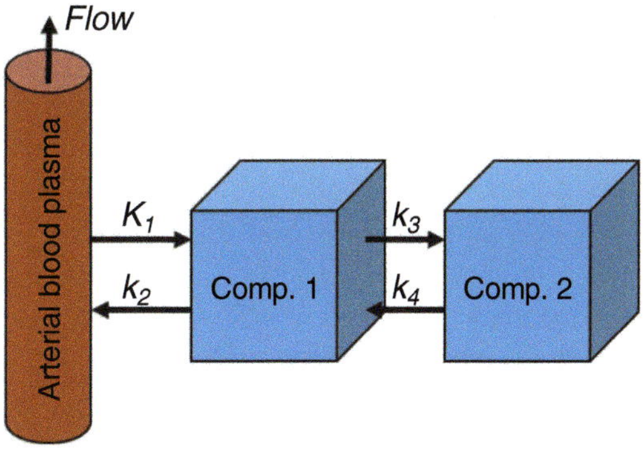

Fig. 19.11 Two-tissue compartment model used for quantification of metabolic rates

The tissue partial volume recovery coefficient (RC) is often assumed constant on the order of 70% and used to correct *K1*. A commonly used alternative is to model the blood partial volume (BPV) fraction in the myocardial TAC as part of the compartmental model, and RC is estimated as (1−BPV) [67]. See Chaps. 14 and 15 for further details.

The simpler Patlak graphical analysis model has also been employed to quantify pharmacokinetics, but without the need to assume a complex compartmental model. With FDG-PET, Patlak analysis is most frequently used to quantify regional myocardial glucose uptake (rMGU) [68]. As with compartmental modeling, a blood ROI is used to sample the arterial blood tracer concentration, while myocardial ROIs sample the tracer concentrations in the myocardial tissue. Parametric maps of glucose uptake rate (*Ki*) can be obtained quickly and account for arterial blood partial volume. A lumped constant must be applied to calibrate FDG uptake to that of glucose which is dependent on the metabolic state of the patient [69], emphasizing the need to control patient glucose and FFA levels.

19.6 Myocardial Inflammation

Inflammatory cells which often accumulate in response to infection also utilize glucose as a primary energy substrate, enabling inflammation imaging using FDG-PET. Preliminary studies indicate that FDM may be a more specific marker of certain macrophage types [49]. In the cardiac PET context, systemic inflammatory disease with cardiac involvement such as myocarditis, sarcoidosis [70], and psoriasis are possible, but only with suppression of glucose utilization by the myocytes. Glucose suppression is achieved using a low-carbohydrate, high-fat diet which upregulate FFA utilization. Myocardial inflammation may present as focal lesions dispersed throughout the myocardium.

Other possible findings with cardiac FDG-PET may include noncardiac inflammation such as aortitis, vasculitis, pneumonia, as well as cancer. With increased use of implanted medical devices, FDG-PET is also increasingly used to detect infections associated with implanted pace makers, cardiac resynchronization therapy devices, cardioverter defibrillators (ICD), and artificial valves. These findings often require the use of fused CT image interpretation to localize the lesion and additional clinical information to differentiate the cause of infection.

19.7 Vascular Inflammation

Sudden rupture of unstable atherosclerotic plaque in the coronary arteries is the process underlying the vast majority of acute coronary syndromes [71]. Detection of these unstable plaques prior to rupture is therefore highly desirable and could result in specific preventive intervention, but requires tools to distinguish unstable from stable lesions. Currently, it is hypothesized that unstable plaques are characterized by a thin fibrous cap, covering a large necrotic core with macrophage and T-lymphocyte infiltration [72] and spotty calcium deposition.

The primary substrate for metabolic activity in macrophages is glucose, primarily due to the anaerobic environment of the plaque; thus, FDG can be used for imaging active inflammation mediated by macrophages within atherosclerotic plaques. FDG plaque imaging has been demonstrated to be feasible in carotid arteries and large systemic arteries [73], but is more challenging in the coronary vasculature due to FDG uptake in the myocardium and the reduced image resolution due to cardiac and respiratory motion blurring. To achieve FDG image contrast between inflammation sites and the surrounding myocardium, a low-carbohydrate, high-fat diet is prescribed prior to imaging to promote fatty acid utilization by the myocytes and downregulating FDG uptake. In preliminary studies, arterial FDG uptake has been related to the rates of cardiac events [74, 75], microemboli [76] and stroke [77].

It is apparent that FDG uptake is a nonspecific marker of inflammation, and there has been increasing interest in other markers of plaque instability. F-18-sodium-fluoride ($Na^{18}F$), a calcium analogue, has recently been demonstrated to detect unstable and recently ruptured plaques, while FDG significantly underperformed in the same patients [78]. Alternative biomarkers for processes such as plaque neovascularization or apoptosis may prove more capable of identifying high-risk/vulnerable plaques [71]. Early research suggests that ^{18}F-FDM (2-deoxy-2-[^{18}F] fluoro-D-mannose) may be a more specific metabolic substrate alternative to FDG for labeling sites of active macrophage aggregation, which may not only indicate the presence of plaques but also their vulnerability to rapture [49].

Other more specific targets have been sought, for the most part in small animal models. The somatostatin receptors have been suggested as specific macrophage targets in atherosclerosis that can be imaged with ^{68}Ga-DOTATATE [79]. Newer compounds include ^{11}C-PK11195 and ^{18}F-FEDAA that target translocator proteins that are upregulated in macrophages [80] are at very early stages of small animal research. ^{64}Cu-CANF-conjugated nanoparticles target natriuretic peptide clearance receptor and have been shown to target atherosclerotic sites with a human feasibility study currently underway (NCT02417688).

19.8 Cell Signaling

In cardiovascular diseases, PET imaging is used to study all aspects of intercellular signaling including neurocrine (neuronal), endocrine (hormonal), paracrine (local endocrine), autocrine (e.g., immune), juxtacrine (cell adhesion), and matricrine (extracellular matrix adhesion) pathways as illustrated in Fig. 19.12.

19.8.1 Neurocrine (ANS, RAAS) and Endocrine (Adrenalin, Angiotensin)

Neuronal signaling in the heart is achieved mainly through the autonomic system, comprised of the sympathetic and parasympathetic nervous systems as shown in Fig. 19.13. Abnormal activation of the sympathetic nervous system (SNS) is commonly found in patients with heart failure; therefore, imaging of SNS neuronal function in the left ventricle myocardium is important in this population. During SNS activation of the "fight-or-flight" response, the neurotransmitter norepinephrine (NE) also known as noradrenaline is released from nerve terminals within the myocardium and the arterial vessel walls, binding to "adrenergic" receptors in the sinoatrial (SA) and atrioventricular (AV) conduction nodes, as well as the arterial vascular endothelium to increase heart rate, contractility, and coronary blood flow while at the same time increasing systemic blood pressure by peripheral vasoconstriction. There are several adrenergic receptor subtypes within the cardiac sympathetic neurons as shown in

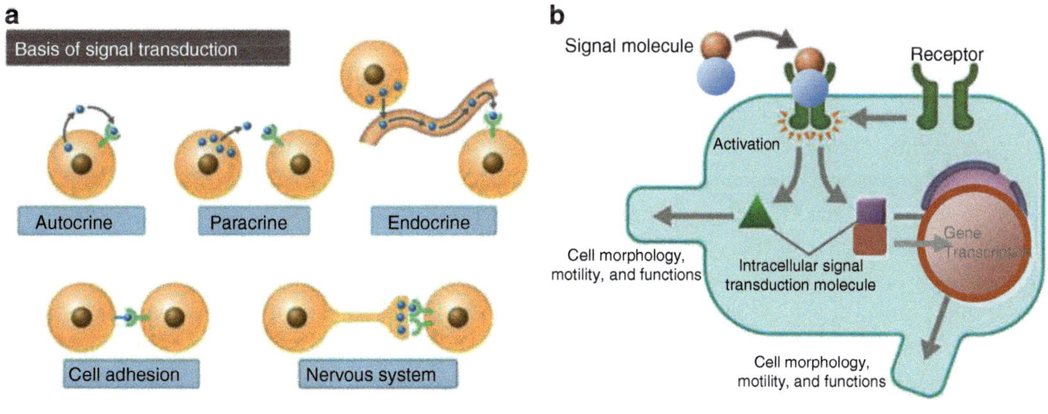

Fig. 19.12 (**a**) Types of intercell cardiac signaling include neurocrine (nerve-to-cell), endocrine (circulating hormone-to-cell), paracrine (local cell-to-cell), autocrine (same cell-to-cell), juxtacrine (cell-to-cell adhesion), and matricrine (extracellular matrix-to-cell adhesion) systems. (**b**) Signaling molecules that are released from the originating source (cell or neuron) diffuse and bind to a specific receptor on the target cell (Adapted from The University of Tokyo/CSLS with permission)

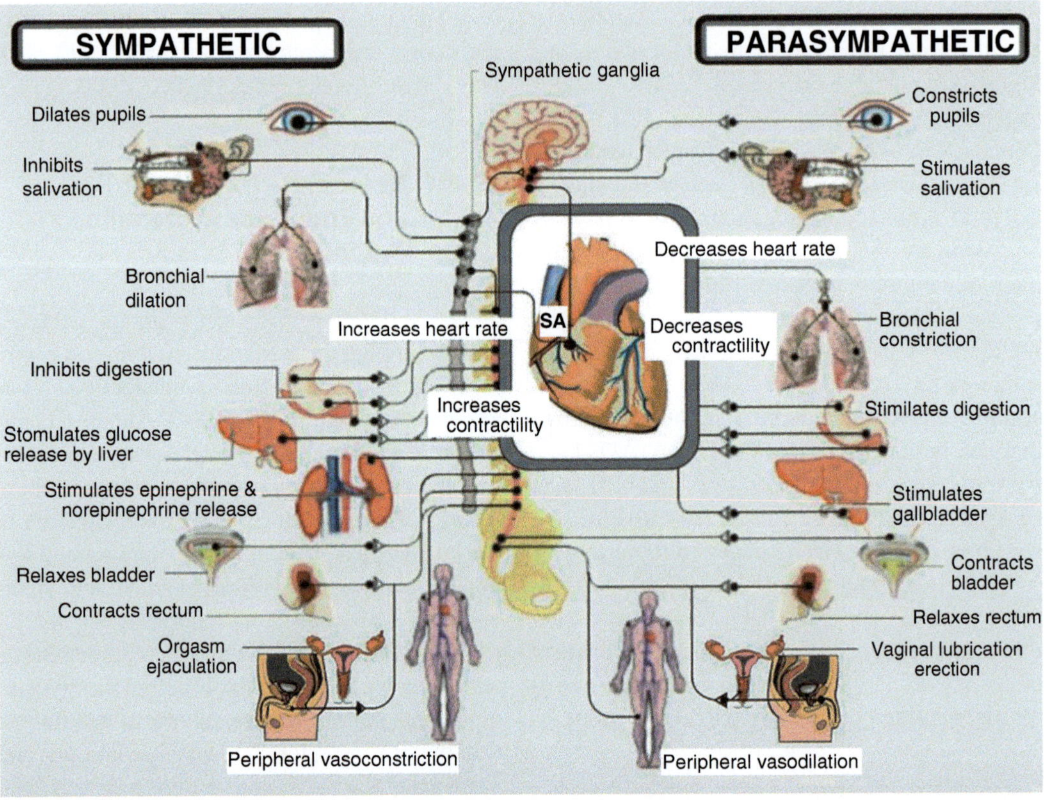

Fig. 19.13 The sympathetic and parasympathetic components of the autonomic nervous system (*ANS*) acting through the sinoatrial (*SA*) node to control heart rate (chronotropy), through the myocardium to control contractility (inotropy) and through the peripheral vasculature to control blood pressure (Source: http://www.qmedical.com/dtr_ans.htm)

Fig. 19.14 and associated PET tracers as listed in Table 19.4. In the normal coronary artery circulation, the vasodilating effect of the beta-adrenergic receptors (βAR) is balanced by the constricting effect of the alpha adrenergic receptors (αAR) to autoregulate blood flow according to the local demands of the heart muscle [82]. ^{11}C-HED is most commonly used to evaluate cardiac sympathetic innervation (nerve density); it enters the nerve terminal via the NE reuptake transporter (NET) and is retained in the synaptic vesicles. The kinetics of HED can be described using a one-tissue compartment model or a simplified model to measure the %/min retention rate (Fig. 19.15). Other ^{11}C- and ^{18}F-labeled tracers are under active development to provide improved quantification of SNS density and function (e.g., less dependent on blood flow) and wider distribution outside of academic research facilities [84]. Sympathetic denervation in ICD patients with advanced ischemic heart disease has been shown to predict the risk of cardiac arrest or sudden death [85].

The cold pressor test (CPT) is often used in clinical research studies to evaluate the vasodilator response to central SNS stimulation (sympathetic stress) as a measure of coronary vascular health [86]; a normal myocardial blood flow increase of 40–50 % is typically observed in response to CPT, whereas the response is absent or even negative (decreased) in patients with advanced atherosclerosis and severe endothelial dysfunction. A secondary endocrine response is also produced by NE (and epinephrine) secretion into the circulating blood by the adrenal glands (Fig. 19.13) in response to sympathetic stress. These circulating catecholamine hormones also act to dilate the coronary vessels by activating the

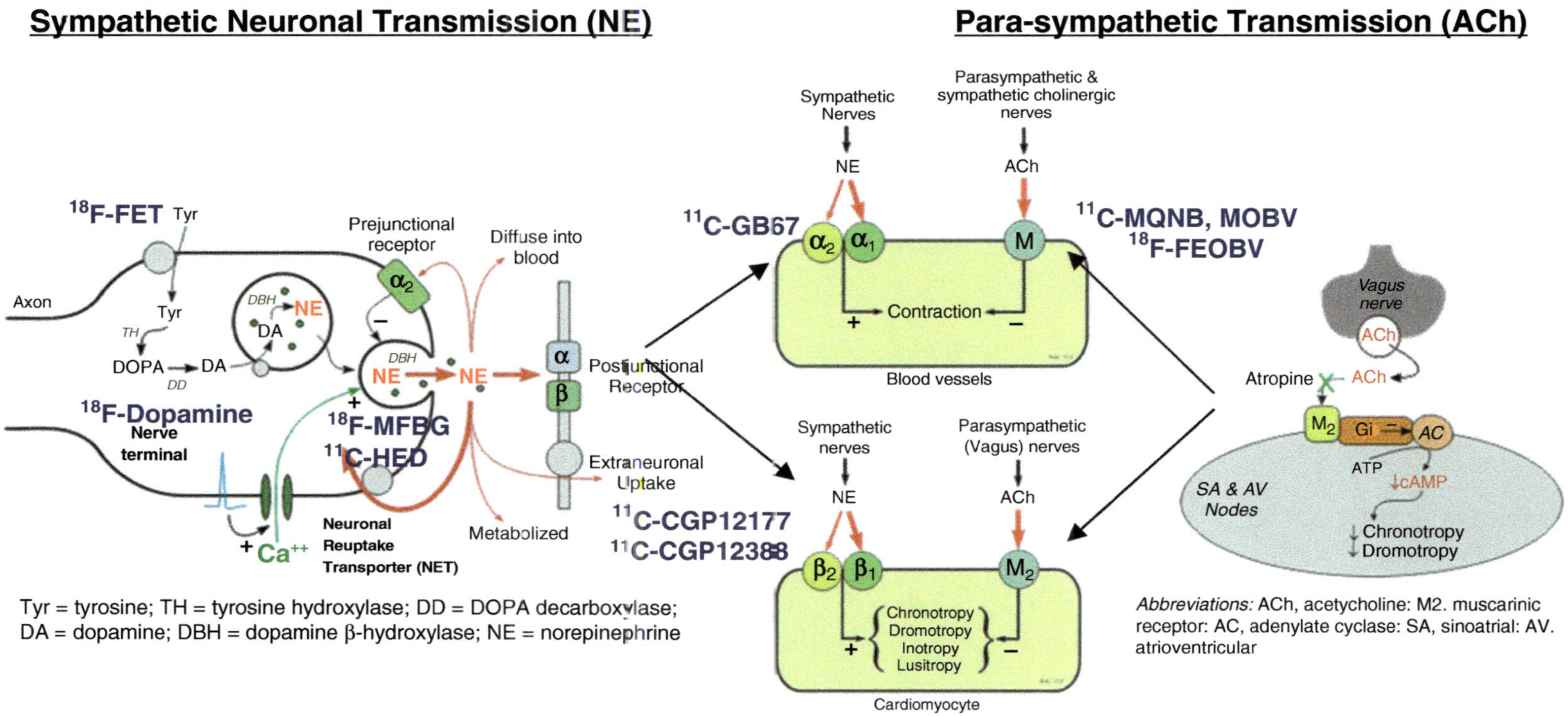

Fig. 19.14 The sympathetic nervous system (*SNS*) uses the neurotransmitter NE to signal the cardiomyocyte and coronary blood vessel actions, whereas the parasympathetic nervous system (*pSNS*) uses ACh acting mainly through the sinoatrial (*SA*) and atrioventricular (*AV*) nodes. Common tracers used to study cardiac autonomic function are shown in *blue*. *Tyr* tyrosine, *TH* tyrosine hydroxylase, *DD* DOPA decarboxylase, *DA* dopamine, *DBH* dopamine β-hydroxylase, *NE* norepinephrine, *Ach* acetylcholine, *M2* muscarinic receptor, *AC* adenylate cyclase, *SA* sinoatrial, *AV* atrioventricular (Modified with permission from cvphysiology.com)

βAR on the vascular endothelium, and their effect on MBF can be measured using any of the validated PET flow tracers (Table 19.3).

Sympathetic stress also causes the liver to release glucose stores into the circulation, thereby prompting the endocrine function of the pancreas to release insulin hormone, which promotes uptake into the heart and other body organs to increase cellular energy levels. Disturbances in insulin-glucose metabolic signaling, e.g., diabetes mellitus, can be investigated using ^{11}C-glucose, ^{18}F-FDG, or other analogues as described in the section on metabolic tracers.

Table 19.4 PET tracers for molecular imaging of neuroreceptors in the heart

PET probe name	Isotope	Biological target
Hydroxyephedrine (HED)	^{11}C	Presynaptic catecholamine reuptake transporter
Epinephrine (Epi)	^{11}C	Presynaptic catecholamine uptake and storage
Phenylephrine (PE)	^{11}C	Presynaptic catecholamine uptake and metabolism
Benzylguanidine (MFBG, LMI-1195)	^{18}F	Presynaptic catecholamine reuptake transporter
Dopamine (DA), tyrosine (Tyr)	^{18}F	Presynaptic sympathetic function
CGP12177, CGP12388	^{11}C	β-Adrenergic receptor
GB67, yohimbine	^{11}C	α-Adrenergic receptor
MQNB, MOBV, OMV, MABV	^{11}C	Muscarinic ACh receptor
FEOBV, FBPT, FBMV	^{18}F	Muscarinic ACh receptor

Adapted from Dobrucki and Sinusas [81] with Permission

Activation of the parasympathetic nervous system (pSNS) generally opposes the effects of the SNS described above, lowering heart rate, contractility, and systemic blood pressure as part of the "rest-and-digest" response. There is high density of parasympathetic nerves in the atrial tissues of the heart, particularly in the SA and AV nodes that regulate heart rate. The PET tracers ^{11}C-MQNB and ^{18}F-FEOBV have been used to evaluate left atrial (LA) innervation in patients and animal models of atrial fibrillation [87].

The recent success of heart failure therapies targeted at the renin-angiotensin-aldosterone system (RAAS), specifically the combination drug neprilysin/angiotensin II type I receptor (AT1R) blocker (ARB) sacubitril/valsartan [88] and similar compounds, is prompting a renewed interest in the use of PET imaging for the management of these patients. The components of the RAAS are shown in Fig. 19.16, with several PET tracers available to probe the endocrine functions through receptor binding and angiotensin-converting enzyme (ACE) activity. The circulating hormone angiotensin II (Ang II) signals a number of cardiovascular responses, including increased blood pressure by activating the AT1 and AT2 receptors in the adrenal glands and peripheral vasculature; however,

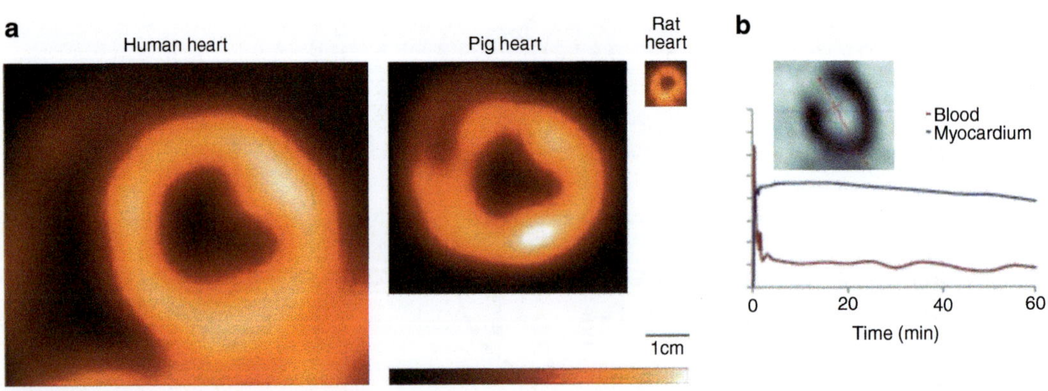

Fig. 19.15 11C-HED PET images showing normal sympathetic innervation in multiple species (**a**), and representative tracer kinetics in the normal rat heart (**b**) (Reproduced with permission from Refs. [8, 83])

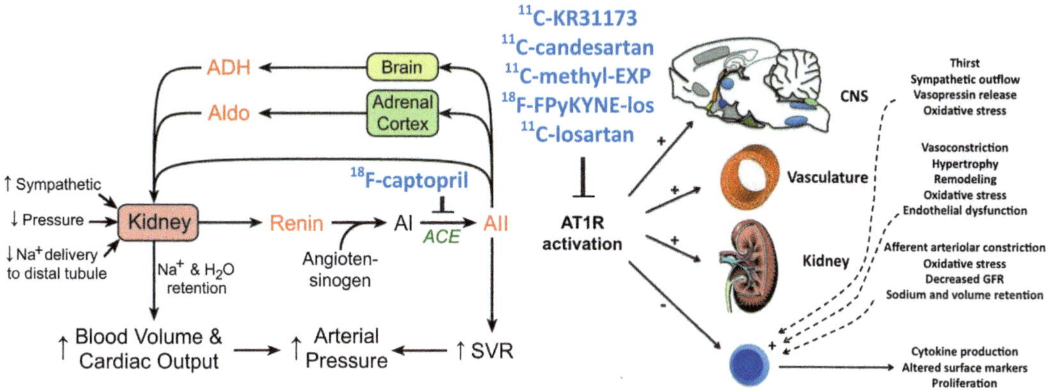

Fig. 19.16 Renin-angiotensin-aldosterone system (*RAAS*) with associated PET tracers (enzyme inhibitors and receptor blockers) shown in *blue* text. Renin is an enzyme secreted by the kidney which converts angiotensinogen to angiotensin I (AI or Ang I) in the blood, which is then converted to angiotensin II (AII or Ang II) by ACE in the lungs. Circulating Ang II signals the adrenal glands to release aldosterone (Aldo), the pituitary gland in the brain to release antidiuretic hormone (ADH), and the peripheral vasculature to constrict (↑SVR), all leading to increased systemic blood pressure (Modified with permission from cvphysiology.com (A) and Harrison and Guzik [89] (B))

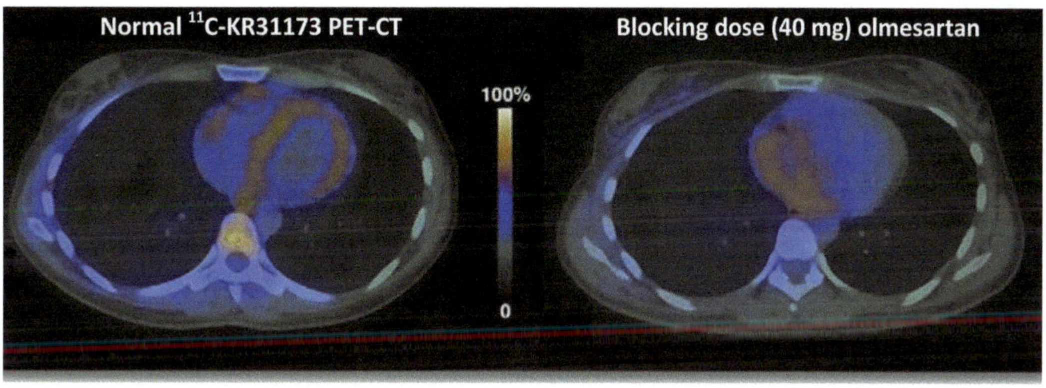

Fig. 19.17 PET-CT images demonstrating AT1 receptor distribution in the left ventricle myocardium of a healthy normal subject using ^{11}C-KR31173 (*left*). Specific binding is demonstrated by blocking the receptors with pre-injection of AT1R antagonist olmesartan (*right*)

there are also AT1 receptors in the heart as shown recently in Fig. 19.17. AT1R-ligand binding and receptor occupancy studies may be useful for dose titration in heart failure to maximize clinical efficacy and minimize unwanted side effects.

19.8.2 Paracrine (e.g., Nitric Oxide) and Autocrine (Immune)

Local cell-to-cell (paracrine) signaling occurs in many parts of the cardiovascular system and is particularly relevant in the pathophysiological development of atherosclerotic plaque as shown in Fig. 19.18. A classic example of this local endocrine signaling is through the messenger molecule nitric oxide (NO). It is produced in vascular endothelial cells by endothelial nitric oxide synthase (eNOS) and diffuses rapidly to the adjacent smooth muscle cells to signal vessel wall relaxation and dilatation. Reduced bioavailability of NO is associated with endothelial dysfunction in early subclinical disease and has also been investigated with the tracer ^{18}F-NOS in cardiac transplant rejection mediated by autocrine signaling of the immune system response [90].

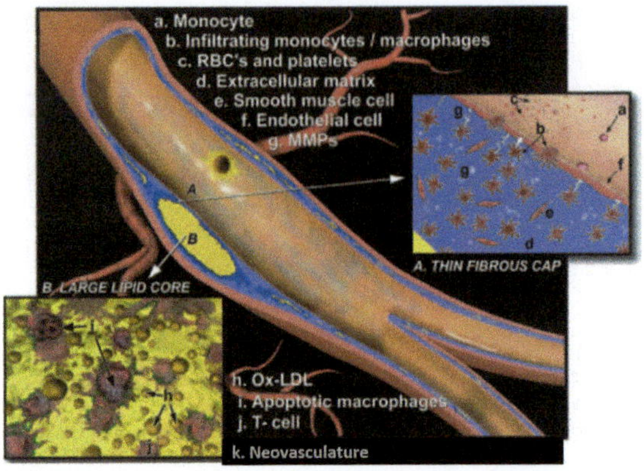

PET probes:

a.	^{18}F reporter-gene probes, ^{68}Ga, ^{64}Cu-nanoparticles (cell labeling)
b.	^{18}F -FDG, ^{11}C-PK1119 (inflammation)
c.	^{18}F-Ap4A, ^{64}Cu-prothrombins (thrombosis)
d, g.	^{18}FB-ML5 (MMP inhibitors, ECM remodeling)
e.	^{82}Rb, ^{13}NH$_3$, H$_2$^{15}O (vascular reactivity)
f.	^{18}F-NOS (NO bioavailability)
h.	^{18}F, ^{64}Cu-liposomes (drug delivery)
i.	^{18}F-annexins (apoptosis), ^{18}F-MISO ^{64}Cu-ATSM, CTS (hypoxia)
j.	^{18}FB-IL2, CXCR4 (cytokines, chemokines)
k.	^{18}F, ^{68}Ga,^{64}Cu-RGD peptide (integrins)
l.	^{18}F- fluoride (hydroxyapatite)

Fig. 19.18 Cell signaling PET probes have been used to examine the molecular processes in the progressive development and rupture of atherosclerotic plaque (Modified from [94])

The inflammatory response of monocyte recruitment and infiltration can be studied using cell labeling techniques that include reporter-probe/gene transfection systems such as the ^{18}FHBG/HSVtk combination [91] or simpler methods such as direct ex vivo labeling with ^{18}FDG and reinjection to evaluate endogenous cell homing to sites of injury or disease. ^{18}FDG uptake by activated macrophages has also been shown to correlate well with histochemical staining by CD68. However, this tracer is rather nonspecific, whereas new tracers targeting macrophages more specifically are under development such as choline (cell membrane formation), octreotate (somatostatin receptors), and PK11195 (benzodiazepine receptor/translocator protein) ligands and analogues [92].

FDG-PET inflammation imaging is finding new applications in areas outside of the vasculature, including sarcoidosis, myocarditis, aortitis, and endocarditis, as well as detection of the local inflammatory response/infections around implanted devices. ^{18}F-fluoride (NaF) uptake has been demonstrated at the site of acute ruptured plaques, reflecting the process of active calcification, and may also be a marker of atherosclerotic plaque that is prone or vulnerable to rupture [78]. This tracer also has potential for application in valvular diseases where calcification is a frequent cause of dysfunction, e.g., in aortic valve stenosis.

A comprehensive listing of cardiovascular imaging tracers can be found in the Molecular Imaging and Contrast Agent Database (MICAD) [93].

19.9 Cardiac PET in Clinical Trials

As demonstrated in this chapter, the role of cardiac PET in clinic is changing. Large-scale, multicenter clinical trials are necessary to evaluate the value of PET for prognosis, diagnosis, therapy planning, and overall disease management costs. These studies are difficult to achieve due to relatively small number of cardiac PET studies currently being performed and the wide range of patient demographics, disease etiologies, therapies, and confounding factors. Therefore, multisite collaboration research is required and is being increasingly applied by the cardiac PET community. Fortunately, cardiac PET imaging protocol standardization between sites is relatively simple to achieve (due to the relative simplicity of the protocols) and validate.

Due to its exquisite sensitivity to detect minute physiologic and increasing number of biomarkers, cardiac PET plays an important role in detecting disease progression and responses to therapies. With wider acceptance, cardiac PET will be increasingly used to evaluate new therapies with the goal of accelerating their development. At time of writing of this chapter, the World

Health Organization International Clinical Trials Registry (via http://www.nhs.uk/) lists 49 clinical trials using cardiac PET which are actively recruiting participants.

19.10 Future Directions

Cardiac PET has developed steadily over the past three decades and continues to evolve. Instrumentation has matured to the point where routine clinical application use is feasible for evaluation of perfusion, functional assessment, and viability. It is expected that myocardial blood flow quantification will become more readily applied, primarily using ^{82}Rb and ^{13}N-ammonia imaging and possibly with ^{18}F-flurpiridaz. The development of more advanced image reconstruction algorithms, particularly those employing more precise time-of-flight information and motion correction, holds the promise of higher effective count statistics which could be leveraged to achieve higher spatial resolution, improved image contrast, reduced image noise, and higher temporal resolution.

Nevertheless, it is the availability of novel tracers that will open the door to new clinical and research applications. Already researchers have begun using PET for stem cell tracking and viability assessment, angiogenesis, apoptosis, and metabolic diseases. With advancements of our understanding in the fields of proteomics, cell signaling, cellular metabolism, and disease processes, we are able to identify more specific molecules for cardiac imaging. Developments in the fields of radiochemistry including faster chemistry and micro-volumes enable production of a wider range of molecules with greater purity. Small animal imaging and rapid translation to human studies have accelerated in vivo characterization and validation of these molecules. Synergetic interaction with experts in multiple disciplines is the key ingredient to achieving future applications.

The emergence of PET-MR hybrid systems is another active field of development. While these systems are currently prohibitively expensive for widespread cardiology, future integrated PET and MR protocols offering comprehensive information (e.g., rest-stress MBF, viability, tissue characterization, angiography, anatomy, and cardiac function from a 1-h imaging session) and appropriate reimbursement may become more common. In the research setting, the demand for PET-MR systems is well established due to comprehensive imaging and the ability to correct PET motion artifacts using MRI motion tracking.

Cardiac small animal PET and PET hybrid imaging has become common for elucidating disease mechanisms, evaluation of therapies, and accelerating development of new imaging targets. The development of new PET tracers is especially benefitting from these developments by accelerating feasibility, radio-distribution and dosimetry studies. The ability to use the same image analysis software and techniques for clinical and small animal PET has further accelerated knowledge translation.

References

1. Dilsizian V, Bacharach SL, Beanlands RS, Bergmann SR, Delbeke D, Gropler RJ, Knuuti J, Schelbert HR, Travin MI. PET myocardial perfusion and metabolism clinical imaging. J Nucl Cardiol. 2009;16(4):651.
2. Burns M. The market for PET radiopharmaceuticals & PET imaging. BIO-Tech Systems, Inc. 2014;370.
3. Cherry SR, Sorenson JA, Phelps ME. Physics in nuclear medicine. 4th ed. Philadelphia: Elsevier/Saunders; 2012.
4. Klein R, Beanlands RSB, deKemp RA. Quantification of myocardial blood flow and flow reserve: technical aspects. J Nucl Cardiol. 2010;17(4):555–70.
5. Huang C, Petibon Y, Ouyang J, Reese TG, Ahlman MA, Bluemke DA, El Fakhri G. Accelerated acquisition of tagged MRI for cardiac motion correction in simultaneous PET-MR: phantom and patient studies. Med Phys. 2015;42(2):1087–97.
6. Ratib O, Nkoulou N. Potential applications of PET/MR imaging in cardiology. J Nucl Med Off Publ Soc Nucl Med. 2014;55 Suppl 2:40S–6.
7. Iqbal B, Currie G, Greene L, Kiat H. Novel radiopharmaceuticals in cardiovascular medicine: present and future. J Med Imaging Radiat Sci. 2014;45(4):423–34.
8. Bengel FM, Higuchi T, Javadi MS, Lautamäki R. Cardiac positron emission tomography. J Am Coll Cardiol. 2009;54(1):1–15.

9. Massoud TF, Gambhir SS. Molecular imaging in living subjects: seeing fundamental biological processes in a new light. Genes Dev. 2003;17(5):545–80.
10. Welling MM, Duijvestein M, Signore A, van der Weerd L. In vivo biodistribution of stem cells using molecular nuclear medicine imaging. J Cell Physiol. 2011;226(6):1444–52.
11. Members C, Klocke FJ, Baird MG, Lorell BH, Bateman TM, Messer JV, Berman DS, O'Gara PT, Carabello BA, Russell RO, Cerqueira MD, Sutton MGSJ, DeMaria AN, Udelson JE, Kennedy JW, Verani MS, Williams KA, Antman EM, Smith SC, Alpert JS, Gregoratos G, Anderson JL, Hiratzka LF, Faxon DP, Hunt SA, Fuster V, Jacobs AK, Gibbons RJ, Russell RO. ACC/AHA/ASNC guidelines for the clinical use of cardiac radionuclide imaging. Circulation. 2003;108(11):1404–18.
12. Loong CY, Anagnostopoulos C. Diagnosis of coronary artery disease by radionuclide myocardial perfusion imaging. Heart. 2004;90 Suppl 5:v2–9.
13. Bateman T, Heller G, Mcghie A, Friedman J, Case J, Bryngelson J, Hertenstein G, Moutray K, Reid K, Cullom S. Diagnostic accuracy of rest/stress ECG-gated Rb-82 myocardial perfusion PET: comparison with ECG-gated Tc-99m sestamibi SPECT. J Nucl Cardiol. 2006;13(1):24–33.
14. Hachamovitch R, Rozanski A, Shaw LJ, Stone GW, Thomson LEJ, Friedman JD, Hayes SW, Cohen I, Germano G, Berman DS. Impact of ischaemia and scar on the therapeutic benefit derived from myocardial revascularization vs. medical therapy among patients undergoing stress-rest myocardial perfusion scintigraphy. Eur Heart J. 2011;32(8):1012–24.
15. Yoshinaga K, Chow BJW, Williams K, Chen L, deKemp RA, Garrard L, Lok-Tin Szeto A, Aung M, Davies RA, Ruddy TD, Beanlands RSB. What is the prognostic value of myocardial perfusion imaging using rubidium-82 positron emission tomography? J Am Coll Cardiol. 2006;48(5):1029–39.
16. Mc Ardle BA, Dowsley TF, deKemp RA, Wells GA, Beanlands RS. Does rubidium-82 PET have superior accuracy to SPECT perfusion imaging for the diagnosis of obstructive coronary disease? J Am Coll Cardiol. 2012;60(18):1828–37.
17. Merhige ME, Breen WJ, Shelton V, Houston T, D'Arcy BJ, Perna AF. Impact of myocardial perfusion imaging with PET and 82Rb on downstream invasive procedure utilization, costs, and outcomes in coronary disease management. J Nucl Med. 2007;48(7):1069–76.
18. Gibbons RJ, Balady GJ, Bricker JT, Chaitman BR, Fletcher GF, Froelicher VF, Mark DB, McCallister BD, Mooss AN, O'Reilly MG, Winters WL, Gibbons RJ, Antman EM, Alpert JS, Faxon DP, Fuster V, Gregoratos G, Hiratzka LF, Jacobs AK, Russell RO, Smith SC. ACC/AHA 2002 guideline update for exercise testing: summary article a report of the American College of Cardiology/American Heart Association Task Force on Practice Guidelines (Committee to Update the 1997 Exercise Testing Guidelines). Circulation. 2002;106(14):1883–92.
19. Dilsizian V, Bacharach SL, Beanlands RS, Bergmann SR, Delbeke D, Dorbala S, Gropler RJ, Knuuti J, Schelbert HR, Travin MI. ASNC imaging guidelines/SNMMI procedure standard for positron emission tomography (PET) nuclear cardiology procedures. J Nucl Cardiol. 2016. [Epub ahead of print].
20. Yoshinaga K, Katoh C, Manabe O, Klein R, Naya M, Sakakibara M, Yamada S, deKemp RA, Tsutsui H, Tamaki N. Incremental diagnostic value of regional myocardial blood flow quantification over relative perfusion imaging with generator-produced rubidium-82 PET. Circ J. 2011;75(11):2628–34.
21. Naya M, Morita K, Yoshinaga K, Manabe O, Goto D, Hirata K, Katoh C, Tamaki N, Tsutsui H. Long-term smoking causes more advanced coronary endothelial dysfunction in middle-aged smokers compared to young smokers. Eur J Nucl Med Mol Imaging. 2011;38(3):491–8.
22. Lynch F, Sweeney M, O'Regan RG, McLoughlin P. Hypercapnia-induced contraction in isolated pulmonary arteries is endothelium-dependent. Respir Physiol. 2000;121(1):65–74.
23. Croteau E, Renaud JM, Archer C, Klein R, DaSilva JN, Ruddy TD, Beanlands RS, deKemp RA. β2-adrenergic stress evaluation of coronary endothelial-dependent vasodilator function in mice using 11C-acetate micro-PET imaging of myocardial blood flow and oxidative metabolism. EJNMMI Res. 2014;4(1):68.
24. Holly TA, Abbott BG, Al-Mallah M, Calnon DA, Cohen MC, DiFilippo FP, Ficaro EP, Freeman MR, Hendel RC, Jain D, Leonard SM, Nichols KJ, Polk DM, Soman P. Single photon-emission computed tomography. J Nucl Cardiol. 2010;17(5):941–73.
25. Knollmann D, Knebel I, Koch K-C, Gebhard M, Krohn T, Buell U, Schaefer WM. Comparison of SSS and SRS calculated from normal databases provided by QPS and 4D-MSPECT manufacturers and from identical institutional normals. Eur J Nucl Med Mol Imaging. 2008;35(2):311–8.
26. Slomka PJ, Nishina H, Berman DS, Akincioglu C, Abidov A, Friedman JD, Hayes SW, Germano G. Automated quantification of myocardial perfusion SPECT using simplified normal limits. J Nucl Cardiol Off Publ Am Soc Nucl Cardiol. 2005;12(1):66–77.
27. Parkash R, deKemp RA, Ruddy TD, Kitsikis A, Hart R, Beauschene L, Williams K, Davies RA, Labinaz M, Beanlands RSB. Potential utility of rubidium 82 pet quantification in patients with 3-vessel coronary artery disease. J Nucl Cardiol. 2004;11(4):440–9.
28. Ziadi MC, Beanlands RSB. The clinical utility of assessing myocardial blood flow using positron emission tomography. J Nucl Cardiol. 2010;17(4):571–81.
29. Ziadi MC, deKemp RA, Williams KA, Guo A, Chow BJW, Renaud JM, Ruddy TD, Sarveswaran N, Tee RE, Beanlands RSB. Impaired myocardial flow reserve on rubidium-82 positron emission tomography imaging predicts adverse outcomes in patients assessed for myocardial ischemia. J Am Coll Cardiol. 2011;58(7):740–8.

30. Dayanikli F, Grambow D, Muzik O, Mosca L, Rubenfire M, Schwaiger M. Early detection of abnormal coronary flow reserve in asymptomatic men at high risk for coronary artery disease using positron emission tomography. Circulation. 1994;90(2):808–17.
31. Johnson NP, Gould KL. Physiological basis for angina and ST-segment change. JACC Cardiovasc Imaging. 2011;4(9):990–8.
32. Johnson NP, Gould KL. Integrating noninvasive absolute flow, coronary flow reserve, and ischemic thresholds into a comprehensive map of physiological severity. JACC Cardiovasc Imaging. 2012;5(4):430–40.
33. Lortie M, Beanlands RSB, Yoshinaga K, Klein R, DaSilva JN, deKemp RA. Quantification of myocardial blood flow with 82Rb dynamic PET imaging. Eur J Nucl Med Mol Imaging. 2007;34(11):1765–74.
34. Johnson NP, Kirkeeide RL, Gould KL. Is discordance of coronary flow reserve and fractional flow reserve due to methodology or clinically relevant coronary pathophysiology? JACC Cardiovasc Imaging. 2012; 5(2):193–202.
35. Pijls NHJ, Fearon WF, Tonino PAL, Siebert U, Ikeno F, Bornschein B, van't Veer M, Klauss V, Manoharan G, Engstrøm T, Oldroyd KG, Ver Lee PN, MacCarthy PA, De Bruyne B. Fractional flow reserve versus angiography for guiding percutaneous coronary intervention in patients with multivessel coronary artery disease. J Am Coll Cardiol. 2010;56(3):177–84.
36. Kini AS, Kim MC, Moreno PR, Krishnan P, Ivan OC, Sharma SK. Comparison of coronary flow reserve and fractional flow reserve in patients with versus without diabetes mellitus and having elective percutaneous coronary intervention and abciximab therapy (from the PREDICT Trial). Am J Cardiol. 2008;101(6): 796–800.
37. Nesterov SV, Han C, Mäki M, Kajander S, Naum AG, Helenius H, Lisinen I, Ukkonen H, Pietilä M, Joutsiniemi E, Knuuti J. Myocardial perfusion quantitation with 15O-labelled water PET: high reproducibility of the new cardiac analysis software (Carimas™). Eur J Nucl Med Mol Imaging. 2009;36(10):1594–602.
38. Bengel FM. Leaving relativity behind. J Am Coll Cardiol. 2011;58(7):749–51.
39. Klein R. Editorial: derivation of respiratory gating signals from ECG signals. J Nucl Cardiol. 2015;23(1):84–6.
40. Hunter CRRN, Hill J, Ziadi MC, Beanlands RSB, deKemp RA. Biodistribution and radiation dosimetry of (82)Rb at rest and during peak pharmacological stress in patients referred for myocardial perfusion imaging. Eur J Nucl Med Mol Imaging. 2015;42(7):1032–42.
41. Packard RRS, Huang S-C, Dahlbom M, Czernin J, Maddahi J. Absolute quantitation of myocardial blood flow in human subjects with or without myocardial ischemia using dynamic flurpiridaz F 18 PET. J Nucl Med. 2014;55(9):1438–44.
42. Schelbert HR. Current status and prospects of new radionuclides and radiopharmaceuticals for cardiovascular nuclear medicine. Semin Nucl Med. 1987; 17(2):145–81.
43. Yoshida K, Mullani N, Gould KL. Coronary flow and flow reserve by PET simplified for clinical applications using rubidium-82 or nitrogen-13-ammonia. J Nucl Med. 1996;37(10):1701–12.
44. deKemp RA, Declerck J, Klein R, Pan X-B, Nakazato R, Tonge C, Arumugam P, Berman DS, Germano G, Beanlands RS, Slomka PJ. Multisoftware reproducibility study of stress and rest myocardial blood flow assessed with 3D dynamic PET/CT and a 1-tissue-compartment model of 82Rb kinetics. J Nucl Med. 2013;54(4):571–7.
45. Tahari AK, Lee A, Rajaram M, Fukushima K, Lodge MA, Lee BC, Ficaro EP, Nekolla S, Klein R, deKemp RA, Wahl RL, Bengel FM, Bravo PE. Absolute myocardial flow quantification with 82Rb PET/CT: comparison of different software packages and methods. Eur J Nucl Med Mol Imaging. 2014;41(1):126–35.
46. Klingensmith WC, Noonan C, Goldberg JH, Buchwald D, Kimball JT, Manson SM. Decreased perfusion in the lateral wall of the left ventricle in PET/CT studies with 13N-ammonia: evaluation in healthy adults. J Nucl Med Technol. 2009;37(4):215–9.
47. Maddahi J, Czernin J, Lazewatsky J, Huang S-C, Dahlbom M, Schelbert H, Sparks R, Ehlgen A, Crane P, Zhu Q, Devine M, Phelps M. Phase I, first-in-human study of BMS747158, a novel 18F-labeled tracer for myocardial perfusion PET: dosimetry, biodistribution, safety, and imaging characteristics after a single injection at rest. J Nucl Med. 2011;52(9):1490–8.
48. Giedd KN, Bergmann SR. Fatty acid imaging of the heart. Curr Cardiol Rep. 2011;13(2):121–31.
49. Tahara N, Mukherjee J, de Haas HJ, Petrov AD, Tawakol A, Haider N, Tahara A, Constantinescu CC, Zhou J, Boersma HH, Imaizumi T, Nakano M, Finn A, Fayad Z, Virmani R, Fuster V, Bosca L, Narula J. 2-deoxy-2-[18F]fluoro-d-mannose positron emission tomography imaging in atherosclerosis. Nat Med. 2014;20(2):215–9.
50. Panneerselvam K, Freeze HH. Mannose enters mammalian cells using a specific transporter that is insensitive to glucose. J Biol Chem. 1996;271(16):9417–21.
51. Herrero P, Dence CS, Coggan AR, Kisrieva-Ware Z, Eisenbeis P, Gropler RJ. l-3-11C-lactate as a PET tracer of myocardial lactate metabolism: a feasibility study. J Nucl Med. 2007;48(12):2046–55.
52. Renstrom B, Rommelfanger S, Stone CK, DeGrado TR, Carlson KJ, Scarbrough E, Nickles RJ, Liedtke AJ, Holden JE. Comparison of fatty acid tracers FTHA and BMIPP during myocardial ischemia and hypoxia. J Nucl Med Off Publ Soc Nucl Med. 1998;39(10):1684–9.
53. DeGrado TR, Kitapci MT, Wang S, Ying J, Lopaschuk GD. Validation of 18F-fluoro-4-thia-palmitate as a PET probe for myocardial fatty acid oxidation: effects of hypoxia and composition of exogenous fatty acids. J Nucl Med Off Publ Soc Nucl Med. 2006;47(1):173–81.
54. Shoup TM, Elmaleh DR, Bonab AA, Fischman AJ. Evaluation of trans-9-18F-fluoro-3,4-Methyleneheptadecanoic acid as a PET tracer for myocardial fatty

acid imaging. J Nucl Med Off Publ Soc Nucl Med. 2005;46(2):297–304.
55. Peterson LR, Gropler RJ. Radionuclide imaging of myocardial metabolism. Circ Cardiovasc Imaging. 2010;3(2):211–22.
56. Mc Ardle BA, Beanlands RSB. Myocardial viability: whom, what, why, which, and how? Can J Cardiol. 2013;29(3):399–402.
57. D'Egidio G, Nichol G, Williams KA, Guo A, Garrard L, deKemp R, Ruddy TD, DaSilva J, Humen D, Gulenchyn KY, Freeman M, Racine N, Benard F, Hendry P, Beanlands RSB, PARR-2 Investigators. Increasing benefit from revascularization is associated with increasing amounts of myocardial hibernation: a substudy of the PARR-2 trial. JACC Cardiovasc Imaging. 2009;2(9):1060–8.
58. Allman KC, Shaw LJ, Hachamovitch R, Udelson JE. Myocardial viability testing and impact of revascularization on prognosis in patients with coronary artery disease and left ventricular dysfunction: a meta-analysis. J Am Coll Cardiol. 2002;39(7):1151–8.
59. Rohatgi R, Epstein S, Henriquez J, Ababneh AA, Hickey KT, Pinsky D, Akinboboye O, Bergmann SR. Utility of positron emission tomography in predicting cardiac events and survival in patients with coronary artery disease and severe left ventricular dysfunction. Am J Cardiol. 2001;87(9):1096–99, A6.
60. Di Carli MF, Davidson M, Little R, Khanna S, Mody FV, Brunken RC, Czernin J, Rokhsar S, Stevenson LW, Laks H. Value of metabolic imaging with positron emission tomography for evaluating prognosis in patients with coronary artery disease and left ventricular dysfunction. Am J Cardiol. 1994;73(8):527–33.
61. Eitzman D, al-Aouar Z, Kanter HL, vom Dahl J, Kirsh M, Deeb GM, Schwaiger M. Clinical outcome of patients with advanced coronary artery disease after viability studies with positron emission tomography. J Am Coll Cardiol. 1992;20(3):559–65.
62. Beanlands RSB, Nichol G, Huszti E, Humen D, Racine N, Freeman M, Gulenchyn KY, Garrard L, deKemp R, Guo A, Ruddy TD, Benard F, Lamy A, Iwanochko RM, PARR-2 Investigators. F-18-fluorodeoxyglucose positron emission tomography imaging-assisted management of patients with severe left ventricular dysfunction and suspected coronary disease: a randomized, controlled trial (PARR-2). J Am Coll Cardiol. 2007;50(20):2002–12.
63. Abraham A, Nichol G, Williams KA, Guo A, deKemp RA, Garrard L, Davies RA, Duchesne L, Haddad H, Chow B, DaSilva J, Beanlands RSB, for the P. 2 Investigators. 18F-FDG PET imaging of myocardial viability in an experienced center with access to 18F-FDG and integration with clinical management teams: the Ottawa-FIVE substudy of the PARR 2 trial. J Nucl Med. 2010;51(4):567–74.
64. Dilsizian V, Bateman TM, Bergmann SR, Prez RD, Magram MY, Goodbody AE, Babich JW, Udelson JE. Metabolic imaging with β-methyl-p-[123I]-iodophenylpentadecanoic acid identifies ischemic memory after demand ischemia. Circulation. 2005;112(14):2169–74.
65. Inaba Y, Bergmann SR. Prognostic value of myocardial metabolic imaging with BMIPP in the spectrum of coronary artery disease: a systematic review. J Nucl Cardiol Off Publ Am Soc Nucl Cardiol. 2010;17(1):61–70.
66. Watabe H, Ikoma Y, Kimura Y, Naganawa M, Shidahara M. PET kinetic analysis – compartmental model. Ann Nucl Med. 2006;20(9):583–8.
67. Hutchins GD, Caraher JM, Raylman RR. A region of interest strategy for minimizing resolution distortions in quantitative myocardial PET studies. J Nucl Med Off Publ Soc Nucl Med. 1992;33(6):1243–50.
68. Gambhir SS, Schwaiger M, Huang SC, Krivokapich J, Schelbert HR, Nienaber CA, Phelps ME. Simple noninvasive quantification method for measuring myocardial glucose utilization in humans employing positron emission tomography and fluorine-18 deoxyglucose. J Nucl Med Off Publ Soc Nucl Med. 1989;30(3):359–66.
69. Bøtker HE, Böttcher M, Schmitz O, Gee A, Hansen SB, Cold GE, Nielsen TT, Gjedde A. Glucose uptake and lumped constant variability in normal human hearts determined with [18F]fluorodeoxyglucose. J Nucl Cardiol. 1997;4(2):125–32.
70. Youssef G, Leung E, Mylonas I, Nery P, Williams K, Wisenberg G, Gulenchyn KY, Dekemp RA, Dasilva J, Birnie D, Wells GA, Beanlands RSB. The use of 18F-FDG PET in the diagnosis of cardiac sarcoidosis: a systematic review and metaanalysis including the Ontario experience. J Nucl Med. 2012;53(2):241–8.
71. Rudd JHF, Narula J, Strauss HW, Virmani R, Machac J, Klimas M, Tahara N, Fuster V, Warburton EA, Fayad ZA, Tawakol AA. Imaging atherosclerotic plaque inflammation by fluorodeoxyglucose with positron emission tomography. J Am Coll Cardiol. 2010;55(23):2527–35.
72. Burke AP, Farb A, Malcom GT, Liang YH, Smialek J, Virmani R. Coronary risk factors and plaque morphology in men with coronary disease who died suddenly. N Engl J Med. 1997;336(18):1276–82.
73. Cocker MS, Mc Ardle B, Spence JD, Lum C, Hammond RR, Ongaro DC, McDonald MA, deKemp RA, Tardif J-C, Beanlands RSB. Imaging atherosclerosis with hybrid [18F]fluorodeoxyglucose positron emission tomography/computed tomography imaging: what Leonardo da Vinci could not see. J Nucl Cardiol. 2012;19(6):1211–25.
74. Arauz A, Hoyos L, Zenteno M, Mendoza R, Alexanderson E. Carotid plaque inflammation detected by 18F-fluorodeoxyglucose-positron emission tomography: pilot study. Clin Neurol Neurosurg. 2007;109(5):409–12.
75. Paulmier B, Duet M, Khayat R, Pierquet-Ghazzar N, Laissy J-P, Maunoury C, Hugonnet F, Sauvaget E, Trinquart L, Faraggi M. Arterial wall uptake of fluorodeoxyglucose on PET imaging in stable cancer disease patients indicates higher risk for cardiovascular events. J Nucl Cardiol Off Publ Am Soc Nucl Cardiol. 2008;15(2):209–17.

76. Moustafa RR, Izquierdo-Garcia D, Fryer TD, Graves MJ, Rudd JHF, Gillard JH, Weissberg PL, Baron J-C, Warburton EA. Carotid plaque inflammation is associated with cerebral microembolism in patients with recent transient ischemic attack or stroke a pilot study. Circ Cardiovasc Imaging. 2010;3(5):536–41.
77. Grandpierre S, Desandes E, Meneroux B, Djaballah W, Mandry D, Netter F, Wahl D, Fay R, Karcher G, Marie P-Y. Arterial foci of F-18 fluorodeoxyglucose are associated with an enhanced risk of subsequent ischemic stroke in cancer patients: a case–control pilot study. Clin Nucl Med. 2011;36(2):85–90.
78. Joshi NV, Vesey AT, Williams MC, Shah ASV, Calvert PA, Craighead FHM, Yeoh SE, Wallace W, Salter D, Fletcher AM, van Beek EJR, Flapan AD, Uren NG, Behan MWH, Cruden NLM, Mills NL, Fox KAA, Rudd JHF, Dweck MR, Newby DE. 18F-fluoride positron emission tomography for identification of ruptured and high-risk coronary atherosclerotic plaques: a prospective clinical trial. Lancet. 2014;383(9918):705–13.
79. Li X, Bauer W, Kreissl MC, Weirather J, Bauer E, Israel I, Richter D, Riehl G, Buck A, Samnick S. Specific somatostatin receptor II expression in arterial plaque: (68)Ga-DOTATATE autoradiographic, immunohistochemical and flow cytometric studies in apoE-deficient mice. Atherosclerosis. 2013;230(1):33–9.
80. Gaemperli O, Shalhoub J, Owen DRJ, Lamare F, Johansson S, Fouladi N, Davies AH, Rimoldi OE, Camici PG. Imaging intraplaque inflammation in carotid atherosclerosis with 11C-PK11195 positron emission tomography/computed tomography. Eur Heart J. 2012;33(15):1902–10.
81. Dobrucki LW, and Sinusas AJ. PET and SPECT in cardiovascular molecular imaging. Nat Rev Cardiol. 2010;7(1):38–47.
82. Schelbert HR. Anatomy and physiology of coronary blood flow. J Nucl Cardiol. 2010;17(4):545–54.
83. Thackeray JT, deKemp RA, Beanlands RS, DaSilva JN. Insulin restores myocardial presynaptic sympathetic neuronal integrity in insulin-resistant diabetic rats. J Nucl Cardiol Off Publ Am Soc Nucl Cardiol. 2013;20(5):845–56.
84. Raffel DM, Chen W, Jung Y-W, Jang KS, Gu G, Cozzi NV. Radiotracers for cardiac sympathetic innervation: transport kinetics and binding affinities for the human norepinephrine transporter. Nucl Med Biol. 2013;40(3):331–7.
85. Fallavollita JA, Heavey BM, Luisi AJ, Michalek SM, Baldwa S, Mashtare TL, Hutson AD, Haka MS, Sajjad M, Cimato TR, and others. Regional myocardial sympathetic denervation predicts the risk of sudden cardiac arrest in ischemic cardiomyopathy. J Am Coll Cardiol. 2014;63(2):141–9.
86. Schindler TH, Zhang X-L, Vincenti G, Mhiri L, Lerch R, Schelbert HR. Role of PET in the evaluation and understanding of coronary physiology. J Nucl Cardiol. 2007;14(4):589–603.
87. Petrou M, Frey KA, Kilbourn MR, Scott PJH, Raffel DM, Bohnen NI, Müller MLTM, Albin RL, Koeppe RA. In vivo imaging of human cholinergic nerve terminals with (−)-5-(18)F-fluoroethoxybenzovesamicol: biodistribution, dosimetry, and tracer kinetic analyses. J Nucl Med Off Publ Soc Nucl Med. 2014;55(3):396–404.
88. McMurray JJV, Packer M, Desai AS, Gong J, Lefkowitz MP, Rizkala AR, Rouleau JL, Shi VC, Solomon SD, Swedberg K, Zile MR. Angiotensin–neprilysin inhibition versus enalapril in heart failure. N Engl J Med. 2014;371(11):993–1004.
89. Harrison DG, Guzik TJ. Studies of the T-cell angiotensin receptor using cre-lox technology an unan-T-cellpated result. Circ Res. 2012;110(12):1543–5.
90. Herrero P, Laforest R, Shoghi K, Zhou D, Ewald G, Pfeifer J, Duncavage E, Krupp K, Mach R, Gropler R. Feasibility and dosimetry studies for 18F-NOS as a potential PET radiopharmaceutical for inducible nitric oxide synthase in humans. J Nucl Med Off Publ Soc Nucl Med. 2012;53(6):994–1001.
91. Sun N, Lee A, Wu JC. Long term non-invasive imaging of embryonic stem cells using reporter genes. Nat Protoc. 2009;4(8):1192–201.
92. Tarkin JM, Joshi FR, Rudd JHF. PET imaging of inflammation in atherosclerosis. Nat Rev Cardiol. 2014;11(8):443–57.
93. National Center for Biotechnology Information (US). Molecular imaging and contrast agent database (MICAD). Bethesda: National Center for Biotechnology Information (US); 2004.
94. Naghavi M, Libby P, Falk E, Casscells SW, Litovsky S, Rumberger J, Badimon JJ, Stefanadis C, Moreno P, Pasterkamp G, Fayad Z, Stone PH, Waxman S, Raggi P, Madjid M, Zarrabi A, Burke A, Yuan C, Fitzgerald PJ, Siscovick DS, de Korte CL, Aikawa M, Airaksinen KEJ, Assmann G, Becker CR, Chesebro JH, Farb A, Galis ZS, Jackson C, Jang I.-K, Koenig W, Lodder RA, March K, Demirovic J, Navab M, Priori SG, Rekhter MD, Bahr R, Grundy SM, Mehran R, Colombo A, Boerwinkle E, Ballantyne C, Insull W, Schwartz RS, Vogel R, Serruys PW, Hansson GK, Faxon DP, Kaul S, Drexler H, Greenland P, Muller J. E, Virmani R, Ridker PM, Zipes DP, Shah PK, Willerson JT. From Vulnerable Plaque to Vulnerable Patient. Circulation. 2003;108(14):1664–72.

PET in Neurological and Psychiatric Disorders: Technologic Advances and Clinical Applications

20

Andreas Matusch and Tina Kroll

Contents

20.1 **Introduction** 486

20.2 **New Aspects of Longstanding Diagnostic Applications** 488

20.3 **Role of [^{18}F]FDG in Neurodegenerative Disease** 489

20.3.1 New Concept of Amyloid Pathology and Alzheimer's Disease (AD) 489

20.3.2 Other Dementias and Mixed Pathology 489

20.3.3 Use and Technical Aspects of [^{18}F]FDG-PET in the Frame of Clinical Trials 490

20.4 **[^{18}F]FDG in Various Conditions** 491

20.4.1 Movement Disorders and Functional Disorders 491

20.4.2 Major Depressive Disorder (MDD) 491

20.4.3 Bipolar Disorder (BD) 493

20.4.4 Schizophrenia 493

20.4.5 Other Neuropsychiatric Disorders 494

20.4.6 Risk Assessment of Carotid Plaques/Chronic Ischemia 494

20.5 **Contribution of [^{18}F]FDG and Other PET Tracers to the Characterization of Epilepsies** 495

20.6 **[^{18}F]F-DOPA and [^{11}C]raclopride** 496

20.7 **rCBF by [^{15}O]H_2O or [^{15}O]CO_2, OEF by [^{15}O]O_2, rCBV by [^{15}O]CO or [^{11}C]CO, $rCMRO_2$, and Tissue Viability by [^{11}C]Flumazenil** 497

20.7.1 General 497

20.7.2 Measuring the Cerebrovascular Reserve ... 497

20.7.3 Preoperative Identification of "Speaking" Brain Tissue 498

20.7.4 Quantifying Damage Extent and Rescue in Stroke 498

20.8 **Amyloid Imaging May Guide Inclusion into Clinical Trials** 499

20.8.1 Generations of Amyloid Tracers 499

20.8.2 White Matter Uptake 499

20.8.3 Uptake Pattern of Amyloid Tracers 500

20.8.4 Validation of Amyloid Tracers 501

20.8.5 Applications of Amyloid Tracers in Clinical Settings/Gray Cases 501

20.8.6 Amyloid PET and/or CSF-Aβ/Tau 502

20.8.7 Amyloid Diagnostics in Clinical Trials 502

20.8.8 Longitudinal Change of Amyloid Tracer Versus [^{18}F]FDG Uptake and Others 503

20.9 **PET as Inclusion/Progression Parameter in Clinical Trials** 503

20.9.1 Longitudinal (Phases IIb and III) Drug Studies: Outcome Parameter 503

20.9.2 Studying Effects of Medical Devices/Various Therapeutic Interventions 504

20.10 **Drug Development: Dose Finding by Occupation/Displacement** 506

20.10.1 P-II Studies of Successful Candidates 506

20.10.2 P-II Studies of Unsuccessful Candidates 506

20.10.3 Post-marketing Receptor/Target Occupation Studies 506

20.11 **Drug Development: Biodistribution of Radiolabeled Candidate Compounds** ... 507

20.11.1 Phase 0 Microdosing or P-I Studies Using Radiolabeled Candidate Drugs 507

A. Matusch, MD (✉) • T. Kroll, MD
Institute of Neuroscience and Medicine (INM-2), Forschungszentrum Jülich, Jülich, Germany
e-mail: a.matusch@fz-juelich.de

M.M. Khalil (ed.), *Basic Science of PET Imaging*, DOI 10.1007/978-3-319-40070-9_20

20.11.2 Compounds Secondarily Used as Radioligands Post-marketing 509

20.12 **Studying Indirect Neurochemical Effects of Acute Pharmaceuticals and Interventions onto Radioligand Targets** 509
20.12.1 Assessing Endogenous Neurotransmitter Release 510
20.12.2 Ketamine 511
20.12.3 Oxytocin 511
20.12.4 Assessing the Kinetics of a Drugs Effect on Perfusion 511

20.13 **Pressing Diagnostic Questions Acceded by Early Investigatory Tracers** 511
20.13.1 Protein Tau and Alpha-Synuclein Markers 511
20.13.2 P-Glycoprotein Imaging 512
20.13.3 Markers of Inflammation 513
20.13.4 Myelin Imaging 513
20.13.5 Astroglia Imaging 514
20.13.6 Open Questions Regarding the Pathophysiology of Neuropsychiatric Disease 514

20.14 **(Patho)Physiological Studies of Neurotransmission** 514
20.14.1 Huntington's Disease (HD) 515
20.14.2 Alzheimer's Disease 515
20.14.3 Schizophrenia 516
20.14.4 Bipolar Disorder, Depression, and Seasonal Affective Disorder 516
20.14.5 Anxiety Disorder 517

20.15 **Targets of Radioligands/ Radiosubstrates** 518
20.15.1 G Protein-Coupled Receptors (GPCR) 518
20.15.2 Ion Channel-Coupled Receptors 523
20.15.3 Enzymes 525
20.15.4 Membrane Transporters 525
20.15.5 Others 526

Conclusion 526

References 527

Abstract

This chapter resumes applications of PET in neurological and psychiatric disease and research. Routine applications and recent developments in [^{18}F]FDG-PET are dealt with, followed by the role of amyloid PET as inclusion parameter in clinical trials. A large series of PET tracers do target neurotransmitter signaling at various steps. This serves as a tool to decipher the pathophysiology of disease as well as to conduct pharmacokinetic and dose-finding studies of new drug candidates. After presenting the different types of experimental approaches, an overview of targets is given that had been imaged thus far by PET in the human brain. Taken together, PET imaging always accompanied and catalyzed the emergence of new technologies – may it be deep brain stimulation or new biomarkers – at the threshold to routine.

20.1 Introduction

From a practical point of view, as mentioned in previous chapters, the virtues of PET over SPECT are the higher sensitivity and broader range of possible radionuclides and radiotracers. Under the dose and time limitations for human imaging, a higher spatial resolution can be realized using PET. For by far most of SPECT methods introduced to clinical routine, there is today a PET analogue available. In some cases even for the identical molecule SPECT and PET isotopologues are available. Therefore, in the range of cyclotrons, SPECT methods may be progressively replaced by PET methods. Especially the neuropsychiatric domain has been fueling PET applications since the beginning. When it comes to neuropharmacological research and drug development, PET is almost unique as in any organic compound a ^{12}C can be replaced by ^{11}C. So, besides pure diagnostic applications, PET has its place at the threshold of drug development, monitoring of molecular targets, as – mostly secondary – outcome parameter/end point in the frame of clinical studies and basic pathophysiological research. When it comes to the upcoming field of multifunctional probes (theranostics) in cancer research and therapy, the reader is referred to Chaps. 4 and 17 and related publications. The same applies for reporter probes for gene therapy and the field of neuro-oncology.

Especially in the brain, PET does not yield direct quantitative measures, but a series of indirect measures has been established. From static data, some quotients can be derived using regional or blood radioactivity concentration as a reference. After dynamic data acquisition, kinetic models can be applied, and several parameters are fitted to the data points. In the case of compartment models, primarily transition rate constants are inferred.

Depending on the molecular behavior, tracer uptake may be characterized by one of the following types or a combination thereof: solely determined by perfusion (such as $[^{15}O]H_2O$), irreversible into a "deep compartment" (such as $[^{18}F]$FDG or $[^{18}F]$DOPA), or, last, reversible (such as $[^{11}C]$flumazenil or $[^{18}F]$altanserin). Kinetic models for each of these have been designed. When a new tracer is established, typically dynamic data are acquired over a rather long time starting from tracer injection, and arterial blood is sampled and fractionated at tenths of time points to constitute an input function. On this data, a dozen of these models are applied, and then one looks which fits best. In subsequent approaches, acquisition time may be shortened and blood sampling simplified or omitted. In case of a reversible tracer kinetics, equilibrium conditions may be obtained a priorily by applying a loading dose of the tracer followed by a continuous maintenance infusion. Background and application of quantitation and modeling are extensively dealt with in Chaps. 13 and 14. Of highest biological and clinical significance are the dimensionless parameters tracer distribution volume and ligand receptor binding potential (*BP*), which best correlates with the ex vivo measure of maximum binding capacity (B_{max} the concentration of all available binding sites also termed receptor density, typically nM). In ideal cases in vivo *BP* equals in vitro $BP = f \times B_{max}/K_D$; with K_D equilibrium dissociation constant of the receptor-ligand complex; *f*, free fraction of radioligand which is not protein bound.

With a special focus on brain PET, a consensus conference in 2007 proposed the following nomenclature of in vivo measures of *BP* [1]: *BP* referenced to the total plasma concentration of intact radioligand is $BP_P = V_T - V_{ND} = K_1 \times k_3/(k_2 \times k_4)$; with $V_T = C_T/C_P$, total distribution volume, quotient of tissue, and plasma radioactivity concentrations; V_{ND}, non-displaceable distribution volume; and k_{1-4}, rate constants of two-compartment model, and K_1 influx constant from blood space. *BP* referenced to the non-displaceable uptake equaling radioactivity concentration in a reference region is $BP_{ND} = V_T/V_{ND} - 1 = \text{DVR} - 1 = k_3/k_4$, with DVR distribution volume ratio.

Other parameters characterizing ligand molecules are the 50% inhibition concentration $IC_{50} = K_i(1 + C/K_D)$ with K_i, inhibition constant [2]; *C*, ligand concentration and the octanol water equilibrium partition quotient $\log P = C_{Octanol}/C_{Water}$; and C_x, ligand concentrations.

As a special constraint, accessibility of brain tissue is restricted by the blood-brain barrier (BBB) if there is no specific channel such as for selected ions and nutrients such as glucose and amino acids or specific endocytosis such as for transferrin. Broad experience leaded to Lipinski's rule of five (RO5) which describes molecular features necessary for high probability solubility and intestinal permeability, also as precondition for BBB passage. The compound should have not more than 5 H-bond donors and 10 H-bond acceptors, a molecular weight smaller than 500, and a log*P* smaller than 5 [3]. A more recent adaption claimed a number of nitrogen plus oxygen atoms (N+O) not exceeding 5 and $\log P - (N+O) > 0$ as predictors of BBB permeability [4].

Even fulfilling these preconditions, molecules which initially penetrated into the endothelial intracellular space may be secondarily secreted back to the capillary via efflux pumps localized in the luminal membrane. Of these the most prominent is permeability-glycoprotein 1 (p-gp, MDR1) coded by the ATP-binding cassette (ABC) transporter gene family. A smaller contribution to drug efflux comes from multidrug resistance protein (MRP4) and breast cancer resistance protein (BCRP). Candidate drugs are nowadays routinely tested as p-gp substrates before entering further in vivo development [5].

Anatomical structures mentioned in this chapter are illustrated in Fig. 20.1. With a special scope on the PET literature, the nonfamiliar reader may retain some definitions: synonyms of the orthogonal directions anterior-posterior are rostral-caudal and of superior-inferior, dorsal-ventral. The plain spanned in lateral and up-down direction is termed coronal, the plain spanned in front-back and up-down direction sagittal, and the plain spanned in lateral and front-back direction axial or longitudinal. Striatum is the sum of caudate nucleus and putamen. The ventral part of the caudate nucleus is also termed nucleus accumbens or ventral striatum. The hippocampus is composed of cornu ammonis (segments CA1–4) and fascia dentata.

20.2 New Aspects of Longstanding Diagnostic Applications

Since the beginning of the PET era in the 1980s, cerebral blood flow and metabolism have been studied using [^{18}F]FDG and [^{15}O]tracers in key neurological conditions such as stroke, epilepsy, or degenerative disease. [^{18}F]FDG and [^{15}O]tracers have also been the diagnostic gold standard in the broad field of neurophysiological and psychological activation studies. Also the dopaminergic system has been acceded by SPECT and PET since a long time. Whenever [^{18}F]FDG is used for serial measurements with partially investigatory purposes, absolute quantitation of regional cerebral metabolic rate of glycolysis (rCMR_{Glc}) is desirable in order not to neglect global effects. Therefore, an arterial input function is required. Here, as an easy alternative to circumvent arterial blood sampling, emission data acquisition from the cardiac blood pool at a thoracic bed position during 35 min following injection is established. Some venous blood samples serve for calibration [6, 7]. Many changes of rCMR_{Glc} due to interventions or disease are global and local. At rest glucose consumption in the brain, in average 29–32 μmol/min/100 g tissue, amounts to about 25 % of that of the total body. The local range spans from 15 to 22 μmol/min/100 g in white matter to 45–50 μmol/min/100 g in the visual cortex [8]. The following sections 3-7 deal with these new aspects of "old" applications. Sections 8-13 present new applications. Sections 14 and 15 give an overview by disease and by target, respectively.

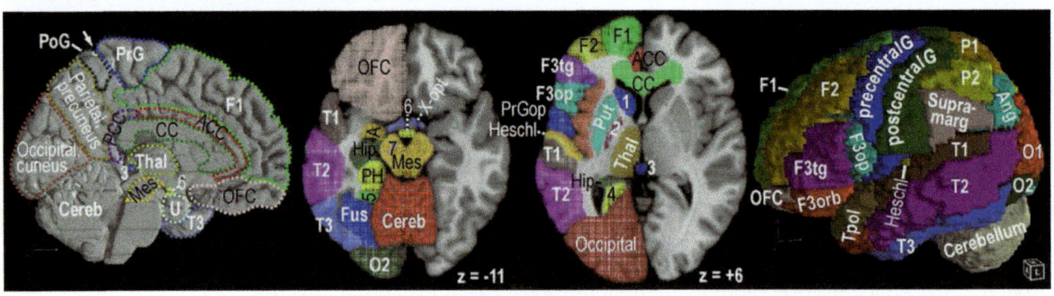

Fig. 20.1 For orientation, macroanatomical structures are delineated on the left hemisphere of the Collin standard brain. Shown are a view from mesial (*left*), two axial sections 11 mm below and 6 mm above the anterior commissure – posterior commissure (ac-pc) plain (*middle*) and a view from lateral (*right*). The set of regions follows the one ("atlas") implemented in the Pmod 3.1 software tool (Pmod, Zürich, Switzerland). *Abbreviations*: *1* caudate nucleus, *2* globus pallidus, *3* epiphysis, *4* lowest extension of the mesial parietal lobe, *5* lingula or gyrus lingualis, *6* corpora mammillaria, *7* substantia nigra (brown stripe inside the mesencephalon), *A* amygdala, *ACC* anterior cingulate cortex, *Ang* angular gyrus, *BA* Brodmann area, *CC* corpus callosum, *Cereb* cerebellum, *F1* superior frontal gyrus, *F2* medial frontal gyrus, *F3* inferior frontal gyrus subdivided into F3orb, pars orbitalis, F3tg, pars triangularis containing BA45, F3op, pars opercularis containing BA44, BA44 and 45 make up the Broca region, *Fus* fusiform gyrus, *Heschl* transversal temporal gyrus, containing the primary acoustic cortex, *Hip* hippocampus composed of fascia dentata and cornu ammonis; Mes, mesencephalon, *O1* superior occipital gyrus, *O2* middle or lateral occipital gyrus, *OFC* orbitofrontal cortex (gyrus rectus and gyrus supraorbitalis), *P1* superior parietal gyrus, *P2* inferior parietal gyrus, *PoG or postcentralG* postcentral gyrus, *PrG or precentralG* precentral gyrus, *PrGop* opercular part of the precentral gyrus, *Put* putamen, *Supramarg* gyrus supramarginalis, *T1* superior temporal gyrus containing at its posterior upper face the Wernicke region (posterior part of BA22), *T2* middle temporal gyrus, *T3* inferior temporal gyrus, *Thal, thalamus* Tpol, temporal pole composed of the rostral parts of T1 and T2, *U* uncus or gyrus uncinatus, *X-opt* chiasma opticum

20.3 Role of [^{18}F]FDG in Neurodegenerative Disease

For more than a decade, [^{18}F]FDG-PET was an in vivo "gold standard" in the differential diagnosis among the different entities of dementia and mild cognitive impairment. However, the advent of reliable pathobiochemical markers, refinement of the neuropsychological phenotype and of MRI acquisition, and analysis techniques fundamentally changed the clinical and diagnostic approach to and concept of neurodegenerative disorder.

20.3.1 New Concept of Amyloid Pathology and Alzheimer's Disease (AD)

Especially for amyloid pathology, cerebrospinal fluid markers and PET amyloid ligand imaging markers have been validated in larger biopsy and autopsy cohorts. This enables diagnosis of prodromal AD (synonym MCI due to AD) in a large quantity of unambiguous cases especially for highly enriched study cohorts. The current concept of the International Working Group (IWG) around Bruno Dubois [9, 10] requests:

1. A gradual deterioration of memory over more than 6 months with an amnestic syndrome where delayed cued recall is compromised
2. A pathophysiological marker, CSF, or amyloid PET
3. A topographical marker, either medial temporal lobe atrophy (assessed by volumetry/morphometry) or hypometabolism in [^{18}F]FDG-PET in parietotemporal regions including posterior cingulum (PCC) and precuneus

CSF is to be sampled in polypropylene tubes to minimize adsorption and displays low $A\beta_{1-42}$ (<550 pg/ml [11]), low ratio $A\beta_{1-42}/A\beta_{1-40}$ (<0.1 [11]), high tau (>614 pg/ml [11]), high serine 181 phospho-tau (>61 pg/ml [12]), and high ratio tau/$A\beta_{1-42}$. Knowledge of the individual status of the apolipoprotein E (APOE) polymorphism (isoforms ε2, ε3, or ε4, whereby ε4 carriers have increased risk of developing AD amounting to 10-30-fold in homozygous) considerably contributes information.

In addition, the familiar genetic mutations of amyloid precursor protein (APP) presenilin 1 or 2 (PS1 or PS2) are highly orientating. In up to 80 % of AD cases, there is a familial genetic background, the penetration of which is not obligatory and may vary in a wide continuum [13].

20.3.2 Other Dementias and Mixed Pathology

One reason for the incomplete specificity (about 94 %) and limited sensitivity (about 84–96 %) of [^{18}F]FDG-PET in the diagnosis of AD is that the pattern of moderate parietotemporal hypometabolism including PCC and precuneus is also found in cognitively normal subjects affected by atherosclerosis, diabetes, and obesity. In non-demented Parkinson's disease (PD), lateral parietal hypometabolism prevailed, whereas in the continuum of PD with dementia (PDD) and Lewy body disease (LBD), hypometabolism was observed in the occipital cortex (BA18) in addition to PCC and precuneus. In LBD, specificity and sensitivity of [^{18}F]FDG PET were estimated at 67 % and 83–99 %, respectively, and in frontotemporal lobe dementia (FTLD) about 89 % and 97–99 % [14, 15].

There is a large spectrum of mixed pathology and overlap in amyloid deposition, dopaminergic deficit (revealing Lewy body pathology), and vascular pathology. Therefore, the evolution goes away from setting a singular diagnostic etiquette rather to determining the contribution of each pathology to a given case using CSF markers, amyloid PET, dopamine transporter (DAT) SPECT or PET, and morphological MRI (searching for macro- and microinfarcts, microbleedings, and perivascular edema).

In FTLD there is less overlap with amyloid pathology. Typically, glucose hypometabolism involves the frontal, anterior temporal, and anterior cingulate cortex. See Fig. 20.2 for different patterns of hypometabolism. A similar frontal pattern can be observed in cases of amyotrophic lateral sclerosis (ALS), also essentially a ubiquitin pathology and of progressive supranuclear palsy (PSP), a tau pathology with accompanying frontal syndrome. In addition, tau radioligands are upcoming, while imaging markers of ubiquitin pathology – coming with disturbance and precipitations of TAR-DNA binding protein 43 (TDP43) and fused in sarcoma protein (FUS) – are not yet in view.

Vascular dementia (VaD) is primarily diagnosed upon the one- or multi-stepwise discontinuous evolution and MRI or cranial computed tomography (cCT). However, metabolic defects or deficits may considerably exceed MRI lesions. As a function of the subcategory of VaD, in multinfarct VaD, an overlapping pattern of multifocal hypometabolism may be observed corresponding to the respective areas of (silent) infarcts or malperfusions. In states of subcortical VaD/multilacunar infarcts/leukoaraiosis, [^{18}F]FDG uptake may be decreased in the basal ganglia, cerebellum, and diffuse cortical areas. Occasionally, the state after so-called "strategic" infarcts, e.g., in the gyrus angularis, inferomedial temporal lobe, dorsomedian thalamus, or basal forebrain, can mimic features of dementia. In the latter cases, [^{18}F]FDG may reveal large cortical areas of deafferentation [16].

20.3.3 Use and Technical Aspects of [^{18}F]FDG-PET in the Frame of Clinical Trials

Notwithstanding, [^{18}F]FDG-PET proved highest sensitivity as a progression marker [17] in longitudinal AD trials studying pharmacological [18–20] and other interventions. Amyloid PET proved unsuitable for this purpose as amyloid ligand binding slowly responds to interventions and amyloid deposition occurs early in the sequence of pathological events. Furthermore, in any atypical or gray cases, [^{18}F]FDG-PET still contributes to the characterization of the neurofunctional state.

In the recent years, a composite index (PALZ) of [^{18}F]FDG-PET-evidenced hypometabolism comprised within the PMOD software package (PMOD, Zurich, Switzerland) has been increasingly used for quantitation purposes in studies. The Minoshima tool (3D-SSP/Neurostat) is

AD, m 61, 2 yrs.
AD f 68, 5 yrs.
FTD, f 55, 3 yrs.
LBD, m 64, 2 yrs.

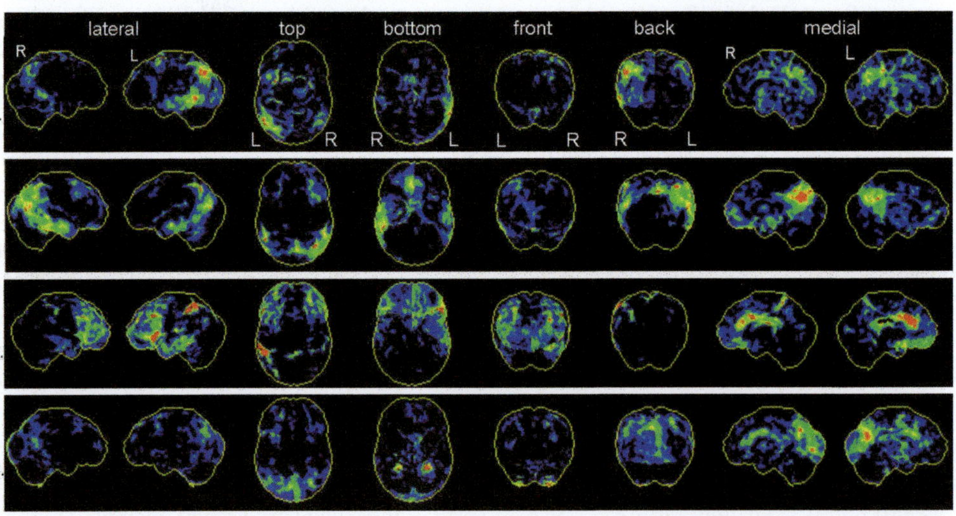

Fig. 20.2 Clinical cases of dementia syndromes assessed by [^{18}F]FDG-PET. Given are orthogonal maximum intensity projections of pixelwise Z-statistics of relative regional cerebral metabolic rates of glucose ($rCMR_{Glc}$). The individual and an age-matched normative control cohort are compared. The decrease versus controls is rainbow color coded, blue codes minor, and red most intense decreases. *AD* Alzheimer dementia, *FTLD* frontotemporal dementia, *LBD* Lewy body dementia. The diagnosis was further confirmed by measurements of amyloid and tau in CSF and clinical follow-up. Given are the individual disease durations

widely established for fast calculation of individual parametric Z-score datasets in comparison to an integrated control cohort. The visualization of Z-scores in maximum intensity projection increases accuracy especially of non-experienced raters (c.f. Fig. 20.2) [21].

The superiority of [^{18}F]FDG-PET over perfusion SPECT using [^{99m}Tc]HMPAO has been clearly evidenced in direct comparison [14].

Usually non-partial volume corrected [^{18}F] FDG-PET are used which reflect the composite of functional compromise and atrophy and thus are more sensitive. In order to identify areas of compensatory relatively upregulated metabolism, partial volume corrected PET were analyzed. In AD, the left and to a less extent right amygdala were identified as sites of highest metabolic compensation, whereas hypometabolism was most overproportional to loss of parenchyma in the PCC [22].

It has to be kept in mind that corticoids, any CNS-depressing drug (e.g., psychotropic, narcotic, sedative, antipsychotic), or state (postsurgical, previous chemo- or radiotherapy) will not only reduce global $rCMR_{Glc}$ but also affect the regional distribution pattern, while stimulants, e.g., caffeine, nicotine, cocaine, and amphetamine, may rather increase global $rCMR_{Glc}$ while activity and sensorial stimuli may increase local $rCMR_{Glc}$ [23].

Nuclear imaging techniques recently have been included into guidelines for the diagnostics of dementia disorders, e.g., of NIH, Alzheimer's association, AHRQ, NICE etc.

20.4 [^{18}F]FDG in Various Conditions

20.4.1 Movement Disorders and Functional Disorders

PET can contribute valuable information in the characterization of various movement disorders such as dystonias, tics, tremors, etc. Especially [^{18}F]FDG may help to differentiate central and peripheral origins. For example, a patient with up to 100 faciobrachial dystonic seizures per day consecutive to an autoimmune encephalitis showed intense bilateral putaminal hypermetabolism [24].

[^{18}F]FDG-PET may contribute additional orientation among atypical parkinsonian syndromes. In corticobasal degeneration, typically highly asymmetrical [^{18}F]FDG uptake is observed with hypometabolism including the cerebral cortex, striatum, and thalamus [23, 25]. In multisystem atrophy, parkinsonian variant (pMSA), there is isolated striatal hypometabolism and in PSP bilateral frontal hypometabolism [23, 25]. See 20.3.2 for PD and LBD.

In several cases, the functional or somatic nature of a symptom is not clear. Here [^{18}F]FDG-PET can reveal, e.g., areas of cortical underfunction. For example, cortical deafferentations after punctiform thalamic infarctions can be detected, and aphasia can be differentiated from a pure functional aphasia in the context of a reactive depressive episode [26]. In a cohort of 11 patients with unilateral pain-related nondermatomal somatosensory deficits, hypometabolism in the contralateral postcentral gyrus, posterior insula, and putamen was observed [27].

20.4.2 Major Depressive Disorder (MDD)

A large meta-analysis on resting state [^{18}F]FDG in depressed episodes within major depressive disorder (MDD) [28] evidenced hypometabolism in the pregenual and posterior cingulum, the BA9 part of middle frontal gyri (or dorsolateral prefrontal cortex, DLPFC) and insula bilaterally, and the left superior temporal gyrus. Hypermetabolism, in turn, was observed bilaterally in the BA10 area situated in the most rostral portion of superior and medial frontal gyrus, in the thalamus and the left caudatus. The outcome of these clinical cohorts is (necessarily) heterogeneous as various and different etiopathologies may underlie MDD. Especially, active inflammatory pathology would rather come with hypermetabolism, while degeneration implies hypometabolism. Subjects may have been scanned at various time points in the course of undulating symptoms, i.e., at the beginning of or during a depressive episode, in the recovery phase, or in (relative) remission. Furthermore, specific activation patterns could be closely correlated to specific individual symptoms so that the final picture may reflect an overlay of symptom correlated (state) and disease or pathology immanent (trait) metabolism/activation.

A series of studies investigated [^{18}F]FDG uptake or perfusion at baseline and after treatment. Whatever type of treatment was applied, findings converged to a compensation of hypofrontality and disappearance of the subgenual anterior cingulate cortex (sgACC) activation in responders.

In detail, selective serotonin reuptake inhibitors (SSRI) increased metabolism in dorsal anterior and posterior cingula, both middle frontal gyri (BA8/9, 46, 47), and the gyrus supramarginalis, while activity in sgACC, parahippocampal gyri, right insula, and left putamen was decreased [28]. In this meta-analysis, 9 [^{18}F]FDG studies were included with 22 patients treated by fluoxetine, 51 patients treated by paroxetine, and 6 by citalopram. Further studies directly compared paroxetine versus interpersonal psychotherapy [29], venlafaxine versus cognitive behavioral therapy [30], and double-blind fluoxetine versus placebo [31]. In all studies prefrontal and dorsal cingulum hypometabolism recovered, while rCMR_{Glc} decreased in sgACC, parahippocampus, and thalamus [31]. In addition, medication involved additional metabolic changes in the striatum [30, 31], brainstem, and hippocampus [31]. A single total sleep deprivation was most effective in normalizing anterior cingulate cortex (ACC) hyperactivity, while left prefrontal hypoperfusion normalized after the final recovery assessed by a third scan [32]. Electroconvulsive therapy increased ACC perfusion in responders (vide infra 4.3.2) [33]. Light therapy has only been assessed in 6 patients insufficient to detect changes in [^{18}F]FDG uptake [34]. A recent [^{18}F]FDG study absolutely quantified $rCMR_{\mathrm{Glc}}$ using a venously calibrated cardiac input function 2 h after the infusion of subanesthetic ketamine (35 mg) or placebo in 21 depressed BD patients. After ketamine, rCMR_{Glc} was nonsignificantly decreased globally by 0.3 % and locally in posterior brain regions such as the lingual and fusiform gyri, occipital cortex, and cerebellum and furthermore in both hippocampi and the left thalamus. The only significant finding was an increase by 2 % in sgACC, the amplitude of which furthermore correlated with the clinical response. The inverse correlation was observed in the right ventral striatum [7].

Conversely, re-induction of depression in remitted patients by nutritional tryptophane depletion was accompanied by a re-apparition of prefrontal hypometabolism [35].

A third type of studies measured the response amplitude of metabolism/perfusion to diverse behavioral, especially emotional stimuli. Positive emotional stimuli elicited less activation in MDD compared to controls in the left posterior orbital gyrus and left cerebellar posterior lobe and more activation in sgACC and inferior frontal gyrus (areas 47 and 11). The response to negative stimuli was increased in the right superior temporal gyrus [28].

A fourth type of analysis aims at extracting predictors for the response to a given type of treatment from baseline scans of those patients where thorough, in-depth, and long-term clinical follow-up is available. Also in view of the abovementioned findings, the sgACC was considered an indicator of treatment response [36] and a promising target for deep brain stimulation in progressive secondarily refractory MDD, which has been realized meanwhile in at least 45 published cases. However, a controlled randomized double-blinded trial was discontinued in 2014 because of inefficiency [37]. Further neuroimaging biomarkers as predictors for differential treatment response are under investigation [38]. Moreover, the response amplitude to a decision-making activation task was higher in the ACC in maniac and lower in the frontal pole of depressed patients versus controls, even more accentuating the corticolimbic divergence.

20.4.3 Bipolar Disorder (BD)

In BD cohorts, during depressive episodes, similar to MDD, prefrontal (DLPFC and dorsal ACC) under-function and over-function of limbic structures within the ACC, anterior temporal cortex, amygdala, and parahippocampus were observed [39]. About 2 dozens of rCMR_{Glc} and r*CBF* studies using PET and SPECT of patients in depressive, euthymic, or maniac state of BD converged toward the following findings: frontal metabolism is low compared to controls in euthymic, lower in depressive, and lowest in maniac state, while ACC metabolism is high compared to controls in depressed, higher in euthymic, and highest in maniac BD patients [40]. This activation pattern was the substance of the (fronto-) corticolimbic theory of mood disorders. Moreover, the amplitude of response to a decision-making task was higher in maniac patients which presented even higher CMR_{Glc} in the ACC and in depressed patients with even lower CMR_{Glc} in the frontal pole [41].

20.4.4 Schizophrenia

Current clinical criteria of schizophrenia, e.g., in the ICD-10 2004 (edited by the World Health Organization), section F20, comprise distortion of thinking, perception, and inappropriate or blunted affects. Specification still relies on the first rank criteria formulated by Kurt Schneider in 1938 [42] which are also termed "positive symptoms": thought echo, thought insertion or withdrawal, thought broadcasting, delusional perception and delusions of control, influence or passivity, and hallucinatory voices commenting or discussing the patient in the third person. "Negative symptoms" may precede and persist after an acute episode and comprise avolition; cognitive, emotional, and speech deficits; and psychomotor poverty. In the DSM V, more general terms are used and further clarification shifted to the footnotes. Schizophrenia is a diagnosis by exclusion of any somatic origin and developmental disorders and excluding especially psychoactive drugs. No instrumental or biochemical test is established so far.

A seminal study investigated resting state [^{18}F]FDG-PET with absolute quantification by an input function of arterialized blood radioactivity concentrations in 26 drug-naive schizophrenic (SZ) patients versus 32 controls. A global reduction of cerebral glucose metabolism by about 5–6 % was observed, particularly in medial and left prefrontal areas BA9 and 10 (−6 %), primary sensory cortex (−8 %), precuneus (−7 %), and both thalami (−10 %), reaching significance here (*T*-value 2.5 and 21) [43].

A comparison of 67 drug-naive first-episode schizophrenic patients and 103 healthy controls in [^{18}F]FDG-PET under activation by a serial verbal learning test revealed dramatic hypometabolism engaging the entire prefrontal, posterior parietal, and lateral temporal cortex, caudate nuclei, and mediodorsal thalamic nuclei. Relative hypermetabolism was detected in the pregenual ACC and anterior temporal lobe, including the gyrus uncinatus. As usual in clinical cohorts, no arterial blood samples were available, and therefore, uptake values were only relative and not absolute. Furthermore, the entire brain and not, i.e., the pons or cerebellum, served as reference region. Therefore, it is probably a technical side effect that relative white matter SUVs were almost globally increased in SZ. Rather, glucose metabolism may have been globally decreased with frontoparietal, caudate, and thalamic accentuation [44].

When it comes to later states of schizophrenia, the bias of medication compromises any comparisons to healthy controls. However, it is of key interest to investigate states dominated by positive symptoms such as delusions, acoustic verbal hallucinations (AVH), mental disorganization, and reality distortion well separated from states of pure negative symptoms. Therefore, it was an innovative approach of a Milan-based group to compare a cohort of patients with negative symptoms with a cohort of BD, treated by similar doses of the same atypical antipsychotics. Drug load was accounted for as covariate. A voxelwise SPM8 comparison of SUV images revealed at best insignificant differences in cortical and gray matter uptake pattern, while relative white matter metabolism was significantly higher compared to BD. This again can be interpreted as sign of globally lower $rCMR_{Glc}$ in negative-symptom schizophrenic patients compared to MDD [45]. Inputs to SPM8 were unreferenced SUV values, but in the intrinsic algorithms of SPM, there are global normalizations at one or two steps in data processing, and a ROI wise measurement of absolute values may have yielded constant white matter $rCMR_{Glc}$.

In schizophrenia research the same patients were scanned during acoustic verbal hallucinations (AVH) and in intervals free of hallucinations. Other studies compared hallucinators and non-hallucinators. Findings converged to activations of primary and secondary acoustic cortices and, surprisingly, not necessarily activation of the Wernicke region but even more of the Broca region, furthermore of supplementary motor cortices, ACC, and striatum, as reviewed by Bossong and Allen [46]. Targeted individualized repetitive transcranial magnetic stimulation (rTMS) onto left temporolateral areas hyperactive during hallucinations could considerably alleviate hallucinatory pathology [47].

20.4.5 Other Neuropsychiatric Disorders

In anxiety-spectrum disorders including specific phobia and social anxiety disorder, a series of activation studies under provocation conditions evidenced hyperperfusion/metabolism of a "fear network" [48] comprising the amygdalae, midbrain (periaqueductal gray) insula, and ACC, while activity in the orbitofrontal cortex (OFC) decreased as a function of fear [49]. In posttraumatic stress disorder, a related pattern was observed but with inconstant and rather inversed behavior of ACC and OFC [49].

In obsessive compulsive disorder (OCD), common findings were glucose hypermetabolism in ACC, caudatus, and OFC. Successful SSRI or cognitive behavioral therapy normalized metabolism in caudatus and OFC [50–52].

In multiple sclerosis, [^{18}F]FDG showed gray matter hypometabolism in MS which longitudinally progressed, and the site of which was well related with dominating symptoms such as thalamic and hippocampal hypometabolism with memory dysfunction and scattered frontal hypometabolism with frontal syndrome [53].

In ALS, if the primary motoneurons are affected, hypometabolism of the motor cortex is observed as a "stripe" sign. Furthermore, frequently frontal glucose hypometabolism is observed [23]. In both, most cases of FTLD and most cases of ALS ubiquitin pathology are observed coming with inclusions of TDP-43 and more rarely of FUS, which can spread into the frontal lobes. In Creutzfeldt-Jakob disease, fronto-parieto-occipital hypometabolism was reported, while temporal [^{18}F]FDG uptake was comparatively preserved [54].

20.4.6 Risk Assessment of Carotid Plaques/Chronic Ischemia

The advent of PET-CT combination enabled also the combination of CT contrast angiography and PET. In such combined datasets acquired after prolonged washout, 90 min after injection of 370 MBq [^{18}F]FDG, it was possible to resolve active and non-active sectors of carotid plaques. The respective target-to-background ratio (TBR) may be further established as sensitive parameter of plaque activity, vulnerability, and inflammation which promises a closer link to the pathomechanism compared to purely morphologic measures of lumen obstruction. [^{18}F]FDG TBR allowed good discrimination of asymptomatic plaques with and without microembolic transcranial Doppler signals registered over 60 min [55]. Also TBR was higher in the 60 symptomatic compared to the 63 asymptomatic patients examined. In a clinical trial of the anti-atherosclerotic drug dalcetrapib, carotid plaque [^{18}F]FDG-PET/CT TBR obtained at baseline and in 3 and 6 months served as longitudinal readout biomarker in 92 patients. Dalcetrapib is a cholesteryl ester transfer protein (CETP) modulator. Unfortunately, none of the plaque measures changed differentially in the verum and placebo group [56]. Smaller precedent studies were concordant [57, 58]. This method could fully exploit its strengths when combined with a measurement of the cerebrovascular reserve such as [^{15}O]H_2O-PET with and without acetazolamide challenge, see 20.7.2.

20.5 Contribution of [^{18}F]FDG and other PET Tracers to the Characterization of Epilepsies

In the clinical workup of epilepsy, the key interest is on focus localization. Highest accuracy can be achieved by comparing measurements of ictal and interictal brain functional state. Beyond electrophysiological techniques such as EEG and MEG, neuroimaging may contribute estimates of focus volume and shape and localize deep foci. In a considerable number of cases, extracranial EEG does not clearly localize the focus; here nuclear medicine techniques are of special value. As (i) the duration of most seizures is short within a time range of about 2 min and (ii) imaging "online" during clonic activity is hardly possible, an ideal tracer for seizure neuroimaging must have a (i) short uptake phase and (ii) a delayed washout behavior, ideally with trapping for several hours. Unfortunately the uptake period of [^{18}F]FDG lasts for 30–45 min [59] so that it is unsuitable for ictal versus interictal comparisons. [^{99m}Tc]ECD (Neurolite™) in turn has proven almost ideal properties – high first-pass tissue extraction followed by metabolic trapping – and allows literally to freeze the functional state following the 60 s postinjection and to acquire the SPECT even 4 h later. This procedure has been established under the acronym of SISCOM (subtraction ictal SPECT coregistered to MRI) yielding spatial resolutions full width of half maximum (FWHM) of about 7 mm [60, 61]. In principle, the higher resolution of PET (FWHM down to 2 mm) could benefit established [^{99m}Tc]tracers (half-life, 6.0 h) when using [^{94m}Tc] (half-life 4.9 h), but, this cyclotron nuclide is rarely available and emits additional gamma at 703, 850, and 871 KeV, warranting special data correction algorithms. As there is no reactor PET nuclide with suitable half-lives – 67.6 h of ^{68}Ga would be too long and 1.3 min of ^{82m}Rb too short – upcoming subtractive ictal versus interictal PET applications will be restricted to very specialized centers and research rather than routine applications. Cases of induced or very frequent seizures may be most suitable for such subtractive PET studies.

The second interest in epilepsy research is imaging the interictal state solely rather with a pathophysiological research purpose than in clinical routine. Only [^{18}F]FDG found some larger dissemination and displays – in negative contrast – areas of interictal hypometabolism usually larger than the epileptogenic focus and of vague delimitation. [^{18}F]FDG-PET/MRI is of special value in the search for focal cortical dysplasias and extra-temporal foci which are not apparent on MRI alone [59]. A recent Spanish study systematically acquired and compared MRI, coregistered [^{18}F]FDG-PET, video-scalp EEG monitoring, [^{99m}Tc]HMPAO-SISCOM, and intracranial EEG in patients with refractory epilepsy [62]. Of all 35 patients, MRI, [^{18}F]FDG-PET, and video-scalp EEG were available. In 11 of 15 patients with an MRI rated normal and in 19 of 20 patients with a lesion visible in MRI, [^{18}F]FDG-PET/MRI could localize lesions concordant with the final EEG focus, making a sensitivity of 86 %. Remarkably, in three cases scalp EEG was discordant with intracranial EEG, while PET was in only one of these. In total intracranial EEG as a gold standard was available in ten cases, in which PET was concordant in eight cases and discordant in one and showed hypometabolism considerably exceeding the focus in another case. SISCOM in turn was acquired in 25 cases. In 16 (64 %) of these, SISCOM was concordant with best EEG findings, while SISCOM was non-localizing or normal in six and discordant in another three cases because of too late injection or artifacts. In 7 of these 25 cases, intracranial EEG as a gold standard were acquired, yielding concordant results in 4 cases, a non-localizing SISCOM in 1 case, and discordant findings in 2 cases, thus making a sensitivity of

57% [62]. This study underlines that a rational diagnostic algorithm should first acquire interictal [18F]FDG-PET which should imperatively be coregistered to MRI and on a second-level SISCOM.

A New England-based study reported on 53 patients with refractory epilepsy which all had [99mTc]ECD-SISCOM injected within 30 s after seizure onset and interictal [18F]FDG-PET but without coregistration to MRI [63]. Upon isolated visual inspection, only 23 (43%) PET showed hypometabolic zones concordant with EEG foci, while 4 were discordant and in 26 cases PET was normal or non-localizing. Forty-seven SISCOMs revealed concordant areas of ictal hyperperfusion, while in the other six, there was discordance to even intracranial EEG. Consequently, of 48 cases with intracranial EEG recordings available, 42 confirmed SISCOM, corresponding to a sensitivity of 88%.

A recent study showed the feasibility of presurgical combined hybrid [18F]FDG-PET/MRI and MR-compatible 256-electrode EEG. Structural MRI, resting state functional MRI correlated to interictal epileptic discharges, PET coregistered to MRI, and electrical source imaging were performed. No MRI acquisition was performed during the about 30 min uptake period of [18F]FDG in order not to stimulate auditory areas. In total, 12 patients were studied; complete datasets of all four modalities were obtained in five patients and partial data in the other. In 8 of 11 patients, [18F]FDG-PET coregistered to MRI-detected focal hypometabolism. Key advantages are simultaneity and thus observation of an identical functional and medication state of the brain, precise coregistration of PET and MR, optionally exact imaging, and easy integration of the electrode positions [64].

For visual interpretation, tilting of 3D datasets not ac-pc but parallel to the temporal lobe may be helpful so that within a double-banana-shaped aspect the contour of the temporal cortex can be followed entirely while minimizing overlay with the orbitofrontal cortex. Partial volume correction and simultaneous acquisition in hybrid systems may further increase the sensitivity of [18F]FDG-PET/MRI.

[11C]flumazenil has been used – as in cerebrovascular disease and stroke – to image the viability of brain tissue. Reduced [11C]flumazenil binding helped to detect epileptic foci in MRI-negative cases and yielded results concordant with EEG, e.g., in 7 of 16 patients [65].

20.6 [18F]F-DOPA and [11C]raclopride

[18F]DOPA as presynaptic marker of dopamine reuptake transporters (DAT) and aromatic L-amino acid decarboxylase (AADC) and [11C]raclopride as postsynaptic D_2 ligand have been established since decades in the differential diagnostics of movement disorders and particularly parkinsonian syndromes and Lewy body disease (LBD). In clinical routine, imaging the dopaminergic system is of particular interest for cases of mixed or unclear pathology, i.e., when there is no clear response to L-DOPA/dopamine agonist treatment and the contribution of a – potentially treatable – dopaminergic deficit to a complex pathology is in question. [18F]DOPA has meanwhile an EU market admission and in addition to the advantages of PET over SPECT is selective for dopaminergic terminals in contrast to the tropane derivative DAT ligands [18F]FP-CIT or [123I]FP-CIT, [123I]β-CIT, and [99mTc]TRODAT which show also some binding to serotonin reuptake transporters (SERT) and norepinephrine reuptake transporters (NET).

As a large panel of neuroactive drugs and especially the agonists used in PD act on D_2R and have long terminal or brain tissue elimination half-lives, imperatively individual washout times have to be respected at least so that cerebral concentrations can be expected below 1/10 K_D. Therefore, a large part of D_2R imaging in clinical routine, also using [123I]IBZM, has to be interpreted with big care. Moreover [11C]raclopride is one of the rare exceptional receptor radioligands which is susceptible to displacement by the endogenous neurotransmitter and suitable for the measurement of transmitter release (c.f. 6.1).

Therefore, [^{11}C]raclopride has been used in a large number of interventional (c.f. 5) and activation studies. In addition to its D_2R binding capacity, [^{11}C]raclopride is well suitable as a perfusion marker, and a first-pass tissue extraction radioligand delivery rate *R1* can be fitted from dynamic datasets. This additional information has been exploited to increase the discriminatory power between PD and multisystem atrophy [66]. Dopamine receptor imaging in PD has been reviewed recently [67].

20.7 rCBF by [^{15}O]H_2O or [^{15}O]CO_2, OEF by [^{15}O]O_2, rCBV by [^{15}O]CO or [^{11}C]CO, rCMRO$_2$, and Tissue Viability by [^{11}C]Flumazenil

20.7.1 General

The circulatory and blood supply state of brain tissue has been characterized by the key parameters cerebral blood flow (CBF, ml/min/100 g of tissue), oxygen extraction fraction (OEF or E, unitless), and cerebral blood volume (CBV, ml/100 g). [^{15}O]H_2O–, [^{15}O]O_2–, and [^{15}O]CO-PET, respectively, are still considered and used as the gold standard for the quick and accurate quantitation thereof. A typical setting involves injection of, e.g., 555 MBq [^{15}O]H_2O and dynamic image acquisition for 80 s. Absolute quantitation necessitates arterial blood sampling to constitute the input function. Traditionally emission scans are acquired over about 80–120 s post start of injection and entirely put into statistical analysis. Recently the influence of length and position of the time interval p.i. selected for analysis was systematically investigated in datasets from a motor task versus baseline. Highest statistical power and thus sensitivity of comparisons could be reached using 20–50 s p.i. for all regions [68]. Rather historical is the steady-state method for measuring CBF by continuous inhalation of constantly delivered [^{15}O]CO_2 which within about 10 min equilibrates into blood. Images were acquired over 20–30 min necessitating very high radioactivity doses but only few arterial blood samples. [^{15}O]O_2 and [^{15}O]CO are applied by single inhalation of a tracer dose which very quickly enters the blood and equilibrates within. Signal acquisition also lasts over about 80 s. For correction, not only full-blood activity but also plasma activity has to be measured. As [^{15}O]O_2 virtually completely binds to hemoglobin, plasma activity almost exclusively accounts for the metabolic product [^{15}O]H_2O and has to be subtracted from the full-blood input function. For calculation of CBF and OEF, the CBV fraction has to be subtracted from the respective time-activity curve [69].

The cerebral metabolic rate of oxygen consumption ($CMRO_2$, in average 3.2 mL/min/100 g, gray matter 6 mL/min/100 g, white matter 2 mL/min/100 g) is a derived parameter: $CMRO_2 = CBF \times OEF$. As an alternative to deriving $CMRO_2$ from a triple tracer experiment using [^{15}O]H_2O, [^{15}O]O_2, and [^{15}O]CO, a kinetic model has been established which allows calculating $CMRO_2$, CBF, and CBV from a single dynamic [^{15}O]O_2 acquisition [70].

In this context, it should be kept in mind that the brain takes about 20 % of the total body basal oxygen consumption and about 15 % of the cardiac output, equaling 750 ml/min and globally 50–55 mL/100 g/min (20 in white matter and 80 in gray matter). The oxygen consumption of the entire brain is 50 mL/min which burn 60 mg/min glucose [26]. Average glucose consumption is estimated at 100 mg/min.

20.7.2 Measuring the Cerebrovascular Reserve

Perfusion measurements, preferentially by [^{15}O]H_2O-PET, are applied in clinical neurology in some situations to support decisions before interventions. Before revascularization interventions (e.g., carotid endarterectomy) in atypical cases or ventricular shunt placement, cerebral hemodynamics and reserve capacity of blood supply may be assessed while comparing scans at baseline and scans under induction of a luxury perfusion in well-perfused regions using acetazolamide [71–73]. Atypical cases comprise, e.g., those with comorbidity or not fulfilling standard time and gravity criteria or cases with complex anomalies of vascular anatomy or arteriovenous malformations. For this indication, also perfusion SPECT can be applied, nowadays preferentially with [^{99m}Tc]ECD which is superior to [^{99m}Tc]HMPAO. [^{99m}Tc]ECD is more stable in vitro; the cerebral distribution is more stable allowing to freeze the state at injection and readout 4 h later and more. The dosimetry is more favorable. However, [^{99m}Tc]ECD to some part reflects cellular metabolic uptake, while [^{99m}Tc]HMPAO purely correlates to blood flow arrival [26]. Thus, images will differ in states of perfusion-metabolic uncoupling. Both tracers slightly underestimate rCBF as first-pass tissue extraction is incomplete versus [^{15}O]H_2O. Luxury perfusion can alternatively be induced by hypercapnia (CO_2) or – more common in myocardial scintigraphy – by adenosine.

20.7.3 Preoperative Identification of "Speaking" Brain Tissue

Before neurosurgical removal of brain tissue or endovascular interventions with unavoidable obliteration of blood vessels, "speaking areas" of the individual brain may be identified by individual activation studies while comparing scans at baseline with scans during a task assumed to involve the operation area and its neighborhood such as motor, speech, recognition, etc. On an individual level, [^{15}O]H_2O-PET is superior to fMRI due to its considerably higher sensitivity, dynamical range, and spatial accuracy [74]. The big advantage of [^{15}O]H_2O-PET is that on an individual level, typically 6–18 tracer injections and scans ("shots") can be performed, yielding high statistical power [74]. Just very recently, PET/MRI combinations offered the possibility to simultaneously acquire [^{15}O]H_2O-PET in combination with blood oxygen level-dependent (BOLD) or arterial spin labeling (ASL) MRI sequences and thus validate the latter. Thereby, e.g., ASL correlated better with [^{15}O]H_2O-PET than did BOLD.

20.7.4 Quantifying Damage Extent and Rescue in Stroke

Classical work studied the perfusion defect in stroke and the extent of the center of irreversibly damaged tissue and the penumbra of salvageable tissue therein. The survival perfusion threshold could be experimentally determined at 17–18 mL/min/100 g for infinity, 15 for 80 min, 10 for 40 min, and 0 mL/min/100 g for 25 min. Large series of [^{15}O]H_2O-PET obtained typically few hours after stroke allowed a classification of a core zone with CBF below 12 mL/min/100 g with regularly infarction on later cCTs, the penumbra with CBF between 12 and 22 mL/min/100 g with some chances of infarction and some chances of recovery, and, third, a solely functionally and temporarily compromised area with CBF > 22 mL/min/100 g. In the penumbra, OEF is compensatorily increased to a maximum, while in irreversibly damaged tissue, OEF is low. OEF thus is the marker of the penumbra. In the subacute phase after ischemic infarct, a luxury hyperperfusion was particularly observed in areas with secondary loss of initially increased OEF [8]. This corresponds to malignant infarction with edematous propensity [8].

PET was at the origin of understanding the pathophysiological cascade after acute ischemia and elaborating the salvageable penumbra concept and deepened the understanding of timing and effect of i.v. thrombolysis. With the advent of MRI technology, at the end of the 1990s, diffusion and perfusion-weighted MRI (PWI and DWI) took the relay [8]. The perfusion-diffusion mismatch thereby corresponds to the penumbra but, however, tends to overestimate it depending on fine-tuning of PWI parameters [75]. When it comes to absolute quantitation of tissue gain and loss, PET and SPECT are still unrivalled. A study assessed the perfusion deficit before thrombolysis by [^{15}O]H_2O-PET and the final infarct size by DWI-MRI 3 weeks later [75]. However in clinical trials on revascularization, they are largely replaced by MRI techniques. As $^{[123]}$ECD SPECT allows to "freeze" the state at injection and the signal can be read out hours later, a cCT and tracer injection can save some minutes time versus MRI before revascularization. [^{18}F]fluoromisonidazole ([^{18}F]FMISO) selectively enriches within hypoxic tissue. The "cold" compound was initially developed as radiosensitizer for tumor therapy. [^{18}F]FMISO has been proposed as an alternative marker of the penumbra with selective enrichment in hypoxic tissue with residual perfusion [8, 76]. However, [^{18}F]FMISO-enriching areas where not as accurately delimited as hyper-OEF areas [8].

The $GABA_A$ ligand [^{11}C]flumazenil ([^{11}C]FMZ) turned out to be a good marker of salvageable tissue within the penumbra and for irreversibly damaged tissue in negative contrast, respectively. Reliable thresholds for core, penumbra, and intact tissue could be set. The PWI-DWI mismatch showed good correlations with [^{11}C]FMZ uptake.

20.8 Amyloid Imaging May Guide Inclusion into Clinical Trials

The development of tracers for cerebral protein deposits of Aβ-amyloid, protein tau, α-synuclein/Lewy bodies, ubiquitin/TDP43, etc., has been driven by the interest in early etiologic therapies. Therefore, the gold standard for evaluation of these tracers cannot be a vague clinical semiology but *postmortem* neuropathological verification and quantitation. In about 20 % of autopsies, a previous purely clinical diagnosis of AD could be falsified. In autopsy series a mixed pathology of Aβ-amyloid and α-synuclein was rather the rule (50–80 %) in the continuum of DLB-PDD, while mixed pathology was rather the exception in frontotemporal lobe dementia (FTLD) where isolated tau was found in about 40 % (FTLD-tau) and isolated TDP-43 in about 60 % of cases (FTLD-U). Isolated α-synuclein pathology was detected in multisystem atrophy (MSA) [77].

20.8.1 Generations of Amyloid Tracers

At the beginning, a series of studies used the first-generation marker of cerebral protein deposits [^{18}F]FDDNP which is not specific and recognizes Aβ and tau [78]. A breakthrough was achieved with the introduction of the 2-phenylbenzothiazole and thioflavin-T derivative [^{11}C]PiB. This compound is virtually Aβ-selective. Unspecific white matter uptake is comparatively low. A high discriminatory power is provided between amyloid carriers and non-carriers, as confirmed by biopsy or autopsy. Still [^{11}C]PiB is the amyloid tracer with the most measurements reported in the literature. In the recent years, three "3rd-generation" [^{18}F]Aβ-amyloid tracers obtained admission to the market after extensive phase I–III validation, including biopsy or autopsy confirmation. These are the 3′-[^{18}F]fluoro-analogue of PiB, [^{18}F]flutemetamol (GE067, GE Healthcare), and the stilbene [^{18}F]florbetabene (Piramal) in the EU and USA and its pyridine analogue [^{18}F]florbetapir (AV45, Amyvid, Eli Lilly) in the USA and UK. An example of [^{18}F]florbetabene PET scans is given in Fig. 20.3. Unfortunately, the white matter uptake of all these three [^{18}F]-tracers is higher than of [^{11}C]PiB, and accordingly the discriminatory power is reduced [77]. A cohort of 10 controls and 10 AD patients received [^{11}C]PiB and [^{18}F]florbetabene subsequently, yielding differences of SUVR of 75 % and 56 % and Cohen's d as a measure of diagnostic discriminatory power of 3.3 and 3.0, respectively [79]. [^{18}F]NAV4694 (Navidea, formerly [^{18}F]AZD4696) which is in advanced P-IIb and P-III development at the threshold to market admission displays considerable lower white matter uptake. [^{18}F]NAV4694, as flutemetamol and PiB, is a heteroaromatic planar analogue of thioflavin-T [80].

20.8.2 White Matter Uptake

As a consequence of unspecific white matter uptake, amyloid imaging is particularly sensitive to motion artifacts. Due to partial volume effects coming with limited spatial resolution, brain areas with high atrophy risk to be rated as unaffected. This is not the case for the hippocampus, which almost regularly displays

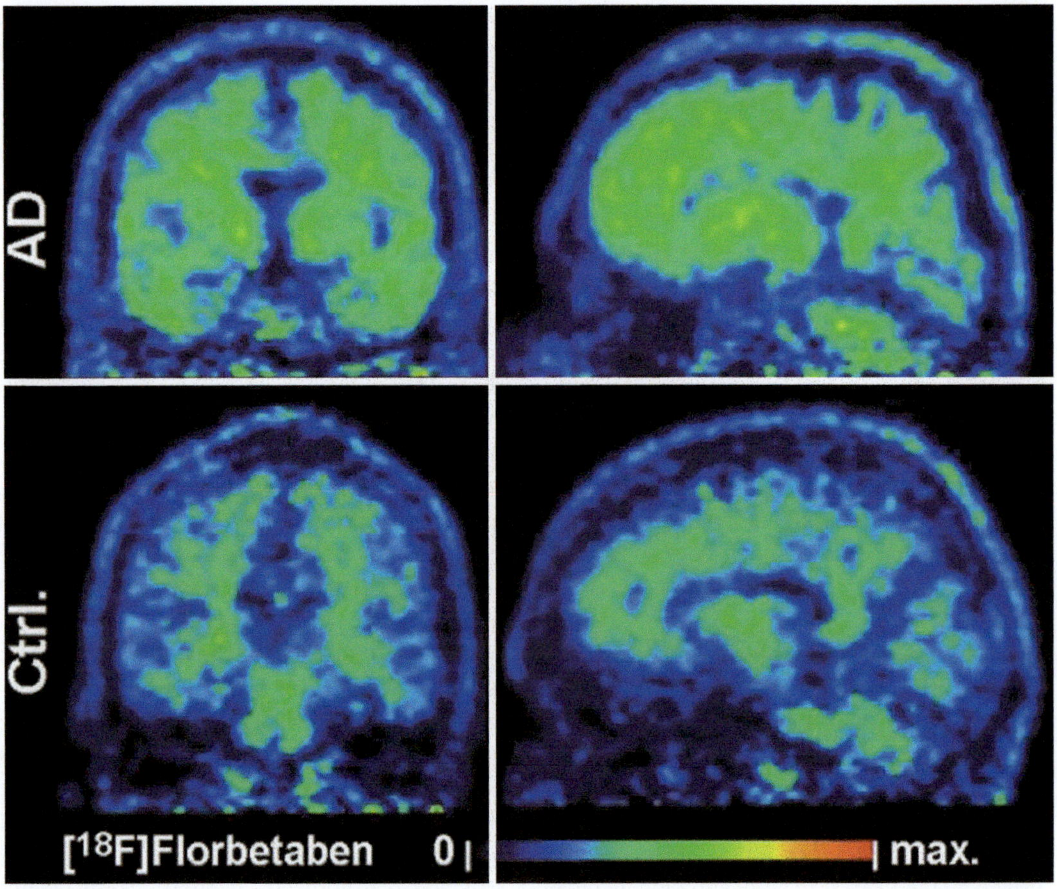

Fig. 20.3 Exemplary PET scans of a 69-year-old AD patient symptomatic since 5 years and a healthy control person aged 22 years using the amyloid ligand [^{18}F]florbetaben, acquired 90–110 min postinjection of 342 MBq and 253 MBq, respectively. Note the gray matter uptake equaling and partially exceeding white matter in AD while there is exclusive white matter uptake in the control

little amyloid deposition and only in state IV in histopathological examinations [81]. For precise detection of very early and localized cortical amyloid deposits, an accurate coregistration of structural MRI and PET is warranted which may best be provided by simultaneous acquisition at hybrid scanners. A high challenge and still matter of debate is also the choice of a (white matter) reference region which is little subdued to longitudinal changes [82]. In healthy controls amyloid tracer uptake reflects white matter distribution with perfect congruency. To turn this shortage into a virtue, amyloid imaging has been proposed for white matter quantitation in MS [83].

20.8.3 Uptake Pattern of Amyloid Tracers

In a typical AD case, homogeneous confluent white and gray matter uptake of the amyloid tracer or even prevailing cortical uptake is observed especially in the precuneus, PCC, lateral parietal lobe, and lateral temporal lobe in nearly perfect congruency to glucose hypometabolism in [^{18}F]FDG scans. Notwithstanding, also in the dorsolateral prefrontal cortex, strong amyloid signals are observed. The comparatively preserved $rCMR_{\mathrm{Gluc}}$ there may be due to lower neuronal vulnerability or compensatory mechanisms such as upregulated cholinergic or dopaminergic signaling [77]. In most cases, visual inspection allows already identifying a positive measurement, but quantitative analysis could considerably improve accuracy [84]. Interpretation should regard APO-ε4 status. The of APO-ε4 genotype is associated with higher amyloid burden. In AD populations >50% are carriers of at least one e4 allel versus 30% and less in control populations.

20.8.4 Validation of Amyloid Tracers

The specificity of amyloid tracers has been validated in large autopsy/biopsy series. Correlations of amyloid load determined in vivo and ex vivo were almost perfect. In the validation European Medicines Agency (EMEA) subcohort of the [^{18}F]flobetaben phase III study, a total of 74 brains were collected. Aβ was histopathologically detected in 47, all of which had a positive PET. Within the 27 Aβ-negative cases, only one had a false-positive PET [85, 86]. Resuming the sum of trials, sensitivity and specificity of [^{18}F]flobetaben are indicated at 98 and 89 % [86].

Furthermore, large series assessed the accuracy of clinical diagnosis of AD based on examination and structural MRI/CT by neuropathological verification. For instance, of 34 patients initially presenting with amnestic MCI and later having converted to dementia, finally 10 (29 %) of cases had non-AD pathology [87].

20.8.5 Applications of Amyloid Tracers in Clinical Settings/Gray Cases

In cognitively normal elderly control populations, about 30 % of amyloid-positive scans were reported, in mild cognitive impairment 60 %, and in clinical AD 80–90 %. Equal numbers were reported from autopsy series [81].

Smaller investigatory studies shed light onto caveats and shortcomings in practical settings especially in front of non-Alzheimer and mixed pathology/gray cases. In a very recent trial, eight FTLD cases showed a [^{18}F]florbetapir SUVR relative to cerebellar cortex of 1.20 in PCC versus 1.31 in 10 controls and 1.94 in 10 AD cases. One FTLD case homozygous for APOE-ε4 was positive; two AD cases and all controls were amyloid negative upon quantitative analysis. Visual inspection alone yielded high uncertainty; only two of the eight FTLD scans were unanimously rated negative by all four raters. All cases were defined clinically and underwent additional diagnostic [^{18}F]FDG-PET; CSF data were not provided [84]. It should be kept in mind that FTLD clinically may manifest as behavioral variant or more rarely as semantic dementia (SD) involving a rather Wernicke-like aphasia with difficulties of object naming and knowing the meaning of single words. SD is mostly associated to TDP43. The genetic background of FTLD is heterogeneous; mutations of the progranulin (GRN), the C9orf72, the TARDP, or the valosin-containing protein (VCP) gene corresponding to subtypes A-D are detected in TDP43 pathology including the overlap with ALS. Also FUS pathology accounts for a continuum of FTLD and ALS. Tau pathology includes strict sense Pick's disease (PiD, with round tau-positive Pick bodies) and the overlap of FTLD with corticobasal degeneration (CBD), PSP and parkinsonism linked to chromosome 17 due to mutations of the microtubule-associated protein tau (MAPT). FTLD-UPS (tau and TDP43-negative ubiquitinated inclusions due to mutations of the CHMP2B gene) and FTLD-ni (no inclusions) account for the smaller number of other FTLD cases [88]. Classical CSF markers tau and 181-phospho-tau are slightly increased and can be even decreased in FTLD irrespective of TDP43 or tau pathology. Aβ is normal in FTLD [88]. Other CSF parameters such as TDP43 in conjunction with [^{18}F]FDG-PET and MRI are under development, e.g., in the prospective LOF cohort [89].

Atypical Alzheimer variants with more focal cortical dysfunction and almost regularly widespread amyloid detection comprise (i) primary progressive nonfluent aphasia, rather resembling a Broca phenotype with agrammatism and apraxia of speech but spared single word comprehension (this type is however grouped to FTLD by some authors and mostly associated to tau pathology [88]), (ii) logopenic progressive aphasia, resembling the conduction aphasia type with impaired single word repetition but spared spontaneous speech production with some phonologic errors, (iii) frontal variant of AD, and (iv) posterior cortical atrophy [10, 90].

In DLB defined clinically – and confirmed by the occurrence of a L-DOPA-sensitive parkinsonian syndrome in the follow-up or DAT imaging – positive amyloid scans were reported in 54 of 92 cases (59 %) coming from 8 studies in the years 2007 and 2012 [91]. Remarkably, also isolated striatal amyloid deposition was observed in DLB-PDD [92]. An equal amount of amyloid binding may not account for an equal contribution to the functional deficit in DLB versus AD, as in DLB-PDD rather diffuse plaques may prevail and in AD rather the more malignant neuritic plaques, which of course cannot be discriminated by imaging [92, 93].

In a cohort of 39 patients with Down syndrome, [^{18}F]FBB PET was positive for amyloid depositions in 90 % aged over 50 years, in 53 % aged 45–49 years, and in 7 % aged 40–45 years [86].

Meanwhile a multitude of diagnostic possibilities came up in the field of dementia and Alzheimer's disease. Ongoing prospective and registry studies and expert panels/study groups such as the "Amyloid Imaging Task Force of the Society of Nuclear Medicine and Molecular Imaging and the Alzheimer's Association" (AITF) or Alzheimer's Disease Neuroimaging Initiative (ADNI) aim to conduct studies and identify most appropriate algorithms for applying sequences of diagnostic tests in front of a given setting of clinical symptoms.

In pure clinical routine, the symptoms are in the foreground, and the question of discriminating AD from FTLD in a case of aphaso-agraphoagnosic symptom in progressed state seems academic. Rather fruitful applications of amyloid diagnostics may be cases of comorbidity where the detection of amyloid pathology implies clinical consequences. In a person affected since decades by major depressive disorder and recent complaints of memory loss, discrimination of depressive pseudodementia from degenerative dementia and discontinuation of antidepressants with anticholinergic side effect plus addition of an AChE inhibitor may be in question. When DLB is suspected, an eventual presynaptic dopaminergic deficit is accessible to effective therapy and may be scanned first (e.g., [^{123}I]ioflupan SPECT) before Aβ. In those cases, it is however the question whether to use CSF or PET diagnostics.

20.8.6 Amyloid PET and/or CSF-Aβ/ Tau

It is of key interest to define indications for performing amyloid PET instead of or in addition to CSF analytics in clinical routine. As of the state of today, it can be stated that CSF has the advantage of multi-analyte capability, able to detect also non-degenerative, e.g., inflammatory pathology, and manometry can be performed upon sampling. Amyloid PET thus may be applied in patients who refuse lumbar puncture or where interruption of antiaggregation/anticoagulation therapy seems risky. The figures of merit of CSF versus PET seem quite comparable: e.g., the ratio t-tau/Aβ1-42 could discriminate autopsy-confirmed cases of FTLD ($n = 30$) from AD ($n = 19$) with 90–100 % sensitivity and 82–96 % specificity [88] compared to 98 and 89 % reported for [^{18}F]FBB (in autopsy 47 AD, 4 normal, 23 diverse other neurodegenerative pathology) [86].

20.8.7 Amyloid Diagnostics in Clinical Trials

In the settings of clinical studies, it is plausible that the combination of amyloid PET and CSF analytics yields higher sensitivity and specificity than any method alone. In the presymptomatic course preceding AD, PET may convert more early than CSF and define the asymptomatic at-risk state of AD. This may be especially the case when localized cortical deposits can be detected in perfectly coregistered PET/MRI hybrid datasets. Both CSF analytics and amyloid PET can separate AD from other pathology with high accuracy but can neither discriminate among other pathologies nor other pathologies from normal cases [88]. Therefore, a key interest of amyloid PET is to clean up FTLD cohorts from contaminations with CSF-negative cases of atypical AD pathology.

Conversely, in recent AD trials, 36 % (14/39) of APOE-ε4-negative subjects and even 7 % (7/115) of APOE-ε4 carriers initially clinically diagnosed as AD revealed to be amyloid negative [94]. Therefore, including only double PET and CSF-positive subjects obviously yields higher enriched cohorts. This may be of special interest, when amyloid-modifying drugs are studied (c.f. 4.2). Thus, amyloid PET is paramount as exclusion marker in FTLD studies and as inclusion marker in AD studies.

20.8.8 Longitudinal Change of Amyloid Tracer Versus [18F] FDG Uptake and Others

Occurrence and levels of biomarkers in AD likely follow a stereotype sequence or cascade as formulated by Jack [58]. Thereby, levels are saturable and follow a sigmoid kinetics which, meanwhile, has been empirically confirmed. Very early in the presymptomatic at-risk phase, $A\beta_{1-42}$ CSF levels decrease, and amyloid PET tracer uptake (SUV) increases. As second step with ongoing neurodegeneration, t-tau and p-tau levels increase and [18F]FDG uptake decreases. Third morphological changes such as hippocampal atrophy occur, and lastly clinical symptoms – first amnestic than aphaso-apraxo-agnostic – arise (c.f. Fig. 20.4). Therefore, the rate of change observed in a given biomarker much depends on the clinico-pathological stage.

However, we guess it noteworthy to give an idea of some annual rates of change observed in pathological cohorts versus controls assembled in Table 20.1

Across several studies, a longitudinal increase of amyloid tracer uptake – however with wide variability in annual rates of change – has been evidenced in MCI, while several studies found stable levels in AD [96, 100–103]. This variability may be due to different stages included in the respective cohorts.

20.9 PET as Inclusion/Progression Parameter in Clinical Trials

Principally in large trials, PET can serve for cross-sectional cohort characterization during inclusion or as a longitudinal progression marker readout and secondary endpoint. Some ongoing AD studies defined amyloid PET as obligatory inclusion parameter (c.f. 2).

20.9.1 Longitudinal (Phases IIb and III) Drug Studies: Outcome Parameter

Amyloid imaging was used to monitor the effect of therapeutic anti-amyloid antibodies. In a phase III study, 2452 patients stratified for APO-ε4 received bapineuzumab or placebo. In subgroups (115 carriers and 39 noncarriers), [11C]PiB PET were obtained at baseline and at week 45 and week 71. Amyloid levels clearly rose over time under placebo and stayed constant under verum in APO-ε4 carriers. In noncarriers, this effect on imaging parameters could only be detected transitorily at week 45. In contrast, clinical benefit was only observed at the disability assessment in dementia (DAD) scale in the mildly affected subgroup (MMSE >20) of noncarriers [94]. As this study was conducted from 2007 to 2012, amyloid PET was not yet a criterion of eligibility, and 13 of the 39 noncarriers were amyloid negative at baseline.

Before and after 1½ years of solanezumab or placebo in a total of 2052 patients, 266 patients

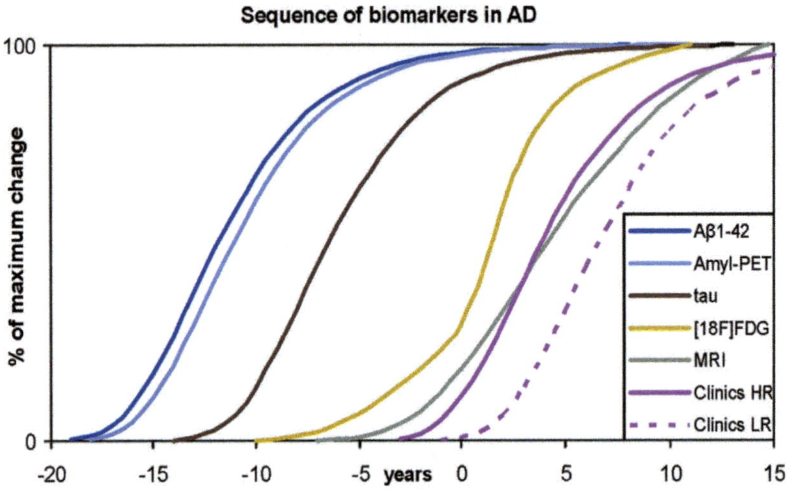

Fig. 20.4 Biomarkers in AD each follow a saturation kinetics and occur in a stereotypic sequence or cascade. Hypothetic plot of the evolution of biomarkers over time scaled from zero equalling normal to 100 % meaning maximum pathological level and time zero denoting phenoconversion/clinical onset (adapted from Jack et al. [81]). It is an open question whether genetic risk factors such as APOE ε4 or familiar variants Alzheimer (APP, PS1, PS2) shift the course of all biomarkers in parallel toward younger age of onset or whether the delay from pathological amyloid markers to neurodegeneration (tau, FDG, MRI) is shortened. *Aβ1-42* tau, CSF parameters, *Amyl-PET* amyloid PET, *clinics HR* clinical symptoms in subjects "high risk" with low compensatory capacity, *clinics LR* clinical course at "low risk" in subjects with high compensatory capacity

received a [^{18}F]florbetapir scan without yielding any significant change vs. placebo. In the entire study population, 59 % were APO-ε4 carriers, while this number was not given for the PET subsample. Details about the PET data are not reported yet [104].

It is highly interesting to see forthcoming refined analyses of these phase III data especially differentiating patients with amyloid-negative versus amyloid-positive scan at baseline and converters versus nonconverters. The spectrum of clinical response may be plotted as a function of baseline amyloid load and of baseline cognitive scores.

In the REAL-PET study, [^{18}F]F-DOPA PET was the key measurement to detect an eventual neuroprotective effect of the D-agonist ropinirole versus L-DOPA [105]; of 162 patients, at least 2 PET within 2 years of follow-up were available, and putaminal [^{18}F]F-DOPA uptake decreased less, by 13 % under ropinirole versus 20 % under L-DOPA. An analysis by voxel-wise statistics revealed also significantly less decline in the substantia nigra. Whether these findings really reflect a higher density and inventory of dopaminergic branches and terminals or are due to less downregulation of DAT under more constant dopaminergic tonus is however questionable [105]; see also 1.2.6.

20.9.2 Studying Effects of Medical Devices/Various Therapeutic Interventions

20.9.2.1 Deep Brain Stimulation

The metabolic effects of deep brain stimulation (DBS) for various indications at various sites have been studied using [^{18}F]FDG. Here acute and chronic effects in the neighborhood of active electrode contacts and at distance have to be discriminated. The best established application, the inhibitory 180 Hz stimulation of the nucleus subthalamicus (STN), in PD has the disadvantage that the intensive [^{18}F]FDG uptake in the thalamus outshines the tiny subjacent STN. A series of novel targets are recently on the way of being established for indications such as refractory depression, obesity,

Table 20.1 Annual rate of change for different AD PET markers

Radioligand	Region or index, parameter	*n*, state	APO-ε4 status +	Follow-up, years	% annual change	Reference
[^{18}F]FDG	PCC, temporal cortex, angular gyrus[a]	104 Ctrl	<27 %	0–3	−0.9	Lo et al. [95]
		203 MCI	<53 %	0–3	−2.3	
		97 AD	<66 %	0–2	−5.0	
[^{18}F]FDG	PCC, temporal, parietal[b]	11 Ctrl	18 %	0–(2–4)	0.6	Ossenkoppele et al. [96]
		12 MCI	67 %	0–(2–4)	−1.4	
		8 AD	75 %	0–(2–4)	−3.5	
[^{11}C]PiB	PCC-*SUVr*[b]	11 Ctrl	18 %	0–(2–4)	0.7	Ossenkoppele et al. [96], identical subjects
		12 MCI	67 %	0–(2–4)	0.9	
		8 AD	75 %	0–(2–4)	−1.3	
[^{11}C]PiB	PCC-*SUVr*	10 MCI	4 +	0–2 2–5	5.3 4.4	Kemppainen et al. [97]
		6 AD,	All +	0–2 2–5	4.7 3.3	
[^{11}C]PiB	GCA-*SUVr*	40 AD	All +	0–0.8 0–1.4	1.6 4.2	Salloway et al. [94], Bapineuzumab
		15 AD	All –	0–0.8 0–1.4	4.0 −2.4	
[^{18}F]florbetapir	Frontal, parietal, temporal ctx, cingulum[c]	14 Ctrl. A–	All –	0–2	0.2	Landau et al. [82]
		37 Ctrl. A+	41 %	0–2	1.8	
		54 eMCI	63 %	0–2	1.1	
[^{18}F]florbetapir	Composite	20 mild AD	n.d.	1.9	−0.6	Roche [98, 99]

In Kemppainen et al. [97] each subject was scanned three times, at the beginning and after 2 and 5 years follow-up. In Salloway et al. [94] each subject was scanned three times at 0, 41, and 71 weeks. Rates of change in the 41–71 weeks interval were too much scattered and therefore not reported here

GCA global cortical average, a composite VOI of anterior and posterior cingulum, frontal, parietal, and lateral temporal gyrus was analyzed with cerebellar vermis and pons as reference, *PCC* posterior cingulate cortex, *A–* amyloid negative, *A+* amyloid positive, *eMCI* early MCI

[a]Reference were vermis and pons

[b]Reference was cerebellar gray matter

[c]Reference was cerebellar white matter

Alzheimer's disease, heroin addiction, Tourette syndrome, etc. Here mostly an about 30 Hz stimulation with stimulatory effect onto the surrounding is chosen. Indeed, PET findings actually seem to confirm a net stimulatory effect on the cube centimeters around the active contacts and also in distant cortical areas and basal ganglia [106, 107]. As psychiatric parameters do not respond as quickly as Parkinson symptoms to changes of stimulation parameters and are influenced by a series of confounders, the potential of PET in optimization of targets and of parameter selection – once an electrode is implanted – is promising.

20.9.2.2 Convulsive Therapy

A large series of metabolic and perfusion studies assessed the response to convulsive therapy for refractory depression mostly in the postictal and in one seminal study also in the ictal phase [108]. It could be demonstrated that the ictal territory after conventional electrode position, dimension, and polarization involved large fronto-parieto-temporal areas. In the immediate postictal phase, there was global cortical depression, while later (than 1 week) frontal metabolism recovered, exceeding the baseline and reaching control levels. The same behavior was observed after seizures induced inductively (termed "magnetic seizure therapy") in the vertex region [109].

20.10 Drug Development: Dose Finding by Occupation/Displacement

20.10.1 P-II Studies of Successful Candidates

The partial D_2- and 5-HT_{2A} antagonist and partial 5-HT_{1A} agonist aripiprazole introduced in 2002 has become a blockbuster among antipsychotics. D_2-receptor occupation at the daily doses 0.5, 1, 2, 10, and 30 mg had been studied using [^{11}C]raclopride. At 1 mg, 54 % of striatal D_2R were occupied, at 10 mg 85 %, and at 30 mg 89 %. Indeed, in most patients, 10 mg/day exert the full antipsychotic effect, and 20 or 30 mg/day contribute no additional effect [110].

The SERT inhibitor and 5-HT_{3A}-antagonist vortioxetine (Lu AA21004) introduced in 2013 – with less affinity on some other 5-HTR – has been dosed at 2.5, 5, 10, 20, and 60 mg before measuring SERT occupancy with [^{11}C]MADAM and [^{11}C]DASB. Both tracers yielded similar saturation curves [111]. The K_D calculated from human PET data was 16.7 nM corresponding to the oral dose of 8.5 mg [112]. Twenty milligrams yielded 90 % occupancy in [^{11}C]DASB PET and 60 mg 70 and 93 % in [^{11}C]MADAM PET [111]. No significant occupancy of 5-HT_{1A}R could be detected after 30 mg over 9 days using [^{11}C]WAY100635 [112].

20.10.2 P-II Studies of Unsuccessful Candidates

Spending enormous effort in the clinical development of candidate compounds, which fail at the end brings some frustration. However, it is encouraging in the aftermath to have certainty that sufficient doses have been applied. So, a well-conducted initial PET dose-finding trial which yielded saturated receptor occupation after a single dose can help to avoid multiple useless subsequent studies at higher doses and eventually multiple dose applications. Some examples are the neuroleptic N-desmethylclozapine, ACP104 which had been studied using D_2R-ligand PET [113] or the allosteric mGluR5 antagonist AZD2066. It was developed for neuropathic pain and depression and was studied at the doses 3.5 mg, 6.9 mg, and 13.5 mg using [^{11}C]ABP688-PET. About 50 % occupation was observed after 6.9 mg and plasma K_i calculated at 1.2 μM [114]. A similar dose-finding study was conducted for the allosteric antagonist AFQ056 developed for levodopa-induced dyskinesias [115]. The mGluR5 negative allosteric modulator STX107 is being studied with [^{11}C]FPEB and [^{11}C]SP203 (NCT01896843).

20.10.3 Post-marketing Receptor/Target Occupation Studies

20.10.3.1 Occupation Studies at Monoamine Receptors

Paradigmatic for this type of PET application was the systematic study of D_2-receptor occupation by typical and atypical neuroleptics using the radioligands [^{11}C]raclopride and [^{18}F]fallypride. A broad series of typical and atypical neuroleptics proved to occupy 65–85 % of D_2R in vivo at therapeutic doses [116]. For most other ligand receptor systems, therapeutic doses are selected that come with receptor occupation in this range, but several exceptions do exist. Clozapine behaved exceptionally as already at 65 % occupancy a ceiling effect was observed [117]. In vitro, receptor-ligand association and dissociation, expressed by the dynamic rate constants K_{on} and K_{off}, was considerably faster in atypical neuroleptics [118]. Additional D_1R occupation was absent in haloperidol and sulpiride but amounted to 36–44 % in flupentixol and 38–52 % in clozapine [117]. The mixed D_2R/D_3R agonist ligand [^{11}C](+)PHNO unexpectedly showed increased BP_{ND} in the D_3-rich structures globus pallidus and substantia nigra after 2.5 weeks treatment with olanzapine and risperidone [119].

As an example of a large series of neuropsychiatric drugs binding to 5-HT_{2A} receptors, we show a case before and after olanzapine and a case after having taken as little as 25 mg amitriptyline (Fig. 20.5). Zolmitriptan in the dose 10 mg caused 4–5 % occupation of 5-HT_{1B}R as measured with [^{11}C]AZ10419369 [120], and only 5-$HT_{1D,F}$R blockade may be retained as mode of action.

20.10.3.2 Occupation Studies at Monoamine Transporters

SERT was occupied to 83 % in $n=7$ subjects after 4 weeks treatment with 20 mg/day of the SSRI paroxetine, whereby a ceiling plateau was reached at 85 % at plasma concentrations exceeding 28 µg/L. The SSRI citalopram yielded 77 % SERT occupation after 4 weeks at 20 mg/day in $n=4$ subjects [121].

NET occupation by quetiapine was shown to amount to 19 and 35 % after 150 mg and 300 mg using (S, S)-[^{18}F]FMeNER-D_2 [122].

Occupation of NET and SERT was studied in monkeys using [^{11}C]MRB and [^{11}C]AFM, respectively. Four different doses of atomoxetine in the range 0.03–3 mg/kg i.v. revealed IC_{50} for NET and SERT at plasma concentrations of 121 and 388 nM [123].

A significant contribution of DAT blockade to the action of bupropion could be ruled out as only 22 % of DAT were occupied at chronic 300 mg/day and plasma levels of 90 µg/L bupropion and 1107 µg/L hydroxyl-bupropion, as demonstrated by [^{11}C]RTI32-PET [124]. So the initial classification of bupropion as NET/DAT inhibitor had to be revised.

20.10.3.3 Occupation Studies at Other Targets

A dose of 450 mg caffeine, corresponding to about 4.5 cups of coffee, caused 50 % displacement of [^{18}F]CPFPX from A_1AR receptors in a 70 kg human [125].

The occupation of acetylcholinesterase by the antagonist galantamine admitted for Alzheimer's disease therapy was studied using [^{11}C]PMP [126]. Doses of 5 mg and 10 mg of donepezil, introduced as acetylcholinesterase inhibitor, occupied 60 and 75 % of σ1-receptors in the brain of 8 volunteers as assessed by [^{11}C]SA4503. The IC_{50} of donepezil was reported at 15 nM. [^{11}C]SA4503 uptake showed a global gray matter distribution [127].

These post-marketing occupation studies help to think over and understand therapeutic strategies. Especially the comprehensive study of D_2-ligand neuroleptics corroborated the abandon of typical neuroleptics in general and appealed for the strict contraindication in Parkinson's disease. They are paramount for the choice of sufficient washout times and further characterization of marketed drugs used as comparators/positive controls in clinical crossover trials. Finally, the sum of data permits a comprehensive overview and enables the understanding of structure, function, and relationship and serves as a basis for in silico modeling.

20.11 Drug Development: Biodistribution of Radiolabeled Candidate Compounds

20.11.1 Phase 0 Microdosing or P-I Studies Using Radiolabeled Candidate Drugs

The FDA "critical path" concept paper from 2004 [128] and Lappin and Garner [129] introduced the concept of microdosing to foster pharmacokinetic studies of drug candidates in humans. The methods in view were explicitly the use of [^{14}C]-labeled compounds and detection by accelerator mass spectrometry – here about 4 KBq is a sufficient dose for a 70 kg human – and use of [^{11}C]- or [^{18}F]-labeled compounds and PET. Microdose was considered a dose undercutting the pharmacological threshold by more than a factor of 100. In absolute terms a microdose should be at least below 100 µg. In contrast to the EMEA, the US Food and Drug Administration (FDA) set an additional absolute threshold of 30 nmol for proteins and peptides.

For a series of drugs meanwhile admitted to the market, PK data – as part of the application dossier – were obtained using PET and innumerable of failed candidates studied by PET.

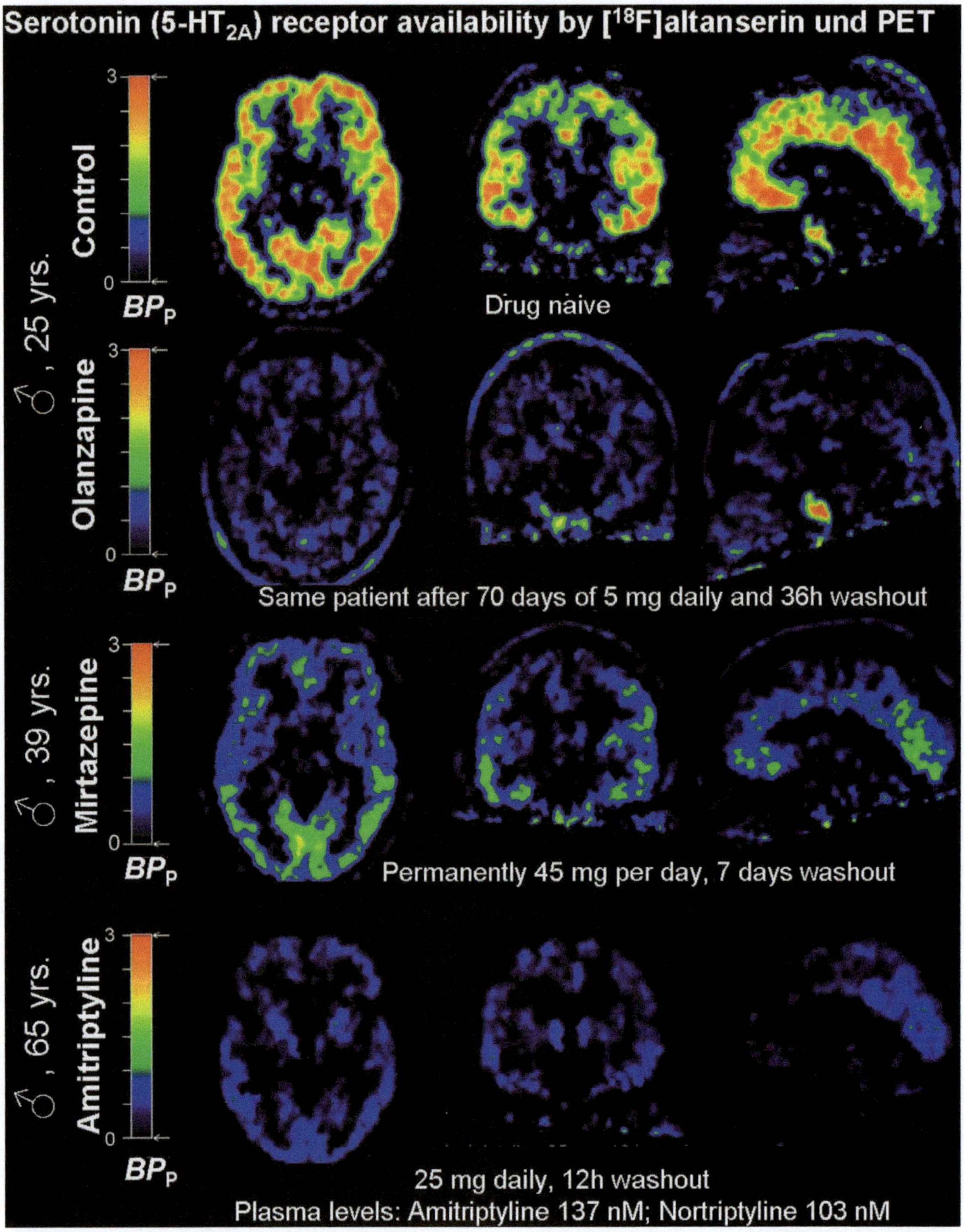

Fig. 20.5 Occupation studies of 5-HT_{2A}-receptors using [^{18}F]altanserin. Images were acquired at distribution equilibrium 120–180 min after the start of a loading bolus followed by a maintenance infusion whereby the bolus equaled the dose infused over 2.1 h (K_{Bol}). Color coded is the binding potential BP_P which is the quotient of specific cerebral (voxel – cerebellar reference region) and plasma radioactivity concentration attributable to parent compound. Of note is the extreme high-affinity and high cerebral persistence of numerous current neuropsychiatric drugs necessitating washout times of several weeks after standard doses. This compromises the interpretation of numerous patient studies and still keeps urgent questions such as the behavior of 5-HT receptors under chronic selective serotonin reuptake inhibitors (SSRI) in the realm of speculations

Candidates admitted to the market
With [^{11}C]zolmitriptan, the intranasal application pathway was studied. Zolmitriptan has been admitted to the market since 1998 and is one of the more potent 5-$HT_{1(B),D,F}$ agonist antimigraine drugs. Nasopharynx deposition decreased to 50 % in 20 min, distribution in the upper abdomen reached 25 %, and a small amount of radioactivity corresponding to a SUV of 0.02, 10 % of blood levels, more than the cerebral blood volume of 3 % would explain, could be detected in the brain. The maximum plasma concentration was attained after 15 min [130].

The biodistribution of [^{11}C]vortioxetine (c.f. Sect. 4.1) was studied in the mini-pig. The BBB penetrance was excellent and uptake highest in the thalamus followed by the cortex, cerebellum, and striatum and slightly lower in the hippocampus [131].

Discontinued candidates or candidates in development
Omigapil – such as rasagiline – is a planar polycyclic propargylamine derivative and promised as inhibitor of the glutaraldehyde-3-phosphate dehydrogenase an anti-apoptotic and neuroprotective action. [^{11}C]omigapil and PET revealed BBB penetrance but an unspecific cerebral distribution pattern [132].

The M1 muscarinic positive allosteric modulator [^{11}C]GSK1034702 displayed good brain penetrance, reaching brain to plasma ratios (V_T) up to 5 and BP_P up to 0.9 and good metabolic stability. The uptake pattern with global enrichment in gray matter with a slight maximum in the amygdalohippocampal region differed from those established for orthosteric M1 antagonist ligands. This may be due to the fact that different receptor populations were labeled, e.g., monomers by the allosteric and dimers by the orthosteric ligand. On the basis of this phase 0/phase 1 PET study, GSK1034702 entered further developmental steps [133].

Inhibitors of the multidrug efflux transporter p-gp are in development in order to increase the concentration of cytostatics in resistant tumors. The biodistribution of tariquidar and elacridar has been studied using their ^{11}C-labeled isotopologues without and with p-gp blockade [134].

Taken together, application of traces of [^{11}C]-labeled candidate drugs is an elegant way to study absorption, distribution, metabolism, and elimination (ADME) in humans without dose exposition. For a typical phase 0/phase I study, only 8–12 volunteers are required.

20.11.2 Compounds Secondarily Used as Radioligands Post-marketing

This is an atypical inverse fate of compounds. Typically well-working neuroreceptor PET radioligands are compounds that failed as drugs such as raclopride, altanserin, MPPF, etc.

[^{11}C]clozapine showed an intense ubiquitous cerebral gray matter uptake of 4.4–6 % ID/kg. The highest binding was in the striatum and insula and the lowest in the hippocampus. After 3½ h, cerebral concentrations had decreased to about 58 %. The excretion was to the largest part, hepatobiliary [135].

Donepezil was the first acetylcholinesterase inhibitor marketed for Alzheimer's disease. Only recently it had been labeled with [^{11}C] to [^{11}C]methoxy-donepezil and proved useful to demonstrate parasympathetic denervation in peripheral organs, such as the small intestine (35 % reduction of uptake) and pancreas (22 % reduction of uptake), in Parkinson's disease thus complementing sympathetic imaging (typically of the myocardium) using [^{123}I] MIBG [136].

20.12 Studying Indirect Neurochemical Effects of Acute Pharmaceuticals and Interventions onto Radioligand Targets

PET is also frequently used not to study the direct drug target but indirect downstream neurochemical effects typically after acute single applications of old or recent candidate drugs. In this context, knowledge of the binding behavior of the radioligand at its target is paramount, especially whether radioligand binding is sensitive or not to changes of endogenous neurotransmitter levels. As an exception rather than the rule, some few neuroreceptor radioligands are sensitive to concentration changes of their endogenous neurotransmitter analogue. Mechanisms may be direct displacement/occupation from/of the binding site, allosteric interactions, or the switch between high- and low-affinity receptor populations, i.e., monomers/dimers/clusters of G protein-coupled receptors (GPCR) high-affinity state or uncoupled low-affinity state receptors and finally rapid changes of receptor concentrations by de novo translation, activation (e.g., by glycosylation) from pre-existing reservoirs, deactivation/degradation, or externalization/internalization. A second line of research looks at the perfusion-metabolic response after acute or chronic drug treatment and has considerably contributed to the understanding of the action of the entire classes of pharmaceuticals such as anesthetics.

20.12.1 Assessing Endogenous Neurotransmitter Release

As a kind of external validation or calibrator, transmitter levels can be directly measured locally by microdialysis in the animal or intraoperatively in humans. With the caveats of artifacts through local tissue lesion and cicatrization around the probe, this method can be seen as gold standard to verify hypothesis derived from indirect observations made by PET. Especially acute pharmacological stimuli which provoke high neurotransmitter release can be validated and compared with changes of radioligand binding potential. For example, 100 % increase in DA release corresponded to about 1 % change of [^{11}C]raclopride BP_{ND} [137].

For assessing neurotransmitter changes due to a challenge by PET, two timing schedules exist. Either two separate measurements with and without stimulus premedication are conducted as occupation experiment. Or, in a displacement experiment, first distribution equilibrium of the radioligand is achieved and then the stimulus applied.

Observations of decreased radioligand receptor availabilities after release of endogenous transmitter are not necessarily a consequence of one step occupation/displacement but also can account for a switch of receptors to different states or populations. For G protein-coupled receptors, the high-affinity Gαβγ-GDP-bound receptive state is well described. Ligand binding causes the exchange of GDP by GTP which hydrolyses the G protein-receptor complex and the trimeric G protein into the subunits Gα-GDP and Gβγ. Without G protein, the receptor is in its low-affinity state. In vitro, the γ-thio or γ-imino analogue of GTP, Gpp(NH)p or GTPγS, respectively, allows to quantitatively transform all receptors into low-affinity state.

Agonist radioligands rather tend to preferentially recognize the high-affinity state of receptors. Allosteric radioligands, e.g., the A_1AR antagonistic ligand [^{18}F]CPFPX, can paradoxically show higher binding to the low-affinity state.

Classically, dopamine release is achieved with amphetamine and serotonin release with fenf–luramine, eventually in combination with SSRI. Extracellular glutamate can be increased by *N*-acetylcysteine, which causes an intra-/extracellular shift via the glial cystine/glutamate anti-porter or by ketamine. Glutamate can be decreased by ceftriaxone which activates the glial GLT1 transporter.

In addition to [^{11}C]raclopride or [^{18}F]fallypride (c.f. 1.4) also the μ-opioid ligands [^{11}C]diprenorphine and [^{11}C]carfentanil [138] and the SERT ligand [^{11}C]DASB [139] proved sensible to endogenous transmitter changes in many studies. Recently, the decrease of mGluR5 radioligand [^{11}C]ABP688 BP_{ND} in response to *N*-acetylcysteine or ketamine could be evidenced [140, 141]. Conversely, decreasing extracellular glutamate levels by stimulation of GL transporters with ceftriaxone was followed by an increase of [^{11}C]ABP688 BP_{ND} [142].

20.12.2 Ketamine

Ketamine, at subanesthetic doses, has been in the focus of psychiatrists since a long time as it induces, e.g., feelings of de-realizations, perceptual changes, and mostly visual hallucinations. As the so induced state was considered as model psychosis, some researchers hoped to better understand the real pathology when looking at a mimicked one. Some years ago, the immediate and impressive antidepressant effect of ketamine infusions was discovered, which usually lasts about 2–3 weeks. Nowadays ketamine for depressions refractory to at least one precedent treatment trial has broadly entered clinical routine. Racemic ketamine (57 mg for a 70 kg person) globally reduced the availability of mGluR5 by 20 % in 7 and by >40 % in three subjects as measured by double [^{11}C]ABP688 PET [143]. S-ketamine at 29 mg yielding plasma concentrations of 135 μg/L did neither influence 5-HT_{2A}R binding as measured by an equilibrium study using [^{18}F]altanserin [144] nor did 8 mg change [^{18}F]fallypride binding to D_2/D_3R [145] nor did racemic ketamine at target controlled infusion yielding a serum concentration of 350 μg/L change [^{11}C]flumazenil binding to the BZD site on $GABA_A$R [146]. Differential brain metabolic effects of R- and S-ketamine were detected [147]. The acute metabolic effect was at 326 μg/L, an absolute increase of thalamic (by 15 %), frontal (by 14 %), and parietal (by13 %) rCMR_{Glc} [148], for the subacute effect (c.f. 1.2.2 and Ref. [7]). Brain perfusion was studied at three different dosages, coming with plasma levels of 37, 132, and 411 μg/L, respectively, that yielded rCBF increases of up to 38 % in ACC, 29 % in the thalamus, 27 % in the putamen, and 25 % in the frontal cortex. $rCMR_{O2}$ was unchanged, and rCBV only increased in the frontal cortex by 4 % [149].

20.12.3 Oxytocin

Intranasal oxytocin (OXT) is today being developed as an add-on drug for psychiatric disease. In the vole rodent, the dopaminergic system as mediator of the cerebral and especially psychosocial effect of oxytocin has been established by (i) autoradiographic detection of high densities of OXT receptors in the entire striatum and (ii) microinjection studies of DA agonists and antagonists before OXT application. However, mechanisms of actions of OXT in humans are still enigmatic. A [^{11}C]raclopride study could not detect any evidence of even slight displacement [150]. An analogue result was obtained with [^{18}F]fallypride. The 5-HT_{1A}R BP_{ND} in the raphé nuclei region increased by 7 % under OXT, as measured by [^{18}F]MPPF. This is the inverse of what was observed in anxiety states, corroborating the additive anxiolytic potential of OXT.

20.12.4 Assessing the Kinetics of a Drugs Effect on Perfusion

Here, the option to obtain serial images in [^{15}O]H_2O-PET is of particular benefit. For example, the kinetics of the perfusional effect of rapid release rizatriptan were studied at baseline and 40, 50, 60, 70, and 80 min after application showed a peak 13 % reduction in CBF at 60 min and return to baseline at 80 min. Spatial distribution of the effect was strictly global [151].

20.13 Pressing Diagnostic Questions Acceded by Early Investigatory Tracers

20.13.1 Protein Tau and Alpha-Synuclein Markers

Currently, tau pathology is missed in as much as 70 % of cases [152]. However, specific treatments for these conditions such as glucagon synthase kinase 3β-inhibitors are coming up. Here, algorithms have to be improved. In order to identify "clean" cases and not to dilute the cohort by AD cases, the exclusion of amyloid pathology is paramount. The first proper tau tracers have shown promising results in humans. For example, in a cohort of 8 clinical probable AD cases, [18F]THK5105 showed significant 21 % (5.8 × SD) higher inferotemporal uptake compared to 8 controls [153]. Moreover, when plotting individual uptake in this region, all 8 AD cases were fully separated from all 8 controls. Also superior temporal and parietal uptake were significantly increased by 17 %, whereas nonspecific white matter uptake in pons and subcortical was perfectly reproducible. The white matter and gray matter contrast was by far not as pronounced as in amyloid imaging. Interestingly, in AD the hippocampal formation which is spared out by amyloid tracers could clearly be labeled by tau tracers [153].

[11C]PBB3 showed a tau-specific pattern and promising qualities in three controls, three AD, and one [11C]PIB-negative patient with corticobasal degeneration. In AD, the highest binding was observed in the hippocampi and ACC with different cortical spread and, interestingly, in both striata, thalami, and PCC of the patient with CBD [154].

[18F]T808 was first tested in 3 controls and 4 mild and 4 severe AD patients and showed considerably higher uptake in the hippocampus in AD at a target-to-cerebellum ratio of 1.22–1.49 versus 0.97–1.06 and one overlap case [155]. Image acquisition was best 80–100 min postinjection, and some uptake in the skull bone pointed to defluorination which may be overcome by premedication with "cold" fluoride. The selectivity of tau over Aβ was >27. More early, [18F]T807 and [18F]THK523 have been successfully assessed in humans. [18F]T808 was of faster kinetics than [18F]T807 and therefore preferable [155].

[11C]BF-227 in vitro showed equal affinity for Aβ and α-synuclein [77] and therefore may serve as lead for more specific α-synuclein probes. In 8 multisystem atrophy (MSA) patients – MSA is the α-synucleinopathy less contaminated by cases of mixed pathology – versus 8 controls, cingular, mediotemporal, motor cortex, and basal ganglia distribution volumes were increased by 15–16 %. In the putamen 18 % were reached, in subcortical white matter 32 %, while in the mesencephalon binding was constant and in the cerebellar cortex by 7 % smaller [156].

20.13.2 P-Glycoprotein Imaging

The transmembrane ATP-binding cassette (ABC) transporter p-glycoprotein (p-gp) accounts for by far the largest part of drug efflux pump capacity across the BBB outward of the brain. BCRP, MDR4, or MRP1 are reported to play only a minor role. P-gp pumps many radioligands and drugs out of the brain and is the reason for their effective net none or low BBB penetration. Overexpression of efflux transporters is particularly relevant for pharmacoresistance of tumors and epilepsies. R-[11C]verapamil has revealed as useful and specific inhibitor/substrate marker for p-gp. [11C]verapamil uptake correlates inversely with p-gp performance. In controls, distribution volumes V_T of about 0.72 were achieved, while under presumed total blockade of p-gp by 225 mg tariquidar before tracer injection followed by a maintenance infusion of another 225 mg over 1 h yielded V_T of about 2.63 in whole brain gray matter [157]. Only in the pituitary, there was very high uptake under both conditions (V_T of 3.66 and 3.06). As parameter most close to p-gp function, the extraction fraction $E = K_1/CBF$ has been proposed. Analogous p-gp radiotracers are [11C]N-desmethyl-loperamide ([11C]dLop) [157] with considerable lower unspecific binding, [11C]phenytoin [158] or [11C]laniquidar [159]. P-gp has recently came into the focus of research as also Alzheimer amyloid $A\beta_{1-42}$ apparently is a substrate as suggested by genetic knockout, pharmacological blockade and induction in hAPP Alzheimer model mice. Medicament-free AD patients displayed significantly higher [11C]verapamil extraction fraction compared to matched controls [160]. P-gp under-function was comparable in AD patients with and without microbleeds [161]. A further practical application of p-gp imaging may be drug refractory epilepsies where high levels of p-gp may have been induced.

20.13.3 Markers of Inflammation

The 18-kD translocator protein (TSPO, formerly termed peripheral benzodiazepine receptor) is expressed on activated microglia and macrophages. These, for instance, infiltrate MS lesions, starting from the perivenous space. After a long era of [^{11}C]PK11195, a series of second-generation PET ligands – such as [^{18}F]PBR111 [162], [^{11}C]PBR28 [163], [^{11}C]DAA1106, [^{18}F]fluoroethyl-DAA1106, or [^{11}C]vinpocetin [164] – have been established which come with higher signal to background ratios. Quantitation could considerably be improved by stratification for the rs6971 TSPO gene polymorphism. The low-affinity haplotype (bearing the Ala147Thr substitution) virtually did not bind the tracers at all. In manifest MS patients, TSPO binding was especially pronounced at the hypercellular edge of T2 hyperintense lesions. Moreover, TSPO tracer uptake was detected in T2-negative areas which displayed reduced magnetization transfer ratio interpreted as preactive lesions. Those could also be detected in patients classified as having clinically isolated syndrome, a term used for a first symptomatic episode at risk for converting into MS. At the same brain locations, T2 hyperintensities showed up in MRI conducted some months later. TSPO radioligand PET thus allows imaging the disease activity attributable to the innate branch of the immune system even before manifesting demyelination [165].

No imaging detection method is so far established for T cells, which constitute less total mass but higher functional relevance [165].

As formulated, e.g., in the classification of Lassmann and Lucchinetti [166], in the majority of MS cases, there is a clear preference of one of several distinct inflammatory mechanisms, i.e., MS is not one but rather three diseases. Furthermore, well-defined autoantigenes can be identified, distinct in each individual case. Distinct antigens are available for therapeutic tolerance induction – a sort of desensitization – e.g., glatiramer acetate and differential action of several therapeutics as function of the pathomechanism is established. Newer theories assume neuronal damage to precede inflammation. Therefore, there is an urgent need for methods allowing in vivo classification of the inflammatory subtype, in vivo detection and quantification of major target antigens in the individual case, and detection of early not yet inflammatory neuronal damage. [^{11}C]PK11195 has also been used to monitor the effect of 1 year treatment with glatiramer acetate.

Apart from MS, microglial activation could also be detected in the caudal brainstem in Parkinson's disease, in the thalamus and motor cortex in motor neuron disease, and in the thalamus, brainstem, cerebellum, and association cortices in Alzheimer's disease [167].

Alternatively to TSPO, cyclooxygenase 1 and 2 (COX 1 and COX2) may be attractive markers of inflammation. COX ligands ([^{11}C]celecoxib, a [^{18}F] derivative of celecoxib and [^{11}C]ketoprofen), thus far, are in preclinical development. Since a long time also adenosine (A_1, A_{2A}) receptors have been discussed, starting from immunohistochemistry findings. Recently, a 37% upregulation was observed in rat experimental HSV1 encephalitis using the A_1AR ligand [^{11}C]MPDX [168].

Taken together, the position of PET in diagnosis and therapeutic monitoring of MS remains highly experimental and did not exceed the level of pilot studies.

In MS CSF is collected routinely for the determination of oligoclonal bands and differential diagnosis of other inflammatory pathologies. However, it is paramount to identify the autoantigen maintaining inflammatory plaques. As the CSF is only the efflux compartment (the "urine" of the brain), there is a high need to directly assess the pathobiochemistry and immunology within the brain parenchyma.

20.13.4 Myelin Imaging

Amyloid tracers such as [^{11}C]PIB or [^{18}F]FBB display comparatively high and homogeneous binding to white matter in healthy volunteers only in installed amyloid pathology. Binding spreads into gray matter where it reaches higher levels. The binding in white matter has been used as a measure of myelin content in MS and might become a marker of the degenerative pathological load and its progression [83]. Some dedicated tracers which also intercalate into the beta-sheath conformation of myelin proteins are in preclinical development, e.g., [^{11}C]CIC and [^{11}C] MeDAS.

αB-crystalline aggregates form in the debris of myelin sheaths and is considered a marker of the demise of oligodendrocytes. However, up to now there is no specific marker.

20.13.5 Astroglia Imaging

MAO-B is exclusively expressed on astrocytes (c.f. 9.4). The irreversible MAO-B ligand N-[^{11}C-methyl]L-deuterodeprenyl ([^{11}C]DED) serves as marker of astrocytosis. Deuterodeprenyl displayed considerably slower association onto MAO-B than did deprenyl, and therefore, its kinetics is not so much limited by perfusion. The quotient [^{18}F]FDG/[^{11}C]DED uptake therefore was sensitive to neuronal cell loss such as in Creutzfeldt-Jakob disease (CJD) [54]. Already [^{18}F]FDG was decreased by two standard deviations (SD) and [^{11}C]DED increased by two SD in the cerebellar, frontal association, inferoparietal, and visual occipital cortex. CJD was confirmed by autopsy in 8 patients. Increased DED uptake was colocalized with [^{11}C]PIB-labeled amyloid deposits in prodromal Alzheimer's [169].

20.13.6 Open Questions Regarding the Pathophysiology of Neuropsychiatric Disease

The neurocognitive effects of the neuropituitary peptides adiuretin/vasopressin (AVP) and oxytocin have come into focus of behavioral neuropsychopharmacological research. Unfortunately, although widespread, the densities OXT1, OXT2, V1a, V1b, and V2 receptors are quite low (below 300 fmol/mg protein) so that a radioligand following classical principles is hardly envisageable.

20.14 (Patho)Physiological Studies of Neurotransmission

Key challenges in assessing the state of neurotransmitter receptors in neuropsychiatric disease are the accuracy of the diagnosis (neuropathological confirmation was available in a small minority of cases), the bias by preexisting medication (which was present in many published studies), and conversely the difficulty to recruit completely drug-naive patients or the impossibility to assess later disease states. This is especially the case for the monoaminergic systems and major psychiatric disease (major depressive disorder, schizophrenia, major forms of (i) personality disorder, (ii) posttraumatic stress disorder, (iii) attention deficit hyperactivity disorder) as here treatment by neuroleptics or antidepressants, almost all with a monoamine antagonistic component is considered as ethical imperative. The same holds true for Parkinson's disease and dopamine agonists.

In the past, the search for diagnostic applications for neurotransmitter radioligands resembled the search for the needle in the haystack. While honestly looking back, contributions to understanding the pathophysiology were very limited in the big majority of studies. Several thousands of patients with more or less well-defined pathology have undergone PET studies. Mostly, only small changes of radioligand binding in the range of 15–30% or lower versus healthy controls were detected. Almost always healthy and diseased populations considerably overlapped, the discriminative power was low, and the interindividual variability was high. Rather the exception than the rule was the striking finding of presynaptic dopaminergic deficit in all PD and of postsynaptic dopaminergic deficit only in atypical PD.

Conversely, it is not surprising to see a degeneration of multiple neurotransmitter (NT) systems in various more or less localized neurodegenerative diseases. For example, a decrease of tenths of NT was observed in the caudate nucleus in Huntington's disease, the cholinergic deficit in Alzheimer's disease had been known for decades from neuropathological studies, and cholinergic drugs had been introduced years before PET studies confirmed comparatively slight reductions of acetylcholinesterase (AChE) and $\alpha_4\beta_2$-nicotinic receptors in AD.

The monoaminergic hypothesis in depression and schizophrenia could not be confirmed in a way that monoaminergic changes would be more than a downstream feature or susceptibility factor in the etiopathology of these diseases.

One of the major drawbacks of especially antagonist receptor radioligands is that they recognize not only the membrane-bound non-refractory high-affinity G protein coupled ready to receive fraction of receptors but the total inventory including the reserve stored at vesicles and refractory receptors. It has to be assumed that from individual to individual, the same net level of signal transduction can be realized with a different total inventory of receptors. The net amount of signal transduction arises from fine-tuning every component of the system. Among these are presynaptic reuptake, synthesis, and storage capacity and postsynaptic total inventory of receptors versus non-refractory membrane-bound receptors ready to receive and transmit a signal.

20.14.1 Huntington's Disease (HD)

As mentioned above, HD has been the subject of PET imaging with almost every second radioligand studied in humans. The big advantage is that (i) by genotyping, the diagnosis can be confirmed with almost 100 % certainty; (ii) there is a well-established relationship between the genetic dose of CAG trinucleotide expansions and the age of disease onset or the extent of pathology at a given age [170], respectively; and (iii) due to the autosomal dominant inheritance and prevalence, numerous premanifest gene carriers have been identified and followed up by specialized centers. Although comparatively rare, HD shares many features of neurodegenerative mass diseases, such as intracellular inclusions of protein aggregates (truncated huntingtine in HD), a temporospatial sequence of cellular dysfunction and death, and unfortunately a lack of curative treatment. Therefore, HD has been considered a model neurodegenerative disease. DAT, VMAT2, D_1R, D_2R [171], and $GABA_AR$ [172] have been found considerably diminished in the striatum, starting already in the presymptomatic stage [171], while A_1AR showed a bimodal behavior with increase in early premanifest and decrease in the manifest state. Also microglial activation has been evidenced [173].

Phosphodiesterase 10a (PDE10a) is almost exclusively localized in the striatum and has turned out as an attractive target and biomarker, as it is highly enriched in the striatal medium spiny neurons preferentially affected by the HD pathology. PDE10a is the subject of ongoing treatment studies and accessible to PET imaging with a well-functioning radioligand, [^{18}F]MNI659. [^{18}F]MNI659 PDE10a binding turned out to be considerably reduced in premanifest gene carriers some years before disease onset. A cohort of 9 affected subjects was scanned twice with a delay of about 1 year. Uptake was 50 % lower versus controls, and annual decreases were 17 % in the caudatus, 7 % in the putamen, and 6 % globus pallidus [174, 175].

20.14.2 Alzheimer's Disease

Using tracers for neurotransmitter systems, the cholinesterase (AChE) has been found considerably decreased in AD using [^{11}C]MP4A, e.g., by 12 % in the amygdala and 23 % in the occipital cortex, while in the cholinergic nucleus basalis of Meynert, a 7 % increase was observed [176]. [^{11}C]PMP is an alternative AChE tracer. The ligand for nicotinic $\alpha_4\beta_2R$ [^{18}F] A85380 shows essentially thalamic and discrete frontotemporal uptake, while parieto-occipital binding is very low. The distribution kinetics of this ligand is extremely slow so that images are acquired, e.g., 6–7 h p.i. One study found BP_{ND} (referenced to a white matter region) decreased by 0.15 and 0.18 (45 % and 54 %) in the temporal cortex of MCI and AD and by 0.3 or 16 % in the thalamus in AD while unchanged in MCI [177]. Another study observed decreases by 5 % and 7 % in the temporal cortex and by 8 % and 10 % in the thalamus, respectively, of [^{123}I]I-A85380 V_T values referenced to plasma radioactivity [178]. [^{11}C]nicotin is an alternative tracer for $\alpha_4\beta_2$R and yielded similar results of decreased binding in MCI and AD with correlations of binding to the performance of attention [179]. [^{11}C]nicotin needs shorter scan time (1 h) but additional measurement of CBF for quantitation by the established kinetic model [179]. [^{18}F]Flubatine has successfully been established in human PET and was metabolically highly stable. A reliable quantification is possible after only 90 min of scan time yielding thalamic BP_{ND} of 3.4 [180].

Few other transmitter systems have been investigated in AD. 5-HT$_{2A}$R were reduced by 69 % temporal and frontal, by 55 % parietal and temporoparietal, and by 35 % occipital in 9 unmedicated AD versus 12 matched controls. It is highly plausible that this reduction exceeds atrophy effects and, to some part, reflects neurochemical changes [181]. Binding of the MAO-B ligand [^{11}C]deprenyl was found increased reflecting astrocytosis [182]. DAT and VMAT2 binding was preserved and therefore enables differential diagnosis to LBD and PD [77], as shown for DAT in phase III of the radiotracer development [183].

Memantine is – at concentrations reached in vivo – an α_7-nicotinic antagonist and has been widely used in AD. Series of neuropsychiatric assessments showed improvement of executive functions but deterioration of memory in healthy volunteers and AD patients [184]. The α7-radioligand [^{11}C]NS14492 has recently been established in mini-pigs showing a parieto-thalamic maximum of uptake. Drug occupancy with two different developmental ligands was studied yielding 60–81 % occupation at 10 mg/kg [185].

20.14.3 Schizophrenia

In view of the legendary efficiency of dopamine (DA) antagonists, it was a surprising finding that D$_2$R and DAT were constant in unmedicated schizophrenic patients as evidenced by resting state [^{11}C]raclopride, [^{123}I]IBZM or [^{18}F]CFT, [^{123}I]FP-CIT, and [^{99m}Tc]TRODAT-1 PET or SPECT studies, respectively. Notwithstanding, resting state [^{18}F]F-DOPA uptake was increased pointing to a selective increase of neuronal aromatic amino acid decarboxylase (AADC) [186]. Furthermore, the amplitude of DA liberation after amphetamine challenge was considerably increased as inferred from measuring D$_2$R occupation with [^{11}C]raclopride [187]. Taken together, this points to an increased DA production, storage, and liberation capacity per presynaptic terminal, at constant number of available terminals. It suggests constant arborization and sprouting of DA neurons.

A study evidenced an upregulation of cannabinoid CB1 receptors using [^{18}F]MK9470 [188] confirming an earlier case report using [^{124}I]AM281 [189].

20.14.4 Bipolar Disorder, Depression, and Seasonal Affective Disorder

A consistent finding in BD was decreased SERT in the brainstem in all cohorts and increased SERT in the thalamus in euthymic or only mildly depressed BD, while thalamic, hippocampal, ACC, and putaminal SERT was decreased in considerably depressed BD [40]. The effect of season, sunlight exposure, and seasonal depression on the serotonergic system was studied in several works [190]. In healthy controls scanned throughout the year by [^{11}C]DASB, cortical and thalamic SERT availability (BP_{ND}) was about 20 % higher in the winter compared to the summer [190, 191]. These findings would be in line with an overtuning of the serotonergic system (c.f. 8.5). However, this dependency was only present in carriers of the S-allele of the 5-HTTLPR polymorphism of the SERT, associated with lower SERT expression and higher susceptibility to mood disorders [191]. Interestingly the S-allele was not directly associated with a poorer response to SSRI but eventually with lower optimal plasma levels of SSRI [192]. Furthermore, the daily sunshine duration inversely correlated with the SERT availability [193]. An analogous study using [^{11}C]McN5652 yielded concordant results [194]. Corticolimbic 5-HT$_{1A}$R were decreased by 20–30 % in a group with lower light exposition in the last 5 days versus a high exposition group [195]. Similarly, higher [^{18}F]F-DOPA uptake was observed in the winter compared to the summer – pointing to higher DAT and higher DOPA synthesis capacity [196] – and D_2R availability was lower in darker times [197]. In MDD, globally 34 % higher cerebral density of MAO-A was detected using [^{11}C]harmin. Seventeen patients with at least 5 months of washout after the last treatment were studied versus 17 matched controls. As MAO-A is localized in neurons and not glia and degrades all monoamines, norepinephrine, dopamine, and serotonin, this finding may reflect increased presynaptic turnover and faster clearance of monoamines or even a higher density of mitochondria. It had been hypothesized that MAO-A elevation may be the primary monoamine lowering process in MDD which seems too simplistic in view of more recent findings. Phosphodiesterase 4 (PDE4), the enzyme degrading the second messenger cAMP, has been proposed as target for antidepressant drugs as some evidence pointed to increased cAMP signaling in MDD. PDE4 was downregulated globally by 22 % in 28 unmedicated MDD patients versus 25 controls as measured using [^{11}C]rolipram-PET [198].

20.14.5 Anxiety Disorder

Social anxiety disorder was investigated in a dual-tracer study by Frick and coworkers. Eighteen medicament-naive, fasted nonsmoking and non-caffeinated patients displayed (i) significantly higher serotonin synthesis rates, as measured by [^{11}C]HTP in the raphé nuclei, dorsal ACC(cg24), and right amygdala; (ii) significantly higher SERT binding potential BP_{ND}, as measured by [^{11}C]DASB, in both thalami, the right striatum, and raphé nuclei, to a lower degree also in the amygdalae versus 18 matched controls [199]; and (iii) positive correlation of anxiety severity and [^{11}C]HTP influx in the right amygdala. An increase in SERT in striatum and cortical regions had also been observed by two other groups [49]. The amplitudes of change were not indicated but appear as about 12 and 20 % in the color-coded illustrations. In other studies a decrease of 5-$HT_{1A}R$ in the raphé nuclei, ACC, amygdala, and sometimes also in insula and OFC was reported as reviewed by Fredrikson [49]. DLPFC 5-$HT_{2A}R$ were positively correlated with harm avoidance personality – an anxiety-prone trait – in healthy controls assessed by [^{123}I]5-I R91150 PET [200]. All these findings would be in line with a constitutive overtuning of the serotonergic system: feedback inhibition of serotonin synthesis is diminished in the raphé nuclei – particularly here and also elsewhere, 5-$HT_{1A}R$ are of somatodendritic localization acting as autoreceptors [201, 202]. Cortical and amygdalar presynaptic uptake and synthesis capacity are increased. Lastly, postsynaptic 5-$HT_{2A}R$ in the cerebrum are increased [202]. Conversely, in a patient who was largely incapable of fear and anxiety because of selective underdevelopment and calcification of the amygdale (Urbach-Wiethe disease), we observed cortical postsynaptic 5-$HT_{2A}R$ globally decreased by 71 %, pointing to a considerable under-tuning of the serotonergic system [203]. In this view the anxiolytic effect of SSRI can also be explained by presynaptic serotonin depletion as chronic effect of SSRI. Also the anxiolytic effect of mirtazapine (combined $5HT_{1A}$ agonist and $5HT_{2A}$, SERT, and NET antagonist) and of buspirone (5-HT_{1A} agonist) is explained by their action on the raphé and other autoreceptors.

In this context, some revision of an old view in the light of new experimental evidence seems warranted: chronic monoaminergic reuptake inhibitors (RI) such as SSRI were repeatedly believed to increase extracellular monoamine concentrations as it is the case after acute application. For example, 45 min after an acute dose of only 10 mg of the SSRI citalopram significant up to 7 % increase in 5-HT_{1A} binding could be observed using [^{11}C]CUMI-101 [204]. However, monoamines are soaked off the extracellular space and the synaptic cleft with high efficiency by glial organic cation transporters (OCT) which remain unblocked under therapy. Therefore, as net steady-state effect of RIs rather depletion in neuronal terminals can be expected. As in glia there is no synapto-vesicular storage, serotonin is rapidly degraded there. Indeed a very well-conducted study in rats receiving chronic citalopram via osmotic minipumps, 6 mg per day per animal yielding plasma levels of 361 nM, over 17 days, analyzed serotonin and metabolites in dissected pieces of brain tissue. Serotonin was significantly decreased to 13 % of the level of the placebo group in ACC, to 70 % in the dorsal, to 42 % in the medial raphé nucleus, to 60 % in the amygdale, and to 38 % in the dorsal hippocampus. Also the 5-hydroxytryptophane content decreased significantly and comparably [205].

Concerning other neurotransmitter systems, [^{11}C]flumazenil and [^{123}I]iomazenil binding to $GABA_A$/BZD-R was found decreased in the temporal pole and prefrontal cortex in anxiety disorder [49]. DAT could be slightly decreased. Two studies found decreased NK_1R (for the endogenous ligand substance P) in the amygdala [49], both using [^{11}C]GR205171 [206].

20.15 Targets of Radioligands/Radiosubstrates

In this section radiotracer targets mentioned above and some more are listed following a classification by biochemical function. If available additional data/remarks/examples are given, otherwise only the respective text subsection is indicated. We restrict on those tracers established in humans and only selected promising preclinical candidates. Further examples of radiopharmaceuticals may be found in Chap. 4 of this book. Full records of any radiotracer may be obtained from the Molecular Imaging and Contrast Agent Database (MICAD) online at www.ncbi.nlm.nih.gov/books/NBK5330 also accessible via www.pubmed.org. Dissociation and inhibitory constants may be obtained from the PDSP Ki Database at http://pdsp.med.unc.edu/pdsp.php. Radioligand/radiosubstrate binding is guided by the protein structure and conformation of their targets. Some particular features of radioligand for particular targets can be understood from protein structure.

20.15.1 G Protein-Coupled Receptors (GPCR)

GPCR are characterized by their 7-transmembrane domain. In their receptive high-affinity state, they bind at their intracellular face a trimeric GTP-hydrolyzing protein (G protein) occupied by GDP (Gαβγ-GDP). Ligand binding leads to the exchange of GDP by GTP and dissociation of the G protein-receptor complex and of the G protein itself into the subunits Gα-GTP and Gβγ. Without G protein, the receptor is in its low-affinity state. Both Gα-GPT and Gβγ act as second messenger at intracellular and membrane-bound secondary targets. Recycling comprises dephosphorylation of Gα-GPT and reconstitution of the receptor – Gαβγ-GDP complex (c.f. 6.1). A series of G-protein subtypes is known, 21 of Gα, 5 of Gβ, and 12 of Gγ. $G\alpha_q$ and $G\alpha_{11}$ activate phospholipase C β_1 and β_4; $G\alpha_{12}$ and $G\alpha_{13}$ activate protein Rho which in turn stimulates Rho-kinase; Gβγ activate phospholipase C β_2 and β_3, phosphatidylinositol –3-kinase, voltage-gated Ca^{2+}-channels, or acetylcholine opened K^+-channels; $G\alpha_S$ stimulates and $G\alpha_i$ inhibits adenylatcyclase. Instead of $G\alpha_{i,\ s,\ q}$ the abbreviations $G_{i,\ s,\ q,}$ etc., are common. The localization of GPCR can be postsynaptic, presynaptic axonal, or presynaptic somatodendritic, and this influences the mode of action, e.g., a frequent feature is feedback inhibition by axonal inhibitory autoreceptors.

By their conformation and amino acid sequence, GPCR can be subdivided into families which traditionally involve classes A-F over all biological organisms. Based on sequence homology studies, Frederikson and coworkers [207] in 2003 alternatively proposed for the human GPCR the GRAFS system which may more adequately meet relevance in humans (c.f. Table 20.2). The structure and size of receptors between families are fundamentally different. A schedule of relationship and homology by amino acid sequence is given in Fig. 20.6. Virtually all GPCR to which PET radioligands are directed belong to the rhodopsin family, such as all monoamine receptors. An important exception is the family of metabotropic glutamate receptors (mGluR).

20.15.1.1 Serotonergic System

A total of 13 GPCR subtypes are described in humans which comprise $5\text{-}HT_{1A,\ B,\ D,\ E,\ F}$, $5\text{-}HT_{2A,\ B,\ C}$, 5-HT4, $5\text{-}HT5_{A,\ B}$, $5\text{-}HT_6$, and $5\text{-}HT_7$. $5\text{-}HT_3$ is an ion channel. $5\text{-}HT_1R$ are G_i/G_0 coupled.

Table 20.2 Phylogenetic families of G protein-coupled receptors

Traditional[a]	GRAFS[a]	GPCR classes according to Fredriksson
A	R	Rhodopsin
B1	S	Secretin
B2	A	Adhesion
C	G	Glutamate (metabotropic)
D		Fungal mating pheromone
E		Cyclic AMP
F	F	Frizzled/smoothened/TAS2

[a]Alternative classifications, "GRAFS" standing for the initials of the five families

5-HT$_{1A}$R

The radioligand [^{18}F]MPPF is currently most frequently used. [^{18}F]MPPF binding is sensitive to changes in serotonin levels in line with log$P$=2.81 and K_D=3.2 nM as the affinity of serotonin on h5HT$_{1A}$R has been measured at K_D=4.7 nM [208]. However, the brain uptake of [^{18}F]MPPF is suboptimal due to a considerable clearance by p-gp. [^{11}C]CUMI-101 is a more recent partial agonist ligand [204]. About 80 human studies were also performed using [^{11}C]WAY100635, which has been labeled at the O-methyl or better at the carbonyl position. Also the [^{18}F]-version, [^{18}F]FCWAY, has been established but underlies defluorination in vivo. WAY100625 is not only a 5-HT$_{1A}$ antagonist but has also D$_4$ agonistic properties [209]. The kinetic modeling of [^{11}C]WAY100625 radiotracers is compromised by its fast degradation to radiometabolites. In line with its high affinity (K_D=0.32 nM) and high lipophilicity (log$P$=2.81), it is not displaceable by endogenous serotonin. The distribution of 5-HT$_{1A}$ is highest in the hippocampus and opercular region.

5-HT$_{1B}$R

[^{11}C]AZ10419369 has been established in humans. 5-HT$_{1B}$R showed a cortico-striatal distribution with clear occipital maximum and only lower binding in the thalamus [120]. This distribution may be one candidate substrate of the propensity of the posterior cerebral region to certain pathology such as the visual aura in migraine. 5-HT$_{1B}$R has been shown as the most relevant presynaptic inhibitory receptor, while the effect of 5HT$_{1A}$R and 5-HT$_{2C}$R was negligible [205]. Alternatively, [^{11}C]P943 has been used in over three human studies [210].

5-HT$_{2A}$R

For imaging these G$_Q$-coupled receptors, mostly [^{18}F]altanserin, [^{11}C]MDL100907, and [^{18}F]setoperone have been used. [^{18}F]altanserin has the disadvantage of a brain-penetrating hydroxyl-metabolite [^{18}F]altanserinol presumably produced by unspecific tissue ketoreductases. [^{18}F]setoperone has in addition to 5-HT$_{2A}$R some affinity to D$_2$R and α_1R. An alternative tracer was [^{123}I]5-I R91150 [200, 210]. [^{11}C]CIMBI36 has recently been introduced into human imaging and yielded BP_{ND} up to 1.5 in the frontal cortex, slightly lower than [^{18}F]altanserin yielding values >2.0. 5-HT$_{2A}$R are of global cortical distribution and absent in the cerebellum and very rare in basal ganglia and hippocampus. Highest densities were found in the primary sensory cortices (BA3, 17, 22, own PET data and [211]). This may corroborate the hallucinogenic potential of the agonist LSD.

5-HT$_4$R

5-HT$_4$R are coupled to G$_S$. 5-HT$_4$R have been proposed as cumulative markers of chronic serotonin levels, with inverse relationship. [^{11}C]SB207145 has been established and proved insensitive to acute citalopram, and binding was 9% lower in carriers of the S-allele of the 5-HTTLPR polymorphism in the promoter region of the gene coding the SERT which comes with lower expression of SERT [212].

5-HT$_6$R have been labeled in humans using [^{11}C]GSK215083 [210].

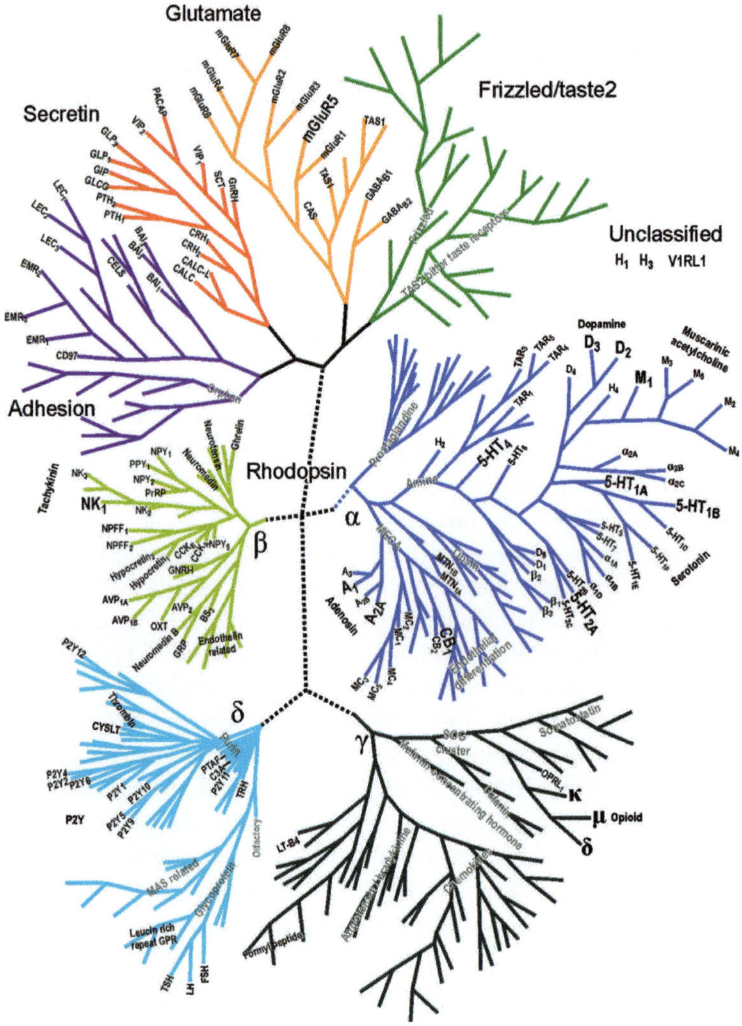

Fig. 20.6 Phylogenetic map of human G protein-coupled receptors (GPCR) calculated according to a maximum parsimony bootstrap method and visualizing gene sequence homology. According to space limitations the association of clusters in the map is not perfectly proportional. Within a cluster, however, the distance on a branch corresponds to the difference in the sequence (Adapted from Fredriksson et al. [207]). Note that GPCR cluster into the families *Glutamate*, *Rhodopsin*, *Adhesion*, *Frizzled/TAS2* and *Secretion* according to the "GRAFS" schedule. The Rhodopsin group, by far the largest and most relevant in pharmacology, is further subdivided into branches α, β, γ, and δ. Names of subbranches are given in *gray color*. In the abbreviations listed in the following, the "R" for receptor was systematically omitted. Receptors of high relevance for neuro-PET are highlighted. *5-HTR*$_{2A}$ 5-hydroxytryptamin (=serotonin) 2A, *α* α-adrenergic, *AVP* arginine-vasopressine, *β* β-adrenergic, *BAI* brain-specific angiogenesis inhibitor, *BS* uterinbombesin, *C3A* complement factor 3, *CALC* calcitonin, *CAS* calcium sensing, *CB* cannabinoid, *CCK* cholecystokinin, *CELS* EGF LAG seven-pass G type, *CRH* corticotropin-releasing hormone, *CYSLT* cysteinyl-leukotriene, *D*$_1$ dopamine-1, *EDN* endothelin related, *EMR* EGF-like module containing, *FSH* follicle-stimulating hormone, *GCG* glucagon, *GIP* gastric inhibitory polypeptide, *GHRH* growth hormone-releasing hormone, *GLP* glucagon-like peptide, *GnRH* gonadotropin-releasing hormone, *GRP* gastrin-releasing peptide, *H* histamine, *LEC* lectomedin, *LH* luteinizing hormone, *LT-B4* leucotrien-B4, *M* muscarinic acetylcholine, *MAS* the MAS oncogene, *MC* melanocortin, *mGluR* metabotropic glutamate, *MTN* melatonin, *NPFF* neuropeptide FF, *NPY* neuropeptide Y, *OPRL1* opioid receptor-like 1, *OXT* oxytocin, *P2Y* purine receptors, *PACAP* pituitary adenylate cyclase-activating protein, *PPY* pancreatic polypeptide, *PrP* prolactin-releasing peptide, *PTAF* platelet activating factor, *PTH* parathyroid hormone, *SCT* secretin, *TAR* trace amine receptor, *TAS1* taste sensing 1, *TRH* thyrotropin-releasing hormone, *TSH* thyroid-stimulating hormone, *VIP* vasoactive intestinal peptide

20.15.1.2 Dopaminergic System

D_xR are grouped into the D1 family with D_1 and D_5 coupled to G_S and localized among others at the "direct-loop" GABAergic striatopallidal projection neurons in the striatal matrix which use dynorphin and substance P as cotransmitter. The D2 family comprises the G_i-coupled D_2 and D_3. D_2 is preferentially localized in striosomes and at the "indirect loop" GABAergic striatopallidal projection neurons which use enkephalin as cotransmitter.

D_1R

[^{11}C]SCH23390 is the classical D_1R model ligand. Also, [^{11}C]NNC112 has been frequently used. Both these antagonist ligands are not influenced by endogenous dopamine even not after amphetamine challenge. Alternative D_1 ligands tested in humans performed poorer in terms of striatum/cerebellum ratio and uptake kinetics. In addition to a clear striatal enrichment, some D_1R occurred in the substantia nigra and very little in the cortex [211].

D_2R/D_3R

Classical ligands are [^{11}C]raclopride and [^{18}F]fallypride with complementary bandwidth of sensitivity; benzamide-type ligands such as [^{11}C]raclopride, [^{18}F]FLB457, or [^{123}I]IBZM are more suitable to quantify high concentrated D_2R in the striatum; and butyrophenone-type ligands such as [^{18}F]fallypride, [^{18}F]desmethoxyfallypride, [^{11}C]N-methylspiperone ([^{11}C]NMSP), and [^{18}F]fluoroethyl-spiperone ([^{18}F]FESP) are better suited for quantifying low concentrated extrastriatal D_2R (see also 1.4 [67]). Also the agonists [^{11}C]NPA and [^{11}C]MNPA have been used in humans [67]. D_2R form functional heterodimers with several other GPCR, e.g., with 5-HT_{2A} or A_{2A}.

[^{11}C](+)PHNO has higher affinity to D_3R and thus preferentially binds to the ventral striatum and globus pallidus [67].

20.15.1.3 Noradrenergic System

Here the G_q or less frequently $G_{12/13}$-coupled α_{1A}, α_{1B}, and α_{1D}, the G_i-coupled postsynaptic autoreceptors α_{2A}, α_{2B}, and α_{2C}, and the G_s-coupled β_1, β_2, and β_3 are described. Among others radioligands established in humans are the α_{2C}-antagonist [^{11}C]ORM-13070 with a prominent striatal (reaching BP_P of 0.7 and V_T of 1.6) and thalamic and a slight cortical distribution beneath absence in the cerebellum [213]. The non-subtype selective α_2R-ligand [^{11}C]yohimbine showed highest uptake cortically in the cingulum and in parietal and occipital cortex with V_T around 0.8, in the striatum and cerebellum with 0.6, and in white matter with 0.46 [214]. Notwithstanding, autoradiography showed – as far as available – selectively high α_2R binding in areas BA3, BA22, and the hippocampus [211] Alpha-1 and beta-adrenoceptor radioligands have not yet surpassed preclinical stage.

20.15.1.4 Cholinergic System

One has to note that central cholinergic neurons release galanin as cotransmitter. Beneath the ion channel nicotinic receptors, at least five isoforms of GP-coupled muscarinic receptors exist.

Muscarinic acetylcholine receptors (M_xR)

Nonselective muscarinic antagonism was the principle of the first antiparkinsonian drugs. Acetylcholine was considered a general counterbalance of dopamine in the striatum, and the essentially anti-tremor action is today believed to relay on cholinergic interneurons which are inhibited by the nigrostriatal dopaminergic projections via D_1R. Nonselective muscarinergic antagonism is also hallucinogen – desired effect of belladonna, thorn apples, and toadstools – and an inconvenient side effect in elderly people especially of almost all tricyclic antidepressants and phenothiazine neuroleptics. M_1R, M_1R, and M_1R are generally coupled to G_q-stimulating PLC.

M_1R occur in high density in the striatum, hippocampus, and in the outer layers of parietal and superior temporal cortex and localize to neurons [211]. (+)-N-[^{11}C]methyl-3-piperidinyl benzilate ([^{11}C]MPB) have recently been introduced to human studies. The highest binding with BP_{ND} up to 5 was observed in the striatum and the occipital cortex; considerable binding in other cortices was absent in the cerebellum. In a cohort of chronic fatigue syndrome, patients producing anti-M1 autoantibodies (AB) binding was

reduced globally by 20 % versus patients without AB and versus controls, while acetylcholine esterase levels measured by [^{11}C]MP4A were constant [215]. Also [^{11}C]benzatropine had been used for M_1R imaging in humans and perfectly reproduced the autoradiographic distribution [216]. For the allosteric agonist [^{11}C] GSK1034702 [133], see 5.1.

M_2R are particularly highly expressed in primary somatosensory areas (BA3, 17, 22), in the striatum, and in the dorsomedian thalamus. Low levels are found in the hippocampus [211, 217]. In the cortex M_2R act stimulatory while in the striatum preferentially as inhibitory autoreceptors. The selective M_2R agonist ligand [^{18}F]FP-TZTP proved metabolically sufficiently stable (41 % parent after 40 min) and sensible to occupation/competition by endogenous acetylcholine, suggested by applications of the acetylcholine esterase inhibitor physostigmine in humans. The native biodistribution showed a uniform gray matter distribution maximal in the striatum and cerebellum, while lowest binding was observed in the thalamus. This is in clear disagreement with autoradiographic data, suggesting bias by brain-penetrating radiometabolites or regionally considerably different levels of acetylcholine [218].

M_4R are coupled to G_i/G_0 and act as inhibitory autoreceptors.

20.15.1.5 Other Receptors of the Rhodopsin Family

Adenosine

Adenosine can act as neuromodulator and leaks to the extracellular space when cells operate beyond their energy homeostasis. It can also originate from extracellular ADP degraded by diphosphatases. [^{18}F]CPFPX [125] and [^{11}C] MPDX are established A_1R ligands and show a ubiquitous gray matter distribution sparing the cerebellum and partially the hippocampus (own PET and autoradiography data). With [^{11}C] TMSX, the striatal distribution of $A_{2a}R$ has been demonstrated. A_1R are coupled to $G_{i1/2/3}$ or G_0, $A_{2A}R$ to G_S. $A_{2A}R$ seem to be particularly "sticky" as they tend to form heterodimers with a series of other GPCR. Less frequent in the CNS are $A_{2B}R$ and A_3R.

Opioid μ-, κ-, δ-, orphan, receptors

The endogenous ligand of μ-R *is* β-endorphin (posttranslationally processed from the prohormone pro-opio-melanocortin, POMC), of *κ-R is* dynorphin from prodynorphin, and of *δ-R* is enkephalin from proenkephalin or alternatively from prodynorphin. All three opioid receptors are coupled to G_i. [^{18}F]fluoroethyl-diprenorphine and [^{11}C]diprenorphine are non-subtype selective strongest available opioid receptor antagonists. [^{11}C]carfentanil is an extremely potent μ-agonist. Already 1 μg are pharmacologically active in humans; therefore, specific activities have to be particularly high to fulfill the tracer criterion. Subjects homozygous for the A allele of the OPMR1 A118G polymorphism had about 20 % higher BP_{ND} for [^{11}C]diprenorphine [219].

Tachykinin receptors

Neurokinin receptors NK_1, NK_2, and NK_3 are G_q coupled and sensitive to the endogenous ligands substance P, neurokinin A, and neurokinin B. [^{11}C]R116301-PET showed highest binding in the striatum, and some few bindings in the frontal, parietal, and temporal cortex, none in thalamus and occipital lobe (c.f. end of 20.14.5).

Cannabinoid receptors

[^{18}F]MK9470 or [^{123}I]AM281 (see 20.14.3).

Histamine receptors

Four isoforms H_1R–H_4R are described. H_1R are coupled to G_q; H_2R to G_S, H_3R, and H_4R couple to G_i. A H_1R ligand established in humans is [^{11}C] doxepin, which shows global gray matter distribution relatively sparing the cerebellum. A series of occupation studies were conducted with classical antihistaminics others determined the antihistaminic side effect of some antipsychotics and antidepressants [220]. Notwithstanding in healthy volunteers single doses of 5 mg levocetirizine and 60 mg fexofenadine lead both to only 8 % H_1R occupation and no sedation [221]. One has to note that serious allergic disorders come with a systemic inflammatory state where the tightness of the BBB is compromised, and usually non-brain-penetrating drugs may penetrate. H_3R could be labeled using [^{11}C]GSK189254. In the putamen V_T values of 70 were reached and 30–37 in amygdalae, cingulum, and insula. In the thalamus, cerebellum, and parietal and occipital cortex, an uptake corresponding to V_T of 20 was observed. Cerebral binding could be reduced to 6–9 after occupation with the full dose and 120 μg of the cold ligand GSK239512 which was also tested at 6 and 14 μg [222]. Already beforehand [^{11}C]MK8278 had been established for H_3R neuroimaging showing predominant striatal uptake (V_T 17, BP_{ND} 2.2) and also significant specific binding in all other gray matter areas in humans (V_T ranging 7–10 and BP_{ND} 0.5–1.2) which could be blocked by a cold candidate drug [223]. The others, H_2R and H_4R, are of considerable low cerebral expression, and no PET neuroimaging has been described.

20.15.1.6 Metabotropic Glutamate Receptors

As mentioned above and in Fig. 20.6, mGluR constitute a completely distinct family of GPCR, characterized by unique conformational features including a comparatively large extracellular and a small intracellular domain. In mGluR two subunits are connected via a disulfide bond to dimers. The dimeric conformation is obligatory for glutamate binding which takes place at the extracellular venus fly trap domain. Rhodopsin-type receptors in turn bind their endogenous ligand in the transmembrane domain. In mGluR, a cysteine-rich repeat domain makes the connection to the canonic 7-transmembrane domain. As the binding pocket is very similar in all subtypes mGluR1-mGluR8, subtype selectivity cannot be assured by orthosteric ligands but via allosteric sites at the cysteine-rich repeat domain. Therefore, only allosteric subtype selective ligands are available which preferentially recognize monomers [224].

mGluR5

For mGluR5 a large series of diaryl-ethinyl derivatives has been synthesized of which [^{11}C] ABP688 has been applied in a series of physiological and pathological conditions in humans. The distribution of [^{18}F]FPEB and [^{18}F]FP203 was studied in healthy volunteers, the latter also in the frame of a dose-finding trial (c.f. 6.1 [142]). MGluR5 had a ubiquitous cortical distribution and was absent in the cerebellum. In basal ganglia mGluR5 levels decreased in the order caudatus, putamen, and thalamus.

20.15.2 Ion Channel-Coupled Receptors

20.15.2.1 Glutamate

The ionotropic glutamate receptors NMDA-, AMPA-, and kainate-R are all heterotetrameric pores, structurally distinct from pentameric nicotinic and $GABA_A$-receptors. While AMPA and Kainate transmit only small cations, Na^+ and K^+, NMDA in open state is also permeable for Ca^{2+}, and it lets pass comparatively large portions of ions until becoming refractory. The tryptophan metabolite kynuric acid acts as endogenous antagonist at glycine site of NMDA-R and at AMPA and kainate-R. No AMPA and no Kainate receptor-ligand has thus far been established in humans.

NMDA-R

NMDA-R are nonselective cation channels with – in addition to the glutamate site on the NR2A subunit – several distinct modulatory binding sites for glycine or D-serine at the NR1 and NR3 subunit leading to signal potentiation and for Zn^{2+} which blocks conductance. As a special feature, in basic state (at −50 to −80 mV membrane voltage), the conductive pore is clogged by a Mg^{2+} cation. A predepolarization is necessary to remove this "lid" and to give free the channel. Two NMDA ligands have recently been established in humans but not yet tested in a larger spectrum of conditions. [^{11}C]CNS5161 showed increased striatal uptake upon L-DOPA application in dyskinetic versus not dyskinetic Parkinson's disease patients [225] and recently favorable dosimetry [226]. Uptake in controls was highest in the thalamus followed by the striatum and frontal and lateral temporal cortex, while it was low in the occipital cortex. This is in contrast to autoradiographic studies showing highest binding in hippocampus, insular, and opercular cortex and particularly low thalamic binding [211, 217]. [^{18}F]GE179 proved advantageous tracer kinetics in 9 healthy volunteers [227]. Another NMDA ligand is [^{11}C]GSK-931145. Efforts to image the glycine binding site of NMDA were undertaken using [^{11}C]AcL703 the cerebral uptake of which was small at 0.6% ID/L but exceeded white matter uptake in cerebellar cortex by a factor of 2 [228].

The following four receptors $GABA_AR$, nAChR, GlycinR, and $5\text{-}HT_3R$ share a heteropentameric structure.

20.15.2.2 Gamma-Amino Butyric Acid, $GABA_A$

Benzodiazepine (BZD) sites at $GABA_A$R-chloride channel

This is the target of the classical ligand [^{18}F]flumazenil which proved as a general viability marker of neuronal tissue (c.f. 20.7). The distribution is of cortical predominance including the cerebellum and highest in the occipital and in the opercular region. Basal ganglia are relatively spared (own data). At the BZD site do also act halogenated gas anesthetics such as halothane, sevoflurane, etc., and the injection anesthetics propofol and etomidate. Besides the BZD site, the $GABA_A$R has distinct binding sites for barbiturates.

20.15.2.3 Nicotinic Acetylcholine Receptors (nAChR)

NAChR are nonselective small cation channels (for Na^+ and K^+) in the shape of a pore composed of five subunits with the general configuration 2αβγδ or 2α3β. The α-subunits bind the ligand and with their isoforms α_1–α_{10} most contribute to ligand selectivity. Of β isoforms 1–4 are known of γ the alternative ε in the muscular nAChR and of δ only one. While α_1 and β_1 are restricted to the muscle, subunits α_2–α_7 and β_2–β_4 occur in the brain. NAChR are the site of action of the agonists nicotine and cytisine.

Nicotinic $\alpha_4\beta_2$R

This is the most frequent nAChR (mostly $2\alpha_4 3\beta_2$) of almost ubiquitous cerebral distribution and target of the partial agonist varenicline used to assist nicotine withdrawal. Particularly high receptor densities were observed in the thalamus and high densities in the mesencephalon. The uptake in cortex was lower with a parietotemporal dorsal-frontal accentuation and lowest occipital and in the dorsal cerebellum. Most PET ligands showed a high white matter uptake [229]. 2-[^{18}F]A85380 (synonym 2-FA), 6-[^{18}F]A85380, [^{123}I]A85380, [^{11}C]nicotine, and recently [^{18}F]flubatine have been used to study AD (c.f. 20.14.2). [^{18}F]AZAN recently entered human use [230]. Seminal studies for understanding kinetics and mechanism of tobacco addiction were conducted using these nAChR radioligands. While acute tobacco/nicotine caused occupation/displacement of/from $\alpha_4\beta_2R$-sites, $\alpha_4\beta_2R$ were upregulated in subacute withdrawal (e.g., 36 h after cessation) by up to 80% everywhere except in the thalamus. A driving interest is here to *a priorily* predict the response to different types of withdrawal treatment. High $\alpha_4\beta_2R$ binding potentials were associated with higher risk of relapse in a study on 81 subjects. In the successfully abstinent group $\alpha_4\beta_2R\text{-}BP_P$ were only 20–29% over normal, while in the group who restarted smoking $\alpha_4\beta_2R$ were upregulated by 66–80% [229].

Nicotinic α_7R

The ligand [^{18}F]ASEM was the first one tested in humans [231]. It showed a global gray matter distribution with BP_{ND} around 1, somewhat lower in the cerebellum and amygdalohippocampal area. [^{11}C]NS14492 is in preclinical development; see 8.2.

20.15.2.4 Others

Glycine receptors (GlR)

GlR are heteropentameric pores similar to nicotinic and $GABA_A$-receptors with conductance for Cl^- anions and thus inhibitory effect in adults.

$5\text{-}HT_3R$ are also pores composed of 5 subunits with conductance for Na^+ and K^+ and thus stimulatory.

P2X purine receptors for ATP an ADP are heterotrimeric pores with conductance for Na^+ and some Ca^{2+}.

For these targets, no radioligand studies in humans are reported yet.

20.15.3 Enzymes

20.15.3.1 Extracellular Enzymes

Acetylcholinesterase

[^{11}C]MP4A and [^{11}C]PMP are well established and were used to study AD (c.f. 20.14.2).

20.15.3.2 Intracellular Enzymes: Signal Transduction

MAO

The distribution of MAO-A in humans is ubiquitous in gray matter, relatively sparing the striatum and with maxima in thalamus, occipital cortex, and brainstem. MAO-B, in turn, is more selectively distributed to the striatum (especially caudate nucleus), thalamus, and ACC. In smokers, both MAOs were considerably decreased, and this effect could be attributed to the tobacco alkaloid harman, which is a MAO inhibitor of slow clearance from tissue. During withdrawal from smoking, MAO levels inversely correlated with plasma harman levels [232].

MAO-A

[^{11}C]chlorgylin, as a "suicide" inhibitor, binds irreversibly. [^{11}C]harmine binds reversibly to MAO-A with $K_D = 2.0$ nM and thus is well suited for occupation/competition studies, i.e., with moclobemide. The same applies for [^{11}C]befloxaton [232]; See also 20.14.4.

MAO-B (c.f. 20.13.5)

Aromatic amino acid decarboxylase (AADC)

AADC catalyzes the last step in the synthesis of dopamine and serotonin and can be measured by modeling [^{18}F]DOPA or [^{11}C]tryptophan scans (c.f. 20.6, 20.14.5 and 20.15.4).

Phosphodiesterase – PDE4

PDE4 can be acceded by [^{11}C]rolipram. It showed a global cortical and thalamic distribution, while binding was low in the central region and mesial temporal lobe and almost absent in the cerebellum [198] (c.f. 20.14.4).

Phosphodiesterase – PDE10

A PDE10 ligand, [^{18}F]MNI659, proved as most sensitive early progression marker in Huntington's disease (c.f. 20.14.1).

Synapto-vesicular protein 2A (SV2A)

SV2A enables the fusion of mature synaptic GABA and glycine vesicles with the membrane as precondition for exocytosis. It revealed as the molecular target of levetiracetam. This widely used broad-spectrum anticonvulsive enhances the efficiency of SV2A. Concerning [^{18}F]UCB-H, the first SV2A ligand tested in humans up today a dosimetry study on five subjects is available which showed good brain penetrance with 1.2 % of injected activity remaining in the brain 2 h postinjection. There seems to be a global cortical distribution, slightly lower in the cerebellum [233].

20.15.4 Membrane Transporters

DAT

Beneath the commercialized and widely distributed [^{123}I]FP-CIT (Ioflupan, DATSCAN), there are also [^{123}I]βCIT, [^{99m}Tc]TRODAT 1, [^{18}F]CFT, [^{11}C]RTI32, and [^{18}F]FP-CIT that have been frequently applied. All these tropane derivatives are not perfectly DAT selective but display some binding to SERT and NET explaining some thalamic, mesencephalic, and amygdala binding in humans, respectively. Therefore, not only dopaminergic treatment but also medication with antidepressants (tricyclic, SSRI, etc.) should be acknowledged for better interpretation. [^{18}F]F-DOPA in contrast is selective for dopaminergic terminals (c.f. 20.6).

SERT or 5-HTT

Here [^{11}C]DASB is reported more stable and selective as [^{11}C]McN5652, [^{11}C]MADAM, or [^{123}I]ADAM. [^{11}C]DASB has a comparably fast tissue uptake kinetics and low plasma protein binding [234]. [^{11}C]DASB is sensitive to changes in serotonin levels. SERT also makes the selectivity of 5-hydroxy-L [β-^{11}C]-tryptophan, ([^{11}C]HTP), or [^{18}F]HTP which is intracellularly decarboxylized by the nonselective AADC and the uptake of which best reflects AADC activity in serotonergic terminals [235]. Irreversible intracellular trapping and thus kinetic modeling are analogous to [^{18}F]F-DOPA [199].

Pretreatment with carbidopa in order to inhibit degradation by peripheral AADC may be given.

NET

[^{123}I]metaiodobenzylguanidine ([^{123}I]MIBG) crosses the NET as "false substrate" and enriches in peripheral sympathetic fibers. It is in widespread clinical use for early recognition of PD and LBD where myocardial sympathetic denervation occurs, and therefore tracer uptake is absent. Some BBB penetrating NET radioligands have been used in human brain PET.

(S, S)-[^{11}C]O-methyl-reboxetine ([^{11}C]MRB) showed almost exclusive uptake in the dorsolateral thalamus and pulvinar, locus coeruleus and raphé nuclei, and hypothalamic regions [236]; BP_{ND} of up to 0.45 are reached.

(S, S)-[^{18}F]FMeNER-D_2 yields a slightly different distribution with also BP_{ND} up to 0.5 in the entire thalamus [122] [^{11}C]MRP (c.f. 20.10.3.2).

Glycine transporter (GlyT1)

For GlyT1 recently the radiotracer [^{18}F]MK6577 has been established in humans, and specificity was proved by an occupation study evidencing a homogenous distribution of unspecific binding. Specific binding was restricted to brainstem, cerebellar nuclei, and thalamus reaching V_T values of 4–8, while cortical V_T did not exceed 40 % of pontine V_T [237]. Similar results had been obtained before using [^{11}C]RO5013853 with V_T values ranging from 0.9 in the cortex to 2.6 in the pons. Here in addition slight uptake in the globus pallidus could be resolved and autoradiography permitted localization to the granular layers of the cerebellar cortex and the fascia dentata as well to selected white matter structures such as the alveus or cerebellar fibers [238].

Vesicular monoamine transporter 2 (VMAT2),

VMAT2 actively pumps monoamines into synaptic vesicles. The substrate selectivity is not strict, and serotonin, dopamine, noradrenalin, and histamine are transported. The isoform VMAT1 is exclusively localized in neuroendocrine cells. [^{11}C]DTBZ yielded a striatal distribution complemented by uptake in the substantia nigra, by the noradrenergic amygdala, and by the serotonergic raphe nuclei. Recently the fluoropropyl-analogue on [^{18}F]FP-DTBZ (synonym [^{18}F]AV133) had been established. DTBZ-PET was used in cohorts of AD, PD, and HD. Apparently VMAT2 is the most stable marker of monoaminergic neurons, little subdued to regulatory changes [239].

20.15.5 Others

18KD translocator protein (TSPO) (c.f. 20.13.3)
Aβ-Amyloid deposits (c.f. 20.8 and 20.9)
Protein-tau (τ) (c.f. 20.13.1)
Alpha-synuclein (c.f. 20.13.1)
P-glycoprotein (p-gp) (c.f. 20.13.2)
Myelin (c.f. 20.13.4)
σ_1-Receptors

σ_1R are intracellular chaperon proteins localized at the endoplasmic reticulum which modulate Ca^{2+} signaling through the IP3 receptor. Fluvoxamine, opipramol, dextromethorphan, haloperidol, and others show affinity for this receptor. The σ_1R ligand [^{11}C]SA4503 is established in humans [127] (c.f. 20.10.3.3).

Estrogen receptors (EstR)

The majority of EstR are transcription factors localized intracellularly. The non-α/β-selective ligand [^{18}F]fluoroestradiol proved promising for the detection of small cerebral metastases of breast cancer [240].

Conclusion

PET since its existence played a pivot role at the junction of basic neuroscience, pathophysiological and preclinical research, and introduction of new treatment methods into clinical routine. In the scope of the inverse way from bedside to bench, PET served to the metabolic and neurochemical characterization of rare, instructive, or new cases. PET accompanied and corroborated the introduction of poststroke thrombolysis, deep brain stimulation, and electroconvulsive therapy. Almost every second central-acting drug is today assessed by PET in the frame of clinical P-0 to P-III trials, for biodistribution and dose finding or as longitudinal readout. PET studies of neurotransmitter systems could corroborate and show the limits of the monoamine hypothesis of psychiatric disease. The same is actually underway concerning the glutamate hypothesis. A very recent ascent of PET applications came with tracers for Aβ-amyloid deposits in the brain. Tracers for tau and α-synuclein are in view. These advances in diagnostics parallel the advent of first etiologic curative treatment options in this field.

Acknowledgment Andreas Bauer is thankfully acknowledged for inspiring, encouraging, and continuously generously supporting this work. Figures 20.2, 20.3, and 20.5 were derived from studies we conducted in the frame of his research group with his support. There are no conflicts of interest to disclose.

References

1. Innis RB, Cunningham VJ, Delforge J, et al. Consensus nomenclature for in vivo imaging of reversibly binding radioligands. J Cereb Blood Flow Metab. 2007;27:1533–9.
2. Cheng Y, Prusoff WH. Relationship between the inhibition constant (K_i) and the concentration which causes 50 per cent inhibition (IC_{50}) of an enzymatic reaction. Biochem Pharmacol. 1973; 22:3099–108.
3. Lipinski CA, Lombardo F, Dominy BW, Feeney PJ. Experimental and computational approaches to estimate solubility and permeability in drug discovery and development settings. Adv Drug Deliv Rev. 2001;46:3–26.
4. Norinder U, Haeberlein M. Computational approaches to the prediction of the blood–brain distribution. Adv Drug Deliv Rev. 2002;54:291–313.
5. Desai A, Sawada G, Watson IA, Raub TJ. Integration of on silico and in vitro tools for scaffold optimization during drug discovery: predicting p-glycoprotein efflux. Mol Pharm. 2013;10:1249–61.
6. Moore DF, Altarescu G, Barker WC, et al. White matter lesions in Fabry disease occur in 'prior' selectively hypometabolic and hyperperfused brain regions. Brain Res Bull. 2003;62:231–40.
7. Nugent AC, Diazgranados N, Carlson PJ, et al. Neural correlates of rapid antidepressant response to ketamine in bipolar disorder. Bipolar Disord. 2014;16:119–28.
8. Heiss WD. Radionuclide imaging of stroke. J Nucl Med. 2014;55:1831–41.
9. Dubois B, Feldman HH, Jacova C, et al. Research criteria for the diagnosis of Alzheimer's disease: revising the NINCDS-ADRDA criteria. Lancet Neurol. 2007;6:734–46.
10. Dubois B, Feldman HH, Jacova C, et al. Revising the definition of Alzheimer's disease: a new lexicon. Lancet Neurol. 2010;9:1118–27.
11. ADx-Neurosciences-Euroimmun-Product-data--sheet. Microtiter ELISA EQ 6511-9601-L, EQ 6521-9601-L, EQ 6531-9601-L. In: http://www.euroimmun.de/fileadmin/template/images/pdf/Alzheimer_PLUS_Tau_und_APOE.pdf; 2014.
12. Wiltfang J, Esselmann H, Bibl M, et al. Amyloid beta peptide ratio 42/40 but not A beta 42 correlates with phospho-Tau in patients with low- and high-CSF A beta 40 load. J Neurochem. 2007;101:1053–9.
13. Cruchaga C, Haller G, Chakraverty S, et al. NIA-LOAD/NCRAD Family Study Consortium. Rare variants in APP, PSEN1 and PSEN2 increase risk for AD in late-onset Alzheimer's disease families. PLoS One. 2012;7:e31039.
14. Davison CM, O'Brien JT. A comparison of FDG-PET and blood flow SPECT in the diagnosis of neurodegenerative dementias: a systematic review. Int J Geriatr Psychiatry. 2014;29:551–61.
15. Tripathi M, Tripathi M, Damle N, et al. Differential diagnosis of neurodegenerative dementias using metabolic phenotypes on F-18 FDG PET/CT. Neuroradiol J. 2014;27:13–21.
16. Kim HJ, Yoon CW, Ye BS, et al. Vascular dementia. In: Dierckx RAJO, Otte A, de Vries EFJ, van Waarde A, Leenders KL, editors. PET and SPECT in neurology. Heidelberg: Springer; 2014.
17. Drzezga A, Lautenschlager N, Siebner H, et al. Cerebral metabolic changes accompanying conversion of mild cognitive impairment into Alzheimer's disease: a PET follow-up study. Eur J Nucl Med Mol Imaging. 2003;30:1104–13.
18. Kadir A, Andreasen N, Almkvist O, et al. Effect of phenserine treatment on brain functional activity and amyloid in Alzheimer's disease. Ann Neurol. 2008;63:621–31.
19. Keller C, Kadir A, Forsberg A, Porras O, Nordberg A. Long-term effects of galantamine treatment on brain functional activities as measured by PET in Alzheimer's disease patients. J Alzheimers Dis. 2011;24:109–23.
20. Landau SM, Harvey D, Madison CM, et al. Alzheimer's Disease Neuroimaging Initiative. Associations between cognitive, functional, and FDG-PET measures of decline in AD and MCI. Neurobiol Aging. 2011;32:1207–8.
21. Minoshima S, Frey KA, Koeppe RA, Foster NL, Kuhl DE. A diagnostic approach in Alzheimer's disease using three-dimensional stereotactic surface projections of fluorine [18F]FDG-PET. J Nucl Med. 2005;36:1238–48.
22. Caroli A, Lorenzi M, Geroldi C, et al. Metabolic compensation and depression in Alzheimer's disease. Dement Geriatr Cogn Disord. 2010;29:37–45.

23. Schöll M, Damian A, Engler H. Fluoredesoxyglucose PET in neurology and psychiatry. PET Clin. 2014;9:371–90.
24. Fidzinski P, Jarius S, Gaebler C, et al. Faciobrachial dystonic seizures and antibodies to Lgi1 in a 92-year old patient: a case report. J Neurol Sci. 2015;347:404–5.
25. Ossenkoppele R, Booij J, Scheltens P, van Berckel BNM. Dementia due to neurodegenerative disease: molecular imaging findings. In: Dierckx RAJO, Otte A, de Vries EFJ, van Waarde A, editors. PET and SPECT in neurology. Heidelberg: Springer; 2014. p. 185–211.
26. Catafau AM. Brain SPECT in clinical practice: part I: perfusion. J Nucl Med. 2001;42:259–71.
27. Egloff N, Sabbione ME, Salathé C, Wiest R, Juengling FD. Nondermatomal somatosensory deficits in patients with chronic pain disorder: clinical findings and hypometabolic pattern in FDG-PET. Pain. 2009;145:252–8.
28. Fitzgerald PB, Laird AR, Maller J, Daskalakis ZJ. A meta-analytic study of changes in brain activation in depression. Hum Brain Mapp. 2008;29:683–95.
29. Brody AL, Saxena S, Stoessel P, et al. Regional brain metabolic changes in patients with major depression treated with either paroxetine or interpersonal therapy: preliminary findings. Arch Gen Psychiatry. 2001;58:631–40.
30. Kennedy SH, Konarski JZ, Segal ZV, et al. Differences in brain glucose metabolism between responders to CBT and venlafaxine in a 16-week randomized controlled trial. Am J Psychiatry. 2007;164:778–88.
31. Mayberg HS, Silva JA, Brannan SK, et al. The functional neuroanatomy of the placebo effect. Am J Psychiatry. 2002;159:728–37.
32. Holthoff VA, Beuthien-Baumann B, Pietrzyk U, et al. Changes in regional cerebral perfusion in depression. SPECT monitoring of response to treatment. Nervenarzt. 1999;70:620–6.
33. Bonne O, Krausz V, Shapira B, et al. Increased cerebral blood flow in depressed patients responding to electroconvulsive therapy. J Nucl Med. 1996;37:1075–80.
34. Cohen RM, Gross M, Nordahl TE, et al. Preliminary data on the metabolic brain pattern of patients with winter seasonal affective disorder. Arch Gen Psychiatry. 1992;49:545–52.
35. Bremner JD, Innis RB, Salomon RM, et al. Positron emission tomography measurement of cerebral metabolic correlates of tryptophan depletion-induced depressive relapse. Arch Gen Psychiatry. 1997;54:364–74.
36. Mayberg HS, Brannan SK, Mahurin RK, et al. Cingulate function in depression: a potential predictor of treatment response. Neuroreport. 1997;8:1057–61.
37. Crowell AL, Garlow SJ, Riva-Posse P, Mayberg HS. Characterizing the therapeutic response to deep brain stimulation for treatment-resistant depression: a single center long-term perspective. Front Integr Neurosci. 2015;9:41.
38. Dunlop BW, Kelley ME, McGrath CL, Craighead WE, Mayberg HS. Preliminary findings supporting insula metabolic activity as a predictor of outcome to psychotherapy and medication treatments for depression. J Neuropsychiatry Clin Neurosci. 2015;27:237–9.
39. Brooks III JO, Hoblyn JC, Woodard SA, Rosen AC, Ketter TA. Corticolimbic metabolic dysregulation in euthymic older adults with bipolar disorder. J Psychiatr Res. 2009;43:497–502.
40. Haarman BCM, van der Lek RFR, Ruhé HG, et al. Bipolar disorders. In: Dierckx RAJO, Otte A, de Vries EFJ, van Waarde A, den Boer JA, editors. PET and SPECT in psychiatry. Heidelberg: Springer; 2014.
41. Rubinsztein JS, Fletcher PC, Rogers RD, et al. decision making in mania: a PET study. Brain. 2001;124:2550–63.
42. Schneider K. Klinische psychopathologie. 15th ed. Stuttgart: Thieme; 2007.
43. Clark C, Kopala L, Li DK, Hurwitz T. Regional cerebral glucose metabolism in never-medicated patients with schizophrenia. Can J Psychiatry. 2001;46:340–5.
44. Buchsbaum MS, Buchsbaum BR, Hazlett EA, et al. Relative glucose metabolic rate higher in white matter in patients with schizophrenia. Am J Psychiatry. 2007;164:1072–81.
45. Altamura AC, Bertoldo A, Marotta G, et al. White matter metabolism differentiates schizophrenia and bipolar disorder: a preliminary PET study. Psychiatry Res. 2013;214:410–4.
46. Bossong MG, Allen P. PET and SPECT findings in patients with hallucinations. In: Dierckx RAJO, Otte A, de Vries EFJ, van Waarde A, den Boer JA, editors. PET and SPECT in psychiatry. Heidelberg: Springer; 2014.
47. Klirova M, Horacek J, Novak T, et al. Individualized rTMS neuronavigated according to regional brain metabolism ([^{18}F]FGD PET) has better treatment effects on auditory hallucinations than standard positioning of rTMS: a double-blind, sham-controlled study. Eur Arch Psychiatry Clin Neurosci. 2013;263:475–84.
48. Shin LM, Liberzon I. The neurocircuitry of fear, stress, and anxiety disorders. Neuropsychopharmacology. 2010;35:169–91.
49. Fredrikson M, Faria V, Furmark T. Neurotransmission: a review of PET and SPECT studies in anxiety disorders. In: Dierckx RAJO, Otte A, de Vries EFJ, van Waarde A, den Boer JA, editors. PET and SPECT in psychiatry. Heidelberg: Springer; 2014.
50. Baxter Jr LR, Phelps ME, Mazziotta JC, et al. Local cerebral glucose metabolic rates in obsessive-compulsive disorder. A comparison with rates in unipolar depression and in normal controls. Arch Gen Psychiatry. 1987;44:800.

51. Brody AL, Saxena S, Schwartz JM, et al. FDG-PET predictors of response to behavioral therapy and pharmacotherapy in obsessive compulsive disorder. Psychiatry Res. 1998;84:1–6.
52. Nordahl TE, Benkelfat C, Semple WE, et al. Cerebral glucose metabolic rates in obsessive compulsive disorder. Neuropsychopharmacology. 1989;2:23–8.
53. de Paula FD, Copray S, Buchpiguel C, Dierckx R, de Vries E. PET imaging in multiple sclerosis. J Neuroimmune Pharmacol. 2014;9:468–82.
54. Engler H, Lundberg PO, Ekbom K, et al. Multitracer study with positron emission tomography in Creutzfeldt-Jakob disease. Eur J Nucl Med Mol Imaging. 2003;30:85–95.
55. Müller HF, Viaccoz A, Fisch L, et al. ^{18}FDG-PET-CT: an imaging biomarker of high-risk carotid plaques. Correlation to symptoms and microembolic signals. Stroke. 2014;45:3561–6.
56. Mani V, Woodward M, Samber D, et al. Predictors of change in carotid atherosclerotic plaque inflammation and burden as measured by 18-FDG-PET and MRI, respectively, in the dal-PLAQUE study. Int J Cardiovasc Imaging. 2014;30:571–82.
57. Marnane M, Merwick A, Sheehan OC, et al. Carotid plaque inflammation on ^{18}F-fluorodeoxyglucose positron emission tomography predicts early stroke recurrence. Ann Neurol. 2012;71:709–18.
58. Rudd JH, Myers KS, Bansilal S, et al. Relationships among regional arterial inflammation, calcification, risk factors, and biomarkers: a prospective fluorodeoxyglucose positron-emission tomography/computed tomography imaging study. Circ Cardiovasc Imaging. 2009;2:107–15.
59. Morales-Chacón LM, Sánchez-Catasús CA, Quincoses OT, Lorigados-Pedre L, Dierckx RAJO. Nuclear medicine neuroimaging and electromagnetic source localization in nonlesional drug-resistant focal epilepsy. In: Dierckx RAJO, Otte A, de Vries EFJ, van Waarde A, Leenders KL, editors. PET and SPECT in neurology. Heidelberg: Springer; 2014. p. 843–60.
60. Hong SB, Tae WS. SISCOM (Subtraction ictal SPECT coregistered to MRI). In: Dierckx RAJO, Otte A, de Vries EFJ, van Waarde A, Leenders KL, editors. PET and SPECT in neurology. Heidelberg: Springer; 2014. p. 829–41.
61. O'Brien TJ, O'Connor MK, Mullan BP, et al. Subtraction ictal SPET co-registered to MRI in partial epilepsy: description and technical validation of the method with phantom and patient studies. Nucl Med Commun. 1998;19:31–45.
62. Fernández S, Donaire A, Serès E, et al. PET/MRI and PET/MRI/SISCOM coregistration in the presurgical evaluation of refractory focal epilepsy. Epilepsy Res. 2015;111:1–9.
63. Desai A, Bekelis K, Thadani VM, et al. Interictal PET and ictal subtraction SPECT: sensitivity in the detection of seizure foci in patients with medically intractable epilepsy. Epilepsia. 2013;54:341–50.
64. Grouiller F, Delattre BM, Pittau F, et al. All-in-one interictal presurgical imaging in patients with epilepsy: single-session EEG/PET/(f)MRI. Eur J Nucl Med Mol Imaging. 2015;42:1133–43.
65. Hammers A, Koepp MJ, Hurlemann R, et al. Abnormalities of grey and white matter [^{11}C]flumazenil binding in temporal lobe epilepsy with normal MRI. Brain. 2002;125:2257–71.
66. Van Laere K, Clerinx K, D'Hondt E, de Groot T, Vandenberghe W. Combined striatal binding and cerebral influx analysis of dynamic ^{11}C-raclopride PET improves early differentiation between multiple-system atrophy and Parkinson disease. J Nucl Med. 2010;51:588–95.
67. Niccolini F, Su P, Politis M. Dopamine receptor mapping with PET imaging in Parkinson's disease. J Neurol. 2014;261:2251–63.
68. Kortekaas R, Georgiadis JR. An investigation of statistical power of [^{15}O]-H_2O PET perfusion imaging: The influence of delay and time interval. In: Dierckx RAJO, Otte A, de Vries EFJ, van Waarde A, Leenders KL, editors. PET and SPECT in neurology. Heidelberg: Springer; 2014. p. 139–48.
69. Mintun MA, Raichle ME, Martin WR, Herscovitch P. Brain oxygen utilization measured with O-15 radiotracers and positron emission tomography. J Nucl Med. 1984;25:177–87.
70. Huang SC, Feng DG, Phelps ME. Model dependency and estimation reliability in measurement of cerebral oxygen utilization rate with oxygen-15 and dynamic positron emission tomography. J Cereb Blood Flow Metab. 1986;6:105–19.
71. Kuhn FP, Warnock G, Schweingruber T, et al. Quantitative H2[^{15}O]-PET in pediatric moyamoya disease: evaluating perfusion before and after cerebral revascularization. J Stroke Cerebrovasc Dis. 2015;25:965–71.
72. Nezu T, Yokota C, Uehara T, et al. Preserved acetazolamide reactivity in lacunar patients with severe white-matter lesions: ^{15}O-labeled gas and H_2O positron emission tomography studies. J Cereb Blood Flow Metab. 2012;32:844–50.
73. Imaizumi M, Kitagawa K, Oku N, et al. Clinical significance of cerebrovascular reserve in acetazolamide challenge -comparison with acetazolamide challenge H2O-PET and Gas-PET. Ann Nucl Med. 2004;18:369–74.
74. Reinges MH, Krings T, Meyer PT, et al. Preoperative mapping of cortical motor function: prospective comparison of functional magnetic resonance imaging and [^{15}O]-H_2O-positron emission tomography in the same co-ordinate system. Nucl Med Commun. 2004;25:987–97.
75. Heiss WD, Grond M, Thiel A, et al. Tissue at risk of infarction rescued by early reperfusion: a positron emission tomography study in systemic recombinant tissue plasminogen activator thrombolysis of acute stroke. J Cereb Blood Flow Metab. 1998;18:1298–307.

76. Alawneh JA, Moustafa RR, Marrapu ST, et al. Diffusion and perfusion correlates of the ^{18}F-MISO PET lesion in acute stroke: pilot study. Eur J Nucl Med Mol Imaging. 2014;41:736–44.
77. Villemagne VL, Fodero-Tavoletti M, Yates P, Masters C, Rowe C. Aβ imaging in aging, Alzheimer's disease and other neurodegenerative conditions. In: Dierckx RAJO, Otte A, Vries EFJ, Waarde A, Leenders KL, editors. PET and SPECT in neurology. Heidelberg: Springer; 2014. p. 213–54.
78. Mason NS, Mathis CA, Klunk WE. Positron emission tomography radioligands for in vivo imaging of Aβ plaques. J Label Compd Radiopharm. 2012;56:89–95.
79. Villemagne VL, Mulligan R, Pejoska S, et al. Comparison of [11C]PiB and [18F]florbetaben for Aβ imaging in aging and Alzheimer's disease. Eur J Nucl Med Mol Imaging. 2012;39:983–9.
80. Cselényi Z, Jönhagen ME, Forsberg A, et al. Clinical validation of ^{18}F-AZD4694, an amyloid-ß-specific PET radioligand. J Nucl Med. 2012;53:415–24.
81. Jack Jr CR, Barrio JR, Kepe V. Cerebral amyloid PET imaging in Alzheimer's disease. Acta Neuropathol. 2013;126:643–57.
82. Landau SM, Fero A, Baker SL, et al. Measurement of longitudinal A-beta change with ^{18}F florbetapir PET and standard uptake values. J Nucl Med. 2015;56:567–74.
83. Stankoff B, Freeman L, Aigrot MS, et al. Imaging central nervous system myelin by positron emission tomography in multiple sclerosis using [methyl-^{11}C]-2-(4′-methylaminophenyl)-6-hydroxybenzothiazole. Ann Neurol. 2011;69:673–80.
84. Kobylecki C, Langheinrich T, Hinz R, et al. ^{18}F-florbetapir PET in patients with frontotemporal dementia and Alzheimer disease. J Nucl Med. 2015;56:386–91.
85. Sabbagh M, Seibyl J, Stephens A, et al. A negative florbetaben PET scan reliably excludes amyloid pathology as confirmed by histopathology in a large phase 3 trial. Piramal Neuraceq Summary of product characteristics. 2014.
86. Sabri O, Seibyl J, Rowe CC, Barthel H. Beta-amyloid imaging with flobetaben. Clin Transl Imaging. 2015;3:13–26.
87. Jicha G, Parisi J, Dickson D, et al. Neuropathologic outcome of mild cognitive impairment following progression to clinical dementia. Arch Neurol. 2006;63:674–81.
88. Irwin DJ, Trojanowski JQ, Grossman M. Cerebrospinal fluid biomarkers for differentiation of frontotemporal lobar degeneration from Alzheimer's disease. Front Aging Neurosci. 2013;5:6.
89. Krudop WA, Kerssens CJ, Dols A, et al. Building a new paradigm for the early recognition of behavioral variant frontotemporal dementia: Late Onset Frontal Lobe Syndrome study. Am J Geriatr Psychiatry. 2014;22:735–40.
90. Reesink FE, Stormezand GN, Dierckx RAJO, De Deyn PP. Nuclear imaging in frontotemporal dementia. In: Dierckx RAJO, Otte A, de Vries EFJ, van Waarde A, editors. PET and SPECT in neurology. Heidelberg: Springer; 2014.
91. Ducksbury R, Whitfield T, Walker S. SPECT/PET findings in Lewy body dementia. In: Dierckx RAJO, Otte A, de Vries EFJ, van Waarde A, Leenders KL, editors. PET and SPECT in neurology. Heidelberg: Springer; 2014. p. 373–415.
92. Bohnen NI, Frey KA. Parkinson dementia: PET findings. In: Dierckx RAJO, Otte A, de Vries EFJ, van Waarde A, Leenders KL, editors. PET and SPECT in neurology. Heidelberg: Springer; 2014. p. 359–72.
93. Burack MA, Hartlein J, Flores HP, et al. In vivo amyloid imaging in autopsy-confirmed Parkinson disease with dementia. Neurology. 2010;74:77–84.
94. Salloway S, Sperling R, Fox NC, et al. Bapineuzumab 301 and 302 Clinical Trial Investigators. Two phase 3 trials of bapineuzumab in mild-to-moderate Alzheimer's disease. N Engl J Med. 2014;370:322–33.
95. Lo RY, Hubbard AE, Shaw LM, et al. Longitudianl change of biomarkers in cognitive decline. Arch Neurol. 2011;68:1257–66.
96. Ossenkoppele R, Tolboom N, Foster-Dingley JC, et al. Longitudinal imaging of Alzheimer pathology using [^{11}C]PIB, [^{18}F]FDDNP and [^{18}F]FDG PET. Eur J Nucl Med Mol Imaging. 2012;39:990–1000.
97. Kemppainen NM, Scheinin NM, Koivunen J, et al. Five-year follow-up of C-11-PIB uptake in Alzheimer's disease and MCI. Eur J Nucl Med Mol Imaging. 2014;41:283–9.
98. Roche HL. SCarlet RoAD, a study of gantenerumab in patients with mild Alzheimer disease. 2015.
99. Frantz N. Clinical trials results and new data analyses in mayloid-related therapies from the Alzheimer's association international conference 2015. In: Association As ed; 2015.
100. Jack Jr CR, Lowe VJ, Weigand SD, et al. Serial PIB and MRI in normal, mild cognitive impairment and Alzheimer's disease: implications for sequence of pathological events in Alzheimer's disease. Brain. 2009;132:1355–65.
101. Villemagne VL, Pike KE, Chetelat G, et al. Longitudinal assessment of Abeta and cognition in aging and Alzheimer disease. Ann Neurol. 2011;69:181–92.
102. Kadir A, Almkvist O, Forsberg A, et al. Dynamic changes in PET amyloid and FDG imaging at different stages of Alzheimer's disease. Neurobiol Aging. 2012;33:198.e1–14.
103. Koivunen J, Scheinin N, Virta JR, et al. Amyloid PET imaging in patients with mild cognitive impairment: a 2-year follow-up study. Neurology. 2011;76:1085–90.
104. Doody RS, Thomas RG, Farlow M, et al. Phase 3 trials of solanezumab for mild-to-moderate Alzheimer's disease. N Engl J Med. 2014;370:311–21.

105. Whone AL, Watts RL, Stoessl AJ, et al. REAL-PET Study Group. Slower progression of Parkinson's disease with ropinirole versus levodopa: The REAL-PET study. Ann Neurol. 2003;54:93–101.
106. Bewernick BH, Hurlemann R, Matusch A, et al. Nucleus accumbens deep brain stimulation decreases ratings of depression and anxiety in treatment-resistant depression. Biol Psychiatry. 2010;67:110–6.
107. Kuhn J, Hardenacke K, Lenartz D, et al. Deep brain stimulation of the nucleus basalis of Meynert in Alzheimer's dementia. Mol Psychiatry. 2015;20:353–60.
108. Ackermann RF, Engel J, Baxter L. Positron emission tomography and autoradiographic studies of glucose utilization following electroconvulsive seizures in humans and rats. Ann N Y Acad Sci. 1986;462:263–9.
109. Kayser S, Bewernick BH, Matusch A, et al. Magnetic seizure therapy in treatment-resistant depression: clinical, neuropsychological and metabolic effects. Psychol Med. 2015;45:1073–92.
110. Yokoi F, Gründer G, Biziere K, et al. Dopamine D2 and D3 receptor occupancy in normal humans treated with the antipsychotic drug aripiprazole (OPC14597): a study using positron emission tomography and [^{11}C]raclopride. Neuropsychopharmacology. 2002;27:248–59.
111. Areberg J, Luntang-Jensen M, Søgaard B, Nilausen DØ. Occupancy of the serotonin transporter after administration of Lu AA21004 and its relation to plasma concentration in healthy subjects. Basic Clin Pharmacol Toxicol. 2012;110:401–4.
112. Stenkrona P, Halldin C, Lundberg J. 5-HTT and 5-HT(1A) receptor occupancy of the novel substance vortioxetine (Lu AA21004). A PET study in control subjects. Eur Neuropsychopharmacol. 2013;23:1190–8.
113. Natesan S, Reckless GE, Barlow KB, Nobrega JN, Kapur S. Evaluation of N-desmethylclozapine as a potential antipsychotic – preclinical studies. Neuropsychopharmacology. 2007;32:1540–9.
114. Kågedal M, Cselényi Z, Nyberg S, et al. A positron emission tomography study in healthy volunteers to estimate mGluR5 receptor occupancy of AZD2066 – estimating occupancy in the absence of a reference region. Neuroimage. 2013;82:160–9.
115. Steffer J. Estimation of regional brain mGluR5 receptor occupancy following single oral doses of the mGluR5 antagonist AFQ056 with positron emission tomography (PET) of [^{11}C]ABP688 in healthy volunteers. In: 3rd Winter Brain Symposium of the Psychogeriatric University Hospital Division of Psychiatry Research of the University of Zurich, Sils Maria; 2007.
116. Farde L, Wiesel FA, Halldin C, Sedvall G. Central D2-dopamine receptor occupancy in schizophrenic patients treated with antipsychotic drugs. Arch Gen Psychiatry. 1988;45:71–6.
117. Farde L, Nordström AL, Wiesel FA, et al. Positron emission tomographic analysis of central D1 and D2 dopamine receptor occupancy in patients treated with classical neuroleptics and clozapine. Relation to extrapyramidal side effects. Arch Gen Psychiatry. 1992;49:538–44.
118. Kapur S, Seeman P. Does fast dissociation from the dopamine d(2) receptor explain the action of atypical antipsychotics?: a new hypothesis. Am J Psychiatry. 2001;158:360–9.
119. Mizrahi R, Agid O, Borlido C, et al. Effects of antipsychotics on D3 receptors: a clinical PET study in first episode antipsychotic naive patients with schizophrenia using [^{11}C]-(+)-PHNO. Schizophr Res. 2011;131:63–8.
120. Varnäs K, Jucaite A, McCarthy DJ, et al. A PET study with [^{11}C]AZ10419369 to determine brain 5-HT1B receptor occupancy of zolmitriptan in healthy male volunteers. Cephalalgia. 2013;33:853–60.
121. Meyer JH, Wilson AA, Ginovart N, et al. Occupancy of serotonin transporters by paroxetine and citalopram during treatment of depression: a [^{11}C] DASB PET imaging study. Am J Psychiatry. 2001;158:1843–9.
122. Nyberg S, Jucaite A, Takano A, et al. Norepinephrine transporter occupancy in the human brain after oral administration of quetiapine XR. Int J Neuropsychopharmacol. 2013;16:2235–44.
123. Ding YS, Naganawa M, Gallezot JD, et al. Clinical doses of atomoxetine significantly occupy both norepinephrine and serotonin transports: implications on treatment of depression and ADHD. Neuroimage. 2014;86:164–71.
124. Meyer JH, Goulding VS, Wilson AA, et al. Bupropion occupancy of the dopamine transporter is low during clinical treatment. Psychopharmacology (Berl). 2002;163:102–5.
125. Elmenhorst D, Meyer PT, Matusch A, Winz OH, Bauer A. Caffeine occupancy of human cerebral A1 adenosine receptors: in vivo quantification with [^{18}F] CPFPX and PET. J Nucl Med. 2012;53:1723–9.
126. Darreh-Shori T, Kadir A, Almkvist O, et al. Inhibition of acetylcholinesterase in CSF versus brain assessed by ^{11}C-PMP PET in AD patients treated with galantamine. Neurobiol Aging. 2008;29:168–84.
127. Ishikawa M, Sakata M, Ichii K, et al. High occupancy of σ_1 receptors in the human brain after single oral administration of donepezil: a positron emission tomography study using [^{11}C]SA4503. Int J Neuropsychopharmacol. 2009;12:1127–31.
128. Food and Drug Administration. Innovation or stagnation: challenge and opportunity on the critical path to new medical products, vol. 1. Washington, DC; U.S. Department of Health and Human Services, Silver Spring, MD, USA, 2004. p. 1.
129. Lappin G, Garner RC. Big physics, small doses: the use of AMS and PET in human microdosing of development drugs. Nat Rev Drug Discov. 2003;2:233–40.
130. Yates R, Sörensen J, Bergström M, et al. Distribution of intranasal C-zolmitriptan assessed by positron emission tomography. Cephalalgia. 2005;25: 1103–9.

131. Andersen VL, Hansen HD, Herth MM, Knudsen GM, Kristensen JL. ^{11}C-labeling and preliminary evaluation of vortioxetine as a PET radioligand. Bioorg Med Chem Lett. 2014;24:2408–11.
132. Ermert J, Stüsgen S, Lang M, Roden W, Coenen HH. High molar activity of [^{11}C]TCH346 via [^{11}C] methyl triflate using the "wet" [^{11}C]CO2 reduction method. Appl Radiat Isot. 2008;66:619–24.
133. Ridler K, Cunningham V, Huiban M, et al. An evaluation of the brain distribution of [^{11}C]GSK1034702, a muscarinic-1 (M_1) positive allosteric modulator in the living human brain using positron emission tomography. EJNMMI Res. 2014;4:66.
134. Bauer M, Karch R, Zeitlinger M, et al. Interaction of ^{11}C-tariquidar and ^{11}C-elacridar with P-glycoprotein and breast cancer resistance protein at the human blood–brain barrier. J Nucl Med. 2013;54:1181–7.
135. Park HS, Kim E, Moon BS, et al. In vivo tissue pharmacokinetics of carbon-11-labeled clozapine in healthy volunteers: a positron emission tomography study. CPT Pharmacometrics Syst Pharmacol. 2015;4(5): 305–11.
136. Gjerløff T, Fedorova T, Knudsen K, et al. Imaging acetylcholinesterase density in peripheral organs in Parkinson's disease with ^{11}C-donezepil PET. Brain. 2015;138:653–63.
137. Tsukada H, Nishiyama S, Kakiuchi T, et al. Is synaptic dopamine concentration the exclusive factor which alters the in vivo binding of [^{11}C]raclopride?: PET studies combined with microdialysis in conscious monkeys. Brain Res. 1999;841:160–9.
138. Bencherif B, Fuchs PN, Sheth R, et al. Pain activation of human supraspinal opioid pathways as demonstrated by [^{11}C]carfentanil and positron emission tomography (PET). Pain. 2002;99:589–98.
139. Lundquist P, Wilking H, Urban Höglund A, et al. Potential of [^{11}C]DASB for measuring endogenous serotonin with PET: binding studies. Nucl Med Biol. 2005;32:129–36.
140. Sandiego CM, Nabulsi N, Lin SF, et al. Studies of the metabotropic glutamate receptor 5 radioligand [^{11}C]ABP688 with N-acetylcysteine challenge in rhesus monkeys. Synapse. 2013;67:489–501.
141. Miyake N, Skinbjerg M, Easwaramoorthy B, et al. Imaging changes in glutamate transmission in vivo with the metabotropic glutamate receptor 5 tracer [^{11}C] ABP688 and N-acetylcysteine challenge. Biol Psychiatry. 2011;69:822–4.
142. Zimmer ER, Parent MJ, Leuzy A, et al. Imaging in vivo glutamate fluctuations with [^{11}C]ABP688: a GLT-1 challenge with ceftriaxone. J Cereb Blood Flow Metab. 2015;35:1169–74.
143. DeLorenzo C, DellaGioia N, Bloch M, et al. In vivo ketamine-induced changes in [^{11}C]ABP688 binding to metabotropic Glutamate receptor Subtype 5. Biol Psychiatry. 2015;77:266–75.
144. Matusch A, Hurlemann R, Rota Kops E, et al. Acute S-ketamine application does not alter cerebral [^{18}F] altanserin binding: a pilot study in humans. J Neural Transm. 2007;114:1433–42.
145. Vernaleken I, Klomp M, Moeller O, et al. Vulnerability to psychotogenic effects of ketamine is associated with elevated D2/3-receptor availability. Int J Neuropsychopharmacol. 2013;16:745–54.
146. Salmi E, Långsjö JW, Aalto S, et al. Subanesthetic ketamine does not affect ^{11}C-flumazenil binding in humans. Anesth Analg. 2005;101:722–5.
147. Vollenweider FX, Leenders KL, Oye I, Hell D, Angst J. Differential psychopathology and patterns of cerebral glucose utilisation produced by (S)- and (R)-ketamine in healthy volunteers using positron emission tomography (PET). Eur Neuropsychopharmacol. 1997;7:25–38.
148. Långsjö JW, Salmi E, Kaisti KK, et al. Effects of subanesthetic ketamine on regional cerebral glucose metabolism in humans. Anesthesiology. 2004;100:1065–71.
149. Långsjö JW, Kaisti KK, Aalto S, et al. Effects of subanesthetic doses of ketamine on regional cerebral blood flow, oxygen consumption, and blood volume in humans. Anesthesiology. 2003;99:614–23.
150. Striepens N, Matusch A, Kendrick KM, et al. Oxytocin enhances attractiveness of unfamiliar female faces independent of the dopamine reward system. Psychoneuroendocrinology. 2014;39:74–87.
151. Okazawa H, Tsuchida T, Pagani M, et al. Effects of 5-HT1B/1D receptor agonist rizatriptan on cerebral blood flow and blood volume in normal circulation. J Cereb Blood Flow Metab. 2006;26:92–8.
152. Frey K. Amyloid imaging in dementia: contribution or confusion? J Nucl Med. 2015;56:331–2.
153. Okamura N, Furumoto S, Fodero-Tavoletti MT, et al. Non-invasive assessment of Alzheimer's disease neurofibrillary pathology using F-18-THK5105 PET. Brain. 2014;137:1762–71.
154. Maruyama M, Shimada H, Suhara T, et al. Imaging of tau pathology in a tauopathy mouse model and in Alzheimer patients compared to normal controls. Neuron. 2013;79:1094–108.
155. Chien DT, Szardenings AK, Bahri S, et al. Early clinical PET imaging results with the novel PHF-tau radioligand [^{18}F]T808. J Alzheimers Dis. 2014;38:171–84.
156. Kikuchi A, Takeda A, Okamura N, et al. In vivo visualization of alpha-synuclein deposition by carbon-11-labelled 2-[2-(2-dimethylaminothiazol-5-yl) ethenyl]-6-[2-(fluoro)ethoxy]benzoxazole positron emission tomography in multiple system atrophy. Brain. 2010;133:1772–8.
157. Bauer M, Karch R, Zeitlinger M, et al. Approaching complete inhibition of P-glycoprotein at the human blood–brain barrier: an (R)-[^{11}C]verapamil PET study. J Cereb Blood Flow Metab. 2015;35:743–6.
158. Mansor MS, Boellaard R, Froklage FE, et al. Quantification of dynamic ^{11}C-Phenytoin PET studies. J Nucl Med. 2015;56:1372–7.
159. Postnov A, Froklage FE, van Lingen A, et al. Radiation dose of the P-glycoprotein tracer ^{11}C-laniquidar. J Nucl Med. 2013;54:2101–3.

160. Deo AK, Borson S, Link JM, et al. Activity of P-glycoprotein, a ß-amyloid transporter at the blood–brain barrier, is compromised in patients with mild Alzheimer disease. J Nucl Med. 2014;55:1106–11.
161. van Assema DM, Goos JD, van der Flier WM, et al. No evidence for additional blood–brain barrier P-glycoprotein dysfunction in Alzheimer's disease patients with microbleeds. J Cereb Blood Flow Metab. 2012;32:1468–71.
162. Colasanti A, Guo Q, Muhlert N, et al. In vivo assessment of brain white matter inflammation in multiple sclerosis with ^{18}F-PBR111 PET. J Nucl Med. 2014;55:1112–8.
163. Oh U, Fujita M, Ikonomidou VN, et al. Translocator protein PET imaging for glial activation in multiple sclerosis. J Neuroimmune Pharmacol. 2011;6:354–61.
164. Vas A, Sóvágó J, Halldin C, et al. Cerebral uptake and regional distribution of [^{11}C]-vinpocetin after intravenous administration to healthy men: a PET study. Orv Hetil. 2002;143:2631–6.
165. Colasanti A, Piccini P. PET imaging in multiple sclerosis: focus on the translocator protein. In: Dierckx R, Otte A, de Vries E, van Waarde A, Leenders KL, editors. PET and SPECT in neurology. Heidelberg: Springer; 2014. p. 757–74.
166. Lucchinetti CF, Brück W, Rodriguez M, Lassmann H. Distinct patterns of multiple sclerosis pathology indicates heterogeneity on pathogenesis. Brain Pathol. 1996;6:259–74.
167. Brooks DJ. PET imaging of translocator protein expression in neurological diseases. In: Dierckx R, Otte A, de Vries E, van Waarde A, Leenders KL, editors. PET and SPECT in neurology. Heidelberg: Springer; 2014. p. 653–67.
168. Paul S, Khanapur S, Boersma W, et al. Cerebral adenosine A1 receptors are upregulated in rodent encephalitis. Neuroimage. 2014;92:83–9.
169. Carter S, Schöll M, Almkvist O, Wall A. Evidence for astrocytosis in prodromal Alzheimer disease provided by ^{11}C deuterium-L-deprenyl: a multitracer PET paradigm combining ^{11}C-Pittsburgh compound B and ^{18}F-FDG. J Nucl Med. 2012;53:37–46.
170. Langbehn DR, Hayden MR, Paulsen JS. CAG-repeat length and the age of onset in Huntington disease (HD): a review and validation study of statistical approaches. Am J Med Genet B Neuropsychiatr Genet. 2010;153B:397–408.
171. Pavese N, Andrews TC, Brooks DJ, et al. Progressive striatal and cortical dopamine receptor dysfunction in Huntington's disease: a PET study. Brain. 2003;126:1127–35.
172. Kunig G, Leenders KL, Sanchez-Pernaute R, et al. Benzodiazepine receptor binding in Huntington's disease: [^{11}C]flumazenil uptake measured using positron emission tomography. Ann Neurol. 2000;47:644–8.
173. Matusch A, Saft C, Elmenhorst D, et al. Cross sectional PET study of cerebral adenosine A1 receptors in premanifest and manifest Huntington's disease. Eur J Nucl Med Mol Imaging. 2014;41:1210–20.
174. Ahmad R, Bourgeois S, Postnov A, et al. PET imaging shows loss of striatal PDE10A in patients with Huntington disease. Neurology. 2014;82:279–81.
175. Russell D, Jennings D, Barret O, et al. Monitoring loss of striatal phosphodiesterase 10a (PDE10a) with [^{18}F]MNI659 and PET: a biomarker of early Huntigton disease (HD) progression. Neurology. 2015;84:S15.004.
176. Herholz K, Weisenbach S, Zündorf G, et al. In vivo study of acetylcholine esterase in basal forebrain, amygdala, and cortex in mild to moderate Alzheimer disease. Neuroimage. 2004;21:136–43.
177. Kendziorra K, Wolf H, Meyer PM, et al. Decreased cerebral a4ß2* nicotinic acetylcholine receptor availability in patients with mild cognitive impairment and Alzheimer's disease assessed with positron emission tomography. Eur J Nucl Med Mol Imaging. 2011;38:515–25.
178. Mitsis EM, Reech KM, Bois F, et al. ^{123}I-5-IA-85380 SPECT imaging of nicotinic receptors in Alzheimer disease and mild cognitive impairment. J Nucl Med. 2009;50:1455–63.
179. Kadir A, Almkvist O, Wall A, Långström B, Nordberg A. PET imaging of cortical ^{11}C-nicotine binding correlates with the cognitive function of attention in Alzheimer's disease. Psychopharmacology (Berl). 2006;188:509–20.
180. Sabri O, Becker GA, Meyer PM, et al. First-in-human PET quantification study of cerebral a4ß2* nicotinic acetylcholine receptors using the novel specific radioligand (−)-[^{18}F]Flubatine. Neuroimage. 2015;118:199–208.
181. Blin J, Baron JC, Dubois B, et al. Loss of brain 5-HT2 receptors in Alzheimer's disease. In vivo assessment with positron emission tomography and [^{18}F]setoperone. Brain. 1993;116:497–510.
182. Gulyás B, Pavlova E, Kása P, et al. Activated MAO-B in the brain of Alzheimer patients, demonstrated by [^{11}C]-L-deprenyl using whole hemisphere autoradiography. Neurochem Int. 2011;58:60–8.
183. McKeith I, O'Brien J, Walker Z, et al. DLB Study Group. Sensitivity and specificity of dopamine transporter imaging with 123I-FP-CIT SPECT in dementia with Lewy bodies: a phase III, multicentre study. Lancet Neurol. 2007;6:305–13.
184. Becker B, Klein EM, Striepens N, et al. Nicotinic acetylcholine receptors contribute to learning-induced metaplasticity in the hippocampus. J Cogn Neurosci. 2013;25:986–97.
185. Ettrup A, Mikkelsen JD, Lehel S, et al. ^{11}C-NS14492 as a novel PET radioligand for imaging cerebral alpha7 nicotinic acetylcholine receptors: in vivo evaluation and drug occupancy measurements. J Nucl Med. 2011;52:1449–56.
186. Howes OD, Kambeitz J, Kim E, et al. The nature of dopamine dysfunction in schizophrenia and what this means for treatment. Arch Gen Psychiatry. 2012;69:776–86.

187. Abi-Dargham A, Gil R, Krystal J, et al. Increased striatal dopamine transmission in schizophrenia: confirmation in a second cohort. Am J Psychiatry. 1998;155:761–7.
188. Ceccarini J, De Hert M, Van Winkel R, et al. Increased ventral striatal CB1 receptor binding is related to negative symptoms in drug free patients with schizophrenia. Neuroimage. 2013;79:304–12.
189. Berding G, Schneider U, Gielow P, et al. Feasibility of central cannabinoid CB1 receptor imaging with [^{124}I]AM281 PET demonstrated in a schizophrenic patient. Psychiatry Res. 2006;147:249–56.
190. Praschak-Rieder N, Willeit M. Imaging of seasonal affective disorder and seasonality effects on serotonin and dopamine function in the human brain. Curr Top Behav Neurosci. 2012;11:149–67.
191. Kalbitzer J, Erritzoe D, Holst KK, et al. Seasonal changes in brain serotonin transporter binding in short serotonin transporter linked polymorphic region-allele carriers but not in long-allele homozygotes. Biol Psychiatry. 2010;67(11):1033–9.
192. Tomita T, Yasui-Furukori N, Nakagami T, et al. The influence of 5-HTTLPR genotype on the association between the plasma concentration and therapeutic effect of paroxetine in patients with major depressive disorder. PLoS One. 2014;9:e98099.
193. Praschak-Rieder N, Willeit M, Wilson AA, Houle S, Meyer JH. Seasonal variation in human brain serotonin transporter binding. Arch Gen Psychiatry. 2008;65:1072–8.
194. Buchert R, Schulze O, Wilke F, et al. Is correction for age necessary in SPECT or PET of the central serotonin transporter in young, healthy adults? J Nucl Med. 2006;47:38–42.
195. Spindelegger C, Stein P, Wadsak W, et al. Light-dependent alteration of serotonin-1A receptor binding in cortical and subcortical limbic regions in the human brain. World J Biol Psychiatry. 2012;13:413–22.
196. Eisenberg DP, Kohn PD, Baller EB, et al. Seasonal effects on human striatal presynaptic dopamine synthesis. J Neurosci. 2010;30:14691–4.
197. Tsai HY, Chen KC, Yang YK, et al. Sunshine-exposure variation of human striatal dopamine D(2)/D(3) receptor availability in healthy volunteers. Prog Neuropsychopharmacol Biol Psychiatry. 2011;35:107–10.
198. Fujita M, Hines CS, Zoghbi SS, et al. Downregulation of brain phosphodiesterase type IV measured with ^{11}C-(R)-rolipram positron emission tomography in major depressive disorder. Biol Psychiatry. 2012;72:548–54.
199. Frick A, Åhs F, Engman J, et al. Serotonin synthesis and reuptake in social anxiety disorder: a positron emission tomography study. JAMA Psychiatry. 2015;72:794–802.
200. Baeken C, Bossuyt A, De Raedt R. Dorsal prefrontal cortical serotonin 2A receptor binding indices are differentially related to individual scores on harm avoidance. Psychiatry Res. 2014;221:162–8.
201. Tohyama Y, Yamane F, Merid MF, Diksic M. Effects of selective 5-HT1A receptor antagonists on regional serotonin synthesis in the rat brain: an autoradiographic study with alpha-[^{14}C] methyl-L-tryptophan. Eur Neuropsychopharmacol. 2001;11:193–202.
202. Hamon M, Lanfumey L, el Mestikawy S, et al. The main features of central 5-HT1 receptors. Neuropsychopharmacology. 1990;3:349–60.
203. Hurlemann R, Schlaepfer TE, Matusch A, et al. Reduced 5-HT(2A) receptor signaling following selective bilateral amygdala damage. Soc Cogn Affect Neurosci. 2008;4:79–84.
204. Selvaraj S, Turkheimer F, Rosso L, et al. Measuring endogenous changes in serotonergic neurotransmission in humans: a [^{11}C]CUMI-101 PET challenge study. Mol Psychiatry. 2012;17:1254–60.
205. Bosker FJ, Tanke MA, Jongsma ME, et al. Biochemical and behavioral effects of long-term citalopram administration and discontinuation in rats: role of serotonin synthesis. Neurochem Int. 2010;57:948–57.
206. Frick A, Ahs F, Linnman C, et al. Increased neurokinin-1 receptor availability in the amygdala in social anxiety disorder: a positron emission tomography study with [^{11}C]GR205171. Transl Psychiatry. 2015;5:e597.
207. Fredriksson R, Lagerström MC, Lundin LG, Schiöth HB. The G-protein-coupled receptors in the human genome form five main families. Phylogenetic analysis, paralogon groups and fingerprints. Mol Pharmacol. 2003;63:1256–72.
208. Riad M, Zimmer L, Rbah L, et al. Acute treatment with the antidepressant fluoxetine internalizes 5-HT1A autoreceptors and reduces the in vivo binding of the PET radioligand [^{18}F] MPPF in the nucleus raphe dorsalis of rat. J Neurosci. 2004;24:5420–6.
209. Chemel BR, Roth BL, Armbruster B, Watts VJ, Nichols DE. WAY-100635 is a potent dopamine D4 receptor agonist. Psychopharmacology (Berl). 2006;188:244–51.
210. Paterson LMKB, Nutt DJ, Pike WW, Knudsen GM. 5-HT radioligands for human brain imaging with PET and SPECT. Med Res Rev. 2013;33:54–111.
211. Zilles K, Palomero-Gallagher N, Schleicher A. Transmitter receptors and functional anatomy of the cerebral cortex. J Anat. 2004;205:417–32.
212. Fisher PM, Holst KK, Mc Mahon B, et al. 5-HTTLPR status predictive of neocortical 5-HT4 binding assessed with [^{11}C]SB207145 PET in humans. Neuroimage. 2012;62:130–6.
213. Lehto J, Scheinin A, Johansson J, et al. Detecting dexmedetomidine-evoked reduction of noradrenaline release in the human brain with the alpha2C adrenoceptor PET ligand [^{11}C]ORM-13070. Synapse. 2016;70:57–65.
214. Nahimi A, Jakobsen S, Munk OL, et al. Mapping α_2 adrenoceptors of the human brain with ^{11}C-yohimbine. J Nucl Med. 2015;56:392–8.

215. Yamamoto S, Ouchi Y, Nakatsuka D, et al. Reduction of [11C](+)3-MPB binding in brain of chronic fatigue syndrome with serum autoantibody against muscarinic cholinergic receptor. PLoS One. 2012;7:e51515.
216. Xie G, Gunn RN, Dagher A, et al. PET quantification of muscarinic cholinergic receptors with [N-11C-methyl]benztropine and application to studies of propofol-induced unconsciousness in healthy human volunteers. Synapse. 2004;51:91–101.
217. Zilles K, Amunts K. Receptor mapping: architecture of the human cerebral cortex. Curr Opin Neurol. 2009;22:331–9.
218. Podruchny TA, Connolly C, Bokde A, et al. In vivo muscarinic 2 receptor imaging in cognitively normal young and older volunteers. Synapse. 2003;48:39–44.
219. Ray R, Ruparel K, Newberg A, et al. Human Mu opioid receptor (OPMR1 A118G) polymorphism is associated with brain mu-opioid receptor bindingh potential in smokers. Proc Natl Acad Sci U S A. 2011;108:9268–73.
220. Sato H, Ito C, Hiraoka K, et al. Histamine H1 receptor occupancy by the new-generation antipsychotics olanzapine and quetiapine: a positron emission tomography study in healthy volunteers. Psychopharmacology (Berl). 2015;232:3497–505.
221. Hiraoka K, Tashiro M, Grobosch T, et al. Brain histamine H1 receptor occupancy measured by PET after oral administration of levocetirizine, a non-sedating antihistamine. Expert Opin Drug Saf. 2015;14:199–206.
222. Ashworth S, Berges A, Rabiner EA, et al. Unexpectedly high affinity of a novel histamine H(3) receptor antagonist, GSK239512, in vivo in human brain, determined using PET. Br J Pharmacol. 2014;171:1241–9.
223. Van Laere KJ, Sanabria-Bohórquez SM, Mozley DP, et al. (11)C-MK-8278 PET as a tool for pharmacodynamic brain occupancy of histamine 3 receptor inverse agonists. J Nucl Med. 2014;55:65–72.
224. Mølck C, Harpsøe K, Gloriam DE, et al. mGluR5: exploration of orthosteric and allosteric ligand binding pockets and their applications to drug discovery. Neurochem Res. 2014;39:1862–75.
225. Ahmed I, Bose SK, Pavese N, et al. Glutamate NMDA receptor dysregulation in Parkinson's disease with dyskinesias. Brain. 2011;134:979–86.
226. Dhawan V, Robeson W, Bjelke D, et al. Human Radiation Dosimetry for the N-Methyl-d-Aspartate Receptor Radioligand 11C-CNS5161. J Nucl Med. 2015;56:869–72.
227. McGinnity CJ, Hammers A, Riaño Barros DA, et al. Initial evaluation of 18F-GE-179, a putative PET Tracer for activated N-methyl D-aspartate receptors. Nucl Med. 2014;55:423–30.
228. Matsumoto R, Haradahira T, Ito H, et al. Measurement of glycine binding site of N-methyl-D-asparate receptors in living human brain using 4-acetoxy derivative of L-703,717, 4-acetoxy-7-chloro-3-[3-(4-[11C]ethoxybenzyl) phenyl]-2(1H)-quinolone (AcL703) with positron emission tomography. Synapse. 2007;61:795–800.
229. Brody AL, Mukhin AG, Mamoun MS, et al. Brain nicotinic acetylcholine receptor availability and response to smoking cessation treatment. A randomized trial. JAMA Psychiatry. 2014;71:797–805.
230. Wong DF, Kuwabara H, Kim J, et al. PET imaging of high-affinity α4β2 nicotinic acetylcholine receptors in humans with 18F-AZAN, a radioligand with optimal brain kinetics. J Nucl Med. 2013;54:1308–14.
231. Wong DF, Kuwabara H, Pomper M, et al. Human brain imaging of α7 nAChR with [18F]ASEM: a new PET radiotracer for neuropsychiatry and determination of drug occupancy. Mol Imaging Biol. 2014;16:730–8.
232. Fowler JS, Logan J, Shumay E, et al. Monoamine oxidase: radiotracer chemistry and human studies. J Labelled Comp Radiopharm. 2015;58:51–64.
233. Bretin F, BahriMA BC, et al. Biodistribution and radiation dosimetry for the novel SV2A radiotracer [18F]UCB-H: first in human study. Mol Imaging Biol. 2015;17:557–64.
234. Huang Y, Hwang DR, Narendran R, et al. Comparative evaluation in nonhuman primates of five PET radiotracers for imaging the serotonin transporters: [11C]McN 5652, [11C]ADAM,[11C] DASB, [11C]DAPA, and [11C]AFM. J Cereb Blood Flow Metab. 2002;22:1377–98.
235. Lundquist P, Blomquist G, Hartvig P, et al. Validation studies on the 5-hydroxy-L-[beta-11C]-tryptophan/PET method for probing the decarboxylase step in serotonin synthesis. Synapse. 2006;59:521–31.
236. Li CS, Potenza MN, Lee DE, et al. Decreased norepinephrine transporter availability in obesity: Positron Emission Tomography imaging with (S, S)-[11C]O-methylreboxetine. Neuroimage. 2013;86:306–10.
237. Joshi AD, Sanabria-Bohorquez S, Bormans G, et al. Characterization of the novel GlyT1 PET tracer [18F] MK6577 in humans. Synapse. 2015;69:33–40.
238. Wong DF, Ostrowitzki S, Zhou Y, et al. Characterization of [11C]RO5013853, a novel PET tracer for the glycine transporter type 1 (GlyT1) in humans. Neuroimage. 2013;75:282–90.
239. Huang CY, Liu CH, Tsao E, et al. Chronic manganism: a long-term follow-up study with a new dopamine terminal biomarker of 18F-FP-(+)-DTBZ (18F-AV-133) brain PET scan. J Neurol Sci. 2015;353:102–6.
240. Khayum MA, Doorduin J, Glaudemans AWJM, Dierckx RAJO, de Vries EFJ. PET and SPECT imaging of steroid hormone receptors. In: Dierckx R, Otte A, de Vries E, van Waarde A, Leenders KL, editors. PET and SPECT in neurology. Heidelberg: Springer; 2014.

Role of PET/CT in Pediatric Malignancy

21

Joe Barfett, Reza Vali, and Amer Shammas

Contents

21.1 **Introduction** 538
21.2 **Functional Versus Anatomic Imaging in Pediatric Malignancy** 538
21.3 **Special Considerations in the Pediatric Population** 540
21.3.1 Radiation Dose 540
21.3.2 Sedation 541
21.3.3 Special Considerations in ^{18}F-FDG PET/CT 541
21.3.4 Isotopes and Radiopharmaceuticals 542
21.3.5 Protocols for Fluorodeoxyglucose PET 542
21.3.6 F18-FDG PET Normal Variants and Pitfalls in Children 543
21.3.7 Standardized Uptake Values 543
21.3.8 Thymus 544
21.3.9 Tonsils 545
21.3.10 Marrow Hyperplasia 545
21.3.11 Brown Fat 545
21.3.12 Posttreatment Change 546
21.3.13 Other Pitfalls 546
21.3.14 Other Radiopharmaceuticals 547
21.4 **Image Fusion** 549
21.5 **Tumors of the Sympathetic Nervous System** 549
21.5.1 Neuroblastoma 549
21.5.2 Pheochromocytoma 553
21.6 **Lymphoma** 554
21.6.1 Hodgkin's Disease 554
21.6.2 Non-Hodgkin's Lymphoma 555
21.6.3 Initial Staging with ^{18}F-FDG PET/CT 556
21.6.4 Evaluation of Therapy Response with ^{18}F-FDG PET/CT 557
21.6.5 Evaluation of Relapse or Recurrence 558
21.6.6 Posttransplant Lymphoproliferative Disorder 558
21.7 **Leukemia** 560
21.8 **Tumors of the Brain and Central Nervous System** 560
21.9 **Osseous and Soft Tissue Malignancy** 562
21.9.1 Osteosarcoma 563
21.9.2 Ewing's Sarcoma 564
21.9.3 Rhabdomyosarcoma 565
21.10 **Nephroblastoma (Wilms' Tumor)** 566
21.11 **Hepatoblastoma** 566
21.12 **Thyroid Malignancy** 567
Conclusion 567
References 568

J. Barfett
Saint Michael Hospital, University of Toronto, Toronto, ON, Canada

R. Vali • A. Shammas (✉)
The Hospital for Sick Children, University of Toronto, Toronto, ON, Canada
e-mail: reza.vali@sickkids.ca; amer.shammas@sickkids.ca

Abstract

Positron emission tomography (PET)/computed tomography (CT) is emerging as an important noninvasive imaging modality for assessing a wide variety of malignancies in both adults and children. However, a different approach may be needed in children than that

M.M. Khalil (ed.), *Basic Science of PET Imaging*, DOI 10.1007/978-3-319-40070-9_21

of adults due to vulnerability of children to radiation, different types of malignancies in pediatric population comparing with adults, and special technical issues and pitfalls in pediatric PET/CT imaging. In this chapter, we discuss special considerations in pediatric PET/CT imaging and explore the use of FDG-PET in pediatric malignancies, including lymphomas, sympathetic nervous system tumors, bone and soft tissue sarcomas, neuroblastomas, and the less-common tumors, such as thyroid cancers, Wilms' tumors, and hepatoblastomas.

21.1 Introduction

Although the incidence of childhood malignancy is quite low, approximately 130 per million children in the United States [1], cancer remains the second most common cause of death in children age 1–14 years [2], second only to accidental death. The International Classification of Childhood Cancer (ICCC) categorizes pediatric malignancy into 12 major groups [3] including leukemias, brain and central nervous system malignancy, lymphomas, soft tissue sarcoma, tumors of the sympathetic nervous system, renal tumors, bone tumors, carcinoma and melanoma, germ cell tumors, retinoblastoma, hepatic tumors, and other or unspecified tumors (Table 21.1). Leukemia, central nervous system cancer, and lymphoma are the three most common forms of childhood cancer, accounting for 30, 20, and 14 % of overall incidence [4]. Outcome in these three particular malignancies has improved markedly in past decades and has contributed to an overall increase in 5-year survival from 58 % in 1977 to 83 % in 2007 [5].

The overall incidence of pediatric malignancy is increasing and has escalated from 0.5 % to approximately 1 % over the past 30 years with most of this increase having occurred in carcinoma, lymphoma, and germ cell tumors [4]. The reasons for this increase are not understood, and the pessimistic natural history of most pediatric cancers weighs against improvements in tracking and documentation of statistics as the sole cause.

Nuclear medicine and specifically positron emission tomography (PET) imaging have played a major role in the improved detection and staging of malignancy [6]. Thus PET/CT imaging is of pivotal importance in all pediatric cancer centers for most malignancies. A wealth of new PET tracers is on the horizon which promises to significantly expand the molecular imaging toolbox [7–9]. (See Chap. 17 for more details about new emerging PET tracers.)

21.2 Functional Versus Anatomic Imaging in Pediatric Malignancy

Although ultrasound is widely used in the initial detection of pediatric malignancy, CT and MR imaging remain the standard of care for the initial staging of most tumors, with the possible exception of leukemia as discussed below. As opposed to "emission tomography" which is common in nuclear medicine, computed tomography is a form of "transmission tomography" relying upon X-rays with energies generally between 60 and 140 keV depending primarily on the body habitus of the patient. As an X-ray imaging modality, CT images the spatial distribution of density, which is often significantly altered by malignancy. In addition, iodinated contrast enables the assessment of both the vascularity and, generally in a nonquantitative fashion, capillary permeability of structures under examination. 4D CT, which can potentially rigorously calculate perfusion and capillary leak in malignancy [10], is seldom used in the pediatric population due to the implicit relatively high radiation exposure and the short time over which that dose is applied. Where iodinated contrast is employed, the tube energy is often set to approximate the 32 keV K-edge of iodine [11] to maximize visibility of the agent as closely as possible while maintaining acceptable image quality. Dual energy CT, an old technique with fairly recent implementation in clinical practice, enables multi-element decomposition and can

Table 21.1 Age-adjusted and age-specific SEER Cancer Incidence Rates, 2005–2009 by the International Classification of Childhood Cancer (ICCC) http://seer.cancer.gov/csr/1975_2009_pops09/results_merged/sect_29_childhood_cancer_iccc.pdf

No.	Type of malignancy	Percentage (%)	0–14[a]	0–19[a]	5-year survival[b]
1	Leukemias	30	51.6	47.1	80.7
2	Brain and CNS tumors	20	42.2	43.1	72.1
3	lymphomas	14	16.6	25.1	90.0
4	Soft tissue sarcomas	7	10.9	12.4	71.0
5	SNS tumors	7	10.2	7.8	75.4
6	Renal tumors	6	7.8	6.3	88.8
7	Osseous tumors	5	7.3	9.2	69.0
8	Carcinomas	3	6.7	17.1	92.7
9	Germ cell tumors	3	5.7	11.9	91.2
10	Retinoblastomas	3	4.1	3.1	97.8
11	Hepatic tumors	1	2.5	2.2	68.2
12	Others	1	0.5	0.5	

[a]Rates are per 1,000,000 and are age adjusted to the 2000 US Std Population (19 age groups – Census P25-1130)
[b]5-Year Relative Survival (Percent), 2002–2008 by International Classification of Childhood Cancer(ICCC) Selected Group and Subgroup and Sex and Age. Benign brain and myelodysplastic syndromes are excluded

potentially supplement structural imaging with "iodine maps" which may offer improved routine assessment of these functional parameters at routine dose [12]. In CT, because the acquisition is so fast, problems such as patient motion or a mistimed contrast bolus which are common in pediatric imaging can only be corrected by repeat scanning which entails a second radiation dose. Low-dose CT is however extensively used in nuclear imaging for anatomic localization and attenuation correction and being an attenuation-based modality carries a technical advantage over MRI in this regard [13].

Conventional MR images the spatial distribution of hydrogen in water molecules using a hydrogen coil and strong magnetic fields. Unlike CT images, which can be acquired in seconds, a complete MRI requires several minutes to sometimes over an hour to acquire depending on the size of the imaging field, number and type of sequences chosen, and whether gadolinium-enhanced images are required. Thus sedation is often necessary in children, in our experience, under the age of 6 even with a skilled technologist. Although exquisite contrast resolution is available in MRI (unlike CT which offers better spatial resolution), MRI does not image tissue density directly and so carries limitations in terms of attenuation correction of nuclear images including PET. These limitations can potentially be overcome with appropriate software [14]. MRI is capable of high-end functional imaging including perfusion imaging, the imaging of molecular motion, intravascular flow assessment, and blood-oxygen-level-dependent (BOLD) imaging and offers numerous extensively described though more experimental techniques such as arterial spin labeling to assess perfusion without contrast, as well as thermometry to assess metabolic activity in the form of heat. It is important to note however that from a clinical point of view, none of these advanced tools has been shown to outperform PET/CT imaging clinically for the staging of disease or assessment of treatment response. Despite the power of MRI particularly in the brain, PET has remained a useful tool in addition to MRI to assess brain tumors for histologic grade, response to therapy, and recurrence [15–17]. In addition, because MRI is affected by signal dropout next to air, metal, or dense calcium, MRI is limited to assess the lung parenchyma, mucosal interfaces, or bone/tissue adjacent to orthopedic hardware [18–20].

Conversely nuclear imaging, especially PET when coupled with CT, excels in these technically challenging situations. In addition, PET images which are limited by problems such as motion artifact can often simply be reacquired without additional dose to the patient. All imaging modalities including CT, MRI, conventional nuclear imaging, and PET should be regarded as complimentary tools in a well-equipped imaging department, each with their own strengths.

21.3 Special Considerations in the Pediatric Population

Obtaining high-quality studies in children is both challenging and rewarding. It is important to understand that in pediatric nuclear medicine, the staff is working with both frightened child and anxious parents. Careful planning (including a flexible scheduling), communication appropriate for the child's stage of development, appropriate injection techniques, paying attention to the imaging environment (including the use of immobilization devices or safety restraints, distraction techniques, and the possibility of sedation when necessary), and a friendly atmosphere are the key factors to deal with children and their parents. In general, it takes about twice as long to complete a procedure on a pediatric patient as on an adult.

21.3.1 Radiation Dose

Although the oncogenic potential of ionizing radiation is a function of age, with younger patients being at higher risk than older patients, the likelihood of secondary malignancy arising as a result of diagnostic medical radiation exposure, even in children, is so low as to be statistically difficult to calculate [21]. Studies published to date claiming an association between medical radiation and cancer are influenced by controversial statistical assumptions or selection bias [6].

Studies assuming a linear no-threshold model of radiation injury deemed to be a conservative view by the International Commission on Radiological Protection and back-projecting atomic bomb and nuclear accident cancer risks are deemed by some authors as inappropriate [6]. These studies are contradicted by many years of high-dose I131 therapy data for hyperthyroidism which has failed to demonstrate any definite increase in cancer risk [22, 23].

Two principles can however be universally agreed upon:

1. Test only when truly medically indicated.
2. When testing, use as low a radiation dose as is reasonably achievable (ALARA).

ALARA applies to technologists and physicians as much as it applies to patients [24].

Although children are more radiosensitive than adults [25], nuclear medicine tracers have an advantage over X-ray imaging techniques such as CT in that the dose is applied over a longer duration [26]. Double-stranded DNA breaks, which are repaired over 1–4 h at diagnostic doses, may not compound with each other as readily in any given cell if a patient is radiated over hours (i.e., ^{18}F-FDG PET), days (i.e., Tc 99m), or weeks (i.e., Ga 67) for any given cumulative dose in mSv [27].

Shorter half-lives result in decreased cumulative dose. It is preferable for diagnostic purposes to avoid isotopes which emit beta or alpha particles, and as such I123 is strongly favored over I131 for scintigraphic applications. PET imaging in general employs shorter half-life tracers than conventional nuclear medicine imaging and benefits, on the whole, from a corresponding dose reduction, particularly where many of the on-site cyclotrons produced short half-life isotopes are concerned. PET dosimetry is discussed in Chap. 3.

An important caveat to the above however is in special populations, for example, children with known mutations inhibiting proper DNA repair. A classic example is retinoblastoma, where patients are so radiosensitive as to avoid sun and X-ray exposure as well as other sources of oxidative injury [28, 29]. In adults, the classic example is BRCA mutation, which is likely associated with increased radiosensitivity [30, 31]. Such special populations do become a major issue in specialized tertiary and quaternary pediatric hospitals. In these patients, there may be particularly aggressive application of ALARA, and MRI with sedation may in some instances be preferable to ionizing radiation exposure.

In 2015, it is no longer reasonable to assume that iodinated contrast media and gadolinium-based contrast agents do not produce oxidative DNA injury [32]. These agents produce the same double-stranded DNA injury as does radiation exposure, alcohol consumption [33], toxin exposure including smoking, and excessive exercise [34], all of which are discouraged in children and young adults.

The pediatric injected dose are usually calculated from the adult dose based on different formulas adjusting for weight ((body mass (kg) × adult dose)/70 kg), body surface area ((BSA (m^2) × adult dose)/1.73 m^2), age (Webster's formula; (age (years) + 7) × (adult dose)/(age (years) + 1)), or the European Association of Nuclear Medicine (EANM) Paediatric Dose Card [35–37]. With the new technology and improved instrumentation, the optimum doses for children should be changed. This was addressed in the new North American consensus guidelines published in 2010 [38]. However, the selection of the appropriate dose depends on the patient population, choice of equipment, specific requirements of the clinical protocols, and the physician's judgment [35]. Thus, deviation from the administered activities listed in the consensus guidelines can be considered appropriate when clinically indicated [35].

21.3.2 Sedation

Pharmacologic sedation can be kept to a minimum with adequate patient preparation, patient and parent education, as well as technologists that are experienced in the care of children. When absolutely necessary, the most commonly used drugs include midazolam, oral chloral hydrate, and pentobarbital [39, 40]. Patients > 15 kg with developmental delay are also most commonly sedated with either midazolam or pentobarbital [39, 40]. Pentobarbital, as all barbiturates, is contraindicated in patients with porphyria. Seizure patients subjected to pentobarbital may require dose adjustments or tapering of dose [40].

In addition to its sedative and anxiolytic effects, benzodiazepines such as midazolam have useful amnestic effect which can be particularly helpful if a patient must be exposed to multiple repeat tests in an imaging department [40]. In general each center will have its own guidelines on the sedation of children. For reference, the American Academy of Pediatrics (AAP) also publishes useful guidelines which guide best practices. Institutional protocols should be developed in collaboration with anesthesiology and include the availability of reversal drugs [39]. The continuing support and availability of anesthesiology is of immense benefit to a nuclear medicine department specializing in the care of children.

Patients with risk factors for anesthesia, including but not limited to airway obstruction, snoring, cardiorespiratory illness of any kind, asthma, intracranial pressure abnormality, or altered neck biomechanics, would benefit the most from real-time monitoring by a qualified anesthetist. Risks such as malignant hyperthermia should also be considered [40]. Playing with the patient; providing a pacifier, bottle, or (preferably non attenuating) toy; the use of distractors including nap time and room decorations; the availability of experienced and qualified technologists; and booking adequate time for imaging of difficult cases will significantly reduce the need for sedation in an imaging department.

21.3.3 Special Considerations in ^{18}F-FDG PET/CT

The use of PET/CT was less frequent than adults for several reasons, including the concern about the radiation dose, less common frequency of children malignancy, and the lack of availability of PET/CT in pediatric centers. However, the usefulness of PET/CT in pediatric malignancy has been shown in many studies during the last decade. Although the basis of PET/CT in children is the same as adult, there are some physiologic variation in ^{18}F-FDG biodistribution and potential pitfalls in pediatric population which are needed to be addressed for correct interpretation of the images. Some of these issues are discussed in this section.

21.3.4 Isotopes and Radiopharmaceuticals

PET isotopes are generally cyclotron produced and have shorter half-lives than their conventional nuclear medicine counterparts. Fluorine 18 (F18), with a half-life of 110 min, is among the longer lived PET tracers. The most common F18 tracer is fluorodeoxyglucose (^{18}F-FDG). ^{18}F-FDG has found numerous applications in the assessment and staging of cancers throughout the body, assessing response to treatment, and is used widely in the assessment of organ metabolism particularly in the heart and brain.

F18′s half-life is long enough to permit offsite production and compounding into a radiopharmaceutical of interest. Other commonly used PET isotopes include N13 (half-life ~10 min) and O15 (half-life ~2 min) which are used in N13 ammonia and oxygen 15 water studies, respectively. The half-life of these isotopes is so short that they necessitate production in an on-site cyclotron. Such cyclotrons have dropped dramatically in price in recent years. Negative ion cyclotrons are entirely self-shielded and have a small footprint in an imaging department. On-site compounding and synthesis of PET tracers can be semiautomated but does usually require dedicated personnel including, ideally, a radiopharmacist.

21.3.5 Protocols for Fluorodeoxyglucose PET

As in adult, reviewing the history, clinical indication, history of diabetes, fasting states, recent infection, patient ability to lie still during the acquisition, and the need for sedation should be reviewed before the study [41]. Patients are instructed to fast and not consume beverages, except for water, for at least 4–6 h before the administration of ^{18}F-FDG to decrease physiologic glucose levels and to reduce serum insulin levels to near basal levels. Insulin levels greatly affect the biodistribution of ^{18}F-FDG, and where ^{18}F-FDG is used, care should be taken to ensure that a patient has not eaten in the 4–6 h preceding a study. Blood glucose should be checked before the administration of ^{18}F-FDG and should be in the range of approximately 3–11 μmol/mL. Diabetic children pose a special problem and may, if they are significantly hyperglycemic, administer a weight-based sliding scale dose of insulin and wait at least an hour prior to injection. It would be better to rebook the case if possible to a day when euglycemia is achieved. Weight, height, and blood glucose concentrations are recorded for all patients.

Image acquisition for the whole body PET scan usually starts approximately 60–90 min after injection of 5.18 MBq/kg (0.14 mCi/kg) ^{18}F-FDG, at doses ranging from 37 MBq (1 mCi) to 370 MBq (10 mCi). Patients were imaged from skull base to mid-thighs (approximately 3 min per bed position). The number of bed positions depends on the size of the patient, and it is usually less than 7 bed positions in small children and 7–10 bed positions for adolescents. In general, the arms are elevated over the head to avoid beam-hardening artifacts over the torso [41]. However, for optimal imaging of the head and neck, the arms should be positioned along the side [41]. The patient should void before the acquisition of the images to limit the radiation dose to the kidneys and bladder and also to be able to lie still on the bed for the acquisition time. Metallic objects and any other unnecessary objects should be removed from the patient whenever possible [41].

Dual-time point ^{18}F-FDG PET imaging usually consists of initial imaging at 60 min after tracer injection and then reimaging later at 2–4 h postinjection. Dual-time point image is based on the premise that ^{18}F-FDG uptake in inflammatory cells usually washes out, while ^{18}F-FDG tends to be retained in malignant cells [42, 43]. Dual-time protocols have been used in pediatric population but for logistic reasons are not frequently applied in practice [44].

In children and adolescents and particularly when the weather is cold, it can be helpful to provide an ambient room for approximately 1 hour prior to injection of ^{18}F-FDG to decrease metabolism in brown fat [45]. Patients who had recently undergone diagnostic CT scans are imaged using a low-dose helical CT scan (in our protocol: 5 mm/slice, 90 kV; 20 and 30 mA for patients weighing <30 and ≥ 30 kg, respectively) prior to the PET scan for attenuation correction and anatomic localization. Diagnostic CT scans were obtained when clinically indicated and when patients do not have a recent CT scan. In those cases, the attenuation correction is calculated based on the correlative diagnostic CT images (in our protocol: 5 mm/slice, 120 kV, and a weight-based range for the mA, with dose modulation).

21.3.6 F18-FDG PET Normal Variants and Pitfalls in Children

The normal distribution of ^{18}F-FDG uptake in children is unique and may differ from that in adults. A number of physiologic variants are commonly seen, including normal physiologic activity in the head and neck, heart, breast, thymus, liver, spleen, gastrointestinal tract, genital system, urinary collecting system, bone marrow, muscles, and brown adipose tissue [46]. Benign lesions with increased ^{18}F-FDG activity are also frequently seen and can be misinterpreted as malignancies [46]. Other parameters such as the standardized uptake value (SUV) can also be different in pediatric population.

21.3.7 Standardized Uptake Values

The standardized uptake value (SUV) is a measurement unique to PET and is defined as attenuation-corrected activity in a region of interest divided by decay-corrected injected activity divided by body mass [47, 48]. It is also important to note that activity in a region of interest does change somewhat with different devices and reconstruction algorithms [49]. Still, standardized uptake value is the key semiquantitative parameter on which PET quantification is based and can be presumed to be reasonably reliable when patients are reimaged on the same device with the same dose of tracer over a time frame such that body weight is reasonably consistent.

SUVmax, or the largest SUV value in an ROI, is often chosen due to its reproducibility between readers (i.e., cancers are generally hotter on PET toward their center of mass, due to both cellular density and partial volume effects). Changes in SUV or SUVmax can indicate the aggressiveness of disease or response to therapy. In general, cancer responding to therapy will show a decrease in SUVmax, with the exception of radiation treatment of tumor which will often go through a short-term hypermetabolic phase followed by a gradual decline (see below). Measurement of SUV in small ROIs can be made less reliable by partial volume effects [50] (see Chap. 15 for further details).

It is important to recognize that fat has a relatively low metabolic rate, and so some authors prefer to normalize to lean body mass or body surface area in the SUV calculation, particularly in obese patients, where normalized to body weight SUV can be artifactually overestimated in non-adipose tissue [48]. The percentage of fat is changing in pediatric patients from 11 % in the newborn to about 26 % during the following 5 months and then decreases gradually until 12 months of age [51]. After that the percentage of fat depends on many factors including diet, physical activity, and genetics [51]. Thus, pediatric SUV normalized to body weight is not exactly the same as that of adults. Moreover, the clinical significance of SUV values in different pathologies and normal versus suspected malignancy reference numbers in children cannot be simply extrapolated from the adult values and should be interpreted cautiously. The optimal method for calculating SUV in children may be different from that used in adults due to the body changes and growth that take place during childhood. Therefore, it has been suggested that, in pediatric patients, SUV calculated on the basis of body surface area would serve as a better metabolic activity marker than would SUV calculated on the basis of body weight.

21.3.8 Thymus

Thymic tissue persists in children and often persists into early adulthood. Thymus is often mildly to moderately ^{18}F-FDG avid on PET and can be mistaken for mediastinal tumor (Fig. 21.1). Thickness of the thymus gland, measured perpendicular to a lobe, should be less than 1.8 cm in children under twenty and 1.3 cm in older patients [52, 53]. The shape of the thymus is quadrilateral during childhood and triangular during adolescence. Morphologic features such as thickness of the gland and its homogeneity are used on either diagnostic or low-dose localizer CT to determine the presence of disease [53].

Thymus uptake of ^{18}F-FDG can increase following chemotherapy which is a frequent consequence of chemotherapy, especially in young patients undergoing chemotherapy for lymphoma, leukemia, or testicular cancer. The reasons for this hyperplasia are debated. An important function of the thymus is to "train" lymphocytes toward adap-

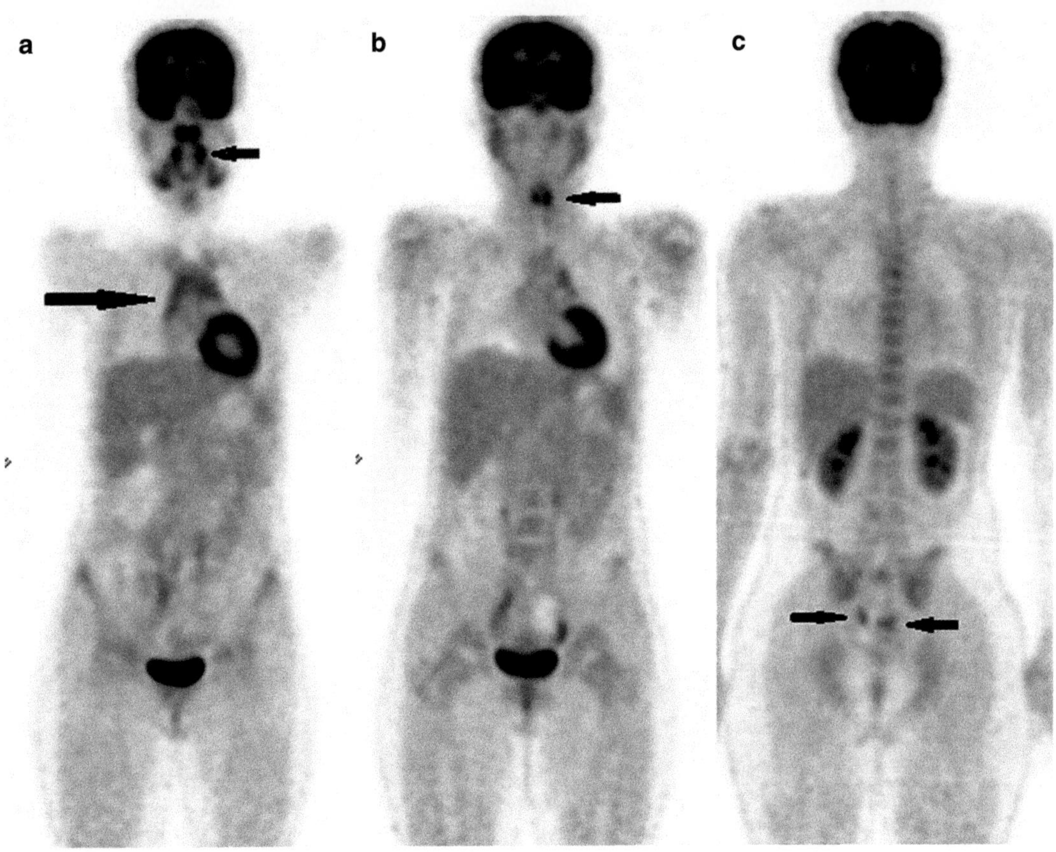

Fig. 21.1 Physiologic activity in a 13-year-old female. (**a**) Physiologic activity in the palatine and lingual (*small arrow*) tonsils and normal uptake in the thymus (*long arrow*). (**b**) Physiologic activity in the vocal cords or muscles in the vocal cord region (*arrow*). (**c**) Normal uptake of the bone marrow. Foci of activity in the pelvic region due to follicular activity of ovaries (*arrows*)

tive immunity. Chemotherapy is associated with decreased white counts and thymus atrophy. Steroids, frequently concomitant with chemotherapy for the treatment of lymphoma, can also induce thymus atrophy which then "rebounds" with subsequent marrow hyperplasia [54].

It can be challenging to differentiate benign from malignant thymus ^{18}F-FDG activity. In general, homogeneous thymic uptake at post-therapy ^{18}F-FDG PET and the absence of uptake at pre-therapy ^{18}F-FDG PET indicate post-therapy thymic hyperplasia. To some extent the SUV of thymus tissue can guide decisions. Brink et al. reported a mean SUV of 2.8 and max of 3.8 in thymic hyperplasia [54]. Ferdinand et al. indicates that thymic SUV >4 warrants further investigation to exclude malignancy [55].

Thymic carcinoma is a rare malignancy in children and in general is associated with significantly increased ^{18}F-FDG uptake. Sasaki et al. reported SUV of 7.2 ± 2.9 in thymus carcinoma, which is in turn significantly higher than activity found in invasive thymoma (3.8 ± 1.3) and noninvasive thymoma (3 ± 1) [56]. Thymoma can therefore not be reliably differentiated from thymus hyperplasia. Morphologic features on CT are helpful in these cases to differentiate benign change from malignancy.

21.3.9 Tonsils

The tonsils are very metabolically active in children and can demonstrate significant ^{18}F-FDG avidity on PET scan (Fig. 21.1). The palatine and lingual tonsils, in part because of their size, are particularly avid. Upper respiratory tract infections can cause tonsillar hypertrophy and increased thymus metabolism. The symmetry of tonsil activity is an important means of differentiating benign from malignant processes [57]. Lymphoma in the head and neck, oropharyngeal malignancy, and posttransplant lymphoproliferative disorder (PTLD) are all associated with increased ^{18}F-FDG activity and can mimic or be difficult to differentiate from normal functioning tonsillar tissue. Comparison to any prior ^{18}F-FDG PET imaging and correlation to CT, ultrasound, or MR imaging can be helpful in the assessment of challenging cases.

21.3.10 Marrow Hyperplasia

Marrow suppression is a frequent complication of chemotherapy with or without colony-stimulating factor administration and can also result from tumor infiltration of bone marrow. After treatment, most often by chemotherapy or steroids, suppressed marrow can subsequently rebound and demonstrate diffuse hypermetabolism, with increased activity on ^{18}F-FDG PET that can be confused for diffuse malignant change [58–60]. Anemia, including thalassemia, medications such as interferon can also cause diffuse increased bone activity and represent an important cause of false-positive findings [61, 62]. Treatment with hematopoietic cytokines such as granulocyte colony-stimulating factor (CSF), hematopoietic growth factor, or erythropoietin can also produce diffuse skeletal ^{18}F-FDG accumulation. Increased activity can persist for up to 3 weeks after the discontinuation of granulocyte CSF treatment. Increased activity in the spleen is also frequently noted in association with increased marrow activity (Fig. 21.2). Normal bone marrow is mildly ^{18}F-FDG avid that is less intense than liver activity (Fig. 21.1).

21.3.11 Brown Fat

Physiologic high uptake from activated adrenergic innervation of adipocytes is a normal variant especially in children. This brown fat, rich in mitochondria, is more common in children than adults and is typically found in the neck, supraclavicular regions, axillae, mediastinum, and paravertebral and perinephric regions. The distribution of brown fat is usually symmetric. However, focal and asymmetric uptake can occur in the neck or mediastinum, leading to false-positive results.

Brown fat because of its ^{18}F-FDG avidity can present a considerable problem in the interpretation

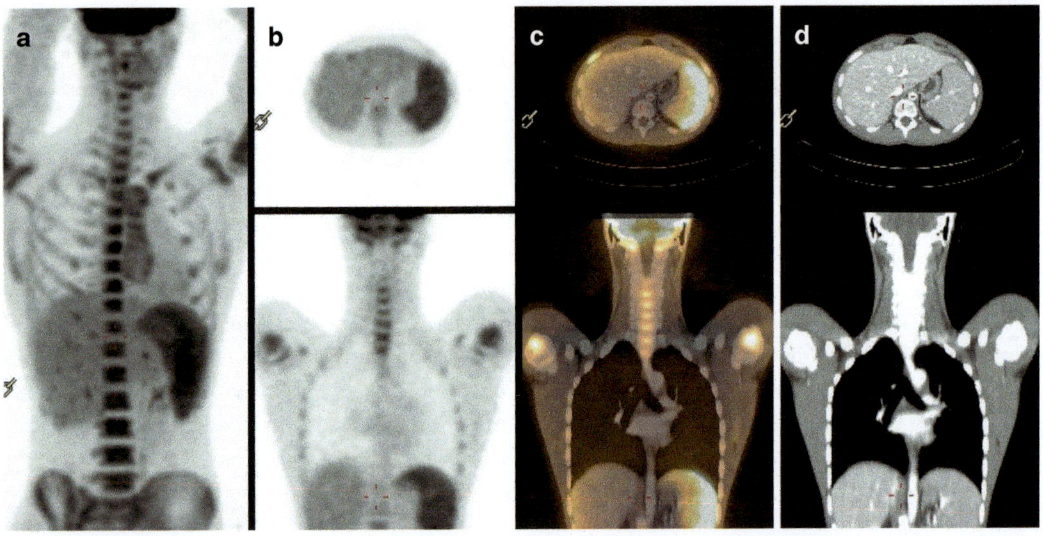

Fig. 21.2 18F-FDG PET/CT in a 17-year-old patient with lymphoma after two cycles of chemotherapy and one day after injection of GCSF. (**a**) Maximum intensity projection (MIP), (**b**) Axial and coronal PET, (**c**) Axial- and coronal-fused PET/CT, and (**d**) CT scan showed marked improvement of the activity previously visualized in the mediastinum (not shown here). Increased activity in the spleen and bone marrow is due to GCSF effect

of ^{18}F-FDG PET studies (Fig. 21.3). The most practical way to control brown fat activity is to control the temperature of the patient before injection and in the period between injection and image acquisition [45, 63]. Some authors have also used medication, most commonly propranolol and diazepam, to decrease activity in brown fat [63].

Fusion imaging with CT enables to differentiate between ^{18}F-FDG uptake corresponding to fat-attenuation tissue at CT and uptake from pathologic causes.

21.3.12 Posttreatment Change

It is generally recommended to wait at least 4–6 weeks after surgery and at least 1–2 weeks after biopsy prior to performing ^{18}F-FDG PET [64]. A shorter interval than this has been associated with physiologic increased uptake in healing tissues which could be mistaken for a false positive. It is important for institutions to develop a practice pattern in conjunction with the treating physician.

Radiation therapy is associated with inflammation and the recruitment of white blood cells which are intensely ^{18}F-FDG avid. Thus, tumors subjected to radiotherapy can demonstrate marked increased ^{18}F-FDG uptake which can persist for weeks. It is ideal to wait 6 weeks after radiation therapy prior to PET imaging to assess response [64]. Reduced bone marrow ^{18}F-FDG uptake can be noted several months after external beam radiation therapy. This phenomenon has been attributed to the replacement of bone marrow by fatty tissue.

21.3.13 Other Pitfalls

If children are significantly active before ^{18}F-FDG administration or in the interval between ^{18}F-FDG administration and imaging, uptake in metabolically active muscles may limit assessment. It is best for patients undergoing ^{18}F-FDG PET imaging to avoid strenuous exercise or vigorous sports in the days which precede imaging. Chewing of gum or sucking pacifier after ^{18}F-FDG injection can cause symmetric intense uptake in the masseter muscles. Uptake in the diaphragm, the crura of the diaphragm, and the intercostal muscles can be detected in children who have been crying during the uptake phase.

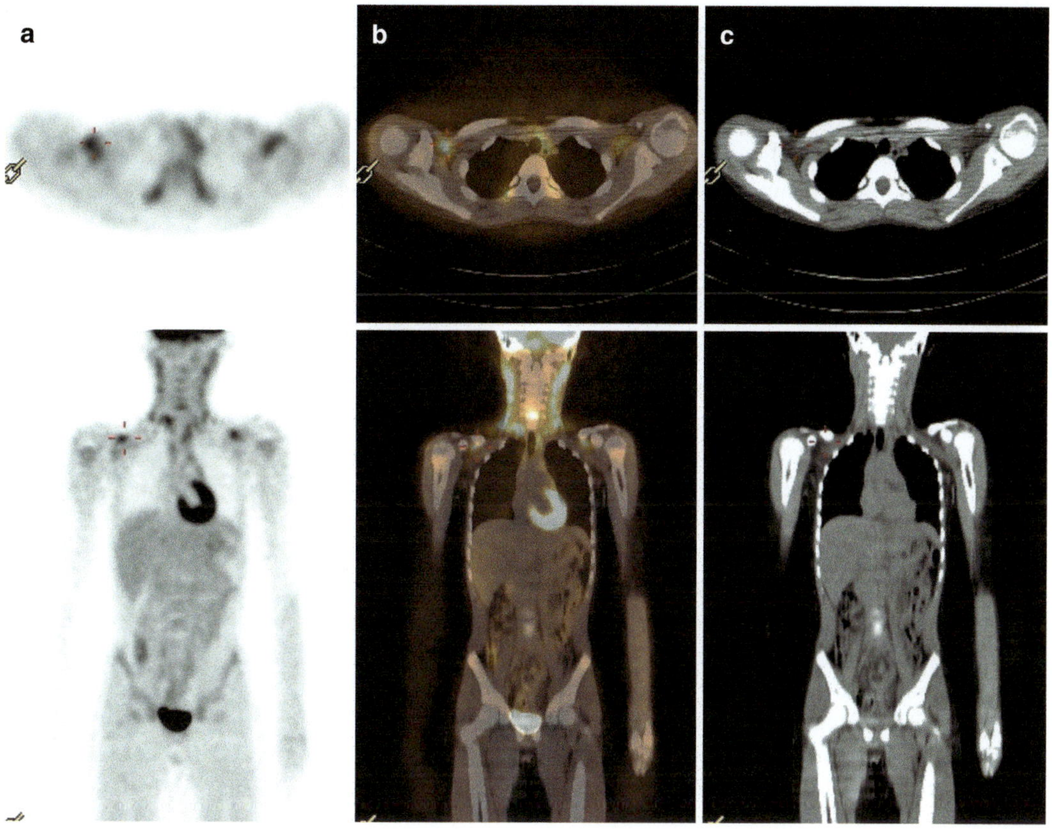

Fig. 21.3 Axial and coronal PET (**a**), fused PET/CT (**b**), and CT (**c**) of 18F-FDG PET/CT in a 12-year-old boy diagnosed with large B-cell lymphoma 3 years before, referred for evaluation of recurrence. Multiple foci of FDG activity are noted in the neck, supraclavicular region, and chest bilaterally corresponding to the hypodense regions on CT due to brown fat uptake. The patient had positive neck lymph nodes, an FDG-avid lesion in the right lung, and lumbar spine involvement which were not shown here

A common source of a false negative in ^{18}F-FDG PET scan is altered biodistribution caused by improper patient preparation. Usually this is due to increased circulating insulin and characterized by decreased uptake in tumor, decreased uptake in the brain, and increased uptake in peripheral skeletal muscle. Repeating the exam may be indicated in such a situation [72].

A second common cause of a false negative is the collision of tumor activity with the normal biodistribution of activity and can be a problem particularly in the genitourinary system on ^{18}F-FDG PET as ^{18}F-FDG is cleared by the kidneys [72]. Visibility of cancers in the genitourinary tract can be limited on ^{18}F-FDG PET. If possible and age appropriate, patients should empty the bladder prior to ^{18}F-FDG PET image acquisition.

21.3.14 Other Radiopharmaceuticals

Studies on the use of other PET tracers beyond ^{18}F-FDG in pediatric population are limited. ^{18}F-sodium fluoride (^{18}F-NaF) has been extensively used in adult for detection of bone metastases in different tumors and can also potentially be useful in pediatric patients [65, 66]. Accumulation of ^{18}F-NaF in the skeletal system is similar to that of 99mTC-MDP based on local blood flow and osteoblastic activity. However, the protein binding is lower allowing for earlier images than conventional bone scan. The extraction of ^{18}F-NaF is also higher than 99mTC-MDP. Thus the image contrast is better with ^{18}F-NaF. PET images also provide better spatial resolution than conventional gamma cameras. However, the radiation dose is higher than the bone scan. The recommended dose of ^{18}F-NaF is approximately 2.2 MBq/kg, with a minimum of 11.1 MBq and a maximum of 148 MBq [67]. Imaging starts 45–60 min after the radiotracer administration. The biodistribution of the tracer is similar to the 99mTC-MDP and depends on the patient's age with more activity in the growth plates.

3′-Deoxy-3′-[F18]-fluorothymidine (^{18}F-FLT) FLT is an analog of thymidine and the uptake reflects cellular proliferation. Thus increased activity with ^{18}F-FLT is more suggestive of tumor proliferation than inflammation. FLT is retained in proliferating tissues and malignant tumors through the activity of thymidine kinase 1 (TK1), an enzyme that is highly expressed during the DNA synthesis phase of the cell cycle [68]. TK1 phosphorylates FLT to form negatively charged FLT-monophosphates which are impermeable to the cell membrane. Since most tumor cells have a much higher TK1 activity than normal cells, the intracellular trapping of FLT and accumulation of radioactivity occurs [68]. Current published literature have demonstrated the feasibility of using FLT PET imaging in patients with lung cancer [69–72], gastrointestinal cancer [73, 74], melanoma [75], lymphoma [76, 77], breast cancer [78, 79], soft tissue sarcomas [80], as well as primary malignant brain tumors in adults and children [81–85]. ^{18}F-FLT has been safely administered to children between the ages of 2–13 years with no observable adverse effects [81–85]. ^{18}F-FLT minimally crosses intact blood–brain barrier [86, 87], thus the high background activity which is typically visualized with ^{18}F-FDG is not seen using ^{18}F-FLT. Published literature related to the use of ^{18}F-FLT PET in the evaluation of CNS tumors in the pediatric population is limited and restricted only to studies involving children with glioblastoma [81–85]. The recommended dose is 5.18 MBq/kg (0.14 mCi/kg) using a minimum dose of 37 MBq (1 mCi) up to a maximum of 370 MBq (10 mCi). Imaging is usually performed 45–60 min after the radiotracer administration.

Tumors have varying degrees of hypoxia. Tumor hypoxia may be related to chaotic vasculature in some tumors or rapid growth in others. It is usually associated with increase angiogenesis and tumor aggressiveness [88, 89]. Studies have shown that tumor hypoxia increases the risk of metastases and decreases the sensitivity to chemo/radiation therapy [90–93]. This may be due to the aggressiveness of the tumor or abnormal vasculature that may diminish delivery of anticancer therapy. Using hypoxia-selective cytotoxins may increase the effect of chemo/radiation therapy [94–97]. Tumor hypoxia has been also reported to be associated with increased risk of recurrence and a poorer prognosis [89, 98]. Detection of hypoxic components of tumors is possible with histologic evaluation. However, due to the patient situation, tumor type, location, etc., surgical resection of tumors is not recommended in all malignancies. Moreover, in some instances, information of hypoxic component of tumor is needed before the surgical resection (e.g., before neoadjuvant treatment in osteosarcoma). Tissue biopsy is inaccurate in these situations since it may not reflect the whole tumor. Imaging is a surrogate marker of histological assessment to detect these hypoxic components as it is noninvasive and repeatable and represents the whole tumor. 1-α-D-(5-deoxy-5-[18 F]-fluoroarabinofuranosyl)-2-nitroimidazole (^{18}F-FAZA) is a 2-nitroimidazole-based molecule that undergoes reductive metabolism under hypoxic conditions, producing reactive intermediates that bind to intracellular macromolecules. Studies in adult population and different tumors have shown that 18F-FAZA is a promising radiotracer for detection of hypoxic components in tumors [96, 99]. The recommended dose is 5.2 MBq/kg (0.14 mCi/kg) using a minimum dose of 37 MBq (1 mCi) up to a maximum of 370 MBq (10 mCi). Imaging is usually performed 2–3 h after the radiotracer administration (hypoxia tracers are reviewed in Chap. 17).

11C-Methionine (11C-METH) is an amino acid PET tracer mainly used in brain imaging tumors. The uptake in brain tumor is probably related to passive diffusion from the altered blood–brain barrier and active uptake by the tumor due to increased amino acid metabolism. Similar to the ^{18}F-FLT, the background activity is very minimal with 11C-METH, allowing detection of small viable brain tumors. The pediatric studies were limited; however, they showed a higher sensitivity of 11C-METH for the detection of viable brain tumor than that of ^{18}F-FDG [100, 101]. The pediatric dose and protocol are not well established. In general, due to the short half-life of C11, imaging will start 20 min after the administration of 5.5 MBq/kg of the radiotracer [101].

68Ga-DOTA-conjugated peptides [68Ga-DOTA0-Tyr3]octreotide (68Ga-DOTATOC, 68Ga-edotreotide), [68Ga-DOTA0-1NaI3]octreotide (68GaDOTA-NOC), and [68Ga-DOTA0-Tyr3]octreotate (68GaDOTA-TATE) have been used to detect somatostatin receptor-positive tumors. Somatostatin receptors are positive in a variety of tumors [102]. The activity administered ranges from 100 to 200 MBq in adults [102]. The exact dose in pediatric patients is not well established; the dose in children should be reduced according to the recommendations of the EANM Paediatric Task Group [102]. Imaging is usually obtained 45–90 min after the radiotracer administration depending on the type of analog used [102].

Other radiotracers like 11C-hydroxyephedrine (HED), 11C-epinephrine, and 18-F-dihydroxyphenylalanine (DOPA) have been also used for sympathetic nervous system and neuroendocrine tumors. 11C-HED is similar to norepinephrine (NE), but unlike NE it is not metabolized and is used for sympathetic nervous tumors imaging [103]. 11C-Epinephrine has been used in pheochromocytoma and neuroblastoma [104]. ^{18}F-DOPA has been also used in pheochromocytoma, hyperinsulinemia, and brain tumors [105].

21.4 Image Fusion

Nuclear medicine image techniques benefit strongly from attenuation correction to mitigate the effects of photon absorption by the patient. Although historically transmission attenuation correction was used for this purpose [106], the widespread dissemination and reduced cost of CT led to the coupling of PET and SPECT to low-dose CT exams for anatomic localization and correction. Attenuation, itself a function of density, is ideally corrected by the density maps produced in CT. Acquisition of CT data with PET data usually minimizes the registration problem.

Increasingly in pediatric nuclear medicine practice, where a diagnostic CT is required, PET imaging can be acquired simultaneously with diagnostic CT on a hybrid device supporting a multi-slice CT scanner [107]. PET/MRI is a more recent development which enables the simultaneous acquisition of PET and MRI data, though at considerable expense and with potentially longer acquisition times. Pediatric centers, which usually have to sedate children undergoing MRI [108], often cite both this fact and the limitations of MRI for attenuation correction as a reason not to opt for a hybrid PET/MRI device. Using multisequence MRI to perform attenuation correction reliably is an area of active investigation, and significant advances have been recently made [109–112].

21.5 Tumors of the Sympathetic Nervous System

21.5.1 Neuroblastoma

Sympathetic nervous system (SNS) tumors account for about 7 % of all pediatric malignancies. Neuroblastoma, including ganglioneuroblastoma, is the most common form of all SNS tumors in children (approximately 97 %). Neuroblastoma (NBL) is a common lesion in young children and unfortunately associated with significant mortality. NBL accounts for 20 % of malignancy in children diagnosed below the age of 1 year and is especially common during the first 3 months of infancy. NBL is the second most common, after brain tumors, solid malignancy in childhood.

The long-term survival of NBL patients remains challenging. Age remains among the most important predictors of survival in NBL patients, with presentation beyond 5 years associated with a 5-year survival of approximately 40%. Survival in younger children, especially less than 1 year, has improved dramatically since 1975, from approximately 35–83% today as a result of improved therapy. Aside from age, stage at diagnosis is a very important prognostic indicator, with complete resection of a local tumor and negative margins indicating a more optimistic long-term prognosis. Molecular and cytogenetic factors including DNA content, proto-oncogenes, and catecholamine synthesis are all linked to prognosis.

The etiology of neuroblastoma is unclear. The predilection of the tumor in infants has implicated genetic factors or in utero toxicity, for example, alcohol [113] or other drug exposure, as potentially playing a role in causation [114, 115]. The effects of maternal substance and/or environmental exposures on the development of neuroblastoma is however controversial [116].

Diagnosis of neuroblastoma is usually enabled by a combination of imaging findings and elevated serum or urine catecholamines. There is a spectrum of catecholamine metabolites including dopamine, homovanillic acid, and vanillylmandelic acid which can be represented in neuroblastoma patients [117].

The natural history of neuroblastoma is quite variable, with some patients demonstrating spontaneous regression and some patients demonstrating differentiation of tumor into mature nonmalignant tissue. Other NBLs demonstrate aggressive behavior despite multimodality treatment and are associated with poor outcomes.

The International Neuroblastoma Staging System (INSS) uses the distribution of disease as evidenced by imaging studies, operability, lymph node metastases, and bone marrow metastases as factors influencing prognosis (Table 21.2). The more recent International Neuroblastoma Risk Group (INRG) system describes 13 potential prognostic factors to categorize patients into four groups (5-year survival of <50%, 50–75%, 75–85%, and >85%) [118].

Metastases are unfortunately common at presentation, and hence multimodality imaging is important in the initial assessment of neuroblastoma [119]. Ultrasound is a frequent first test in a child with typical symptoms of abdominal mass, pain, anemia, fever, weight loss, paraneoplastic syndrome, and occasionally blindness. Ultrasound is usually followed by diagnostic CT or MRI. With positive biochemistry, scintigraphy is generally employed I123 MIBG for definitive workup [120, 121].

Table 21.2 International Neuroblastoma Staging System (INSS)

Stage	Description
1	Localized tumor with complete gross excision (with or without microscopic residual disease) with no ipsilateral lymph nodes involvement
2a	Localized tumor with incomplete gross excision and no ipsilateral lymph involvement
2b	Localized tumor with or without complete gross excision, with ipsilateral lymph nodes involvement
3	Unresectable unilateral tumor crossing the midline (with or without regional lymph node involvement); or localized unilateral tumor with contralateral regional lymph node involvement; or midline tumor with bilateral extension which is unresectable or with positive lymph nodes
4	Any primary tumor with involvement of distant lymph nodes, bone, bone marrow, liver, skin, and/or other organs (except as defined for stage 4S)
4s	Localized primary tumor (as defined for stage 1, 2A, or 2B), with metastases limited to the skin, liver, and/or bone marrow (limited to infants 1 year of age)

MIBG scintigraphy has been extensively described for the workup of NBL and remains standard of care at even quaternary pediatric oncology centers [120, 121]. MIBG has been used in prognostication and in assessment of response to therapy, with a decrease or absence of MIBG activity following therapy indicative of a good prognosis. Similarly, as bone metastases are quite common in NBL, the Tc 99m MDP bone scan has been used extensively for the assessment of osseous metastases [122]. However, in approximately 10% of cases, NBL is not MIBG avid (Fig. 21.4).

$^{18}F-FDG\,PET$ has shown utility in NBL patients, and both the primary tumor and metastases may be ^{18}F-FDG avid (Fig. 21.5), even in

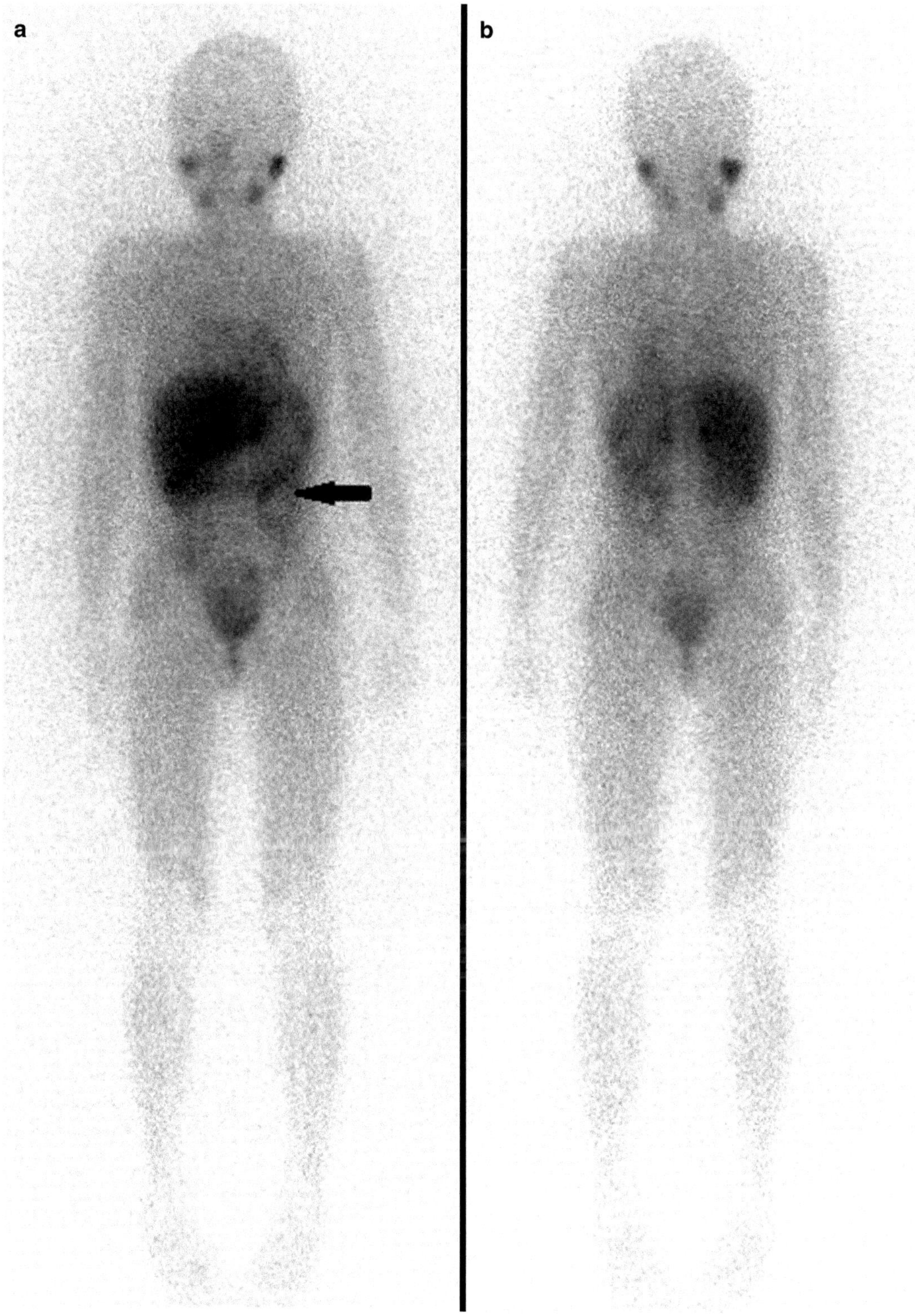

Fig. 21.4 Twelve-year-old male with neuroblastoma in the left abdomen. (**a**) Anterior and (**b**) posterior MIBG scan showed mild MIBG activity in the region of the tumor (*arrow*). The liver uptake was inhomogeneous with no definite focal increased activity

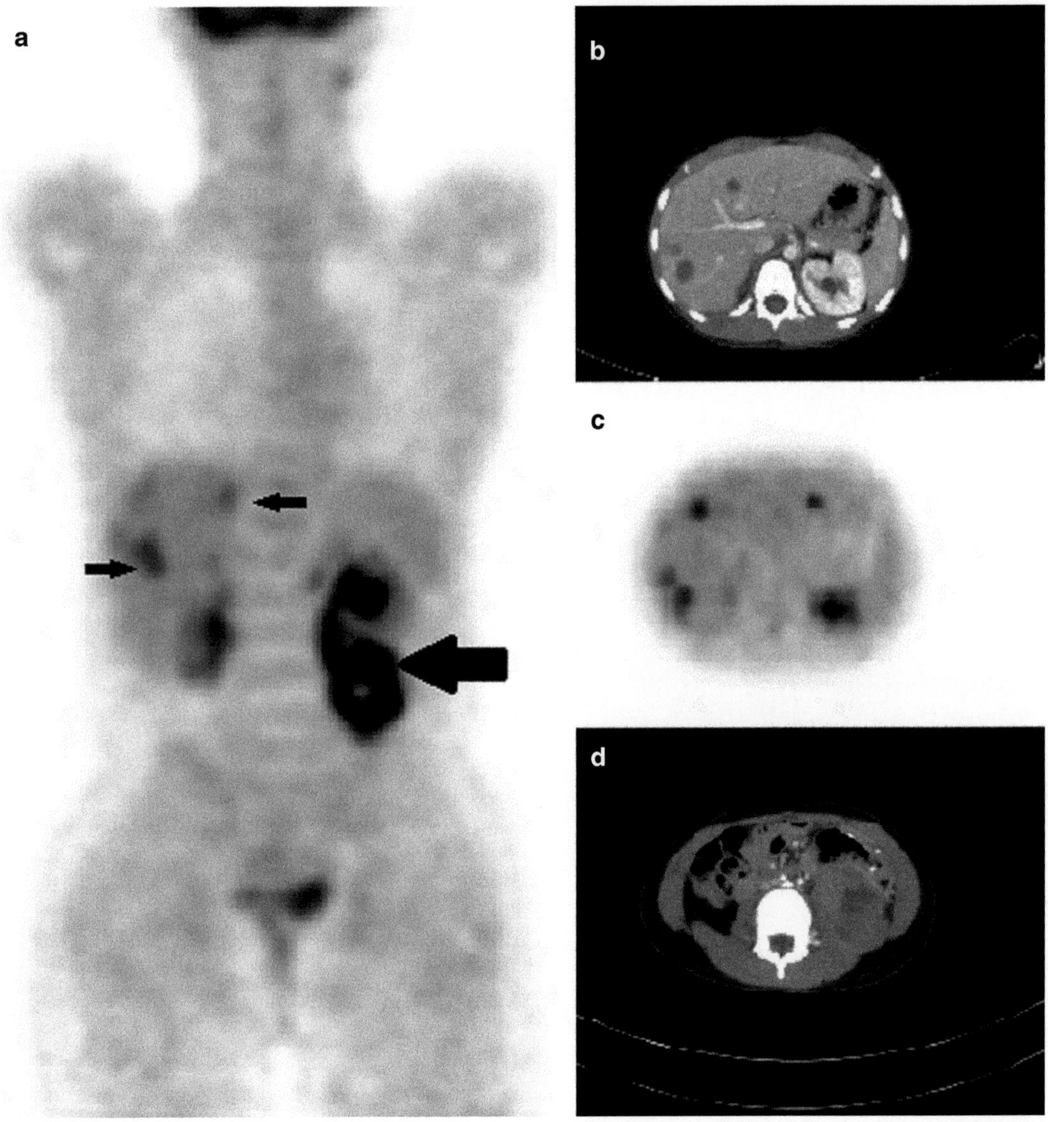

Fig. 21.5 18F-FDG PET/CT in the same patient as described in Fig. 21.3, with a left paravertebral mass with very mild MIBG uptake. (**a**) Coronal PET showed a heterogenous intense uptake in the left abdominal paravertebral lesion as well as multiple foci of increased activity in the liver suggestive of metastases. A superimposed infectious process in the liver could not be excluded. Biopsy proved the diagnosis of metastatic neuroblastoma. (**b**) Axial CT from the upper abdomen and (**c**) axial PET showed multiple lesions in the liver. (**d**) Axial CT from the abdomen shows the left abdominal paravertebral mass

occasional MIBG-negative NBL. A study of 60 patients by Sharp et al. comparing ^{18}F-FDG to I123 MIBG documented the superiority of ^{18}F-FDG for early-stage disease and the potential benefits of MIBG for evaluation of higher-stage disease [123]. MIBG demonstrated superiority for the evaluation of stage 4 disease. In addition, ^{18}F-FDG can provide helpful information in cases of mildly MIBG avid tumor at major decision points in therapy, such as prior to bone marrow transplantation or major surgery (Figs. 21.4 and 21.5). ^{18}F-FDG is advantageous in that the test can be performed in one day. The other benefits of ^{18}F-FDG are the higher photon energy and the better attenuation correction characteristics of PET in abdominal imaging, especially in obese patients. In another study by Choi et al. on 30 neuroblastoma patients, ^{18}F-FDG PET was more sensitive than CT in the evaluation of distant lymph node involvement [124].

$^{18}F-FDG$ does however have important caveats. Firstly, ^{18}F-FDG can be a nonspecific tracer, showing uptake in inflammatory lesions or any of the false positives indicated above. Secondly, ^{18}F-FDG has been shown to be less useful than MIBG for the evaluation of osseous/bone marrow disease [123]. There is some evidence however that ^{18}F-FDG can have better accuracy for the detection of soft tissue metastases than MIBG [103, 125]. Thus, until larger studies can be performed, ^{18}F-FDG and MIBG are perhaps best considered complimentary tools in NBL.

11C-Hydroxyephedrine, the PET equivalent of MIBG, has been used in a small number of patients and was found to be comparable though potentially limited in the assessment of perihepatic disease due to high background activity in the liver on hydroxyephedrine PET [103]. ^{18}F-FDOPA is another tracer which has shown considerable promise in NBL, with Piccardo et al. showing higher sensitivity in FDOPA compared to paired I123 MIBG in 28 scans over 19 patients [126]. FDOPA detected distant lesions in 94 % of cases rather than 65 % of cases with MIBG. Management was hence changed in 9/28 or 32 % of scans.

NBL does demonstrate somatostatin receptors and hence gallium 68 DOTA is of potential in PET imaging. Ga 68 DOTATOC has been shown to be superior to planar indium 111 octreotide in a series of neuroendocrine tumors [127]. In a small series, Ga 68 DOTATOC PET was found to have a sensitivity (97.2 %) superior to MIBG (90.7 %) [128], a result which will hopefully be confirmed in a larger study.

21.5.2 Pheochromocytoma

The pheochromocytoma arises from chromatin cells of the adrenal medulla or, occasionally, from extra-adrenal paraganglionic tissue. Approximately 85 % of cases arise from the adrenal medulla. The organ of Zuckerkandl and ganglionic tissue surrounding the kidney can also give rise to pheochromocytoma. The pheochromocytoma is much more common in adolescents than children, with 11 years being the mean age of presentation.

When pheochromocytoma arises in children, it is often in association with a genetic syndrome, most commonly von Hippel–Lindau, multiple endocrine neoplasia, neurofibromatosis 1, and familial paraganglioma syndrome [129, 130]. Thus, the presentation of a child with pheochromocytoma should prompt further investigation for other abnormalities within the spectrum of these syndromes and might include further imaging of the head, thyroid, skeleton, and abdomen [130, 131].

Elevated levels of circulating plasma catecholamines or urine catecholamines in the correct clinical presentation are essentially diagnostic [132]. Paraganglioma, conversely, is less likely to be associated with biochemical abnormality, and so in syndromes where both pheochromocytoma and paraganglioma may be present, a negative serum or urine catecholamine level should not dissuade from further imaging including imaging of the sympathetic nervous system [131].

Ultrasound, CT, and/or MRI is often employed in the initial evaluation of pheochromocytoma, with signal and enhancement characteristics of the latter being essentially diagnostic in the correct clinical and biochemical context [131]. MIBG imaging, usually bound to I123, confirms the diagnosis and is used to evaluate for any additional sites of involvement or distant metastatic disease [133]. Approximately 90 % of pheochromocytomas are MIBG avid.

Although pheochromocytoma is usually ^{18}F-FDG avid (Fig. 21.6), some lesions will not accumulate ^{18}F-FDG, and hence where PET is performed, an adrenergic PET imaging agent such as 11C hydroxyephedrine may be preferable where available to a glucose analog [134]. Pheochromocytomas frequently express somatostatin receptors and thus excellent preliminary results have also been obtained with gallium 68 DOTA somatostatin analogs in a limited literature [135].

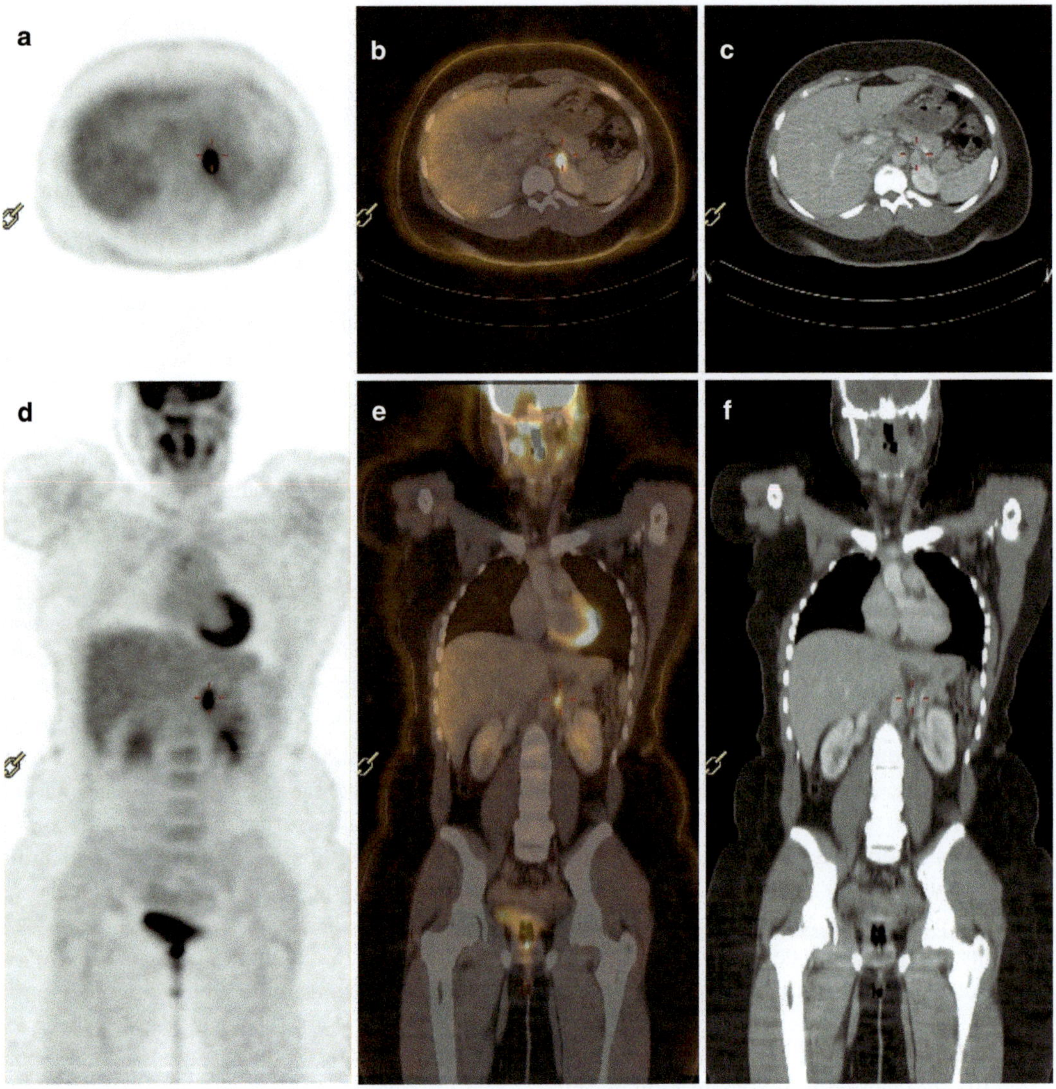

Fig. 21.6 Axial PET (**a**), fused PET/CT (**b**), and CT (**c**), coronal PET (**d**), fused PET/CT (**e**), and CT (**f**) of 18F-FDG PET/CT in an 18-year-old female, clinically and biochemically suspicious for recurrence or metastases of pheochromocytoma. Right suprarenal pheochromocytoma was resected a year ago. A focal intense FDG activity is noted in the left suprarenal region corresponding to the soft tissue density on the CT suggestive of pheochromocytoma. No other FDG-avid lesions were detected to suggest metastasis

21.6 Lymphoma

Lymphoma is the third most common type of childhood malignancy after leukemia and brain tumors, accounting for approximately 15 % of pediatric cancers. The peak age is 15–19 years old. Lymphoma makes up almost 24 % of the childhood malignancy for the age 15–19, while it accounts only 3 % of the pediatric cancers below the age of 5. Lymphoma is categorized into Hodgkin's disease (HD) and non-Hodgkin's lymphomas (NHL).

21.6.1 Hodgkin's Disease

HD is more common in young adults. It is more common in 15–30 years of age. The other peak age for HD is >55 years old. The 5-year survival is more than 90 % for the patient younger than 20 years old. The exact etiology of HL is not well known. Both genetic predisposition and environmental factor (prior viral infection) have been suggested to be responsible for HD. According to the Revised European–American Lymphoma Update of the WHO classification, HD is categorized into two main groups: (1) nodular lymphocyte predominant Hodgkin's lymphoma (NLPHL) and (2) classical HD.

NLPHL accounts for approximately 10 % of all HD and has a very good prognosis. It frequently involves the cervical and axillary lymph nodes; mediastinal and extra-nodal involvements are rare. Classical HD is categorized into four histologic subtypes:

1. Nodular sclerosis: the most common type in North America and Western Europe; approximately 70 % of cases, with good prognosis
2. Mixed cellularity: the second most common in North America and Western Europe and probably most common in underdeveloped areas; characterized by pleomorphic cellular infiltrate of plasma cells, eosinophils, lymphocytes, histiocytes, and Reed–Sternberg cells; has intermediate prognosis
3. Lymphocyte rich: characterized by small lymphocytes with occasional and probably atypical form of Reed–Sternberg cells (lymphocytic–histiocytic); has a good prognosis
4. Lymphocyte depleted: rare in children; more common in HIV patient and positive EBV; has the worst prognosis

21.6.2 Non-Hodgkin's Lymphoma

NHL is more common in younger children. The 5-year survival is approximately 72 %. The incidence of NHL is less variable with age in children comparing with HD. Congenital immunodeficiency disorders (CIDs) and HIV are reported to be associated with an increased risk of NHL. NHLs are a heterogeneous group of disease, usually with higher proliferative neoplastic cells and aggressive behavior compared with the HD [136]. NHL can be categorized into many subgroups. The major subgroups are:

1. Burkitt and Burkitt-like lymphomas (more common in 5–14 years old; often occur in the abdomen)
2. Lymphoblastic lymphoma precursor T (usually mediastinal)
3. Anaplastic large cell lymphoma
4. Diffuse large B-cell lymphoma (DLBCL; most common subtype among 15–19-year-olds)
5. Follicular lymphoma

The NHLs can also categorize into slow-growing types (e.g., follicular lymphoma), more aggressive types (e.g., DLBC), and fast-growing types (e.g., Burkitt and Burkitt-like lymphomas).

The clinical presentation varies and depends on the type of lymphoma, location, and systemic presentations. Peripheral lymphadenopathy is the most common finding. Cough or shortness of breath secondary to the mediastinal mass, B symptoms (fever, weight loss, anorexia, and night sweats), tiredness, pruritus, neurologic symptoms, anemia, and bone pain are other sign and symptoms. Clinical history, physical examination, laboratory tests, chest X-ray, and CT scans are among the initial evaluation. Histopathology will confirm the diagnosis. Accurate staging of disease is important for prognosis and treatment management. On one hand, it is necessary to use appropriate intensive chemotherapy and radiotherapy (especially for HD) to achieve a good response, and on the other hand, it is essential to avoid unnecessary treatment to minimize the complications of therapy [137, 138]. For HD, Ann Arbor staging or Cotswold classification (a modification of Ann Arbor) is usually used, and for NHLs of the children, St. Jude Children's Research Hospital is the preferred staging system (Tables 21.3 and 21.4).

Nuclear medicine has an important role in evaluation of lymphoma. Bone scan with ^{99m}Tc-MDP is useful in detection of bone metastasis especially in HD. 67Ga citrate scan has been used for a long time as functional imaging modality for the staging and response to therapy with a sensitivity and specificity of approximately 80 % and 90 %, respectively [139]. ^{67}Ga scan is more positive in high-grade B-cell or Burkitt lymphoma [140]. Due to increased radiation exposure, lower resolution, and the need to image the patient for a longer time, ^{67}Ga scan has been replaced by ^{18}F-FDG PET/CT for initial staging and evaluation of response and recurrence in children.

Table 21.3 Hodgkin's disease staging

Stage	Description
Stage I	A single lymph node group involvement or localized involvement of an extralymphatic organ
Stage II	More than one lymph node group involvement or localized involvement of an extralymphatic organ (all on the same side of the diaphragm)
Stage III	Involvement of lymph nodes on both sides of the diaphragm with or without localized involvement of an extralymphatic organ
Stage IV	Diffuse involvement of one or more extralymphatic organs

Table 21.4 St. Jude's staging for childhood NHL staging

Stage	Description
Stage I	Single tumor outside the lymph nodes or nodal involvement in one group of lymph nodes (not in the mediastinum or abdomen)
Stage II	A single extra-nodal tumor with regional node involvement
	More than one group of nodes on the same side of the diaphragm
	Two extra-nodal tumors on the same side of the diaphragm
	A primary gastrointestinal tract tumor with or without involvement of associated mesenteric nodes and can be completely resected by surgery
Stage III	Two single extra-nodal tumors or two or more nodal groups on the opposite sides of the diaphragm
	All the primary chest tumors
	Unresectable extensive primary intra-abdominal disease
	All paraspinal or epidural tumors
Stage IV	Central nervous system and/or bone marrow involvement

21.6.3 Initial Staging with ^{18}F-FDG PET/CT

21.6.3.1 Hodgkin's Disease

Classic HD is strongly ^{18}F-FDG avid in more than 97 % of cases [141, 142] (Fig. 21.7). The ^{18}F-FDG avidity is slightly lower in NLPHL [143]. London et al. found a sensitivity and specificity of 98 and 99.6 % for ^{18}F-FDG PET/CT at initial staging of HD compared with 77 and 98.7 % for conventional anatomical modalities [144]. The high sensitivity and specificity of ^{18}F-FDG PET/CT at initial staging of HD are also confirmed by other authors [145, 146]. ^{18}F-FDG PET/CT has a higher sensitivity than bone marrow biopsy in both adults and children [147–149]. This is probably due to the biopsy site which is usually done from posterior iliac spine. The bone marrow involvement may be patchy or multifocal on ^{18}F-FDG PET/CT [148]. The sensitivity of ^{18}F-FDG PET/CT is lower than chest CT scan for the lung lesions especially if the nodules are less than 5 mm in size [146]. ^{18}F-FDG PET/CT can also be useful for radiotherapy planning. In a study by Girinsky et al., pre-chemotherapy ^{18}F-FDG PET data were essential for correctly implementing the involved-node radiotherapy concept [150]. The other purpose of initial study is to have a baseline for the evaluation of response to therapy. ^{18}F-FDG PET/CT at initial evaluation may be also of interest to guide biopsy [146, 151].

21.6.3.2 Non-Hodgkin's Lymphoma

The risk of bone marrow involvement and presentation at a higher stage (usually stage 3 or 4) is higher in NHL than HD [149, 152]. The aggressive form of NHL is more prevalent in pediatric population than adults; thus, the risk of false-negative ^{18}F-FDG PET study in pediatric NHL is very low [153, 154]. However, since involvement of the brain, kidneys, abdomen, and diffuse bone marrow is relatively common in different types of NHL, the accuracy of ^{18}F-FDG PET/CT may be affected by the physiologic uptake in these organs [155, 156]. Based on the Revised Response Criteria for Malignant Lymphoma (RRCML), ^{18}F-FDG PET is recommended (although is not mandatory yet) at diagnosis, for routine evaluation of

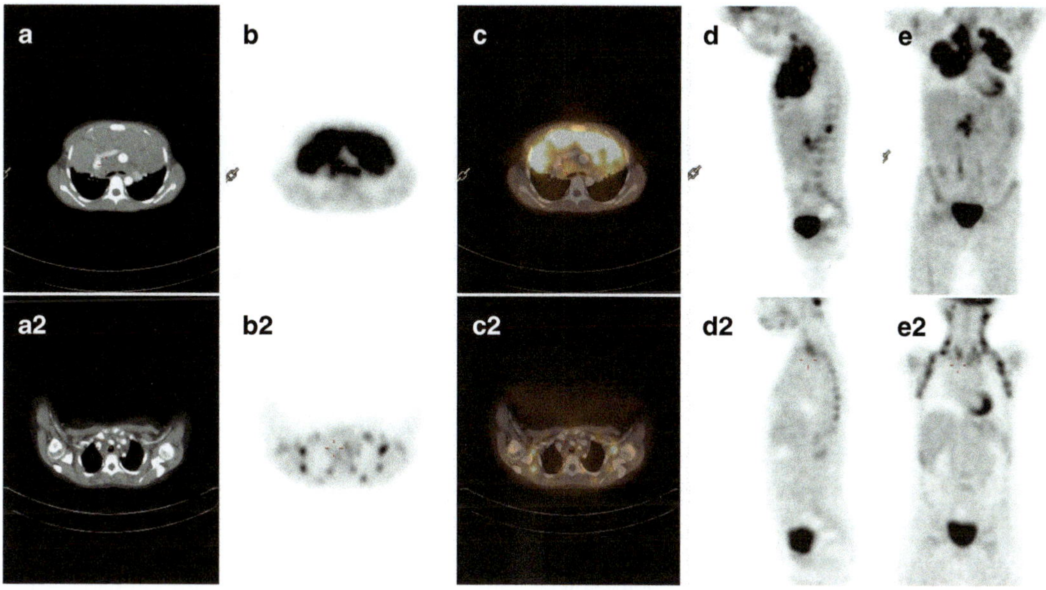

Fig. 21.7 Eight-year-old female with a bulky anterior mediastinal mass diagnosed with Hodgkin's lymphoma. (**a**) Axial CT, (**b**) axial PET, (**c**) axial-fused PET/CT, (**d**) sagittal PET, and (**e**) coronal PET from the 18F-FDG PET/CT performed at initial diagnosis showed a large FDG-avid mass in the anterior mediastinum with multiple foci of increased FDG activity in the supraclavicular regions, spleen, T12, and abdominal lymph nodes (only the anterior mediastinal mass is shown here). The patient is upstaged based on the PET result. After two doses of chemotherapy, (**a2**) axial CT, (**b2**) axial PET, (**c2**) axial-fused PET/CT, (**d2**) sagittal PET, and (**e2**) coronal PET showed marked improvement with minimal residual activity in the mediastinum less than the liver activity suggestive of very good response to therapy. Note is made of multiple foci of FDG activity in the neck and chest corresponding to the hypodense areas on the CT due to brown fat uptake

^{18}F-FDG-avid lymphomas which are curable [157]. There are many reports in which the extranodal involvement is missed by conventional CT scan, particularly in anaplastic large cell lymphomas, DLBC, and Burkitt lymphoma [155, 158, 159]. ^{18}F-FDG PET/CT is also very accurate to detect splenic lesions [145, 160].

21.6.4 Evaluation of Therapy Response with ^{18}F-FDG PET/CT

21.6.4.1 Hodgkin's Disease

^{18}F-FDG PET has an important role in response assessment following chemotherapy in lymphoma even early after a course of therapy (Fig. 21.7). CT scan is a reliable method for staging and restaging of lymphoma. However, the specificity for evaluation of response to therapy is relatively low, especially in patients with bulky disease before treatment [161]. 18F-^{18}F-FDG PET has a high negative predictive value for detection of hypermetabolic tissue after treatment which makes it a reliable method to exclude the presence of any viable residual tumor or recurrence [162].

According to RRCML, although ^{18}F-FDG PET is recommended after completion of chemotherapy, it is not routinely recommended during the therapy [157]. However, the early interim ^{18}F-FDG PET seems to have a prognostic value for therapy response and recurrence [163, 164]. In the EuroNet-PHL-C1 trial (EudraCT 2006-000995-33) that started in 2007, patients will receive the standard treatment including radiotherapy when there is residual viable tissues on the ^{18}F-FDG PET scan after two cycles of chemotherapy [153]. Those with a negative ^{18}F-FDG PET do not receive the radiotherapy at the end of chemotherapy [153, 165]. It should be emphasized that the exact criteria for interpretation of

^{18}F-FDG PET findings after two cycles of chemotherapy have not been fully established, and many factors may affect the interpretation including the time of study, type of tumor, and type of chemotherapy [153]. In a recent study published in New England Journal of Medicine on 602 patients (53.3 % male; median age, 34 years) with Hodgkin's disease, PET scan was performed in 571 patients after third cycles of chemotherapy. The results of PET were negative in 426 of these patients (74.6 %); 420 of those patients were randomly enrolled in two study groups (209 received radiotherapy, and 211 did not receive any further therapy). The results of this study did not show the non-inferiority of the strategy of no further treatment after chemotherapy with regard to progression-free survival based on the PET findings. Moreover, both groups (i.e., with negative PET results after three cycles of chemotherapy), regardless of receiving radiotherapy or not, had a very good prognosis [166].

21.6.4.2 Non-Hodgkin's Lymphoma

Because of limited resolution of PET system and higher prevalence of neoplastic cells in an NHL tumor than HD, a negative PET study at the end of chemotherapy does not necessarily mean there is no viable residual tissue. The interim response to chemotherapy (after two cycle) has probably more prognostic value in this respect [153]. This is important to differentiate those patients who need more intensified chemotherapy versus those who need less therapy to avoid therapy complications [167]. In NHL, a negative interim ^{18}F-FDG PET scan is indicative of a good response and good prognosis [6, 168]. However, this is not confirmed in all types of NHL. In a study by Bakhshi et al., neither interim ^{18}F-FDG PET nor interim CT scan could predict survival [169]. Further studies in different types of NHL in pediatric are needed to clarify the exact role of PET in therapy response of NHL.

21.6.5 Evaluation of Relapse or Recurrence

^{18}F-FDG PET/CT has a sensitivity of 90–100 % to detect residual tissue after therapy. However, the specificity is relatively low with approximately 16–18 % of the cases. False-positive results are due to fibrosis, abdominal wall hernia, inflammation, thymus, and HIV-associated lymphadenopathy [170]. In order to avoid false-positive result due to post-therapeutic inflammation, the study should be done at least 3 weeks after chemotherapy and 2–3 months after radiotherapy. A negative ^{18}F-FDG PET study is a strong indicator of the absence of relapse, while a positive study sometimes warrants further investigation with other imaging modalities or biopsy to confirm the recurrence or relapse [6, 162] (Fig. 21.8).

In summary, ^{18}F-FDG PET is recommended for staging of lymphoma at diagnosis and evaluation of treatment response after completion of therapy. ^{18}F-FDG PET will probably play more roles in the future for the evaluation of therapy response during the treatment (between cycles 1 and 4) and for monitoring the patients, planning the radiation field, and biopsy planning.

21.6.6 Posttransplant Lymphoproliferative Disorder

Posttransplant lymphoproliferative disorder (PTLD) is a relatively uncommon but serious complication of both solid organ and bone marrow transplantation [171, 172]. PTLD comprises of a heterogeneous group of lymphoproliferative diseases, ranging from benign hyperplasia to malignant lymphoma [173]. It is the most common malignancy affecting children after transplantation [174]. The risk of PTLD is higher in children than in adults, probably because of the greater incidence of Epstein–Barr virus (EBV) infection [175, 176]. The overall mortality rate is relatively high [177, 178], but prognosis is likely better in children than in adults [179].

PTLD can be categorized into four major histopathologic types:

(a) Early lymphoid hyperplasia/infectious mononucleosis-type lesions
(b) Polymorphic PTLD

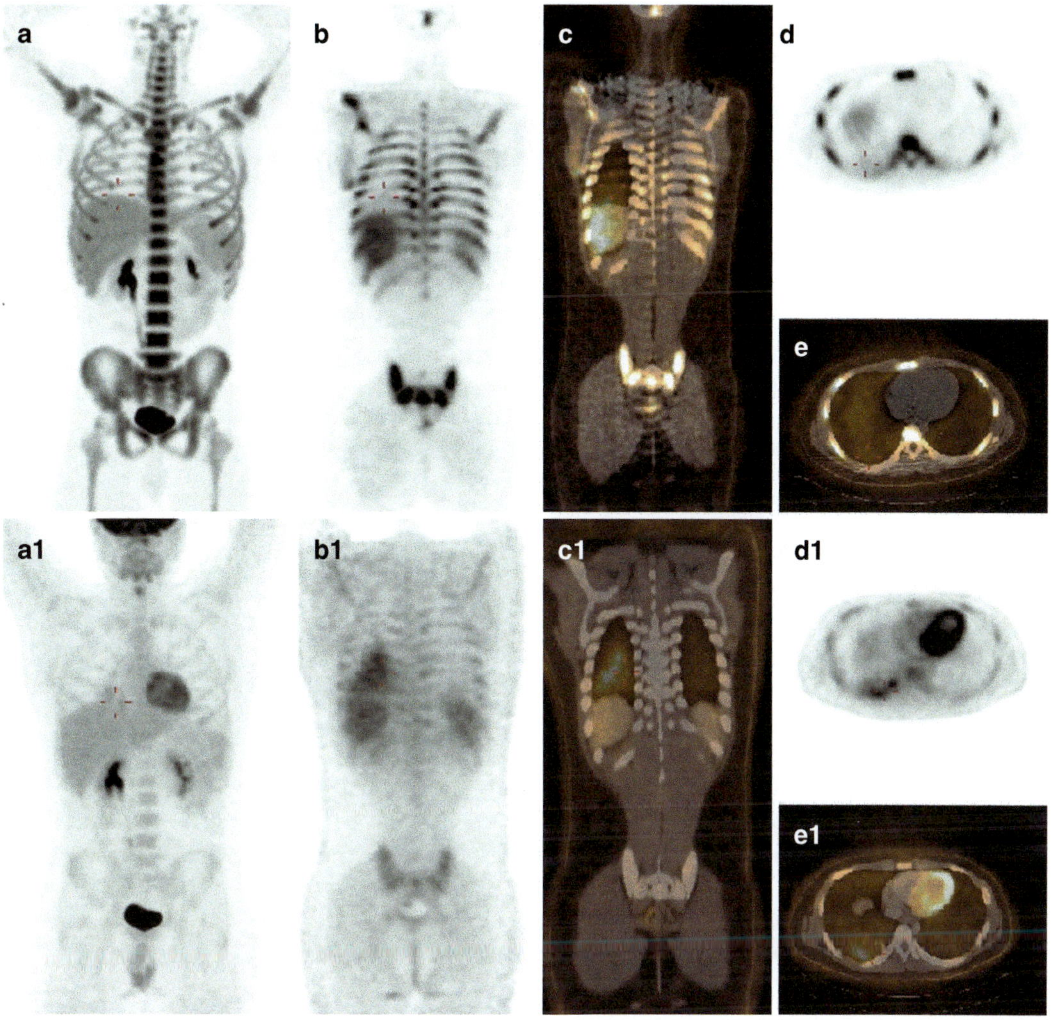

Fig. 21.8 Fifteen-year-old male with Hodgkin's disease after two cycles of chemotherapy. 18F-FDG PET/CT showed mild hilar uptake (not shown here) as well as mild activity in the right basal lung likely due to infection (shown in (**a1**) MIP, (**b1**) coronal PET, (**c1**) coronal-fused PET/CT, (**d1**) axial PET, and (**e1**) axial-fused PET/CT). The right basal lung did not show any increased activity on 18F-FLT (shown in (**a**) MIP, (**b**) coronal PET, (**c**) coronal-fused PET/CT, (**d**) axial PET, and (**e**) axial-fused PET/CT) suggestive of infection rather than tumoral involvement. Note intense activity in the bone marrow on 18F-FLT scan

(c) Monomorphic PTLD, including types 1 and 2, with type 1 including diffuse large B-cell lymphoma (DLBCL), Burkitt lymphoma, and plasma cell myeloma/plasmacytoma-like lesions and type 2 including peripheral and hepatosplenic T-cell lymphomas
(d) Classical Hodgkin-type lymphomas [180]

Although PTLD may occur at any time, it is more common in the first year after transplantation and declines over time [178]. The diagnosis of PTLD is based on histopathology confirmation in following clinical and biochemical suspicion.

Evaluation of the extent of disease is important for the patient treatment management ranging from immunosuppressive therapy during the early phase or surgery on localized lesions to systemic chemotherapy in patients with monomorphous and classical Hodgkin lymphoma-type PTLD. Children with PTLD are usually staged according to the St. Jude staging system of non-Hodgkin's lymphoma (Table 21.4). Computerized tomography (CT), bone marrow biopsy, and, occasionally, magnetic resonance imaging (MRI) are often used to stage the disease.

Recently ^{18}F-FDG PET/CT showed promising results for staging and response to therapy in PTLD both in adults [181–187] and children [183, 184, 188]. Takehana et al. showed that ^{18}F-FDG PET/CT is useful in the management of patients with PTLD since both nodal and extra-nodal lesions demonstrated intense ^{18}F-FDG uptake in children [184]. In this study, one of the potential benefits of ^{18}F-FDG PET/CT was the ability to detect occult lesions not visualized on other imaging modalities, particularly extra-nodal lesion. Other studies showed the usefulness of ^{18}F-FDG PET/CT to evaluate response to therapy in children [183, 188] (Fig. 21.9). Further prospective studies are needed to define the exact role of ^{18}F-FDG PET/CT in staging, response to therapy, and prognosis in pediatric PTLD.

21.7 Leukemia

Leukemias account for 25 % of childhood malignancy and are therefore the most common cause of childhood cancer. Acute lymphoid leukemia (ALL) is the most common form representing approximately 75 % of cases, while acute myeloid leukemia (AML) accounts for most of the remainder. The incidence of ALL peaks at 2–4 years, while AML is most common in neonates or adolescents. There is a Caucasian preponderance.

Ionizing radiation exposure and genetic predisposition have been implicated in the development of ALL. Today ALL has a reasonably good prognosis, particularly in children age 1–10, with overall survival of approximately 80–90 %. Improved treatments are responsible for the dramatic improvements in survival in what was generally a fatal disease in the 1970s. AML carries a more guarded prognosis. Multiple factors have been implicated in the development of AML including genetic predisposition, radiation, medications, and environmental exposures.

The skeleton is commonly involved in leukemia; however imaging is generally not indicated prior to treatment and does not significantly alter management. PET/CT with ^{18}F-FDG usually demonstrates increased skeletal activity due to a combination of tumor infiltration and marrow hyperplasia [189]. ^{18}F-FDG PET has been described to investigate relapse where clinically appropriate or to assess the complications of bone marrow transplant [190]. Caution has been advised in the interpretation of ^{18}F-FDG PET for the workup of ALL in patients receiving high-dose steroid therapy [191], as steroid can alter the biodistribution of ^{18}F-FDG.

21.8 Tumors of the Brain and Central Nervous System

Cancers of the central nervous system make up the most common solid tumors in children and constitute the second most common pediatric malignancy, accounting for 16–20 % of all cancers in children and adolescents. Brain tumors, unfortunately, remain the leading cause of death in children with cancer. Astrocytoms, including the aggressive poorly differentiated astrocytoma, account for 52 % of childhood pediatric malignancies, which primitive neuroectodermal tumors (PNETs) account for 21 % (Fig. 21.10), other tumors of glial origin for 15 %, and ependymomas for 9 % (Table 21.5). Astrocytoma is the most common supratentorial brain tumor in children, many of which can be low grade, and hence there is particular interest and utility in deducing tumor histology from functional imaging. In the third ventricle, hypothalamic gliomas, craniopharyngiomas, and germ cell tumors are most common. In the posterior fossa, medulloblastoma, cerebellar astrocytoma, ependymoma, and brain stem glioma are the most common malignancies. In general, with the major exception of the juvenile pilocytic astrocytoma, the prognosis for central nervous system malignancy in children is poor and is particularly poor in infants with PNET or ependymoma.

Imaging of pediatric brain malignancy is a particularly strong example of the complimentary aspects of all neuroimaging modalities. MRI, with exquisite contrast resolution, is standard in the workup of these patients, as is CT for the

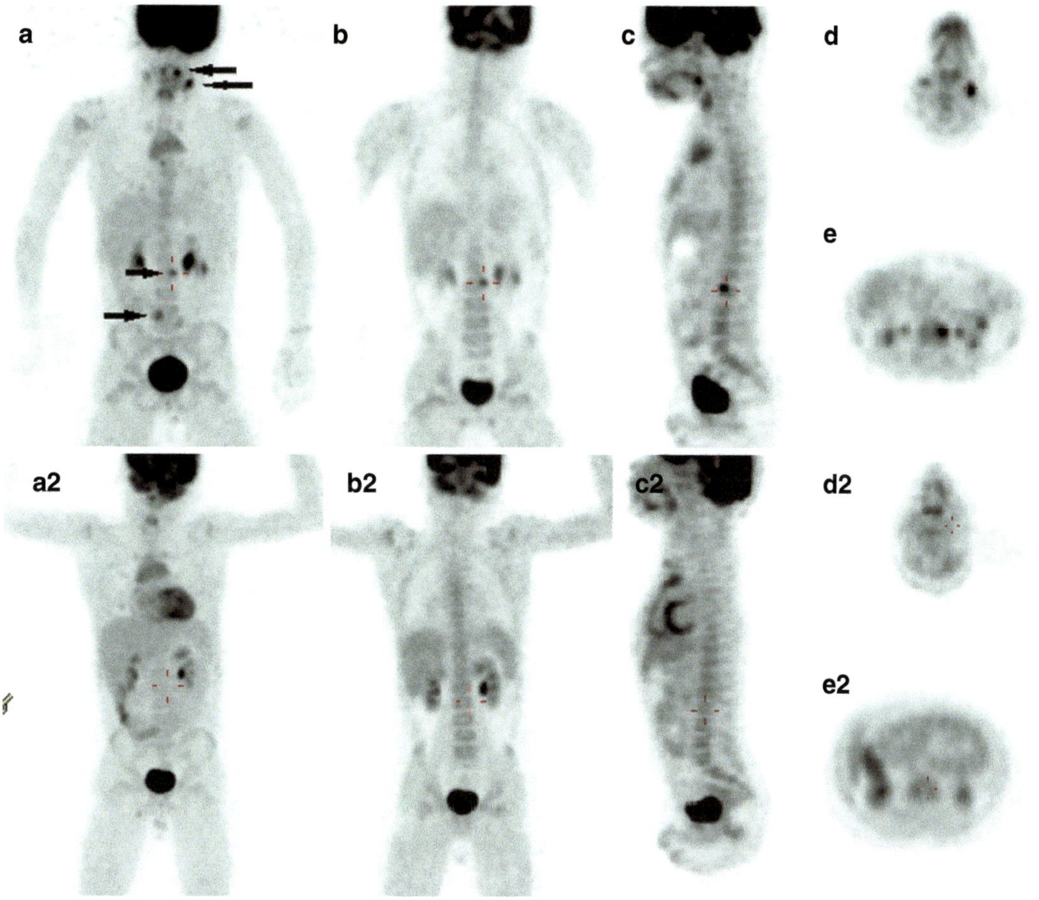

Fig. 21.9 A 7-year-old boy with the diagnosis of PTLD in the tonsils 1 year after lung transplant. 18F-FDG PET/CT was performed to evaluate the extent of the disease. (**a**); MIP image showed multiple foci of increased activity in the tonsil, a neck lymph node, spine, and abdomen (*arrows*). (**b**) Coronal PET, (**c**) sagittal PET, and (**e**) axial PET showed the spine lesion. (**d**) Axial PET showed the neck lymph node. 45 days later after a trial of decreased immune-suppression therapy, the lesions were resolved suggestive of a good response to therapy (see (**a2**) MIP, (**b2**) coronal PET, (**c2**) sagittal PET, (**d2**), axial PET from the neck, and (**e2**) axial PET from the abdomen, after reduced immune-suppression therapy)

evaluation of calcifications and for rapid perioperative assessment. Nuclear medicine continues to find a niche in clinical practice to assess cellular metabolism in these lesions and in adjacent brain parenchyma which often suffers from post-therapeutic change.

PET tracers have been extensively described in the workup of brain and spine malignancy. ^{18}F-FDG PET has been, due to its wide availability, the most widely studied tracer. ^{18}F-FDG activity in a brain tumor has been shown to correlate to histologic grade which in turn influences prognosis [192–194], assesses recurrent tumor [195], as well as determines whether a low-grade tumor is undergoing transition to higher grade [195, 196]. ^{18}F-FDG however suffers to some extent from nonspecificity, as well as uptake in normal brain tissue. Hence an extensive literature has developed in predominantly C11-labeled amino acids in PET imaging [15, 101] as well as choline [197]. C11 methionine is commonly used, and because it is not taken up by brain tissue, it provides excellent target to background ratio and can be used for initial staging/grading, to guide surgery (usually fused to CT or MRI), to assess response to treatment, and to differentiate

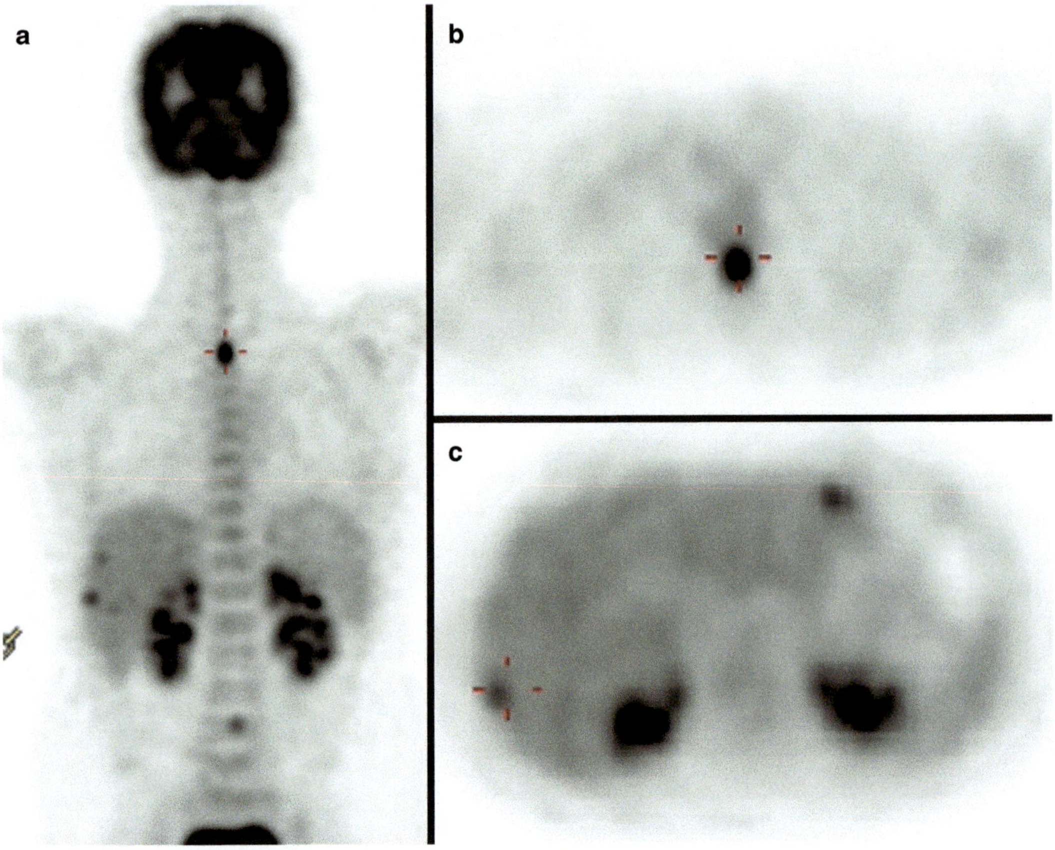

Fig. 21.10 Eleven-year-old boy with PNET. 18F-FDG PET/CT showed multiple FDG-avid lesions in the liver ((**a**) coronal PET and (**c**) axial PET), brain (not shown here), spinal cord ((**a**) coronal PET and (**b**) axial PET), and right iliac crest (nor shown here) suggestive of metastatic disease. Biopsy from the liver lesions confirmed the diagnosis of metastatic PNET

residual/recurrent tumor from scar or other therapeutic changes [198–200].

Since corticosteroids, chemotherapy, and radiation therapy all change cerebral glucose uptake, evaluation of response to chemotherapy with ^{18}F-FDG PET is not very straightforward in pediatric brain tumors [6]. Since ^{18}F-FDG PET and MR spectroscopy have a complementary role in the assessment of brain tumor metabolic activity, the introduction of integrated PET/MR scanners may open new windows for the clinical value of ^{18}F-FDG PET imaging in pediatric brain tumors [6, 201]. Other radiotracers such as ^{18}F-FLT or ^{18}F-DOPA are probably more useful for pediatric brain tumor imaging [82].

21.9 Osseous and Soft Tissue Malignancy

Ewing's sarcoma and osteosarcoma together constitute approximately 6 % of childhood malignancy. The 5-year survival of children with primary bone cancer is improving, with one author citing an increase in survival from 49 % in 1984 to 63 % in 1994. The 5-year survival rate today is generally at or greater than 70 %. The incidence of osteosarcoma is approximately twice that of Ewing's sarcoma, with the incidence of these cancers beginning at age 5 and increasing to peak at approximately age 18.

Table 21.5 WHO histopathologic classification of CNS tumors

Tumor origin	Tumor cell type (examples)
Neuroepithelial tissue	*Astrocytic tumors* (astrocytoma, anaplastic astrocytoma, pilocytic astrocytoma, pleomorphic xanthroastrocytoma, subependymal giant cell astrocytoma)
	Oligodendroglial tumors (oligodendroglioma, anaplastic oligodendroglioma)
	Ependymal tumors (ependymoma, anaplastic ependymoma, myxopapillary ependymoma)
	Neuronal tumors (gangliocytoma, ganglioma, desmoplastic infantile neuroepithelioma, dysembryoplastic neuroepithelial tumor)
	Choroid plexus tumors (choroid plexus papilloma, choroid plexus carcinoma)
	Pineal tumors (pineocytoma, pineoblastoma)
Embryonal origin	*Primary neuroectodermal tumors* (medulloblastoma, neuroblastoma, ependymoblastoma)
	Other embryonal cells (medulloepithelioma, neuroblastoma, ependymoblastoma)
Germ cell	*Germinoma*
	Embryonal carcinoma
	Endodermal sinus tumor
	Choriocarcinoma
	Teratoma
	Mixed germ cell tumors
	Ependymoblastoma
Tumors in the sella turcica	*Pituitary adenoma*
	Craniopharyngioma

21.9.1 Osteosarcoma

The peak incidence of osteosarcoma in children is between 11 and 18 years, with a 5-year survival of between 70 and 80%. Survival has improved with a combination of neoadjuvant chemotherapy and aggressive surgery. Osteosarcoma is thought to originate in primitive bone-forming mesenchymal stem cells and often arises from the metaphyseal aspect of long bones. The distal femur and proximal tibia/fibula account for half of cases. An association with ionizing radiation, Paget's disease, and genetic susceptibility has been hypothesized. Advances in surgery have improved functional outcome, though surgical resection is still often disfiguring.

Table 21.6 Surgical staging for osteosarcoma

Stage	Description
Stage IA	Low grade, intra-compartmental
Stage IB	Low grade, extra-compartmental
Stage IIA	High grade, intra-compartmental
Stage IIB	High grade, extra-compartmental
Stage III	With metastases

The detection of distant metastases is the most important component of the imaging workup as metastases strongly negatively influence prognosis. Grading of the tumor is the next most important aspect of the workup, including the detection of any extension of tumor outside the anatomic compartment. The majority of osteosarcomas are high grade but remain confined to one anatomic compartment. Children and adolescents commonly present with pain and swelling.

Musculoskeletal plain film is usually followed by MRI for initial diagnosis, which is generally followed by biopsy correlation, bone scan including SPECT of the thorax, and CT of the thorax, abdomen, and pelvis. Plain films often show an aggressive lesion with expansion of the bone and extensive periosteal reaction. MRI of the affected bone is crucial in determining the extent of local spread and the presence of skip lesions. The CT thorax and bone scan SPECT detect metastatic disease to the thorax. Lung and bone are the two most common sites of metastases in osteosarcoma. The surgical staging system of osteosarcoma is provided in Table 21.6.

Prior to the more widespread implementation of ^{18}F-FDG PET, Tc 99m MDP was often the tracer of choice for total body scan in the osteosarcoma patient. Primary tumor is generally hyperemic on blood flow and pool images and intensely MDP avid on delayed skeletal phase images. Both distant bone and lung metastases are generally MDP avid [202]. Occasionally, bone scan shows changes of associated hypertrophic osteoarthropathy when lung disease is present. Radiotherapy has limited role in the therapy of osteosarcoma for curative intent and is hence reserved for inoperable tumors. Irradiated osteosarcomas can remain MDP avid for months after therapy, and hence other tracers such as ^{18}F-FDG PET or thallium 201 are preferred for this indication. Thallium 201 is an excellent tracer to stage and assess response to treatment in osteosarcoma, as is Tc 99m sestamibi in a more limited literature, where failure of appropriate response tends to indicate more aggressive surgery [203, 204].

$^{18}F-FDG\,PET$ was described in a prospective study by Volker et al. in 46 patients (Ewing = 23, osteosarcoma = 11, rhabdomyosarcoma = 12) to demonstrate that ^{18}F-FDG PET was as accurate as the combination of all other modalities including MRI and conventional nuclear imaging [205]. Although CT showed better sensitivity to lung metastases (100 % vs. 25 %), PET was superior to all modalities for the detection of metastatic adenopathy (95 % vs 25 %) and osseous lesions (90 % vs. 57 %). A combination of MDP bone scan and ^{18}F-FDG PET was shown to have a higher sensitivity (100 %) for the detection of bone metastases compared to ^{18}F-FDG PET (92 %) or bone scan (74 %) alone [206]. ^{18}F-FDG PET may be of less value than conventional tracers in predicting response to chemotherapy, as a study by Huang et al. demonstrated a tumor necrosis rate of 22 % by ^{18}F-FDG PET compared to 55 % necrosis on pathology in the same series of ten patients [207]. Thus, though some authors have had better success [208, 209], ^{18}F-FDG PET may underestimate response to therapy and should be used with caution for this indication in the osteosarcoma patient.

Fluorine-18-labeled sodium fluoride (^{18}F-NaF) has also been used in pediatrics in different clinical indications. The biodistribution of ^{18}F-NaF is similar to that of ^{99m}Tc-MDP [67]. However, there are some advantages with ^{18}F-NaF PET compared with the conventional bone scan. First, the extraction of the ^{18}F-NaF by bone is faster than ^{99m}Tc-MDP due to its lower protein binding. Thus, it allows for earlier imaging. Secondly, the extraction of the radiotracer is greater than MDP, so the target to background ratio is higher. Finally, the resolution of PET system is better than that of conventional gamma cameras. All these factors allow for obtaining higher-quality images with ^{18}F-NaF PET. Although there are many reports showing promising results with ^{18}F-NaF PET/CT to detect bone metastases in different tumors in adults, to our knowledge, there is no report focusing on using ^{18}F-NaF in detecting bone metastases in children. However, it seems that it can be very useful in children especially for tumors with lesser uptake on bone scan such as LCH. Further studies are needed to evaluate the exact role of ^{18}F-NaF PET/CT in pediatric oncology. The radiation absorbed dose is similar or only slightly more than that of ^{99m}Tc-MDP bone scan [67].

21.9.2 Ewing's Sarcoma

Ewing's sarcoma is the second most common bone tumor in children, representing 3 % of childhood malignancies, and represents a family of small round cell tumors. Ewing's sarcoma can occur in intraosseous or extraosseous form or as a peripheral primitive neuroectodermal tumor, neuroepithelioma, or Askin tumor. Ewing's most likely originates from neural crest cells and can arise in either the appendicular or axial skeleton. There is a predilection to Caucasians.

The overall 5-year survival for Ewing's is 70 %, with younger children demonstrating better overall survival than older children or adults. Approximately 25 % of patients have distant metastases at the time of treatment. Prognosis is a function of resectability of the primary (i.e., appendicular versus axial skeletal involvement), presence of distant metastases, and response to chemotherapy. The lymph nodes, bone, and lungs are the most common sites of distant metastases, though any organ can be affected.

The diagnosis is usually made by tissue biopsy after a lesion is worked up by X-ray and MRI. MRI is warranted to assess the entire bone occupied by tumor for skip lesions. Bone scan demonstrates a more homogenous pattern of uptake than the generally more heterogenous uptake seen in osteosarcoma. The distribution of tumor is generally more diaphyseal or metadiaphyseal compared to osteosarcoma which is usually situated at the metaphysis. Diagnostic chest CT is the modality of choice for the assessment of lung metastases [205].

Bone metastases are ultimately detected in 33–45 % of patients who were free of metastatic disease at presentation. Thus serial ^{18}F-FDG PET scans or bone scans are usually performed in the first 2 years after diagnosis to detect any occult disease. Erlemann et al. demonstrated that assessment of the primary tumor on MRI provided a more accurate assessment of therapeutic response than did bone scan (85 % versus 50 %) and thus if bone scan does not demonstrate improvement with therapy, MRI is indicated for further assessment [210]. Definite decrease in MDP uptake at the tumor site does indicate response.

Although as in osteosarcoma, ^{18}F-FDG PET has value equal or exceeding conventional tracers for the initial staging of Ewing's sarcoma, for Ewing in particular ^{18}F-FDG PET does not have value for the assessment of response to treatment [211]. Both responders and nonresponders can have decreased ^{18}F-FDG activity at tumor sites. As in osteosarcoma, CT thorax has greater sensitivity than ^{18}F-FDG PET for the detection of pulmonary metastases, and so diagnostic CT thorax is needed in addition to PET/CT if the CT component of the PET is not of diagnostic quality [205].

21.9.3 Rhabdomyosarcoma

Rhabdomyosarcoma (RMS) is an aggressive tumor demonstrating bimodal peaks of incidence between the ages of 2–5 years and 15–19 years (Table 21.7). The survival rate has improved from 20 % in the 1960s to 70 % today, mainly due to accurate imaging of the local disease extension and effective surgical resection. There is a role for radiotherapy in the treatment of local disease. Distant metastases are associated with poor prognosis. Other factors associated with poor prognosis include unfavorable sites of primary disease such as the meninges, bladder/prostate, retroperitoneum, extremities, and abdomen, as well as alveolar type, poorly differentiated histology, large tumor size (i.e., > 5 cm), nodal involvement, elderly age, and local/nodal or bone mets. RMS accounts for 4–8 % of malignancy in children less than 15 years old. The etiology of RMS is poorly understood with some association documented between incidence and other genetic diseases including neurofibromatosis 1, Gorlin syndrome, retinoblastoma syndrome, Costello syndrome, Rubinstein–Taybi syndrome, and Beckwith–Wiedemann. Maternal substance abuse has also been linked to the development of RMS.

^{18}F – FDG PET has been described for the workup of RMS. ^{18}F-FDG uptake widely varies

Table 21.7 TNM Staging of rhabdomyosarcoma

Stage	Description
Stage I	T1 or T2 (a or b), N0/1/x and M0 and in favorable site: head and neck (excluding parameningeal), orbit, genitourinary (non-bladder/non-prostate), biliary tract
Satge II	T1 or T2 a (not b), N0 or Nx (not N1) and M0; site: bladder and/or prostate, extremity, cranial parameningeal, other areas including trunk, retroperitoneum, etc.
Satge III	T1 or T2 a, N1, M0 in bladder and/or prostate or T1 or T2b, N0 or N1 or Nx, M0 in extremity, cranial parameningeal, and others including trunk, retroperitoneum, etc., except the biliary tract
Stage IV	M1 (irrespective of T and N and the site of tumor)

T1 = Confined to anatomic site of origin ((a) if diameter is ≤ 5 cm; (b) if diameter is > 5 cm)
T2 = Extension and/or invasion to surrounding tissue ((a) if diameter is ≤ 5 cm; (b) if diameter is > 5 cm)
N0 = Regional nodes not clinically involved
N1 = Regional nodes clinically involved by tumor
Nx = Clinical status of regional nodes unknown (especially sites where lymph node evaluation is not possible)
M0 = No distant metastasis
M1 = With distant metastasis

in RMS [212]. Increased ^{18}F-FDG activity at the site of primary tumor is associated with poor differentiation and hence overall more aggressive tumor and worse prognosis [213, 214]. ^{18}F-FDG also shows excellent sensitivity to the detection of local disease and distance metastases, including metastatic adenopathy and bone metastases. Several authors have shown ^{18}F-FDG PET to be superior in terms of the accurate detection of distance metastases to a combination of conventional modalities including CT, MRI, and bone scintigraphy [94, 215]. The exception is in the detection of pulmonary metastases, to which ^{18}F-FDG PET can be insensitive. Therefore, diagnostic CT is indicated in the RMS patient. ^{18}F-FDG PET is also capable of accurately detecting recurrent disease or relapse where there has been prior treatment.

21.10 Nephroblastoma (Wilms' Tumor)

The Wilms' tumor is the most common form of pediatric renal malignancy, accounting for 95 % of renal cancers in children and 6 % of all childhood cancer (Table 21.8). The peak age of incidence for Wilms' tumor is 3–4 years, and the cancer is generally felt to most commonly affect children less than years old. Due to a slow indolent growth pattern, earlier detection, and aggressive surgical management, the 5-year survival rate of children with Wilms' tumor is approximately 90 %. The etiology of Wilms' tumor is unknown and likely sporadic; however a minority of cases (~5 %) are associated with genetic defects including Beckwith–Wiedemann, Denys–Drash, and Perlman syndromes. When metastases are present, the lung and liver are most commonly involved.

Table 21.8 Staging system used for Wilms' Tumor

Stage	Description
Stage I	Tumor limited to kidney (completely excised)
Stage II	Tumor extends beyond the kidney (but is completely removed)
Stage III	More than one of the following criteria must be met:
	1. Unresectable primary tumor
	2. Lymph node involvement
	3. Positive surgical margins
	4. Tumor spillage involving peritoneal surfaces either before or during surgery or transected tumor thrombus
Stage IV	Hematogenous metastases
Stage V	Bilateral renal involvement at initial diagnosis

The workup of Wilms' tumor at time of presentation usually includes an initial abdominal ultrasound followed by CT scan with contrast. Patients often present with an asymptomatic abdominal mass; however it can also present with abdominal pain, hypertension, fever, hematuria, anemia, and weight loss. The extent of local invasion and venous extension is generally determined by conventional imaging modalities such as ultrasound and CT. ^{18}F-FDG PET, because of renal excretion of ^{18}F-FDG and consequent poor target to background, can be less useful than conventional imaging for the assessment of the primary renal mass. ^{18}F-FDG PET/CT however may have some role in the assessment of liver and lung metastases or other distant spread [216]. One author has used ^{18}F-FDG PET to assess response to therapy [217].

21.11 Hepatoblastoma

The hepatoblastoma and hepatoma are the two most common hepatic malignancies in children, with hepatoblastoma occupying the majority (~2/3) of cases. Hepatoma occupies most of the remaining cases. Hepatic malignancy is uncommon in children, representing approximately 1 % of childhood cancer.

Hepatoblastoma is most common in children under the age of 5 years. The pathophysiology of hepatoblastoma is not well characterized, likely in part due to the rarity of the tumor. With a combination of aggressive surgery, chemotherapy, and sometimes radiotherapy, the 5-year survival rate for hepatoblastoma is 60 %.

Hepatocellular carcinoma generally affects children over the age of 10, and due to a combination of local aggressiveness and metastatic spread prior to detection, it is associated with a more pessimistic prognosis.

The liver normally demonstrates mild diffuse ^{18}F-FDG activity. Fatty infiltration, which is not uncommon in children, can demonstrate ^{18}F-FDG accumulation which can be confused with malignancy. Conventional imaging modalities such as ultrasound, CT, and MRI are generally used more extensively than PET for the workup of hepatic tumors. Where ^{18}F-FDG PET has been utilized, increased ^{18}F-FDG uptake is associated with more aggressive tumor grade and poor prognosis [218, 219]. There has been meaningful progress in the combination of ^{18}F-FDG uptake and alpha fetoprotein to detect recurrence of tumor after therapy [218]. A decrease in ^{18}F-FDG uptake in a tumor post-therapy is associated with response [219]. In addition, if alpha fetoprotein is negative, ^{18}F-FDG PET can be used for a systemic screening for poorly differentiated distant metastases in a manner analogous to thyroid malignancy [219].

The PET literature in pediatric hepatic malignancy is limited, partially due to the rarity of the tumor, and consists primarily of small case series. There would be significant benefit to the future examination of larger series of cases.

21.12 Thyroid Malignancy

Thyroid cancer is the most common type of endocrine cancer accounting for 1–1.5 % of all pediatric malignancies. Thyroid cancer is very rare in early childhood; the peak age is in the 15–19-year-old group. The majority of thyroid cancers are of differentiated type, mainly papillary (85 %) and to a lesser extent follicular cancer (10 %). The exact cause is unknown; however, there are many risk factors that may increase the risk of thyroid cancers, including ionizing radiation, family history of thyroid cancer, female gender, and sex hormones. The incidence is higher in females; however, the prognosis is slightly worse in males.

131-I has a major role in the management of the thyroid cancer for both diagnosis and ablation therapy. The role of PET in thyroid cancer is limited to the cases of negative iodine scan and positive serum thyroglobulin level. The spectrum of well differentiated to undifferentiated thyroid cancer corresponds to the spectrum of iodine versus ^{18}F-FDG avidity, respectively [220]. That is, while well-differentiated thyroid cancers are generally hot on iodine scintigraphy, more clinically aggressive undifferentiated tumors tend to be hot on ^{18}F-FDG PET. Thus, ^{18}F-FDG PET is generally the imaging tool of choice for the workup of a patient with elevated or rising thyroglobulin where iodine imaging has been negative [221, 222]. In this clinical scenario, it has been the author's experience that metastatic adenopathy can demonstrate ^{18}F-FDG avidity, and hence morphologic features on corresponding CT are important to assess along with activity.

The incidence of medullary thyroid cancer is very rare in children (about 2 % of thyroid cancers). The information about the diagnosis and treatment of medullary thyroid cancer in children is very limited and is usually extrapolated from the adult data. Laboratory examination (serum calcitonin level, CEA measurement, etc.), ultrasound, CT scan, 99mTc(pentavalent)-DMSA study, ^{18}F-FDG PET/CT, and ^{18}F-DOPA PET/CT have been used to detect and follow up lesions [223, 224].

Conclusion

Combined ^{18}F-FDG PET/CT is being used more frequently in the evaluation of various malignancies in pediatric patients including lymphomas, soft tissue tumors, and bone sarcomas. PET/CT can provide valuable information that is not apparent on anatomical imaging for staging and monitoring response to therapy. The growing evidence supports the continued investigation of PET and PET/CT imaging in the management and surveillance of pediatric malignancies.

Using ^{18}F-FDG PET/CT in children requires an awareness of the technical and logistical issues unique to children such as sedation or anesthesia. Adequate preparation of patients and families is essential. A thorough knowledge and understanding of the normal distribution of ^{18}F-FDG uptake in children, normal variants of pediatric ^{18}F-FDG PET/CT, and artifacts are necessary for accurate image interpretation of pediatric PET/CT imaging that differs from those of adults.

With the introduction of new imaging techniques such as PET/MR or diffusion MRI, it is expected to have an emerging role in pediatric oncology imaging with lower radiation burden compared to PET/CT. However, the exact role and value are not well established yet and further investigation is needed. Newer radiotracers such as ^{68}Ga-DOTA, ^{18}F-DOPA, ^{18}F-FAZA, and ^{18}F-FLT may be used in specific pediatric tumors. ^{18}F- NaF can be used for skeletal imaging in malignant disease. Tumor receptor imaging has the potential to improve tumor detection and characterization.

References

1. Davidoff AM. Pediatric oncology. Semin Pediatr Surg. 2010;19(3):225–33.
2. Siegel R, Naishadham D, Jemal A. Cancer statistics, 2012. CA Cancer J Clin. 2012;62(1):10–29.
3. Steliarova-Foucher E, et al. International classification of childhood cancer, third edition. Cancer. 2005;103(7):1457–67.
4. Steliarova-Foucher E, et al. Trends in childhood cancer incidence in Europe, 1970–99. Lancet. 2005;365(9477):2088.
5. SEER NCI. The Survival, Epidemiology, and End Result Program: SEER stats fact sheet: thyroid cancer. National Cancer Institute. 2014. http://seer.cancer.gov/statfacts/html/thyro.html.
6. Uslu L, et al. Value of 18F-FDG PET and PET/CT for evaluation of pediatric malignancies. J Nucl Med. 2015;56(2):274–86.
7. Gulyas B, Halldin C. New PET radiopharmaceuticals beyond FDG for brain tumor imaging. Q J Nucl Med Mol Imaging. 2012;56(2):173–90.
8. Persson M, et al. 68Ga-labeling and in vivo evaluation of a uPAR binding DOTA- and NODAGA-conjugated peptide for PET imaging of invasive cancers. Nucl Med Biol. 2012;39(4):560–9.
9. Fernandes E, et al. Positron emitting tracers in preclinical drug development. Curr Radiopharm. 2012;5(2):90–8.
10. Prezzi D, Khan A, Goh V. Perfusion CT imaging of treatment response in oncology. Eur J Radiol. 2015;84:2380–5.
11. Coursey CA, et al. Dual-energy multidetector CT: how does it work, what can it tell us, and when can we use it in abdominopelvic imaging? Radiographics. 2010;30(4):1037–55.
12. Lee YH, et al. Spectral parametric segmentation of contrast-enhanced dual-energy CT to detect bone metastasis: feasibility sensitivity study using whole-body bone scintigraphy. Acta Radiol. 2015;56(4):458–64.
13. Brady SL, Shulkin BL. Ultralow dose computed tomography attenuation correction for pediatric PET CT using adaptive statistical iterative reconstruction. Med Phys. 2015;42(2):558–66.
14. Schafer JF, et al. Simultaneous whole-body PET/MR imaging in comparison to PET/CT in pediatric oncology: initial results. Radiology. 2014;273(1):220–31.
15. Dunkl V, et al. The usefulness of dynamic O-(2-18F-fluoroethyl)-L-tyrosine PET in the clinical evaluation of brain tumors in children and adolescents. J Nucl Med. 2015;56(1):88–92.
16. Misch M, et al. (18)F-FET-PET guided surgical biopsy and resection in children and adolescence with brain tumors. Childs Nerv Syst. 2015;31(2):261–7.
17. Fraioli F, et al. 18F-fluoroethylcholine (18F-Cho) PET/MRI functional parameters in pediatric astrocytic brain tumors. Clin Nucl Med. 2015;40(1):e40–5.
18. Kurihara Y, et al. MRI of pulmonary nodules. AJR Am J Roentgenol. 2014;202(3):W210–6.
19. Loeffelbein DJ, et al. PET-MRI fusion in head-and-neck oncology: current status and implications for hybrid PET/MRI. J Oral Maxillofac Surg. 2012;70(2):473–83.
20. Buckwalter KA, Lin C, Ford JM. Managing postoperative artifacts on computed tomography and magnetic resonance imaging. Semin Musculoskelet Radiol. 2011;15(4):309–19.
21. Hendee WR, O'Connor MK. Radiation risks of medical imaging: separating fact from fantasy. Radiology. 2012;264(2):312–21.
22. Dobyns BM, et al. Malignant and benign neoplasms of the thyroid in patients treated for hyperthyroidism: a report of the cooperative thyrotoxicosis therapy follow-up study. J Clin Endocrinol Metab. 1974;38(6):976–98.
23. Ron E, et al. Cancer mortality following treatment for adult hyperthyroidism. Cooperative Thyrotoxicosis Therapy Follow-up Study Group. JAMA. 1998;280(4):347–55.
24. Fahey FH, Treves ST, Adelstein SJ. Minimizing and communicating radiation risk in pediatric nuclear medicine. J Nucl Med. 2011;52(8):1240–51.
25. Preston DL, et al. Studies of mortality of atomic bomb survivors. Report 13: solid cancer and noncancer disease mortality: 1950–1997. Radiat Res. 2003;160(4):381–407.
26. Turner HC, et al. Effect of dose rate on residual gamma-H2AX levels and frequency of micronuclei in X-irradiated mouse lymphocytes. Radiat Res. 2015;183(3):315–24.

27. Pouliliou S, Koukourakis MI. Gamma histone 2AX (gamma-H2AX) as a predictive tool in radiation oncology. Biomarkers. 2014;19(3):167–80.
28. Huda W. Radiation risks: what is to be done? AJR Am J Roentgenol. 2015;204(1):124–7.
29. Ng AK, et al. Secondary malignancies across the age spectrum. Semin Radiat Oncol. 2010;20(1):67–78.
30. Fridlich R, et al. BRCA1 and BRCA2 protect against oxidative DNA damage converted into double-strand breaks during DNA replication. DNA Repair (Amst). 2015;30:11–20.
31. Drooger JC, et al. Diagnostic and therapeutic ionizing radiation and the risk of a first and second primary breast cancer, with special attention for BRCA1 and BRCA2 mutation carriers: a critical review of the literature. Cancer Treat Rev. 2015; 41(2):187–96.
32. Piechowiak EI, et al. Intravenous iodinated contrast agents amplify DNA radiation damage at CT. Radiology. 2015;275:692–7. doi:10.1148/radiol.14132478.
33. Lacaille H, et al. Comparison of the deleterious effects of binge drinking-like alcohol exposure in adolescent and adult mice. J Neurochem. 2015; 132(6):629–41.
34. Heydenreich J, et al. Reliability of a fully automated interpretation of gamma -H2AX foci in lymphocytes of moderately trained subjects under resting conditions. J Nutr Metab. 2014;2014:478324.
35. Gelfand MJ. Dose reduction in pediatric hybrid and planar imaging. Q J Nucl Med Mol Imaging. 2010;54(4):379–88.
36. Accorsi R, Karp JS, Surti S. Improved dose regimen in pediatric PET. J Nucl Med. 2010;51(2):293–300.
37. Lassmann M, et al. The new EANM paediatric dosage card. Eur J Nucl Med Mol Imaging. 2007;34(5):796–8.
38. Gelfand MJ, et al. Pediatric radiopharmaceutical administered doses: 2010 North American consensus guidelines. J Nucl Med. 2011;52(2):318–22.
39. American Academy of P, et al. Guidelines for monitoring and management of pediatric patients during and after sedation for diagnostic and therapeutic procedures: an update. Pediatrics. 2006;118(6): 2587–602.
40. Arlachov Y, Ganatra RH. Sedation/anaesthesia in paediatric radiology. Br J Radiol. 2012;85(1019): e1018–31.
41. Delbeke D, et al. Procedure guideline for tumor imaging with 18F-FDG PET/CT 1.0. J Nucl Med. 2006;47(5):885–95.
42. Shen G, et al. Potential performance of dual-time-point 18F-FDG PET/CT compared with single-time-point imaging for differential diagnosis of metastatic lymph nodes: a meta-analysis. Nucl Med Commun. 2014;35(10):1003–10.
43. Shen G, et al. Diagnostic value of dual time-point 18 F-FDG PET/CT versus single time-point imaging for detection of mediastinal nodal metastasis in non-small cell lung cancer patients: a meta-analysis. Acta Radiol. 2015;56:681–7.
44. Costantini DL, et al. Dual-time-point FDG PET/CT for the evaluation of pediatric tumors. AJR Am J Roentgenol. 2013;200(2):408–13.
45. Zukotynski KA, et al. Constant ambient temperature of 24 degrees C significantly reduces FDG uptake by brown adipose tissue in children scanned during the winter. Eur J Nucl Med Mol Imaging. 2009;36(4): 602–6.
46. Shammas A, Lim R, Charron M. Pediatric FDG PET/CT: physiologic uptake, normal variants, and benign conditions. Radiographics. 2009;29(5): 1467–86.
47. Keyes Jr JW. SUV: standard uptake or silly useless value? J Nucl Med. 1995;36(10):1836–9.
48. Ghanem MA, Kazim NA, Elgazzar AH. Impact of obesity on nuclear medicine imaging. J Nucl Med Technol. 2011;39(1):40–50.
49. Krak NC, et al. Effects of ROI definition and reconstruction method on quantitative outcome and applicability in a response monitoring trial. Eur J Nucl Med Mol Imaging. 2005;32(3):294–301.
50. Boellaard R, et al. Effects of noise, image resolution, and ROI definition on the accuracy of standard uptake values: a simulation study. J Nucl Med. 2004;45(9):1519–27.
51. Bemben MG, et al. Age-related variability in body composition methods for assessment of percent fat and fat-free mass in men aged 20–74 years. Age Ageing. 1998;27(2):147–53.
52. Nakahara T, et al. FDG uptake in the morphologically normal thymus: comparison of FDG positron emission tomography and CT. Br J Radiol. 2001;74(885):821–4.
53. Francis IR, et al. The thymus: reexamination of age-related changes in size and shape. AJR Am J Roentgenol. 1985;145(2):249–54.
54. Brink I, et al. Increased metabolic activity in the thymus gland studied with 18F-FDG PET: age dependency and frequency after chemotherapy. J Nucl Med. 2001;42(4):591–5.
55. Ferdinand B, Gupta P, Kramer EL. Spectrum of thymic uptake at 18F-FDG PET. Radiographics. 2004;24(6):1611–6.
56. Sasaki M, et al. Differential diagnosis of thymic tumors using a combination of 11C-methionine PET and FDG PET. J Nucl Med. 1999;40(10): 1595–601.
57. Heusner TA, et al. Incidental head and neck (18) F-FDG uptake on PET/CT without corresponding morphological lesion: early predictor of cancer development? Eur J Nucl Med Mol Imaging. 2009;36(9):1397–406.
58. Elstrom RL, et al. Enhanced marrow [18F]fluorodeoxyglucose uptake related to myeloid hyperplasia in Hodgkin's lymphoma can simulate lymphoma involvement in marrow. Clin Lymphoma. 2004;5(1):62–4.
59. Knopp MV, et al. Bone marrow uptake of fluorine-18-fluorodeoxyglucose following treatment with hematopoietic growth factors: initial evaluation. Nucl Med Biol. 1996;23(6):845–9.

60. Trout AT, et al. Optimizing the interval between G-CSF therapy and F-18 FDG PET imaging in children and young adults receiving chemotherapy for sarcoma. Pediatr Radiol. 2015;45:1001–6.
61. Aflalo-Hazan V, et al. Increased FDG uptake by bone marrow in major beta-thalassemia. Clin Nucl Med. 2005;30(11):754–5.
62. Plantade A, et al. Diffusely increased F-18 FDG uptake in bone marrow in a patient with acute anemia and recent erythropoietin therapy. Clin Nucl Med. 2003;28(9):771–2.
63. Hong TS, et al. Brown adipose tissue 18F-FDG uptake in pediatric PET/CT imaging. Pediatr Radiol. 2011;41(6):759–68.
64. Lin EC, Alavi A. PET and PET/CT: a clinical guide. 2nd ed. New York: Thieme Medical Publishers Inc.; 2009.
65. Bhargava P, Hanif M, Nash C. Whole-body F-18 sodium fluoride PET-CT in a patient with renal cell carcinoma. Clin Nucl Med. 2008;33(12):894–5.
66. Even-Sapir E, et al. Assessment of malignant skeletal disease: initial experience with 18F-fluoride PET/CT and comparison between 18F-fluoride PET and 18F-fluoride PET/CT. J Nucl Med. 2004;45(2): 272–8.
67. Segall G, et al. SNM practice guideline for sodium 18F-fluoride PET/CT bone scans 1.0. J Nucl Med. 2010;51(11):1813–20.
68. Bading JR, Shields AF. Imaging of cell proliferation: status and prospects. J Nucl Med. 2008;49 Suppl 2:64S–80.
69. Buck AK, et al. Clinical relevance of imaging proliferative activity in lung nodules. Eur J Nucl Med Mol Imaging. 2005;32(5):525–33.
70. Everitt S, et al. Imaging cellular proliferation during chemo-radiotherapy: a pilot study of serial 18F-FLT positron emission tomography/computed tomography imaging for non-small-cell lung cancer. Int J Radiat Oncol Biol Phys. 2009;75(4):1098–104.
71. Yamamoto Y, et al. Correlation of 18F-FLT and 18F-FDG uptake on PET with Ki-67 immunohistochemistry in non-small cell lung cancer. Eur J Nucl Med Mol Imaging. 2007;34(10):1610–6.
72. Yap CS, et al. Evaluation of thoracic tumors with 18F-fluorothymidine and 18F-fluorodeoxyglucose-positron emission tomography. Chest. 2006;129(2): 393–401.
73. Kameyama R, et al. Detection of gastric cancer using 18F-FLT PET: comparison with 18F-FDG PET. Eur J Nucl Med Mol Imaging. 2009;36(3): 382–8.
74. Yamamoto Y, et al. Detection of colorectal cancer using 18F-FLT PET: comparison with 18F-FDG PET. Nucl Med Commun. 2009;30:841–5.
75. Cobben DC, et al. 3′-18F-fluoro-3′-deoxy-L-thymidine: a new tracer for staging metastatic melanoma? J Nucl Med. 2003;44(12):1927–32.
76. Buck AK, et al. Molecular imaging of proliferation in malignant lymphoma. Cancer Res. 2006;66(22): 11055–61.
77. Herrmann K, et al. Early response assessment using 3′-deoxy-3′-[18F]fluorothymidine-positron emission tomography in high-grade non-Hodgkin's lymphoma. Clin Cancer Res. 2007;13(12):3552–8.
78. Kenny L, et al. Imaging early changes in proliferation at 1 week post chemotherapy: a pilot study in breast cancer patients with 3′-deoxy-3′-[18F]fluorothymidine positron emission tomography. Eur J Nucl Med Mol Imaging. 2007;34(9):1339–47.
79. Pio BS, et al. Usefulness of 3′-[F-18]fluoro-3′-deoxythymidine with positron emission tomography in predicting breast cancer response to therapy. Mol Imaging Biol. 2006;8(1):36–42.
80. Buck AK, et al. Imaging bone and soft tissue tumors with the proliferation marker [18F]fluorodeoxythymidine. Clin Cancer Res. 2008;14(10):2970–7.
81. Choi SJ, et al. [18F]3′-deoxy-3′-fluorothymidine PET for the diagnosis and grading of brain tumors. Eur J Nucl Med Mol Imaging. 2005;32(6):653–9.
82. Gilles R, et al. (18)F-fluoro-L-thymidine-PET for the evaluation of primary brain tumours in children: a report of three cases. Nucl Med Commun. 2010;31(6):482–7.
83. Hatakeyama T, et al. 11C-methionine (MET) and 18F-fluorothymidine (FLT) PET in patients with newly diagnosed glioma. Eur J Nucl Med Mol Imaging. 2008;35(11):2009–17.
84. Saga T, et al. Evaluation of primary brain tumors with FLT-PET: usefulness and limitations. Clin Nucl Med. 2006;31(12):774–80.
85. Tripathi M, et al. Comparative evaluation of F-18 FDOPA, F-18 FDG, and F-18 FLT-PET/CT for metabolic imaging of low grade gliomas. Clin Nucl Med. 2009;34(12):878–83.
86. Shields AF. Positron emission tomography measurement of tumor metabolism and growth: its expanding role in oncology. Mol Imaging Biol. 2006;8(3): 141–50.
87. Shields AF, et al. Imaging proliferation in vivo with FLT and positron emission tomography. Nat Med. 1998;4(11):1334–6.
88. Vaupel P, Mayer A. Hypoxia in cancer: significance and impact on clinical outcome. Cancer Metastasis Rev. 2007;26(2):225–39.
89. Harrison LB, et al. Impact of tumor hypoxia and anemia on radiation therapy outcomes. Oncologist. 2002;7(6):492–508.
90. Molls M, et al. Relevance of oxygen in radiation oncology. Mechanisms of action, correlation to low hemoglobin levels. Strahlenther Onkol. 1998;174 Suppl 4:13–6.
91. Hockel M, et al. Association between tumor hypoxia and malignant progression in advanced cancer of the uterine cervix. Cancer Res. 1996;56(19):4509–15.
92. Hockel M, et al. Hypoxia and radiation response in human tumors. Semin Radiat Oncol. 1996;6(1):3–9.
93. Bottaro DP, Liotta LA. Cancer: out of air is not out of action. Nature. 2003;423(6940):593–5.
94. Dorie MJ, Brown JM. Modification of the antitumor activity of chemotherapeutic drugs by the hypoxic

cytotoxic agent tirapazamine. Cancer Chemother Pharmacol. 1997;39(4):361–6.
95. Papadopoulou MV, Bloomer WD. NLCQ-1 (NSC 709257): exploiting hypoxia with a weak DNA-intercalating bioreductive drug. Clin Cancer Res. 2003;9(15):5714–20.
96. Beck R, et al. Pretreatment 18F-FAZA PET predicts success of hypoxia-directed radiochemotherapy using tirapazamine. J Nucl Med. 2007;48(6):973–80.
97. von Pawel J, et al. Tirapazamine plus cisplatin versus cisplatin in advanced non-small-cell lung cancer: a report of the international CATAPULT I study group. Cisplatin and tirapazamine in subjects with advanced previously untreated non-small-cell lung tumors. J Clin Oncol. 2000;18(6):1351–9.
98. Brizel DM, et al. Oxygenation of head and neck cancer: changes during radiotherapy and impact on treatment outcome. Radiother Oncol. 1999;53(2):113–7.
99. Grosu AL, et al. Hypoxia imaging with FAZA-PET and theoretical considerations with regard to dose painting for individualization of radiotherapy in patients with head and neck cancer. Int J Radiat Oncol Biol Phys. 2007;69(2):541–51.
100. O'Tuama LA, et al. Two-phase [11C]L-methionine PET in childhood brain tumors. Pediatr Neurol. 1990;6(3):163–70.
101. Utriainen M, et al. Metabolic characterization of childhood brain tumors: comparison of 18F-fluorodeoxyglucose and 11C-methionine positron emission tomography. Cancer. 2002;95(6):1376–86.
102. Virgolini I, et al. Procedure guidelines for PET/CT tumour imaging with 68Ga-DOTA-conjugated peptides: 68Ga-DOTA-TOC, 68Ga-DOTA-NOC, 68Ga-DOTA-TATE. Eur J Nucl Med Mol Imaging. 2010;37(10):2004–10.
103. Shulkin BL, et al. PET hydroxyephedrine imaging of neuroblastoma. J Nucl Med. 1996;37(1):16–21.
104. Sisson JC, Shulkin BL. Nuclear medicine imaging of pheochromocytoma and neuroblastoma. Q J Nucl Med. 1999;43(3):217–23.
105. Hoegerle S, et al. Pheochromocytomas: detection with 18F DOPA whole body PET--initial results. Radiology. 2002;222(2):507–12.
106. deKemp RA, Nahmias C. Attenuation correction in PET using single photon transmission measurement. Med Phys. 1994;21(6):771–8.
107. Biermann M, et al. Is there a role for PET-CT and SPECT-CT in pediatric oncology? Acta Radiol. 2013;54(9):1037–45.
108. Srinivasan M, Bhaskar S, Carlson DW. Variation in procedural sedation practices among Children's Hospitals. Hosp Pediatr. 2015;5(3):148–53.
109. Martinez-Moller A, Nekolla SG. Attenuation correction for PET/MR: problems, novel approaches and practical solutions. Z Med Phys. 2012;22(4):299–310.
110. Roy S, et al. PET attenuation correction using synthetic CT from ultrashort echo-time MR imaging. J Nucl Med. 2014;55(12):2071–7.
111. Berker Y, Kiessling F, Schulz V. Scattered PET data for attenuation-map reconstruction in PET/MRI. Med Phys. 2014;41(10):102502.
112. Yip S, et al. Sensitivity study of voxel-based PET image comparison to image registration algorithms. Med Phys. 2014;41(11):111714.
113. Kinney H, Faix R, Brazy J. The fetal alcohol syndrome and neuroblastoma. Pediatrics. 1980;66(1):130–2.
114. Kramer S, et al. Medical and drug risk factors associated with neuroblastoma: a case–control study. J Natl Cancer Inst. 1987;78(5):797–804.
115. Michalek AM, et al. Gravid health status, medication use, and risk of neuroblastoma. Am J Epidemiol. 1996;143(10):996–1001.
116. Bunin GR, et al. Neuroblastoma and parental occupation. Am J Epidemiol. 1990;131(5):776–80.
117. Strenger V, et al. Diagnostic and prognostic impact of urinary catecholamines in neuroblastoma patients. Pediatr Blood Cancer. 2007;48(5):504–9.
118. Maris JM. Recent advances in neuroblastoma. N Engl J Med. 2010;362(23):2202–11.
119. Kushner BH. Neuroblastoma: a disease requiring a multitude of imaging studies. J Nucl Med. 2004;45(7):1172–88.
120. Olivier P, et al. Guidelines for radioiodinated MIBG scintigraphy in children. Eur J Nucl Med Mol Imaging. 2003;30(5):B45–50.
121. Lonergan GJ, et al. Neuroblastoma, ganglioneuroblastoma, and ganglioneuroma: radiologic-pathologic correlation. Radiographics. 2002;22(4):911–34.
122. Howman-Giles RB, Gilday DL, Ash JM. Radionuclide skeletal survey in neuroblastoma. Radiology. 1979;131(2):497–502.
123. Sharp SE, et al. 123I-MIBG scintigraphy and 18F-FDG PET in neuroblastoma. J Nucl Med. 2009;50(8):1237–43.
124. Choi YJ, et al. (18)F-FDG PET as a single imaging modality in pediatric neuroblastoma: comparison with abdomen CT and bone scintigraphy. Ann Nucl Med. 2014;28(4):304–13.
125. Taggart DR, et al. Comparison of iodine-123 metaiodobenzylguanidine (MIBG) scan and [18F] fluorodeoxyglucose positron emission tomography to evaluate response after iodine-131 MIBG therapy for relapsed neuroblastoma. J Clin Oncol. 2009;27(32):5343–9.
126. Piccardo A, et al. Comparison of 18F-dopa PET/CT and 123I-MIBG scintigraphy in stage 3 and 4 neuroblastoma: a pilot study. Eur J Nucl Med Mol Imaging. 2012;39(1):57–71.
127. Pashankar FD, O'Dorisio MS, Menda Y. MIBG and somatostatin receptor analogs in children: current concepts on diagnostic and therapeutic use. J Nucl Med. 2005;46 Suppl 1:55S–61.
128. Kroiss A, et al. Functional imaging in phaeochromocytoma and neuroblastoma with 68Ga-DOTA-Tyr3-octreotide positron emission tomography and 123I-metaiodobenzylguanidine: a clarification. Eur J Nucl Med Mol Imaging. 2012;39(3):543.

129. De Krijger RR, et al. Frequent genetic changes in childhood pheochromocytomas. Ann N Y Acad Sci. 2006;1073:166–76.
130. Pacak K, et al. Biochemical diagnosis, localization and management of pheochromocytoma: focus on multiple endocrine neoplasia type 2 in relation to other hereditary syndromes and sporadic forms of the tumour. J Intern Med. 2005;257(1):60–8.
131. Pacak K, Eisenhofer G, Grossman A. The incidentally discovered adrenal mass. N Engl J Med. 2007;356(19):2005.
132. Pacak K, et al. Pheochromocytoma: recommendations for clinical practice from the First International Symposium. October 2005. Nat Clin Pract Endocrinol Metab. 2007;3(2):92–102.
133. Havekes B, et al. Update on pediatric pheochromocytoma. Pediatr Nephrol. 2009;24(5):943–50.
134. Trampal C, et al. Pheochromocytomas: detection with 11C hydroxyephedrine PET. Radiology. 2004;230(2):423–8.
135. Janssen I, et al. Superiority of [68Ga]-DOTATATE PET/CT to other functional imaging modalities in the localization of SDHB-associated metastatic pheochromocytoma and paraganglioma. Clin Cancer Res. 2015;21:3888–95.
136. Brugieres L, Minard V, Patte C. Lymphomas in children and adolescents. Rev Prat. 2012;62(4):453–8.
137. Bhatia S, et al. High risk of subsequent neoplasms continues with extended follow-up of childhood Hodgkin's disease: report from the Late Effects Study Group. J Clin Oncol. 2003;21(23):4386–94.
138. Prasad PK, et al. Long-term non-cancer mortality in pediatric and young adult cancer survivors in Finland. Pediatr Blood Cancer. 2012;58(3):421–7.
139. Howman-Giles R, Stevens M, Bergin M. Role of gallium-67 in management of paediatric solid tumours. Aust Paediatr J. 1982;18(2):120–5.
140. Sty JR, Kun LE, Starshak RJ. Pediatric applications in nuclear oncology. Semin Nucl Med. 1985;15(2):171–200.
141. Elstrom R, et al. Utility of FDG-PET scanning in lymphoma by WHO classification. Blood. 2003;101(10):3875–6.
142. Rigacci L, et al. Positron emission tomography in the staging of patients with Hodgkin's lymphoma. A prospective multicentric study by the Intergruppo Italiano Linfomi. Ann Hematol. 2007;86(12): 897–903.
143. Jerusalem G, et al. Whole-body positron emission tomography using 18F-fluorodeoxyglucose compared to standard procedures for staging patients with Hodgkin's disease. Haematologica. 2001;86(3):266–73.
144. London K, et al. 18F-FDG PET/CT in paediatric lymphoma: comparison with conventional imaging. Eur J Nucl Med Mol Imaging. 2011;38(2): 274–84.
145. Hutchings M, et al. Position emission tomography with or without computed tomography in the primary staging of Hodgkin's lymphoma. Haematologica. 2006;91(4):482–9.
146. Kabickova E, et al. Comparison of 18F-FDG-PET and standard procedures for the pretreatment staging of children and adolescents with Hodgkin's disease. Eur J Nucl Med Mol Imaging. 2006;33(9):1025–31.
147. Moulin-Romsee G, et al. (18)F-FDG PET/CT bone/bone marrow findings in Hodgkin's lymphoma may circumvent the use of bone marrow trephine biopsy at diagnosis staging. Eur J Nucl Med Mol Imaging. 2010;37(6):1095–105.
148. Pelosi E, et al. FDG-PET in the detection of bone marrow disease in Hodgkin's disease and aggressive non-Hodgkin's lymphoma and its impact on clinical management. Q J Nucl Med Mol Imaging. 2008;52(1):9–16.
149. Purz S, et al. [18F]Fluorodeoxyglucose positron emission tomography for detection of bone marrow involvement in children and adolescents with Hodgkin's lymphoma. J Clin Oncol. 2011;29(26): 3523–8.
150. Girinsky T, et al. Is FDG-PET scan in patients with early stage Hodgkin lymphoma of any value in the implementation of the involved-node radiotherapy concept and dose painting? Radiother Oncol. 2007;85(2):178–86.
151. Hermann S, et al. Staging in childhood lymphoma: differences between FDG-PET and CT. Nuklearmedizin. 2005;44(1):1–7.
152. Muslimani AA, et al. The utility of 18-F-fluorodeoxyglucose positron emission tomography in evaluation of bone marrow involvement by non-Hodgkin lymphoma. Am J Clin Oncol. 2008;31(5):409–12.
153. Kluge R, et al. FDG PET/CT in children and adolescents with lymphoma. Pediatr Radiol. 2013;43(4):406–17.
154. Weiler-Sagie M, et al. (18)F-FDG avidity in lymphoma readdressed: a study of 766 patients. J Nucl Med. 2010;51(1):25–30.
155. Abramson SJ, Price AP. Imaging of pediatric lymphomas. Radiol Clin North Am. 2008;46(2):313–38, ix.
156. Toma P, et al. Multimodality imaging of Hodgkin disease and non-Hodgkin lymphomas in children. Radiographics. 2007;27(5):1335–54.
157. Cheson BD, et al. Revised response criteria for malignant lymphoma. J Clin Oncol. 2007;25(5): 579–86.
158. Cahu X, et al. 18F-fluorodeoxyglucose-positron emission tomography before, during and after treatment in mature T/NK lymphomas: a study from the GOELAMS group. Ann Oncol. 2011;22(3):705–11.
159. Karantanis D, et al. 18F-FDG PET and PET/CT in Burkitt's lymphoma. Eur J Radiol. 2010;75(1): e68–73.
160. Rini JN, et al. 18F-FDG PET versus CT for evaluating the spleen during initial staging of lymphoma. J Nucl Med. 2003;44(7):1072–4.

161. Seam P, Juweid ME, Cheson BD. The role of FDG-PET scans in patients with lymphoma. Blood. 2007;110(10):3507–16.
162. Rhodes MM, et al. Utility of FDG-PET/CT in follow-up of children treated for Hodgkin and non-Hodgkin lymphoma. J Pediatr Hematol Oncol. 2006;28(5):300–6.
163. Furth C, et al. Early and late therapy response assessment with [18F]fluorodeoxyglucose positron emission tomography in pediatric Hodgkin's lymphoma: analysis of a prospective multicenter trial. J Clin Oncol. 2009;27(26):4385–91.
164. Kostakoglu L, et al. PET predicts prognosis after 1 cycle of chemotherapy in aggressive lymphoma and Hodgkin's disease. J Nucl Med. 2002;43(8): 1018–27.
165. Kluge R, Korholz D. Role of FDG-PET in staging and therapy of children with Hodgkin lymphoma. Klin Padiatr. 2011;223(6):315–9.
166. Radford J, et al. Results of a trial of PET-directed therapy for early-stage Hodgkin's lymphoma. N Engl J Med. 2015;372(17):1598–607.
167. Duhrsen U, et al. Positron emission tomography guided therapy of aggressive non-Hodgkin lymphomas--the PETAL trial. Leuk Lymphoma. 2009;50(11):1757–60.
168. Depas G, et al. 18F-FDG PET in children with lymphomas. Eur J Nucl Med Mol Imaging. 2005;32(1): 31–8.
169. Bakhshi S, et al. Pediatric nonlymphoblastic non-Hodgkin lymphoma: baseline, interim, and post-treatment PET/CT versus contrast-enhanced CT for evaluation--a prospective study. Radiology. 2012;262(3):956–68.
170. Lavely WC, et al. FDG PET in the follow-up management of patients with newly diagnosed Hodgkin and non-Hodgkin lymphoma after first-line chemotherapy. Int J Radiat Oncol Biol Phys. 2003;57(2): 307–15.
171. Burns DM, Crawford DH. Epstein-Barr virus-specific cytotoxic T-lymphocytes for adoptive immunotherapy of post-transplant lymphoproliferative disease. Blood Rev. 2004;18(3):193–209.
172. Blaes AH, Morrison VA. Post-transplant lymphoproliferative disorders following solid-organ transplantation. Expert Rev Hematol. 2010;3(1):35–44.
173. Taylor AL, Marcus R, Bradley JA. Post-transplant lymphoproliferative disorders (PTLD) after solid organ transplantation. Crit Rev Oncol Hematol. 2005;56(1):155–67.
174. Feng S, et al. Tumors and transplantation: the 2003 Third Annual ASTS State-of-the-Art Winter Symposium. Am J Transplant. 2003;3(12):1481–7.
175. Dharnidharka VR, et al. Post-transplant lymphoproliferative disorder in the United States: young Caucasian males are at highest risk. Am J Transplant. 2002;2(10):993–8.
176. Shapiro R, et al. Posttransplant lymphoproliferative disorders in adult and pediatric renal transplant patients receiving tacrolimus-based immunosuppression. Transplantation. 1999;68(12):1851–4.
177. Leblond V, et al. Lymphoproliferative disorders after organ transplantation: a report of 24 cases observed in a single center. J Clin Oncol. 1995;13(4):961–8.
178. Opelz G, Dohler B. Lymphomas after solid organ transplantation: a collaborative transplant study report. Am J Transplant. 2004;4(2):222–30.
179. Gallego S, et al. Post-transplant lymphoproliferative disorders in children: the role of chemotherapy in the era of rituximab. Pediatr Transplant. 2010;14(1): 61–6.
180. Campo E, et al. The 2008 WHO classification of lymphoid neoplasms and beyond: evolving concepts and practical applications. Blood. 2011;117(19): 5019–32.
181. Bianchi E, et al. Clinical usefulness of FDG-PET/CT scan imaging in the management of posttransplant lymphoproliferative disease. Transplantation. 2008;85(5):707–12.
182. Dierickx D, et al. The accuracy of positron emission tomography in the detection of posttransplant lymphoproliferative disorder. Haematologica. 2013;98(5):771–5.
183. O'Conner AR, Franc BL. FDG PET imaging in the evaluation of post-transplant lymphoproliferative disorder following renal transplantation. Nucl Med Commun. 2005;26(12):1107–11.
184. Takehana CS, et al. (18)F-FDG PET/CT in the management of patients with post-transplant lymphoproliferative disorder. Nucl Med Commun. 2014;35(3):276–81.
185. Bakker NA, et al. PTLD visualization by FDG-PET: improved detection of extranodal localizations. Am J Transplant. 2006;6(8):1984–5.
186. Noraini AR, et al. PET-CT as an effective imaging modality in the staging and follow-up of post-transplant lymphoproliferative disorder following solid organ transplantation. Singapore Med J. 2009;50(12):1189–95.
187. Panagiotidis E, et al. (18)F-fluorodeoxyglucose positron emission tomography/computed tomography in diagnosis of post-transplant lymphoproliferative disorder. Leuk Lymphoma. 2014;55(3):515–9.
188. von Falck C, et al. Post transplant lymphoproliferative disease in pediatric solid organ transplant patients: a possible role for [18F]-FDG-PET(/CT) in initial staging and therapy monitoring. Eur J Radiol. 2007;63(3):427–35.
189. Su K, et al. Diffuse homogeneous bone marrow uptake of FDG in patients with acute lymphoblastic leukemia. Clin Nucl Med. 2013;38(1):e33–4.
190. Endo T, et al. Localized relapse in bone marrow of extremities after allogeneic stem cell transplantation for acute lymphoblastic leukemia. Am J Hematol. 2004;76(3):279–82.
191. Sharp SE, Gelfand MJ, Absalon MJ. Altered FDG uptake patterns in pediatric lymphoblastic lymphoma patients receiving induction chemotherapy

that includes very high dose corticosteroids. Pediatr Radiol. 2012;42(3):331–6.
192. Stanescu L, et al. FDG PET of the brain in pediatric patients: imaging spectrum with MR imaging correlation. Radiographics. 2013;33(5):1279–303.
193. Kruer MC, et al. The value of positron emission tomography and proliferation index in predicting progression in low-grade astrocytomas of childhood. J Neurooncol. 2009;95(2):239–45.
194. Borgwardt L, et al. Increased fluorine-18 2-fluoro-2-deoxy-D-glucose (FDG) uptake in childhood CNS tumors is correlated with malignancy grade: a study with FDG positron emission tomography/magnetic resonance imaging coregistration and image fusion. J Clin Oncol. 2005;23(13):3030–7.
195. Glantz MJ, et al. Identification of early recurrence of primary central nervous system tumors by [18F]fluorodeoxyglucose positron emission tomography. Ann Neurol. 1991;29(4):347–55.
196. Hanson MW, et al. FDG-PET in the selection of brain lesions for biopsy. J Comput Assist Tomogr. 1991;15(5):796–801.
197. Giovannini E, et al. Clinical applications of choline PET/CT in brain tumors. Curr Pharm Des. 2015;21(1):121–7.
198. Torii K, et al. Correlation of amino-acid uptake using methionine PET and histological classifications in various gliomas. Ann Nucl Med. 2005;19(8):677–83.
199. Ceyssens S, et al. [11C]methionine PET, histopathology, and survival in primary brain tumors and recurrence. AJNR Am J Neuroradiol. 2006;27(7):1432–7.
200. Van Laere K, et al. Direct comparison of 18F-FDG and 11C-methionine PET in suspected recurrence of glioma: sensitivity, inter-observer variability and prognostic value. Eur J Nucl Med Mol Imaging. 2005;32(1):39–51.
201. Hipp SJ, et al. Molecular imaging of pediatric brain tumors: comparison of tumor metabolism using (1)(8)F-FDG-PET and MRSI. J Neurooncol. 2012;109(3):521–7.
202. Gilday DL, Ash JM, Reilly BJ. Radionuclide skeletal survey for pediatric neoplasms. Radiology. 1977;123(2):399–406.
203. Rosen G, et al. Serial thallium-201 scintigraphy in osteosarcoma. Correlation with tumor necrosis after preoperative chemotherapy. Clin Orthop Relat Res. 1993;293:302–6.
204. Ramanna L, et al. Thallium-201 scintigraphy in bone sarcoma: comparison with gallium-67 and technetium-MDP in the evaluation of chemotherapeutic response. J Nucl Med. 1990;31(5):567–72.
205. Volker T, et al. Positron emission tomography for staging of pediatric sarcoma patients: results of a prospective multicenter trial. J Clin Oncol. 2007;25(34):5435–41.
206. Byun BH, et al. Comparison of (18)F-FDG PET/CT and (99 m)Tc-MDP bone scintigraphy for detection of bone metastasis in osteosarcoma. Skeletal Radiol. 2013;42(12):1673–81.
207. Huang TL, et al. Comparison between F-18-FDG positron emission tomography and histology for the assessment of tumor necrosis rates in primary osteosarcoma. J Chin Med Assoc. 2006;69(8):372–6.
208. Mansky PJ, et al. Treatment of metastatic osteosarcoma with the somatostatin analog OncoLar: significant reduction of insulin-like growth factor-1 serum levels. J Pediatr Hematol Oncol. 2002;24(6):440–6.
209. Kong CB, et al. (1)(8)F-FDG PET SUVmax as an indicator of histopathologic response after neoadjuvant chemotherapy in extremity osteosarcoma. Eur J Nucl Med Mol Imaging. 2013;40(5):728–36.
210. Erlemann R, et al. Response of osteosarcoma and Ewing sarcoma to preoperative chemotherapy: assessment with dynamic and static MR imaging and skeletal scintigraphy. Radiology. 1990;175(3):791–6.
211. Gaston LL, et al. 18F-FDG PET response to neoadjuvant chemotherapy for Ewing sarcoma and osteosarcoma are different. Skeletal Radiol. 2011;40(8):1007–15.
212. Tateishi U, et al. Comparative study of FDG PET/CT and conventional imaging in the staging of rhabdomyosarcoma. Ann Nucl Med. 2009;23(2):155–61.
213. Klem ML, et al. PET for staging in rhabdomyosarcoma: an evaluation of PET as an adjunct to current staging tools. J Pediatr Hematol Oncol. 2007;29(1):9–14.
214. Adler LP, et al. Noninvasive grading of musculoskeletal tumors using PET. J Nucl Med. 1991;32(8):1508–12.
215. Ricard F, et al. Additional benefit of F-18 FDG PET/CT in the staging and follow-up of pediatric rhabdomyosarcoma. Clin Nucl Med. 2011;36(8):672–7.
216. Moinul Hossain AK, et al. FDG positron emission tomography/computed tomography studies of Wilms' tumor. Eur J Nucl Med Mol Imaging. 2010;37(7):1300–8.
217. Qin Z, et al. Use of 18F-FDG-PET-CT for assessment of response to neoadjuvant chemotherapy in children with Wilms tumor. J Pediatr Hematol Oncol. 2015;37:396–401.
218. Wong KK, et al. The use of positron emission tomography in detecting hepatoblastoma recurrence--a cautionary tale. J Pediatr Surg. 2004;39(12):1779–81.
219. Mody RJ, et al. FDG PET for the study of primary hepatic malignancies in children. Pediatr Blood Cancer. 2006;47(1):51–5.
220. Ciarallo A, et al. Value of fluorodeoxyglucose PET/computed tomography patient management and outcomes in thyroid cancer. PET Clin. 2015;10(2):265–78.
221. Asa S, et al. The role of FDG-PET/CT in differentiated thyroid cancer patients with negative iodine-131 whole-body scan and elevated anti-Tg level. Ann Nucl Med. 2014;28(10):970–9.

222. Elboga U, et al. F-18 FDG PET/CT imaging in the diagnostic work-up of thyroid cancer patients with high serum thyroglobulin, negative I-131 whole body scan and suppressed thyrotropin: 8-year experience. Eur Rev Med Pharmacol Sci. 2015;19(3): 396–401.
223. Beheshti M, et al. The value of 18F-DOPA PET-CT in patients with medullary thyroid carcinoma: comparison with 18F-FDG PET-CT. Eur Radiol. 2009;19(6):1425–34.
224. Howe TC, et al. Role of Tc-99m DMSA (V) scanning and serum calcitonin monitoring in the management of medullary thyroid carcinoma. Singapore Med J. 2008;49(1):19–22.

Role of PET/CT in Radiotherapy Treatment Planning

22

Maria Picchio, Elena Incerti, and Nadia Di Muzio

Contents

22.1	**Introduction**	578
22.1.1	Lung Cancer	581
22.1.2	Head and Neck Cancers	583
22.1.3	Esophageal Cancers	585
22.1.4	Breast Cancer	585
22.1.5	Lymphomas	587
22.1.6	Myelomas	588
22.1.7	Brain Tumors	590
22.1.8	Gynecological Malignancies	592
22.1.9	Colorectal Cancer	594
22.1.10	Prostate Cancer	596
22.1.11	Imaging Hypoxia in Radiotherapy	598
Conclusions		599
References		599

M. Picchio (✉) • E. Incerti
Department of Nuclear Medicine, IRCCS San Raffaele Scientific Institute, Milan, Italy
e-mail: picchio.maria@hsr.it; incerti.elena@hsr.it

N. Di Muzio
Department of Radiation Oncology, IRCCS San Raffaele Scientific Institute, Milan, Italy
e-mail: dimuzio.nadia@hsr.it

Abstract

This chapter focuses on the rationale, target validation, dose prescription verification and evaluation, and recent clinical achievements in the field of integrating positron emission tomography imaging into radiotherapy treatment planning. Application of functional imaging to radiotherapy is a rapidly expanding field with the development of new modalities and techniques. Functional imaging of positron emission tomography in conjunction with radiotherapy provides new avenues toward the clinical application of dose painting as a new radiotherapy strategy delivering optimized dose redistribution according to the functional imaging information to further improve tumor control.

New biological imaging methodologies mainly based on positron emission tomography/computed tomography, magnetic resonance imaging, and magnetic resonance spectroscopy imaging, in conjunction with radiotherapy, make dose painting possible. It can be used to draw a three-dimensional map of radiobiological relevant parameters as its inherent potential to trace the real target volume, consisting of tumor cells that require a therapeutic dose to control the disease. Positron emission tomography/computed tomography is outstanding and widely used in daily clinical practice. It offers molecular biological information on the tumor microenvironment in addition to anatomical imaging

M.M. Khalil (ed.), *Basic Science of PET Imaging*, DOI 10.1007/978-3-319-40070-9_22

and shows significant biological heterogeneity of tumors, such as metabolism, proliferation, hypoxia, radioresistance cell density, and perfusion.

Index Acronyms

3D	Three dimensional
AC	Attenuation correction
ACE	11C-acetate
AMT	Alpha-[11C]methyl-L-tryptophan
ART	Adaptive radiotherapy
ATSM	Copper-64 diacetyl-bis (N4-methylthiosemicarbazone)
BTV	Biological target volume
CECT	Contrast-enhanced computed tomography
CH	Chemotherapy
CHO	11C/18F-choline
CMR	Complete metabolic response
CRC	Colorectal carcinoma
CRT	Chemo radiation therapy
CT	Computed tomography
CTV	Clinical target volume
DLBCL	Diffuse large B-cell lymphoma
DPBC	Dose painting by contours
DPBN	Dose painting by numbers
EBRT	External beam radiation therapy
EORTC	European Organization for Research and Treatment of Cancer
EP	Extramedullary plasmacytoma
FAZA	18F-fluoroazomycinarabinoside
FDA	Food and Drug Administration
FDG	18F-fluorodeoxyglucose
FDOPA	18F-3,4-dihydroxy-6-^{18}F-fluoro-l-phenylalanine
FES	18F-fluoroestradiol
FET	18F-fluoro-ethyl-tyrosine
FIGO	International Federation of Gynecology and Obstetrics
FL	Follicular lymphoma
FLIPI	Follicular Lymphoma International Prognostic Index
FLT	18F-fluorothymidine
FMISO	18F-fluoromisonidazole
GTV	Gross tumor volume
HL	Hodgkin's lymphoma
HNC	Head and neck cancers
IMAT	Intensity-modulated arc therapy
IMRT	Intensity-modulated radiation therapy
INRT	Involved node radiation therapy
ISRT	Involved site radiation therapy
LARC	Locally advanced rectal cancer
LC	Lung cancer
LN	Lymph node
LRC	Locoregional control
MET	11C-methionine
MM	Multiple myeloma
MRI	Magnetic resonance imaging
NHL	Non-Hodgkin's lymphoma
NPV	Negative predictive value
NSCLC	Non-small-cell lung cancer
OAR	Organ at risk
OS	Overall survival
PCa	Prostate cancer
pCR	Pathological complete response
PET	Positron emission tomography
PMR	Partial metabolic response
PP	Paraprotein
pPR	Pathological partial response
PPV	Positive predictive value
PTV	Planning target volume
RC	Renal cancer
RECIST	Response criteria in solid tumor
RIWGRC	Revised IWG response criteria
ROI	Region of interest
RT	Radiation therapy
SBP	Solitary bone plasmacytoma
SBRT	Stereotactic body radiation therapy
SIB	Simultaneous integrated boost
SMD	Stable metabolic disease
SP	Solitary plasmacytoma
SUV	Standardized uptake values
T1-gad	Gadolinium-enhanced T1 weighted
TCP	Tumor control probability
TVD	Target volume delineation

22.1 Introduction

Radiation oncology plays an important role in cancer management [1–3]. Radiation therapy (RT) and diagnostic radiology have always enjoyed a close relationship. Advances in diagnostic imaging have resulted in parallel changes in the planning of RT. In parallel, RT treatment planning and delivery have benefited from new technology and techniques. Intensity-modulated radiation therapy (IMRT) techniques have been developed to allow higher doses to be delivered in a highly conformal manner. IMRT is based on the use of numerous radiation beams with optimized nonuniform intensities resulting from inverse treatment planning, which can achieve much better dose conformity than conventional RT techniques. The net effect is that IMRT is usually capable of delivering a dose pattern that uniformly irradiates the target while sculpting and redistributing the dose outside the target to reduce irradiation of critical organs. A direct consequence of this more conformal method of treatment planning and delivery is that volumes must be more precisely defined. Radiation oncologists have had to rethink what is absolutely required to be within the irradiated volume and what can be safely spared. Therefore, much attention recently has been focused on which are the appropriate volumes and how they are generated via segmentation or contouring. Image-guided techniques allow for these treatments to be delivered accurately on a daily basis and are able to appropriately control for target motion within the body, whether it is due to respiration or distension/emptying of organs.

In the era of high precision RT, accurate tumor volume delineation regarding tumor boundaries, shape, and volume is crucial. Quantification is necessary for characterizing partial metabolic response (PMR) or stable metabolic disease (SMD). The European Organization for Research and Treatment of Cancer (EORTC) and positron emission tomography (PET) response criteria in solid tumors (PERCIST) criteria for quantifying response yield very similar response classifications of patients [4]. For target volume selection and delineation, anatomic imaging modalities such as computed tomography (CT) and magnetic resonance imaging (MRI) remain the most widely used modalities. CT is widely available, does not have geometric distortion, and provides intrinsic information on the electronic densities of various tissues. However, CT lacks contrast resolution for normal soft tissue structures and tumor extent, which has led to significant inter- and intra-observer variations in delineation of the gross tumor volume (GTV) in lung, head and neck, esophageal, and prostate cancer and gynecologic and brain tumors. MRI has been shown to be more accurate than CT for evaluating the soft tissue or bone extent of nasopharynx, prostate, and brain tumors with smaller interobserver variations in delineation of the GTV. However, for pharyngeal-laryngeal tumors, both MRI and CT have limitations with significant interobserver variability in target volume delineation [5, 6].

Over the last few decades, molecular imaging, particularly PET, has been widely used for cancer diagnosis, staging, restaging, monitoring therapy response, and RT planning [7, 8] (Figs. 22.1 and 22.2). As a highly sensitive and accurate nuclear medicine imaging technology based on molecular biology, PET has a unique ability to assess the functional and biochemical processes of the tissues, which are potentially altered in the earliest stages of diseases. PET detects changes often before anatomical or structural changes have occurred or evident on MRI/CT. It compares normal and abnormal tissues at a functional rather than morphological level. PET promises to improve the target definition by defining a metabolically active biological target volume (BTV). The advent of hybrid PET/CT scanners has allowed hardware fusion of functional and anatomic imaging; this provides better localization of the functional imaging and decreases the interobserver variations in identifying target volumes, which has proven to be a major advance for RT planning.

18F-fluorodeoxyglucose (FDG) is the most commonly used and the only oncologic PET tracer approved by the Food and Drug Administration (FDA) for routine clinical use. More than 90 % of oncologic PET imaging is performed by FDG-PET due to the increased metabolism of glucose by tumor cells in most cancers. In addition to diagnosis, staging, restaging, and monitoring response to cancer treatment, FDG-PET can be useful for selection or delineation of RT target volumes [9]. However, FDG is not a tumor-specific substance; its accumulation

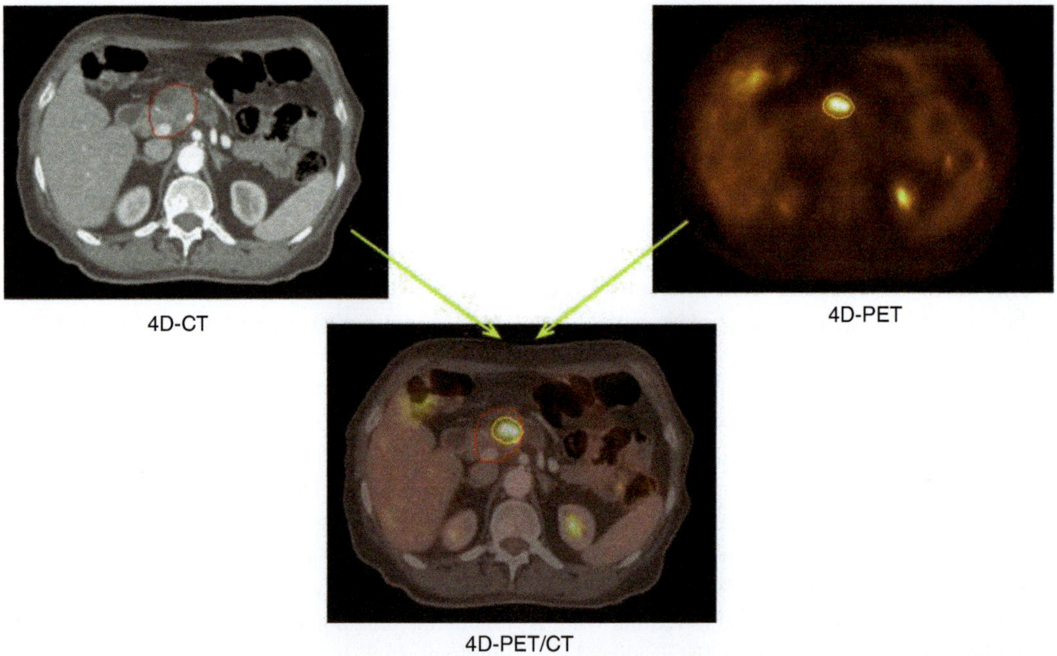

Fig. 22.1 Image fused 4D-PET/CT of patient with pancreatic tumor for radiotherapy planning. Standard planning target volume (STD-PTV) is correlated with 4D-CT image (*red outlines*) and 4D-planning target volume (4D-PTV) with 4D-PET image (*yellow outlines*). The use of information obtained from 4D studies allows the definition of target volumes as 4D-PTV reduced compared to those obtained with STD-PTV

in benign lesions, such as inflammation, may cause false-positive results which lead to low tumor specificity.

In addition to glucose, amino acids and choline have also shown increased tumor consumption and tumor specificity. Radiolabeled radiotracers, such as 11C-methionine (MET) and 11C/18F-labelled choline (CHO), may in fact have significant potential for tumor detection in organ sites with an undesirable FDG-PET background such as with brain tumor or in tumors with low intrinsic FDG uptake, such as prostate cancer (PCa). Also, 11C-acetate (ACE) acts as a probe of tissue metabolism through entry into catabolic or anabolic metabolic pathways as mediated by acetyl-coenzyme A, and it is also a useful PET tracer for various cancer types, such as lung cancer (LC), hepatocellular carcinoma, renal cancer (RC), PCa, and astrocytomas, which makes it a potential substitute for FDG in target volume selection and delineation in RT planning [10, 12–14].

In RT treatment, it is reported that there is a strong correlation between locoregional control (LRC) and overall survival (OS) [15–18]. A straightforward way to improve local tumor control, as proved by large bodies of evidence, is to increase the radiation dose further [19, 20]. Current treatment prescriptions are already close to patient tolerance making it nearly impossible to raise the dose prescription of the whole target tumor. New biological imaging methodologies such as PET can be used to draw a three-dimensional (3D) map of radiobiological relevant parameters as its inherent potential to trace the real target volume – volume consisting of tumor cells that requires a therapeutic dose to control the disease. The RT prescription usually takes larger target region to some primary dose and then boosts the GTV (including high-uptake regions) to a higher dose. The primary and boost doses are typically planned for spatially homogeneous delivery to their respective target regions. There has been also increasing clinical interest in

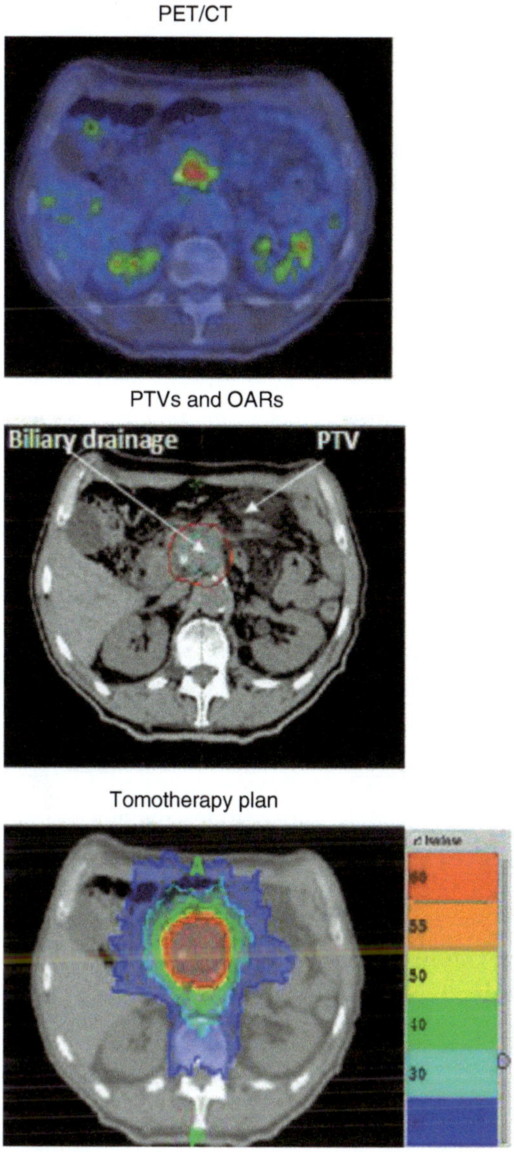

Fig. 22.2 Patient with pancreatic adenocarcinoma (histological grade: T4N0) previously treated with chemotherapy (5-FU). Helical tomotherapy planned on planning target volume (*PTV*) based on PET/CT image with the dose of 60 Gy, 2 Gy/f

delivering a nonhomogeneous dose to the target based on FDG-PET uptake, with the aim of improving LRC [21].

An increased precision of target subvolume localization by using PET/CT information plus a therapeutic dose delivered by dose painting may have an additional effect to improve LRC and further reduce the potential of tumor recurrence.

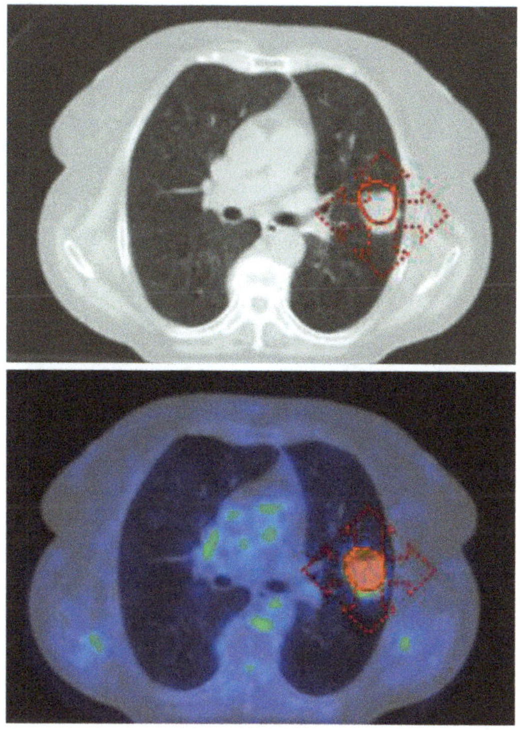

Fig. 22.3 PET/CT images contoured with organ motion in patient with lung cancer for radiotherapy treatment planning

Metabolic PET can provide information that impact RT planning in several ways, by detecting a tumor that is missed by CT or MRI, by detecting additional tumor regions outside the tumor volume as defined by CT or MRI, and by showing subregions with increased or altered metabolism within the GTV that could be preferentially targeted and treated with escalated radiation doses.

22.1.1 Lung Cancer

LC is the leading cause of cancer death in both men and women. Eighty percent of LC is non-small-cell lung cancer (NSCLC). While difficult to treat, the best opportunity to cure NSCLC is by radical surgical resection in the early stages of disease. RT is a key treatment modality in the curative treatment of patients with LC (Figs. 22.3 and 22.4). Recent progress in combined modality treatments incorporating chemotherapy (CH) and

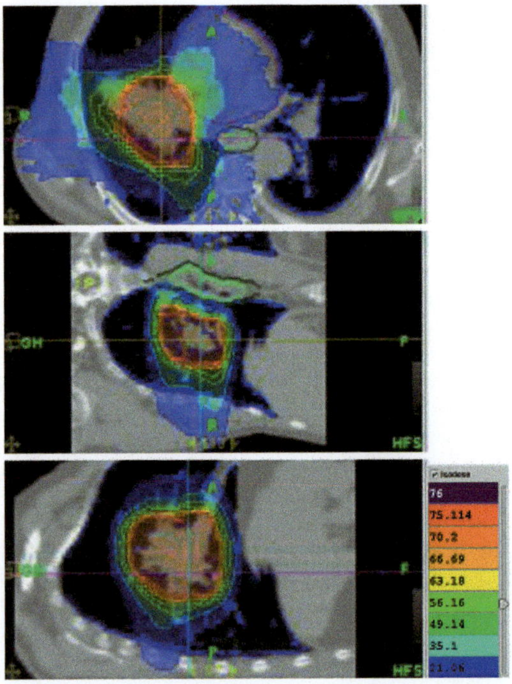

Fig. 22.4 Tomotherapy treatment planned in an 88-year-old man with lung cancer. The plan has 39 fractions defined for a planned delivery of 70.2 Gy. This dose was given on area in *red line* and is defined as planned target volume

radiation, with or without surgery, as well as technical advances in radiation delivery, has led to significant improvements in treatment outcomes. Accurate evaluation of lymph node (LN) metastases is crucial for planning curative RT.

FDG-PET has been widely used in evaluation of patients with LC. The overall sensitivity, specificity, and accuracy of FDG-PET for detection of LC are very high for primary, residual, and recurrent disease. FDG-PET scan is more sensitive than CT in detection of LN involvement and distant metastases in NSCLC [9, 22]. Changes in the target volumes of over 20 % and stage alteration of 20–50 % have been consistently observed when FDG-PET was incorporated in target volume delineation (TVD). Most prominent changes are often associated with the presence of atelectasis in the treated areas, or the identification of additional LN disease, which may be difficultly visualized on CT [23–29]. In addition, incorporation of FDG-PET in the delineation of regional LN disease may lead to a decrease in the LN-GTV. This has been demonstrated in patients with N2-N3 disease by van Der Wel et al., who showed a PET-related decrease of the LN-GTV from 13.7 ± 3.8 to 9.9 ± 4.0 cm^3 ($p = 0.011$) [29]. It led to significant decrease in radiation dose to the esophagus (V55 decreased from 30.6 ± 3.2 to 21.9 ± 3.8 %, $p = 0.004$) and the normal lungs (V20 decreased from 24.9 ± 2.3 to 22.3 ± 2.2 %, $p = 0.012$). As a result, dose escalation from 56.0 ± 5.4 to 71.0 ± 13.7 Gy ($p = 0.038$) became feasible, which led to improved tumor control probability (TCP), that is, the probability that a given dose of radiation will provide tumor control or eradication considering the specific biological cells of the tumor, from 14.2 ± 5.6 to 22.8 ± 7.1 % ($p = 0.026$) without accounting for geometric misses, and improved TCP from 12.5 to 18.3 % when it is accounted.

These findings further demonstrate the advantage of incorporating FDG-PET information in TVD especially for stage III NSCLC, which makes dose escalation possible. The theoretical dose escalation level was addressed in many planning studies. Different dose-painting strategies to shape the radiation dose according to the functional image information have been proposed recently: dose escalation and dose redistribution. Dose escalation applies an additional dose to the functional subvolumes of the target, whereas dose redistribution consists of increasing the dose to the radioresistant areas while reducing the dose to the rest of the tumor in a way to keep the mean dose constant.

There are two strategies for the realization of dose escalation: dose painting by contours (DPBC) and dose painting by numbers (DPBN). DPBN intends to increase the additional dose gradually, according to the local PET voxel intensities, while a homogeneous dose of BTV which contoured by a threshold created in PET image is given in DPBC. For both DPBC and DPBN plans, strict planning constraints set for the organ at risk (OAR) should be complied. In addition, as the feasibility of technique is largely proved [30–36], both are therefore considered clinically acceptable and alternatives for boosting subvolumes.

MacManus et al. reported that metabolic response correlated well with RT outcome. Complete metabolic response (CMR) predicted good RT outcome: 1-year survival for CMR and non-CMR patients was 93 % and 47 %, respectively, and 2-year survival was 62 % and 30 %, respectively [37]. Additionally, PET/CT scans have been shown to detect distant metastases that are missed by conventional scans, which is of obvious benefit to patients who may require additional treatment [38].

Respiratory motion can have a significant impact on static oncological PET/CT imaging where standardized uptake values (SUV) and/or volume measurements are important. The impact is highly dependent upon motion amplitude, lesion location and size, attenuation map, and respiratory pattern. To overcome the motion effect, motion compensation techniques may be necessary in clinical practice to improve the tumor quantification for determining the response to therapy or for RT treatment planning. PET/CT imaging of the lung and abdomen region is generally affected by patient respiratory motion, which can lead to underestimation of maximum SUV (SUV_{max}) of a region of interest (ROI), overestimation of tumor volume, and mismatched PET and CT images that yield attenuation correction (AC) errors, registration errors, and tumor mislocalization [39]. It has been reported that various respiratory motion correction methods can cause tumor SUV_{max} to increase as much as 159 % and tumor volume to decrease as much as 43 % compared to those of the conventional measurement in patient studies [40, 41].

Currently hypoxia is deeply evaluated with the use of different PET tracers such as 18F-fluoromisonidazole (FMISO), 18F-fluoroazomycinarabinoside (FAZA), and copper-64 diacetyl-bis (N4-methylthiosemicarbazone) (ATSM). A crucial advantage of PET imaging for studying tumor hypoxia is its capacity to provide in vivo 3D images of the distribution of positron emitting tracers that selectively bind to hypoxic tissue in a safe and noninvasive manner [42]. Postema et al. published results using FAZA in NSCLC patients reporting an incidence of baseline hypoxia in 7 of 13 patients (54 %) [43].

22.1.2 Head and Neck Cancers

Oncologic imaging plays an important role in head and neck cancers (HNC) in detection, staging, restaging, and therapy response assessment of these tumors. Accurate staging at the time of diagnosis is critical for selecting the appropriate treatment strategy. Unfortunately, at the time of initial diagnosis, more than 50 % of patients already present with regional LN metastases or even distant metastases. In this population, RT plays a critical role when surgery is contraindicated. However, radical treatment is associated with increased toxicity, particularly when concomitant CH or altered fractionation strategies are used. A meta-analysis of both combined chemoradiation (CRT) and altered fractionation confirmed significant LRC and survival benefits overall but were unable to demonstrate a survival benefit in the >70 age group [44].

FDG-PET can provide important complementary information for RT planning in HNC (Fig. 22.5), and its role has been reviewed in several publications [45–48]. Although there are some contradictory results [49, 50], many clinical studies have shown that the uptake of FDG, usually measured as the SUV_{max}, is a significant predictor of prognosis for many tumor sites, including HNC [51–53]. Moreover, high FDG uptake is correlated with increased local failure and shorter survival [54–56]. The precise mechanism causing tumors with higher SUV values to present a poorer treatment response is unknown. Tumors with a high SUV may:

(i) consist of a higher tumor cell density or greater tumor/stroma cell ratio [57]
(ii) be more metabolically active and consequently exhibit a higher proliferation rate
(iii) be more hypoxic [58, 59]
(iv) exhibit a higher DNA repair capacity [60]

or some combination of these options.

The vast majority of recurrences seem to be the result of insufficient dose delivered to portions of selected target volumes. Therefore, dose painting becomes a compelling strategy if a spatial variation in LRC can be established. Based

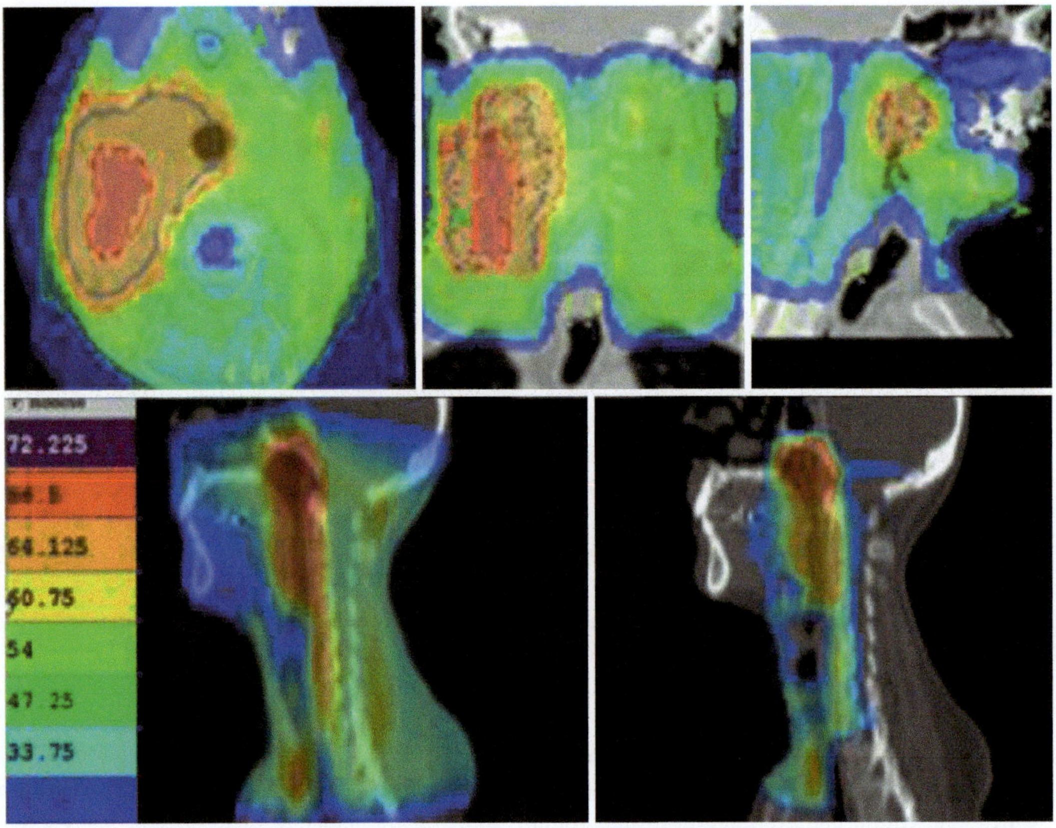

Fig. 22.5 Radiotherapy treatment planning in a patient affected by head and neck cancer. Helical tomotherapy radiation treatment was delivered with the simultaneous integrated boost approach at different dose escalated to metabolic sub volume. A boost – 69 Gy – was given on FDG-PET-positive volume (*red area*); clinical target volume and clinical negative neck received 66 Gy (*orange area*) and 54 Gy (*green area*), respectively

on clinical outcomes, the FDG-avid region in a tumor is recognized as a possible target for dose escalation. Several planning and optimization studies have assessed the feasibility of dose boosting on a subvolume of a tumor, based on a FDG-PET image, using IMRT [36, 61]. Some clinical data suggest that to reach equal response rates, FDG-avid tumors are likely to require at least 10–30 % more dose than FDG non-avid tumors. However, due to the confounding effect of tumor volume/T-stage and other prognostic factors, tests of the estimated dose-modifying effect, using high-quality prospective clinical trial data, are needed.

Changes in the tumor and surrounding normal tissues during RT for HNC support treatment adaptations [62–64]. Adaptive radiotherapy (ART) appears to be superior over nonadaptive treatment: it increases minimum doses in the target structures and decreases the cumulative maximum dose in dose-painted areas. It also readjusts the dose-painting patterns. However, there is a disagreement over benefits of ART [65, 66] that originates from variations in timing and frequency of adaptive procedures, methods of plan adjustments to anatomical and biological changes, and methods of dose accumulation.

FDG-PET/CT can play various roles in the treatment of HNC including staging, restaging, and defining BTV for high-dose RT boost. Potentially, the GTV can be changed on the basis of PET information, facilitating sparing of nearby normal tissues and allowing dose escalation to relatively small subvolumes. In addition, biological imaging using FDG-PET may identify areas of tumor spread not recognized by morphological imaging, potentially improving the accuracy of GTV definition [67, 68].

22.1.3 Esophageal Cancers

The incidence of esophageal cancer ranks in the top ten worldwide with a relatively high mortality rate. Esophageal cancers consist primarily of two subtypes, adenocarcinoma (comprising 50–80 % of all esophageal cancer cases) and squamous cell carcinoma (comprising most of the remaining cases).

RT is one of the primary treatments for esophageal cancer. Combined CH and RT has proven superior to either therapy alone as primary treatment for esophageal cancer. Esophageal IMRT is associated with significantly better OS, LRC, and noncancer-related death compared with 3D conformal RT [69]. There are no prospective data yet, but retrospective series suggest that treatment is well tolerated and may allow delivery of a higher tumor dose, of significant interest for the treatment of medically inoperable elderly patients [70].

FDG-PET is not generally used for the initial diagnosis of esophageal cancer due to significant FDG uptake in inflammatory esophagitis, Barrett's esophagus, and other benign diseases. FDG-PET plays also a limited role in the evaluation of regional LN disease in patients with esophageal cancer but has a high sensitivity for evaluation of local recurrence and a high sensitivity and specificity for detection of distant disease occurring outside the initial surgical field [71, 72].

Accurate delineation of GTV is a prerequisite for a successful treatment of this cancer with RT. In esophageal cancer, the determination of cephalic and caudal tumor extent by CT is rather uncertain. Drudi et al. found that the lengths of esophageal carcinoma measured by CT scan and esophagogram corresponded to the lengths of surgical specimens in only 32 % and 59 % of cases, respectively. Therefore, methods to increase the accuracy of TVD are needed. Several studies have reported that PET/CT could improve primary tumor and LN detection [73]. Furthermore, clinicopathological studies in surgically treated patients showed that CT scanning is reasonably good in showing radial tumor extent but poor in assessing longitudinal extent and that CT is often inaccurate when it is used to estimate the extent of LN involvement. PET is better than CT in showing tumor longitudinal extent. PET may be the only way to estimate the lower tumor border when an endoscope cannot be passed through a stenosed esophagus. Therefore, integrated PET/CT imaging aids the estimation of more accurate tumor volume and the distinction of precise anatomical barriers.

In a prospective trial of PET for RT planning in esophageal cancer, Leong et al. [74] showed that PET has a significant impact on GTV by identifying unsuspected LN involvement. Moureau-Zabotto et al. [75] showed that the addition of PET information to CT-based RT planning altered GTV values in 19 of 34 patients (56 %); GTV was reduced in 12 and increased in 7 (21 %). Han et al. [76] reported that an SUV cutoff of 2.5 provided an accurate estimation of GTV length. Vali et al. [77] reported that the use of a threshold of approximately 2.5 may be considered the best strategy for the delineation of GTV in esophageal cancer.

The use of FDG-PET/CT has been shown to change target volumes contoured by radiation oncologists in a considerable proportion of patients (20–90 %) with consequent changes in treatment planning [78, 79].

22.1.4 Breast Cancer

Breast cancer is the most common cancer in female patients and carries a significant risk for recurrence and metastases. Breast cancer is the second leading cause of death in women. For localized cancers, the 5-year survival rate is more than 96 %, but survival decreases dramatically with regional or distant metastatic disease. Strategies in managing breast cancer include various combinations of surgery, RT, and CH regimens. RT is mainly applied in three areas:

(i) adjuvant RT after breast surgery
(ii) RT for isolated recurrence after surgery
(iii) RT for metastatic disease

Breast cancer has several known characteristics that determine aggressiveness and can be used as therapeutic targets as well as a means for monitoring responsiveness to therapy. Published reports are limited in assessing the utility of FDG-

PET in breast cancer RT planning [72]. At present, FDG-PET has not shown significant utility in RT planning after breast-conserving surgery. Whole breast irradiation after breast-conserving surgery is one of the standard treatments for the patients with early-stage breast cancer [80, 81]. After the whole breast irradiation, additional boost to the tumor bed has demonstrated considerable improvement in local control rate [82, 83]. In the modern era, CT-based planning has been used to individualize treatment and tailor RT treatment fields to encompass the breast and draining lymphatic while minimizing dose to the heart, lungs, and spinal cord. 3D planning has also enabled more accurate demarcation of the lumpectomy cavity at depth rather than relying solely on the surgical scar at the skin's surface.

Preoperative PET/CT may provide the more reliable diagnostic tool to localize the tumor bed in breast cancer RT (Fig. 22.6). Other studies reported that the FDG-PET/CT can improve the delineation of lumpectomy cavity for partial breast irradiation. The PET/CT-derived planning target volumes (PTVs) are larger than the CT-derived PTVs and are not well-covered dosimetrically by CT-based treatment plans. A PET/CT-based treatment plan covers both PET/CT and CT PTVs with only a modest increase in the dose to the normal tissue, being able to influence treatment planning for partial breast irradiation [84]. While the importance of RT technique in preventing locoregional recurrence has been previously established in other malignancies such as cervical and HNC [85, 86], no studies have systematically examined the importance of RT field design with modern imaging modalities and treatment planning in preventing locoregional recurrence in breast cancer patients.

In patients with clinical stages II and III, PET/CT was documented to be superior to conventional imaging modalities for the detection of extra-axillary regional metastatic LN (infraclavicular, supraclavicular, and internal mammary LNs) and distant metastases [87–92]. The role of FDG-PET is especially prominent in the management of oligometastatic disease; a state of limited metastatic spread of disease is potentially curable with local therapy. This is an area

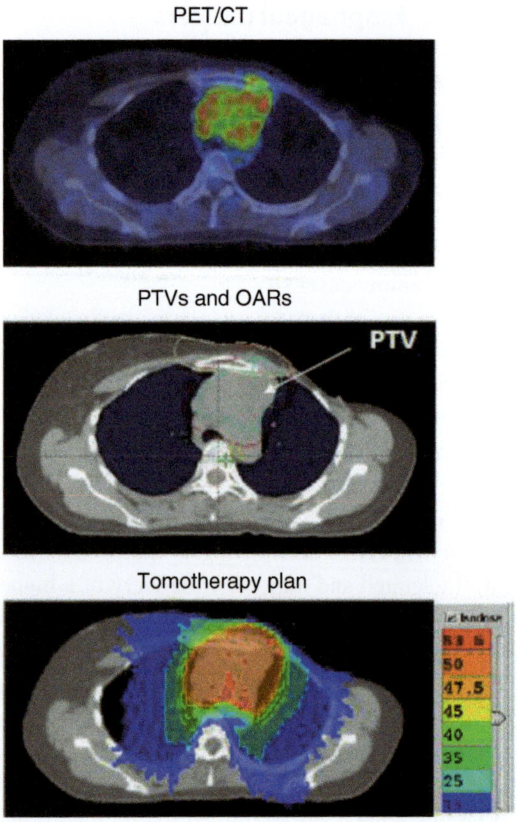

Fig. 22.6 A 50-year-old woman with metastatic breast cancer previously treated with hormone therapy and chemotherapy. Patient performed radiotherapy on left breast, supraclavicular fossa, internal mammary lymph node (1991), and chest wall (2003). At follow-up control patient presents recurrence in mediastinal lymph node. Helical tomotherapy was planned on planning target volume (*PTV*) based on PET/CT image with a dose of 60 Gy, 2 Gy/fraction

in which RT is emerging as an important treatment modality [93].

Novel tracers, such as CHO, 18F-fluoroestradiol (FES), 18F-fluorothymidine (FLT), and progesterone-receptor in breast cancer, have the potential to add meaningful biomarkers to clinical imaging and treatment trials, to study tumor molecular physiology with the potential to improve diagnosis, treatment selection, drug development, and pharmacodynamic monitoring of the effects of treatment. These tracers are likely to move closer to clinical use and to become a useful tool for personalized treatment [94].

22.1.5 Lymphomas

Lymphomas often respond well to therapy, and survival rates are generally 90 % or higher when diseases are detected at early stages, making it one of the most curable forms of cancer [95]. The primary therapeutic modalities are CH and RT, as surgery does not often play a role in the management of this disease. Accurate imaging is crucial to treatment strategy, and FDG-PET has become a useful imaging modality in the staging and treatment evaluation algorithm for lymphoma by providing unique metabolic information.

Most of the existing evidence in the literature on the contribution of PET/CT in lymphoma staging comes from studies performed in Hodgkin's lymphoma (HL). PET/CT proved to be more sensitive and specific than other conventional modalities, including CT, for the evaluation of extent of LN and extra-LN disease. Stage variation occurs in nearly 25 % of patients, mostly to upstage disease, leading to a change in treatment strategy in nearly 10–15 % of them [96]. The role of a contrast-enhanced CT (CECT) performed simultaneously in the same diagnostic session with the PET scan is still a subject of debate. PET/CECT may be useful in patients with abdominal and pelvic involvement for delineating LN from adjacent bowel loops and vasculature [97].

Prognostic value of PET/CT in baseline staging also has been reported in follicular lymphoma (FL), which is the most common indolent (slow-growing) form of non-Hodgkin's lymphoma (NHL) (grade 3 more specifically). Le Dortz et al. found that a score value ≥2, whatever the Follicular Lymphoma International Prognostic Index (FLIPI) score, was the only predictive factor in multivariate analysis on treatment outcome.

In conclusion, PET/CT is strongly recommended before treatment onset for patients in routine staging workup in most lymphoma subset with the exception of marginal extra-LN lymphoma, cutaneous lymphoma, and small lymphocytic lymphoma [98]. In HL, FDG-PET enables an early evaluation of the metabolic changes occurring during the induction treatment as early as after the first [99], the second [100–103], and the third [104] cycle of CH (interim PET). In this regard, PET/CT yielded highly promising results as a surrogate of chemosensitivity for predicting tumor response and progression-free survival (PFS), with a sensitivity and specificity of 43–100 % and 67–100 %, respectively [105], even superseding the prognostic role of the International Prognostic Score [106].

In April 2009 at a workshop on interim PET in lymphoma, simple and reproducible rules have been proposed for interim PET visual interpretation [107, 108], and these criteria have been recently retrospectively validated [109]. Briefly, the adopted rules include the following statements:

(i) visual assessment is preferred, but SUV determination can be used in some cases
(ii) interim-PET interpretation should always be made by comparing the single foci of FDG uptake to those recorded in the baseline study
(iii) intensity of FDG uptake should be graded according to a five-point scale in which two reference organs, the mediastinal blood pool structures and liver, are used to define different grades of FDG uptake

Two recent meta-analysis, reviewing 34 studies comprehensive of 882 HL and 604 diffuse large B-cell lymphoma (DLBCL-NHL) patients, showed that FDG-PET performed after treatment is highly predictive of treatment outcome in terms of PFS and OS both in HL and DLBCL patients with and without residual masses, with a higher sensitivity for HL and a higher specificity for DLBCL [110, 111]. Despite the good response to therapy, a residual mass can be demonstrated by radiological means in up to 80 % of HL and up to 40 % of NHL patients after completion of treatment [112, 113], even if only less than half of these masses will harbor residual disease. In advanced-stage HL, before the advent of functional imaging for treatment response evaluation, involved field RT was proposed for LN lesions or residual masses, as an integral part of a combination CH for HL, in particular ABVD (doxorubicin, bleomycin, vinblastine, and dacarbazine) treatment [114].

More recently, PET/CT performed at the end of treatment for lymphoma proved effective in discriminating residual active disease from fibrotic masses, with a sensitivity of 43–100 % and a specificity of 67–100 % [111]. Not surprisingly, the negative predictive value (NPV) of the end-treatment PET depends on the efficacy of the administered CH, as high as 94 % after an aggressive regimen, such as bleomycin, etoposide, doxorubicin, cyclophosphamide, vincristine, procarbazine, and prednisone (BEACOPP) escalated in advanced-stage HL or as low as 75 % after the low-intensity regimen vincristine, epidoxorubicin, bleomycin, cyclophosphamide, etoposide, prednisone (VEBEP) [115]. Another relevant role played by post-CH PET scan is to guide RT both in HL and DLBCL. Accurate TVD has become an essential component of radiation field design, owing to treatment strategies that now incorporate reduced radiation field sizes and targeted conformal therapies [116, 117]. In particular, radiation using involved node RT (INRT) or involved site RT (ISRT) restricts RT to the initially involved LNs with a margin, thus requiring more precision in identifying involved disease. FDG-PET information for defining target volumes for RT planning has also drawn great interest and has significant value in monitoring response to therapy and predicting outcomes for patients with lymphoma. Pretreatment PET is required for the application of ISRT or INRT principles to early-stage HL and NHL [116, 118, 119], even if it is unfortunately often logistically difficult to acquire a PET study in pre-CH phase. ISRT similarly restricts RT to the initially involved LN but allows for a larger margin to account for uncertainties [116].

Multiple studies have demonstrated that target volume alterations can occur when PET is obtained at the time of simulation for HL. Few studies, however, have specifically examined PET for radiation planning in a predominantly NHL population including other hematologic malignancies. The implications on TVD may differ for HL and NHL. Most studies examining the use of PET for radiation planning in HL have fused pretreatment PET scans obtained in the treatment position to posttreatment CT simulation scans because PET is often negative at the completion of CH. In NHL, patients are often referred for definitive therapy; in that case, they are likely to have positive PET at time of radiation. Although sensitivity and specificity of PET is well defined in HL, its utility is more controversial for low-grade NHL [120–122].

Consistent data from multiple studies have established the role of post-therapy FDG-PET imaging for the prediction of recurrent HL and DLBCL [123]. An NPV and a positive predictive value (PPV) of 80 and 100 % were reported, respectively, for FDG-PET in the identification of residual aggressive NHL after completion of first-line CH [124, 125]. More recently, it was emphasized that end-of-treatment PET was highly predictive of PFS and OS, regardless of interim PET result in early-stage HL and performed better than interim PET in the low-risk HL population [101, 126]. The revised IWG response criteria incorporated FDG-PET to accurately assess end-therapy persistent masses in both NHL and HL. Filippi et al. investigate the role of RT in patients affected with primary mediastinal B-cell lymphoma (PMBCL) with residual FDG-PET-positive disease after rituximab CH, and their result indicates that approximately 50 % of PMBCL patients show residual disease at FDG-PET scan after CRT. RT is able to convert to CR approximately 85 % of these patients, but those with a Deauville score of 5 (10 %) appear at high risk of progression and death, and they might be candidates for intensified programs [127].

22.1.6 Myelomas

Multiple myeloma (MM) is a hematologic neoplasm characterized by bone marrow invasion of a neoplastic clone of plasma cells, presence of bone lytic lesions, and extramedullary organ invasion in later stages of the disease. The disease course is heterogeneous with a patient survival ranging from a few months to more than a decade. In this perspective, a still unfilled need exists for reliable prognostic tool identification in order to predict the individual disease outcome in a single-patient basis. As in other solid and hematologic cancers, one of the most important prognostic factors is tumor dissemination (or stage) at baseline; the most frequently involved organ is the bone and bone marrow [128, 129].

The MM staging system was introduced in 1975 by Durie and Salmon to allow patient stratification with different tumor bulk by calculating the measurable theoretical myeloma cell mass. MM is yet incurable, and local therapies are frequently used to treat MM-induced lesions in the palliative setting and solitary osseous or extra-osseous plasmacytomas in the definitive setting. RT is used to treat bone pain, to manage areas at risk for pathologic fracture, and to sterilize residual disease after surgery. MM is highly responsive to RT owing to its radiosensitivity, with clinical response rates as high as 97 % [130–132]. However, the emergence in the last decade of new imaging techniques, such as FDG-PET/CT and MRI, has provided new insights on tumor spread at disease onset and gradually revolutionized staging system developing a more integrating clinical and imaging approach, the Durie/Salmon PLUS myeloma staging.

Sensitivity of FDG-PET/CT proved very high for detection of extraskeletal lesions, while MRI outperforms FDG-PET/CT for detecting bone and bone marrow invasion by disease, especially for spine and pelvic localizations. PET/CT detected bone lesions mainly on the basis of their increased metabolic activity instead of any anatomical alteration. Moreover, it provided an accurate identification of tumor viability that is useful for treatment planning and monitoring. FDG-PET/CT proved a powerful prognosticator in MM: metabolic target volume measurement at baseline and longitudinal studies aimed at assessing the role of minimal residual disease detection by FDG-PET/CT are the most innovative aspect of functional imaging in this disease [133].

Solitary plasmacytoma (SP) is potentially curable malignant neoplasms of plasma cell lineage, often accompanied by a serum paraprotein (PP) or by urinary free light chain (Bence-Jones protein) excretion. They comprise approximately 10 % of all plasma cell tumors, occurring as either solitary bone plasmacytoma (SBP) or as extramedullary plasmacytoma (EP) [134, 135]. Although RT can result in local control rates in excess of 80 % in both SPB and EP [136, 137], MM will ultimately develop in 50–70 % [138–141] and <50 % [135, 140, 142, 143] of patients with SBP and EP, respectively. The majority of SBP will progress to MM within 3–4 years [144]. Prognostic factors for progression of SBP to MM include older age [145], increasing tumor size [146], and persistence of PP after RT [147].

The frequent progression of SP to MM after definitive RT suggests that the staging workup has been insufficiently sensitive to detect occult systemic disease at presentation. FDG-PET/CT can play a useful role in the evaluation of patients with SP who are candidates for definitive RT or who have been treated with RT (Fig. 22.7). PET influenced the initial clinical management in 35 % of patients who underwent staging PET scans as part of their workup before definitive RT. There is some indication in the literature that PET may be useful for response assessment in MM, but there is little information on response assessment on SP [148]. Persistence of FDG uptake for some months after RT in an irradiated SP does not necessarily indicate a bad prognosis or by itself constitute an indication for further treatment. In the absence of new lesions or a rising PP level, a period of observation may be the most appropriate course of action. PET can reliably image known deposits of malignant plasma cell disorders and can image new sites of disease that are not apparent using other imaging modalities such as CT or MRI [149].

Schirrmeister et al. [150, 151] reported that PET influenced patient management in 4 (27 %) of 15 cases of SP, by changing diagnosis or by accurately restaging disease. In patients with SP and negative PP levels, biochemical studies may not be useful for monitoring disease status after

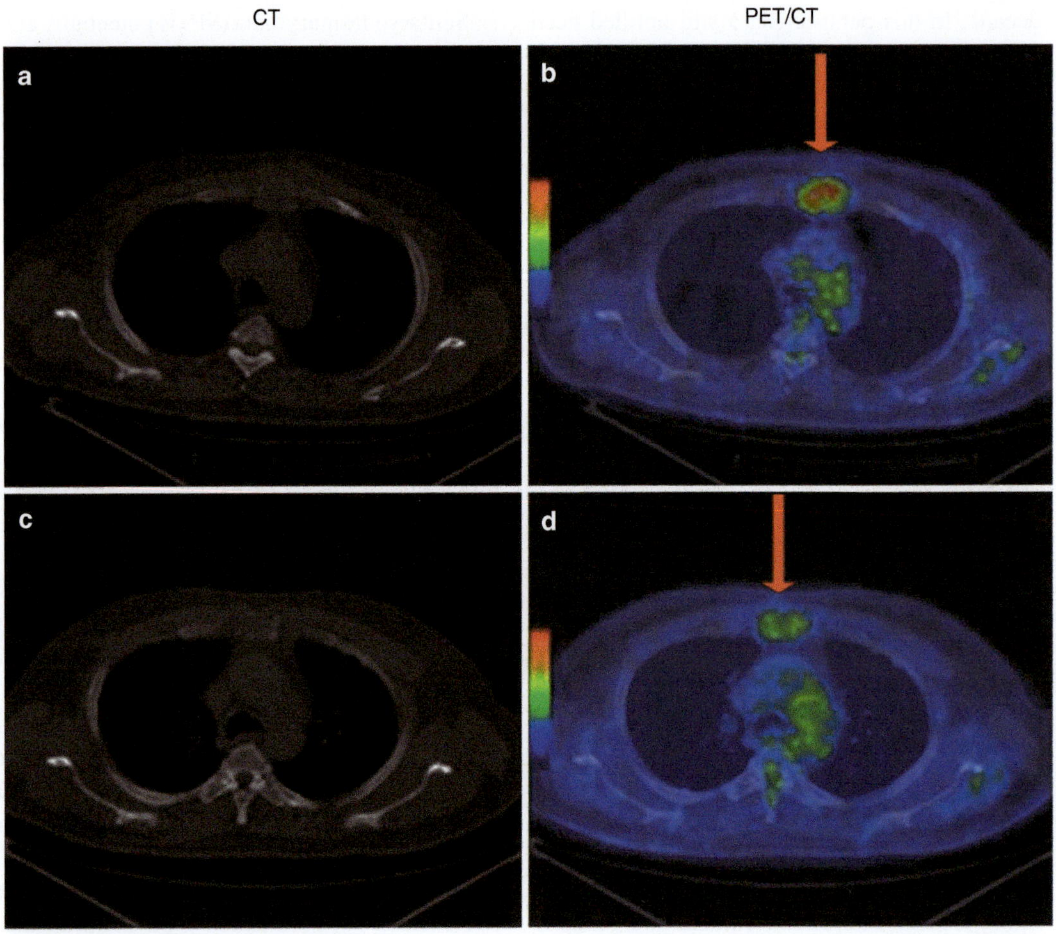

Fig. 22.7 Patient with sternal solitary bone plasmacytoma undergone to radiotherapy treatment (30 Gy/10 fractions). The comparison between CT and PET/CT before (**a**, **b**) and after (**c**, **d**) radiotherapy treatment showed minimal residual uptake (*red arrow*) on the treated lesion

local RT. In a rise of PP after therapy, imaging may distinguish local from distant disease progression. PET/CT images can be directly imported into planning systems for contouring at the RT workstation, facilitating 3D BTV determination. PET can provide clear images of the extent of soft tissue extension of SP, even when the tumor edge is isodense with surrounding normal tissue on CT, and may be the best modality for planning treatment of a boosting dose of RT to the GTV after an initial wider field treatment. Most series report the use of doses in the 40–50 Gy range.

The radiation target volume for SP typically includes the whole affected bone and any soft tissue extension. It is common practice to treat a smaller volume around the GTV with a boosting dose after an initial dose has been given to a wider field. There is evidence for a dose-response effect for local control. Frassica et al. [138] reported a series in which 11 % of SPB cases developed local recurrences following treatment with a median dose of 39.75 Gy, but no cases of local failure occurred if ≥45 Gy was used. Mendenhall et al. [152], in a review of 81 cases, reported a 94 % local control rate with ≥40 Gy vs. a 69 % control rate with doses <40 Gy.

22.1.7 Brain Tumors

Brain tumors include all tumors that arise inside the cranium, especially gliomas, which are inherently serious and life-threatening because of their invasive and infiltrative character in the limited space of the intracranial cavity. Surgery, CH, and RT are the main treatment modalities for gliomas. RT as a primary treatment modality is mainly reserved for the inoperable cases; however, it is often employed in an adjuvant setting, particularly if there is residual tumor left behind after surgical resection.

RT continues to play an important role in the treatment of brain tumors. As an initial step in RT planning, patients undergo a CECT scan in the treatment position. MRI has been used to improve the accuracy of outlining tumors owing to the superiority of MR in identifying intracranial anatomic structures.

Standard planning for RT relies on both gadolinium-enhanced T1-weighted (T1-Gad) and T2-weighted fluid-attenuated inversion recovery sequences to image the contrast-enhancing portion of the tumor and peritumoral edema, respectively. By introducing MR fusion to CT planning, MR increased the clinical target volume (CTV) compared with that seen on CT and felt that the integration of MR data with CT information was of significant practical value in treatment planning. In the RT of high-grade gliomas, the target volume is identified using postoperative CT and MRI with intravenous contrast. The area of T1-Gad MRI is often used to define the extent of GTV radiologically. However, several pathologic studies have shown that the contrast enhancement may not represent the outer tumor border because infiltrating glioma cells can be identified well beyond the area of enhancement [153]. Gadolinium contrast enhancement is also a nonspecific sign of blood-brain barrier disruptions and cannot accurately differentiate nonspecific postsurgical changes from residual tumor [154].

Normal brain cells consume large amounts of glucose due to their high metabolic demand; therefore, FDG-PET alone is not suitable for brain tumor evaluation. Multimodality images including MRI or CT and FDG-PET are essential for accurate evaluation of brain tumors. However, due to increased proliferation and protein synthesis, brain tumors also have increased amino acid uptake and upregulated amino acid transporters. Radiolabeled amino acid and its analogs are a class of tumor imaging agents that may be more suitable for tumors with high FDG background imaging.

PET imaging with MET, FLT, and CHO is a good option for functional imaging in brain tumor RT planning. MET, 18F-fluoro-ethyl-tyrosine (FET), and 18F-3,4-dihydroxy-6-^{18}F-fluoro-l-phenylalanine (FDOPA) have been comparatively studied and produce very similar quality images for brain tumors [155], except that there is normal physiologic uptake of FDOPA in the basal ganglia. Uptake of MET and FET does not accumulate in normal anatomic structures of the brain. In a prospective study of the treatment of primary glioblastomas, poor coverage of MET uptake (which was not used for TVD) was associated with an increased risk of noncentral recurrence [156]. However, a prospective study of patients treated using FET-PET target volumes showed the observed pattern of failure to be predominantly central [157].

Uptake of FET has been used to delineate radiation boost volumes. In a phase II trial of dose escalation for glioblastomas, a simultaneous integrated boost of 72 Gy in 30 fractions delivered to an FET-PET-defined PTV, concurrent with 60 Gy in 30 fractions delivered to a traditional MRI-defined PTV, did not lead to a survival benefit [158]. In a retrospective series relating the results of MRI and FET-PET to the outcome of biopsy, Pauleit et al. found a higher sensitivity and specificity of combined MRI and FET-PET for biopsy selection as compared to MRI only [159]. Data previously published by Niyazi et al., showed that targets delineated by means of FET uptake were 30 % larger than those solely based on MRI [160]. Piroth et al. conducted a phase II trial investigating the possible benefit of FET adapted local dose escalation [161]. In their cohort ($n = 22$), the FET-PET volume was almost twice as large as the Gad-enhanced MRI volume. Both groups used fixed LN thresholds of 1.5 and 1.6, respectively. Moreover, Grosu et al. published data of improved but enlarged target volumes for both meningioma and glioma when integrating MET-PET into the planning procedure [162].

Creating the PTV without integrating FET-PET would have resulted in missing a mean volume proportion of 17 % of the FET-positive tissue. However, to date, there is no evidence from prospective randomized and controlled trials that inclusion of this volume would convert into a clinical benefit. If all FET-positive lesions are considered to be tumor tissue not visible in MRI, it is essential to include these regions into the target volume. Knowing that most glioma recurrences are located within or at the margin of the initial RT field, this finding may emphasize the importance of conducting FET-PET/CT prior to RT. Currently, a randomized controlled trial evaluating MRI-based contouring in comparison to FET-PET for recurrent glioma is being planned under the auspices of the German Neuro-Oncology Group.

Biologically based treatment planning with FDOPA-PET may also be possible because there is a correlation between FDOPA uptake, cell density, and cell proliferation in newly diagnosed tumors [163]. FDOPA provides equivalent visual and quantitative SUV information to MET but offers a significantly longer physical half-life of 18F (109 min) compared with 11C (20 min). This is significant, as 11C tracers can be used only at institutions with an on-site cyclotron, limiting their use to essentially large academic centers and not generally applicable in practice. Normal uptake of FDOPA in the basal ganglia can present challenges when trying to distinguish between normal brain and adjacent tumor, which is absent with FET-PET uptake. Pafundi et al. reported that FDOPA-PET may more accurately identify regions of higher-grade/higher-density disease in patients with astrocytoma and will have utility in guiding stereotactic biopsy and RT targeting [164]. Future studies will investigate the role of FDOPA-PET with relative cerebral volume in perfusion MRI for targeting the most aggressive disease components and to determine whether biologically based treatment planning with FDOPA-PET/CT can improve outcomes for high-grade gliomas.

Finally, the amino acid PET tracer alpha-[11C]methyl-L-tryptophan (AMT) is transported in tumor tissue by the L-type amino acid transporter but is not incorporated into proteins [165]. Instead, AMT is utilized by the kynurenine immunomodulatory pathway [166, 167]. Under pathologic conditions, induction of this pathway's rate-limiting enzyme, indoleamine 2,3-dioxygenase, leads to increased metabolism of tryptophan and thus AMT accumulation via the kynurenine pathway [168, 169]. This pathway plays an important role in brain tumor pathogenesis [170]. Christensen et al., found that retrospectively created GTVs based on preoperative AMT-PET, either alone or in conjunction with postoperative MRI findings, demonstrating significant discordance with the standard clinical high-risk GTV generated via T1-Gad findings alone. Importantly, there was no significant difference in volumetric size of the GTVs determined by AMT-PET relative to those determined by MRI alone. Despite this, the investigational AMT volume offered superior coverage of the volume of initial progression when compared to the standard MRI-based GTV. Ideally, increased accuracy of GTV definition would allow for smaller empiric safety margins for microscopic spread that determines the CTV.

These findings and the associated methodology need to be prospectively confirmed and refined in a larger patient population, which will also allow inclusion of known predictors of glioblastoma progression, prior to attempts to affect clinical outcome with PET-driven escalation of therapy fields.

22.1.8 Gynecological Malignancies

The potential role of PET was largely recognized and integrated into the RT treatment for some gynecological malignancies (Fig. 22.8). In particular FDG-PET has been demonstrated to be useful in patients with cervical cancer candidate to RT; preliminary data suggest a potential use also in patients with endometrial cancer, uterine sarcoma, and ovarian cancer. In cervical cancer stage IB1-IIA, patients may be treated with either radical hysterectomy or CRT, which is associated with similar cure rates [171]. In accuracy unfortunately, most of the present diagnostic modalities have limitations leading to discrepancies between pre- and postoperative evaluation and staging [172]. This may result in the necessity to refer patients to chemo-RT following radical hysterectomy. Several studies have demonstrated a high incidence of short- and long-term side effects of combined therapy (i.e., surgery and RT), as compared to RT alone, with no significant benefit in OS.

There are a few major indications for referring patients to RT following surgery. The first indication occurs when positive LN is diagnosed during the postoperative pathological examination. This may be due to the relatively low sensitivity of MRI, PET/CT, and CT scans in detecting pelvic and para-aortic affected small LN (40–70 %)

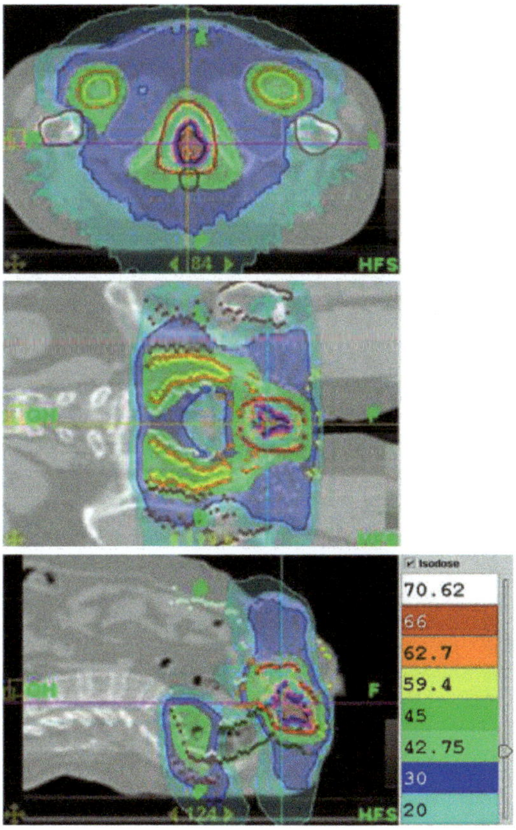

Fig. 22.8 Patient with vaginal tumor relapse performed tomotherapy treatment on pelvis and inguinal lymph node with simultaneous integrated boost to 66 Gy/28 fractions and showed a complete response at 11 months (data not shown)

[172]. PET/CT has been extensively used for LN assessment during the last decade and has proved valuable in accurate assessment of LN metastases. Various studies reported the specificity, sensitivity, PPV, and NPV of PET/CT for diagnosis of extracervical lesions to be 94–100 %, 60–77 %, 90 %, and 74 %, respectively, with an accuracy of 94 % [173]. Other indications include high tumor grade, tumor invasion into the cervical stroma, lymph and vascular space invasion, and involved or close margins.

Few studies have investigated the utility of SUV_{max} in patients with cervical cancer. In a large study involving 240 patients, Kidd et al. and Grigsby et al. showed a correlation between SUV_{max} and tumor grade. Other studies have attempted to establish the use of SUV_{max}, in para-aortic LN as a predictor of recurrence and death [173]. Others have attempted to correlate SUV_{max} at the primary tumor site with outcome and with recurrence [174]. Some have attempted to identify SUV_{max} cutoff values for predicting treatment response and prognosis. This is now used by some medical centers in order to estimate residual tumor following primary RT [175, 176]. To date, however, no studies have attempted to adjust treatment modality based on SUV_{max}. PET/CT in the primary evaluation of operable cervical cancer can help in the optimal selection of patients for surgery such that multimodality treatment with its attendant increase in morbidity is avoided.

For International Federation of Gynecology and Obstetrics (FIGO) stages IIB to IVA cervical cancer, CRT is the standard treatment [177]. A randomized trial showed that hysterectomy after CRT does not increase toxicity and improves LRC [178]. For tumors larger than 4 cm, there might be a survival benefit in favor of extrafascial hysterectomy after CRT [178]. IMRT and intensity-modulated arc therapy (IMAT) have major advantages compared to conventional RT. There is proof of improved cause-specific survival and significantly reduced dose received by small bowel, rectum, bladder, and bone marrow [179]. The implementation of IMAT has been facilitated by incorporating MRI and FDG-PET/CT in the RT planning [180, 181]. MRI is considered almost as a necessity in modern RT planning for cervical cancer, although the American College of Radiology Imaging Network Intergroup study recognized the low accuracy of MRI to diagnose minimal parametrial extent [182]. Recently, Vincens et al. published their experience with MRI performed on 44 patients treated with CRT, brachytherapy, and subsequent surgery for FIGO IB2-II cervical cancer. Their results demonstrate that surgery is safe after CRT and that MRI performs excellent in predicting resectability of the tumor. The sensitivity, specificity, and NPV for MRI concerning the end point "no residual disease or only isolated cells" was 80%, 55%, and 83%, respectively [183].

It is well known that FDG-PET/CT is superior in detecting LN to CT alone leading to improved coverage of target volumes and modified radiation fields in 20% of patients [184]. SUV_{max} at diagnosis has been reported to predict disease-free survival and OS [175]. Post-therapy FDG uptake is inversely correlated with cause-specific survival and OS [185]. The use of FDG-PET/CT during RT to predict outcome is not unequivocally proven [186]. There is mounting evidence that FDG-PET/CT has an increasing role in the management of ovarian cancer, with its main indication to detect tumor recurrence in presence of rising CA-125 serum values and negative conventional imaging studies. The benefits of the use of FDG-PET/CT in these settings have been largely reported, with a sensitivity of more than 90% in detecting occult metastases. Zimny et al. documented that FDG-PET/CT preceded the conventional diagnosis by a median of 6 months in patients considered clinically free of disease [187]. It has been recently reported in a prospective multicenter with a cohort of 90 patients the impact of FDG-PET/CT in suspected recurrent ovarian cancer, affecting disease management decisions in 60% of the cases with a much higher detection rate compared to conventional imaging [188].

22.1.9 Colorectal Cancer

Colorectal carcinoma (CRC) is the third most common cause of malignancy in both men and women and the second most common cause of death in the Western world. Rectal cancer is challenging because of its unique anatomical characteristics (i.e., partial covering by peritoneum), critical position, and therapeutic options (aimed at preserving pelvic floor integrity, sphincter continence, and genitourinary functions) [189]. The study of rectal cancer showed that CRT provides preoperative best results in terms of local control and toxicity compared with postoperative CRT. The preoperative CRT has thus become standard of care in the treatment of advanced but operable rectal cancer [190].

Two recent phase III trials have shown that the addition of 5-fluorouracil to preoperative RT improves local control and roughly triples the pathological complete response (pCR) rate compared to RT alone [191, 192]. The obtaining of a pCR is of great importance because it is strongly associated with a good prognosis [193]. The rate of pCR is now considered the primary focus of many studies of phases II and III. In an attempt to improve the pCR rate and the overall progress of the disease, researchers have associated with the RT new drugs such as capecitabine, oxaliplatin, irinotecan, raltitrexed, or "targeted agents" such as bevacizumab, cetuximab, or gefitinib. Most patients are subject to significant shrinkage of the primary tumor during CRT, and recent results suggest that the degree of response during CRT according to both morphologic and functional parameters may be predictive of good outcome after surgery. The idea of exploiting tumor shrinkage to condense an adaptive boost to the residual tumor could permit a larger dose escalation without significantly increasing toxicity [194].

To find a better therapeutic approach, PET was also considered. FDG-PET/CT evaluates the metabolic activity being useful in the process of staging, restaging, and assessment of response to treatment [195]. In a meta-analysis of 3080 patients with CRC from 111 datasets, Kinkel et al. [196] found that the mean weighted sensitivity for detecting hepatic metastases was 55% for ultrasound, 72% for CT, 76% for MRI, and 90% for FDG-PET. A prospective study of 73 patients with liver metastatic CRC [197] showed that CECT missed extrahepatic disease in 33%

of the cases, whereas PET/CT failed to detect disease in only 11 % of the cases. A limitation associated with PET/CT is inability to distinguish between chronic infection and tumor because as both associated with increased FDG uptake. In addition, in a number of small studies analyzing the ability of PET/CT and MRI to detect subcentimeter liver metastases, MRI resulted superior than PET/CT with a higher sensitivity and specificity for detection, particularly with the use of newer MR hepatobiliary-specific contrast agents [198]. Hence, MRI appears to be the modality of choice for detecting hepatic metastases smaller than 10 mm.

Some studies also document the positive impact of PET/CT on tumor delineation for RT planning in rectal cancer [199, 200]. The PET-derived GTV strongly correlated with the CT-derived GTV ($r_2=0.84$; $p<0.01$) and with the volume determined by subsequent anatomic-pathologic analysis ($r_2=0.77$; $p<0.01$). The use of PET/CT-derived GTV allowed external beam therapy to adequately cover N1 LN stations in the perirectal soft tissues. Studies of GTV delineation by MRI compared with PET/CT have shown that MRI tends to overestimate GTV. However, the clinical significance of GTV variance between MRI and PET on management has yet to be established [200, 201]. In patients with rectal cancer, preoperative hypofractionated RT results in an improved local tumor control, whereas preoperative treatment with CRT results in a significant down staging of the tumor [202]. In 15–30 % of the patients being preoperatively treated with CRT, even complete tumor regression is observed 6–8 weeks after completion of the CRT [203]. Patients with a pCR after preoperative treatment with CRT have better long-term outcome than patients presenting with a pathological partial response (pPR). pCR might be indicative of a prognostically favorable biological tumor profile with a lower probability for local or distant recurrence and improved survival.

An important strategy to improve local tumor control might be escalating the radiation dose, in view of the fact that a higher radiation dose has been shown to yield a higher local control rate. However, the increase of radiation dose is limited by the toxicity to surrounding normal tissues. One possibility to achieve a higher radiation dose to the tumor without additional damage to normal tissues would be to increase the dose to particular subparts of the tumor based on the intra-tumor heterogeneity visualized using functional imaging [204]. There is a growing interest in nonuniform dose distribution techniques like dose painting or subvolume boosting to increase the rate of local tumor control [205]. Selective irradiation of tumor subvolumes of potentially radioresistant regions within the tumor along with a decrease in radiation dose to less resistant regions could even increase local tumor control rates with equal or decreased levels of side effects. However, before the potential of nonuniform dose distributions can be used in clinical practice for rectal cancer patients, the regions in the tumor with an increased resistance to treatment should be defined accurately. Especially for subvolume boosting with RT, accurate knowledge about the orientation and location of the tumor is required prior to each RT fraction.

For rectal cancer, pCR after preoperative treatment with CRT was found to result in better long-term outcome, a low probability for local and distant recurrence, as well as improved survival when compared to the patients presenting with a pPR. Relationships between residual metabolic uptake and long-term outcome and the probability for recurrence have not yet been proven for rectal cancer. Therefore, a multicentric study on response prediction for rectal cancer is started using multivariate analysis with nomograms [206]. Preliminary results show that one of the criteria found to be highly predictive for the probability on distant metastases and local recurrence within 5 years was the presence of residual (PET-positive) disease after preoperative treatment with CRT. One of the limitations of FDG-PET-based response monitoring is the increased FDG uptake in (peritumoral) inflammatory cells induced by RT treatment [203]. For the patients with a visually observed peritumoral inflammatory response on the PET images, the inflammatory response was also reported by the pathologist after examination of the resected specimen. High FDG uptake regions within rectal tumors prior to

CRT can identify the location of the residual metabolic active areas after treatment. If those zones may be located with high accuracy, dose escalation in high FDG uptake zones within the tumor is expected to result in a higher rate of local tumor control or even a pCR after preoperative treatment with CRT [207].

FDG-PET/CT is a reliable technique for the assessment of response to CRT in locally advanced rectal cancer (LARC); the combination of the visual and semiquantitative analysis increases the diagnostic validity, in order to consider the most conservative surgical treatment [208]. The prognostic and predictive impact of FDG-PET/CT baseline in patients with LARC treated with neoadjuvant CRT as an alternative approach was documented [209]. Furthermore, Calvo et al. [210, 211] assessed that FDG-PET may be useful in assessing the response of CRT in LARC and suggested that the initial SUV_{max} may be of prognostic value with regard to the outcome of the patient in the long term. Denecke et al. [212] published that FDG-PET is superior to CT and MRI in predicting response to preoperative treatment of LARC. Furthermore, the feasibility of the inclusion of MRI and FDG-PET/CT, performed before, during, and after chemo preoperative RT in treatment planning in the course of therapy was also demonstrated [213].

22.1.10 Prostate Cancer

PCa is an age-related disease and is most common in men age 65 and older. The natural history of PCa is very slow, and typically, patients with early-stage disease are asymptomatic. However, advanced-stage PCa with metastases is life-threatening. Hormonal therapy, surgery, and RT are the mainstays of PCa treatment. For RT planning in PCa patients, accurate mapping of the primary tumor, LN, and possible distant metastatic sites is critical for delivering an effective treatment while minimizing treatment-associated morbidity. The specificity of CHO-PET/CT in the detection of primary PCa has shown in numerous studies to be limited due to its limited potential in differentiating between benign prostatic lesions and PCa [214]. Nevertheless, CHO-PET/CT has been reported as a promising imaging biomarker in PET/CT imaging for RT planning in primary PCa by enabling identification of dominant intraprostatic regions, and a boost dose can be delivered (range 84–100 Gy); in particular, simultaneous integrated boost (SIB) IMRT, which might improve tumor control in comparison to a standard IMRT plan, allows dose escalation to intraprostatic regions with only minor increases in the probability of normal tissue complications in OAR [215]. SIB was defined in some studies as a tumor-to-background uptake value ratio of >2 [216], in others as a threshold value of 60% of the CHO SUV_{max} that was also the best threshold showing the highest overlap between the PET volume and histopathology [217].

SUV_{mean} and SUV_{max} were dependent on prognostic risk factors such as T-stage and Gleason score. More aggressive PCa (with high Gleason scores) can be more readily detected using CHO-PET/CT. This has also been shown for MRI and MR spectroscopy [218–220].

CHO-PET signals for the prostate provided adequate spatial information for delineation of the whole prostate for external beam radiation therapy (EBRT). However, CHO-PET signals within the prostate present limitations for defining subvolumes for internal boost because of insufficient differentiation between normal prostate tissue and cancer. The use of CHO-PET/CT for RT planning in the primary setting with respect to irradiation of LN metastases is difficult due to limitations in CHO-PET/CT for LN staging. It was reported a limited sensitivity of 60% for the detection of LN metastases [221] due to a false-positive findings in the presence of inflammatory changes [222]. Thus, detection of every single LN metastases is challenging [223], which limits its feasibility for irradiation of single LN. PET/CT prior to RT might be useful in high-risk PCa to detect LN metastases which might be included in the conventional irradiation field (instead of irradiation of single LN).

RT is commonly used in the treatment of primary and metastatic PCa lesions [224–226] (Fig. 22.9). Among various imaging modalities available for localizing the site of recurrence, the use of CHO-PET/CT has proved to be a valuable tool for restaging patients with PCa with biochemical failure and particularly for detecting LN recurrences in providing better results than conventional imaging modalities, even in those with low serum PSA values [227, 228]. Some studies validated by open pelvic/retroperitoneal lymphadenectomy have shown good specificity and PPV of CHO-PET/CT in restaging LN metastases [229]. Several studies have investigated the potential value of CHO-PET/CT-guided RT in patients with PCa recurrence [11], especially pertaining to local and LN recurrence reporting a biochemical relapse-free survival of 40% with a median follow-up of 2-years [230] and 75 % with median 3.8-years follow-up after salvage RT [231]. In the majority of patients (84 %), no or mild late side effects were observed [232]. In addition, the majority of the authors reported that 18F- labelled CHO-PET/CT planning could be helpful in dose escalation allowing boost doses higher than 60 Gy to metastatic LN regions [232]. Stereotactic body RT was investigated to treat limited LN recurrences, as detected by CHO-PET with good results: 3-year follow-up, OS, disease-free survival, and local control rates were 92%, 17%, and 90%, respectively [233]. In addition SRT has shown the best results with respect to the outcome in patients with a PSA level <1 ng/ml in those with biochemical recurrence after RP [234].

Taking into account the limited lesion-based sensitivity of CHO-PET/CT for detecting LN

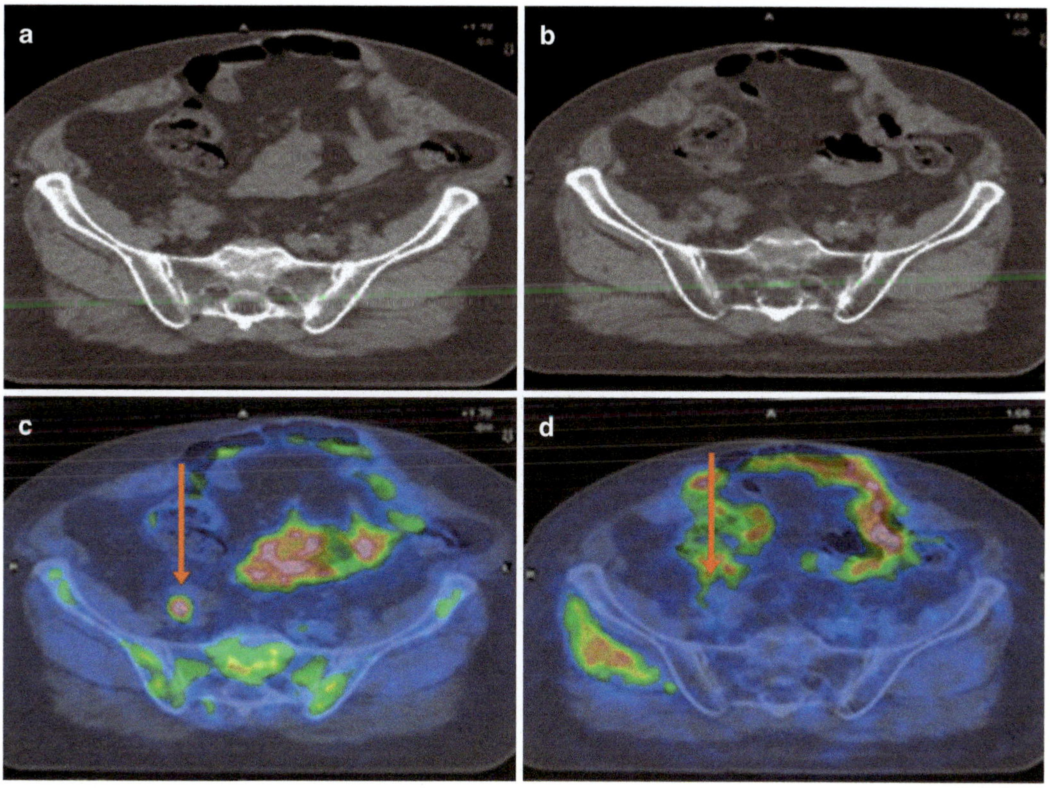

Fig. 22.9 11C-choline PET/CT performed in patient with prostate cancer recurrence as a guide for treatment planning. Helical tomotherapy high dose moderately hypofractionated (67.2 Gy/28 fractions) was performed on common iliac lymph node (*red arrow*) resulted positive at 11C-choline PET/CT (**a**, **c**). Four months after treatment 11C-choline PET/CT could detect a complete metabolic response (**b**, **d**)

recurrence as well as its inability to identify micrometastases due to its limited spatial resolution, the approach which includes lymphatic drainage in the irradiation field with an additional boost to PET-positive LN seems to be conceptually more useful than irradiation of single LN. However, there are very few data on the irradiation of oligometastases in recurrent disease [235–237].

Radiation can be delivered with external beam radiation therapy (EBRT) or stereotactic body RT (SBRT). EBRT is usually delivered to wider volumes using 3D Conformal RT or IMRT. IMRT is now commonly employed in radical or post-prostatectomy setting, in particular if a pelvic LN irradiation is necessary. As far as salvage setting is concerned, prophylactic irradiation of pelvic LN area might play a potential role owing to the risk of occult LN metastases. The role of adjuvant RT after salvage surgery for a LN relapse has been investigated with promising results as prognostic role [230, 238]. The utility of CHO-PET/CT for patient stratification prior to RT in differentiating between patients with local disease and those with systemic disease has been assessed. Since an early diagnosis of recurrent PCa and the exact localization of the site of recurrence (local recurrence, LN involvement, or systemic recurrence including bone metastases which is related to a poor prognosis) have a direct influence on therapeutic strategy, CHO-PET/CT can aid in detection and localization of recurrent PCa for disease management and selection of individualized therapy strategies.

In addition to 11C- labelled CHO, also 18F-labelled CHO [239, 240] and ACE [241], may be considered in planning RT of PCa patients. 18F-labelled CHO presents a very similar behavior to 11C- labelled CHO in PCa patients. The most striking difference between the two tracers is the urinary elimination that is high for 18F- labelled CHO, being an important disadvantage for imaging prostate region. Conversely, 18F- labelled CHO imaging has the advantage of a longer half-life (approximately 110 min vs. 20 min of 11C-labelled CHO) allowing transportation from one single cyclotron center to several PET centers. In studies of RT dose escalation, 18F- labelled CHO has been used to delineate GTV and to generate the PTV in patients with intraprostatic lesion, attempting to reduce irradiation dose to the bladder and the rectum. A recent meta-analysis about the diagnostic performance of 18F- labelled CHO and 11C- labelled CHO-PET/CT in the LN staging of PCa showed a pooled sensitivity of 49.2 % (95 % confidence interval [CI], 39.9–58.4) and a pooled specificity of 95 % (95 % CI, 92–97.1) [242].

Analogously, ACE also is a valuable PET tracer for imaging PCa, being used both for primary PCa and metastatic sites. The role of ACE as an image guide for RT planning has been evaluated in patients with intracapsular PCa with promising results [243]. However, data are still limited to establish its clinical role in RT planning.

22.1.11 Imaging Hypoxia in Radiotherapy

Hypoxia in tumors occurs because the oxygen demands exceed the oxygen supply. The growth and development of solid tumors requires the formation of a functional vascular supply, which evolves from the normal host vascular network by the process of angiogenesis. Although chronic hypoxia obviously depends on a diffusion limitation of oxygen, the actual distance from the blood vessel at which it exists can be highly variable, and even cells next to the blood vessel can be at intermediate levels of hypoxia and show a reduced radiation sensitivity [244, 245]. The most obvious way is to identify those patients whose tumors contain significant levels of hypoxia and thus require some additional treatment to overcome the hypoxic cell-induced radiation resistance. Another potential application of imaging would be in using it to decide the radiation dose delivered to the tumor [246]. Two strategies have been suggested [21, 247]: one strategy simply involves increasing the radiation dose homogenously to the GTV, in which a substantial hypoxic fraction has been identified. However, raising the dose uniformly has the potential to increase the dose to the surrounding normal tissue and thereby to increase proportionally the risk for adverse reactions. The second strategy uses hypoxia imaging data to define a BTV. In this situation, one could then keep the total radiation dose constant, but redistribute the dose within the GTV, thus raising the dose to the hypoxic areas with a compensatory dose-reduction to the non-hypoxic regions.

Hypoxia is one of the most important prognostic factors in RT of several types of cancer, for example, HNC, sarcoma, and cancer of the cervix uteri, influencing long-term survival as well as local tumor control [248–250]. A variety of methods for measuring oxygen levels in tumor tissue and assessing hypoxia have been developed [251, 252]. A promising noninvasive method for measuring hypoxia is PET with FMISO showing specific uptake in hypoxia [58, 253, 254]. An analysis of FMISO kinetics and uptake prior to RT in HNC revealed a prognostic value of typical kinetic patterns [255, 256].

More recently, FAZA has been proposed as hypoxia radiotracer; FAZA was improved with respect to FMISO for its behavior, such as lower lipophilicity than that of FMISO [257]. As a consequence, FAZA rapidly enters cells where it is readily available for accumulation in hypoxic tissues and shows more rapid clearance from non-target tissues [258].

An alternative range of compounds for hypoxia imaging has been developed based on ATSM being the most extensively evaluated, with applications in tumor and myocardial hypoxia imaging [259–261]. Importantly, ATSM has shown greater sensitivity to changes in tissue oxygen concentration than FMISO [262]. PET tracers, and particularly nitroimidazoles, are probably the most proper method to directly identify the presence of hypoxia. Conversely, those based on blood perfusion provide indirect measurements thus being less specific. Although PET imaging with specific hypoxia tracers are very promising, clinical data confirming their role in predicting patient outcome are still needed. In addition, there is also the need to establish the clinical role of the use of hypoxia tracers for increasing radiation dose delivered to hypoxic tumor subvolumes, representing this topic a relevant clinical implication in radiation oncology.

Conclusions

During the last 20 years, the continuous technological progress has revolutionized the role of PET scan also in radiation oncology. Moving from its original role for tumor staging and restaging PET/CT has become a crucial modality for tumor prognostication: as a new tool for tumor volume and spread measurement at baseline and for treatment tailoring. Challenges for its use with MRI in a single-shot scan (PET/MRI) with the use of innovative PET tracers are opening new frontiers for the radiation medical imaging research. In parallel, technologic advances in RT planning and delivery have made highly conformal and accurate treatments a reality. Integration of PET into RT planning is thus a natural evolution of both technologies, as a method of accurate target definition both at the beginning and at the end of treatment but also during potentially adaptive treatment that is dependent on tumor response.

References

1. Das SK, Ten Haken RK. Functional and molecular image guidance in radiotherapy treatment planning optimization. Semin Radiat Oncol. 2011;21(2):111–8.
2. Shi X, et al. PET/CT imaging-guided dose painting in radiation therapy. Cancer Lett. 2014;355(2):169–75.
3. Kunkler IH, et al. Review of current best practice and priorities for research in radiation oncology for elderly patients with cancer: the International Society of Geriatric Oncology (SIOG) task force. Ann Oncol Off J Eur Soc Med Oncol/ESMO. 2014;25(11):2134–46.
4. Wahl RL, et al. From RECIST to PERCIST: evolving considerations for PET response criteria in solid tumors. J Nucl Med Off Pub Soc Nucl Med. 2009;50 Suppl 1:122S–50.
5. Gregoire V, et al. PET-based treatment planning in radiotherapy: a new standard? J Nucl Med Off Pub Soc Nucl Med. 2007;48 Suppl 1:68S–77.
6. Chiti A, Kirienko M, Grégoire V. Clinical use of PET-CT data for radiotherapy planning: what are we looking for? Radiother Oncol. 2010;96(3):277–9.
7. Zhu A, Lee D, Shim H. Metabolic positron emission tomography imaging in cancer detection and therapy response. Semin Oncol. 2011;38(1):55–69.
8. Pinkawa M, Eble MJ, Mottaghy FM. PET and PET/CT in radiation treatment planning for prostate cancer. Expert Rev Anticancer Ther. 2011;11(7):1033–9.
9. Ford EC, et al. 18F-FDG PET/CT for image-guided and intensity-modulated radiotherapy. J Nucl Med Off Pub Soc Nucl Med. 2009;50(10):1655–65.

10. Picchio M, et al. Clinical evidence on PET/CT for radiation therapy planning in prostate cancer. Radiother Oncol J Eur Soc Therapeutic Radiol Oncol. 2010;96(3):347–50.
11. Picchio M, et al. (11)C-Choline PET/CT as a guide to radiation treatment planning of lymph-node relapses in prostate cancer patients. Eur J Nucl Med Mol Imaging. 2014;41(7):1270–9.
12. Liu WS, et al. The role of pretreatment FDG-PET in nasopharyngeal carcinoma treated with intensity-modulated radiotherapy. Int J Radiat Oncol Biol Phys. 2012;82(2):561–6.
13. Higashi K, et al. 11C-acetate PET imaging of lung cancer: comparison with 18F-FDG PET and 99mTc-MIBI SPET. Eur J Nucl Med Mol Imaging. 2004;31(1):13–21.
14. Hellwig D, et al. Diagnostic performance and prognostic impact of FDG-PET in suspected recurrence of surgically treated non-small cell lung cancer. Eur J Nucl Med Mol Imaging. 2006;33(1):13–21.
15. Auperin A, et al. Meta-analysis of concomitant versus sequential radiochemotherapy in locally advanced non-small-cell lung cancer. J Clin Oncol Off J Am Soc Clin Oncol. 2010;28(13):2181–90.
16. Schaake-Koning C, et al. Radiosensitization by cytotoxic drugs. The EORTC experience by the Radiotherapy and Lung Cancer Cooperative Groups. Lung Cancer. 1994;10 Suppl 1:S263–70.
17. Machtay M, et al. Higher biologically effective dose of radiotherapy is associated with improved outcomes for locally advanced non-small cell lung carcinoma treated with chemoradiation: an analysis of the Radiation Therapy Oncology Group. Int J Radiat Oncol Biol Phys. 2012;82(1):425–34.
18. Machtay M, et al. Defining local-regional control and its importance in locally advanced non-small cell lung carcinoma. J Thorac Oncol Off Pub Int Assoc Study Lung Cancer. 2012;7(4):716–22.
19. Bradley J. A review of radiation dose escalation trials for non-small cell lung cancer within the Radiation Therapy Oncology Group. Semin Oncol. 2005;32(2 Suppl 3):S111–3.
20. Aerts HJ, Lambin P, Ruysscher DD. FDG for dose painting: a rational choice. Radiother Oncol J Eur Soc Therapeutic Radiol Oncol. 2010;97(2):163–4.
21. Bentzen SM, Gregoire V. Molecular imaging-based dose painting: a novel paradigm for radiation therapy prescription. Semin Radiat Oncol. 2011;21(2):101–10.
22. Pommier P, et al. Impact of (18)F-FDG PET on treatment strategy and 3D radiotherapy planning in non-small cell lung cancer: a prospective multicenter study. Am J Roentgenol. 2010;195(2):350–5.
23. Nestle U, et al. Comparison of different methods for delineation of 18F-FDG PET-positive tissue for target volume definition in radiotherapy of patients with non-small cell lung cancer. J Nucl Med Off Pub Soc Nucl Med. 2005;46(8):1342–8.
24. Erdi YE, et al. Radiotherapy treatment planning for patients with non-small cell lung cancer using positron emission tomography (PET). Radiother Oncol J Eur Soc Therapeutic Radiol Oncol. 2002;62(1):51–60.
25. Ceresoli GL, et al. Role of computed tomography and [18F] fluorodeoxyglucose positron emission tomography image fusion in conformal radiotherapy of non-small cell lung cancer: a comparison with standard techniques with and without elective nodal irradiation. Tumori. 2007;93(1):88–96.
26. Yin LJ, et al. Utilization of PET-CT in target volume delineation for three-dimensional conformal radiotherapy in patients with non-small cell lung cancer and atelectasis. Multidiscip Respir Med. 2013;8(1):21.
27. Mah K, et al. The impact of (18)FDG-PET on target and critical organs in CT-based treatment planning of patients with poorly defined non-small-cell lung carcinoma: a prospective study. Int J Radiat Oncol Biol Phys. 2002;52(2):339–50.
28. Bradley J, et al. Impact of FDG-PET on radiation therapy volume delineation in non-small-cell lung cancer. Int J Radiat Oncol Biol Phys. 2004;59(1):78–86.
29. van Der Wel A, et al. Increased therapeutic ratio by 18FDG-PET CT planning in patients with clinical CT stage N2-N3M0 non-small-cell lung cancer: a modeling study. Int J Radiat Oncol Biol Phys. 2005;61(3):649–55.
30. Troost EG, et al. 18F-FLT PET/CT for early response monitoring and dose escalation in oropharyngeal tumors. J Nucl Med Off Pub Soc Nucl Med. 2010;51(6):866–74.
31. Witte M, et al. Dealing with geometric uncertainties in dose painting by numbers: introducing the DeltaVH. Radiother Oncol J Eur Soc Therapeutic Radiol Oncol. 2011;100(3):402–6.
32. Deveau MA, et al. Feasibility and sensitivity study of helical tomotherapy for dose painting plans. Acta Oncol. 2010;49(7):991–6.
33. Thorwarth D, Alber M. Implementation of hypoxia imaging into treatment planning and delivery. Radiother Oncol J Eur Soc Therapeutic Radiol Oncol. 2010;97(2):172–5.
34. Vanderstraeten B, et al. [18F]fluoro-deoxy-glucose positron emission tomography ([18F]FDG-PET) voxel intensity-based intensity-modulated radiation therapy (IMRT) for head and neck cancer. Radiother Oncol J Eur Soc Therapeutic Radiol Oncol. 2006;79(3):249–58.
35. Rickhey M, et al. A biologically adapted dose-escalation approach, demonstrated for 18F-FET-PET in brain tumors. Strahlentherapie und Onkologie Organ der Deutschen Rontgengesellschaft … [et al]. 2008;184(10):536–42.
36. Berwouts D, et al. Three-phase adaptive dose-painting-by-numbers for head-and-neck cancer: initial results of the phase I clinical trial. Radiother Oncol J Eur Soc Therapeutic Radiol Oncol. 2013;107(3):310–6.

37. Mac Manus MP, et al. Metabolic (FDG-PET) response after radical radiotherapy/chemoradiotherapy for non-small cell lung cancer correlates with patterns of failure. Lung Cancer. 2005;49(1):95–108.
38. Greco C, et al. Current status of PET/CT for tumour volume definition in radiotherapy treatment planning for non-small cell lung cancer (NSCLC). Lung Cancer. 2007;57(2):125–34.
39. Nehmeh SA, Erdi YE. Respiratory motion in positron emission tomography/computed tomography: a review. Semin Nucl Med. 2008;38(3):167–76.
40. Nehmeh SA, et al. Effect of respiratory gating on quantifying PET images of lung cancer. J Nucl Med Off Pub Soc Nucl Med. 2002;43(7):876–81.
41. Nehmeh SA, et al. Effect of respiratory gating on reducing lung motion artifacts in PET imaging of lung cancer. Med Phys. 2002;29(3):366–71.
42. Trinkaus ME, et al. Imaging of hypoxia with 18F-FAZA PET in patients with locally advanced non-small cell lung cancer treated with definitive chemoradiotherapy. J Med Imaging Radiat Oncol. 2013;57(4):475–81.
43. Postema EJ, et al. Initial results of hypoxia imaging using 1-alpha-D: –(5-deoxy-5-[18F]-fluoroarabinofuranosyl)-2-nitroimidazole (18F-FAZA). Eur J Nucl Med Mol Imaging. 2009;36(10):1565–73.
44. Pignon JP, et al. Meta-analysis of chemotherapy in head and neck cancer (MACH-NC): an update on 93 randomised trials and 17,346 patients. Radiother Oncol J Eur Soc Therapeutic Radiol Oncol. 2009;92(1):4–14.
45. Arens AI, et al. FDG-PET/CT in radiation treatment planning of head and neck squamous cell carcinoma. Q J Nucl Med Mol Imaging Off Pub Italian Assoc Nucl Med. 2011;55(5):521–8.
46. Romesser PB, et al. Superior prognostic utility of gross and metabolic tumor volume compared to standardized uptake value using PET/CT in head and neck squamous cell carcinoma patients treated with intensity-modulated radiotherapy. Ann Nucl Med. 2012;26(7):527–34.
47. Newbold K, Powell C. PET/CT in radiotherapy planning for head and neck cancer. Front Oncol. 2012;2:189.
48. Kirienko M, et al. Prognostic value of pre-therapy (18)FDG PET/CT for the outcome of (18)FDG PET-guided SIB-IMRT in patients with head and neck cancer. Eur J Nucl Med Mol Imaging. 2012;39:S201–2.
49. Vesselle H, et al. Fluorodeoxyglucose uptake of primary non-small cell lung cancer at positron emission tomography: new contrary data on prognostic role. Clin Cancer Res Off J Am Assoc Cancer Res. 2007;13(11):3255–63.
50. Agarwal M, et al. Revisiting the prognostic value of preoperative (18)F-fluoro-2-deoxyglucose ((18)F-FDG) positron emission tomography (PET) in early-stage (I & II) non-small cell lung cancers (NSCLC). Eur J Nucl Med Mol Imaging. 2010;37(4):691–8.
51. Torizuka T, et al. Prognostic value of 18F-FDG PET in patients with head and neck squamous cell cancer. Am J Roentgenol. 2009;192(4):W156–60.
52. Machtay M, et al. Pretreatment FDG-PET standardized uptake value as a prognostic factor for outcome in head and neck cancer. Head Neck. 2009;31(2):195–201.
53. Halfpenny W, et al. FDG-PET. A possible prognostic factor in head and neck cancer. Br J Cancer. 2002;86(4):512–6.
54. Castaldi P, et al. Can "early" and "late"18F-FDG PET-CT be used as prognostic factors for the clinical outcome of patients with locally advanced head and neck cancer treated with radio-chemotherapy? Radiother Oncol J Eur Soc Therapeutic Radiol Oncol. 2012;103(1):63–8.
55. Kunkel M, et al. Radiation response non-invasively imaged by [18F]FDG-PET predicts local tumor control and survival in advanced oral squamous cell carcinoma. Oral Oncol. 2003;39(2):170–7.
56. Xie P, et al. Prognostic value of 18F-FDG PET/CT before and after radiotherapy for locally advanced nasopharyngeal carcinoma. Ann Oncol Off J Eur Soc Med Oncol/ESMO. 2010;21(5):1078–82.
57. Herholz K, et al. Correlation of glucose consumption and tumor cell density in astrocytomas. A stereotactic PET study. J Neurosurg. 1993;79(6):853–8.
58. Rajendran JG, et al. Hypoxia and glucose metabolism in malignant tumors: evaluation by [18F]fluoromisonidazole and [18F]fluorodeoxyglucose positron emission tomography imaging. Clin Cancer Res Off J Am Assoc Cancer Res. 2004;10(7):2245–52.
59. Zimny M, et al. FDG – a marker of tumour hypoxia? A comparison with [18F]fluoromisonidazole and pO2-polarography in metastatic head and neck cancer. Eur J Nucl Med Mol Imaging. 2006;33(12):1426–31.
60. Jain VK, et al. Effects of 2-deoxy-D-glucose on glycolysis, proliferation kinetics and radiation response of human cancer cells. Int J Radiat Oncol Biol Phys. 1985;11(5):943–50.
61. Vercauteren T, et al. Deformation field validation and inversion applied to adaptive radiation therapy. Phys Med Biol. 2013;58(15):5269–86.
62. Castadot P, et al. Adaptive functional image-guided IMRT in pharyngo-laryngeal squamous cell carcinoma: is the gain in dose distribution worth the effort? Radiother Oncol J Eur Soc Therapeutic Radiol Oncol. 2011;101(3):343–50.
63. Hansen EK, et al. Repeat CT imaging and replanning during the course of IMRT for head-and-neck cancer. Int J Radiat Oncol Biol Phys. 2006;64(2):355–62.
64. Bhide SA, et al. Weekly volume and dosimetric changes during chemoradiotherapy with intensity-

modulated radiation therapy for head and neck cancer: a prospective observational study. Int J Radiat Oncol Biol Phys. 2010;76(5):1360–8.
65. Ho KF, et al. Monitoring dosimetric impact of weight loss with kilovoltage (kV) cone beam CT (CBCT) during parotid-sparing IMRT and concurrent chemotherapy. Int J Radiat Oncol Biol Phys. 2012;82(3):e375–82.
66. Height R, et al. The dosimetric consequences of anatomic changes in head and neck radiotherapy patients. J Med Imaging Radiat Oncol. 2010;54(5):497–504.
67. Romesser PB, et al. A prognostic volumetric threshold of gross tumor volume in head and neck cancer patients treated with radiotherapy. Am J Clin Oncol. 2012;37(2):154–61.
68. Picchio M, et al. Predictive value of pre-therapy (18) F-FDG PET/CT for the outcome of (18)F-FDG PET-guided radiotherapy in patients with head and neck cancer. Eur J Nucl Med Mol Imaging. 2014;41(1): 21–31.
69. Lin SH, et al. Propensity score-based comparison of long-term outcomes with 3-dimensional conformal radiotherapy vs intensity-modulated radiotherapy for esophageal cancer. Int J Radiat Oncol Biol Phys. 2012;84(5):1078–85.
70. Chen YJ, et al. Helical tomotherapy for radiotherapy in esophageal cancer: a preferred plan with better conformal target coverage and more homogeneous dose distribution. Med Dosim Off J Am Assoc Med Dosim. 2007;32(3):166–71.
71. Rohren EM, Turkington TG, Coleman RE. Clinical applications of PET in oncology. Radiology. 2004;231(2):305–32.
72. Krause BJ, Schwarzenbock S, Souvatzoglou M. FDG PET and PET/CT. Recent Results Cancer Res. Fortschritte der Krebsforschung. Progres dans les recherches sur le cancer. 2013;187:351–69.
73. Drudi S, et al. Esophagogram and CT vs endoscopic and surgical specimens in the diagnosis of esophageal carcinoma. Radiol Med. 2002;103(4):344–52.
74. Leong T, et al. A prospective study to evaluate the impact of FDG-PET on CT-based radiotherapy treatment planning for oesophageal cancer. Radiother Oncol J Eur Soc Therapeutic Radiol Oncol. 2006;78(3):254–61.
75. Moureau-Zabotto L, et al. Impact of CT and 18F-deoxyglucose positron emission tomography image fusion for conformal radiotherapy in esophageal carcinoma. Int J Radiat Oncol Biol Phys. 2005;63(2):340–5.
76. Han D, et al. Comparison of (18)F-fluorothymidine and (18)F-fluorodeoxyglucose PET/CT in delineating gross tumor volume by optimal threshold in patients with squamous cell carcinoma of thoracic esophagus. Int J Radiat Oncol Biol Phys. 2010;76(4):1235–41.
77. Vali FS, et al. Comparison of standardized uptake value-based positron emission tomography and computed tomography target volumes in esophageal cancer patients undergoing radiotherapy. Int J Radiat Oncol Biol Phys. 2010;78(4):1057–63.
78. van Heijl M, et al. Influence of ROI definition, partial volume correction and SUV normalization on SUV-survival correlation in oesophageal cancer. Nucl Med Commun. 2010;31(7):652–8.
79. Hatt M, et al. Impact of partial-volume effect correction on the predictive and prognostic value of baseline 18F-FDG PET images in esophageal cancer. J Nucl Med Off Pub Soc Nucl Med. 2012;53(1): 12–20.
80. Clarke M, et al. Effects of radiotherapy and of differences in the extent of surgery for early breast cancer on local recurrence and 15-year survival: an overview of the randomised trials. Lancet. 2005; 366(9503):2087–106.
81. Fisher B, et al. Twenty-year follow-up of a randomized trial comparing total mastectomy, lumpectomy, and lumpectomy plus irradiation for the treatment of invasive breast cancer. N Engl J Med. 2002;347(16): 1233–41.
82. Romestaing P, et al. Role of a 10-Gy boost in the conservative treatment of early breast cancer: results of a randomized clinical trial in Lyon, France. J Clin Oncol Off J Am Soc Clin Oncol. 1997;15(3):963–8.
83. Bartelink H, et al. Impact of a higher radiation dose on local control and survival in breast-conserving therapy of early breast cancer: 10-year results of the randomized boost versus no boost EORTC 22881-10882 trial. J Clin Oncol Off J Am Soc Clin Oncol. 2007;25(22):3259–65.
84. Ford EC, et al. Comparison of FDG-PET/CT and CT for delineation of lumpectomy cavity for partial breast irradiation. Int J Radiat Oncol Biol Phys. 2008;71(2):595–602.
85. Li XA, et al. Variability of target and normal structure delineation for breast cancer radiotherapy: an RTOG Multi-Institutional and Multiobserver Study. Int J Radiat Oncol Biol Phys. 2009;73(3):944–51.
86. Beadle BM, et al. Patterns of regional recurrence after definitive radiotherapy for cervical cancer. Int J Radiat Oncol Biol Phys. 2010;76(5):1396–403.
87. Segaert I, et al. Additional value of PET-CT in staging of clinical stage IIB and III breast cancer. Breast J. 2010;16(6):617–24.
88. Groheux D, et al. The yield of 18F-FDG PET/CT in patients with clinical stage IIA, IIB, or IIIA breast cancer: a prospective study. J Nucl Med Off Pub Soc Nucl Med. 2011;52(10):1526–34.
89. Aukema TS, et al. Detection of extra-axillary lymph node involvement with FDG PET/CT in patients with stage II-III breast cancer. Eur J Cancer. 2010;46(18):3205–10.
90. Fuster D, et al. Preoperative staging of large primary breast cancer with [18F]fluorodeoxyglucose positron emission tomography/computed tomography compared with conventional imaging procedures. J Clin Oncol Off J Am Soc Clin Oncol. 2008; 26(29):4746–51.

91. Heusner TA, et al. Breast cancer staging in a single session: whole-body PET/CT mammography. J Nucl Med Off Pub Soc Nucl Med. 2008;49(8):1215–22.
92. Groheux D, et al. Effect of (18)F-FDG PET/CT imaging in patients with clinical stage II and III breast cancer. Int J Radiat Oncol Biol Phys. 2008;71(3):695–704.
93. Kruse V, et al. Serum tumor markers and PET/CT imaging for tumor recurrence detection. Ann Nucl Med. 2013;27(2):97–104.
94. Linden HM, Dehdashti F. Novel methods and tracers for breast cancer imaging. Semin Nucl Med. 2013;43(4):324–9.
95. Ferme C, et al. Chemotherapy plus involved-field radiation in early-stage Hodgkin's disease. N Engl J Med. 2007;357(19):1916–27.
96. Cheson BD. Role of functional imaging in the management of lymphoma. J Clin Oncol Off J Am Soc Clin Oncol. 2011;29(14):1844–54.
97. Pinilla I, et al. Diagnostic value of CT, PET and combined PET/CT performed with low-dose unenhanced CT and full-dose enhanced CT in the initial staging of lymphoma. Q J Nucl Med Mol Imaging Off Pub Italian Assoc Nucl Med. 2011;55(5): 567–75.
98. Barrington SF, et al. Role of imaging in the staging and response assessment of lymphoma: consensus of the International Conference on Malignant Lymphomas Imaging Working Group. J Clin Oncol Off J Am Soc Clin Oncol. 2014;32(27):3048–58.
99. Kostakoglu L, et al. FDG-PET after 1 cycle of therapy predicts outcome in diffuse large cell lymphoma and classic Hodgkin disease. Cancer. 2006;107(11):2678–87.
100. Hutchings M, et al. FDG-PET after two cycles of chemotherapy predicts treatment failure and progression-free survival in Hodgkin lymphoma. Blood. 2006;107(1):52–9.
101. Zinzani PL, et al. Early interim 18F-FDG PET in Hodgkin's lymphoma: evaluation on 304 patients. Eur J Nucl Med Mol Imaging. 2012;39(1):4–12.
102. Gallamini A, et al. The predictive value of positron emission tomography scanning performed after two courses of standard therapy on treatment outcome in advanced stage Hodgkin's disease. Haematologica. 2006;91(4):475–81.
103. Cerci JJ, et al. 18F-FDG PET after 2 cycles of ABVD predicts event-free survival in early and advanced Hodgkin lymphoma. J Nucl Med Off Pub Soc Nucl Med. 2010;51(9):1337–43.
104. Hutchings M, et al. Prognostic value of interim FDG-PET after two or three cycles of chemotherapy in Hodgkin lymphoma. Ann Oncol Off J Eur Soc Med Oncol/ESMO. 2005;16(7):1160–8.
105. Terasawa T, et al. Fluorine-18-fluorodeoxyglucose positron emission tomography for interim response assessment of advanced-stage Hodgkin's lymphoma and diffuse large B-cell lymphoma: a systematic review. J Clin Oncol Off J Am Soc Clin Oncol. 2009;27(11):1906–14.
106. Gallamini A, et al. Early interim 2-[18F]fluoro-2-deoxy-D-glucose positron emission tomography is prognostically superior to international prognostic score in advanced-stage Hodgkin's lymphoma: a report from a joint Italian-Danish study. J Clin Oncol Off J Am Soc Clin Oncol. 2007;25(24):3746–52.
107. Gallamini A, et al. Interim positron emission tomography scan in Hodgkin lymphoma: definitions, interpretation rules, and clinical validation. Leuk Lymphoma. 2009;50(11):1761–4.
108. Meignan M, Gallamini A, Haioun C. Report on the first international workshop on interim-PET-scan in lymphoma. Leuk Lymphoma. 2009;50(8):1257–60.
109. Biggi A, et al. International validation study for interim PET in ABVD-treated, advanced-stage hodgkin lymphoma: interpretation criteria and concordance rate among reviewers. J Nucl Med Off Pub Soc Nucl Med. 2013;54(5):683–90.
110. Zijlstra JM, et al. 18F-fluoro-deoxyglucose positron emission tomography for post-treatment evaluation of malignant lymphoma: a systematic review. Haematologica. 2006;91(4):522–9.
111. Terasawa T, et al. 18F-FDG PET for posttherapy assessment of Hodgkin's disease and aggressive Non-Hodgkin's lymphoma: a systematic review. J Nucl Med Off Pub Soc Nucl Med. 2008; 49(1):13–21.
112. Radford JA, et al. The significance of residual mediastinal abnormality on the chest radiograph following treatment for Hodgkin's disease. J Clin Oncol Off J Am Soc Clin Oncol. 1988;6(6):940–6.
113. Surbone A, et al. Residual abdominal masses in aggressive non-Hodgkin's lymphoma after combination chemotherapy: significance and management. J Clin Oncol Off J Am Soc Clin Oncol. 1988;6(12):1832–7.
114. Canellos GP. Residual mass in lymphoma may not be residual disease. J Clin Oncol Off J Am Soc Clin Oncol. 1988;6(6):931–3.
115. Engert A, et al. Reduced-intensity chemotherapy and PET-guided radiotherapy in patients with advanced stage Hodgkin's lymphoma (HD15 trial): a randomised, open-label, phase 3 non-inferiority trial. Lancet. 2012;379(9828):1791–9.
116. Specht L, et al. Modern radiation therapy for Hodgkin lymphoma: field and dose guidelines from the international lymphoma radiation oncology group (ILROG). Int J Radiat Oncol Biol Phys. 2014;89(4):854–62.
117. Girinsky T, Ghalibafian M. Radiotherapy of hodgkin lymphoma: indications, new fields, and techniques. Semin Radiat Oncol. 2007;17(3):206–22.
118. Girinsky T, et al. Is FDG-PET scan in patients with early stage Hodgkin lymphoma of any value in the implementation of the involved-node radiotherapy concept and dose painting? Radiother Oncol J Eur Soc Therapeutic Radiol Oncol. 2007;85(2):178–86.
119. Zelenetz AD, et al. Non-Hodgkin's lymphomas, version 3.2012. J Natl Compr Canc Netw. 2012;10(12): 1487–98.

120. Blum RH, et al. Frequent impact of [18F]fluorodeoxyglucose positron emission tomography on the staging and management of patients with indolent non-Hodgkin's lymphoma. Clin Lymphoma. 2003; 4(1):43–9.
121. Jerusalem G, et al. Whole-body positron emission tomography using 18F-fluorodeoxyglucose compared to standard procedures for staging patients with Hodgkin's disease. Haematologica. 2001; 86(3):266–73.
122. Jerusalem G, et al. Positron emission tomography (PET) with 18F-fluorodeoxyglucose (18F-FDG) for the staging of low-grade non-Hodgkin's lymphoma (NHL). Ann Oncol Off J Eur Soc Med Oncol/ ESMO. 2001;12(6):825–30.
123. Hueltenschmidt B, et al. Whole body positron emission tomography in the treatment of Hodgkin disease. Cancer. 2001;91(2):302–10.
124. Spaepen K, et al. Prognostic value of positron emission tomography (PET) with fluorine-18 fluorodeoxyglucose ([18F]FDG) after first-line chemotherapy in non-Hodgkin's lymphoma: is [18F]FDG-PET a valid alternative to conventional diagnostic methods? J Clin Oncol Off J Am Soc Clin Oncol. 2001;19(2):414–9.
125. Spaepen K, Mortelmans L. Evaluation of treatment response in patients with lymphoma using [18F] FDG-PET: differences between non-Hodgkin's lymphoma and Hodgkin's disease. Q J Nucl Med Mol Imaging Off Pub Italian Assoc Nucl Med. 2001;45(3):269–73.
126. Filippi AR, et al. Interim positron emission tomography and clinical outcome in patients with early stage Hodgkin lymphoma treated with combined modality therapy. Leuk Lymphoma. 2013;54(6):1183–7.
127. Filippi AR, et al. Radiation therapy in primary mediastinal B-cell lymphoma with positron emission tomography positivity after rituximab chemotherapy. Int J Radiat Oncol Biol Phys. 2013;87(2):311–6.
128. Kyle RA, Rajkumar SV. Criteria for diagnosis, staging, risk stratification and response assessment of multiple myeloma. Leukemia. 2009;23(1):3–9.
129. Durie BG. The role of anatomic and functional staging in myeloma: description of Durie/Salmon plus staging system. Eur J Cancer. 2006;42(11):1539–43.
130. Mose S, et al. Role of radiotherapy in the treatment of multiple myeloma. Strahlentherapie und Onkologie Organ der Deutschen Rontgengesellschaft ... [et al]. 2000;176(11):506–12.
131. Leigh BR, et al. Radiation therapy for the palliation of multiple myeloma. Int J Radiat Oncol Biol Phys. 1993;25(5):801–4.
132. Shin SM, et al. Feasibility and efficacy of local radiotherapy with concurrent novel agents in patients with multiple myeloma. Clin Lymphoma Myeloma Leuk. 2014;14(6):480–4.
133. Fonti R, et al. Metabolic tumor volume assessed by 18F-FDG PET/CT for the prediction of outcome in patients with multiple myeloma. J Nucl Med Off Pub Soc Nucl Med. 2012;53(12):1829–35.
134. Hernandez JA, Land KJ, McKenna RW. Leukemias, myeloma, and other lymphoreticular neoplasms. Cancer. 1995;75(1 Suppl):381–94.
135. Knowling MA, Harwood AR, Bergsagel DE. Comparison of extramedullary plasmacytomas with solitary and multiple plasma cell tumors of bone. J Clin Oncol Off J Am Soc Clin Oncol. 1983;1(4):255–62.
136. Bolek TW, Marcus Jr RB, Mendenhall NP. Solitary plasmacytoma of bone and soft tissue. Int J Radiat Oncol Biol Phys. 1996;36(2):329–33.
137. Jyothirmayi R, et al. Radiotherapy in the treatment of solitary plasmacytoma. Br J Radiol. 1997; 70(833):511–6.
138. Frassica DA, et al. Solitary plasmacytoma of bone: Mayo Clinic experience. Int J Radiat Oncol Biol Phys. 1989;16(1):43–8.
139. Holland J, et al. Plasmacytoma. Treatment results and conversion to myeloma. Cancer. 1992;69(6): 1513–7.
140. Liebross RH, et al. Solitary bone plasmacytoma: outcome and prognostic factors following radiotherapy. Int J Radiat Oncol Biol Phys. 1998;41(5):1063–7.
141. Dimopoulos MA, et al. Curability of solitary bone plasmacytoma. J Clin Oncol Off J Am Soc Clin Oncol. 1992;10(4):587–90.
142. Alexiou C, et al. Extramedullary plasmacytoma: tumor occurrence and therapeutic concepts. Cancer. 1999;85(11):2305–14.
143. Strojan P, et al. Extramedullary plasmacytoma: clinical and histopathologic study. Int J Radiat Oncol Biol Phys. 2002;53(3):692–701.
144. Mayr NA, et al. The role of radiation therapy in the treatment of solitary plasmacytomas. Radiother Oncol J Eur Soc Therapeutic Radiol Oncol. 1990;17(4):293–303.
145. Bataille R, Sany J. Solitary myeloma: clinical and prognostic features of a review of 114 cases. Cancer. 1981;48(3):845–51.
146. Tsang RW, et al. Solitary plasmacytoma treated with radiotherapy: impact of tumor size on outcome. Int J Radiat Oncol Biol Phys. 2001;50(1):113–20.
147. Wilder RB, et al. Persistence of myeloma protein for more than one year after radiotherapy is an adverse prognostic factor in solitary plasmacytoma of bone. Cancer. 2002;94(5):1532–7.
148. Mulligan ME. Imaging techniques used in the diagnosis, staging, and follow-up of patients with myeloma. Acta Radiol. 2005;46(7):716–24.
149. Orchard K, et al. Fluoro-deoxyglucose positron emission tomography imaging for the detection of occult disease in multiple myeloma. Br J Haematol. 2002;117(1):133–5.
150. Schirrmeister H, et al. Initial results in the assessment of multiple myeloma using 18F-FDG PET. Eur J Nucl Med Mol Imaging. 2002;29(3):361–6.
151. Schirrmeister H, et al. Positron emission tomography (PET) for staging of solitary plasmacytoma. Cancer Biother Radiopharm. 2003;18(5):841–5.

152. Mendenhall CM, Thar TL, Million RR. Solitary plasmacytoma of bone and soft tissue. Int J Radiat Oncol Biol Phys. 1980;6(11):1497–501.
153. Kelly PJ, et al. Imaging-based stereotaxic serial biopsies in untreated intracranial glial neoplasms. J Neurosurg. 1987;66(6):865–74.
154. Gross MW, et al. The value of F-18-fluorodeoxyglucose PET for the 3-D radiation treatment planning of malignant gliomas. Int J Radiat Oncol Biol Phys. 1998;41(5):989–95.
155. Chen W. Clinical applications of PET in brain tumors. J Nucl Med Off Pub Soc Nucl Med. 2007;48(9):1468–81.
156. Lee IH, et al. Association of 11C-methionine PET uptake with site of failure after concurrent temozolomide and radiation for primary glioblastoma multiforme. Int J Radiat Oncol Biol Phys. 2009;73(2):479–85.
157. Weber DC, et al. Recurrence pattern after [(18)F] fluoroethyltyrosine-positron emission tomography-guided radiotherapy for high-grade glioma: a prospective study. Radiother Oncol J Eur Soc Therapeutic Radiol Oncol. 2009;93(3):586–92.
158. Piroth MD, et al. Integrated boost IMRT with FET-PET-adapted local dose escalation in glioblastomas. Results of a prospective phase II study. Strahlentherapie und Onkologie Organ der Deutschen Rontgengesellschaft ... [et al]. 2012;188(4):334–9.
159. Pauleit D, et al. O-(2-[18F]fluoroethyl)-L-tyrosine PET combined with MRI improves the diagnostic assessment of cerebral gliomas. Brain J Neurol. 2005;128(Pt 3):678–87.
160. Niyazi M, et al. FET-PET for malignant glioma treatment planning. Radiother Oncol J Eur Soc Therapeutic Radiol Oncol. 2011;99(1):44–8.
161. Astner ST, et al. Effect of 11C-methionine-positron emission tomography on gross tumor volume delineation in stereotactic radiotherapy of skull base meningiomas. Int J Radiat Oncol Biol Phys. 2008;72(4):1161–7.
162. Grosu AL, et al. L-(methyl-11C) methionine positron emission tomography for target delineation in resected high-grade gliomas before radiotherapy. Int J Radiat Oncol Biol Phys. 2005;63(1):64–74.
163. Fueger BJ, et al. Correlation of 6-18F-fluoro-L-dopa PET uptake with proliferation and tumor grade in newly diagnosed and recurrent gliomas. J Nucl Med Off Pub Soc Nucl Med. 2010;51(10):1532–8.
164. Pafundi DH, et al. Biopsy validation of 18F-DOPA PET and biodistribution in gliomas for neurosurgical planning and radiotherapy target delineation: results of a prospective pilot study. Neuro Oncol. 2013;15(8):1058–67.
165. Diksic M, et al. A new method to measure brain serotonin synthesis in vivo. I. Theory and basic data for a biological model. J Cereb Blood Flow Metab Off J Int Soc Cereb Blood Flow Metab. 1990;10(1):1–12.
166. Chugani DC, et al. Imaging epileptogenic tubers in children with tuberous sclerosis complex using alpha-[11C]methyl-L-tryptophan positron emission tomography. Ann Neurol. 1998;44(6):858–66.
167. Chugani DC, Muzik O. Alpha[C-11]methyl-L-tryptophan PET maps brain serotonin synthesis and kynurenine pathway metabolism. J Cereb Blood Flow Metab Off J Int Soc Cereb Blood Flow Metab. 2000;20(1):2–9.
168. Juhasz C, et al. In vivo uptake and metabolism of alpha-[11C]methyl-L-tryptophan in human brain tumors. J Cereb Blood Flow Metab Off J Int Soc Cereb Blood Flow Metab. 2006;26(3):345–57.
169. Batista CE, et al. Imaging correlates of differential expression of indoleamine 2,3-dioxygenase in human brain tumors. Mol Imaging Biol Off Pub Acad Mol Imaging. 2009;11(6):460–6.
170. Adams S, et al. The kynurenine pathway in brain tumor pathogenesis. Cancer Res. 2012;72(22): 5649–57.
171. Waggoner SE. Cervical cancer. Lancet. 2003;361(9376):2217–25.
172. Amit A, et al. PET/CT in gynecologic cancer: present applications and future prospects – a clinician's perspective. Obstet Gynecol Clin North Am. 2011;38(1):1–21, vii.
173. Yen TC, et al. Standardized uptake value in para-aortic lymph nodes is a significant prognostic factor in patients with primary advanced squamous cervical cancer. Eur J Nucl Med Mol Imaging. 2008;35(3):493–501.
174. Chung HH, et al. Preoperative [18F]FDG PET/CT maximum standardized uptake value predicts recurrence of uterine cervical cancer. Eur J Nucl Med Mol Imaging. 2010;37(8):1467–73.
175. Kidd EA, et al. The standardized uptake value for F-18 fluorodeoxyglucose is a sensitive predictive biomarker for cervical cancer treatment response and survival. Cancer. 2007;110(8):1738–44.
176. Xue F, et al. F-18 fluorodeoxyglucose uptake in primary cervical cancer as an indicator of prognosis after radiation therapy. Gynecol Oncol. 2006;101(1): 147–51.
177. Lukka H, et al. Concurrent cisplatin-based chemotherapy plus radiotherapy for cervical cancer – a meta-analysis. Clin Oncol. 2002;14(3):203–12.
178. Keys HM, et al. Radiation therapy with and without extrafascial hysterectomy for bulky stage IB cervical carcinoma: a randomized trial of the Gynecologic Oncology Group. Gynecol Oncol. 2003;89(3): 343–53.
179. Portelance L, et al. Intensity-modulated radiation therapy (IMRT) reduces small bowel, rectum, and bladder doses in patients with cervical cancer receiving pelvic and para-aortic irradiation. Int J Radiat Oncol Biol Phys. 2001;51(1):261–6.
180. Wolfson AH. Magnetic resonance imaging and positron-emission tomography imaging in the 21st century as tools for the evaluation and management

of patients with invasive cervical carcinoma. Semin Radiat Oncol. 2006;16(3):186–91.
181. Vandecasteele K, et al. Intensity-modulated arc therapy with simultaneous integrated boost in the treatment of primary irresectable cervical cancer. Treatment planning, quality control, and clinical implementation. Strahlentherapie und Onkologie Organ der Deutschen Rontgengesellschaft ... [et al]. 2009;185(12):799–807.
182. Mitchell DG, et al. Early invasive cervical cancer: tumor delineation by magnetic resonance imaging, computed tomography, and clinical examination, verified by pathologic results, in the ACRIN 6651/ GOG 183 Intergroup Study. J Clin Oncol Off J Am Soc Clin Oncol. 2006;24(36):5687–94.
183. Vincens E, et al. Accuracy of magnetic resonance imaging in predicting residual disease in patients treated for stage IB2/II cervical carcinoma with chemoradiation therapy: correlation of radiologic findings with surgicopathologic results. Cancer. 2008;113(8):2158–65.
184. Gupta T, Beriwal S. PET/CT-guided radiation therapy planning: from present to the future. Indian J Cancer. 2010;47(2):126–33.
185. Grigsby PW, et al. Posttherapy [18F] fluorodeoxyglucose positron emission tomography in carcinoma of the cervix: response and outcome. J Clin Oncol Off J Am Soc Clin Oncol. 2004;22(11):2167–71.
186. Bjurberg M, et al. Prediction of patient outcome with 2-deoxy-2-[18F]fluoro-D-glucose-positron emission tomography early during radiotherapy for locally advanced cervical cancer. Int J Gynecol Cancer Off J Int Gynecol Cancer Soc. 2009;19(9):1600–5.
187. Zimny M, Siggelkow W. Positron emission tomography scanning in gynecologic and breast cancers. Curr Opin Obstet Gynecol. 2003;15(1):69–75.
188. Fulham MJ, et al. The impact of PET-CT in suspected recurrent ovarian cancer: A prospective multi-centre study as part of the Australian PET Data Collection Project. Gynecol Oncol. 2009;112(3):462–8.
189. Tagliabue L. The emerging role of FDG PET/CT in rectal cancer management: is it time to use the technique for early prognostication? Eur J Nucl Med Mol Imaging. 2013;40(5):652–6.
190. Sauer R, et al. Preoperative versus postoperative chemoradiotherapy for rectal cancer. N Engl J Med. 2004;351(17):1731–40.
191. Bosset JF, et al. Chemotherapy with preoperative radiotherapy in rectal cancer. N Engl J Med. 2006;355(11):1114–23.
192. Ortholan C, et al. Role of radiotherapy with surgery for T3 and resectable T4 rectal cancer: evidence from randomized trials. Dis Colon Rectum. 2006;49(3):302–10.
193. Capirci C, et al. Prognostic value of pathologic complete response after neoadjuvant therapy in locally advanced rectal cancer: long-term analysis of 566 ypCR patients. Int J Radiat Oncol Biol Phys. 2008;72(1):99–107.
194. Passoni P, et al. Feasibility of an adaptive strategy in preoperative radiochemotherapy for rectal cancer with image-guided tomotherapy: boosting the dose to the shrinking tumor. Int J Radiat Oncol Biol Phys. 2013;87(1):67–72.
195. Cohade C, et al. Direct comparison of (18)F-FDG PET and PET/CT in patients with colorectal carcinoma. J Nucl Med Off Pub Soc Nucl Med. 2003;44(11):1797–803.
196. Kinkel K, et al. Detection of hepatic metastases from cancers of the gastrointestinal tract by using noninvasive imaging methods (US, CT, MR imaging, PET): a meta-analysis. Radiology. 2002;224(3):748–56.
197. Selzner M, et al. Does the novel PET/CT imaging modality impact on the treatment of patients with metastatic colorectal cancer of the liver? Ann Surg. 2004;240(6):1027–34; discussion 1035–6.
198. Seale MK, et al. Hepatobiliary-specific MR contrast agents: role in imaging the liver and biliary tree. Radiographics Rev Pub Radiol Soc North Am. 2009;29(6):1725–48.
199. Patel DA, et al. Impact of integrated PET/CT on variability of target volume delineation in rectal cancer. Technol Cancer Res Treat. 2007;6(1):31–6.
200. Paskeviciute B, et al. Impact of (18)F-FDG-PET/CT on staging and irradiation of patients with locally advanced rectal cancer. Strahlentherapie und Onkologie Organ der Deutschen Rontgengesellschaft ... [et al]. 2009;185(4):260–5.
201. Braendengen M, et al. Delineation of gross tumor volume (GTV) for radiation treatment planning of locally advanced rectal cancer using information from MRI or FDG-PET/CT: a prospective study. Int J Radiat Oncol Biol Phys. 2011;81(4):e439–45.
202. Janssen MH, et al. Evaluation of early metabolic responses in rectal cancer during combined radiochemotherapy or radiotherapy alone: sequential FDG-PET-CT findings. Radiother Oncol J Eur Soc Therapeutic Radiol Oncol. 2010;94(2):151–5.
203. Janssen MH, et al. Accurate prediction of pathological rectal tumor response after two weeks of preoperative radiochemotherapy using (18) F-fluorodeoxyglucose-positron emission tomography-computed tomography imaging. Int J Radiat Oncol Biol Phys. 2010;77(2):392–9.
204. Petit SF, et al. [(1)(8)F]fluorodeoxyglucose uptake patterns in lung before radiotherapy identify areas more susceptible to radiation-induced lung toxicity in non-small-cell lung cancer patients. Int J Radiat Oncol Biol Phys. 2011;81(3):698–705.
205. Lambin P, et al. The ESTRO Breur Lecture. From population to voxel-based radiotherapy: exploiting intra-tumour and intra-organ heterogeneity for advanced treatment of non-small cell lung cancer. Radiother Oncol J Eur Soc Therapeutic Radiol Oncol. 2009;96(2):145–52.
206. van Stiphout RG, et al. Nomogram predicting response after chemoradiotherapy in rectal cancer using sequential PETCT imaging: a multicentric

prospective study with external validation. Radiother Oncol. 2014;113(2):215–22.
207. van den Bogaard J, et al. Residual metabolic tumor activity after chemo-radiotherapy is mainly located in initially high FDG uptake areas in rectal cancer. Radiother Oncol J Eur Soc Therapeutic Radiol Oncol. 2011;99(2):137–41.
208. Murcia Durendez MJ, et al. The value of 18F-FDG PET/CT for assessing the response to neoadjuvant therapy in locally advanced rectal cancer. Eur J Nucl Med Mol Imaging. 2013;40(1):91–7.
209. Lee SJ, et al. Clinical implications of initial FDG-PET/CT in locally advanced rectal cancer treated with neoadjuvant chemoradiotherapy. Cancer Chemother Pharmacol. 2013;71(5):1201–7.
210. Calvo FA, et al. 18F-FDG positron emission tomography staging and restaging in rectal cancer treated with preoperative chemoradiation. Int J Radiat Oncol Biol Phys. 2004;58(2):528–35.
211. Calvo FA, et al. (18)F-FDG PET/CT-based treatment response evaluation in locally advanced rectal cancer: a prospective validation of long-term outcomes. Eur J Nucl Med Mol Imaging. 2013;40(5):657–67.
212. Denecke T, et al. Comparison of CT, MRI and FDG-PET in response prediction of patients with locally advanced rectal cancer after multimodal preoperative therapy: is there a benefit in using functional imaging? Eur Radiol. 2005;15(8):1658–66.
213. Roels S, et al. Biological image-guided radiotherapy in rectal cancer: challenges and pitfalls. Int J Radiat Oncol Biol Phys. 2009;75(3):782–90.
214. Farsad M, Schwarzenbock S, Krause BJ. PET/CT and choline: diagnosis and staging. Q J Nucl Med Mol Imaging Off Pub Italian Assoc Nucl Med. 2012;56(4):343–53.
215. Pinkawa M, et al. Dose-escalation using intensity-modulated radiotherapy for prostate cancer – evaluation of the dose distribution with and without 18F-choline PET-CT detected simultaneous integrated boost. Radiother Oncol J Eur Soc Therapeutic Radiol Oncol. 2009;93(2):213–9.
216. Pinkawa M, et al. Dose-escalation using intensity-modulated radiotherapy for prostate cancer – evaluation of quality of life with and without (18)F-choline PET-CT detected simultaneous integrated boost. Radiat Oncol. 2012;7:14.
217. Park H, et al. Validation of automatic target volume definition as demonstrated for 11C-choline PET/CT of human prostate cancer using multi-modality fusion techniques. Acad Radiol. 2010;17(5):614–23.
218. Zakian KL, et al. Correlation of proton MR spectroscopic imaging with gleason score based on step-section pathologic analysis after radical prostatectomy. Radiology. 2005;234(3):804–14.
219. Ikonen S, et al. Magnetic resonance imaging of clinically localized prostatic cancer. J Urol. 1998;159(3):915–9.
220. Picchio M, et al. Imaging biomarkers in prostate cancer: role of PET/CT and MRI. Eur J Nucl Med Mol Imaging. 2015;42(4):644–55.
221. Schiavina R, et al. 11C-choline positron emission tomography/computerized tomography for preoperative lymph-node staging in intermediate-risk and high-risk prostate cancer: comparison with clinical staging nomograms. Eur Urol. 2008;54(2):392–401.
222. Hacker A, et al. Detection of pelvic lymph node metastases in patients with clinically localized prostate cancer: comparison of [18F]fluorocholine positron emission tomography-computerized tomography and laparoscopic radioisotope guided sentinel lymph node dissection. J Urol. 2006;176(5):2014–8; discussion 2018–9.
223. Schwarzenbock S, Souvatzoglou M, Krause BJ. Choline PET and PET/CT in primary diagnosis and staging of prostate cancer. Theranostics. 2012;2(3):318–30.
224. Heidenreich A, et al. EAU guidelines on prostate cancer. Part II: treatment of advanced, relapsing, and castration-resistant prostate cancer. Eur Urol. 2014;65(2):467–79.
225. De Bari B, et al. The "PROCAINA (PROstate CAncer INdication Attitudes) Project" (Part II) – a survey among Italian radiation oncologists on radical radiotherapy in prostate cancer. Radiol Med. 2013;118(7):1220–39.
226. Alongi F, et al. The PROCAINA (PROstate CAncer INdication Attitudes) Project (Part I): a survey among Italian radiation oncologists on postoperative radiotherapy in prostate cancer. Radiol Med. 2013;118(4):660–78.
227. Picchio M, Castellucci P. Clinical indications of C-choline PET/CT in prostate cancer patients with biochemical relapse. Theranostics. 2012;2(3):313–7.
228. Giovacchini G, et al. [C]Choline PET/CT predicts survival in hormone-naive prostate cancer patients with biochemical failure after radical prostatectomy. Eur J Nucl Med Mol Imaging. 2015;42(6):877–84.
229. Suardi N, et al. Open prostatectomy and the evolution of HoLEP in the management of benign prostatic hyperplasia. Minerva urologica e nefrologica Italian J Urol Nephrol. 2009;61(3):301–8.
230. Incerti E, et al. Radiation Treatment of Lymph Node Recurrence from Prostate Cancer: Is 11C-Choline PET/CT Predictive of Survival Outcomes? J Nucl Med. 2015;56(12):1836–42.
231. Souvatzoglou M, et al. Influence of (11)C-choline PET/CT on the treatment planning for salvage radiation therapy in patients with biochemical recurrence of prostate cancer. Radiother Oncol J Eur Soc Therapeutic Radiol Oncol. 2011;99(2):193–200.
232. Wurschmidt F, et al. [18F]fluoroethylcholine-PET/CT imaging for radiation treatment planning of recurrent and primary prostate cancer with dose escalation to PET/CT-positive lymph nodes. Radiat Oncol. 2011;6:44.
233. Casamassima F, et al. Efficacy of eradicative radiotherapy for limited nodal metastases detected with

choline PET scan in prostate cancer patients. Tumori. 2011;97(1):49–55.
234. Stephenson AJ, et al. Predicting the outcome of salvage radiation therapy for recurrent prostate cancer after radical prostatectomy. J Clin Oncol Off J Am Soc Clin Oncol. 2007;25(15):2035–41.
235. Decaestecker K, et al. Surveillance or metastasis-directed Therapy for OligoMetastatic Prostate cancer recurrence (STOMP): study protocol for a randomized phase II trial. BMC Cancer. 2014;14:671.
236. Ost P, et al. Metastasis-directed therapy of regional and distant recurrences after curative treatment of prostate cancer: a systematic review of the literature. Eur Urol. 2015;67(5):852–63.
237. Gandaglia G, et al. Impact of the site of metastases on survival in patients with metastatic prostate cancer. Eur Urol. 2014;68(2):325–34.
238. Fodor A, et al. Toxicity and efficacy of salvage 11C-Choline PET/CT-guided radiation therapy in patients with prostate cancer lymph nodal recurrence. BJU Int. 2016.
239. Husarik DB, et al. Evaluation of [(18)F]-choline PET/CT for staging and restaging of prostate cancer. Eur J Nucl Med Mol Imaging. 2008;35(2):253–63.
240. Soyka JD, et al. Clinical impact of 18F-choline PET/CT in patients with recurrent prostate cancer. Eur J Nucl Med Mol Imaging. 2012;39(6):936–43.
241. Vees H, et al. 18F-choline and/or 11C-acetate positron emission tomography: detection of residual or progressive subclinical disease at very low prostate-specific antigen values (<1 ng/mL) after radical prostatectomy. BJU Int. 2007;99(6):1415–20.
242. Evangelista L, et al. Utility of choline positron emission tomography/computed tomography for lymph node involvement identification in intermediate- to high-risk prostate cancer: a systematic literature review and meta-analysis. Eur Urol. 2013;63(6):1040–8.
243. Seppala J, et al. Carbon-11 acetate PET/CT based dose escalated IMRT in prostate cancer. Radiother Oncol J Eur Soc Therapeutic Radiol Oncol. 2009;93(2):234–40.
244. Hockel M, Vaupel P. Biological consequences of tumor hypoxia. Semin Oncol. 2001;28(2 Suppl 8):36–41.
245. Hockel M, Vaupel P. Tumor hypoxia: definitions and current clinical, biologic, and molecular aspects. J Natl Cancer Inst. 2001;93(4):266–76.
246. Busk M, Horsman MR. Relevance of hypoxia in radiation oncology: pathophysiology, tumor biology and implications for treatment. Q J Nucl Med Mol Imaging Off Pub Italian Assoc Nucl Med. 2013;57(3):219–34.
247. Sovik A, et al. Radiotherapy adapted to spatial and temporal variability in tumor hypoxia. Int J Radiat Oncol Biol Phys. 2007;68(5):1496–504.
248. Brizel DM, et al. Tumor hypoxia adversely affects the prognosis of carcinoma of the head and neck. Int J Radiat Oncol Biol Phys. 1997;38(2):285–9.
249. Moon EJ, et al. The potential role of intrinsic hypoxia markers as prognostic variables in cancer. Antioxid Redox Signal. 2007;9(8):1237–94.
250. Langen KJ, Eschmann SM. Correlative imaging of hypoxia and angiogenesis in oncology. J Nucl Med Off Pub Soc Nucl Med. 2008;49(4):515–6.
251. Olive PL, Vikse C, Trotter MJ. Measurement of oxygen diffusion distance in tumor cubes using a fluorescent hypoxia probe. Int J Radiat Oncol Biol Phys. 1992;22(3):397–402.
252. Olive PL, Aquino-Parsons C. Measurement of tumor hypoxia using single-cell methods. Semin Radiat Oncol. 2004;14(3):241–8.
253. Maftei CA, et al. Comparison of (immuno-)fluorescence data with serial [(1)(8)F]Fmiso PET/CT imaging for assessment of chronic and acute hypoxia in head and neck cancers. Radiother Oncol J Eur Soc Therapeutic Radiol Oncol. 2011;99(3):412–7.
254. Eschmann SM, et al. Prognostic impact of hypoxia imaging with 18F-misonidazole PET in non-small cell lung cancer and head and neck cancer before radiotherapy. J Nucl Med Off Pub Soc Nucl Med. 2005;46(2):253–60.
255. Eschmann SM, et al. Hypoxia-imaging with (18) F-Misonidazole and PET: changes of kinetics during radiotherapy of head-and-neck cancer. Radiother Oncol J Eur Soc Therapeutic Radiol Oncol. 2007;83(3):406–10.
256. Thorwarth D, et al. A kinetic model for dynamic [18F]-Fmiso PET data to analyse tumour hypoxia. Phys Med Biol. 2005;50(10):2209–24.
257. Chitneni SK, et al. Molecular imaging of hypoxia. J Nucl Med Off Pub Soc Nucl Med. 2011;52(2):165–8.
258. Piert M, et al. Hypoxia-specific tumor imaging with 18F-fluoroazomycin arabinoside. J Nucl Med Off Pub Soc Nucl Med. 2005;46(1):106–13.
259. Vavere AL, Lewis JS. Examining the relationship between Cu-ATSM hypoxia selectivity and fatty acid synthase expression in human prostate cancer cell lines. Nucl Med Biol. 2008;35(3):273–9.
260. Holland JP, Lewis JS, Dehdashti F. Assessing tumor hypoxia by positron emission tomography with Cu-ATSM. Q J Nucl Med Mol Imaging Off Pub Italian Assoc Nucl Med. 2009;53(2):193–200.
261. Valtorta S, et al. Comparison of 18F-fluoroazomycin-arabinofuranoside and 64Cu-diacetyl-bis(N4-methylthiosemicarbazone) in preclinical models of cancer. J Nucl Med Off Pub Soc Nucl Med. 2013;54(7):1106–12.
262. Lewis JS, et al. Evaluation of 64Cu-ATSM in vitro and in vivo in a hypoxic tumor model. J Nucl Med Off Pub Soc Nucl Med. 1999;40(1):177–83.

Index

A
Acceptance testing
  bed motion, 247–248
  count rate performance, 243–244
  image quality, 245–246
  image registration, 248
  image uniformity, 246–247
  imaging performance, 247
  intrinsic background coincidence, 245
  NEMA, 240–241
  PET/MRI, 249
  quantification, 247
  scatter fraction, 241–243
  sensitivity, 244
  spatial resolution, 241–242
  test results, 240
Alpha-[11C]methyl-L-tryptophan (AMT), 592
Alzheimer's disease (AD), 515–516
Anxiety disorder, 517–518
Atom
  atomic mass unit, 9–11
  atomic number, 9
  binding energy, 10–11
  Bohr model, 8
  building blocks, 7
  history, 7–8
  mass and energy, 9
  mass defect, 11
  nomenclatures, 9
  nuclear stability, 12–13
  physical and chemical properties, 6
  quantum mechanics model, 8–9
Auger electron, 23–24
Automatic exposure control (AEC), 49
Avalanche photodiode (APD), 207–209
Average CT (ACT)
  end-inspiration, 389
  4D-CT imaging, 388
  GE scanner, 387
  radiation therapy, 389–392
  slow-scan, 387, 389
  transmission rod sources, 387
  whole-body, 389

B
Binding potential (BP), 341–343
Biokinetic analyses
  animal data, 67–69
  design, 66–67
  human data, 69–70
  radioactive decay, 70
Biomolecules
  aluminium fluoride, 90
  antibodies, 88
  boronic acids/esters, 89
  diagnostic imaging agents, 87–88
  1,3-dipolar cycloaddition, 88–89
  direct nucleophilic fluorination, 88
  ^{18}F-glycosylation reaction, 88
  ^{18}F-labelled alkynes, 89
  ^{18}F-maleimide, 88
  ^{18}F-SFB, 88
  lysine residues, 88
  N-terminal primary amino groups, 88
  serum albumin, 89
  Si-FA, 89
Bipolar disorder (BD), 493
Bohr model, 8
Brain tumor
  amino acid, 591
  AMT, 592
  11C-MET and FLT, 591
  FDOPA, 592
  intracranial ana-tomic structures, 591
  invasive and infiltrative character, 590–591
  radiation boost volumes, 591
  randomized and controlled trials, 592
  T1-Gad, 591
Breast cancer, 435–437, 585–586

C
Cancer
  angiogenesis, 406–408
  apoptosis, 410–411
  bone metabolism, 416–417
  cellular proliferation, 411–413
  chemokine receptor, 417
  EGFR, 414

M.M. Khalil (ed.), *Basic Science of PET Imaging*, DOI 10.1007/978-3-319-40070-9

Cancer (*cont.*)
 FDG
  amino-acid metabolism, 404
  natural amino acids, 404, 405
  synthetic amino acids, 404–405
  and tumour biology, 401–403
 hypoxia, 408–410
 MRI, 401
 multidrug resistance, 417–418
 phospholipid metabolism, 405–406
 somatostatin receptors, 415–416
Carbon-11
 ^{11}C-carbonylation, 92
 clinical oncology and neurology, 91
 ^{11}C-methylation, 91–92
 ^{11}C-tracer and ^{18}F-tracer, 90
 organometallic Grignard reagents, 93
 synthons, 90–91
Cardiac imaging
 carbohydrate metabolism, 467–468
 cell signaling
  autocrine, 477–478
  endocrine, 473–477
  neurocrine, 473–477
  paracrine, 477–478
  types of, 473
 clinical trials, 478–479
 coronary anatomy, 453
 ECG-gated imaging, 464, 465
 FA imaging, 471
 FFA, 468–469
 instrumentation, 453–454
 left ventricle myocardium, 452
 motion artifacts, 452
 MPI
  ^{62}Cu-PTSM, 467
  ^{18}F-flurpiridaz, 465, 467
  intensity, 467
  ^{13}N-ammonia, 465
  ^{15}O-water, 465
  properties, 465, 466
  ^{82}Rb-PET, 456, 464, 467
 myocardial inflammation, 472
 oxidative metabolism, 469
 quantification, 471–472
 SPECT, 453
 stress
  cold pressor test, 458
  interpretation, 458–459
  MBF, 460–464
  MFR, 460–464
  pharmacologic agents, 456, 457
 tracers, 454–456
 vascular inflammation, 472–473
 viability, 469–471
Central slice theorem, 261–262
Cervical cancer, 441
Chromogenic technique, 110
^{11}C-methionine (11C-METH),
  548–549
 appearance, 121
 bacterial endotoxins, 122
 chemical purity, 122
 enantiomeric purity, 123
 pH, 122
 radiochemical identity, 121–122
 radiochemical purity, 123
 radionuclidic purity, 122, 123
 residual solvents, 123
 sterility, 122
Coincidence mode, 174–175
Coincidence timing window, 181–182
Cold pressor test (CPT), 474
Colorectal cancer, 439–441
Colorectal carcinoma (CRC), 594–596
Compartmental modeling
 binding potential, 341–343
 blood flow, 339
 data analysis, 324–325
 definition and assumptions, 325–326
 impulse input function, 329
 impulse response function, 329, 330
 input function
  continuous infusion, 346–347
  dispersion function, 345
  HPLC, 344
  IRF, 329, 330
  left ventricle, 345
  perfusable tissue fraction, 346
  reference region model, 347–349
 in vitro receptor binding experiment, 340–341
 linearization
  Logan plot, 334–335
  1TC model, 333–326, 334–327
  Patlak plot, 336–337
  spectral analysis, 337–338
 oxygen consumption, 339
 parameter estimation
  Gauss-Newton approach, 331
  impulse response fraction, 333
  Marquardt-Levenberg algorithm, 331
  nonlinear fitting, 332
  TAC, 329, 331
  weighted least squares problem, 331
  weighting factor, 331–332
 partition coefficient, 340
 response functions, 329
 TAC, 343–344
 3TC model, 328–329
 2TC model, 327–328, 332, 333
Compton effect, 11, 24
Computed tomography dose index (CTDI), 50–53
Computed tomography (CT) technology
 attenuation scan, 61
 dose metrics
  CTDI, 50–53
  DLP, 55
  dose distribution, 50–51
  effective dose, 57–60
  helical scanning, 50

MSAD, 50–51
parameters, 49
projection radiography, 49–50
scanned length and equilibrium dose, 56–57
SSDE, 56–57
volume CTDI, 53–55
weighted CTDI, 52–54
wide-beam scanners, 55–56
DRLs, 59, 60
exposure factors, 47
factors, 48–49
gantry, 46
helical/spiral scanning, 46
image reconstruction, 47–48
quality control, 61–62
radiation exposure, 47
scanner model, 47–48
tube rotation, 47
whole-body scan, 61
x-ray, 46–47
z-axis, 46
Correction techniques. *See* Motion artifacts
Count-rate performance, 182
Current good manufacturing practice (CGMP)
aspects, 148–149
batch production, 153
breakdown *vs.* malfunction, 157
complaint handling, 159
components, containers, and closures, 152–153
control record, 153
distribution, 158–159
equipment, 152
facilities, 151–152
finished-product testing, 155–156
incomplete product testing, 157
laboratory controls, 154–155
master production, 153
out-of-specification result, 157–158
packaging and labeling, 158
part 212 regulation, 149–150
parts 210 and 211 regulation, 149
patient-care issue, 158
personnel and resources, 150–151
process verification, 154
QA, 150, 151
QC, 150
radiochemical identity/purity test, 158
radiochemical yield limit, 153–154
records, 159
rejection and reprocessing, 158
reserve sample, 157
specific activity, 158
sterility testing, 156

D
Data acquisition
imaging workflow, 218–219
object motion, 219–222
patient study, 218
time-based acquisition system, 218
Data correction
acquisition pro-cess, 275–276
attenuation correction, 276
normalization, 276
scattered and random events, 276–277
Deep brain stimulation (DBS), 504–505
Deformable image registration (DIR), 291
Denoising methods, 296
Depression, 516–517
Detection limit (LOD), 116–117
Detector and system calibration
energy, 237
gain adjustments, 237
recorded events, 236–237
system normalization, 238–240
timing, 237–238
tube balancing, 237
Diagnostic reference levels (DRLs), 59, 60
DIRART, 291
Direct conversion detector, 194
Dose length product (DLP), 55
Dose metrics
CTDI, 50–53
DLP, 55
dose distribution, 50–51
effective dose, 57–60
helical scanning, 50
MSAD, 50–51
parameters, 49
projection radiography, 49–50
scanned length and equilibrium dose, 56–57
SSDE, 56–57
volume CTDI, 53–55
weighted CTDI, 52–54
wide-beam scanners, 55–56
DREES, 293

E
Electromagnetic (EM) radiation
duality principle, 5–6, 11
electric and magnetic field, 4
electromagnetic spectrum, 4–5
wave and particle, 5
Electronic collimation, 174–175
Electrophilic fluorination, 82–83
EMA, 134–135
Energy resolution, 181
Epidermal growth factor receptor (EGFR), 414
Esophageal cancer, 585
Events, 175–176
Ewing's sarcoma, 564–565
Expectation–maximization (EM) algorithm, 267–268

F
Facility design
brick/block construction, 38–39
clinical staff, 39
equipment suppliers, 39
mobile scanner, 40–41
optimisation, 43–46
rest bays and control room, 40
shielding calculation
corridors, 42
critical points, 42
instantaneous dose rates, 41–42
lead and concrete, 41
occupancy, 42
thickness of barriers, 40–41
transmission factors, 41
shielding materials, 40
staff dose, 44–46
staff exposure, 40, 42–43
FDG-6-phosphate (FDG6P), 287
18F-3,4-dihydroxy-6-18 F-fluoro-l-phenylalanine (FDOPA), 592
^{18}F-fluorobenzoate (^{18}F-SFB), 88
^{18}F-2-fluoro-2-deoxy-d-glucose (FDG), 401–403, 579–580
^{18}F-fluorodeoxyglucose (^{18}F-FDG)
appearance of, 117
bacterial endotoxins, 120
chemical purity, 119–120
pH, 119
quality control tests, 117–118
quality requirements, 117
radiochemical identity, 119
radiochemical purity, 120–121
radionuclidic identity, 118–119
radionuclidic purity, 120
residual solvents, 120
sterility, 120
Field of view (FOV), 184, 234
Fluorine-18
biomolecules (*see* Biomolecules)
electrophilic fluorination, 82–83
fluoro-organic drugs, 81
nucleophilic reaction (*see* Nucleophilic fluorination)
unnatural fluorine atom, 81–82
Food and Drug Administration (FDA)
CGMP (*see* Current good manufacturing practice (CGMP))
compounded and noncompounded drugs, 147–148
definition, 147
drug product, 147
imaging, 147
inspection program
coverage selection, 167
issues, 167–169
types, 166–167
production *vs.* practice of pharmacy, 148
USP<823>
aseptic operation, 165
batch and lot, 162
components, materials, and supplies, 164
controls and acceptance, 165–166
facilities and equipment, 164
labeling, 166
organization, 161–162
part 212, 160–161
process and operational controls, 164
process verification, 165
QA, 163
QC, 163
radioactive drug, 162
reprocessing, 166
revision process, 161
SNM, 161
stability, 165
strength, 163
USP 32nd 823, 159–160
validation, 163
verification, 163
Free fatty acids (FFA), 468–469
^{18}F-sodium fluoride (^{18}F-NaF), 547–548

G
Gadolinium-enhanced T1-weighted (T1-Gad), 591
^{68}Ga-edotreotide
appearance, 123
bacterial endotoxins, 125
chemical purity, 125
monograph tests, 123–124
pH, 125
radiochemical identity, 124
radiochemical purity, 126
radionuclidic identity, 124–125
radionuclidic purity, 125–126
residual solvents, 125
sterility, 125
Gallium-68
advantages, 94
applications, 94
bifunctional chelators, 95
chromatography-based post-processing procedure, 94
disadvantages, 94
DOTA, 95–96
half-life, 94
hard Lewis acid, 94–95
HBED-CC, 97
NOTA, 95–96
TRAP-Pr, 96–97
Gamma model, 270
Gas chromatography (GC), 113–114
Gas-filled detector
dose calibrator, 29–31
Geiger-Mueller region, 29
ionization chamber, 29–30
ionization region, 28
ion pairs, 28
proportional region, 28–29
recombination, 28

Gel-clot technique, 110
Gibb's effect, 360
Good manufacturing practice (GMP)
challenges, 137–138
clinical trial, 131
components, 136
documentation, 131–132
drug development
clinical studies, 133
EMA, 134–135
preclinical development, 132
toxicology, 132–133
equipment, 136
European Clinical Trials Directive, 138
European Pharmacopoeia, 129–130
ICH, 130
magistral formula, 131
marketing authorisation, 130–131
materials, 136
official preparation, 131
personnel, 136
pharmaceutical regulation, 128
PIC/S, 129
QbD, 140–141
QMS, 137
qualified person, 130
radionuclidic impurities, 135
radiopharmaceuticals, 138–139
regulatory agencies, 128–129
risk assessment, 139–140
SOPs, 136–137
G protein-coupled receptors (GPCR)
cholinergic system, 521–522
conformation and amino acid, 518
dopaminergic system, 521
metabotropic glutamate receptors, 523
noradrenergic system, 521
rhodopsin family, 522–523
serotonergic system, 518–520
Gynaecological cancer, 441–443

H
Hardware fusion, 380
Head and neck cancers (HNC), 583–584
Headspace gas chromatography (HSGC), 113–114
Hepatoblastoma, 566–567
High-performance liquid chromatography (HPLC), 111–112
Huntington's disease (HD), 515
Hypoxia, 598–599

I
Image reconstruction
backprojection filtering, 261, 263–264
central slice theorem, 261–262
data correction
acquisition pro-cess, 275–276
attenuation correction, 276
normalization, 276
scattered and random events, 276–277
data formation and storage, 260–261
image calibration, 277
line integral model, 261–262
model-based statistical reconstruction
clinical datasets, 264
image noise, 274
image property measurement, 274–275
image resolution, 273–274
MAP estimator (*see* Maximum-a-posteriori (MAP) estimator)
maximum likelihood, 267–270
noise model, 265–266
system model, 266–268
parametric reconstruction, 279–280
3D data, 263–265
TOF, 277–279
Independent Gaussian model, 270
Instrumentation
coincidence processor, 230
data acquisition, 180
dataflow, 230–231
detector design, 178–180
detector flood maps, 231–233
photosensor, 178
scintillation detector, 176, 178
signal processing, 180
sinogram
crosshatch pattern, 235
detector controller, 235–236
detector failure, 235–236
electronics, 235–236
FOV, 234
image reconstruction, 233–234
LOR, 233–234
uni-form cylinder phantom, 235
visual inspection, 236
system design, 180
TOF, 230
Intensity-volume histogram (IVH), 286–287
International Conference on Harmonisation (ICH), 130
International Neuroblastoma Staging System (INSS), 550
Ion channel-coupled receptors
$GABA_A$, 524
glutamate, 523–524
glycine receptors, 524
nAChR, 524

L
Leukemia, 560
Line integral model, 261–262
Line of response (LOR), 233–234
Locoregional control (LRC), 580–581
Lung cancer (LC), 581–583

Lymphoma, 432, 434–435, 587–588
  ^{18}F-FDG
    initial staging, 556–557
    relapse/recurrence, 558
    response assessment, 557–558
  Hodgkin's disease, 554–555
  non-Hodgkin's lymphoma, 555–556
  PTLD, 558–560

M
Major depressive disorder (MDD), 491–492
Marketing authorisation (MA), 130–131
Markov random field (MRF), 271
Maximum-a-posteriori (MAP) estimator
  anatomical prior, 271–272
  non-convex function, 271
  prior function
    Gibbs distribution, 270–271
    independent Gaussian and Gamma model, 270
    MRF, 271
    regularization function, 269–270
    smoothness/anatomical information, 270
    total variation, 271
  reconstruction algorithm, 272–273
Maximum likelihood (ML), 267–270
MIASYS, 289
Morphological features, 287
Motion artifacts
  application, 380
  average CT
    end-inspiration, 389
    4D-CT imaging, 388, 393–394
    GE scanner, 387
    radiation therapy, 389–392
    slow-scan, 387, 389
    transmission rod sources, 387
    whole-body, 389
  brain images, 380, 381
  causes of, 380, 382, 383
  4D-PET, 392–394
  hardware fusion, 380
  heart and liver, 380, 381
  misregistration
    breathing trace, 384
    end-expiration phases, 383, 384
    frequency, 385–387
    lungs, 385, 386
    photopenic region, 383, 384
    respiration-induced artifacts, 383
    skinfold artifacts, 385
Multidrug resistance (MDR), 417–418
Multimodality PET/CT
  attenuation correction, 184–186
  fusion imaging, 183
  hardware approach, 183–185
  limitations and issues, 187–189
  low-dose, 187, 189–190
  randoms correction, 187
  scatter correction, 186–187
Multimodality PET/MR, 193–194
Multiple myeloma (MM), 588–590
Multiple slice average dose (MSAD), 50–51
Multi-target correction (MTC) method, 364, 366, 367
Myocardial blood flow (MBF), 460–464
Myocardial flow reserve (MFR), 460–464
Myocardial perfusion imaging (MPI)
  ^{62}Cu-PTSM, 467
  ^{18}F-flurpiridaz, 465, 467
  intensity, 467
  ^{13}N-ammonia, 465
  ^{15}O-water, 465
  properties, 465, 466
  ^{82}Rb-PET, 456, 464, 467

N
Nephroblastoma, 566
Neuroblastoma (NBL)
  11C-hydroxyephedrine, 553
  diagnosis, 550
  etiology, 550
  ^{18}F-FDG, 550, 552, 553
  history, 550
  INSS, 550
  long-term survival, 549–550
  metastases, 550
  MIBG scintigraphy, 550, 551
Neuroendocrine tumour (NET), 415–416
Neurological disorder
  acetylcholinesterase, 507
  acute pharmaceuticals and interventions
    ketamine, 511
    neurotransmitter release, 510
    oxytocin, 511
    perfusional effect, 511
  amyloid imaging
    clinical settings, 501–502
    clinical trials, 502–503
    CSF-Aβ/ Tau, 502
    vs. [^{18}F] FDG uptake, 503
    generations, 499
    uptake pattern, 500–501
    validation, 501
    white matter uptake, 499–500
  anatomical structures, 487, 488
  binding potential, 487
  blood-brain barrier, 487
  convulsive therapy, 505–506
  [^{11}C] raclopride, 496–497
  DBS, 503–504
  diagnostic, 488
  early investigatory tracers
    alpha-synuclein markers, 511–512
    astroglia imaging, 514
    inflammation, markers of, 513
    myelin imaging, 513–514
    pathophysiology, 514
    P-glycoprotein imaging, 512
    protein tau, 511–512

estrogen receptors, 526
extracellular enzymes, 525
[18F]DOPA, 496–497
[18F]FDG
ALS, 494
Alzheimer's disease, 489
amyloid pathology, 489
anxiety-spectrum disorders, 494
bipolar disorder, 493
carotid plaques/chronic ischemia, 494–495
clinical trials, 490–491
dementias, 489
epilepsy, 495–496
FTLD, 489–490
functional disorders, 491
MDD, 491–492
movement disorders, 491
multiple sclerosis, 494
OCD, 494
schizophrenia, 493–494
VaD, 490
GPCR
cholinergic system, 521–522
conformation and amino acid, 518
dopaminergic system, 521
metabotropic glutamate receptors, 523
noradrenergic system, 521
rhodopsin family, 522–523
serotonergic system, 518–520
ion channel-coupled receptors, 523–524
kinetic models, 487
membrane transporters, 525–526
monoamine receptors, 506–507
monoamine transporters, 507
neurotransmission
anxiety disorder, 517–518
bipolar disorder, 516–517
depression, 516–517
diagnosis, 514
Huntington's disease, 515
monoaminergic hypothesis, 515
schizophrenia, 516
outcome parameter, 503–504
P-II Studies, 506
radiolabeled candidate drugs, 507–509
radioligands post-marketing, 509
rCBF, OEF, and [11C] flumazenil
cerebrovascular reserve, 497–498
circulatory and blood supply, 497
$CMRO_2$, 497
"speaking" brain tissue, 498–499
Nicotinic Acetylcholine Receptors (nAChR), 524
Nitrogen-13, 93
N,N´-Bis[2-hydroxy-5-(carboxyethyl)-benzyl] ethylenediamine-N,N´-diacetic acid (HBED-CC), 97
Noise model, 265–266
Non-small cell lung cancer (NSCLC), 372
Nucleophilic fluorination
aliphatic fluorination, 84–86
aromatic fluorination, 86–87
niobium target, 84
radiotracers, 83–84
TBA, 84
water/acetonitrile solution, 84

O

Obsessive compulsive disorder (OCD), 494
Oesophageal cancer, 438–439
Oncology
breast cancer, 435–437
clinical trials, 443
colorectal cancer, 439–441
FDG-PET, 430–431
gynaecological cancers, 441–443
head and neck cancer, 437–438
lung cancer, 431–433
lymphomas, 432, 434–435
oesophageal cancer, 438–439
thyroid cancer, 438
Ordered subsets EM (OSEM), 268–269
Organ-specific imaging, 194
Osteosarcoma, 563–564
Ovarian cancer, 441–443
Overall survival (OS), 580–581
Oxygen-15, 93
Oxytocin (OXT), 511

P

Parametric reconstruction, 279–280
Partial volume correction (PVC)
cardiology, 364, 367, 371–372
classification methods, 370–371
clinical implications, 359
co-registration, 369
correction approaches, 370
correction methods, 370
data generation, 363–364
deconvolution, 360–361
definition, 359–360
motion, 361
neurology, 366, 368, 369, 372
oncology, 364–366, 372–373
PSF, 356, 358, 359
PVE, 356–358
region-based, 361–364
resolution, 366–368
sampling, 370
segmentation, 369–370
spill-in and spill-out, 356, 357
tissue fraction effect, 358–359
voxel-based, 362–364
Partition coefficient, 340
Patlak graphical method, 307–309

Pediatric malignancy
brain and central nervous system, 560–563
brown fat, 545–546
^{18}F-FDG, 541–543, 546–547
fluorodeoxyglucose, 542–543
functional *vs.* anatomic imaging, 538–539
hepatoblastoma, 566–567
image fusion, 549
isotopes, 542
leukemia, 560
lymphoma (*see* Lymphoma)
marrow hyperplasia, 545
nephroblastoma, 566
osseous and soft tissue malignancy
Ewing's sarcoma, 564–565
osteosarcoma, 563–564
RMS, 565–566
posttreatment changes, 546
radiation dose, 540–541
radiopharmaceuticals
1C-hydroxyephedrine, 549
11C-Methionine, 548–549
3'-Deoxy-3'-[F18]-fluorothymidine, 548
^{18}F-NaF, 547–548
F18's half-life, 542
68Ga-DOTA-conjugated peptides, 549
tumor hypoxia, 548
sedation, 541
SNS (*see* Sympathetic nervous system (SNS))
SUV, 543–544
thymus, 544–545
thyroid cancer, 567
tonsils, 545
PET response criteria in solid tumors (PERCIST), 316
Pharmaceutical Inspection Cooperation Scheme (PIC/S), 129
Photomultiplier tube (PMT), 178, 207
Point spread function (PSF), 266–268, 356, 358, 359
Positron annihilation, 174
Positron emission tomography/magnetic resonance (PET/MR)
acceptance testing, 249
crystal
APD, 207–209
atlas-based attenuation correction, 215–216
data acquisition, 218–222
gradient field, 210
high-field strength magnet, 211
high temporal resolution, 224
image quantitative accuracy, 213–215
image segmentation, 216–218
liver disease, 223
magnetic field, 210
magnetic shielding, 211
multimodal hybrid imaging, 224
myocardial blood flow and flow reserve, 223–224
neurology and psychia-try, 223
patient man-agement, 222–223
PMT, 207
radioactive trans-mission sources, 214
SiPM, 205, 209–210
small animal hybrid system, 212–214
soft tissue contrast, 223
superior contrast resolution, 223
technical and clinical advantages, 221–222
template-based attenuation correction, 215
transmis-sion coil, 210–211
PET/CT, 200–201
system design
block detector, 207
challenges, 203, 205–206
data acquisition, 202–203
detector blocks, 203
fringe magnetic field, 206
GE healthcare, 203, 205
larger-bore magnet, 203
manufacturers, 203, 205
model implementation, 201–202
sequential system, 201–202
Siemens Verio 3-T MRI scanner, 203–204
solid-state semi-conductor photodetector, 206–207
steel/mu-metal, 206
Posttransplant lymphoproliferative disorder (PTLD), 558–560
Processing and analysis
characteristics, 294
CT/MR, 289–291
dynamic features, 287–288
FDG-PET, 286
outcome models, 296–297
radiotherapy
biological target, 291–295
radiomics, 291–292, 296
robustness and stability, 295–296
static features, 286–289
Prostate cancer (PCa), 596–598
Psychiatric disorders. *See* Neurological disorder

Q

Qualified person (QP), 130
Quality assurance (QA), 150, 151, 163
Quality by design (QbD), 140–141
Quality control (QC), 150, 163
analytical techniques
accuracy, 116
characteristics, 116
linearity, 116
LOD, 116–117
LOQ, 116–117
precision, 116
range, 116
robustness, 117
specificity, 116
types, 115
chemical purity, 108–109
^{11}C-methionine
appearance, 121
bacterial endotoxins, 122

chemical purity, 122
enantiomeric purity, 123
pH, 122
radiochemical identity, 121–122
radiochemical purity, 123
radionuclidic purity, 122, 123
residual solvents, 123
sterility, 122
^{18}F-FDG
appearance of, 117
bacterial endotoxins, 120
chemical purity, 119–120
pH, 119
quality control tests, 117–118
quality requirements, 117
radiochemical identity, 119
radiochemical purity, 120–121
radionuclidic identity, 118–119
radionuclidic purity, 120
residual solvents, 120
sterility, 120
^{68}Ga-edotreotide
appearance, 123
bacterial endotoxins, 125
chemical purity, 125
monograph tests, 123–124
pH, 125
radiochemical identity, 124
radiochemical purity, 126
radionuclidic identity, 124–125
radionuclidic purity, 125–126
residual solvents, 125
sterility, 125
gamma spectrometry, 107
amplification and digitization, 114
radionuclides, 114–115
radiopharmaceutical field, 114
gas chromatography, 113–114
half-life, 107
HPLC, 111–112
monographs, 106
parameters, 109–110
pH control, 107
radiochemical purity, 108
radionuclidic purity, 108
positron-emitting radionuclide, 107
separation methods, 110–111
TLC, 112–113
visual inspection, 107
Quality management system (QMS), 137
Quantitation
biological factors, 314
blood glucose level, 314–315
definition, 304–305
dynamic imaging
cardiac imaging, 306
data acquisition, 306
data analysis, 307
neurology, 306–307
Patlak graphical method, 307–309
pharmacokinetic model, 306
vs. static, 309–310
F18-flurodeoxyglucose, 304
motion artifact, 313–314
physical and technical/instrumental factors, 313
response monitoring, 315–317
spectrum of, 305
static imaging
vs. dynamic, 309–310
F18-FDG, 305–306
SUV
activity concentration, 310
advantages, 310
disadvantages, 311
efficiency and user-input levels, 310
lesion contouring methods, 310
lesion segmentation task, 310
normalized injected activity, 310
variants, 311–312
TLG, 312–313
tumor texture analysis, 317–318
Quantitation limit (LOQ), 116–117
Quantum mechanics model, 8–9

R

Radiation dosimetry
biokinetic analyses
animal data, 67–69
design, 66–67
human data, 69–70
radioactive decay, 70
dose calculation, 66
effective dose, 71–72
organ dose, 71
patient-individualized dosimetry, 72–74
pregnant patient, 74–75
sample dose estimates, 72–73
Radiation physics
atom
atomic mass unit, 9–11
atomic number, 9
binding energy, 10–11
Bohr model, 8
building blocks, 7
history, 7–8
mass and energy, 9
mass defect, 11
nomenclatures, 9
nuclear stability, 12–13
physical and chemical properties, 6
quantum mechanics model, 8–9
compton effect, 11, 24
detection and measurement
gas-filled detector, 28–31
neutrons, 33–34
scintillation detectors, 31–33
solid state detector, 34–35
well counter, 30–31

Radiation physics (*cont.*)
electromagnetic radiation
duality principle, 5–6, 11
electric and magnetic field, 4
electromagnetic spectrum, 4–5
wave and particle, 5
excitation and ionization, 23
linear attenuation coefficient, 25–26
mass attenuation coefficient, 25–26
pair production, 25
photoelectric effect, 23–24
radioactivity
alpha decay, 18–19
beta minus decay, 19–20
electron capture, 21–22
isomeric transition, 22–23
positron decay, 20–21
radioactive decay, 22–23
radionuclides
exposure rate constant, 27–28
half-life, 27
positron emitters, 26–27
radiopharmaceuticals
charged particle accelerator, 14–17
diagnosis, 13
fission reaction/neutron, 13–14
fluoro-2-deoxyglucose, 13
positron emitters, 13
radioisotopes, 13
saturation yield, 17–18
specific activity, 17
therapeutic applications, 13
Radiation therapy (RT)
brain tumor
amino acid, 591
AMT, 592
11C-MET and FLT, 591
FDOPA, 592
intracranial ana-tomic structures, 591
invasive and infiltrative character, 590–591
radiation boost volumes, 591
randomized and controlled trials, 592
T1-Gad, 591
breast cancer, 585–586
CRC, 594–596
esophageal cancer, 585
FDG, 579–580
4D-PET/CT, 579–581
gynecological malignancies, 592–594
HNC, 583–584
hypoxia, 598–599
LRC, 580–581
lung cancer, 581–583
lymphomas, 587–588
MM, 588–590
OS, 580–581
prostate cancer, 596–598
Radioactive decay, 70
Radioactivity
alpha decay, 18–19
beta minus decay, 19–20
electron capture, 21–22
isomeric transition, 22–23
positron decay, 20–21
radioactive decay, 22–23
Radionuclides
exposure rate constant, 27–28
half-life, 27
positron emitters, 26–27
Radiopharmaceuticals
carbon-11
^{11}C-carbonylation, 92
clinical oncology and neurology, 91
^{11}C-methylation, 91–92
^{11}C-tracer and ^{18}F-tracer, 90
organometallic Grignard reagents, 93
synthons, 90–91
charged particle accelerator, 14–17
diagnosis, 13
fission reaction/neutron, 13–14
fluorine-18
biomolecules (*see* Biomolecules)
electrophilic fluorination, 82–83
fluoro-organic drugs, 81
nucleophilic reaction (*see* Nucleophilic fluorination)
unnatural fluorine atom, 81–82
fluoro-2-deoxyglucose, 13
gallium-68
advantages, 94
applications, 94
bifunctional chelators, 95
chromatography-based post-processing procedure, 94
disadvantages, 94
DOTA, 95–96
half-life, 94
hard Lewis acid, 94–95
HBED-CC, 97
NOTA, 95–96
TRAP-Pr, 96–97
oxygen-15 and nitrogen-13, 93
positron emitters, 13
radioisotopes, 13
radionuclides, 80–82
saturation yield, 17–18
specific activity, 17
therapeutic applications, 13
RECIST, 316
Reference region model, 347–349
Region-based voxel-wise correction (RBV), 360
Rhabdomyosarcoma (RMS), 565–566
Routine quality assurance
annual tests, 251
clinical trials, 251, 253
daily tests, 249–252
monthly/quarterly tests, 251
Row-action maximum likelihood algorithm (RAMLA), 269

S

Scatter fraction (SF), 241–243
Schizophrenia, 493–494

Scintillation crystal
APD, 207–209
atlas-based attenuation correction, 215–216
data acquisition, 218–222
gradient field, 210
high-field strength magnet, 211
high temporal resolution, 224
image quantitative accuracy, 213–215
image segmentation, 216–218
liver disease, 223
magnetic field, 210
magnetic shielding, 211
multimodal hybrid imaging, 224
myocardial blood flow and flow reserve, 223–224
neurology and psychia-try, 223
patient man-agement, 222–223
PMT, 207
radioactive trans-mission sources, 214
SiPM, 205, 209–210
small animal hybrid system, 212–214
soft tissue contrast, 223
superior contrast resolution, 223
technical and clinical advantages, 221–222
template-based attenuation correction, 215
transmis-sion coil, 210–211
Scintillation detectors, 31–33
Seasonal affective disorder, 516–517
Sensitivity, 180
Siemens Verio 3-T MRI scanner, 203–204
Silicon-based ^{18}F-fluoride acceptor (Si-FA), 89
Silicon photomultiplier (SiPM), 179, 193, 205, 209–210
Single-photon emission computed tomography (SPECT), 453
Single slice rebinning (SSRB), 263–265
Sinogram
crosshatch pattern, 235
detector controller, 235–236
detector failure, 235–236
electronics, 235–236
FOV, 234
image reconstruction, 233–234
LOR, 233–234
uni-form cylinder phantom, 235
visual inspection, 236
Size-specific dose estimate (SSDE), 56–57
Society of Nuclear Medicine (SNM), 161
Solid state detector, 34–35
Solitary plasmacytoma (SP), 589
Somatostatin (SST), 415–416
Spatial resolution, 180–182, 241–242
Specific activity (SA), 324
Standardized uptake value (SUV), 543–544
activity concentration, 310
advantages, 310
disadvantages, 311
efficiency and user-input levels, 310
lesion contouring methods, 310
lesion segmentation task, 310
normalized injected activity, 310
variants, 311–312
Standard Operating Procedures (SOPs), 136–137
Standard uptake value (SUV) descriptors, 286
Stress
cold pressor test, 458
interpretation, 458–459
MBF, 460–464
MFR, 460–464
pharmacologic agents, 456, 457
Sympathetic nervous system (SNS)
neuroblastoma
11C-hydroxyephedrine, 553
diagnosis, 550
etiology, 550
^{18}F-FDG, 550, 552, 553
history, 550
INSS, 550
long-term survival, 549–550
metastases, 550
MIBG scintigraphy, 550, 551
pheochromocytoma, 553–554

T

Tetrabutylammonium (TBA), 84
Texture, 287–288
Thin-layer chromatography (TLC), 112–113
Thyroid cancer, 438, 567
Time-activity curve (TAC), 324–325, 460
Time-of-flight (TOF)
bench-top measurement, 191
benefits, 191–193
BGO-based scanner, 190
clinical improvement, 190
coincidence detector, 176–177
image reconstruction, 277–279
instrumentation, 230
lutetium-based scanner, 190
Poisson count statistics, 190
resurgence, 190–191
system timing resolution, 190
Tissue fraction effect, 358–359
Tofts model, 288
Total lesion glycolysis (TLG), 286, 312–313
Total variation (TV), 271
1,4,7-Triazacyclononane-1,4,7-tris [methyl(2-carboxyethyl)phosphinic acid] (TRAP-Pr), 96–97
Tumor texture analysis, 317–318
Turbidimetric technique, 110
Two Fourier rebinning algorithms of time-of-flight data (FORET), 278–279

V

Vascular dementia (VaD), 490
Volume CTDI ($CTDI_{vol}$), 53–55

W

Weighted CTDI ($CTDI_w$), 52–54
Wilms' tumor, 566

CPI Antony Rowe
Chippenham, UK
2017-03-01 21:35

Manuals of Practice of the Water Environment Federation

The WEF Technical Practice Committee (formerly the Committee on Sewage and Industrial Wastes Practice of the Federation of Sewage and Industrial Wastes Associations) was created by the Federation Board of Control on October 11, 1941. The primary function of the Committee is to originate and produce, through appropriate subcommittees, special publications dealing with technical aspects of the broad interests of the Federation. These publications are intended to provide background information through a review of technical practices and detailed procedures that research and experience have shown to be functional and practical.

Manuals and Reports on Engineering Practice

(As developed by the ASCE Technical Procedures Committee, July 1930, and revised March 1935, February 1962, and April 1982)

A manual or report in this series consists of an orderly presentation of facts on a particular subject, supplemented by an analysis of limitations and applications of these facts. It contains information useful to the average engineer in his everyday work, rather than findings that may be useful only occasionally or rarely. It is not in any sense a "standard," however; nor is it so elementary or so conclusive as to provide a "rule of thumb" for nonengineers.

Furthermore, material in this series, in distinction from a paper (which expresses only one person's observations or opinions), is the work of a committee or group selected to assemble and express information on a specific topic. As often as practicable, the committee is under the direction of one or more of the Technical Divisions and Councils, and the product evolved has been subjected to review by the Executive Committee of the Division or Council. As a step in the process of this review, proposed manuscripts are often brought before the members of the Technical Divisions and Councils for comment, which may serve as the basis for improvement. When published, each work shows the names of the committees by which it was compiled and indicates clearly the several processes through which it has passed in review, in order that its merit may be definitely understood.

In February 1962 (and revised in April 1982) the Board of Direction voted to establish a series entitled "Manuals and Reports on Engineering Practice," to include the Manuals published and authorized to date, future Manuals of Professional Practice, and Reports on Engineering Practice. All such Manual or Report material of the Society would have been refereed in a manner approved by the Board Committee on Publications and would be bound, with applicable discussion, in books similar to past Manuals. Numbering would be consecutive and would be a continuation of present Manual numbers. In some cases of reports of joint committees, bypassing of Journal publications may be authorized.

Contents

List of Figures xxiii
List of Tables xxvii
Preface xxix

Chapter 1 Introduction—Fernando Pasquel 1

1.0 THE IMPORTANCE OF STORMWATER CONTROL MEASURE MAINTENANCE 1
2.0 MANUAL OVERVIEW 4
3.0 HOW TO USE THIS MANUAL 6
4.0 FUNDING OPERATIONS AND MAINTENANCE ACTIVITIES 7
5.0 TERMINOLOGY 8
6.0 REFERENCES 8

Chapter 2 Program Development and Regulatory Framework—Jason T. Sanson, PE; Anwer Ahmed, PE, DWRE, & Maya Carrasquillo, PhD 11

1.0 INTRODUCTION 11
2.0 MAINTENANCE DRIVERS 12
- 2.1 Regulatory Drivers 13
- 2.2 Land Development 13
- 2.3 Performance 13

3.0 ROLES OF REGULATORY AGENCIES 15
- 3.1 Federal 15
- 3.2 State 15
- 3.3 Local 16
- 3.4 Stormwater Control Measure Inspection During Construction 16
- 3.5 Private and Public Parties 18

4.0 PROGRAM DEVELOPMENT 19
4.1 Overview 19
4.2 Extent and Level of Service 19
4.3 Program Models and Functions 20
4.3.1 Program Components 20
4.3.2 Scoping the Maintenance Program 23
4.4 Program Organization 24
4.5 Program Funding 24
4.5.1 Stormwater Fees 26
4.5.2 Loans Programs 26
4.5.3 Grant Funding 26
4.6 Training 26
5.0 RESILIENCE CONSIDERATIONS IN OPERATIONS AND MAINTENANCE 27
6.0 SAMPLE MAINTENANCE AGREEMENTS 28
7.0 REFERENCES 30

Chapter 3 Design and Construction Maintenance Considerations—Andy Sauer, PE, ENV SP; Lauren Moore, PE, ENV SP; & Brenda Macke, PE, CFM, PMP 31
1.0 INTRODUCTION 31
2.0 DESIGN CONSIDERATIONS: DESIGN WITH MAINTENANCE IN MIND 35
2.1 Establishing the Functional Performance With Design 35
2.2 The Designer Perspective 36
2.3 Function and Potential Fail Points 39
2.4 Designing for Potential Fail Points 40
3.0 MAINTENANCE NEEDS DURING CONSTRUCTION 40
3.1 Control and Protection Measures 41
3.1.1 Perimeter Controls 42
3.1.2 Surface Controls 44
3.1.3 Enclosed System Control 45
3.1.4 Stabilization Control 46
3.2 Phasing of Construction: Plan, Communicate, Plan 48
3.2.1 Location Considerations 49
3.2.2 Stormwater Control Function and Fail Points 50

3.2.3 Control, Protection, and Sequencing Plan, and Specification Development 51
3.2.4 Construction Timing and Execution Constraints 56
3.3 Construction Responsibilities 58
3.3.1 Construction Responsibilities and Oversight 58
3.3.2 Training of the Construction Worker—Developing Skilled Stormwater Control Measure Labor 59
4.0 REFERENCE 61

Chapter 4 Conventional Stormwater Control Measures and Green Infrastructure Maintenance—Shandor Szalay & Kevin Flynn 63
1.0 INTRODUCTION 64
1.1 Maintenance Goals 64
1.1.1 Sustained Function 64
1.1.2 System Longevity 65
1.1.3 Aesthetics 66
1.1.4 Balancing Maintenance Level of Service 66
1.1.5 Public and Worker Safety 68
1.2 Key Processes 68
1.2.1 Vegetation and Soil Associations and Feedback 68
1.2.2 Hydraulics, Erosion, and Sedimentation 71
1.2.3 Structural Deterioration 72
2.0 MAINTENANCE TO OPTIMIZE PERFORMANCE AND LONGEVITY 74
2.1 Maintaining Health Vegetation and Soils 74
2.2 Managing Erosion and Sedimentation Processes 75
2.1.1 Minimizing Erosion, Scour, and Settlement 76
2.2.2 Managing Sedimentation and Clogging 76
2.3 Maintaining Structural Components 76
3.0 SPECIAL CONSIDERATIONS 77
3.1 Considerations for Infiltrating Systems 77
3.2 Considerations for Slow-Release Systems 78
3.3 Considerations for Proprietary/Manufactured Devices 78

4.0 MAINTENANCE SUMMARY BY STORMWATER CONTROL MEASURES TYPE 79
4.1 Surface Practices 79
4.1.1 Forebays 79
4.1.1.1 Routine Maintenance 81
4.1.1.2 Common Problems 82
4.1.2 Dry Basins 82
4.1.2.1 Routine Maintenance 83
4.1.2.2 Common Problems 84
4.1.3 Wet Basins 84
4.1.3.1 Routine Maintenance 84
4.1.3.2 Common Problems 85
4.1.4 Wetlands (Including Subsurface Gravel Wetlands) 88
4.1.4.1 Routine Maintenance 88
4.1.4.2 Common Problems 89
4.1.5 Bioretention Filters 90
4.1.5.1 Routine Maintenance 91
4.1.5.2 Common Problems 92
4.1.6 Infiltration Basins 93
4.1.6.1 Routine Maintenance 94
4.1.6.2 Common Problems 95
4.1.7 Surface Sand Filters 96
4.1.7.1 Routine Maintenance 96
4.1.7.2 Common Problems 97
4.1.8 Swales and Strips 97
4.1.8.1 Routine Maintenance 98
4.1.8.2 Common Problems 99
4.2 Subsurface Practices 100
4.2.1 Drain Inlet Inserts and Manufactured Filters 101
4.2.1.1 Routine Maintenance 102
4.2.1.2 Common Problems 102
4.2.2 Vaults and Swirl Concentrators 102
4.2.3 Oil and Water Separators 103
4.2.3.1 Routine Maintenance 104

4.2.3.2 Common Problems 104
4.2.3.3 Special Considerations 104
4.2.4 Infiltration/Retention Trenches and Vaults 105
4.2.5 Dry Wells 106
4.2.5.1 Routine Maintenance 106
4.2.5.2 Common Problems 106
4.3 Cisterns and Rain Barrels 107
4.3.1 Routine Maintenance 109
4.3.2 Common Problems 109
4.4 Landscaped Roofs (Green Roofs) 110
4.4.1 Routine Maintenance 111
4.4.2 Common Problems 112
4.5 Permeable Pavement 113
4.5.1 Routine Maintenance 113
4.5.2 Common Problems 114
5.0 REFERENCES 116

Chapter 5 Inspection and Maintenance During and After Construction (Protocols)— Ed Othmer & Maureen Kerner, PE 119
1.0 OVERVIEW OF INSPECTION AND MAINTENANCE PROTOCOLS 121
2.0 TYPES OF STORMWATER CONTROL MEASURES AND COMPONENTS 124
2.1 STORMWATER CONTROL MEASURE TYPES 124
2.1.1 Basins 125
2.1.2 Swales and Strips 125
2.1.3 Filters 126
2.1.4 Infiltrators 127
2.1.5 Gross Pollutant Traps and Mechanical Operations 128
2.2 Stormwater Control Measure Components 129
3.0 INSPECTION AND MAINTENANCE PREPARATION 129
3.1 Health and Safety 129
3.2 Site Location and Access 131

3.3 Permits and Approvals 131
3.4 Personnel Education and Training 132
4.0 DURING CONSTRUCTION PROTOCOLS 133
4.1 Inspections 134
4.1.1 Verification of Proper Stormwater Control Measures 134
4.1.2 Verification of Location and Contributing Drainage Area 135
4.1.3 Verification of Size and Configuration 135
4.1.4 Verification of Elevations, Grades, and Dimensions 135
4.1.5 Verification of Conformance With Plans and Specifications 135
4.1.6 Verification of Structure Safety 136
4.1.7 Verification of Maintainability 136
4.1.7.1 Verification of Accessibility 137
4.1.7.2 Verification of Durability 137
4.1.8 Verification of Noncompaction 138
4.1.9 Verification of Structural Integrity 138
4.1.10 Verification of Soil/Filter Media 138
4.1.11 Verification of Hydraulic Performance 139
4.1.12 Verification of Plant Establishment 139
4.1.13 As-Built Drawings, Inspection Documentation, and Records Management 140
5.0 POSTCONSTRUCTION PROTOCOLS 140
5.1 Inspections 141
5.1.1 Inspect for Debris and Litter 142
5.1.2 Inspect for Sediment Accumulation 142
5.1.3 Inspect Vegetation 143
5.1.4 Inspect for Erosion 144
5.1.5 Inspect for Settling 144
5.1.6 Inspect Structural Features 145
5.1.7 Inspect Permanent Pool 146
5.1.8 Inspect for Damage/Malfunction of Mechanical, Electrical, Pneumatic, and Hydraulic Components 146

5.1.9 Inspect Porous Pavement 148
5.1.10 Inspect Media 148
5.1.11 Inspect for Evidence/Presence of Nuisance Conditions and Animals 149
5.1.11.1 Inspect for Undesirable Plant Communities 149
5.1.11.2 Inspect for Water Quality Degradation 150
5.1.11.3 Inspect for Water Bird Damage 150
5.1.12 Inspect for Vectors 150
5.1.13 Inspect for Snow and Ice 151
5.1.14 Inspect for Miscellaneous Site Damage 152
5.2 Routine Maintenance Protocols 152
5.2.1 Debris and Litter Removal Control 152
5.2.2 Sediment Removal and Disposal 153
5.2.3 Vegetation Maintenance 153
5.2.3.1 Weed Control 154
5.2.3.2 Mowing 154
5.2.3.3 Dead and Damaged Vegetation Removal 155
5.2.3.4 Pruning and Trimming 155
5.2.3.5 Soil Management 155
5.2.3.6 Reseeding and Replanting 156
5.2.3.7 Mulching 158
5.2.3.8 Watering 158
5.2.4 Minor Erosion 158
5.2.5 Settling Repair 159
5.2.6 Structure Maintenance 160
5.2.6.1 Pretreatment Device, Inlets, Outlet Structures, Chambers, and Subsurface Structures 160
5.2.6.2 Screens and Trash Racks 161
5.2.6.3 Pipes 161
5.2.6.4 Standing Water 162
5.2.6.5 Permanent Pool 162

5.2.7 Mechanical, Electrical, Pneumatic, and Hydraulic Maintenance 162

5.2.7.1 Valves, Orifices, and Aerators 162

5.2.7.2 Pumps and Switches 164

5.2.8 Porous Pavement Cleaning and Winter Maintenance 164

5.2.9 Media Maintenance 166

5.2.10 Nuisance Control 168

5.2.10.1 Animals 168

5.2.10.2 Water Birds 168

5.2.10.3 Undesirable Plant Communities 169

5.2.10.4 Water Quality Degradation 169

5.2.11 Vector Management 170

5.2.12 Snow and Ice Removal 171

5.2.13 Miscellaneous Site Damage 171

5.3 Nonroutine/Emergency Maintenance Protocols 171

5.3.1 Structural Repairs 172

5.3.2 Mechanical Equipment Repairs 172

5.3.3 Dam, Embankment, and Slope Repairs 172

5.3.4 Dewatering 172

5.3.5 Pond Maintenance 173

5.3.6 Fence Repair 173

5.3.7 Elimination of Woody Vegetation 173

5.3.8 Spills 173

5.4 Aesthetic Maintenance 176

5.4.1 Graffiti Removal 176

5.4.2 Vegetation Maintenance 176

5.4.3 Overall Site Maintenance 176

6.0 PRIORITIZING CORRECTIVE MAINTENANCE 177

7.0 MAINTENANCE THRESHOLD INDICATORS 177

8.0 CHECKLISTS 177

9.0 REFERENCES 210

10.0 SUGGESTED READINGS 211

Chapter 6 **Asset Management and Tools— Mark Van Auken & Maureen Kerner, PE** 213

1.0 OVERVIEW OF ASSET MANAGEMENT 213

1.1 Needs 213

1.2 Definitions 214

1.3 Benefits 215

1.4 History 215

1.5 United States Environmental Protection Agency 10-Step Asset Management Process 217

2.0 EVALUATE CURRENT STATE OF ASSETS 219

2.1 Types of Assets 219

2.2 Asset Characteristics 219

2.3 Asset Organization 221

2.4 Gathering Asset Information 222

3.0 IDENTIFY THE APPROPRIATE LEVEL OF SERVICE 225

4.0 EVALUATE CRITICAL ASSETS 226

5.0 EVALUATE INVESTMENT STRATEGIES 231

5.1 Categorizing Assets for Operations and Maintenance or Capital Programs 232

5.2 Identifying Other Program Costs 233

5.3 Gathering Cost Data 233

5.4 Optimizing Operations and Maintenance Investments 235

5.5 Optimizing Capital Investments 236

6.0 EVALUATE LONG-TERM FUNDING OPTIONS 241

6.1 Funding Strategies 241

6.2 Documenting the Asset Management Plan 243

7.0 ADAPTIVE MANAGEMENT 244

7.1 Strategies 244

7.2 Tracking Performance Over Time 245

7.3 Feedback 245

7.4 Update of Asset Management Program 246

8.0 REFERENCES 247

Chapter 7 Personnel, Equipment, and Cost Considerations—Fernando Pasquel & Shandor Szalay 251

1.0 PERSONNEL AND EQUIPMENT REQUIREMENTS 251

1.1 Surface Inspection and Maintenance 252

1.1.1 Crew Requirements 252

1.1.2 Equipment 253

1.1.3 Materials 254

1.2 Subsurface Inspection and Maintenance 254

1.2.1 Crew Requirements 254

1.2.2 Equipment and Materials 255

1.3 Porous Pavement Inspection and Maintenance 256

1.3.1 Crew Requirements 256

1.3.2 Equipment 256

1.3.3 Materials 256

1.4 Nonroutine and Specialty Maintenance 257

1.4.1 Crew Requirements 257

1.4.2 Equipment 257

1.4.3 Materials 258

2.0 BUDGETING CONSIDERATIONS FOR OPERATIONS AND MAINTENANCE PROGRAMS 258

2.1 Budget Components 258

2.2 Estimating/Budgeting Program Costs 260

2.2.1 Factors Affecting Budget Estimates 260

2.2.2 Estimating Life-Cycle Costs 265

3.0 MAINTENANCE CAPITAL IMPROVEMENT PROGRAM 266

4.0 REFERENCES 268

5.0 SUGGESTED READING 269

Chapter 8 Maintenance Scheduling—Brian Currier & Kirk Van Rooyan 271

1.0 INTRODUCTION 271

1.1 Maintenance Scheduling Scenarios 272

1.1.1 Regularly Scheduled or Routine Maintenance 272

1.1.2 Postinspection Ad-Hoc Maintenance 272

1.1.3 *Maintenance During Inspection* 272

1.1.4 *Emergency or Nonroutine Maintenance* 273

1.1.5 *Inspection During Maintenance* 273

2.0 CONSIDERATIONS, PRIORITIES, AND TOOLS FOR SCHEDULING MAINTENANCE 273

2.1 Considerations for Setting Schedules for Activities, Crews, Equipment, and Routes 273

2.1.1 *Predictability of Maintenance Activity* 274

2.1.2 *Availability of Workforce and Equipment* 274

2.1.3 *Availability of Maintenance Products and Materials* 275

2.1.4 *Seasonal Workload* 275

2.1.5 *Seasonal Species Conflicts* 276

2.1.6 *Seasonal Access* 276

2.1.7 *Logistics and Work Schedules* 276

2.1.8 *Regional Factors* 277

2.2 Prioritization 277

2.3 Scheduling Tools 278

3.0 ADAPTIVE MANAGEMENT PROCESS TO OPTIMIZE SCHEDULING 278

4.0 REFERRAL TO THE DESIGN PROFESSIONAL 280

5.0 REFERENCES 281

Chapter 9 Operations and Maintenance Forms, Logs, and Reporting—Aiza Jose-Sanchez, Eric Caldwell, Jordan Duncan, & Kelia Smoot 283

1.0 IMPORTANCE OF TRACKING AND REPORTING INSPECTIONS AND MAINTENANCE 284

1.1 Importance of Inspections and Maintenance During Construction 284

1.2 Importance of Inspections and Maintenance During Operation 287

2.0 COMPONENTS OF STANDARD OPERATING PROCEDURES FOR THE SUCCESSFUL OPERATIONS AND MAINTENANCE OF STORMWATER CONTROL MEASURES 292

2.1 Coordination, Responsibilities, and Communication Protocols 292
2.2 Health and Safety Plans and Incident/Near-Miss Reporting 293
2.3 Data Collection, Processing, Reporting, and Recordkeeping 294
2.3.1 Data Collection 294
2.3.2 Reporting and Processing 294
2.3.3 Recordkeeping 295
2.4 Public Outreach 295
2.5 Enforcement 296
3.0 CONSIDERATIONS FOR THE DEVELOPMENT OF INSPECTION FORMS 297
3.1 Stormwater Control Measure Inventory and Relevant Information 298
3.2 Importance of Rainfall Data 300
3.3 Tools, Databases, and Systems Utilized for Inventory and Data Management 301
3.4 Typical Stormwater Control Measure Concerns During Construction 301
3.4.1 Vegetated Swales and Strips 301
3.4.2 Basins 302
3.4.2.1 Dry Basins 302
3.4.2.2 Wet Basins 302
3.4.2.3 Swirl Concentrators and Vaults 302
3.4.3 Filters 303
3.4.3.1 Media Filters 303
3.4.3.2 Bioretention Filters 303
3.4.3.3 Inlet Basket 304
3.4.3.4 Landscaped Roofs 304
3.4.4 Infiltration 304
3.4.4.1 Infiltration Trench 304
3.4.4.2 Infiltration Basin 305
3.4.4.3 Pervious Pavement 305

3.4.5 Catch Basins 306
3.4.6 Gross Pollutant Controls 306
3.5 Typical Stormwater Control Measure Concerns During Operation 307
3.5.1 Vegetated Swales and Strips 307
3.5.2 Basins 308
3.5.2.1 Dry Basins 308
3.5.2.2 Wet Basins 309
3.5.2.3 Swirl Concentrators and Vaults 309
3.5.3 Filters 310
3.5.3.1 Media Filters 310
3.5.3.2 Bioretention Filters 310
3.5.3.3 Inlet Basket 310
3.5.3.4 Landscaped Roofs 311
3.5.4 Infiltration 311
3.5.4.1 Infiltration Trench 311
3.5.4.2 Infiltration Basin 311
3.5.4.3 Pervious Pavement 312
3.5.5 Catch Basins 312
3.5.6 Gross Pollutant Controls 312
4.0 SAMPLE INSPECTION AND MAINTENANCE REPORTING FORMS 313
4.1 Inspection Forms During Construction 313
4.2 Inspection Forms During Operations and Maintenance 314
5.0 SUMMARY 316
6.0 REFERENCES 344

Chapter 10 Case Studies—Fernando Pasquel; Victoria Chou, PE; Lisa Treese; & Brenda Macke, PE, CFM, PMP 347
1.0 INTRODUCTION 348
2.0 CASE STUDY 1—KANSAS CITY, MO 349

2.1 Stormwater Management Program Overview 349
2.1.1 General Program 349
2.1.2 Operations and Maintenance Activities 350
2.2 Types of Stormwater Control Measures 350
2.2.1 Public Stormwater Control Measures 351
2.2.2 Private Stormwater Control Measures 351
2.3 Maintenance of Stormwater Control Measures 352
2.3.1 Performance of Inspection and Maintenance Activities 352
2.3.2 Lessons Learned 352
2.3.2.1 Green Solutions 352
2.3.2.2 Green Stewards 353
2.3.2.3 Construction Contractor Maintenance 354
2.4 Inspection and Maintenance Responsibilities and Recordkeeping 354
2.4.1 Public Practices 354
2.4.1.1 Maintenance Frequencies and Reporting 354
2.4.1.2 Responsible Parties 355
2.4.1.3 Recordkeeping 358
2.4.2 Private Practices 360
2.4.2.1 Maintenance Frequencies and Reporting 360
2.4.2.2 Responsible Parties 361
2.4.2.3 Recordkeeping 362
2.5 Funding Inspections and Maintenance 362
2.5.1 Public Practices 362
2.5.1.1 Funding Mechanisms 362
2.5.1.2 Summary of Annual Costs 362
2.5.2 Private Practices 363
2.5.2.1 Funding Mechanisms 363
2.5.2.2 Summary of Annual Costs 363
2.6 Challenges and Future Initiatives 364
2.6.1 Asset Management 364

2.6.2 *In-House Maintenance* 364
2.6.3 *Contracted Assistance* 364
2.6.4 *Green Stewards* 365
2.6.5 *Overall Operations and Maintenance Program Planning* 365
3.0 CASE STUDY 2—CITY OF LANCASTER, PA 365
3.1 Stormwater Management Program Overview 365
3.2 Types of Stormwater Control Measures 367
3.3 Maintenance of Stormwater Control Measures 367
3.3.1 *Inspection and Maintenance Activities* 367
3.3.2 *Lessons Learned* 367
3.4 Inspection and Maintenance Responsibilities and Recordkeeping 368
3.4.1 *Maintenance Frequencies and Reporting* 368
3.4.2 *Recordkeeping* 369
3.5 Funding Inspections and Maintenance 369
3.5.1 *Public Practices* 369
3.5.2 *Private Practices* 369
3.6 Challenges and Future Initiatives 370
4.0 CASE STUDY 3—PHILADELPHIA WATER DEPARTMENT 370
4.1 Stormwater Management Program Overview 370
4.2 Types of Stormwater Control Measures 371
4.3 Maintenance of Stormwater Control Measures 372
4.3.1 *Inspection and Maintenance Activities* 372
4.3.2 *Lessons Learned* 372
4.4 Inspection and Maintenance Responsibilities and Recordkeeping 373
4.4.1 *Public Practices* 373
4.4.1.1 *Maintenance Frequencies and Reporting* 373
4.4.1.2 *Recordkeeping* 373
4.4.2 *Asset Management Considerations* 374
4.5 Funding Inspections and Maintenance 374

4.6 Challenges and Future Initiatives 374
4.6.1 *Inspection and Maintenance Challenges* 374
4.6.2 *Future Initiatives to Ensure Continued Performance* 376
5.0 REFERENCES 377
6.0 SUGGESTED READING 377

Index 379

List of Figures

3.1 Expectation of Maintenance Tasks Through Project Life Cycle 32

3.2 Key Characteristics of the Contributing Area 33

3.3 Functional Performance Relationship to Location 37

3.4 Silt Fence Perimeter Control Example for Stormwater Control Measure Control and Protection 43

3.5 Erosion Control Log Perimeter Control Example for Stormwater Control Measure Control and Protection 43

3.6 Permeable Liner (Geotextile) Surface Control Example for Stormwater Control Measure Control and Protection 44

3.7 Bypass Piping Enclosed System Control Example for Stormwater Control Measure Control and Protection 45

3.8 Weir Plate Enclosed System Control Example for Stormwater Control Measure Control and Protection 46

3.9 Ground Cover Stabilization Control Example for Stormwater Control Measure Control and Protection 47

3.10 Hydraulic Application Stabilization Control Example for Stormwater Control Measure Control and Protection 47

3.11 Erosion Control Blanket Stabilization Control Example for Stormwater Control Measure Control and Protection 48

3.12 Water Features Primary Function: Control, Protection, and Sequencing Considerations 51

3.13 Infiltration/Filtration Primary Function: Control, Protection, and Sequencing Considerations 52

3.14 Vegetation Features Primary Function: Control, Protection, and Sequencing Considerations 53

3.15 Water Reuse Primary Function: Control, Protection, and Sequencing Considerations 54

3.16 Screening/Hydromechanics Primary Function: Control, Protection, and Sequencing Considerations 55

3.17 Control and Protection Plan Minimum Requirements 56

3.18 Control and Protection Specification Minimum Requirements 56

3.19 Construction Timing and Execution Constraints 57

3.20 Recommended Verification Checks During Construction 60

4.1 Conceptualized Relationships Between Maintenance Unit Costs for Right-of-Way (ROW) and Off-ROW Systems Along a Gradient of Urban Density and Project Size 67

4.2 Vegetation-Soil Feedback Processes 69

6.1 Key WRF Asset Management Products 216

6.2 U.S. EPA/WERF 10-Step Integrated Planning Process 218

6.3 Effect of Probability and Consequence of Failure on Risk 228

6.4 Asset Management Program Support of Operations and Maintenance and Capital Improvement Plan. 232

6.5 Examples of Metrics, Definitions, and Targets to Use in Optimizing O&M Investments. 236

6.6 Asset Management Components That Support a Methodical Approach for Project Identification 237

6.7 Identifying Capital Improvement Projects Using Asset Management Information. 238

6.8 Defining Failure Modes and Management Strategies to Inform Project Identification 239

6.9 Using BRE and CLR Scores to Validate Projects 240

6.10 Prioritizing Projects Using Factors and Weights 240

6.11 Prioritizing Projects Using Project Risk and CIP Budget. 241

8.1 Adaptive Management Process to Determine Optimal Maintenance Scheduling. 279

9.1 Swirl Concentrator and Rain Garden During Construction Installation 286

9.2 Gross Pollutants Screens at Outfall. Heavy Debris Accumulation Shows Need of Routine or Preventive Maintenance (left); Gross Pollutant Screen Shows Stenciling Marking; the 60% Stenciling Mark Shows the Debris Level at Which the Catch Basin Will Need Routine or Preventive Maintenance (right). 290

9.3 Scouring and Erosion at Outlet Flume and Inflow Lines from Two Wet Ponds Requiring Corrective Maintenance. 291

9.4 Signage Utilized to Provide Outreach for a "Complete Street" or "Green Infrastructure Street" Project—Each Element of Green Infrastructure Is Explained for the General Public at the "Complete Street" Project Site 297

9.5 Installation of an Infiltration Basin. 305
9.6 Excessive Vegetation Dry Basin 308
9.7 Riprap Failure and Beginning of Erosion at Inlets of a Wet Pond. 309
9.8 SCM Construction Inspection Form. 317
9.9 Vegetated Swale and Vegetated Strip Inspection Form 319
9.10 Dry Basin Inspection Form. 321
9.11 Wet Basin Inspection Form. 323
9.12 Media Filter Inspection Form. 325
9.13 Bioretention Filter Inspection Form 328
9.14 Inlet Basket Inspection Form 330
9.15 Landscaped Roof Inspection Form. 331
9.16 Infiltration Trench and Infiltration Basin Inspection Form 332
9.17 Pervious Pavement Inspection Form. 335
9.18 Catch Basin Inspection Form 337
9.19 Swirl Separators and Vault Inspection Form. 339
9.20 Gross Pollutant Screens Inspection Form 342
10.1 KC Water Green Infrastructure Maintenance Mechanisms. . . . 351
10.2 GSI Practices 351
10.3 KC Water Projected Green Infrastructure Asset Growth (2020–2027). 353
10.4 Green Stewards Program as Source of Qualified Potential Employees 357
10.5 Green Infrastructure Asset Components and Maintenance Activity Relationship. 359
10.6 Proportional Costs by Category for 2020 KC Water Green Infrastructure Maintenance, Inspection, Coordination, and Administration 363

List of Tables

1.1 SCM Categories and Types 8

2.1 Other Regulatory Drivers That Influence Post-Construction Stormwater 14

3.1 Categories of Stormwater Control Measures 34

3.2 Relationship Between Primary Function and General Category of Stormwater Control Measure 35

4.1 Summary of Common Maintenance Activities for Surface and Subsurface Practices 80

4.2 Summary of Maintenance Activities, Frequency, and Timing for Subsurface Practices 101

4.3 Summary of Routine Maintenance for Cisterns and Rain Barrels 108

4.4 Summary of Routine Maintenance for Landscaped Roofs 111

4.5 Summary of Routine Maintenance for Permeable Pavement 114

5.1 Erosion Control Methods and Mechanisms 159

5.2 Permanent Pool Fluctuation Diagnosis and Solution 163

5.3 Maintenance Prioritization System 177

5.4 Basin Components 178

5.5 Swale and Strip Components 180

5.6 Filter Components 181

5.7 Infiltrator Components 184

5.8 Gross Pollutant Traps and Mechanical Operations and Components 186

5.9 SCM Inspection Requirements 188

5.10 Inspections and Maintenance Indicators for Basins 190

5.11 Inspections and Maintenance Indicators for Swales and Strips 196

5.12 Inspections and Maintenance Indicators for Filters 198

5.13 Inspections and Maintenance Indicators for Infiltrators 203

5.14 Inspections and Maintenance Indicators for Gross Pollutant Devices and Mechanical Operations 208

6.1 Examples of Typical Stormwater Asset Categories and Types 220
6.2 Typical Asset Information for Bioretention Facility 220
6.3 Example Asset Hierarchy 221
6.4 Comparison of Asset Management Tools 222
6.5 U.S. EPA Stormwater Asset Management Resources 223
6.6 Example Mobile Applications That Support Asset Management Activities for Water Utilities 224
6.7 Level of Service Comparison 226
6.8 Common Triple Bottom Line Elements 229
6.9 Sample Community Asset Risk Scoring Comparison 231
6.10 Stormwater Capital, Operations and Maintenance, and Life-Cycle Costs 234
8.1 Matrix of Activity Types and Potential Crew and Equipment Assignments 274
8.2 Typical Inspection and Maintenance Schedule for Vegetation Management and Mulching by Generalized Climate Conditions 277
10.1 Green Infrastructure Maintenance Providers and Footprint Served. 352

Preface

The effectiveness of stormwater management programs depends largely on how well and how safely stormwater control measures (SCMs) perform over time. Nationwide, the largest challenge of stormwater programs is ensuring long-term performance of SCMs and stormwater systems. In addition, as these programs evolve, the number of SCMs is increasing rapidly. In fact, some communities and utilities in urban areas have tens of thousands of SCMs that have been constructed as part of land development projects or to solve flooding and water quality problems. Many SCMs are also built to address stormwater and combined sewer system regulatory compliance requirements.

The importance of maintenance and the significant numbers of SCMs have created the need for guidance on how stormwater programs must adapt to address evolving SCM design and maintenance requirements, climate change and resilience, and integration of asset management concepts to reduce long-term program costs. Furthermore, successful implementation of SCMs requires good design, proper construction, and perhaps more importantly long-term maintenance. There are several manuals and publications that provide information on maintenance needs in specific geographies or for specific SCMs, but the intent of this publication is to create one comprehensive manual.

The manual was developed as a companion to *Design of Urban Stormwater Controls* (WEF et al., 2012). *Urban Stormwater Controls Operation and Maintenance* describes the importance of incorporating maintenance considerations to the design and construction of SCMs, as well as sharing best practices on the implementation of maintenance programs. The manual also addresses program and regulatory requirements and includes a description of the elements of an inspection and maintenance program, as well as the skill sets needed in modern maintenance crews. Within this manual, users will find a compendium of best practices for inspection and maintenance (protocols), as well as forms and checklists, stormwater asset management considerations, and information on maintenance personnel, equipment, scheduling, and cost considerations. Case studies are presented to illustrate these concepts in large and small utilities/municipalities. You will find all you need to know about stormwater maintenance in this manual.

The manual is targeted to designers of stormwater controls (designing with maintenance in mind) as well as operations and maintenance staff. Senior managers of utilities and municipalities will also benefit from information on program development, costs, staffing and equipment considerations, and funding for operations and maintenance. Manual users will understand the need to take a long-term view of maintenance.

Authors' and reviewers' efforts were supported by the following organizations:

Arcadis U.S., Inc.
Burns & McDonnell
City of Lancaster Department of Public Works
Office of Water Programs at California State University, Sacramento
Philadelphia Water Department

1

Introduction

1.0	THE IMPORTANCE OF STORMWATER CONTROL MEASURE MAINTENANCE	1
2.0	MANUAL OVERVIEW	4
3.0	HOW TO USE THIS MANUAL	6
4.0	FUNDING OPERATIONS AND MAINTENANCE ACTIVITIES	7
5.0	TERMINOLOGY	8
6.0	REFERENCES	8

1.0 THE IMPORTANCE OF STORMWATER CONTROL MEASURE MAINTENANCE

Stormwater runoff is one of the fastest growing sources of pollution in many waterways across the United States (Water Environment Federation Stormwater Institute [WEF SWI], 2021), and stormwater management remains one of the greatest challenges to meeting water quality standards (U.S. EPA, 2021). The pollution consists of nutrients, sediments, metals, motor oil, lawn and garden care products, trash, and anything else that washes from streets and developed parcels into local streams and lakes, and eventually into bays, estuaries, and oceans. In addition, unmanaged stormwater also causes significant flooding and erosion. Stormwater control measures (SCMs; sometimes known as best management practices, BMPs, or green infrastructure) help address the stormwater quality and quantity challenges and provide the following benefits:

- SCMs play a critical role in reducing pollution and protecting the nation's waterways, as well as protecting downstream areas from flooding, erosion, and water quality degradation.
- SCMs are used to manage combined sewer systems (CSSs), and the information in this manual will help in addressing the requirements of

the first of the nine minimum controls, Proper Operation and Regular Maintenance Programs, to reduce the effects of combined sewer overflows (CSOs) on receiving waters, and prevent flooding and sewer backups.

- The SCMs are also key components of resilience and flood risk management strategies and can be a catalyst for climate change adaptation and economic development in urban areas.

Therefore, it is important that SCMs continue to perform over time, and the only way to ensure long-term performance is to have a well-established stormwater maintenance component in a utility's or community's stormwater program. The following are needs and issues that can be addressed by proper operation and maintenance of SCMs:

Aging Stormwater Infrastructure Needs. The Water Environment Federation (WEF) Stormwater Institute conducted in 2020 the second National Municipal Separate Storm Sewer System (MS4) Needs Assessment Survey (WEF SWI, 2021). In this survey, Aging Infrastructure was the top program challenge and the top driver for planning and investment decisions. The maintenance approach, protocols, and tools described in this manual will assist in improving the performance and longevity of SCMs and ultimately the effectiveness of stormwater management programs that depend primarily on how well and how safely SCMs perform.

Evolving SCM Design and Maintenance Needs. Maintenance of SCMs has changed considerably as the design of traditional SCMs (e.g., basins or ponds, infiltration trenches, etc.) has changed, and newer SCMs (e.g., green infrastructure practices, such as bioretention and green roofs, and manufactured devices, such as screens, nets, and swirls concentrators) are implemented. For example, in the past most basins had trickle ditches to concentrate flow from small storms, had short grass as the main vegetative component, and in most cases, had no sediment forebays. Now, most basins have diverse vegetative components, multiple flow paths for the inflow to reach the outfall structure, and sediment forebays, or other pretreatment devices to facilitate maintenance. In addition, new SCMs such as green infrastructure and manufactured devices have been used for the last 25 years, and their design continues to change because of failures, design improvements, and new technologies.

Finally, real-time controls have been introduced in the last 5 to 10 years creating new components (e.g., valves and gates that are activated remotely, solar panels, or electric components, etc.) that require even new maintenance procedures. As the type and design of SCMs evolve, stormwater programs also must evolve, creating a need for guidance on how these programs need to adapt to address new maintenance requirements and incorporate asset management concepts to reduce long-term program costs.

Stormwater MS4 Permits Maintenance Requirements. The effectiveness of a stormwater management program depends largely on how well and how safely stormwater controls perform over time. In addition, the long-term performance of SCMs is linked to the frequency of inspections and proactive maintenance. As a result, stormwater MS4 permit conditions for industrial, construction, and municipal permittees require that pollution prevention, construction, and postconstruction SCMs be adequately inspected and maintained (NRC, 2008). Stormwater programs with effective tracking systems will typically be able to ensure that SCMs and the stormwater system are inspected periodically, and maintenance is conducted by responsible public or private entities. Communities and utilities or any state or local entity (e.g., Department of Public Works, Department of Transportation, Department of Environmental Engineering, Drainage Department, etc.) conducting SCM maintenance activities are responsible through their MS4 permits to ensure that SCMs are maintained properly to facilitate their continued function and performance over time.

SCM Ownership and Private and Public Maintenance. Most SCMs are simple to operate and maintain if there are appropriate maintenance protocols and funding to conduct inspections and maintenance. However, SCMs are becoming more complex, and special skills and knowledge are required to properly maintain them. Regardless of the complexity of the operation and maintenance requirements, all SCMs are part of the local stormwater infrastructure, and this implies that ideally SCMs should be owned and maintained by the public agency responsible for the stormwater system. However, this is seldom true (Watershed Management Institute, 1997).

Many local governments and utilities rely on private property owners or homeowner associations for the maintenance of SCMs and associated assets mainly because of cost. A large portion of the stormwater infrastructure is constructed by developers to comply with development regulations, and local public works or stormwater departments are not ready or do not have adequate funding to take on operations and maintenance responsibilities for that infrastructure. However, as stormwater infrastructure grows and ages, many private owners and entities are also not ready or do not have funds for maintenance, and unfortunately often maintenance is not a priority for them, and SCMs fail. Some communities (e.g., Prince William County, VA, Montgomery County, MD, etc.) have taken over maintenance of selected SCMs as part of the implementation of stormwater utilities. Some cities, like Austin and Seattle, assume responsibility for long-term maintenance of SCMs in residential areas (NRC, 2008). The use of maintenance agreements to ensure that private property owners maintain SCMs in their properties has been standardized for newer SCMs, and this will enhance long-term performance.

The different models of SCM ownership and maintenance responsibilities described above require a good tracking system and clear inspection and maintenance protocols to ensure that SCMs are properly maintained. All SCMs require active routine and nonroutine maintenance to continue to provide stormwater quantity/volume control and water quality benefits.

2.0 MANUAL OVERVIEW

The purpose of this manual is to present best practices that will facilitate development of maintenance programs and incorporation of maintenance consideration in the design and construction of SCMs. This manual also provides stormwater maintenance protocols, forms, reporting, and asset management tools, as well as information on personnel, equipment, and costs to assist in the planning of maintenance activities. In addition, this manual provides maintenance guidance needed by maintenance agency staff (state, municipal, or utility) to adapt to evolving maintenance requirements for SCMs and climate change. Last, this manual presents several case studies that illustrate the evolving nature of stormwater operations and maintenance programs.

This manual responds to the need to address program and regulatory requirements, and includes a description of the elements of an inspection and maintenance program, as well as the skill sets needed in modern maintenance crews. The manual includes information useful to communities and utilities, and any state or local entity conducting maintenance activities of SCMs.

This manual was written by a dedicated group of volunteer authors with experience in government, academia, maintenance contracting, and consulting. The authors gathered information from a multitude of sources (e.g., federal, state, regional, and local) in the attempt to provide a national resource that is useful in all regions of the United States and beyond. It is the authors' hope that this manual fills the gap for a consistent and succinct source of information on the evolving operation and maintenance needs of SCMs. This manual uses the same nomenclature as and complements the publication titled *Design of Urban Stormwater Controls* (WEF et al., 2012).

This manual is divided into ten chapters, each of which addresses important topics regarding operations and maintenance of stormwater control measures as follows:

- **Chapter 1, Introduction.** Describes the importance of stormwater maintenance and provides an overview of this manual and suggestions on how to use it. In addition, this chapter presents information on funding for maintenance and the terminology used to help standardize the multitude of terms currently used in the stormwater sector.

- **Chapter 2, Program Development and Regulatory Framework.** Provides information of the regulatory context that, in many instances, drives the development of stormwater programs and, more specifically, the operations and maintenance roles and components of those programs. In addition, this chapter provides considerations on how to integrate resilience and future climate change programs in operations and maintenance (O&M) programs and how to make SCMs more resilient through maintenance activities.
- **Chapter 3, Design and Construction Maintenance Considerations.** Describes the need to design SCMs with maintenance in mind and presents key design issues that affect long-term maintenance. The chapter also describes maintenance needs during construction to minimize the effects of erosion and sediment on SCMs, as well as the importance of communications during the design and construction phases.
- **Chapter 4, Conventional SCMs and Green Infrastructure Maintenance.** Presents maintenance goals applicable to SCM O&M programs and key processes found on SCMs that need to be sustained. This chapter also summarizes maintenance activities that are needed to optimize SCM performance and provides special considerations to preserve functions of infiltrating systems, slow-release systems, and proprietary/manufactured devices. The chapter ends with a maintenance summary for each type of surface and subsurface SCMs, including routine maintenance activities and common problems.
- **Chapter 5, Inspection and Maintenance During and After Construction (Protocols).** This chapter provides general protocols for inspection and maintenance procedures and practices of SCMs, and describes the different types of SCMs and their components that require maintenance. This chapter also presents guidance on activities to be considered before inspection and maintenance commences. Detailed maintenance routine and nonroutine protocols to be used during construction and postconstruction, as well as checklists to guide maintenance activities, are provided. In addition, this chapter provides guidance on prioritizing corrective actions and thresholds that trigger maintenance. The chapter ends with checklists, equipment, and tools needed for the inspection and maintenance of SCMs.
- **Chapter 6, Asset Management and Tools.** Provides an overview of stormwater asset management and guidance on how to evaluate the current state of assets, as well as identification of levels of service

and evaluation of critical assets. The chapter also describes evaluation of investment strategies and long-term funding options. The chapter ends with an overview of adaptive management concepts for maintenance.

- **Chapter 7, Personnel, Equipment, and Cost Considerations.** Provides information on personnel and equipment requirements, and typical crew requirements for routine surface, subsurface, and permeable pavement SCMs. The chapter also provides brief information on nonroutine crew, equipment, and materials requirements. The chapter includes budgeting considerations for O&M programs, including budget components, estimating program costs, in-house vs. contracted labor, tracking of O&M costs, and development of a maintenance capital improvement program.
- **Chapter 8, Maintenance Scheduling.** Describes the importance of scheduling and provides information on maintenance scheduling scenarios. The chapter also presents considerations, priorities, and tools for scheduling maintenance. In addition, the chapter describes an adaptive management process to optimize scheduling and suggestions on when to engage design professionals to address or improve SCMs and reduce maintenance burdens.
- **Chapter 9, O&M Forms, Logs, and Reporting.** Presents information on tracking and reporting inspections and maintenance along with sample maintenance forms and logs. The chapter also includes consideration for developing inspection forms and examples of inspections and reporting forms.
- **Chapter 10, Case Studies.** Four case studies are presented representing large, midsize, and small communities at different stages of implementation.

3.0 HOW TO USE THIS MANUAL

Audience and Intent. This manual is targeted to designers of SCMs and O&M staff in charge of developing and implementing maintenance programs. In addition, maintenance crews conducting inspection and maintenance activities can use the checklists, fact sheets, and inspections forms and logs provided in Chapters 5 and 9 of this manual.

The manual's intent is to assist designers by providing information and considerations that facilitate design and construction of SCMs by keeping maintenance in mind. The manual also provides program-level insights to assist municipal and utility leaders in the development and implementation of O&M programs. The manual summarizes best O&M practices to support practitioners who are conducting O&M activities in the field and processing data in the office.

4.0 FUNDING OPERATIONS AND MAINTENANCE ACTIVITIES

Obtaining funding for O&M activities can be a significant problem for public agencies because of the competing demands for limited funds. In addition, according to the National Research Council, one of the weakest parts of most stormwater management programs is the lack of information about, and funding to support, the long-term maintenance of SCMs (NRC, 2008). Furthermore, the majority of municipal stormwater programs do not have adequate plans or resources in place for the long-term maintenance of SCMs (NRC, 2008). To overcome these problems, a dedicated source of revenue for the stormwater program, including maintenance of stormwater systems and SCMs, is recommended. WEF has resources on methods to develop and implement funding mechanisms, including the following publications:

- *User-Fee-Funded Stormwater Programs* (WEF, 2013) provides details for the establishment of stormwater utilities.
- *Green Infrastructure Implementation* (WEF, 2014) provides information on program development and overcoming implementation barriers. This publication also includes a chapter on financing strategies that describes the different funding mechanisms that are available for green infrastructure and stormwater programs in general.

Maintenance of private SCMs in commercial or industrial sites is generally not a problem if the stormwater program has clear policies and maintenance procedures, as well as enforcement procedures. Commercial/industrial property owners typically have a maintenance budget and staff or contractors who can conduct maintenance activities. However, finding funds to maintain SCMs for residential property owners and homeowner associations can be problematic. Grants and assistance programs can facilitate funding of maintenance activities in residential areas, but ownership and maintenance by the local municipality or agency (with or without contractor support) will always be the preferred alternative to ensure that O&M activities are conducted in a professional manner. Additional information on O&M program funding is provided in Chapter 2 and long-term funding options in Chapter 6. A high-level discussion on maintenance cost considerations is presented in Chapter 7.

TABLE 1.1 SCM Categories and Types

SCM Category	SCM Types	
Basins	• Dry basins • Cisterns and rain barrels • Wetlands • Oil/water separators	• Wet basins • Vaults and swirl concentrators • Forebays
Swales, Strips, Stream Restoration	• Swales • Level spreaders	• Vegetated strips • Stream restoration
Filters	• Surface and subsurface sand filters • Landscaped/vegetated roofs • Manufactured filters (boxes)	• Bioretention • Drain inlet inserts • Subsurface gravel wetlands
Infiltrators	• Infiltration basins • Dry wells	• Infiltration trenches and vaults • Permeable pavement
Gross Pollutant Traps	• Screens • Baskets • Hoods	• Nets • Racks

5.0 TERMINOLOGY

This manual uses the term "SCMs" to describe BMPs, stormwater facilities, low-impact development, green infrastructure, and manufactured devices, such as screens, nets, and swirls concentrators. The use of SCMs is consistent to the recommended terminology of the National Research Council report (NRC, 2008) and the terminology and nomenclature used in the companion manual, *Design of Urban Stormwater Controls* (WEF et al., 2012). There are many other names and terminology used in the stormwater sector to describe stormwater infrastructure. WEF and ASCE/EWRI continue to use SCMs as the preferred term, and the authors hope that this manual will contribute to the standardization of the use of this term.

Table 1.1. SCM Categories and Types, presents the nomenclature used in this manual. It has been adapted from the *Design of Urban Stormwater Controls* (WEF et al., 2012).

6.0 REFERENCES

National Research Council. (2008). *Urban stormwater management in the United States*. The National Academies Press.

U.S. Environmental Protection Agency. (2021). Stormwater management and green infrastructure research. https://www.epa.gov/water-research/stormwater-management-and-green-infrastructure-research

Water Environment Federation. (2013). *User-fee-funded stormwater programs.*

Water Environment Federation. (2014). *Green infrastructure implementation.*

Water Environment Federation Stormwater Institute. (2021). *2020 National municipal separate storm sewer system (MS4) needs assessment survey results.*

Water Environment Federation, American Society of Civil Engineers, & Environmental & Water Resources Institute. (2012). *Design of urban stormwater controls* (WEF Manual of Practice No. 23, ASCE/EWRI Manuals and Reports on Engineering Practice No. 87). Water Environment Federation.

Watershed Management Institute. (1997). *Institutional aspects of urban runoff management: A guide for program development and implementation.*

2

Program Development and Regulatory Framework

1.0 INTRODUCTION 11
2.0 MAINTENANCE DRIVERS 12
2.1 Regulatory Drivers 13
2.2 Land Development 13
2.3 Performance 13
3.0 ROLES OF REGULATORY AGENCIES 15
3.1 Federal 15
3.2 State 15
3.3 Local 16
3.4 Stormwater Control Measure Inspection During Construction 16
3.5 Private and Public Parties 18
4.0 PROGRAM DEVELOPMENT 19
4.1 Overview 19
4.2 Extent and Level of Service 19
4.3 Program Models and Functions 20
4.3.1 Program Components 20
4.3.2 Scoping the Maintenance Program 23
4.4 Program Organization 24
4.5 Program Funding 24
4.5.1 Stormwater Fees 26
4.5.2 Loans Programs 26
4.5.3 Grant Funding 26
4.6 Training 26
5.0 RESILIENCE CONSIDERATIONS IN OPERATIONS AND MAINTENANCE 27
6.0 SAMPLE MAINTENANCE AGREEMENTS 28
7.0 REFERENCES 30

1.0 INTRODUCTION

Over the past 40 years, cities large and small have responded to development growth with various stormwater controls, and unfortunately most controls have gone without maintenance since their installation. Typically, anything that is constructed will need routine inspection and maintenance to ensure the useful life is met. Stormwater control measures (SCMs) are no different, and whether gray, green, or proprietary they need regular attention. The effect on the environment is dependent on the stormwater control's ability to reduce the risk of flooding and effectively remove pollutants before releasing the stormwater back into the environment.

The maintenance of early generations of SCMs primarily involved keeping conveyance systems like storm sewers, culverts, and ditches open and flowing. As communities have grown, so has the need to inspect, maintain, and operate their SCMs. No matter how effective SCMs may be, none can be expected to continue functioning effectively without regular maintenance and inspections.

The new generation of SCMs have developed in response to extended detention for water quality; surface water impairment because of pollutant loading and regulations are main drivers for improving maintenance. Water quality treatment brought additional features to traditional practices such as stormwater control basins and an entirely new set of control measures such as bioretention, infiltration, permeable pavements, and flow-through practices (Northeast Ohio Storm Water Training Council, 2017).

The responsibility for operations and maintenance (O&M) of SCMs lies, in most cases, with the owner of the SCM. Typically, the owner of the property on which the SCM is constructed is the owner of the control measure and is legally obligated to operate and maintain the control measure. Inspection and maintenance programs are developed to provide owners a structure to identify who is responsible, what is entailed in the responsibility to maintain SCMs, how to inspect and maintain SCMs, and how to build resiliency into their program.

It takes a lot of time and great deal of effort to develop a stormwater maintenance program. It is not enough just to design and construct SCMs properly. Long-term maintenance is important to ensure that the SCM will perform as designed throughout its life. No maintenance or inadequate maintenance are the main deficiencies in most local stormwater programs, and the deferred maintenance may ultimately cause the SCM to fail, causing it to become a nuisance, pose safety concerns, or induce stress on the receiving stream. Therefore, developing and implementing an effective maintenance program is essential (Hirschman & Kosco, 2008).

2.0 MAINTENANCE DRIVERS

The four areas that tend to drive the need for SCM maintenance are regulatory requirements, newly developed or redeveloped land, funding for local stormwater programs, and performance of SCMs.

While stormwater management has become popular over the past few decades, communities across the country are striving to build programs to effectively manage stormwater and meet regulatory requirements of the Clean Water Act (CWA), Phases I and II of the National Pollutant Discharge Elimination System (NPDES) municipal stormwater permit program (Hirschman & Kosco, 2008).

2.1 Regulatory Drivers

Table 2.1 lists regulatory drivers that may influence postconstruction stormwater.

2.2 Land Development

A result of unprecedented growth throughout the United States is stormwater runoff. The transition from pervious to impervious surfaces, combined with various pollutants in stormwater, have led to water quality degradation in virtually all urban streams.

As communities grow, there is a balancing act between maximizing the opportunities and benefits associated with growth while minimizing the environmental effects of development. A community's geography, ecosystem, infrastructure, and the way a community grows is affected when decisions are made at an executive level with little discussion on how stormwater will be managed and how SCMs are going to be maintained.

Incorporating long-term stormwater maintenance in a community's overall master plan can effectively help balance development decisions with environmental protection. The barrier, however, is where and how to engage in development decisions. If stormwater management and long-term maintenance are included in initial planning, managers of the stormwater program can influence what is in a master plan and how the plan can develop for the overall environmental health of a community.

2.3 Performance

A great number of SCMs are installed throughout the country every year including wet ponds, constructed stormwater wetlands, bioretention, infiltration practices, permeable pavement, swales, and rainwater harvesting systems. Unfortunately, many of these SCMs fail as a result of lack of maintenance or even outright neglect. Probable reasons for neglect include lack of inventory, insufficient communication, unclear responsibilities, lack of knowledge, financial barriers, and decentralized measures.

TABLE 2.1 Other Regulatory Drivers That Influence Post-Construction Stormwater (Hirschman & Kosco, 2008)

Regulatory Driver	Link With Post-Construction Stormwater
	Federal
NPDES Stormwater Permits for Construction	Applies to stormwater discharges from sites with disturbance of 1 acre or greater. Requires control of sediment and erosion and other wastes at the site. Operators must develop and implement a Stormwater Pollution Prevention Plan (SWPPP). Provides opportunity for local program to coordinate construction and post-construction phases in plan review, inspection, and maintenance. The maintenance of SCMs is required in municipal separate storm sewer system (MS4) permits.
Combined Sewer System: Long-Term Control Plan (NPDES)	Requires plan to address and minimize overflows from combined systems to U.S. waters. Some communities have both an MS4 and a combined sewer system, and management practices should be coordinated. For instance, practices that limit the volume of stormwater discharges can also help reduce the incidence of CSOs [combined sewer overflows]. In addition, treatment practices such as street sweeping and catch basin cleaning can reduce floatables and sediment in CSOs.
Total Maximum Daily Load (TMDL)	Addresses impaired waters through a program that develops TMDLs. A TMDL is a calculation of the maximum amount of a pollutant that a water body can receive and still meet water quality standards. Post-construction programs specify stormwater practices, retrofits, and/or site-based load limits for development and redevelopment that can address the pollutant(s) identified in the TMDL.
Federal Wetland Permits (Section 404)	Regulates the discharge of dredged and fill material into U.S. waters, including wetlands. Stormwater practices that negatively affect streams and wetlands require permitting and are subject to denial. May push programs and site choices into low-impact development strategies to avoid effects. Stormwater plans may have to be coordinated with mitigation plans required through the wetland permitting process.
Coastal Zone Management Program (CZMP)	Sets out planning goals and milestones for designated coastal zones. Stormwater controls should be coordinated with state-specific CZMPs, which may include SCM performance standards. Nonstructural measures, such as wetland and marsh protection, can be incorporated into stormwater strategy to mesh with CZMP objectives.

(continued)

TABLE 2.1 Other Regulatory Drivers That Influence Post-Construction Stormwater (*continued*)

Regulatory Driver	Link With Post-Construction Stormwater
	State
State Erosion and Sediment Control and Stormwater Programs	Provides performance and/or technology standards for construction stormwater plans and facilities. In most cases, requires coordination between construction and post-construction program elements, such as plan reviews and inspections.
State Scenic River, Open Space, Reforestation, and Resource Protection Programs	Where present, includes state-specific goals with link to stormwater management, such as setbacks from particular rivers.
	Regional
Specific Regional Efforts (e.g., Chesapeake Bay, Great Lakes, and Puget Sound)	Where present, provides regional plans and programs that may have goals, objectives, and/or standards that influence a local stormwater program.
	Local
Existing Codes for Erosion Control, Stormwater, Zoning, Subdivision, and Standing Water and Weeds (Nuisance)	Establishes local rules for development density, streets, setbacks, and so on. These codes assist in planning, design, and maintenance of SCMs.
Greenway, Open Space, and Recreation Plans	Provides planning framework that offers opportunity for coordination between stormwater and planning (e.g., riparian restoration in conjunction with greenway development, stormwater demonstration sites at public parks).

3.0 ROLES OF REGULATORY AGENCIES

3.1 Federal

From a federal level, the CWA is the governing policy that institutes the NPDES permit directing municipalities throughout the country to meet water quality standards for stormwater. A municipal separate storm sewer system (MS4) is permitted authorization to discharge under the NPDES and remain in compliance with the Federal Water Pollution Control Act and their State Water Pollution Control Act.

3.2 State

The role of the state, in delegated MS4 states, is to issue permits and enforce the requirements, including inspection and maintenance requirements.

In states without delegation authority (Massachusetts, New Hampshire, New Mexico, District of Columbia, U.S. territories, and on federal and tribal lands), U.S. Environmental Protection Agency (U.S. EPA) issues and enforces the permit requirements. The MS4 community may declare regulations governing the quantity and quality of stormwater discharges from premises within the community's corporation limits and where applicable, from premises outside of the corporation limits, which are tributary to the sewer system of the MS4. The MS4 community is regularly inspected by the U.S. EPA to ensure the O&M program for the SCMs are implemented as outlined in the issued permit.

3.3 Local

Stormwater is challenging as municipalities expand, and it is important to focus on reducing the risk of flooding, streambank erosion, and water quality degradation that is caused by stormwater runoff in all watersheds. Local municipalities implement policy to design, construct, inspect, and maintain SCMs to address stormwater management concerns. To carry out the policies, municipalities can develop a process, which includes a design manual to ensure consistency with design standards, inspection, and maintenance requirements, which include as-built surveys, facility inspection and maintenance, and maintenance and access easement requirements to allow for maintenance in and around stormwater facilities. Also, consistency in the inspection procedures, requirements, and approvals is important for a local program to be successful.

3.4 Stormwater Control Measure Inspection During Construction

SCMs for construction are designed to control runoff from construction sites during storm events before being discharged into watercourses, lakes, and/or wetlands. The requirements for construction best management practices (BMPs) are intended to adequately reduce sediment and related pollutants contained in construction stormwater runoff. In general, a Stormwater Pollution Prevention Plan (SWPPP or SWP3) is required for qualifying development sites and must be submitted with the construction plans as part of the development plan approval process (City of Columbus, 2012).

First and foremost, the local stormwater program needs to identify their inspection staff. There are a few different ways to achieve the proper staffing levels:

1. Existing inspectors in the building or utility department,
2. Dedicated postconstruction SCM inspectors,

3. Subconsultants or subcontractors retained by the local stormwater program, and
4. Subconsultants or subcontractors retained by the owner/developer.

The following is a good example of an inspection during the construction process presented in *Managing Stormwater in Your Community: A Guide for Building an Effective Post-Construction Program* (Hirschman & Kosco, 2008).

Before construction, the owner/developer must receive approved plans to construct the SCMs, and all appropriate financial responsibility must be confirmed.

A preconstruction meeting should be held before any construction activity. The meeting should review the SCMs to be installed, critical construction milestones, and the sequence of construction.

Project site visits and inspections should be conducted according to an established inspection schedule. These routine inspections can be conducted on a regular basis (e.g., weekly, biweekly) or at important milestones.

The contractors should be aware of postconstruction features that might need to be protected during site work. Contractors should be aware of both structural and nonstructural SCMs approved for the site.

Many postconstruction SCMs cannot be installed until drainage areas are stabilized with vegetation. Infiltration and bioretention facilities are particularly sensitive to sediment loads during construction. Other postconstruction SCMs, such as ponds, are likely to be converted from erosion control basins, and conversion should take place only after the erosion control phase is complete. The inspector must communicate clearly to the contractor about the timing and scheduling for the installation of postconstruction SCMs. This might take place as different phases of the project are stabilized.

Once site conditions are adequate, per the inspector's verbal or written communication, the contractor should install the postconstruction SCMs according to the approved plans and specifications.

Although inspectors cannot be on site during the entire SCM installation process, it is critical that inspections take place at critical milestones. These milestones might include

- Grading for postconstruction SCMs;
- Modifications to embankments, risers, and spillways;
- Construction of forebays or pretreatment cells;
- Placement of underdrain systems;

- Testing and installation of soil or filtering media; or
- Planting, final grading, final stabilization.

Once SCM installation is complete, as verified by the inspector, the applicant's design consultant prepares an as-built plan for each SCM based on actual site conditions. The inspector and the plan reviewer both sign off on the as-built plan, and any discrepancies are noted.

Once the inspector has confirmed that the SCM is properly installed per the plans and specifications and is in good working order, the relevant portion of the performance bond can be released. It is best to observe and document the operation of an established SCM before releasing any bond.

Once SCM installation is complete, the stormwater program can transfer the project documentation to the appropriate staff to use for the long-term inspection and maintenance.

3.5 Private and Public Parties

There are three general approaches that local programs can use to implement a stormwater maintenance program (Hirschman & Kosco, 2008).

A private maintenance approach consists of private landowners performing both routine maintenance and major structural repairs for SCMs on their property. Placing maintenance responsibility in the hands of individual property owners, homeowners associations, and businesses removes the local program from physically maintaining the SCMs; however, by their state permit, they are accountable and act as an enforcement agency to make sure the private property owners provide continuous maintenance.

A local program maintenance means the local program is responsible for SCM maintenance. This approach is not popular among MS4 communities, primarily because it is costly, it requires extensive staffing, and it presents an administrative burden on the program. This approach, however, has advantages. Enforcement issues can be avoided, and the local program has more control over when and how maintenance takes place. In general, this approach requires local programs to collect and manage detailed information about each SCM, maintain a team of dedicated staff, and secure funding.

A blend of public and private maintenance, the most common approach for local programs, provides maximum flexibility for assigning maintenance responsibilities. Programs using this approach are typically shifting some maintenance activities from homeowners associations and other private parties to local programs because the private entities have proved incapable of performing all maintenance activities. Often, a particular problem or high-profile complaint to elected officials causes the shift to occur.

4.0 PROGRAM DEVELOPMENT

4.1 Overview

This section provides an overview of the elements considered essential in developing a robust program for O&M of SCMs. These apply to any stormwater program, municipal, or Department of Transportation (DOT), but each program is different, and not all elements will necessarily apply to all programs. It is essential to establish and clearly communicate the goals of the program, as well as the means to achieve those. The overall SCM maintenance program will include the extent of program coverage; applicable policies; combined inspection, recordkeeping, and reporting responsibilities for applicable permits; differentiation between routine maintenance activities or those driven by inspections; in-house vs. contracted services; and integration with the municipality's or DOT's overall asset management program. These topics are covered in detail in subsequent chapters of this book.

4.2 Extent and Level of Service

The extent of service (EOS) focuses on the stormwater program as a whole and considers citizen safety and welfare, regulatory requirements, and environmental concerns of the municipality or DOT. For the purposes of this manual, the EOS defines the stormwater system components, such as SCMs, maintained by the municipality or DOT and the jurisdictional areas that fall under the program, such as:

1. SCMs located in municipal or DOT properties and rights-of-way that are owned and operated by that municipality or DOT.
2. SCMs located outside municipal- or DOT-owned properties and rights-of-way but within permanent easements legally accepted by the municipality or DOT.
3. SCMs located outside municipal or DOT-owned properties and rights-of-way but within areas where services are provided to citizens or another entity through a legally binding service agreement.

The level of service (LOS) defines the service quality for an activity, such as the frequency and type of action desired to maintain operation of the stormwater management system in accordance with the EOS. The LOS may be prescribed or guided by the asset management program for routine maintenance, repair, rehabilitation, or replacement for the stormwater system. Annual operation, maintenance, and capital expenditure decisions are determined by the LOS. It is recommended that the EOS/LOS policy be written and approved by the appropriate governing bodies.

4.3 Program Models and Functions

4.3.1 Program Components

Operation and maintenance are a challenge and when not addressed properly can lead to failure of SCMs and high costs associated with restoration. Maintenance plans and strategies will vary depending on the SCMs. Proper maintenance is essential to maximizing the environmental, social, and economic benefits of green infrastructure as well as ensuring that projects perform as expected. Establishing written plans and procedures ensure proper long-term maintenance and are critical components to the success of any green infrastructure project. Below are ways to ensure that SCMs are maintained over the long term.

- Identify Staff Resources for Inspection and Maintenance. A municipality needs to determine if SCM inspections and maintenance can be accomplished with existing staff, if additional staff needs to be hired, if specialized training is needed, or if it would be more cost effective to hire an experienced contractor. Consider which municipal departments have the equipment and skill sets to inspect and maintain specific SCMs (e.g., parks or public works for green infrastructure). Training may be needed for both municipal staff and contractors who perform inspections and maintenance.
- Identify Maintenance Triggers. It is important to identify common problems that require nonroutine maintenance to aid inspectors in the field. Such maintenance triggers include excess sediment accumulation, trash and debris, overgrown vegetation, dead or diseased vegetation, signs of erosion, structural damage, or standing water present more than 72 hours after a rainstorm.
- Update Standard Operating Procedures. If municipalities have standard operating procedures for routine landscape and infrastructure maintenance, they should be updated to incorporate SCM maintenance triggers and remedial actions. Additionally, if contractors are used to maintain practices, include specific language in contracts that require training of maintenance crews. Maintenance schedules should be set for each type of practice, and a tracking system should be in place to ensure that maintenance is performed as prescribed.
- Secure Funding for Maintenance. Maintenance of SCMs is an ongoing need and will require dedicated funding. Sources of funding typically

pursued for green infrastructure projects, such as state and federal grants and loans, cannot be used for ongoing maintenance. Local funding sources such as tax revenue or utility fees can provide a stable source of funding for maintenance of green infrastructure practices.

- Enlist the Help of Volunteers. Some routine maintenance, such as removing trash and weeds from SCMs, can be accomplished by partnering with neighborhood organizations, greenway groups, or garden clubs to leverage their funds/volunteers.
- Procure Equipment. Municipalities and utilities should also consider the equipment needed to maintain SCMs and determine if additional equipment is needed. Most of the necessary equipment is typical of general landscape maintenance, as shown below. Note that heavy equipment is discouraged for routine maintenance because it can cause soil compaction, which reduces the effectiveness of the practices.
- Ordinances. The ordinance is the pillar of a local stormwater program, and it provides legal foundation for all other program elements, including design standards, development review procedures, easement requirements, inspections, maintenance, and enforcement. As a local regulation, the ordinance must have political support, and should remain simple and readable for the widest possible audience.
- Easement and Access. Easements should be provided to the local stormwater program allowing access to operate and maintain the SCMs. If necessary, a property owner shall provide an easement that includes the area of the SCM; its appurtenances, such as forebay(s), benches, risers, outlet pipes; a minimum width around the perimeter of the SCM; and a dedicated access easement that allows access to the SCM from the nearest public right-of-way. For facilities that are owned and maintained by a homeowners association, the local stormwater program shall be given access to the SCM for any infrastructure conveying stormwater to the public storm sewer system. When establishing and agreeing to easement limits, the local stormwater program should keep in mind the type of required maintenance equipment and their ability to maneuver and operate in the easement.
- Long-Term Maintenance Plan. A maintenance plan for SCMs that are to be maintained by an entity other than the local stormwater program (e.g., homeowners association) should be reviewed and approved by the local stormwater program to ensure they meet all the O&M requirements at the time the development plan is approved.

  The maintenance plans can be a standalone document that identifies (1) the entity responsible for inspection and maintenance responsibilities,

(2) maintenance tasks to be performed, (3) inspection and maintenance schedules, and (4) a plan showing all access and maintenance easements.

The following is a list of minimum requirements for SCM maintenance in the City of Columbus, Ohio (2012).

1. Inspection of all permanent structures
2. Debris/clogging control through appropriate removal and disposal
3. Vegetation control (mowing, harvesting, wetland plants)
4. Erosion repair
5. Nonroutine maintenance including pollutant and sediment removal and the "rejuvenation" or replacement of filters and appropriate soils
6. Disposal of collected pollutants, sediments, and filter media in accordance with local, state, and federal regulations
7. Mosquito monitoring and abatement, encompassing inspections for conditions conducive to mosquito breeding, routine (e.g., vegetation control, debris, and sediment removal) and nonroutine (e.g., restoration of grade to eliminate ponding) activities to address these conditions, and conditions where the use of insecticides may be warranted. The insecticides used to control mosquitoes should be non-persistent and biodegradable. It is recommended to use EPA registered insecticides in accordance with product labels.

- Long-Term Maintenance Inspection and Reporting. The owner of the SCMs, its administrators, executors, successors, heirs, or assigns is responsible for maintaining the SCMs in good working condition acceptable to the local stormwater program and in accordance with the schedule of long-term maintenance activities provided in the approved stormwater maintenance plan.

  The local stormwater program must hold the owner of the SCM responsible for performing periodic inspections of the SCMs at a frequency stipulated in the approved stormwater maintenance plan. Inspections shall cover all elements for the stormwater control facility as defined in the stormwater maintenance plan. A maintenance inspection log is to be kept on the property where the SCM is located and be accessible by the local stormwater program upon request, and the Maintenance Inspection Report should be required to be submitted annually to the local stormwater program by the end of each calendar year.

- Monitoring the SCMs. If a local program is going to invest a lot of money, resources, and time into making sure SCMs are designed, constructed, and inspected, they will want to determine if their efforts are working as planned. A crucial part of this process is developing a system that consistently and quantitatively measures the program's performance.

  This iterative process ensures that even if the initial goals established for a program prove to be unachievable, the program can adjust and continue to move forward. In addition, if some actions, projects, or approaches do not achieve their stated aims or are not cost effective, adjustments can be made as the program evolves. This process is necessary to achieve improvements in water quality and aquatic habitats. Finally, it supports the documentation of program efforts, which can be helpful in both annual reporting and regulatory inspection and audit procedures.

Other considerations for a comprehensive maintenance program include

- Distinguishing between routine and inspection-driven maintenance and procedures for each.
- Procedures for handling complaints and emergency maintenance.
- Procedures for proper maintenance of proprietary systems.
- Inspection and maintenance manual for the SCMs approved by the municipality or DOT. For other SCMs, a separate maintenance plan will be necessary.
- Maintenance management system that ties into the overall asset management program for the municipality or DOT.
- Recordkeeping and reporting procedures.

4.3.2 Scoping the Maintenance Program

It is best to understand where the program needs to start, and one of the best ways to do it is to inventory the existing and anticipated future SCMs. An important part of the inventory is assessing the physical and regulatory condition of the system. The physical condition includes the stability and functionality of SCMs and conveyances. The regulatory condition addresses whether SCMs and conveyances are located within easements, have proper maintenance access, and are covered by maintenance agreements or covenants.

Identifying the responsible party for the SCMs is one of the most important policy decisions, and the question may have multiple answers. For instance, the local government or an associated utility may be responsible for SCMs on public land and within public rights-of-way, but maintenance for SCMs on private land may be a shared responsibility. This decision may depend on the status of easements, maintenance agreements, and whether maintenance tasks are aesthetic or structural.

The level of service will need to be defined to determine the frequency and scope of maintenance on each SCM. The level of service may depend on the location, amount of area draining to it, current condition of the SCM, or resident complaints. A process will need to be established to ensure the private or public owner of the SCM knows how to address the level of service and to determine who will handle the structural maintenance versus the routine maintenance. The structural maintenance will typically require heavy equipment to repair outlets, sewers, and catch basins, whereas routine maintenance is removing accumulated trash and debris and managing vegetative growth.

4.4 Program Organization

The stormwater program must work for you, and as such, there are no typical models for how it may be organized. For it to be effective, it is important to have a clear division of responsibilities by departments or division within a municipality or DOT for the main functions that a stormwater program must perform. For example, the stormwater program including the director and key staff may reside within the Watershed Management Department but the Parks Department maintains green infrastructure and the Public Works Department is responsible for maintenance and rehabilitation of the stormwater infrastructure within the public right-of-way. Outside stakeholders, such as a nonprofit foundation, may be responsible for workforce development or maintenance of stormwater infrastructure, such as wetlands and bioretention areas used as public amenities. For DOTs, interjurisdictional agreements with adjacent local governments are frequently needed for maintenance of stormwater infrastructure within the state highways rights-of-way. Such agreements should clearly define the extent and level of service, recordkeeping, and reporting requirements for regulatory compliance or other needs.

4.5 Program Funding

There are currently several sources available for financing stormwater management; however, each currently comes with its own set of benefits and challenges. Common funding mechanisms for stormwater management can include property taxes (e.g., municipal general fund), state and federal grants, bonds, loans, permit fees, and connection fees. The most widely used strategy is the municipal general fund, and while it provides more of an ongoing funding source, it does not account for full contribution of stormwater runoff, nor does it include tax-exempt properties. Grants and loans are often unsustainable and provide only a one-time source of funding. For utilities, stormwater fees are also common sources of funding to support maintenance and are typically based on the amount of impervious surface area on the property as the main contributor of stormwater runoff (Central Massachusetts Regional Planning Commission, n.d.).

Recommendations from the U.S. EPA March 2020 report *Evaluating Stormwater Infrastructure Funding and Financing* include primarily strategies to educate and garner more support for local, regional, and federal stormwater funding.

1. Allocate new federal stormwater funding, which emphasizes the need for more federal investment for stormwater infrastructure given the current and future needs to address failing infrastructure and system stresses as a result of climate change, population increases, and so on.
2. Provide stormwater funding education and technical assistance, which highlights the need to educate the public and elected officials on stormwater funding needs as critical to the successful implementation of and community support for funding solutions.

More innovative financing strategies for stormwater projects have been supported as well, that allow for various economic co-benefits and support from private investment. Such strategies include the following (White-Newsome, 2020):

1. Watershed Improvement Districts, where property owners receive reductions in their drainage charges through offsets from SCM projects built on behalf of the district.
2. Environmental Impact Bonds, private investments that operate on a "pay for success" financing model to help projects achieve environmental and socioeconomic goals.
3. Joint Benefits Authority, a funding mechanism that allows multiple government agencies or departments to jointly plan, implement, and fund projects that produce a range of co-benefits.

Community-based public private partnerships, which are often used for funding of large-scale green infrastructure projects, can also provide additional sources of funding and support a more tangible commitment to long-term maintenance and sustainability of stormwater systems (Lueckenhoff & Brown, 2016).

4.5.1 Stormwater Fees

Stormwater fees are a source of funding for communities to generate a revenue stream to address the increasing investment needed to maintain new SCMs that come with new growth and to meet the demands of repair and maintenance of existing SCMs. A stormwater utility fee is a useful way to fund the needs for SCM inspection and O&M. Stormwater fees are typically levied on landowners based on the potential for their property to generate runoff (e.g., based on the size of the property and the amount of development on the property).

4.5.2 Loans Programs

Some states like the Iowa Department of Natural Resources make SCM loans available as a source of low-cost financing to homeowners, developers, or businesses for long-term/voluntary practices that manage stormwater quality. The applicant must designate and have a commitment from the entity responsible for the long-term maintenance of the stormwater quality practices. Not all state and local government entities provide loans to pay for maintenance activities.

4.5.3 Grant Funding

Although not all grant funding available can be used for O&M for SCMs, federal funding programs, such as the America's Water Infrastructure Act of 2018 amended Section 221 of the CWA, which reauthorized the Sewer Overflow and Stormwater Reuse Municipal Grants program, may be utilized to pay for stormwater capital improvements to free up general funds to pay for SCM O&M.

4.6 Training

One of the major challenges in O&M is developing capacity to maintain the systems. The need to provide adequate training for stormwater for both gray and green systems has allowed for various guidelines, training programs, and opportunities for local workforce development to emerge.

The New York State Department of Environmental Conservation (2017) has identified a stormwater maintenance hierarchy that consists of three tiers of technical responsibility regarding maintaining the various stormwater management practices (SMPs):

1. Level 1: Owners and Untrained Staff
2. Level 2: Trained Municipal Staff
3. Level 3: Qualified Professionals

Level 1 primarily consists of residents, property owners, and managers, homeowners association representatives, interns, volunteers, and so on. This tier represents individuals with no formal and/or limited training for stormwater maintenance activities but who have the capability to complete routine inspections and maintenance activities through available information such as guidance manuals. This level represents the majority of maintenance activities; however, there are more complex maintenance challenges that require Level 2 intervention.

Level 2 consists primarily of municipal and utility employees, and landscape contractors who have completed training on stormwater inspection and O&M. This tier prioritizes routine inspections and maintenance, and responding to specific problems that Level 1 personnel are unable to address.

Level 3 includes professional engineers, landscape architects, plumbers, and other certified professionals who possess specific skills for direct inspection and maintenance of SMPs beyond the capacity of Level 2.

Certification programs like the National Green Infrastructure Certification Program (NGICP) provide training courses and a certification for entry-level workers in the construction, inspection, and maintenance of green stormwater infrastructure based on international best management standards (NGICP, 2020). This type of training prioritizes skills most applicable to Level 2 maintenance personnel. The NGICP is also part of a larger workforce development strategy to provide candidates with at least a high school diploma or equivalent with technical skills in the green workforce to make a livable wage.

5.0 RESILIENCE CONSIDERATIONS IN OPERATIONS AND MAINTENANCE

Climate change effects on stormwater are most associated with the damages experienced through severe flooding, erosion, infrastructure failure, saltwater intrusion, public health, and increased economic costs. While flooding in stormwater has often been the focal point of climate mitigation strategies, focus on water quality through green infrastructure and low-impact development have also been adopted as strategies to combat the effects of climate change.

Most strategies around climate change fall into one of two categories—mitigation or adaptation. Mitigative efforts prioritize preventive measures for addressing climate change such as emissions reduction strategies, or specifically in the case of stormwater, building more green infrastructure and green space to support infiltration. Adaptive strategies involve adjustments to current and future climate effects.

Most strategies to develop resilience in stormwater consider mitigative approaches and relate mostly to land use policy and green infrastructure implementation. Because stormwater maintenance rests at the end of the system's life cycle, the capacity to develop climate resilience is contingent on adopted strategies in the planning and implementation phases of a project. However, there are adaptations to O&M of stormwater that can be considered, including the following:

1. Increased inspections of systems to adjust for capacity and overflows.
2. Hybrid gray-green solutions whereas green infrastructure is incorporated to address on-site treatment in a mostly gray stormwater system.
3. Adopting standards for on-site runoff retention of stormwater.
4. For green infrastructure, using plants (with appropriate research) that are mosquito deterrents to minimize public health risks to certain diseases of which mosquitoes are known vectors.

Additional strategies for building climate resilience of stormwater operations provide nontechnical adaptive measures. These strategies include building local workforce capacity to support increased inspection and maintenance needs, which prioritizes the economic and social dimensions of sustainability that support the environmental and technical aspects of resiliency as well. As climate effects intensify, building social and economic resilience will also prove to be a critical component of managing stormwater systems.

The abovementioned strategies, as previously stated, are intended to support more mitigative approaches to build climate resilience for stormwater. However, the importance of developing resilience at every stage of the system life cycle cannot be overstated, and maintenance adaptations are an equally vital component to building stormwater resilience.

6.0 SAMPLE MAINTENANCE AGREEMENTS

Ensuring proper maintenance of stormwater infrastructure and SCMs is critical for optimizing system performance. Proper maintenance procedures are both system- and site-specific; however, to ensure proper maintenance, maintenance agreements should include several key elements. Key elements of a standard O&M agreement include the following:

1. Responsible party, such as private owners, homeowners associations, a government agency or utility, or another private or public entity.
2. Proof of financial responsibility.
3. Legal description of the real estate and service area for which the agreement applies.
4. Inspection and maintenance agreement signed by the developer or system owner.
5. Location maps showing the location of the property and an accurate location of each stormwater management practice affected by the agreement for owner and municipality to locate systems as needed.
6. Long-term maintenance plan to include a description of the stormwater system and its components, inspection priorities, inspection schedule for each system component, and a schematic for each stormwater system (Indiana Office of Community & Rural Affairs, n.d.).

Additionally, a comprehensive list of the different stormwater systems and SCMs within the service area and the necessary maintenance requirements for each should also be incorporated within this maintenance agreement. This level of specificity provides additional clarity for all parties responsible for the O&M of each system.

The subsequent section includes several sample maintenance agreements that can be used as a reference, including the key elements included for each specific locale in addition to those already highlighted above.

1. Stormwater Equipment Manufacturers Association—Draft Stormwater Maintenance Agreement

   https://stormwater.wef.org/2012/12/swema-draft-maintenance-agreement-for-stormwater-controls/

2. Maricopa County, Arizona

   https://www.maricopa.gov/DocumentCenter/View/6772/Operation-and-Maintenance-Manual-Template-PDF

3. Stormwater Management Practices Maintenance Agreement. (Undated). *Indiana Office of Community and Rural Affairs.*

   https://www.in.gov/ocra/files/Appendix-J-Maintenance-Agreement.pdf

7.0 REFERENCES

Central Massachusetts Regional Planning Commission. (n.d.). *Funding stormwater management: Strategies to support stormwater management at the municipal level.* http://www.cmrpc.org/sites/default/files/Documents/CDAP/stormwater%20wrap%20up_secured.pdf

City of Columbus. (2012). *Stormwater drainage manual.* Department of Public Utilities, Division of Sewerage and Drainage. Columbus, OH.

Hirschman, D., & Kosco, J. (2008). *Managing stormwater in your community: A guide for building an effective post-construction program.* EPA Publication No: 833-R-08-001. Center for Watershed Protection, Ellicott City, MD.

Indiana Office of Community & Rural Affairs. (n.d.). https://www.in.gov/ocra/

Lueckenhoff, D., & Brown, S. (2016, October 13). Financing integrated green stormwater infrastructure to improve community health, resiliency—Getting the best deal for the money! *Bloomberg BNA: Daily Environment Report,* No. 198. https://www.epa.gov/sites/default/files/2016-10/documents/bloomberg_bna_financing_gi_greeninfoct2016.pdf

National Green Infrastructure Certification Program. (2020). About NGICP. https://ngicp.org/about/

New York State Department of Environmental Conservation. (2017). *Maintenance guidance: Stormwater management practices.*

Northeast Ohio Storm Water Training Council. (2017). *Maintaining stormwater control measures: Guidance for private owners & operators.* Burton, OH.

U.S. Environmental Protection Agency. (2020, March 30). *EFAB report: Evaluating stormwater infrastructure funding and financing.* https://www.epa.gov/sites/default/files/2020-04/documents/efab-evaluating_stormwater_infrastructure_funding_and_financing.pdf

White-Newsome, J.L. (2020). Initiative takes on water systems, climate change, and inequity. *Water Online.* https://www.wateronline.com/doc/initiative-takes-on-water-systems-climate-change-and-inequity-0001

3

Design and Construction Maintenance Considerations

1.0 INTRODUCTION 31
2.0 DESIGN CONSIDERATIONS: DESIGN WITH MAINTENANCE IN MIND 35
2.1 Establishing the Functional Performance With Design 35
2.2 The Designer Perspective 36
2.3 Function and Potential Fail Points 39
2.4 Designing for Potential Fail Points 40
3.0 MAINTENANCE NEEDS DURING CONSTRUCTION 40
3.1 Control and Protection Measures 41
3.1.1 Perimeter Controls 42
3.1.2 Surface Controls 44
3.1.3 Enclosed System Control 45
3.1.4 Stabilization Control 46
3.2 Phasing of Construction: Plan, Communicate, Plan 48
3.2.1 Location Considerations 49
3.2.2 Stormwater Control Function and Fail Points 50
3.2.3 Control, Protection, and Sequencing Plan, and Specification Development 51
3.2.4 Construction Timing and Execution Constraints 56
3.3 Construction Responsibilities 58
3.3.1 Construction Responsibilities and Oversight 58
3.3.2 Training of the Construction Worker—Developing Skilled Stormwater Control Measure Labor 59
4.0 REFERENCE 61

1.0 INTRODUCTION

Designing and constructing stormwater control measures (SCMs) requires the consideration of the primary function of the stormwater control and the maintenance needed to preserve that function. Unlike gray infrastructure that is strongest the day it is built, SCMs require routine proactive maintenance tasks to first establish the functional performance and then to continually maintain or improve the performance (Figure 3.1). Without maintenance the function will degrade and ultimately fail. Considering maintenance needs during the design, and then through the development of contract documents for construction, is critical to initially establish the functional performance and set up the infrastructure for success.

Establishing the functional performance of an SCM starts with the data used during design, and the performance calculations used in the design and the input data and drainage information. The designer must reasonably estimate the amount of runoff (volume), the peak discharge rate of the runoff, and the water quality of the runoff to anticipate the effect to the overall function. This, in turn, affects the amount of required maintenance for the SCM. Consider an SCM's contributing area (i.e., watershed), the physical characteristics of that area, and the design rainfall event assumed to fall onto the contributing area (Figure 3.2).

- Existing and future **land use** of the contributing area directly affect the runoff potential. For example, an older residential area in the Midwest will have more grass and leaf material that will accumulate in the stormwater control. The designer should consider the potential clogging of the infiltration function. *What can the designer include to anticipate this future maintenance?*
- The **size and the slope** of the contributing area affect the volume of runoff generated and the rate of the peak discharge. The designer should consider the resulting potential for erosion, and how this volume and rate of runoff could affect the function of the vegetative features. *What can the designer include to anticipate this future maintenance needed to (a) establish the functional performance of the plants, and (b) continually improve the vegetated features?*

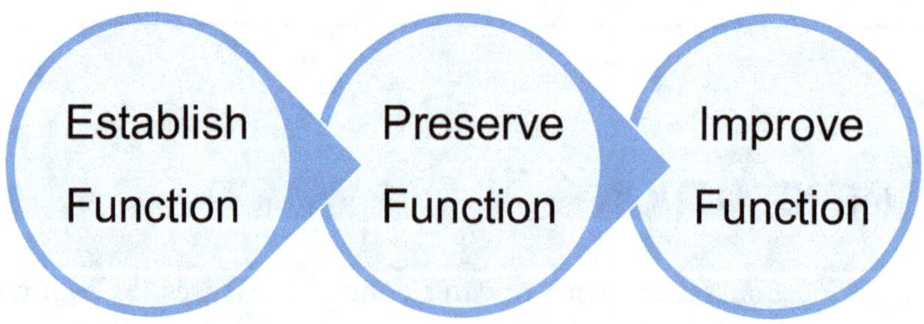

FIGURE 3.1 Expectation of Maintenance Tasks Through Project Life Cycle (Reprinted with permission from Burns & McDonnell Engineering Company, Inc.)

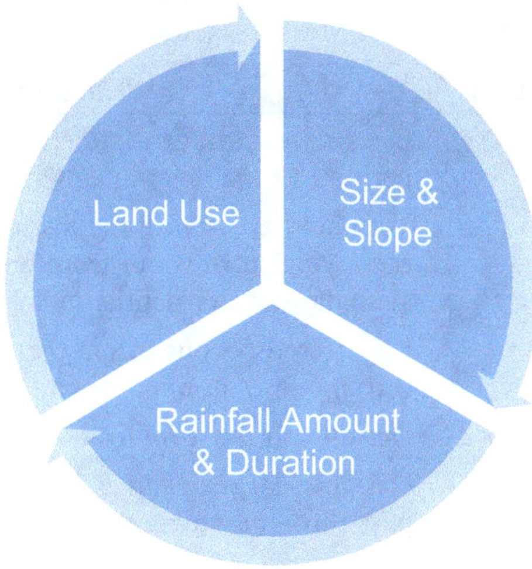

FIGURE 3.2 Key Characteristics of the Contributing Area (Reprinted with permission from Burns & McDonnell Engineering Company, Inc.)

- The **rainfall amount and duration** will determine the size of the stormwater control. The National Oceanic and Atmospheric Administration precipitation frequency data server is a good source of intensity and duration data. For example, designing a stormwater control to a larger rainfall amount could result in increased depth of the control and steeper side slopes to achieve the needed storage volume. The designer should consider how steeper side slopes could slough, generating sediment. The designer should also consider how an increased depth could affect compaction of the bottom soils because of the weight of the impounded water. Both circumstances affect the infiltration function and potentially the water quality function of a water feature. *What can the designer include to anticipate this future maintenance?*

These considerations provide a basis for why it is important to design stormwater controls that capture the right amount of runoff to optimize functional performance. The designer must understand the runoff conditions and quality of the water to plan for maintenance activities that establish the functional performance of the infrastructure.

As established in the Water Environment Federation (WEF) and the American Society of Civil Engineers/Environmental & Water Resources Institute (ASCE/EWRI) manual, *Design of Urban Stormwater Controls* (2012), there are five general categories of stormwater controls that are grouped by common characteristics. They are: (1) Basins, (2) Swales and Strips, (3) Filters, (4) Infiltrators, and (5) Gross Pollutant Traps (GPTs) (see Table 3.1).

TABLE 3.1 Categories of Stormwater Control Measures (Adapted from WEF et al., 2012)

Stormwater Control Measure Category	Definition
Basins	Dry or wet storage that detains stormwater for a period of time that varies with type and design
Swales and Strips	Vegetated areas with the distinct purpose of conveying stormwater from one point to another at shallow water depths
Filters	Engineered porous media that stormwater flows through into an underdrain
Infiltrators	Design volume is infiltrated to the native soil
Gross Pollutant Traps (GPTs)	Designed large openings that allow stormwater to pass through while removing large solids, such as litter, leaves, and plastics

Table 3.1 provides a general definition of the stormwater controls, which is further described in Chapter 4, Section 2.4 of *Design of Urban Stormwater Controls* (WEF et al., 2012).

These general SCM categories can then be regrouped by the primary function that each category provides (Table 3.2), capturing the significant role that this function provides in urban hydrology. The primary function needs to be fully understood to plan, evaluate, and include maintenance considerations in the design phase. These primary functions are:

- Water Features—Retention and ponding of water at the surface
- Infiltration/Filtration—Movement of water through a media or dense vegetation
- Vegetation Features—Plant-soil-water system that sustains vegetation and promotes deep infiltration
- Water Reuse—Temporary storage of runoff for nonpotable uses such as irrigation
- Screening/Hydromechanics—Mechanical screening or hydrodynamic processes

Understanding the primary function allows the designer to optimize stormwater controls to meet water quality and quantity goals for a given application. Considering these aspects in the siting of stormwater controls, a designer can anticipate how these functions could be affected through the construction process and into the establishment of the functional performance. Decisions and practices during construction of the SCM will then be directly affected if that functional performance is established in a means

TABLE 3.2 Relationship Between Primary Function and General Category of Stormwater Control Measure (Reprinted with permission from Burns & McDonnell Engineering Company, Inc.)

Primary Function of Stormwater Control Measure	Category of Stormwater Control Measure				
	Basins	Swales & Strips	Filters	Infiltrators	Gross Pollutant Traps
Water Features	X				
Infiltration/Filtration		X	X	X	
Vegetation Features	X	X		X	
Water Reuse	X		X		X
Screening/Hydromechanics			X		X

that can be preserved and/or improved over time with routine maintenance. Establishing the functional performance of an SCM's primary function is a responsibility held jointly between a designer and a contractor. Design decisions and construction practices must have maintenance in mind.

2.0 DESIGN CONSIDERATIONS: DESIGN WITH MAINTENANCE IN MIND

2.1 Establishing the Functional Performance With Design

Stormwater control measure design requires an approach that anticipates future changes, whether that be land use changes or rainfall pattern changes, to build stormwater infrastructure that is more resilient for the community. This approach must anticipate contributing land area changes and the site-specific maintenance activities that influence the primary function of the SCM.

The designer cannot predict the future or necessarily control construction; however, calculation assumptions and design decisions can be made that reduce the risk of failed function. The functional performance of an SCM is primarily and directly related to its **location**. Consider:

- *How is rainfall runoff getting to the proposed location of the SCM? Is it moving toward the location using the existing land topography? Does it require pipes to convey rainfall runoff to it?* A designer using the topography of the land to bring water to the SCM reduces the dependency on a pipe system for function. The pipe system requires additional maintenance activities.

- *Where does the SCM "sit" in the overall watershed?* If the SCM is at the top of the watershed, or within that "first block," it may be easier for the designer to use that natural topography to collect stormwater. In the middle of the watershed, additional contributing areas converge, and the footprint of the SCM grows. This increased footprint could require additional maintenance activities. For example, how do larger rainfall events bypass the SCM (or does the SCM manage this rainfall)? SCMs in the middle of the watershed begin to blend both at-grade and underground elements to function for a wide range of rainfall events. In the lower portions of the watershed, stormwater has likely already been captured in a pipe system. SCMs built in these locations are designed to manage rainfall runoff that is generated primarily upstream and could be in-line with the pipe and/or channel system, or off-line. These controls are typically more focused on flood control, and not on the most frequent rainfall events.
- *What is the land use today? Tomorrow?* The effect of land use can be estimated through hydrologic calculations, using the most current rainfall data reflective of a respective community's most frequent events and assumptions related to the contributing area's imperviousness. Rainfall design events vary, and the goal for SCMs is typically to design for a range of events. A designer must anticipate the changes upstream in a drainage area, and how that may affect the function of the SCM over time. This may come in the form of considerations for more accessible sediment clean-out points, or vegetation selection based on a community's neighborhood or area plan landscape design requirements.

Assessing location and anticipating the effects of this location on the long-term primary function of the SCM requires the designer to consider the planning, design, construction, and maintenance activities from multiple perspectives (Figure 3.3). It is the designer's responsibility to anticipate these effects to establishing the functional performance of the SCM, and to the routine maintenance activities that will continually preserve and improve the performance of the infrastructure.

2.2 The Designer Perspective

Designers of SCMs have the ultimate challenge. The designer must use the most current available data and information to develop construction documents that will be used by three different audiences over the life of the SCM:

1. An owner, to operate the stormwater infrastructure asset, monitoring the function.

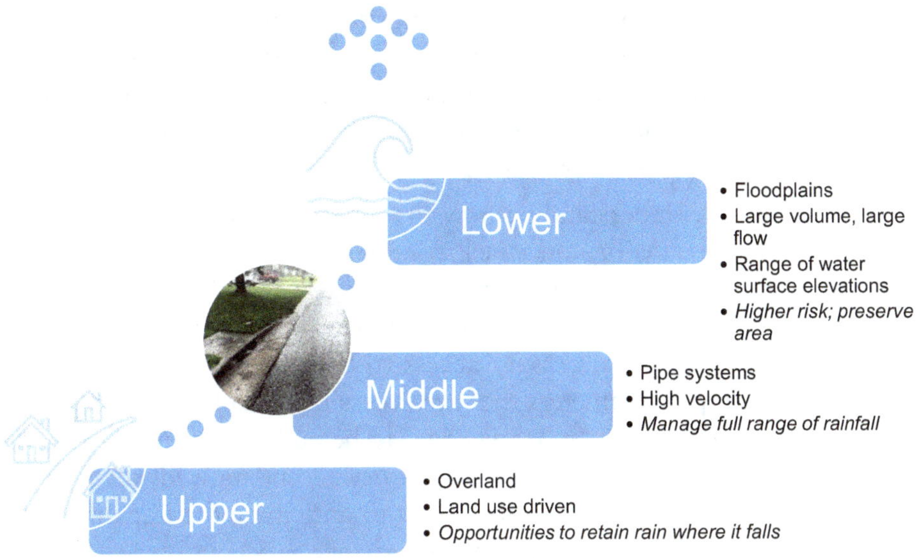

FIGURE 3.3 Functional Performance Relationship to Location (Reprinted with permission from Burns & McDonnell Engineering Company, Inc.)

2. A contractor, to build the stormwater infrastructure, establishing the function.
3. A maintenance team, to perform the day-to-day tasks on stormwater infrastructure assets to preserve and/or improve the function.

This requires a unique perspective; gone are the days when the designer's influence ended at construction. Now, this influence stretches into how the SCM functions through establishment of performance and into long-term management of rainfall events.

Open communication and collaboration between designer and owner. The designer's perspective requires defined decision points from an owner when design begins. These decisions begin with defining anticipated roles and responsibilities for both initial maintenance activities to establish the functional performance and long-term maintenance activities to preserve the function.

- *Example 1.* Understanding how the owner intends to support the establishment and future care of vegetation can help the designer prescribe temporary measures to protect the SCM facility both during construction and at final completion. The designer can be prescriptive, providing guidance for when the temporary measures should be installed and removed, and ideas on how to inspect and supplement these measures to establish the performance of the primary function. Developing appropriate tools to support these measures, such as a maintenance manual, or mapping references, can be planned for by the designer and developed in a manner that supports the owner's operation of the infrastructure.

- *Example 2.* Understanding how the owner intends to perform long-term, routine maintenance tasks, and what those tasks are, assists the designer in identifying critical components where these tasks are necessary to preserve and enhance the function of the SCM. This could include designing necessary access to below-grade components, or specifying pipe diameters that are accessible with the owner's equipment. Or, defining a "mowing edge" to be built, to ultimately help the maintenance team define areas that need to be mowed, versus areas to be left alone. The designer needs to anticipate these maintenance activities and work directly with the owner to account for each activity in the design, and how this maintenance activity would be communicated through the owner to the maintenance team.
- *Example 3.* Understanding how the owner intends to monitor and inspect activities during construction, and the role of the contract documents in these activities, will assist the designer in developing drawings and specifications to assist the contractor in building this functional performance. The designer needs to understand the balance of allowing flexibility versus being prescriptive. The designer also needs to understand and be familiar with product and material availability, and how each would be sourced by the contractor, stored during construction, and then phasing of placement. Even with limited contractor experience in building SCMs, the designer can communicate the importance that primary function plays through the contract documents, and the attention to detail in development of these documents.

The roles and responsibilities of maintenance tasks for SCMs do not begin with final completion of the project; on the contrary, these tasks begin during the construction process to establish the functional performance. Therefore, it is vital that the contractor understand how use of the site during construction, and construction means and methods ultimately influence the function of the SCM. The designer can specify some items in the construction documents to assist in communicating the criticality of protecting the SCM; for example, a focus on controlling erosion and sediment on the interior of a site by providing recommended phasing of construction and phased erosion and sediment control plan sheets. Or, identifying areas where heavy equipment cannot be driven. Or, even more critical, providing detailed material specifications for the SCM components, to contractually guide sourcing, delivery, storage, placement, and inspection at the project site.

2.3 Function and Potential Fail Points

Primary function is the common characteristic that groups various SCMs together. During the design stage, potential fail points where this primary function would be compromised should be identified by the designer. Potential fail points are often most readily identified through the specific site-design characteristics for the SCM. These characteristics include

- ***Retaining water.*** A site designed to retain water likely manages a larger contributing area, which presents its own challenges when considering fail points. A designer must consider how water is conveyed to the SCM, as well as the components that provide for this permanent pool to function. For a wetland, special consideration should be paid to the nuances of establishing the vegetation in this permanent pool, as it is critical to the ***water feature's*** function. The volume of stormwater and what is carried in that runoff (e.g., sediment and fine aggregate) are critical management points for the designer to manage during construction through both temporary and permanent design measures.
- ***Infiltration or filtration.*** The primary function of SCMs that either **infiltrate or filtrate** is that water must "move through" the facility. A designer must consider how this "movement" could be affected during construction, most typically by the quality of the material installed, which is governed by the material specification. The secondary consideration affecting that primary function during construction is protecting that "movement" by considering what is carried in the stormwater runoff (sediment and fines) conveyed to the SCM.
- ***Establish thriving vegetation.*** For SCMs with **vegetation**, the establishment of the vegetation and maintenance of these features are critical to the function of the facility. The designer must consider how to effectively plan for and manage the planting windows and plant-species-specific establishment to provide maximum functional performance. The vegetation plays an integral role in deep infiltration through matured root systems, and uptake through evapotranspiration, working with the soil, aggregate, and piping systems. Therefore, designing to promote to growth of these root systems is essential. For root systems to establish maturity, it is important to control invasive species whose shallow roots can inhibit this growth and "choke out" the preferred plant.

- ***Reusing Water.*** Water collected by SCMs, such as in cisterns or rain barrels, may present the opportunity to reuse for irrigation of other vegetated features on the site, or other nonpotable uses if allowed by regulations. The designer should consider the volume of stormwater in these applications, and how this range and fluctuation can be managed by the facility. The schedule for installation of these facilities may be a key consideration during the construction process, as coordination between a building contractor and a site contractor is necessary to optimize function.
- ***Screening/Hydromechanics.*** Mechanical SCMs can provide specialized treatment and removal of sediment and/or fines, as well as other constituents that may be unique to a given site. These SCMs can also be located at the downstream point in a system, providing treatment before discharging to a water body. For some of these SCMs, the volume of runoff is directly tied to how the system functions; for others, the regular maintenance is critical to retain the screening and filtering function of these facilities. A designer must consider when the primary function of these SCMs needs to be online related to other functions of the site and consider temporary measures that might be needed to preserve that function.

2.4 Designing for Potential Fail Points

Designing for these potential fail points requires the primary function of the SCM to be the continued focus. Designers should approach this by evaluating function at the site and through the watershed in two ways: (1) *Anticipate* these fail points and *incorporate* preferred methods of addressing in a phased approach in construction documents; and (2) *Anticipate* the temporary and long-term maintenance needs during construction to retain the function of these critical features. Design, specification, and communication of adequate stormwater control and protection are essential in preserving the primary function of SCMs during construction.

3.0 MAINTENANCE NEEDS DURING CONSTRUCTION

Construction is almost always unpredictable. As designers it is easy to fall into the trap of planning for the ideal scenario but failing to consider the realities of practical construction means and methods that make this ideal nearly impossible to achieve. For instance, most SCM specifications that currently exist contain a blanket statement to divert stormwater from an SCM until the upstream area is fully stabilized. While this is certainly the most preferable case, it is not always practical when taking into consideration the location, natural topography, contributing area, climate, and weather conditions that affect other construction activities around the SCM. In this case, specification of stormwater control and protection measures and appropriate sequencing of construction becomes a critical step to transition from design to construction reality.

While the plans and specifications that make up the construction documents are indisputably the most critical communication tool between the designer and the contractor, it is equally as important for the two parties to communicate and coordinate the nuances of the design so that expectations and interpretations of the construction documents are clear from the start. This requires planning, communicating, and replanning throughout the construction period. This planning process must take into consideration the location, the primary function, and possible fail points of the SCM and its components, the constraints of construction timing, and execution means/methods.

It is important to understand the roles and responsibilities for each aspect of a construction phasing plan and schedule. This means understanding the role of the prime contractor, their subcontractors, and the transition points between the work of each of those parties. This may require training and education for all the contractors and subcontractors that will be working in or around the SCM. It also means having clear communication and authority expectations between the contractor and those overseeing the work—whether that is the owner, inspector, or designer.

Ultimately, the goal of this concerted effort is to construct, protect, and maintain the SCM and its components effectively to establish the system's initial primary functional performance. The following subsections will discuss control and protection measures, phasing of construction, and construction responsibilities to assist in achieving this goal. Construction is the responsibility of the contractor and the designer, planning for and implementing both temporary and permanent maintenance measures to establish the SCM's functional performance.

3.1 Control and Protection Measures

The control and protection of the SCM components from the beginning of construction until the system is fully established is the primary maintenance need, setting the facility up for success. Stormwater control and protection is not a new concept for the design and construction industry. U.S. Environmental Protection Agency Clean Water Act requirements have regulated stormwater runoff from construction sites using erosion and sediment control measures under the National Pollutant Discharge and Elimination System program since 1987. However, the way those measures can be applied to protect SCMs during construction requires a different perspective. Traditional erosion and sediment control practices focus on managing stormwater runoff that is *leaving* the construction site. Control and protection measures address management of erosion and sediment *within* the construction site, protecting that primary function of the SCM.

One of the leading causes of failure for an SCM is clogging of the aggregate, soil, or piping components of the system *during* construction activities, compromising the establishment of the functional performance of **infiltration or filtration** and **vegetation features**. Erosion and sediment control measures can be utilized within and around the SCM to protect these components during construction. The location and layout of the site before, during, and after construction will dictate the type or combination of measures that are most appropriate, as well as "when" and "how" the measures are implemented. These measures can be anticipated during design, and then refined and adapted during construction.

3.1.1 Perimeter Controls

Perimeter controls establish a physical barrier around the footprint of the SCM to block stormwater and/or catch soil and sediment to limit clogging and damage to the SCM components. Multiple perimeter controls can be applied together to provide more resilient defense from failure. Some common types of perimeter controls include

- ***Silt Fence:*** one of the most common types of erosion and sediment control consisting of a vertical barrier of geotextile fabric placed around the perimeter of the SCM. It is important that the silt fence be properly trenched and anchored to prevent bypass under the perimeter (Figure 3.4).
- ***Erosion Control Logs:*** also commonly referred to as wattles, a form of inlet protection that can be applied linearly around the perimeter of the SCM to block loose soil, sediment, and debris. Common types of erosion control logs include coconut coir, straw, wood, and compost-filled filter socks (Figure 3.5).
- ***Soil Berm:*** construction of a temporary compacted soil berm around the perimeter of the SCM to divert water around the site. Soil berms are most appropriate for sites designed primarily offline with an alternative drainage path around and downstream of the facility. Soil berms are likely not sufficient for SCMs in sump conditions or along

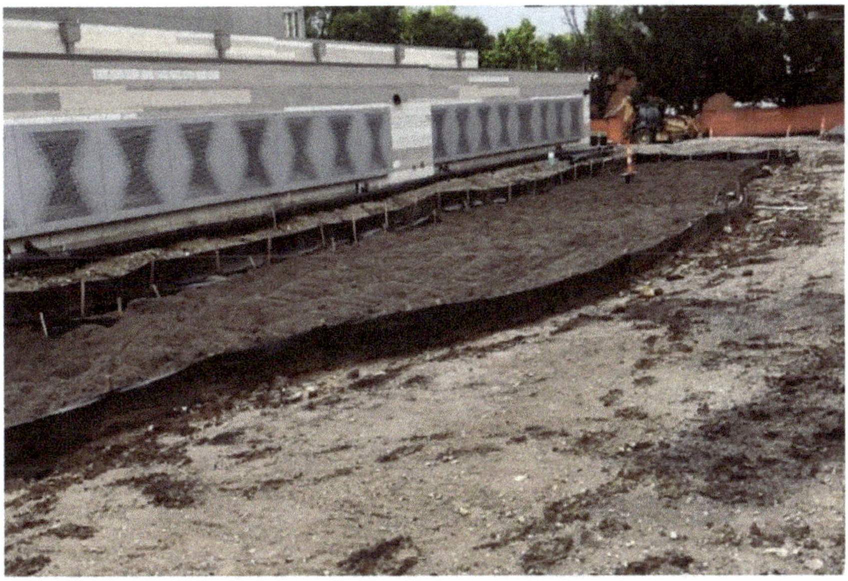

FIGURE 3.4 Silt Fence Perimeter Control Example for Stormwater Control Measure Control and Protection (Reprinted with permission from Burns & McDonnell Engineering Company, Inc.)

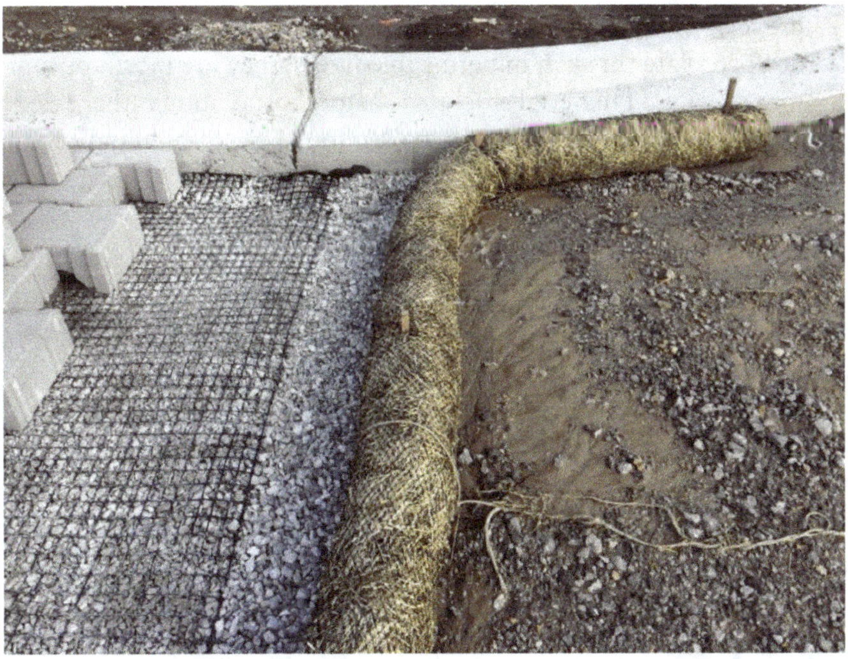

FIGURE 3.5 Erosion Control Log Perimeter Control Example for Stormwater Control Measure Control and Protection (Reprinted with permission from Burns & McDonnell Engineering Company, Inc.)

the primary overland drainage path that will experience higher stormwater flows that risk overtopping or failure of the soil berm.

3.1.2 Surface Controls

Surface control practices are temporary permeable or impermeable coverings to protect the soil and or aggregate material while exposed and vulnerable during construction. Because permeable and impermeable liners are commonly used as a component of the SCM design, it is typically a readily available, inexpensive solution for control and protection. Liners should be staked or anchored into the surrounding soil, such that debris is not able to pass underneath the protective cover. While numerous manufactured products exist that are suitable for surface control applications, they are generally categorized as permeable (geotextile) or impermeable liners:

- ***Permeable Liner:*** a geotextile that allows water to percolate through the liner while filtering sediment to protect the underlying media (Figure 3.6). Permeable liners (geotextile) can be temporarily placed over the surface of aggregate or soil media to protect it until the next layer or vegetation is ready to place.
- ***Impermeable Liner:*** impermeable membrane, or geomembrane that prevents water from migrating through the liner. Because water cannot percolate through impermeable liners, they are most appropriate for covering of material stockpiles before installation rather than covering the SCM surface postinstallation, to avoid ponding of stormwater on the surface.

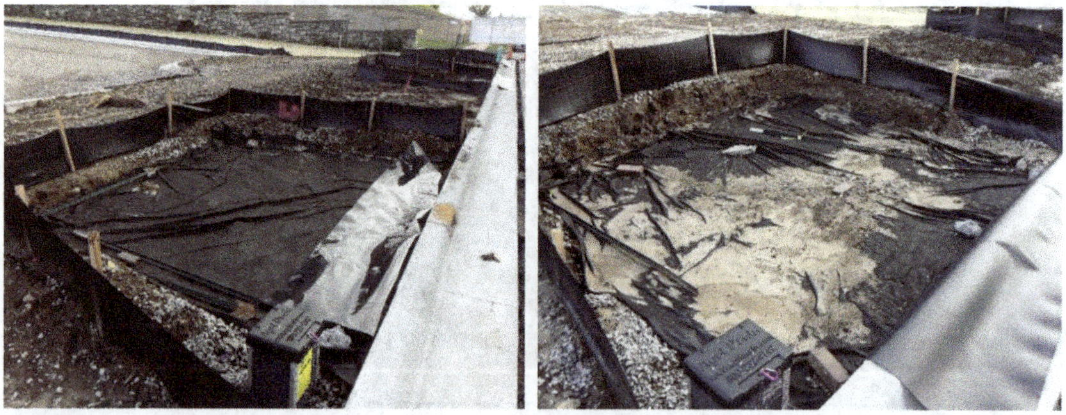

FIGURE 3.6 Permeable Liner (Geotextile) Surface Control Example for Stormwater Control Measure Control and Protection (Reprinted with permission from Burns & McDonnell Engineering Company, Inc.)

3.1.3 Enclosed System Control

Stormwater management for enclosed systems discharging to an SCM can be achieved by providing control and protection at inlet and outlet points, or temporary diversion of flows around the SCM:

- ***Inlet Protection:*** prevents sediment from entering an enclosed storm system by filtering runoff before entering the inlet. Erosion control logs discussed in Section 3.1.1 are all forms of traditional inlet control measures.
- ***Bypass Piping:*** temporary pipe extending from the outlet point of the enclosed system contributing to the SCM and discharging to an appropriate location downstream (Figure 3.7). Bypass piping for a subsurface enclosed system typically includes temporary connections to existing drainage systems not connected to the SCM. Surface systems, such as roof drains and discharging storm sewers at the surface, can connect flexible piping to the discharge point that extends around and downstream of the SCM.

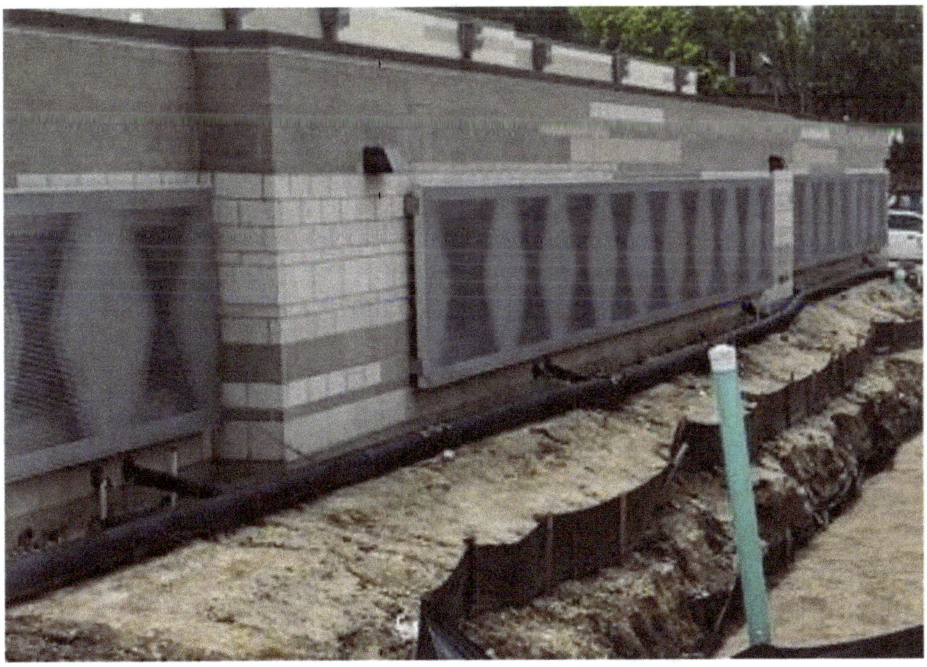

FIGURE 3.7 Bypass Piping Enclosed System Control Example for Stormwater Control Measure Control and Protection (Reprinted with permission from Burns & McDonnell Engineering Company, Inc.)

- ***Weir Plate***: temporary plate installed at the end of the enclosed pipe system to limit the velocity and quantity of stormwater reaching the SCM during construction (Figure 3.8).

3.1.4 Stabilization Control

This type of control is appropriate for establishment of temporary or permanent vegetation immediately surrounding the SCM. It is highly recommended to implement perimeter controls around the SCM in conjunction with stabilization controls. The following are common examples of stabilization controls:

- ***Ground Covers:*** protective layer applied to the soil surface for the establishment of temporary or permanent vegetation (Figure 3.9). Typical ground covers include straw, compost, and various mulches.
- ***Hydraulic Applications:*** homogenous application of soil amendments, mulch, tackifying agents, bonded fiber matrix, and liquid co-polymers onto soil (Figure 3.10).

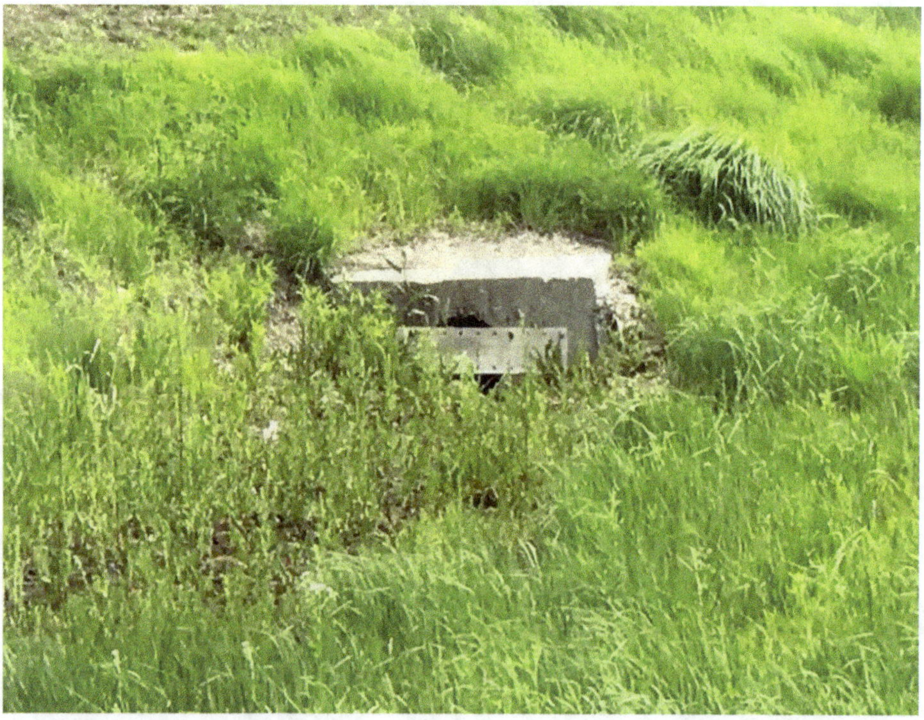

FIGURE 3.8 Weir Plate Enclosed System Control Example for Stormwater Control Measure Control and Protection (Reprinted with permission from Burns & McDonnell Engineering Company, Inc.)

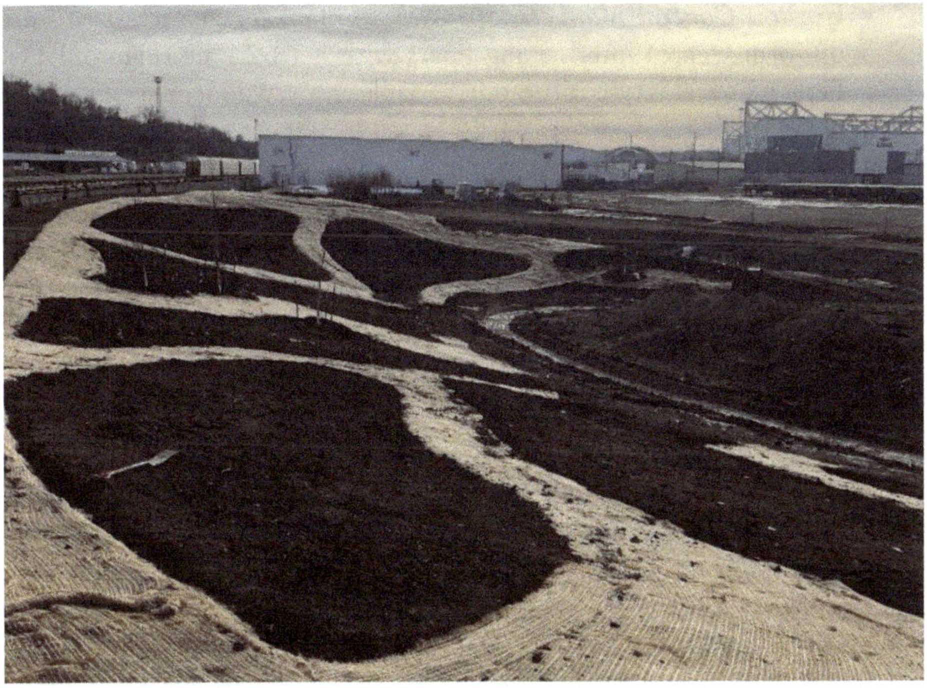

FIGURE 3.9 Ground Cover Stabilization Control Example for Stormwater Control Measure Control and Protection (Reprinted with permission from Burns & McDonnell Engineering Company, Inc.)

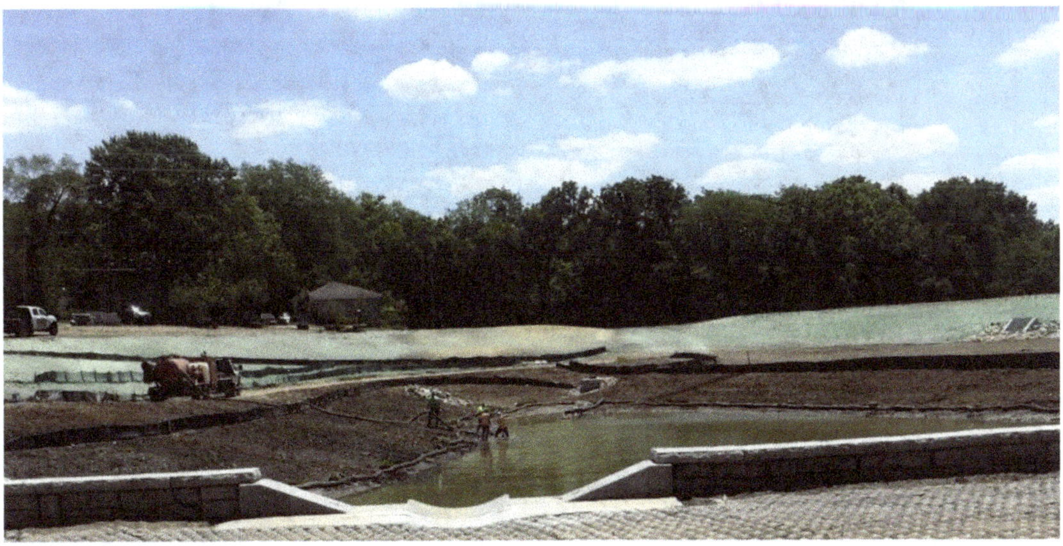

FIGURE 3.10 Hydraulic Application Stabilization Control Example for Stormwater Control Measure Control and Protection (Reprinted with permission from Burns & McDonnell Engineering Company, Inc.)

- ***Erosion Control Blankets:*** open-weave blankets characterized by a uniform web of interlocking fibers with net backing (Figure 3.11). Fiber material is typically biodegradable straw, wood, or coconut fiber material.
- ***Turf-Reinforcement Mats (TRMs):*** three-dimensional synthetic fiber mats used for permanent soil stabilization. TRMs may include biodegradable components, but typically are nondegradable because of the synthetic fibers, filaments, nettings, and/or wire mesh that are processed into the three-dimensional reinforcement matrix.

3.2 Phasing of Construction: Plan, Communicate, Plan

As part of the construction plans, the designer should develop a control and protection plan specific to the project's SCM. The control and protection plan should specify the critical areas for continued protection during construction as well as sequencing of construction all while keeping the establishment of the functional performance in mind. The plan must take into consideration the **location** and site layout of the SCM as well as its primary

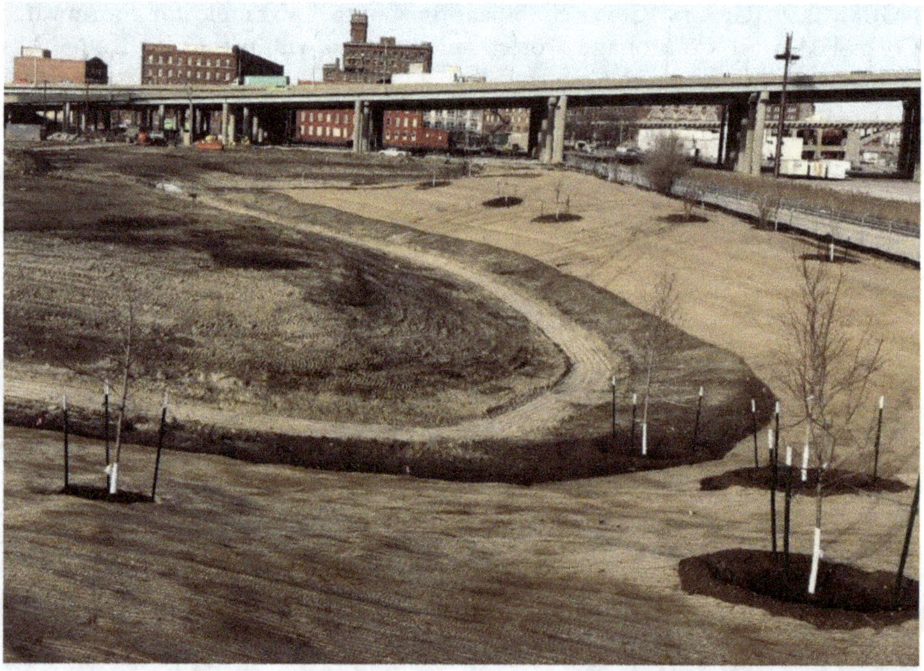

FIGURE 3.11 Erosion Control Blanket Stabilization Control Example for Stormwater Control Measure Control and Protection (Reprinted with permission from Burns & McDonnell Engineering Company, Inc.)

function and fail points. These plans will serve as the initial discussion point between the designer and contractor during the preconstruction phase.

The preconstruction phase is the time for the designer, contractor, and owner to collaborate on the plan and sequencing requirements, potential issues or roadblocks related to construction schedule, and means and methods, and how best to mitigate those issues without affecting the function of the SCM. Communication and willingness to adapt to each other's considerations and constraints is key. It is critical during this phase to also engage the subcontractors for the project in construction conversations, specifically, the crews that will be doing the work on the SCM. This may require multiple methods and meetings to educate the work site on the intended function of these features. This focus on communication and planning at the onset of construction is critical in building an SCM project, where constructing to the details and specifications are instrumental in the success of the facility.

3.2.1 Location Considerations

Just as the designer must anticipate future changes when considering the functional design of the stormwater control, the function must also be considered when defining the phasing of its construction. Determining the ideal sequencing and scheduling of activities for construction of the SCM requires the same thought process as the detailed design, only this time the designer must consider the implications and function *before* the SCM is completed. This means taking into consideration how the location and function of the *individual* components of the stormwater control may be affected by the contributing area and construction activity before they have the stability to function as a system. The key consideration here is developing a plan for minimizing the amount of stormwater and sediment reaching the SCM. Revisiting the location considerations from a preconstruction perspective can assist in this process:

- *How is rainfall runoff getting to the proposed location of the stormwater control before construction begins?* If the existing natural topography allows stormwater to naturally collect at the site, the designer's approach to controlling these effects will differ than if stormwater will ultimately be piped to the SCM. If the site receives overland flow, the designer should plan for more perimeter-type controls to protect the site. Whereas, if the stormwater is conveyed via an existing or future piped system, flows can be diverted using enclosed system controls.

- *Where does the SCM "sit" in the overall watershed?* The amount of stormwater the control measure is designed to receive will play a significant role in the frequency at which control and protection measures need to be maintained and replaced. A site receiving higher velocity runoff and larger quantities of flow will require more substantial control measures and more frequent maintenance.
- *What is the land use today? Tomorrow?* The type and stability of the contributing area affects the type and amount of detrimental material that may reach the site during construction. For a roadside application with curbing, more simple inlet control measures may be sufficient to block trash and sediment coming from the street. Whereas, for a large open site with more mass grading needs will likely require perimeter, surface, and stabilization controls. In an older urban area, sedimentation may also be a result of asphalt or concrete degradation.

The movement of stormwater runoff to the stormwater control, the stability and type of land it is running over, and the amount of stormwater reaching the site before and during construction are the primary factors affecting the type and frequency of control and protection measures needed. However, the need for higher and lower level of protection varies when considering the primary function of the SCM and the fail points that can be detrimental to that long-term function.

3.2.2 Stormwater Control Function and Fail Points

The function and fail points of each type of SCM require different considerations for control and protection, sequencing, and maintenance needs during construction. For instance, infiltrators and filters are highly sensitive to compaction and sedimentation, while basins with permanent pool features likely require compaction for proper retention capabilities. These factors all contribute to considerations in development of the control and protection plan and in construction sequencing.

Water Features. Typical design elements of SCMs containing water features and associated control, protection, and sequencing considerations for each are shown in Figure 3.12.

Infiltration/Filtration. Typical design elements of infiltration/filtration type SCMs and associated control, protection, and sequencing considerations for each are shown in Figure 3.13.

Vegetation Features. Typical design elements of SCMs with vegetation features and associated control, protection, and sequencing considerations for each are shown in Figure 3.14.

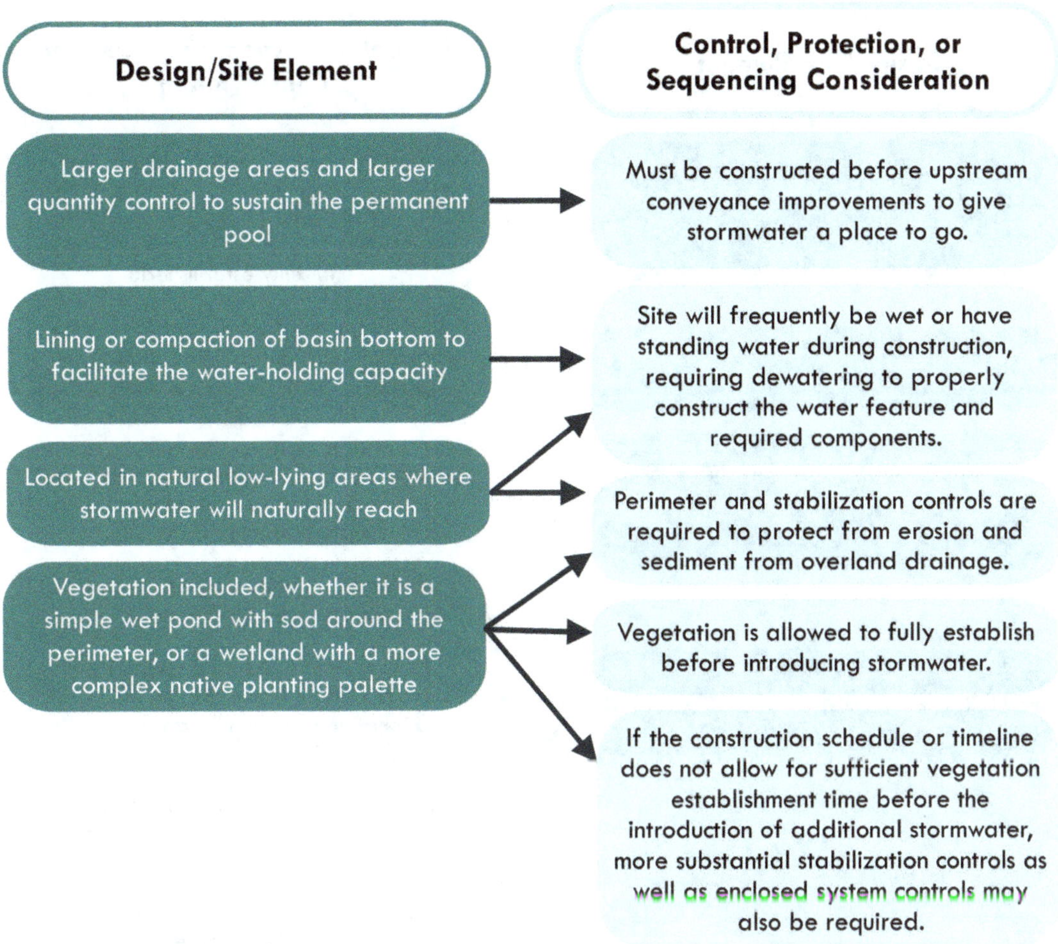

FIGURE 3.12 Water Features Primary Function: Control, Protection, and Sequencing Considerations (Reprinted with permission from Burns & McDonnell Engineering Company, Inc.)

Water Reuse. Typical design elements of water reuse features and associated control, protection, and sequencing considerations for each are shown in Figure 3.15.

Screening/Hydromechanics. Typical design elements of SCMs with screening/hydromechanics features and associated control, protection, and sequencing considerations for each are shown in Figure 3.16.

3.2.3 Control, Protection, and Sequencing Plan, and Specification Development

The construction drawings and technical specifications represent the contractual requirements the contractor commits to with their bid. Because of

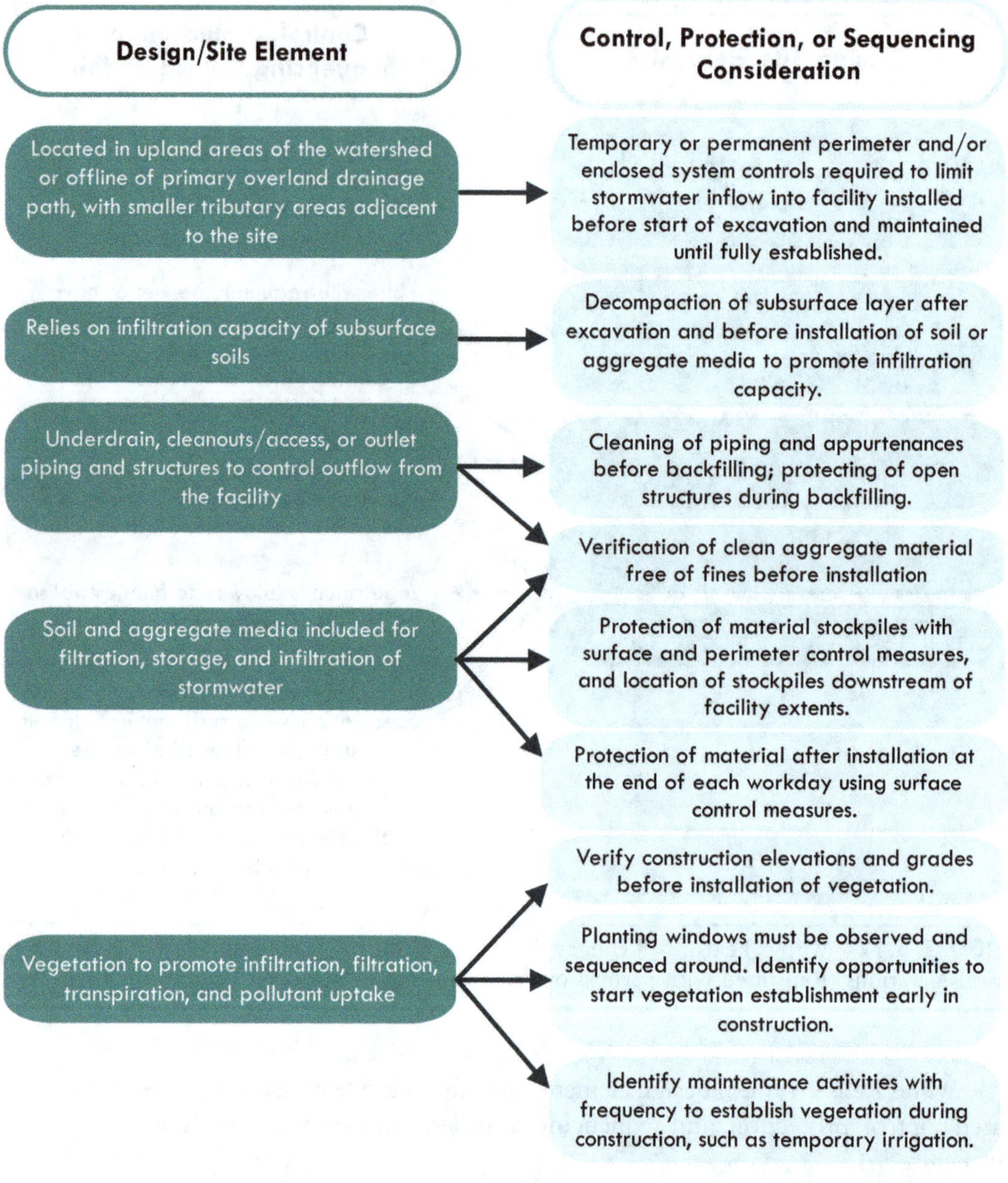

FIGURE 3.13 Infiltration/Filtration Primary Function: Control, Protection, and Sequencing Considerations (Reprinted with permission from Burns & McDonnell Engineering Company, Inc.)

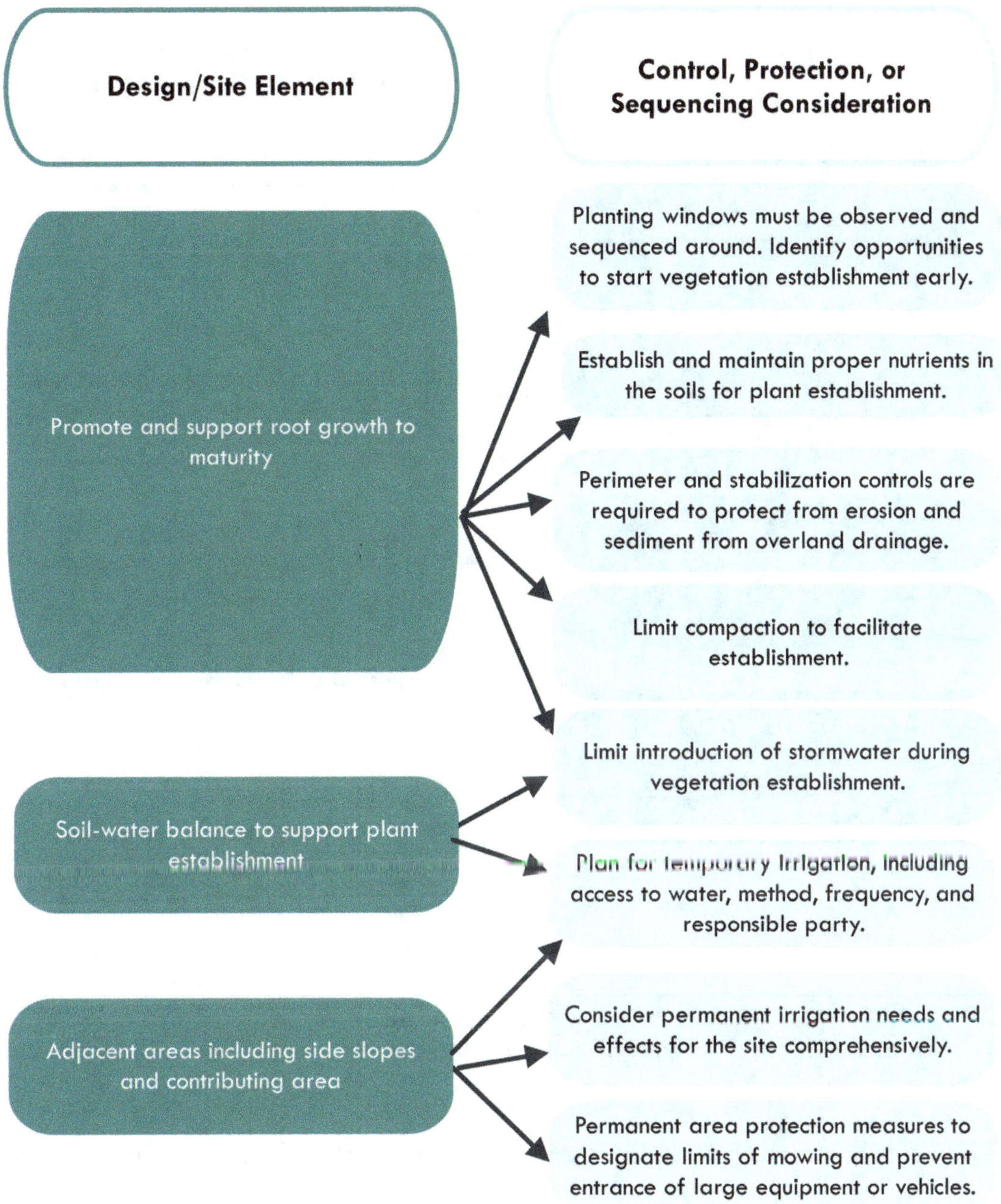

FIGURE 3.14 Vegetation Features Primary Function: Control, Protection, and Sequencing Considerations (Reprinted with permission from Burns & McDonnell Engineering Company, Inc.)

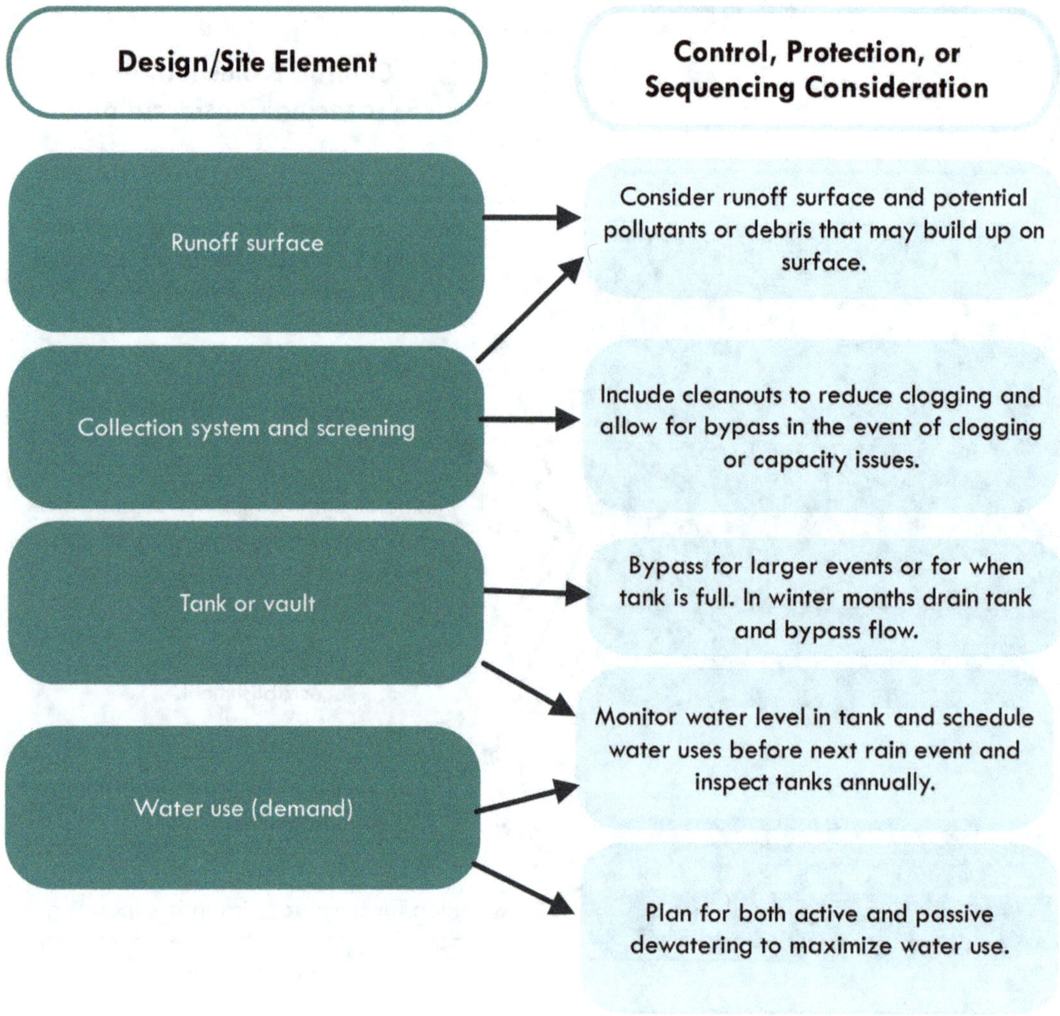

FIGURE 3.15 Water Reuse Primary Function: Control, Protection, and Sequencing Considerations (Reprinted with permission from Burns & McDonnell Engineering Company, Inc.)

this, it is recommended to include a control, protection, and sequencing plan as part of these contract documents.

The control and protection plan should provide the contractor with information on the key SCM areas and components requiring protection during construction, the type of protection that is expected and acceptable, and the requirements for installation, replacement, and removal of those measures. This is also an ideal location to include sequencing and construction phasing requirements, as related to the SCM and the surrounding improvements. Figure 3.17 provides recommended items to include, at a minimum, on the control and protection plan.

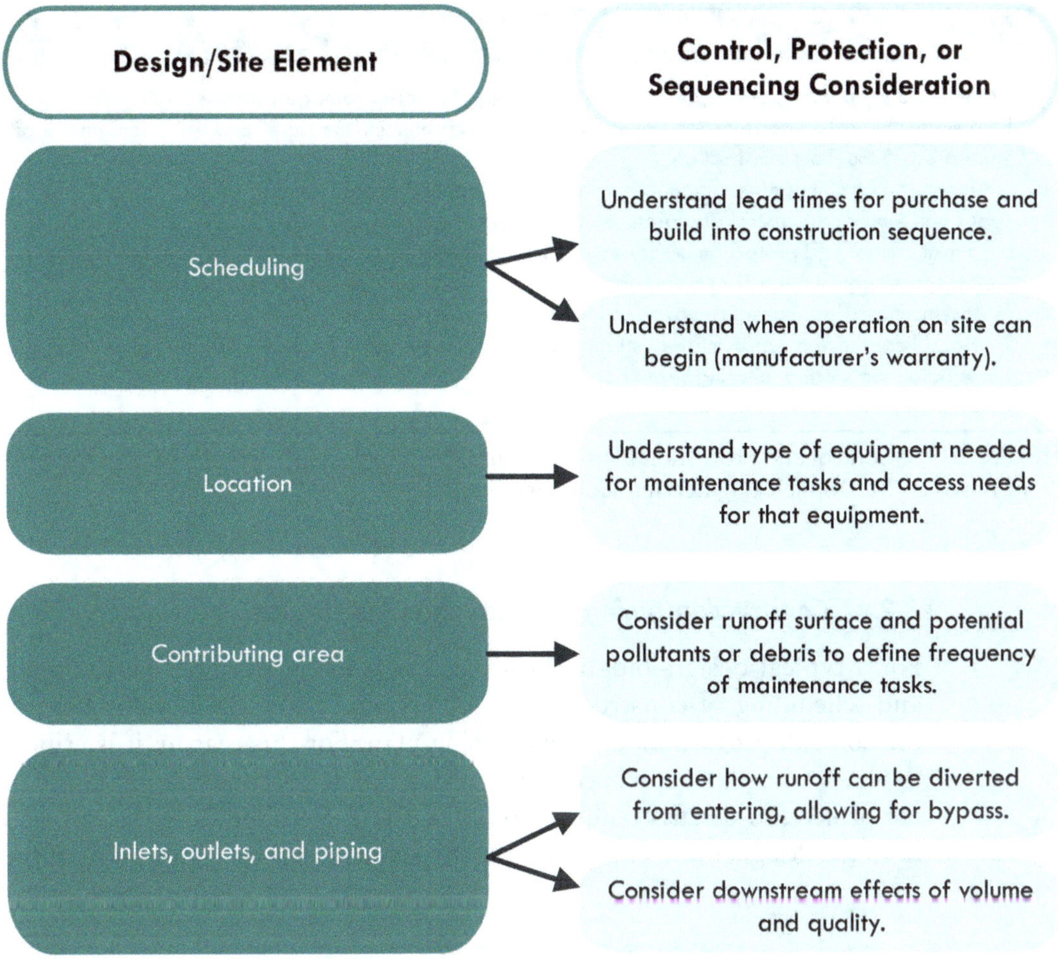

FIGURE 3.16 Screening/Hydromechanics Primary Function: Control, Protection, and Sequencing Considerations (Reprinted with permission from Burns & McDonnell Engineering Company, Inc.)

The construction specifications provide the opportunity for the designer to include more detail on the material, installation, and maintenance requirements of the control and protection measures. Additionally, this is where the designer can include submittal requirements for any items that require verification before, during, and following construction, setting the expectation for the contractor. Figure 3.18 provides recommended items to include in the control and protection specifications.

While the plans and specifications are important for defining contractual obligations of the contractor, it is also essential for these to be adaptive, leaving room for modifications and additional control requirements that are likely to be needed when construction requires a change of course.

Control & Protection Plan

- Existing and proposed topographic information to fully illustrate drainage patterns on the site
- Stormwater control measure areas requiring control and protection measures and limitations on use of those areas throughout construction
- Stormwater control measure components requiring control and protection measures
- Types and location of control and protection measures required
- Details of control and protection measures required, including acceptable material and installation
- Maintenance requirements for control and protection measures, including timing for installation, replacement, and permanent removal
- Tree and vegetative areas outside of stormwater control measure to be protected during construction
- Construction sequencing/phasing requirements

FIGURE 3.17 Control and Protection Plan Minimum Requirements (Reprinted with permission from Burns & McDonnell Engineering Company, Inc.)

3.2.4 Construction Timing and Execution Constraints

For a typical design–bid–build project, it is likely that the exact timing and scheduling of construction is not known during the development of the control, protection, and sequencing plan. For this reason, it is critical to review the plans and specifications during the preconstruction phase of the project, to discuss realistic conditions and considerations for the site. Both the designer and contractor perspective are critical at this point of the

Control & Protection Specifications

- Purpose of the specification section to provide control of stormwater collection, conveyance, and runoff to the stormwater control measure installations within the site and to protect the stormwater control measure during construction and through establishment and maintenance periods
- Definitions or designations for acceptable (and unacceptable) uses of the stormwater control measure areas during construction, including requirements for mitigation of the areas if damaged, compacted, or contaminated
- Material requirements for acceptable control and protection measures to be used,
- Site preparation and installation requirements for control and protection measures to be used
- Requirements for maintenance and disposal of control and protection materials throughout construction
- Submittal requirements for control and protection measures such as stormwater control measure specific construction schedules, a runoff management plan for stormwater on the site, and a site access and utilization plan

FIGURE 3.18 Control and Protection Specification Minimum Requirements (Reprinted with permission from Burns & McDonnell Engineering Company, Inc.)

project's life cycle. The best thing a designer can do at the beginning of construction is to develop a relationship with the contractor that acknowledges each party's strengths: the designer knows the intended function and critical components of the SCM better than anyone; the contractor knows the ins and outs of how to actually build the components, and the constraints that go along with construction. Plan based on the optimal conditions for the establishment of the functional performance of the stormwater control, communicate that plan with the contractor before construction begins, allow the contractor to in turn communicate their plan for construction, and finally identify where the designer and contractor sequencing plans contradict. It is essential that the designer communicate the critical design and fail points of the system in a way that is meaningful to the contractor. It is equally as important that the designer consider the contractor's means and methods for what is practical for the site. With the expertise of both parties in mind, replan based on the reality of the constraints at hand. The most common timing and executing constraints during construction include access to the site, low and high temperatures appropriate for different aspects of the work, appropriate planting windows for the vegetation specified, and the effect and amount of rain during the regional wet season (Figure 3.19).

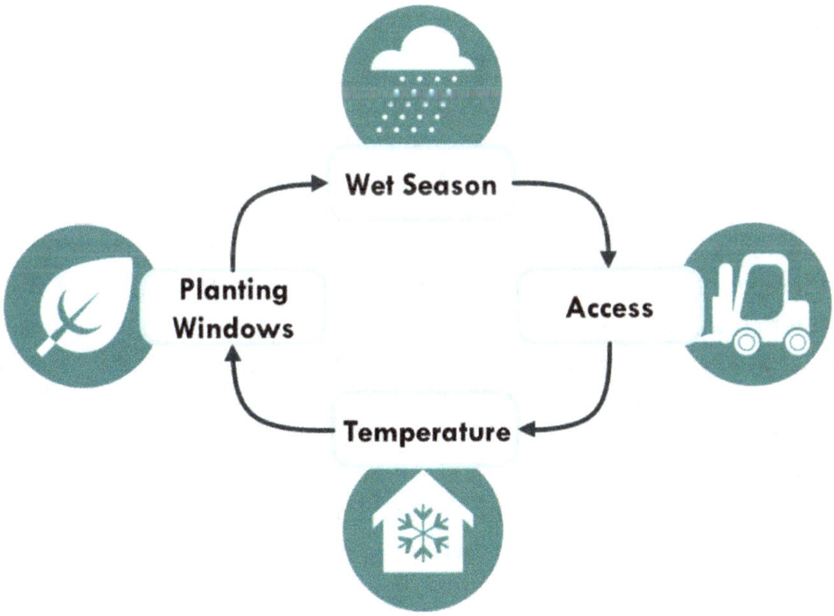

FIGURE 3.19 Construction Timing and Execution Constraints (Reprinted with permission from Burns & McDonnell Engineering Company, Inc.)

3.3 Construction Responsibilities

Execution of a construction project often takes an army. Clear expectation and roles for the contractor, subcontractor, owner, inspector, and designer need to be clearly defined at the start of construction. It is critical that the entire team address the following:

1. Who is responsible for each aspect of the work?
2. Which team members have the required training and experience to perform the work?
3. Which team members have the required training and experience to oversee the work?
4. Who coordinates questions?
5. Who has authority to make decisions/provide direction?

3.3.1 Construction Responsibilities and Oversight

While the role and level of involvement may vary from project to project depending on the contracts in place, the construction project team typically includes the following roles:

1. Owner
2. Contractor
3. Subcontractor(s)
4. Designer
5. Inspector

The owner is typically the overarching decision-maker on the project, and any changes to the work must ultimately be approved by the owner before proceeding. Sometimes owner responsibility can be delegated to the designer, such as to review submittals and to provide support on field issues that arise. While the inspector can be under either the owner or the designer umbrella, the inspector's role is to oversee the work and verify that it is being conducted per the contract documents. The contractor is ultimately responsible for the work being completed and the functional performance of the SCM at the end of construction.

Often SCM components are installed by a subcontractor. The subcontractor's responsibility is tied to respective trade experience. For instance, a piping subcontractor may be installing the underdrain, cleanouts, and outlet structure components while the general grading subcontractor is responsible for the excavation of the overall SCM footprint and grading of slopes draining toward the facility. Then, the concrete subcontractor may be responsible for installing the curbing that defines the perimeter of the SCM. The landscaping subcontractor may then be responsible for filling the excavated SCM with soil and aggregate media before planting. Each of these hand-off points between subcontractors represent weaknesses in the quality of the overall installation and potential failures in adequate control and protection of the SCM. It is critical that the prime contractor provides oversight before, during, and after each transition of work and that the prime contractor is ultimately held responsible for any deficiencies that arise. It is important that each subcontractor understands the components they are expected to control and protect from subsequent work. It is recommended that verification and checks by the inspector and/or designer as well as the contractor be implemented between each step to narrow down issues and points of failure that may arise during subsequent steps (Figure 3.20).

3.3.2 Training of the Construction Worker—Developing Skilled Stormwater Control Measure Labor

Specifications often contain quality assurance and quality control (QAQC) parameters that include training, certification, and/or experience requirements for the contractor completing different aspects of the work. For instance, concrete installers often must meet American Concrete Institute certification for jobs that include flatwork and finishing. Similar training and certification can be required for SCMs through the National Green Infrastructure Certification Program, or through similar regional and local programs. It is important not only that these QAQC requirements are verified at the start of the project, but that the trained and/or certified personnel is always on site while work is ongoing.

Construction workers who are trained and experienced with SCM construction are important in avoiding common mistakes that can lead to failure of the facility to perform. These mistakes are often overlooked by contractors inexperienced in SCM functional performance, as they conflict with more typical construction techniques and materials. Understanding and communicating the key functions of the SCM can help construction workers building the project identify potential issues before they become failures. The following are key considerations during construction that a contractor with training or experience in SCM construction should be able to identify:

- **Subgrade Preparation:** While in typical construction subgrade preparation often includes compaction requirements, it is common that SCM projects specify limiting or even decompaction of subgrade to promote infiltration. It is important to clearly communicate areas of

Prior to Excavation

- Verify staked extents of stormwater control measure match plan dimensions
- Verify critical tie-in elevations match existing grades in construction plans
- Verify who is responsible for installation of perimeter controls

Prior to Installation of Aggregate Media

- Conduct pre-construction infiltration tests in bottom of excavated footprint
- Verify stockpile location is not upstream of stormwater control measure footprint
- Verify aggregate media is clean, washed and free of fines
- Check delivery ticket to verify aggregate media meets approved submittal
- Verify who is responsible for perimeter and surface controls

Prior to Installation of Piping/Structures

- Verify installed aggregate material is still clean and no sedimentation has occurred
- Verify aggregate is installed to depth(s) per plan
- Verify piping/structure material, size and dimensions match approved submittal
- Verify who is responsible for perimeter, surface, and enclosed system control

Prior to Installation of Soil Media

- Verify piping and structure locations and elevations installed per plan
- Verify aggregate material is still clean and no sedimentation has occurred
- Verify aggregate is installed to depth(s) per plan
- Verify stockpile location is not upstream of stormwater control measure footprint
- Check delivery ticket to verify soil media meets approved submittal
- Verify piping and structures are covered so not clogged with soil media during filling
- Verify who is responsible for perimeter, surface controls and enclosed system controls

Prior to Installation of Mulch and Vegetation

- Conduct post-construction infiltration test to verify soil/aggregate media not clogged during placement
- Verify soil media depth and finished grade elevation of stormwater control measure installed per plans
- Verify adjacent and side slopes are graded per plan
- Verify who is responsible for perimeter and stabilization controls
- Verify who is responsible for watering and vegetative maintenance until establishment

FIGURE 3.20 Recommended Verification Checks During Construction (Reprinted with permission from Burns & McDonnell Engineering Company, Inc.)

the project that should limit compaction, and those that require it to establish functional performance.

- **Aggregate Material:** Likely aggregate materials used within SCMs are specified to be "clean, washed, and free of fines." However, most common construction aggregates used in pavement-type work *require* fines for compaction and stability. Because of this, a typical construction worker without experience or training in SCM construction will likely not notice a problem with unwashed aggregate being installed. It is important for the contractor and inspector to know and verify the washing procedures of the supplier result in clean aggregate meeting the specification requirements.
- **Elevations:** The key function of all SCMs is to provide stormwater management, meaning that stormwater must be able to get to and be stored in the SCM. Because SCMs can take many forms, the nuances that differ from the typical application of these features are critical to the function of the practice. For instance, in a typical planter bed mulch is mounded up from the adjacent area, whereas an SCM requires the footprint to be depressed and likely includes a depth to reserve for ponding. Additionally, pavements and curbing are typically sloped to channelize and convey stormwater runoff away from a site, whereas with SCMs these site features are likely shown to drain toward the facilities.
- **Control and Protection:** The entire SCM and all its components can be installed correctly, but failure to adequately control and protect the facility until the job is complete can ultimately result in failure of functional performance. A contractor trained in SCM construction should be able to identify site risks that threaten the integrity of the installation, such as unstable grades, unprotected stockpiles, material, and equipment storage. They should also be able to identify when the measures currently in place require maintenance or replacement. Mitigation of these risks will save significant project time and budget, and ultimately assist in establishing that functional performance.

4.0 REFERENCE

Water Environment Federation, American Society of Civil Engineers/ Environmental & Water Resources Institute. (2012). *Design of urban stormwater controls* (WEF Manual of Practice No. 23; ASCE/EWRI Manuals and Reports on Engineering Practice No. 87). Water Environment Federation.

4

Conventional Stormwater Control Measures and Green Infrastructure Maintenance

1.0 INTRODUCTION 64
1.1 Maintenance Goals 64
1.1.1 Sustained Function 64
1.1.2 System Longevity 65
1.1.3 Aesthetics 66
1.1.4 Balancing Maintenance Level of Service 66
1.1.5 Public and Worker Safety 68
1.2 Key Processes 68
1.2.1 Vegetation and Soil Associations and Feedback 68
1.2.2 Hydraulics, Erosion, and Sedimentation 71
1.2.3 Structural Deterioration 72
2.0 MAINTENANCE TO OPTIMIZE PERFORMANCE AND LONGEVITY 74
2.1 Maintaining Health Vegetation and Soils 74
2.2 Managing Erosion and Sedimentation Processes 75
2.1.1 Minimizing Erosion, Scour, and Settlement 76
2.2.2 Managing Sedimentation and Clogging 76
2.3 Maintaining Structural Components 76
3.0 SPECIAL CONSIDERATIONS 77
3.1 Considerations for Infiltrating Systems 77
3.2 Considerations for Slow-Release Systems 78
3.3 Considerations for Proprietary/Manufactured Devices 78
4.0 MAINTENANCE SUMMARY BY STORMWATER CONTROL MEASURES TYPE 79
4.1 Surface Practices 79
4.1.1 Forebays 79
4.1.1.1 Routine Maintenance 81
4.1.1.2 Common Problems 82
4.1.2 Dry Basins 82
4.1.2.1 Routine Maintenance 83
4.1.2.2 Common Problems 84
4.1.3 Wet Basins 84
4.1.3.1 Routine Maintenance 84
4.1.3.2 Common Problems 85
4.1.4 Wetlands (Including Subsurface Gravel Wetlands) 88
4.1.4.1 Routine Maintenance 88
4.1.4.2 Common Problems 89

4.1.5 *Bioretention Filters* 90
4.1.5.1 *Routine Maintenance* 91
4.1.5.2 *Common Problems* 92
4.1.6 *Infiltration Basins* 93
4.1.6.1 *Routine Maintenance* 94
4.1.6.2 *Common Problems* 95
4.1.7 *Surface Sand Filters* 96
4.1.7.1 *Routine Maintenance* 96
4.1.7.2 *Common Problems* 97
4.1.8 *Swales and Strips* 97
4.1.8.1 *Routine Maintenance* 98
4.1.8.2 *Common Problems* 99
4.2 Subsurface Practices 100
4.2.1 *Drain Inlet Inserts and Manufactured Filters* 101
4.2.1.1 *Routine Maintenance* 102
4.2.1.2 *Common Problems* 102
4.2.2 *Vaults and Swirl Concentrators* 102
4.2.3 *Oil and Water Separators* 103
4.2.3.1 *Routine Maintenance* 104
4.2.3.2 *Common Problems* 104
4.2.3.3 *Special Considerations* 104
4.2.4 *Infiltration/Retention Trenches and Vaults* 105
4.2.5 *Dry Wells* 106
4.2.5.1 *Routine Maintenance* 106
4.2.5.2 *Common Problems* 106
4.3 Cisterns and Rain Barrels 107
4.3.1 *Routine Maintenance* 109
4.3.2 *Common Problems* 109
4.4 Landscaped Roofs (Green Roofs) 110
4.4.1 *Routine Maintenance* 111
4.4.2 *Common Problems* 112
4.5 Permeable Pavement 113
4.5.1 *Routine Maintenance* 113
4.5.2 *Common Problems* 114
5.0 REFERENCES 116

1.0 INTRODUCTION

This chapter provides a review of maintenance for conventional stormwater control measures (SCMs), including green infrastructure. Green infrastructure measures focus on distributed controls that are vegetated or incorporate infiltration. These include bioretention filters and infiltration basins. Conventional stormwater controls include a range of additional technologies like wet and dry basins and subsurface vaults. While this chapter provides additional focus on green infrastructure, many of the concepts presented can apply to conventional SCMs.

1.1 Maintenance Goals

1.1.1 Sustained Function

One of the primary goals of any stormwater infrastructure maintenance is to provide sustained and reliable function over time. In most cases, this means maintaining clear hydraulic flow paths into and out of the system, ensuring that piping, hydraulic control structures, pretreatment devices, and infiltration surfaces are functioning properly, and creating and promoting favorable conditions for vigorous vegetation development and establishment. Execution of routine maintenance activities are critical to maintaining function, as is a periodic functional assessment of the system. These functional tests measure system function directly, rather than inferring function from the condition of observed components. Functional tests such as water level monitoring during simulated or real runoff events, and plant surveys that quantify plant cover, are critical to benchmarking function and to identifying sustained declines in function that may indicate the need for corrective action.

Even when faithfully performing routine maintenance, some decline in system function may occur without corrective action, particularly for right-of-way (ROW) systems and those receiving high sediment loading. Thus, when maintaining for sustained function, periodic functional testing and observation after significant rain events is critical to identify any functional issues and to diagnose the need for corrective maintenance. Common functional issues may include increased bypass as a result of clogging of inflow conveyance systems, inadequate infiltration or storage because of clogging of infiltration surfaces or filling of surface or subsurface storage areas with fine sediment, clogging of hydraulic control structures, lack of storage volume as a result of sediment accumulation, deterioration of outlets and hydraulic controls that changes hydraulic performance, and poor vegetative health because of soil degradation, sedimentation, and erosion. In some cases, corrective action can be implemented to correct the problem and restore a properly functioning system, where in other cases the level of functional loss may require either site decommissioning, or partial or full replacement. In these instances, it is critical to document the design, siting, or technology selection choices that led to underperformance issues, so that adjustments to future implementation approach may be made.

1.1.2 System Longevity

Partial or full system replacement costs can significantly escalate life-cycle costs. By contrast, extending system longevity is a powerful means to lower life-cycle costs and a therefore key focus for any long-term maintenance program. While many processes such as structural deterioration can contribute to premature replacement, perhaps the most important processes that can accelerate system failure is sedimentation and attendant clogging of storage areas and infiltration surfaces. Sedimentation rates are highly variable from site to site based on a variety of factors, including hydraulic loading ratio (the ratio of the drainage area to the footprint area of the SCM), drainage area conditions that affect sediment loading, and pretreatment efficacy. Similarly, some SCM designs and technologies are particularly susceptible to the effects of sedimentation. For instance, infiltration systems may be particularly vulnerable to sedimentation if the system-wide walls are lined, thus preventing lateral exfiltration in the case of clogging of the infiltration surface, and if stone storage is utilized versus open pipe or chamber storage. Generally, these systems should not be sited in high sediment loading environments without extensive pretreatment systems. Also, maintenance and inspection frequency may need to be increased for these types of systems to identify evidence of system performance decline and to ensure proper functioning of pretreatment systems such as inlet filters and forebays.

1.1.3 Aesthetics

Maintenance must be executed at a frequency to achieve the aesthetic expectations of the SCM-owner/operation. These expectations must be clearly defined at the start of the maintenance program, and ideally considered as part of the design process.

Aesthetic expectations can vary significantly by owner/operator, by SCM location, and by SCM type and scale. For example, the aesthetic expectations for smaller, vegetated SCMs located in the right-of-way or other highly visible public spaces, such as sidewalk-scale bioretention filters, are typically heavily influenced by public/community expectations. By contrast, aesthetic expectations for larger scale SCMs (e.g., dry basins, wet basins, wetlands, etc.) may be significantly different, even in public settings, as aesthetic issues such as trash accumulation and unruly vegetation may be perceived differently (i.e., less negatively) when observed in the context of these larger scale SCMs.

Maintaining visual appeal is an important component of public acceptance for some SCMs, and the expectations of the public may in some situations drive the maintenance level of service and maintenance frequency required rather than the SCM functional maintenance needs (see Section 1.1.4). Many aesthetic issues can also indicate functional (see Section 1.1.1) and/or safety (see Section 1.1.5) problems. For example, poor condition of vegetation may be related to drainage or sedimentation issues.

1.1.4 Balancing Maintenance Level of Service

Maintenance budgets are, like most budgets, constrained. Therefore, it is critical to understand the required level of service needed to properly maintain system function over time and to maintain community acceptance. In many urban settings, trash accumulation and vegetation performance issues can contribute to aesthetic issues that undermine community acceptance.

These phenomena have been observed in many urban communities and may "force" municipalities to implement a higher level of service that is required to maintain system function and longevity. In these situations, partnering with local nonprofits, workforce development programs, or community development corporations can be a good strategy for bridging gaps between level of service expectations and budgetary allocations.

Level of service is also an important consideration when looking at full life-cycle cost. Increasing the frequency of certain maintenance activities can prevent system decline, reduce replacement costs, and extend practice service life. These activities may be particularly important for infiltrating systems that contain buried stone storage, particularly those located under sidewalks and other paved surfaces.

One strategy for balancing costs and level of service begins with the understanding that stormwater management systems, even in the same jurisdiction, may have different maintenance needs depending on the system siting, configuration, and design (Figure 4.1). For instance, rain gardens located in park or suburban settings managing roof runoff may have profoundly different maintenance requirements than similar systems located within the ROW in dense urban environments.

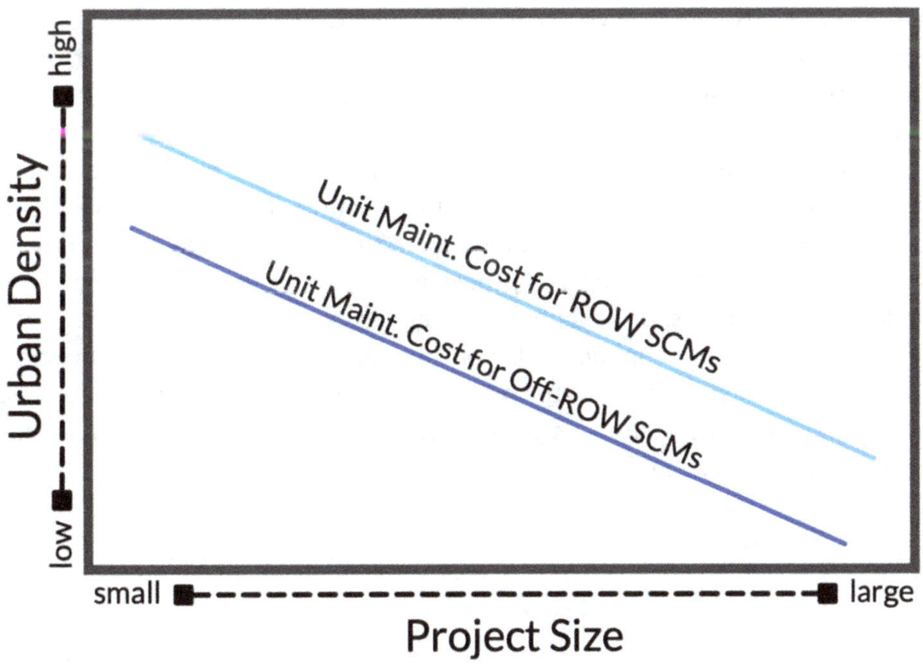

FIGURE 4.1 Conceptualized Relationships Between Maintenance Unit Costs for Right-of-Way (ROW) and Off-ROW Systems Along a Gradient of Urban Density and Project Size (Reprinted with permission from AKRF, Inc.)

Maintenance program managers take advantage of these differences to allow for flexibility in maintenance frequency, rather using a "one size fits all" approach. This type of approach starts with understanding the range of technologies, settings, and designs across an asset portfolio and adapting maintenance regime to various asset types based on maintenance-relevant criteria. Collecting best management practice–specific data on customer/resident complaints, functional performance, and maintenance level of effort can help to identify needs for adjusting maintenance frequency to respond to real-world conditions. These data can also help to identify systems that are chronically underperforming and need to be either decommissioned or substantially reconfigured to reduce long-term costs. By contrast, systems with below average maintenance costs may provide insight into design and siting strategies to guide future implementation efforts.

1.1.5 Public and Worker Safety

Ensuring the safety of both the public and maintenance staff must be set as goals of all maintenance programs. For the public, this requires the establishment of routine inspection and maintenance procedures that identify and immediately address any and all safety hazards, as well as proactively identify potential future hazards if issues were to go unaddressed. Examples of safety hazards include vegetation that obstructs vehicular and pedestrian sight lines, potential tripping hazards associated with unsecured or damaged structures, sharps or other hazardous objects disposed of in or around SCMs, and so on.

To ensure the safety of workers, a program-specific Health and Safety Plan (H&SP) must be established and implemented. H&SPs should include requirements for personnel training and certifications, use of personal protective equipment, and specific processes and procedures to ensure daily safety of personnel such as daily Job Safety Assessments. Site-specific safety protocols are also recommended. This may also include routine inspection and maintenance procedures to ensure the function of SCM safety features, such as safety benches for wet ponds and other basins and worker fall protection systems for landscaped roofs (green roofs).

1.2 Key Processes

1.2.1 Vegetation and Soil Associations and Feedback

Although vegetated SCM performance is context-dependent and multifaceted, most vegetated SCMs rely on effective infiltration at the soil interface as well as through the soil profile. This is most evident when evaluating green stormwater infrastructure (GI) practices such as bioretention filters, but also applies to vegetation in ponds and other vegetated SCMs. As such, surface infiltration rate is a key indicator of performance, which in turn facilitates the growth and health of plantings within vegetated SCMs. Surface infiltration, the velocity at which water initially enters and drains downward through the uppermost soil layer, depends on many interconnected physical, biological, and chemical characteristics (Horton, 1933, 1941; Philip, 1957). These characteristics influence soil structure and plant health, which, in turn, collectively regulate surface infiltration and, consequently, affect system function (Figure 4.2).

Vegetation-soil interactions occur at a range of spatial scales—above and below the surface—and mediate many of the processes that affect infiltration rate. Two forces—gravity and capillary action—are primarily responsible for infiltration rates. Factors that influence the net effects of these forces therefore determine the infiltration rate of a system and dictate vegetated SCM performance. Macropores are soil cavities that enable rapid infiltration by providing preferential flow channels through which fluids drain downward by gravity. Micropores, by contrast, are implicated in infiltration by capillary action and play an important, but secondary, role in controlling infiltration rates.

Erosion and compaction disrupt and disturb vegetation and reduce infiltration as a result of structural changes in soil (Gregory, Dukes, & Jones, 2006; Castellano & Valone, 2007). Scouring and direct rainfall on bare soil, which causes soil particle detachment, can also clog macro- and micropores and seal the soil surface. Ultimately, this reduces infiltration rates and inhibits

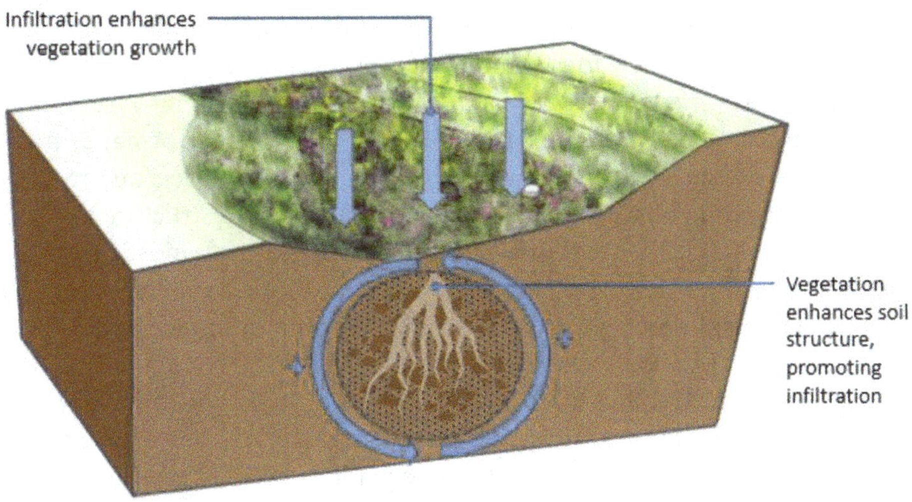

FIGURE 4.2 Vegetation-Soil Feedback Processes (Reprinted with permission from AKRF, Inc.)

plant colonization (Pimentel et al., 1995; Pimentel & Kounang, 1998). While severe soil erosion and surface seal formation often arise from a lack of plant roots (Gyssels et al., 2005) and canopy cover (Morin & Benyamini, 1977; Lado, Paz, & Ben-Hur, 2004), soil degradation also perpetuates conditions that disfavor the growth of vegetation. This is because terrestrial plants require a certain level of soil porosity and moisture retention to access water and nutrients. Under these conditions, a positive feedback loop emerges, highlighting the reciprocal relationship between vegetation and soil that undergirds vegetated SCM function.

Below ground, physical and chemical processes and biological activity affect soil properties and infiltration rates. Plants exude organic compounds in the root zone (rhizosphere), and organic detritus provides carbon-rich substrates from which fungi and microbes produce stabilizing compounds (Schmidt et al., 2011). Organic matter content improves infiltration by maintaining soil structure, which is important for the preservation of preferential flow paths (Boyle, Frankenberger, Jr., & Stolzy, 1989; Ekwue, 1990).

At a larger scale, the presence of roots in soil increases shear strength of the soil matrix, which reduces erodibility. The soil-root matrix has emergent strength—it resists erosive forces and structural damage more effectively than either root or soil can alone (Ghestem et al., 2014). Roots and rhizosphere biota such as invertebrates and fungi also modify soil architecture and increase infiltration rates by facilitating the formation of preferential flow pathways for the downward flow water (Angers & Caron, 1998). These interactions offer an alternative version of vegetation-soil positive feedback loops that confer vegetated SCM performance *benefits* rather than accelerate vegetated SCM performance decline.

Vegetated SCM maintenance should facilitate and amplify beneficial vegetation-soil feedback loops and suppress detrimental feedback loops. Depending on context, however, maintenance practices can also have unintended consequences. Natural processes that promote performance goals should be encouraged yet balanced with other values tied to vegetated SCMs.

Leaf litter and plant detritus, which help maintain soil structure and preserve macropores critical for surface infiltration, are often removed from the top layer of soil for aesthetic reasons as a part of routine maintenance. This may unintentionally increase erosion, scour, and compaction, which depresses infiltration rates (Adekalu, Olorunfemi, & Osunbitan, 2007). Similarly, when soils are compacted, tilling creates conditions necessary for deep root penetration by increasing soil porosity, yet excessive tilling can inadvertently destroy beneficial soil structure and stymie plant growth. Thus, the effects of maintenance on performance and resilience may be highly situational. This presents the challenge of balancing values—stakeholders' aesthetic expectations and vegetated SCM performance goals—that potentially compete.

1.2.2 Hydraulics, Erosion, and Sedimentation

Increases in urbanization and land development are associated with a greater percentage of impervious cover and have altered the hydrologic cycle, local hydraulic forces, and sedimentation regimes. These large-scale changes have increased volumes of runoff, increased peak discharge, and increased transport of sediment and pollutants (NJ Pinelands Commission, 2001; National Research Council, 2008). Green stormwater infrastructure and SCMs use vegetation, soil, and built structures to re-create natural conditions that allow for enhanced infiltration rates, stormwater retention, and water quality improvements. From a maintenance perspective, however, they can also be conceptualized as tools to centralize maintenance needs by concentrating the negative effects of high stormwater flows and related consequences (landscape and water quality degradation).

GI and SCMs are engineered to intercept as much runoff as possible and accumulate nonpoint source pollutants (e.g., total suspended solids [TSS]) found in stormwater. At a local scale, projects alter the existing grade, add or remove materials according to hydraulic properties, and frequently utilize structures such as curb cuts, aprons, and channels to direct flow into GI and SCM systems. While these hydraulic modifications enable GI and SCMs to maximize stormwater capture, they also introduce factors that can necessitate maintenance.

The ability to manage high runoff volumes and concentrated sediments both defines and undermines GI and SCM performance. Green stormwater infrastructure and SCMs improve water quality, mitigate stormwater volume, and control stormwater flowrates. Often such practices make use of confined areas to manage large volumes of stormwater and sediments in a condensed period of time. While this is part of what makes GI an efficient approach to managing stormwater, GI and SCMs often host harsh environments that oppose the long-term goals of performance and resilience. Over time, these factors reduce the capacity for a system to infiltrate, filter, and detain stormwater.

Green infrastructure exposes soil to myriad stresses such as intermittent drought, flooding, and deposition of fine sediments, which can fundamentally alter soil structure. This is an important aspect of GI longevity. Soil structure, which consists of form, stability, and resilience, both influences and is influenced by green infrastructure functional capacity, maintenance regimes, and performance over time. Soil form is the product of particle size distribution and factors that give rise to overall soil texture including mineral composition, air space, moisture content, and biological material (Kay, 1997). Because texture refers largely to fractions of sand, silt, and clay, however, it shapes functional characteristics like surface infiltration rate and water storage capacity. Soils with a high percent of fine material (i.e., clay and silt) tend to have lower infiltration rates (Parr & Bertrand, 1960). Consequently, the accumulation of fine sediment in GI systems decreases infiltration rates filling preferential flow pathways, which are necessary for rapid and deep infiltration through soil. When this occurs, soil stability and resilience can decline as the soil matrix is increasingly unable to maintain and regain previous form during and after exposure to stressors and disturbances (Kay, 1997).

Fine sediments can also fill voids in subsurface gravel storage and reduce volume available for water storage. Subsurface detention basins may be particularly affected by accumulation of fines compared to rain gardens because they lack a surface pretreatment layer of vegetation (Jenkins, Wadzuk, & Welker, 2010). Even measures designed specifically to mitigate the negative effects of fine materials on performance can be rendered nonfunctional. For example, suspended sediment can clog pretreatment systems that are designed to protect subsurface water storage capacity. Clogging of stormwater infiltration practices can ultimately have serious detrimental water quality consequences as decreased infiltration can lead to increased sewer overflows (Bergman et al., 2010).

Strategic designs, engineered devices, and routine maintenance practices can anticipate and mitigate the effects and challenges associated with capturing stormwater. A variety of strategies have been implemented to reduce the quantity of sediments entering GI and SCMs. Sediment forebays are well-established strategies for reducing sedimentation in dry ponds and wetlands (New York City Department of Environmental Conservation, 2018). In urban and ultra-urban settings where space is limited, sediment pretreatment devices are often installed to remove fine particles before they can enter a system. Filtration with vegetative strips and porous pavements can also reduce velocity of stormwater runoff, remove pollutants, and facilitate surface infiltration (Shammaa & Zhu, 2001). Protective matting, vegetation and vegetated strips, and rocks also dissipate the energy of influent stormwater and lessen the erosive forces of water.

1.2.3 Structural Deterioration

Various components that may make up SCM both in GI and non-GI practices can fail or deteriorate with time and affect system performance and functionality. This can range from outlet control structures in a conventional extended detention basin, to curb cut energy dissipaters in GI installations. It is important that structural components be checked periodically during routine maintenance for signs of deterioration. Many times what is visible from a routine check can indicate issues that cannot be fully seen without specialty equipment. For example, standing water long after the designed drain down in a rain garden may indicate clogged subsurface underdrains, or compacted stormwater soil.

Structural deterioration of SCMs could include, but is not limited to, collapsed, caved, or cracked piping, disconnected or missing trash racks, torn pretreatment filter devices, settlement of concrete structures (inlets, manholes, riser pipes, curbing), erosion of subsoils below energy and velocity dissipaters, erosion/undermining of berms and basin slopes, constructed and natural forebays, rust/degradation of gabion baskets, cracking/damage to cleanouts/observation wells, and mechanical wear of proprietary devices.

Materials used in the constructions of the structures will break down with time and stress. While concrete does harden and gain strength with time, as concrete hardens, it also becomes more brittle, which can lead to surface spalling. Exposure to sea water, extreme temperature fluctuations, and heavy loading can accelerate concrete degradation processes. Although water against concrete surface in SCMs will not cause major deterioration for long periods of time, flowing water can erode the surface much faster, exposing aggregate and hastening the rate of deterioration. Metals will oxidize, and the surface may discolor or become pitted; however, generally metal life spans, with proper maintenance, will last the life of the practice if they are robust enough for the tasks for which they are installed. If not maintained, coated metals will eventually succumb to flaking or scratching that expose the bare material, leading to corrosion. Hard plastics can become brittle when exposed to sunlight for prolonged periods. When installed beneath the surface, they are protected from photodegradation. Construction equipment moving over shallow installations can cause bowed or cracked plastic pipe if not properly protected. Many times root intrusion will find perforations in drainage pipe, working in and growing, expanding, and causing cracking. In some instances root intrusion will only cause clogging; however, this may in turn lead to plastic pipe failures. Plastic pipe installed in shallow systems and filled with water as a result of clogging can be subject to freeze-thaw stress causing failure.

Moving water is inherently destructive, and deterioration of some structural elements of SCMs is inevitable. Routine inspection and maintenance, as well as existing protocols for nonroutine maintenance, can preempt and reduce needs for repairs and/or replacements. When repairs and/or replacements are necessary, the elements that deteriorate will not be of the magnitude that would be considered major repair or replacement.

Performance of SCMs can be reduced from physical issues such as collapsed distribution lines, underdrains, failing pretreatment, settlement, and erosion. Maintenance and corrective action of these items may restore performance, and well planned and deployed routine maintenance is the best tool to combat physical issues as they become apparent. However, not taking corrective action can result in the system losing functionality entirely. Seemingly small structural deterioration issues left unattended for long periods of time will require a greater effort to correct and be more costly to control. The best course of action is to frequently inspect, maintain, and repair minor issues before they become major issues. For example, clogging within a conventional inflow point, such as a trench drain, conveyance pipe, riser, or catch basin, may lead to the inflow circumventing and undermining other previously sound structures. Generally, with frequent inspection and deployment of maintenance, clogged conditions at inflow points will be avoided or drastically reduced. If there was some clogging issue that happens to suddenly occur, frequent inspection could identify it, and a repair could be carried out before the issue becomes more severe.

2.0 MAINTENANCE TO OPTIMIZE PERFORMANCE AND LONGEVITY

2.1 Maintaining Health Vegetation and Soils

Green infrastructure and other types of vegetated SCMs, particularly those in highly exposed urban environments, such as roadway margins, may provide challenging conditions for the maintenance of healthy vegetation and high performing engineered soils. Types of challenges may include temperature extremes (Hatfield & Prueger, 2015), high salinity (Zhu, 2002), pollution, litter, drought, flooding/inundation, and sedimentation. To preserve their integrity, and therefore maintain long-term system function, maintenance is necessary.

Soil and vegetation maintenance attempts to anticipate and counteract the effects of such aforementioned challenges to achieve optimal GI and vegetated SCM performance. Maintenance activities are based on seasonal changes and vulnerability of vegetation and soils. Early season maintenance should protect target species and soil surfaces during establishment. Target vegetation and soil are susceptible to degradation at the beginning of the growing season, before emergence, and during summer months, which often have weather extremes. At such times of the year, maintenance should seek to create conditions necessary for beneficial feedback loops between vegetation and soil.

Maintaining healthy vegetation to promote beneficial feedback loops through regular maintenance may involve mulching, watering, pruning, and controlling for weeds and pests. A bare soil surface threatens soil structure in GI and other vegetated SCMs, will be susceptible to erosion and seal formation, and provides space for opportunistic nontarget species to establish and potentially outcompete target species for space, light, nutrients, and so on. Fresh mulch should be applied at the start of the growing season to reduce compaction, protect soil surface, and suppress weed growth. The addition of fresh mulch in the summer can also help to stabilize moisture levels during these periods. Watering as necessary encourages plant growth and better establishment. Application of the correct herbicides can be used to control weeds and before target species emergence. Pesticides can curtail insects that may be detrimental to the target species. Vegetation should be treated to remove, eradicate, or diminish pests and/or disease.

When it comes to vegetation maintenance for optimal GI and vegetated SCM performance, ensuring vegetation emergence and growth is not the only priority. Seasonal pruning also helps maintain balance in vegetative community. Selective pruning that removes lower limbs of trees and shrubs is important to allow sufficient light to filter down to other plants. Pruning is also important to maintain GI and vegetated SCM function, as overgrown woody plants can sometimes inhibit the entry of stormwater into the system and can collect trash/debris, which facilitates clogging. As vigorous vegetation growth is critical to erosion control, evapotranspiration, and pollutant removal, maintenance staff should however not overprune and allow vegetation to develop and grow where possible. Vegetation maintenance also includes maintenance practices that promote site aesthetics and ensure safety. This includes maintaining sight lines and preventing encroachment of plants onto the sidewalks.

2.2 Managing Erosion and Sedimentation Processes

While GI and SCMs are designed, in part, to capture and collect fine-grained sediments, maintenance is required to remove accumulated sediments and clear the surface of sediment layers that may block installed soils that are designed to percolate water well (rain garden media, and high sand content soils). Previously trapped sediments reduce capacity for a system to capture incoming sediments and reduce the volume available to store runoff before slow release or soil infiltration. They can also clog highly porous media, further reducing infiltration. In the absence of routine maintenance, sedimentation processes can approach an equilibrium in which incoming sediment load equals the outgoing sediment load. However, a clogging sediment layer would likely remain, clogging desirable media that filters and percolates while hindering performance, rendering the system as a pass-through for sediment.

Hydraulics and sediment transport regimes may determine the level of maintenance required to achieve a desired performance standard for given GI technology. The operations and maintenance (O&M) of ultra-urban GI and

SCMs presents a particularly vexing challenge as a result of space limitations, high runoff volumes, and high concentrations of sediments. For example, the negative effects of sediment accumulation are especially accentuated in ROW practices compared to GI/SCMs that are designed in open areas because the accumulation takes place across a concentrated area and volume.

2.1.1 Minimizing Erosion, Scour, and Settlement

To combat erosion, scour, and settlement, proper design and installation, including thorough and accountable construction oversight, generally will curtail the majority of early issues that are found at GI/SCMs. Once the site is installed properly and functioning as designed, continual maintenance can find and correct most other issues. Frequent inspection and maintenance can point to particular issues early, allowing faster and simpler fixes, and many times they are less costly.

Specific maintenance activities that can minimize erosion, scour, and settlement involve maintaining inflow points for function. Items such as velocity and energy dissipaters, pretreatment filters, riprap, and forebays need to be kept in good order. The proper function of these devices allows for sediment to drop out, velocities of incoming flows and energy to be decreased, and the system to be protected. In some cases, energy dissipaters prone to continual failure may need to be expanded or redesigned.

2.2.2 Managing Sedimentation and Clogging

Over time, sedimentation will occur, regardless of ongoing inspection and maintenance. Although proper O&M will minimize the effects and stretch the cycle of management, and therefore make the eventual work easier to carry out, it will need to be done periodically.

Managing sedimentation and clogging will depend on the type of SCM/GI, although generally it involves removing sediment, scarifying surface media, maintaining/fortifying inflow protection, maintaining healthy vegetation, maintaining pretreatment devices, maintaining forebays and filter media, and ensuring the system is functioning as intended.

2.3 Maintaining Structural Components

Structural components associated with SCMs may include, but not be limited to, various precast concrete structures for conveyance, flow control and storage, piping, trench drains, headwalls/end walls, risers, weir walls, check dams, concrete channels, manholes and other access structures, forebays and energy dissipaters, infrastructure associated with real-time controls (e.g., solar panels, telemetry equipment, etc.), curbing, porous and traditional paving surfaces, and retaining walls. While routine maintenance of conveyance, flow control, and storage components is required to manage sedimentation and clogging (see Section 2.2.2), periodic inspection and timely as needed repairs to or replacement of structural components is an important strategy toward ensuring the performance and longevity of SCMs. For example, small structural defects, such as cracks in concrete structures, can exacerbate and worsen relatively quickly over a series of runoff events or freeze-thaw cycles, and what could have been a simple repair can escalate into the complete failure of an SCM or conveyance system.

Maintenance staff should be prepared, at minimum, to address minor structural issues that do not require specialized equipment as part of routine maintenance events. This may include patching small areas of pavement, filling small cracks in structures (typically 0.4 m [18 in.] in length or less), replacing access lids/covers and grates, resetting paver stones, and so on. More significant structural defects or those that would require specialized equipment to repair should be evaluated on a case-by-case basis by a trained professional. This may include larger cracks (greater than 0.4 m in length) or damage to concrete structures, structural defects in pipes, cracking of subsurface storage components such as vaults and arches, and so on.

3.0 SPECIAL CONSIDERATIONS

3.1 Considerations for Infiltrating Systems

Infiltrating systems refer to SCMs that retain and treat stormwater, typically through a filtering media such as engineered soil or clean stone, before infiltrating water into the underlying soil. These systems can involve vegetated components or may be buried underground. In either case, sedimentation and clogging of filtering media and of the interface between the SCM and the underlying soil can result in system failure. Pretreatment of stormwater to reduce sediment loading to the SCM, typically via settling or filtration, is critical to the longevity of infiltrating systems. Types of pretreatment systems/strategies include forebays, filter strips, swales, geotextile filter bags, inlet sumps, hoods/traps and other pipe protection devices, and proprietary settling and filter systems. Pretreatment systems must be properly designed/sized for expected stormwater flowrates and sediment loads, and maintained regularly.

In addition to effective pretreatment, stabilization of the upstream watershed/contributing drainage area is critical to ensuring function of infiltrating SCMs, even if pretreatment measures are in place. Erosion occurring in contributing drainage areas should be identified as part of routine SCM inspection and addressed as quickly as possible. During active construction activities within the upstream watershed, infiltrating SCMs need to be either kept offline completely or property protected with appropriately sized erosion and sediment control measures in addition to permanent pretreatment devices. Structural failure or damage to components of stormwater conveyance systems also presents a significant risk to infiltrating SCMs and should be repaired as quickly as possible (see Section 2.3). For example, broken pipes or structures exposed to subsurface elements can result in the accelerated transport of soil/sediment to infiltration surfaces.

3.2 Considerations for Slow-Release Systems

Slow-release systems refer to SCMs that detain and slowly release stormwater back to a sewer system or open water as the principal mode of stormwater management. These systems can involve vegetated components or may be buried underground. In either case, proper maintenance of conveyance systems that deliver runoff to and away from storage areas is critical. Maintenance of the storage area itself is also critical, as proper performance hinges on maintaining sufficient storage to avoid overflow during design storm events. As mentioned above, sedimentation of the storage area, particularly for buried gravel storage, which cannot be easily cleaned, and for systems draining catchments with high sediment loading, is a particularly challenging and costly mode of failure. Loss of storage volume may be detected if rain events significantly smaller than the intended design storm or simulated runoff tests at subdesign storm rates produce significant system overflow.

Slow-release systems often rely on a small diameter water quality orifice to achieve prescribed release rates. In some cases, orifices can be as small as 13 mm (0.5 in.). In such cases, small amounts of sediment, debris, and even biofilm can cause positive feedback mechanisms that result in partial or full restriction of the orifice. In these cases, the system may back up or produce overflow at low rates of inflow or may be slow to drain. Routine observation of system performance after rain events and via simulated runoff testing can identify these performance issues. Manual inspection and cleaning of the orifice should also be performed during routine maintenance, even if the orifice is draining via an underdrain with media filtration.

3.3 Considerations for Proprietary/Manufactured Devices

Proprietary or manufactured devices may be used for pretreatment of pollutants before discharge into a more traditional SCW or GI practice. Pollutants collected by these devices may include floatables, heavy metals, sediment, and hydrocarbons. Particular attention to appropriate disposal methods must be considered for the water used during maintenance of these practices.

Maintenance for proprietary or manufactured devices may require specialized training, or even specialized equipment, to complete. It is important to consider any modifications to existing maintenance procedures that will be required for SCM practices using these devices. While performing maintenance, it is important to have guidelines provided by the manufacturer available in the field. Additionally, maintenance of certain devices may benefit by having a representative of the manufacturer present on site for assistance. This could consist of conducting a manufacturer-led training session once construction of a practice is complete, or on-site visits for specialized, less frequent maintenance.

Replacing parts of proprietary or manufactured devices, especially filtration systems and filtration media, will require that the same or an equivalent product will be available for the intended lifespan of the practice. This may be difficult in the event that the manufacturer is no longer in business or is no longer producing the product.

Proprietary or manufactured devices are often designed to satisfy release rates set forth by a state's environmental agency. Replacement of proprietary filtration media may affect the release rate, and therefore the compliance, of a practice. This issue should be considered when selecting replacement media. Maintenance staff are directed to independently verified maintenance resources for a variety of proprietary manufactured treatment devices available through the State of Washington Department of Ecology emerging stormwater treatment technologies program website and the NJ Corporation for Advanced Technology website.

4.0 MAINTENANCE SUMMARY BY STORMWATER CONTROL MEASURES TYPE

Typical maintenance activities for surface and subsurface practices are summarized in Table 4.1.

4.1 Surface Practices

4.1.1 Forebays

Forebays, also called sediment forebays, are pools or excavated depressions located immediately down-gradient of the stormwater inflow point(s) of an SCM. Forebays are typically used as pretreatment for SCMs (e.g., stormwater wetlands) because they dissipate the energy of influent runoff,

TABLE 4.1 Summary of Common Maintenance Activities for Surface and Subsurface Practices (Reprinted with permission from AKRF, Inc.)

Maintenance Activity	Category	Applicability
Sediment, trash, and debris removal	Surface	Forebays, sand filter, swales and strips, bioretention filters, dry basin, wet basins, wetlands, infiltration basins
	Subsurface	Drain inlet inserts, manufactured filters and vaults, and swirl concentrators; dry wells
Replanting and Reseeding	Surface	All vegetated SCMs
	Subsurface	N/A
Watering	Surface	Herbaceous vegetation and shrubs, sedums, and succulents
	Subsurface	N/A
Removal of dead or damaged vegetation	Surface	All vegetated SCMs
	Subsurface	N/A
Pruning and trimming	Surface	All vegetated SCMs
	Subsurface	N/A
Mowing	Surface	Forebays, sand filter, swales and strips, and bioretention filters
	Subsurface	N/A
Weeding and Pest Management	Surface	All vegetated SCMs
	Subsurface	N/A
Mulching	Surface	Swales and strips, infiltration basins, and bioretention filters
	Subsurface	N/A
Power wash (or similar deep clean)	Surface	N/A
	Subsurface	Drain inlet inserts and filters
Flushing/jetting	Surface	N/A
	Subsurface	Subsurface piping to/from various SCMs
Vault flood/flush	Surface	N/A
	Subsurface	Infiltration/retention trenches and vaults
Oil coalescing plate maintenance	Surface	N/A
	Subsurface	Oil and water separators
Absorbent pad maintenance or replacement	Surface	N/A
	Subsurface	Oil and water separators

reducing erosion and settling sediments, pollutants, and debris before entering a larger SCM. This concentrates maintenance needs within a smaller, more easily accessible area (i.e., the forebay) and reduces the need for maintenance requiring more skilled labor and/or heavy machinery within the main SCM.

4.1.1.1 Routine Maintenance

Because forebays are designed to impound sediments, pollutants, trash, and debris, routine maintenance is essential. If excessive material is allowed to accumulate in a forebay, forebay performance may decline. Failure to remove sediments and other debris in a timely manner may result in resuspension and conveyance of material into the SCM down-gradient, thereby reducing available storage volume and undermining water quality objectives. Routine maintenance is therefore critical to ensure forebay performance, minimizing nonroutine maintenance costs and maximizing SCM longevity.

Sediment, Trash, and Debris Removal. Rates of sediment, trash, and debris accumulation in forebays may vary seasonally and are potentially heavily influenced by siting and design characteristics such as vegetative cover and land use within the contributing drainage area. Forebays should be inspected for accumulated sediment, debris, and trash every 1 to 3 months. Observed floatables should be removed if possible to limit entry into the down-gradient SCM. Sediments should typically be removed using an excavator every few years and/or once sediments measure almost a meter, or several feet, in depth. While quarterly inspection (minimum) and maintenance every few years are recommended to ensure forebay temporary storage capacity is kept available, an adaptive management approach that accounts for local and seasonal variability is recommended.

Methods for sediment removal may differ depending on forebay design characteristics. The bottom floor of forebays are typically stabilized with stone or concrete to reduce erosion and facilitate sediment removal with heavy equipment. However, if the bottom floor is vegetated, hand-removal of accumulated material may be necessary.

Vegetation Maintenance. While forebays are often not vegetated, some designs include vegetation to promote sedimentation. As a result of high sediment loading and hydraulic stress, vegetation within forebays can be particularly difficult to maintain. Vegetation maintenance in forebays also includes management of target vegetation and removal of nontarget vegetation. Grass and other grass-like plants, which can tolerate periodic inundation and dry periods, are typically used in forebays. Vegetation should be cut to between 0.1- and 0.2-m (4- and 8-in.) lengths each month. Larger herbaceous or woody plant species should be removed because they reduce the storage capacity available for water and accumulated sediments. Nontarget vegetation should be removed using manual methods (e.g., hand-pulling). Aquatic-safe herbicides and preemergent weed controls are sometimes used to suppress weeds and reduce manual weeding efforts. There are numerous, aquatic-safe algaecides and glyphosate products available on the market. There are also products that directly target weeds such as Aquathol® Super K, or products that prevent sunlight penetration such as Aquashade® Plus, which work to control underwater growth. To preempt nontarget vegetation establishment, weeding activities should be timed to remove nontarget plant species before they flower and set seed, thereby mitigating seed spread.

4.1.1.2 Common Problems

Rapid Sedimentation. Rapid accumulation of sediments in forebays may sometimes occur, potentially reducing settling efficiency and requiring more frequent maintenance. Frequent inspection, data collection on key performance indicator and maintenance needs, and an adaptive management approach are recommended to address rapid sedimentation.

Erosion and Poor Vegetation Establishment. While forebays should be designed to be stable in all expected conditions, unusually severe storms may produce high influent velocities capable of damaging earthen sides and stripping vegetation. For vegetated forebays, scouring damage is of particular concern after seeding or soon after planting vegetation. Geotextile blankets are often used to lessen shear forces and protect new vegetation. Hydroseeding (i.e., applying seed in a slurry of water, wood fiber mulch, and fertilizer) with a tackifier may be used to lessen scouring forces and promote vegetation growth by maintaining contact between seeds and/or soil. Signs of erosion should be monitored during periodic inspections and addressed proactively.

4.1.2 Dry Basins

Dry basins are detention basins that do not have a permanent pool of water or wetland conditions. Flow discharge from the basin is controlled by an outlet control structure with a low flow outlet such as an orifice, and high flow outlets through which flow from heavier storm are conveyed. Most dry basins constructed within the last 25 years include extended detention functions, which provide some level of detention and filtration for smaller storms. Older basins may lack this function. Some dry basins may be designed for infiltration and are covered in the infiltration basins section of this chapter. These SCMs may or may not have underdrains and can vary in size to manage small or large drainage areas. Dry basins may be vegetated using turf grass or meadow vegetation such as wildflowers and warm season grasses.

4.1.2.1 Routine Maintenance

Maintenance may consist of cleaning sedimentation from pretreatment forebays (see also forebays section), emptying or replacing inlet filter inserts, vegetative maintenance, conveyance cleaning or flushing, dissipater repair and cleaning, and trash and debris cleanup.

Vegetation. Vegetation should be inspected regularly. Invasive species and the establishment of nontarget vegetation should be addressed promptly if observed. Nontarget vegetation should be removed using manual methods (e.g., hand-pulling) unless use of herbicide is approved. To preempt nontarget vegetation establishment, weeding activities should be timed to remove nontarget plant species before they flower and set seed, thereby mitigating seed spread. Outlet control structures should be clear of vegetation blocking water flow. Forebays should be kept free of nontarget vegetation.

Sediment, Trash, and Debris Removal. Regular removal of sediments and debris from pretreatment and inflow-outflow points is critical to maintaining long-term function. Regular removal of any accumulation around outlet control structures is also required to maintain proper drawdown rates. Rates of accumulation of sediment, debris, and trash are context dependent, and the frequency of maintenance required to ensure performance will vary among systems and therefore should occur on an as-needed basis. If the practice is intended to provide infiltration, the infiltrating surface will need to be inspected for sediments clogging the media (see infiltration basins section, this chapter, for more detail).

Subsurface. Cleaning of inflow and outflow conveyance structures and piping should be performed as needed. Cleaning frequency, provided surface components are well cared for, will generally be infrequent, perhaps every few years in most conditions. Closed circuit television (CCTV) inspection of the subsurface piping should be carried out before and after piping cleaning. Pipes are typically cleaned using hydraulic jetting equipment. When conducting jetting, flushing water should be collected downstream, and should not be disposed of within the basin as it will contain high amounts of suspended sediments.

Structural. System pretreatment, conveyance, dissipaters, risers, cleanouts, observation wells, and outfalls need to be routinely inspected during routine maintenance for proper condition and functionality. Guidance on fixing significant structural defects is beyond the scope of routine maintenance work, although routine maintenance does typically cover minor structural repairs.

4.1.2.2 Common Problems

Erosion. Erosion on basin slopes may occur, particularly if slopes are exposed to concentrated runoff and are not well vegetated. Generally, eroded areas should be filled with topsoil, compacted, seeded, and stabilized using erosion fabric. Signs of erosion should be monitored during routine inspections and addressed proactively to prevent more costly, time-consuming repairs. Areas of frequent erosion should be investigated for design or construction issues. Source control or more extensive regrading and reseeding/replanting may be needed in these areas. If erosion issues persist, the use of rock-lined channels or other hard armoring approaches may be needed.

4.1.3 Wet Basins

Wet basins are constructed stormwater management ponds, which consist of a permanent pool of water and perimeter vegetation. Wet basins provide peak flow attenuation, short- and long-term stormwater storage, and removal of pollutants such as total suspended solids, phosphorus (particulate-bound and dissolved forms), total nitrogen, and heavy metals. In addition, wet basins can also help mitigate urban heat island effects, provide habitat for wildlife and aesthetic value, and may improve air quality.

4.1.3.1 Routine Maintenance

Wet basin maintenance addresses functional, aesthetic, and safety objectives. Maintenance activities are generally concentrated at the vegetated perimeter, system inflow and outflow points, and occasionally within stormwater storage basin.

Sediment, Trash, and Debris Removal. Regular removal of sediments and debris from pretreatment, inflow and outflow, and the storage area is central to the prevention of clogging and overall performance and longevity of wet basins. At a minimum, inspection and maintenance to address clogging at outflow points should occur multiple times per year and after every storm greater than 25 mm (1 in.). Rates of accumulation may vary seasonally and are potentially heavily influenced by siting and design characteristics such as vegetative cover and land use within the contributing drainage area. More frequent removal of sediments and debris may be required on an as-needed basis. Over the long term, wet basins must be dredged using heavy equipment.

Vegetation Maintenance. Vegetation maintenance frequency and activities change over the lifespan of a wet basin. Newly planted vegetation should be watered daily for the first 2 months and then regularly (as-needed) for up to 2 years to ensure for successful establishment. Watering is particularly important in drier summer months. Once established, vegetation should be inspected regularly for signs of disease or distress. In general, watering, fertilizing, and mowing of perimeter buffer vegetation are not needed in a mature wet basin.

Invasive species and the establishment of nontarget vegetation should be addressed promptly if observed. Monocultures (i.e., dense growth of a single plant species) may indicate presence of nuisance aquatic vegetation that can outcompete target vegetation. Nontarget vegetation should be removed using manual methods (e.g., hand-pulling) unless the use of herbicide is approved. Aquatic safe herbicides and preemergent weed controls are sometimes used to suppress weed controls and reduce manual weeding efforts. To preempt nontarget vegetation establishment, weeding activities should be timed to remove nontarget plant species before they flower and set seed, thereby mitigating seed spread. Small shallow wet basins may be more susceptible to invasive species than larger, deeper wet basins.

While preventing the establishment of invasive and/or nontarget plant species is an important functional and aesthetic goal, some volunteer colonization and shifting of plant species distributions postinstallation is expected and acceptable. This is especially important to consider in wetlands because actual hydroperiods may differ from the designed hydroperiod. Depending on the duration and extent of inundation, vegetation may need to be replanted and/or supplemented following initial establishment to reflect these differences between observed and designed conditions.

4.1.3.2 Common Problems

Clogging. Inflows and outflows to wet ponds are areas of concentrated flow and thus may be particularly vulnerable to clogging. Frequent inspection and pretreatment maintenance are critical to the prevention of severe clogging. While there is no substitute for direct inspection, ponding depth can also provide useful information about the state of inflow and outflow points. Unexpectedly shallow ponding depth and signs of short-circuiting, particularly after periods of rain, may indicate blockage at one or more inflow points. Conversely, unexpectedly deep ponding may indicate that slow-release outflow points are clogged. If clogging is detected, inflow and/or outflow points may need to be cleaned manually or using a vacuuming and hydraulic jetting. Repeated clogging may be a sign of a design or construction issue.

Erosion. While wet basins are often equipped with forebays to reduce the velocity of influent stormwater, severe storms may produce high influent velocities capable of eroding basin sides and stripping vegetation. Scouring damage is of particular concern after seeding or soon after planting vegetation. Geotextile blankets are often used to lessen shear forces and protect new vegetation. Hydroseeding (i.e., applying seed in a slurry of water, wood fiber mulch, and fertilizer) with a tackifier may be used to lessen scouring forces and promote vegetation growth by maintaining contact between seeds and/or soil. Flatter basin side slopes can also reduce erosion during large storms and during maintenance activities, particularly if heavy machinery is used. Signs of erosion should be monitored during regular inspections and addressed proactively. Erosion at outfalls should be monitored and reported as observed, particularly on the downstream end of a wet basin. Any particular energy dissipating device or material immediately downstream, such as riprap, may be susceptible to erosive forces, and this must be addressed before the condition worsens.

Algae Blooms and Cyanobacteria. Presence of stagnant, high-nutrient (i.e., phosphorus- and nitrogen-containing compounds), and shallow water may result in the proliferation of algae and cyanobacteria, as well as floating and rooting macrophytes. Dense blooms of algae can create large mats of floating, decayed algae capable of producing anoxic conditions that can kill fish and other aquatic organisms. This is particularly problematic during the summer and warm, wet periods. In addition to creating foul odor and unsightly conditions, cyanobacteria and algae blooms can pose a significant public health hazard.

Prevention of excess algae growth is primarily achieved by limiting resource inputs that support algae blooms and cyanobacteria. Preserving an undisturbed (i.e., unmowed) vegetated perimeter around the wet basin is one effective way to filter and absorb nutrients. In addition, quantities of influent nutrient concentrations may be reduced by discouraging the feeding of waterfowl and encouraging pet owners to pick up animal waste. Maintaining sufficient ponding depth to reduce light penetration to the bottom of a practice is also an effective way to control levels of algae and cyanobacteria.

Repeated algae blooms may not be able to be controlled by reducing inputs and may require periodic treatment using algaecides such as copper sulfate, or barley straw. Periodic winter drawdown can also reduce the proliferation of algae and aquatic weeds. Additionally, some wet ponds may benefit from the addition of aeration systems to promote oxygenation. In addition to improving conditions for aquatic life, aeration systems can be effective in preventing the release of phosphorus from bottom sediments under anoxic conditions. Additives such as alum, which removes phosphorus from the water column and "seals" bottom sediments to prevent the anoxic release of phosphorus, can also be helpful in preventing algal blooms, particularly when high rates of internal loading are suspected. Care must be taken, however, as the use of alum may affect the pH and influence the aquatic environment. Finally, pond dredging can be a useful and needed intervention to increase depth (reducing the proliferation of rooted aquatic plants) and remove phosphorus-rich bottom sediments.

Mosquitoes. Mosquito control is of particular concern because of public health risks and annoyance. Because wet basins sustain a permanent pool of water, the presence of mosquitoes may be unavoidable (Minnesota Pollution Control Agency, 2016). Wet basins can, nevertheless, be designed, constructed, and maintained to reduce mosquito populations. Maintenance practices that sustain constant inflows and outflows and maintain consistent water levels (greater than 1.2 m [4 ft] deep) can help prevent the establishment of mosquito habitat and, therefore, control mosquito populations. Ponding that is shallower than the design standard may not only sustain mosquito breeding activity but should also be investigated as a sign of potential underground leakage. Dense aquatic vegetation should also be removed as it may favor mosquito egg-laying and larvae survival while disfavoring natural mosquito predators. The Mosquito and Vector Control Association of California (mvcac.org) provides an abundant wealth of resources that can be referenced for additional mosquito control and response.

Managers can take active steps to facilitate mosquito predation. Mosquito larvicides containing the bacteria Bti (*Bacillus thuringiensis israelensis*) or Bs (*Bacillus sphaericus*) can be deployed as effective control measures that do not directly harm birds, fish, mammals, or amphibians (Marin/Sonoma Mosquito and Vector Control District, 2015). Bat boxes provide roosting sites for bats, which may also reduce mosquito populations through predation (Reiskind & Wund, 2009). In the event of large mosquito outbreaks, approved insecticides that do not pose risks to humans or the environment may also be used (U.S. EPA, 2005).

Safety Issues. Permanent pools of water in wet basins can pose safety hazards, particularly to small children. Routine inspections should observe drain down times, assess whether baseline water levels are safe, and evaluate safety of basin steepness (no steeper than 3:1 is recommended). If drain down times are longer than expected, potential outflow clogging should investigated. Protective fencing, dense surrounding vegetation, and flatter basin slopes may also be effective methods to enhance safety. These can be installed as part of a long-term O&M program if not included in the original design.

Leaks. While wet basins are designed to maintain a permanent pool of water at all times, basin liners can develop leaks. If a leak is detected, excavation may be required to resolve the issue. Such maintenance tasks are beyond the scope of this manual.

Settling and Subsidence. Observation of significant settling or subsidence may indicate subsurface conditions, such as voids or sinkholes that are beyond the scope of this manual.

4.1.4 Wetlands (Including Subsurface Gravel Wetlands)

Stormwater wetlands are constructed wetland systems designed for both short- and long-term stormwater control. Stormwater wetlands incorporate native plants and ecological processes to:

- Detain stormwater runoff and attenuate peak flows through controlled release back to a centralized stormwater conveyance system or open waterbody;
- Remove and transform pollutants such as total suspended solids, nitrogen, phosphorus, and heavy metals via physical, chemical, and biological processes; and
- Provide habitat for wildlife and become aesthetic assets to the community.

4.1.4.1 Routine Maintenance

Wetland maintenance primarily addresses functional, aesthetic, ecological, and safety objectives. Maintenance activities are generally concentrated at the sediment forebay, vegetated areas, system inflow and outflow points, and the stormwater storage basin.

Sediment, Trash, and Debris Removal. Because stormwater wetlands are constructed, in part, to slow the velocity of water and remove pollutants, sediments, organic debris, and litter invariably accumulate and require removal. Routine inspection and maintenance should be performed quarterly to document and address potential performance issues before they develop into problems with escalated costs.

Stormwater wetlands typically contain sediment forebays (also called forebays), which are designed to settle and trap suspended solids before they enter the system. Sediment forebays are easily accessible design features that capture sediments, trash, and debris immediately down-gradient of the system inflow point, streamlining routine inspection and maintenance and reducing the frequency of more costly and intensive maintenance within the stormwater wetland. While sediment, trash, and debris removal occurs primarily in sediment forebays, floating trash and debris may accumulate in the stormwater wetland and should be removed each month.

Excessive sedimentation within the stormwater wetland (i.e., beyond the sediment forebay pretreatment) poses a more serious challenge that requires special maintenance. This may occur if sediment pretreatment is full or damaged or if stormwater flows and sediment concentrations are significantly greater in magnitude than design conditions. If large amounts of sediments are deposited within the system, heavy machinery may be needed to remove accumulated material. Unaddressed, excessive sedimentation may reduce system capacity for volume control and lead to bank destabilization by harming target upland plant species. In stormwater wetlands with subsurface gravel systems, accumulated sediments can also clog void spaces, potentially reducing the storage capacity of the entire system. If this occurs, engineering oversight may be necessary to remediate the issue.

Vegetation Maintenance. Invasive and/or noxious plant species can threaten the performance and longevity of stormwater wetlands. While aggressive and opportunistic plants may provide structural stability, resilience to high amounts of disturbance, and effective pollutant removal, they also may outcompete target plant species and reduce biodiversity. This can have severe, system-level consequences. Monocultures of invasive plant species can result in a loss of stormwater management function as excessive vegetation blocks flow into or out of the system. In addition, monocultures can provide habitat for mosquitoes and remove habitat that hosts natural mosquito predators. Loss of target plant species diversity also diminishes value of stormwater wetlands as aesthetic amenities (Hunt & Lord, 2006).

Removal of invasive plant species can be challenging. In many cases, the coverage of the invasives may be so extensive, and the physical characteristics of the plant species may be that they are large and dense, making it impractical to eliminate or remove by hand as a feasible option. If deemed necessary, licensed professionals may apply approved herbicides in an attempt to eradicate undesirable plant species. Routine inspection and maintenance are important to document and remove invasive plant populations before they are out of control. In some instances, heavy machinery may be required to remove nontarget plants species from wetlands.

While preventing the establishment of invasive and/or nontarget plant species is an important functional and aesthetic goal, some volunteer colonization and shifting of plant species distributions postinstallation is expected and acceptable. This is especially important to consider in wetlands because actual hydroperiods may differ from the designed hydroperiod. Depending on the duration and extent of inundation, vegetation may need to be replanted and/or supplemented following initial establishment to reflect these differences between observed and designed conditions.

4.1.4.2 Common Problems

Mosquitoes. Mosquito control in wetlands is of particular concern because of public health risks and annoyance. While stormwater wetlands can be designed, constructed, and maintained to reduce mosquito populations, the presence of mosquitoes is unavoidable (Minnesota Pollution Control Agency, 2016). For this reason, maintenance practices prevent the establishment of mosquito habitat by sustaining constant inflows and outflows and maintaining consistent water levels (0.9 m [>3 ft] in depth) will help keep mosquito populations at bay.

Stormwater wetland managers can take steps to facilitate mosquito predation. Mosquito larvicides containing the bacteria Bti (*Bacillus thuringiensis israelensis*) or Bs (*Bacillus sphaericus*) can also be deployed as effective control measures that do not directly harm birds, fish, mammals, or amphibians. Bat boxes provide roosting sites for bats, which may reduce mosquito populations through predation. In the event of a large mosquito outbreaks, approved insecticides that do not pose risks to humans or the environment may also be used. The Mosquito and Vector Control Association of California (mvcac.org) provides an abundant wealth of resources that can be referenced for additional mosquito control and response.

Erosion. Erosion can also cause structural damage to embankments and forebays, which can create unsafe conditions and threaten performance. Remediation may demand substantial maintenance. High flowrates entering a wetland may scour vegetation, destabilize slopes, and compromise the structural integrity of flow control structures. Scouring damage is of particular concern after seeding or soon after planting vegetation. Geotextile blankets are often used to lessen shear forces and protect new vegetation. Hydroseeding (i.e., applying seed in a slurry of water, wood fiber mulch, and fertilizer) with a tackifier may be used to lessen scouring forces and promote vegetation growth by maintaining contact between seeds and/or soil. As full-system remediation may be quite costly and disruptive, signs of erosion should be monitored during monthly inspections and addressed proactively.

Safety Issues. Permanent pools of water in wet basins can pose safety hazards, particularly to small children. Routine inspections should observe drain down times, assess whether baseline water levels are safe, and evaluate safety of basin steepness (no steeper than 3:1 is recommended). If drain down times are longer than expected, potential outflow clogging should investigated. Protective fencing, dense surrounding vegetation, and flatter basin slopes may also be effective methods to enhance safety.

Settling and Subsidence. Observation of significant settling or subsidence may indicate subsurface conditions, such as voids or sinkholes that are beyond the scope of this manual.

4.1.5 Bioretention Filters

Bioretention filters are basins or linear features intended to store and filter stormwater using surface storage, vegetation (typically native grasses, forbs, and woody shrubs), and engineered soil media. Bioretention filters typically include pretreatment features, such as forebays, or are located downstream of pretreatment swales or strips intended to capture sediment before it reaches the bioretention filter surface. The surface storage of a bioretention filter is designed to store runoff until it can drain through the bioretention filter surface, which typically consists of a layer of mulch and a layer of soil media that is designed to remove stormwater pollutants such as sediment, nutrients, and metals. Some studies (e.g., Dietz & Clausen, 2006) have reported enhanced metals removal with the use of a mulch layer versus systems with soil media only. Underlying the soil media is a layer of stone and an underdrain system used to convey the filtered stormwater to the downstream receiving waterbody, sewer system, or another SCM (typically rate/flood control system). Surface storage of bioretention filters may also be drained by riser structures, weirs, and/or spillways during larger or more intense rain events.

4.1.5.1 Routine Maintenance

Sediment, Trash, and Debris Removal. Routine maintenance of bioretention filters focuses in part on the removal of accumulated sediment, trash, and debris as well as the upkeep of structures that may include risers, headwalls, weirs, and spillways. Removal of trash, sediment, and debris is critical to filter performance, vegetation health, and aesthetics. Removal of accumulated trash, sediment, and debris from forebays or upstream pretreatment systems (e.g., inlet filters, catch basin sumps, swales and strips, etc.) to prevent this material from reaching the bioretention filter surface is critical to prevent clogging of the filter surface over time and for sustained vegetation performance, as sediment can smother plantings and increase mortality. Sediment, debris, and trash loading will vary significantly based on drainage area characteristics, type and configuration of upstream pretreatment features, and the hydraulics within and directly upstream of the surface storage of the bioretention filter. For urban systems, particularly areas draining streets that lack street sweeping, monthly or even biweekly removal may be needed. For more suburban applications, quarterly removal may be sufficient. Sediment, trash, and debris removal may be difficult in high grasses. Periodic mowing may help to facilitate this work. Sediment removal within underdrain systems is important to the proper hydraulic function of the bioretention filter; these systems should be routinely inspected, and sediment should be removed as needed using hydraulic cleaning techniques.

Vegetation Maintenance. Bioretention filters rely on vegetation to provide some filtration but also to stabilize and prevent erosion of the filter surface and to enhance system aesthetics. Vegetation care, therefore, is critical to the long-term success of bioretention filters, particularly during the first 1 or 2 years after planting/seeding. Vegetation care includes routine watering during the establishment period. Frequent watering may be needed (once a week or more frequently), particularly during the late summer. Vegetative care also includes weeding of invasive and nontarget species and replanting and reseeding areas with poor cover. Spring mulching may also be desirable to suppress weeds and promote moisture retention, but is not recommended as long-term cover. For most bioretention filters, vegetated coverage of at least 85% with target species should be established as a basic performance goal, and vegetation care should be implemented with this goal in mind, adjusting the approach (species selection, etc.) as needed to attain target cover.

Vegetation care in certain environments may also include an aesthetic component. For instance, bioretention filters along roadways within residential or commercial corridors may have higher aesthetic expectations and may require more frequent trash removal, mulching, structural pruning of shrubs, and cutbacks of tall grasses to control site lines, and create more formal aesthetic, as well as deadheading of seed heads to prevent volunteer establishment. In less formal settings, spreading of more aggressive planted species, as well as volunteer establishment of common natives, can be allowed and even encouraged.

4.1.5.2 Common Problems

Sedimentation. Sedimentation in bioretention filters can cause a reduction in filtration capacity, and thus extend surface drain down times, as well as cause vegetation failure and aesthetic issues. Sedimentation tends to occur at stormwater inflow points but can also occur anywhere throughout the filter surface. Persistent or rapid sedimentation may indicate the need for more frequent cleaning of pretreatment features or in some situations design modifications may be needed, which could include the introduction of new or additional sediment pretreatment measures.

Upstream construction activities can also be a significant source of sediment. Coordination with contractors to ensure the installation of proper erosion and sediment control measures can help to protect bioretention filters from sedimentation. Severe sedimentation that results in clogging and extended surface drain down times may require partial or full replacement of the top 50 to 150 mm (2 to 6 in.) of filter media as well as replanting of vegetation.

Erosion. Erosion is a common problem in bioretention filters. Concentrated flows at inflow points, particularly if an energy dissipation device is not provided or is insufficiently sized, combined with poor vegetative establishment can produce erosion of the filter surface. Erosion can also commonly occur downstream of surface overflow features such as weirs and spillways.

Differential settlement of the filter surface can over time lead to channelized flow and associated erosion. The filter surface should routinely be inspected for evidence of channelized flow, such as debris lines, concentrated sediment accumulation, or matted down vegetation, and the surface should be leveled and stabilized to prevent further channelization and gully formation.

If left unaddressed, minor erosion issues can develop into severe erosion, which can compromise the stability of bioretention filter basin embankments and other structural features. Minor erosion problems can typically be fixed with the replacement and appropriate compaction filter media or embankment fill material and the installation/replacement of vegetation.

Poor Vegetation Establishment. The establishment of robust vegetation in bioretention filters is critical for long-term function. In addition to routine vegetation care, repeated areas of poor germination or establishment may require additional interventions to determine the cause of the problem and potential remedies. These may include soil testing to determine the need for soil amendments, or remediation of persistent erosion or sedimentation issues that may result from construction or design issues. Adjustment of species selection and/or the use of larger plant material can help to address trouble spots. Improper planting or seeding, installation outside of recommended planting times, poor quality planting material, insufficient watering, and establishment care can all contribute to the poor plant performance.

4.1.6 Infiltration Basins

Infiltration basins are surface practices intended to store and infiltrate stormwater using surface storage, vegetation (typically native grasses, forbs, and woody shrubs), and engineered soil media. Infiltration basins typically include pretreatment features, such as forebays, or are located downstream of pretreatment swales or strips intended to capture sediment before it reaches the infiltration surface. Surface storage of an infiltration basin is designed to store runoff until it can drain through the surface and the infiltration column and into the subsoil below. The infiltration column may consist of either native soil or a layer of engineered soil media designed to remove stormwater pollutants such as sediment, nutrients, and metals. Some infiltration basins will have a layer of stone below the soil for additional stormwater storage. Surface storage of infiltrations may be drained by riser structures, weirs, and/or spillways during larger or more intense rain events that exceed the infiltration rate of the native soil below.

4.1.6.1 Routine Maintenance

Sediment, Trash, and Debris Removal. Routine maintenance of infiltration basins focuses on the removal of accumulated sediment, trash, and debris as well as the upkeep of structures that may include risers, headwalls, weirs, and spillways. Removal of trash, sediment, and debris is critical to infiltration performance, vegetation health, and aesthetics. Removal of accumulated trash, sediment, and debris from forebays or upstream pretreatment systems (e.g., inlet filters, catch basin sumps, swales and strips, etc.) to prevent this material from reaching the infiltration surface is critical to prevent clogging of the surface over time and for sustained vegetation performance, as sediment can smother plantings and increase mortality. Sediment, debris, and trash loading will vary significantly, based on drainage area characteristics, type and configuration of upstream pretreatment features, and the hydraulics within and directly upstream of the surface storage of the infiltration basin. For urban systems, particularly areas draining streets that lack street sweeping, monthly or even biweekly removal may be needed. For more suburban applications, quarterly or annual removal may be sufficient. Sediment, trash, and debris removal may be difficult in high grasses. Periodic mowing may help to facilitate this work.

Vegetation Maintenance. Infiltration basins may rely on vegetation to provide some filtration of sediment but also to stabilize and prevent erosion of the infiltration surface, enhance/promote soil permeability, and infiltration through their root structures, and to enhance system aesthetics. Vegetation care, therefore, is critical to the long-term success of infiltration basins, particularly during the first 1 or 2 years after planting/seeding. Vegetation care includes routine watering during the establishment period. Frequent watering may be needed (once a week or more frequently), particularly during the late summer. Vegetative care also includes weeding of invasive and nontarget species and replanting and reseeding areas with poor cover. Spring mulching may also be desirable to suppress weeds and promote moisture retention, but it is not recommended as long-term cover. For most infiltration basins, vegetated coverage of at least 85% with target species should be established as a basic performance goal, and vegetation care should be implemented with this goal in mind, adjusting the approach (species selection, etc.) as needed to attain target cover. Vegetation care in certain environments may also include an aesthetic component. In less formal settings, spreading of more aggressive planted species, as well as volunteer establishment of common natives, can be allowed and even encouraged.

4.1.6.2 Common Problems

Sedimentation. Sedimentation in infiltration basins can cause a reduction in surface infiltration capacity, and thus extend surface drain down times, as well as cause vegetation failure and aesthetic issues. Sedimentation tends to occur at stormwater inflow points but can also occur anywhere throughout the basin surface. Persistent or rapid sedimentation may indicate the need for more frequent cleaning of pretreatment features, or in some situations design modifications may be needed, which could include the introduction of new or additional sediment pretreatment measures.

Upstream construction activities can also be a significant source of sediment. Coordination with contractors to ensure the installation of proper erosion and sediment control measures can help to protect infiltration basins from sedimentation. Severe sedimentation that results in clogging and extended surface drain down times may require partial or full replacement of the top 50 to 150 mm (2 to 6 in.) of soil as well as replanting of vegetation.

Erosion. Erosion is a common problem in infiltration basins. Concentrated flows at inflow points, particularly if an energy dissipation device is not provided or is insufficiently sized, combined with poor vegetative establishment, can produce erosion of the infiltration surface. Erosion can also commonly occur downstream of surface overflow features such as weirs and spillways.

Differential settlement of the basin surface can over time lead to channelized flow and associated erosion. The infiltration surface should routinely be inspected for evidence of channelized flow, such as debris lines, concentrated sediment accumulation, or matted down vegetation, and surface should be leveled and stabilized to prevent further channelization and gully formation.

If left unaddressed, minor erosion issues can develop into severe erosion, which can compromise the stability of basin embankments and other structural features. Minor erosion problems can typically be fixed with the replacement and appropriate compaction filter media or embankment fill material and the installation/replacement of vegetation.

Poor Vegetation Establishment. The establishment of robust vegetation in infiltration basins may help promote long-term function. In addition to routine vegetation care, repeated areas of poor germination or establishment may require additional interventions to determine the cause of the problem and potential remedies. These may include soil testing to determine the need for soil amendments, or remediation of persistent erosion or sedimentation issues that may result from construction or design issues. Adjustment of species selection and/or the use of larger plant material can help to address trouble spots. Improper planting or seeding, installation outside of recommended planting times, poor quality planting material, insufficient watering, and establishment care can all contribute to the poor plant performance.

4.1.7 Surface Sand Filters

Surface sand filters are stormwater management filtration practices consisting of a sand filtration bed at or near the ground surface. Other components may include vegetation around the perimeter of the sand layer (generally the sand layer is free of vegetation) for erosion control or additional filtration, underdrains and/or outlet control structures, inflow dissipaters, spillways, pretreatment, and a forebay. A surface sand filter system may include additional storage to attenuate stormwater in combination with the pollutant removal. Stormwater is directed to the sand bed, where the sand bed filters the stormwater before conveying back to the downstream network. However, some designs may also allow for infiltration to the soil below or may include both filtration and release as well as infiltration functions. Surface sand filters can be a variety of sizes, with one or more cells arranged separately or in series. Systems may be designed to appear as an open layer of sand or may be overlain with vegetation and/or soil media.

4.1.7.1 Routine Maintenance

Surface sand filter routine maintenance consists of frequent cleaning and maintenance of visible components, and occasionally cleaning of subsurface components. Over long periods of time, sand media may clog and no longer percolate, or percolate too slowly, requiring full or partial replacement. Sand filters typically provide easy access to surface components that regularly gather debris and sediments from incoming flows. These features, including forebays, dissipaters, and vegetative or mechanical pretreatment systems, need to be maintained regularly as needed to extend the useful life of the sand media.

Vegetation. Vegetation should be inspected periodically throughout the growing season. Although the sand layer is the primary focus of this SCM type, any vegetation that may be surrounding the practice must be maintained. Vegetation growing toward or within the sand bed should be cut back or removed. Invasive species and the establishment of nontarget vegetation should be addressed promptly if observed. Nontarget vegetation should be removed using manual methods (e.g., hand-pulling) unless use of herbicide is approved. Aquatic-safe herbicides and preemergent weed controls are sometimes used to suppress weed controls and reduce manual weeding effort. To preempt nontarget vegetation establishment, weeding activities should be timed to remove nontarget plant species before they flower and set seed, thereby mitigating seed spread.

Sediment, Trash, and Debris Removal. Regular removal of sediments and debris from pretreatment, inflow and outflow, and the sand bed is central to the prevention of clogging and overall performance and longevity of surface sand filters. Rates of accumulation of sediment, debris, and trash are context dependent, and the frequency of maintenance required to ensure the design performance of a system will vary among systems, and therefore, should occur on an as-needed basis. Failure to remove accumulated sediments may result in sediments prematurely degrading the filtration efficiency of the sand media, and may result in the need for full or partial sand replacement.

Subsurface Maintenance. Cleaning of inflow and outflow conveyance should be performed as needed. With good care of surface components, the frequency of subsurface cleaning generally should be infrequent, perhaps every few years. The CCTV inspection of the subsurface piping should be carried out before and immediately after cleaning. Cleaning of conveyance systems is typically performed using hydraulic jetting techniques.

Structural. System pretreatment, conveyance, dissipaters, cleanouts, observation wells, and outfalls need to be routinely inspected during regular cleaning maintenance for proper condition and functionality.

4.1.7.2 Common Problems

Clogging. Fine sediment will accumulate within sand media over time. As a result, the efficacy of the sand filter will diminish. Reduced rates of filtration can cause standing water or increased rates of system overflow and bypass. Although the rate at which this occurs can be reduced with routine maintenance and inspection, sand media replacement will be required eventually. If clogging is observed, testing to determine if subsurface conveyance systems or control structures are clogged or if the media itself is clogged should be implemented before developing remedial action plan. If clogging within the sand media is determined to be present, removal and replacement of approximately 75 mm (3 in.) of sand media may be sufficient to restore system function. However in more severe cases, full depth replacement of the sand media layer may be needed. However, because the cost of full depth replacement may not be significantly higher than partial replacement, full depth replacement is an attractive option in many cases.

4.1.8 Swales and Strips

Swales and strips consist of linear vegetated features intended to convey or filter stormwater, often as a pretreatment measure upstream of a primary storage SCM. Swales are channel-like features used primarily for conveyance, although pollutant removal via vegetated filtration is also typically achieved/desired. Swales are routinely exposed to concentrated flows of stormwater that often have erosive velocities. Swales can be lined with a variety of vegetation, but typically include turf grasses or native meadow mixtures. Swales may include subsurface gravel storage components to promote storage and infiltration and may include sand/gravel/or geotextile liners to limit settling and migration of fines from the subgrade. Swales may include porous check dams to promote temporary ponding and infiltration. Swales may be lined with turf reinforcement matting or, in some cases, the swale bottom may include a rock or river stone strip.

Filters consist of strips of vegetation, typically dense meadow-like plantings including native grasses and forbs, through which stormwater is introduced. Filters are typically oriented perpendicular to flow and are not used for conveyance over long distances. In most cases, stormwater is introduced to filters via sheet flow, commonly using a level spreader or similar device to spread the flow over the full length of the filter.

4.1.8.1 Routine Maintenance

Sediment, Trash, and Debris Removal. As with many SCMs, routine maintenance of both swales and strips focuses in part on the removal of accumulated sediment, trash, and debris. Removal of this material is critical to vegetation health, infiltration performance (if desired), and aesthetics. As swales and strips are often used as pretreatment, significant accumulation of trash, sediment, and debris often occurs within these systems. Routine removal of sediment deposits in particular is critical for vegetation performance, as sediment can smother plantings and increase mortality. These effects may be particularly acute in swales with check dams that promote settling, and less pronounced in wider filter strips receiving diffuse sheet flow. Sediment, debris, and trash loading to swales and strips will vary significantly based on drainage area characteristics, vegetation characteristics, as well as the hydraulics within the swales or strip. For urban systems, particularly areas draining streets that lack street sweeping, monthly or even biweekly removal may be needed. For more suburban applications, quarterly removal may be sufficient. Sediment, trash, and debris removal may be difficult in high grasses. Periodic mowing may help to facilitate this work.

Vegetation Maintenance. Most swales and strips rely heavily on vegetation to provide filtration and control erosion and sedimentation. Vegetation care, therefore, is critical to the long-term success of swales and strips, particularly during the first 1 or 2 years after planting/seeding. Vegetation care includes routine watering during the establishment period. Frequent watering may be needed (once a week or more frequently), particularly during the late summer. Vegetative care also includes weeding of invasive and nontarget species and replanting and reseeding areas with poor cover. Spring mulching may also be desirable to suppress weeds and promote moisture retention, but is not recommended in swales with significant flow velocity or along swale sides, and is not recommended as long-term cover. For most swales and strips, vegetated coverage of at least 85% with target species should be established as a basic performance goal, and vegetation care should be implemented with this goal in mind, adjusting the approach (species selection, etc.) as needed to attain target cover. Vegetation care in certain environments may also include an aesthetic component. For instance, swales along roadways within residential or commercial corridors may have higher aesthetic expectations and may require more frequent trash removal, mulching, structural pruning of shrubs, and cutbacks of tall grasses to control site lines, and create more formal aesthetic, as well as deadheading of seed heads to prevent volunteer establishment. In less formal settings, spreading of more aggressive planted species, as well as volunteer establishment of common natives, can be allowed and even encouraged.

4.1.8.2 Common Problems

Erosion. Erosion is a common problem in both swales and strips. In swales, concentrated flows combined with poor vegetative establishment can produce erosion on the swale bottom. Erosion downstream of check dams is also common, particularly if a stone splash pad or other hardened energy dissipation device is not provided or is insufficiently sized. Discharge of stormwater from piped flow into swales is another erosion hot spot, particularly if armoring is insufficient. If left unaddressed, minor erosion issues can develop into severe erosion, which can include gully erosion and the headward migration of nick points and head cuts. This type of erosion can be difficult to control and repair and may require a temporary diversion of flow to reestablish stable conditions. Minor erosion problems can typically be fixed with compacted soil, seeding or plugging, and the application of erosion blanket. Soil fill should be placed in compacted lifts, scarified before seeding. Seed should be tamped to ensure good soil contact and erosion blanket stapled using manufacturer staple patterns to ensure good soil contact. Blankets should be selected based on modeling of expected velocity and shear stress, and may include straw fiber or coconut fiber blankets. More aggressive erosion can be curtailed with armoring (riprap or other hardened energy dissipation devices) of inflow and discharge points by adding or increasing the size and scope of the armoring.

Erosion is less common in strips, given the diffuse flow of stormwater that commonly flows through these practices. However, sheet flow can quickly result in channelized flow if level spreaders conveying flow into the strip become settled or as a result of slight dips in grade within the strip. Strips should be inspected thoroughly for evidence of channelized flow and associated erosion. Evidence can include debris lines, concentrated sediment accumulation, or matted down vegetation. Because many strips are vegetated using high meadow grasses, erosion problems can be difficult to spot from the filter edge. So inspectors need to systematically inspect the strip to identify minor areas of erosion. These areas can be fixed with soil fill, seeding, and erosion blankets, as described above for swales, and should be aggressively addressed to prevent gully formation. Level spreaders should also be checked and periodically releveled as needed to ensure sheet flow.

Poor Vegetation Establishment. The establishment of robust vegetation in swales and strips is critical for long-term function. In addition to routine vegetation care described above, repeated areas of poor germination or establishment may require additional interventions to determine the cause of the problem and potential remedies. These may include soil testing to determine the need for soil amendments, or remediation of persistent erosion or sedimentation issues that may result from construction or design issues. Adjustment of species selection and/or the use of larger plant material can help to address trouble spots. Improper planting or seeding, installation outside of recommended planting times, poor quality planting material, insufficient watering, and establishment care can all contribute to the poor plant performance.

Sedimentation. Sedimentation can be a persistent issue in a variety of SCMs, contributing to vegetation failure, aesthetic issues, and loss of flow and infiltration capacity. In swales, sedimentation tends to occur in areas of high sediment loading and/or wide, mildly sloping swales or those with check dams. Sedimentation may also occur at the margins of swales, at the slope toe, where velocity and shear stress are lower compared with conditions in the center of the channel. This can lead to concentration of the flow into the channel center, increasing flow velocity and inducing erosion. This can in turn lead to additional sedimentation issues upstream. Persistent or rapid sedimentation may indicate the need for design modifications, which could include the removal of check dams, adjustment of swale dimensions, or the introduction of sediment pretreatment measures. Upstream construction activities can also be a significant source of sediment. Coordination with contractors to ensure the installation of proper erosion and sediment control measures can help to protect swales and strips from sedimentation.

4.2 Subsurface Practices

Typical maintenance activities, timing, and frequencies for subsurface practices are summarized in Table 4.2.

TABLE 4.2 Summary of Maintenance Activities, Frequency, and Timing for Subsurface Practices (Reprinted with permission from AKRF, Inc.)

Maintenance Activity	Maintenance Timing and Minimum Frequency	Applicable SCM Type(s)
Sediment, trash, and debris removal	Monthly or as needed	Drain inlet inserts
	Quarterly initially, adjust to as needed	Manufactured filters and vaults and swirl concentrators; dry wells
	As sump space accumulates	Oil and water separators
Power wash (or similar deep clean)	Annually initially or as needed when clogging observed	Drain inlet inserts
Flushing/Jetting	Annually (initially), adjusted to as observed (CCTV)	Subsurface piping
Vault flood/flush	As needed and determined from CCTV inspection	Infiltration/retention trenches and vaults
Oil coalescing plate maintenance	As needed	Oil and water separators
Absorbent pad maintenance or replacement	6 months minimally or more frequently as needed	Oil and water separators

4.2.1 Drain Inlet Inserts and Manufactured Filters

Drain inlet inserts and filters consist of manufactured devices (e.g., Flexstorm, etc.) that are placed within inlets, generally just underneath the grate surface, and can capture and filter sediments, oils and greases, or other pollutants. These devices can be retrofitted to fit nearly any type of inlet design. Typical inlet insert devices are made of a woven geotextile material manufactured from a durable and flexible plastic and sewn into a bag-like shape. These devices act as a type of fine screen to strain sediment and debris from the incoming stormwater. Once the bag is filled with sediment, overflow space built into the hardware allows flow to bypass the bag. Hardware generally consists of stainless steel, aluminum, or galvanized bracketry that sits on the inlet frame beneath the grate surface. A clamping space or hooks affixes the bag to the frame. Other less typical variants consists of fine filter material with cartridges or inserts (e.g., Streamfilter™, StormEXX®), which capture fine sediments or hydrocarbons. Some filters are incorporated into inlet filter systems, and filter material that captures hydrocarbons typically work by use of sorbent material placed in a skimmer or in a boom within the existing device. Other systems are standalone technologies housed in concrete vaults or manholes (e.g., Jellyfish®, etc.). These types of filters may be removed and cleaned, or disposed and replaced when damaged or clogged beyond repair.

4.2.1.1 Routine Maintenance

Inlet inserts require frequent maintenance. Regularly scheduled maintenance to empty the insert is needed to provide continued functionality. Maintenance personnel should refer to the manufacturer's recommended frequency and procedures to aid in establishing a baseline maintenance regime. When removing filters and inserts, removal of the inlet grate is necessary. After removal of the grate, the insert frames can then be lifted up and out of their resting position and placed on a nearby tarp to avoid contaminating surfaces. The inlet filter is then tipped or flipped over to empty the sediment/debris contents onto the tarp. Once emptied, the inlet filter is reinstalled, and the grate is repositioned. Sediment is removed from the site for offsite disposal. Torn or damaged bags or frames must be replaced as needed. Commonly, inserts are cleaned during inlet vacuum cleaning, as would be carried out during vacuum truck inlet cleaning. Inserts with fine sediment filters or hydrocarbon filters generally must be replaced once the filter media has absorbed its capacity of designed filtered material. Occasionally, cartridge type inserts can be removed for heavy cleaning off site by use of pressure washer or similar methods. Manufacturer's recommendations should be followed in determining a required inspection and replacement frequency for manufactured media-based inlet inserts.

4.2.1.2 Common Problems

Damage. Inlet inserts can be damaged by sharp objects (for woven inserts), burn holes (for plastic-based insert material), or improper installation. Damaged inserts need to be replaced to ensure continued performance. Damaged frames could potentially cause a condition where the entire unit falls into the inlet sump; therefore, damaged frames need prompt replacement. Last, maintenance personnel should be cautious not to damage bags with picks or shovels in trying to break up frozen material during cleaning over winter months.

Clogging. Inserts may clog over time, whether they are filter bags or fine sediment/hydrocarbon type filters. If they clog, generally the system will continue to function as normal as a result of overflow bypass built into the insert design. However, this will allow unfiltered stormwater into the downstream SCM.

4.2.2 Vaults and Swirl Concentrators

Vaults and swirl concentrators are proprietary manufactured devices designed to store, filter, or capture incoming floatables, heavy metals, oils, debris, and TSS. Generally, these systems are manufactured of precast concrete or preformed (plastic or fiberglass) structures that are ordered to fit client design criteria and are installed by setting in place as a unit by crane or earthwork equipment. They work by various principles, but generally these include hydrodynamic separation and gravitational settling. They may be installed as a single unit or may be arranged in a series of multiple units. Vaults and swirl concentrators vary in size to manage a wide variety of flowrates.

Maintenance of vaults and swirl concentrators typically involves opening the device and dredging or vacuuming the structure clear of collected material. This is typically performed through a maintenance hatch or port, or a cover such as a manhole cover. Manufacturers of individual system types provide specific information concerning access and sediment removal procedures. The frequency of maintenance will vary highly, based on the sizing of the device to the drainage area, the land use of the drainage area, and the functionality and efficiency of the device. Generally, the frequency of cleanout will be less frequent than routine maintenance of surface SCMs.

Subsurface Maintenance. As these devices are structural, and generally installed below grade, routine maintenance can be categorized as subsurface maintenance. As such, in instances where entry into the unit is required, confined space certification and precautions should be taken. As maintenance of vaults and swirl concentrators is often performed using a vacuum truck, this work should be combined with pipe jetting, inlet cleaning, and other similar work to reduce overall costs.

Pretreatment Maintenance. Pretreatment installed upstream of the device will help reduce the need and frequency for maintenance and may be a manufacturer recommendation. Therefore, pretreatment maintenance should be considered in the routine maintenance of these type of devices and should be expected to be more frequent than maintenance of the vault or swirl concentrator itself.

4.2.3 Oil and Water Separators

Oil and water separators include a variety of pretreatment devices used to remove hydrocarbons and similar floatable pollutants from stormwater runoff. Oil and water separators are typically used in situations with high potential for oil spills and/or high concentrations of other petroleum products in stormwater runoff such as high traffic areas, parking lots, and auto repair shops. Oil and water separators can take a range of forms, from a simple down-turned elbow in a catch basin to parallel plates that coalesce oil droplets and provide enhanced separation. Selection of specific oil and water separators, and therefore associated maintenance practices, depends on anticipated runoff flow and concentrations of petroleum products.

4.2.3.1 Routine Maintenance

While oil and water separators are typically designed for long-term operation, they require periodic inspection and maintenance. High volumes of stormwater can reduce capture efficiency and create a need for more frequent maintenance of oil and water separators. Consequently, such devices should be maintained before, and checked frequently during, the wet season. At a minimum, oil and water separators should be inspected and maintained every 6 months.

Sediment and Oil Removal. Maintenance of oil and water separators typically consists of sediment, standing water, and oil/residuals removal. If the accumulated sediment at the bottom of an oil and water separator vault exceeds 15 cm (6 in.) (specific limits may vary regionally), maintenance is required. Vacuum trucks and oil absorbing materials (typically proprietary polymer blends) are most commonly used to remove sediments and trapped oil, respectively. After removing water, sediments, and floating oil residue, clean water should be used to refill the oil and water separator vault.

Oil Coalescing Plate/Absorbent Pad Maintenance. Oil and water separator maintenance activities may depend on the design of the device(s) used. Many oil and water separators have oil absorbent pads that must be replaced after approximately 6 months of use. Other devices have oil coalescing plates, which may be cleaned using a low pressure hose and oil absorbing materials. The frequency of replacement or cleaning needs may vary depending on site characteristics.

4.2.3.2 Common Problems

Trash and Floatables. Trash and other floatables can significantly interfere with the function of an oil and water separator and reduce effluent water quality. Frequent inspection and prompt removal of floatables is critical. Pretreatment directly up-gradient of the inflow point to an oil and water separator is recommended.

Structural Damage. Structural damage such as cracks, pipe damage, and/or access ladder deterioration sometimes occur. While maintenance to address such issues is beyond the scope of this manual, they pose potential safety risks and compliance issues.

4.2.3.3 Special Considerations

Oil and water separator maintenance often requires special consideration because of removal and transportation of oil, sludge, and other petroleum products. During routine maintenance, concentrated petroleum products are removed and must be disposed of in accordance with hazardous waste regulations. In addition, if manned entry is required to clean a device, a qualified cleaning technician with proper training in confined space entry may be needed.

4.2.4 Infiltration/Retention Trenches and Vaults

Infiltration/retention trenches and vaults consist of subsurface storage trenches built on site or may also include manufactured devices placed below grade that store, attenuate, or infiltrate stormwater. Built on-site trenches generally consist of a subsurface storage bed of highly porous media that can support loading, such as 20-mm (0.75-in.) clean stone aggregate. They could be installed in an area with or without planned usage above, such as a parking lot or a playground. The stone may or may not be lined with an impervious liner on one or more sides. Typically, if the storage is designed to infiltrate, the bottom grade of the storage media will not be wrapped with an impermeable liner. Overflow/outlet control devices built into the system commonly include underdrain piping and overflow weirs built into concrete control structures. Infiltration/retention trenches and vaults are commonly fed by networks of distribution piping and catch basins (inlets).

Similar to vaults and swirl concentrators, there are a number of vendors with structural manufactured devices that can be placed below grade to create highly efficient void space, allowing stormwater to collect and attenuate, and/or infiltrate. These devices may be made of concrete, such as the Contech Terre Arch®, or metal or plastic, such as the NDS StormChamber® or ACF R-Tank®. These devices functionally replace porous media and may have similar system designs to include distribution or underdrain piping.

Maintenance of stone storage beds that retain or infiltrate is generally limited to flushing the piping and maintaining pretreatment. Maintenance of manufactured products is typically tied to manufacturer recommendations and guidelines, and may involve inspection below grade, flushing of piping, pretreatment cleaning, or flooding to resuspend sediments for flushing.

Subsurface. For stone beds, jetting of distribution and underdrain lines should be done as needed. CCTV inspection is typically performed before cleaning to assess the need for cleaning. Following cleaning, a post inspection CCTV inspection is typically performed to determine the effectiveness of jetting work. Inspection frequency should be at least annually, although drainage area characteristics and the presence of pretreatment will affect intervals. For manufactured devices, the same guidance for cleaning piping applies, although systems with large voids may require a flood and flush task per the manufacturer to cause sediments on the infiltration layer to become temporarily suspended before flushing.

Pretreatment. Pretreatment often plays an important role in keeping the infiltrating surfaces clean and functional. Pretreatment devices may consist of inlet filter bags, cartridge filters, or any combination of manufactured structural devices designed for pretreatment. To ensure the infiltrating surfaces remain clean and functioning, a steady regime of pretreatment maintenance should be a top priority for these type of SCMs.

4.2.5 Dry Wells

Dry wells are stone-filled seepage pits that are designed to collect rainwater from roof gutters, convey it underground, and enable absorption into surrounding soil away from buildings. Key dry well components include roof gutter/downspouts, overflow downspouts, underground piping with a surface observation well, and crushed stone storage.

4.2.5.1 Routine Maintenance

Typical maintenance of dry wells consists of removing leaves, debris, and sediment from surface features (i.e., roof gutters/downspouts and overflow downspouts).

Routine cleaning of surface components is commonly performed multiple times per year and is a simple but effective way to avoid more costly maintenance and/or replacement of subsurface components.

Maintain Roof Gutters and Downspouts. Leaves and debris should routinely be removed from roof gutters and downspouts from April to November. Removal is especially critical during leaf fall and other periods with high production of organic debris (e.g., seeds, pollen), which may accumulate and clog conveyance structures and/or enter stone storage if unaddressed. During such periods, frequent (e.g., weekly) inspection and maintenance may be required. Pretreatment devices such as downspout strainers and roof gutter guards are often used to prevent leaves and debris from entering conveyance structures and facilitate removal by hand or with common tools such as brooms or rakes. Leaves and debris should be removed regularly from pretreatment devices to allow rainwater to easily enter the system and prevent decomposing organic debris from passing through strainer/gutter guard holes, which may be coarsely sized.

4.2.5.2 Common Problems

Clogging. Because dry wells contain exposed/semiexposed roof gutters on the surface and subsurface piping, clogging is a fairly common issue. Signs of clogging include

- Overflowing roof gutters;
- Standing water around the dry well that persists longer than the designed drawdown period (48–72 hours); and/or

- Unexpected/unusually high flow out of overflow downspouts (e.g., at the beginning of a storm or during a small storm).

Overflowing roof gutters typically indicate clogging along the gutter line and/or a downspout blockage. Blockages may be removed by hand or, if the blockage is particularly extensive or compacted, with a handheld drum auger. Persistent standing water and premature or unusually high flows through the overflow spout may be signs that underground pipe or stone storage are clogged with leaves or sediment. Hydraulic jetting can help remove clogs in underground pipes but frequently allowing clogged conditions will accumulate debris and sediments, clogging perforations in underground pipes and filling the storage media with fine sediments, resulting in the need for costly maintenance and/or replacement in the future. Routine maintenance of roof gutters and downspouts is the most cost-effective strategy to reduce clogging.

Erosion at Overflow Downspouts. Dry wells are equipped with overflow downspouts designed to discharge excess water during large storm events. Discharge onto bare ground or soft, pervious surfaces may result in erosion. To mitigate this, managers should consider adding stones or other impervious material as energy dissipaters at the overflow downspout.

Gutter Ice Damage. Snow and ice may cause roof gutter damage during winter months (particularly in the Northeast and Midwest). Roof gutters should be inspected frequently from November to March, particularly if there has been heavy snow and/or precipitation followed by freezing and thawing cycles. Clogged gutters can cause roof gutter backups, which may result in potentially damaging ice dams and buildup. In some instances, the weight of ice and snow may cause roof gutters to sag or detach, creating performance and safety concerns. Severely damaged roof gutters may require replacement.

Observation Well Cap Damage. Dry wells are typically equipped with observation wells. Observation well caps are exposed above the ground surface, allowing for easy access during inspections and making the structures vulnerable to damage. Damage may be of particular concern if observation wells are surrounded by fast-growing vegetation that must be mowed frequently. Care should be taken to avoid observation wells during mowing and string trimming. Highly visible stone or flagging to clearly identify observation wells may help avoid potential damage.

4.3 Cisterns and Rain Barrels

Cisterns and rain barrels include a variety of surface and subsurface tanks designed to store stormwater either for reuse or slow release. Rain barrels are typically small in size and deployed in residential settings, often in connection with education programs. Cisterns, by contrast, are typically much larger in size. Cisterns and rain barrels are made of a variety of materials including plastic, wood, and metal. In addition to the main storage tank, cisterns and rain barrel systems also include conveyance systems to capture and transmit flow into the cistern and rain barrel. Cistern and rain barrel systems also commonly include an intake structure, pumping systems, active controls, and conveyance piping. The conveyance piping will transmit flow to reuse distribution systems, water treatment and disinfection systems, first-flush diverters, or chambers. There is no overflow structure or orifice to convey excess flow back to the sewer system. Cisterns may also be equipped with a low flow or water quality orifice to provide slow release of all or a portion of stored flow in accordance with water quality standards and regulations. Routine maintenance activities and maintenance frequencies are summarized in Table 4.3.

TABLE 4.3 Summary of Routine Maintenance for Cisterns and Rain Barrels (Reprinted with permission from AKRF, Inc.)

Maintenance Activity	Maintenance Timing and Frequency	Notes
Sediment, trash, and debris removal	Annually. Some cisterns may need less frequent cleaning if roof sediment loads are low. If cleaning is needed more than annually, consider source control.	Empty tank before sediment removal and wash down. Accumulated material is typically removed using a vactor truck. Because mobilization is typically for an entire day, look to combine with inlet cleaning or pipe jetting.
Clean intake screens and pretreatment devices	Three times per year	
Drain down, tank cleaning, and line flushing	At least once every two years. If high levels of biofilm or algae are observed, or if odors are detected, consider source control or enhanced pretreatment	Vactor truck may be needed to remove residual water below low flow drain. Combine with sediment removal for efficiency.
Structural tank and pipe inspection using CCTV	Annually	Combine with tank cleaning and sediment removal for efficiency.
Winterization	Annually	Full drain down for tanks that are above frost line and not heat traced.

4.3.1 Routine Maintenance

Routine maintenance of cisterns and rain barrels includes periodic removal of accumulated sediment and debris that accumulates within the cistern tank. The frequency of removal will be highly driven by the sediment and debris loading characteristics of the contributing watershed and the hydraulic loading ratio, and may range from once every few months to several years. Accumulated material is commonly removed using a vacuum truck or similar vacuum-based removal. Regular inspections should be performed to establish the required cleaning frequency and to check for changes in loading rates.

In addition to sediment removal, full drain down and cleaning of the primary storage area, as well as flushing of incoming conveyance lines, should be performed periodically. Cisterns and rain barrels also commonly contain intake screens to prevent the introduction of particulates into distribution systems and to prevent clogging of the primary orifice or control structure. Frequent inspection of intake screens may be required to maintain proper functioning of these systems, particularly in higher loading environments.

In addition to removal of debris from the main storage area, other routine inspection and maintenance items include inspection and, if needed, cleaning of conveyance systems, hydraulic control structures, and pumps and controls. Annually, a structural inspection of the storage systems and conveyance systems should be performed using CCTV or similar remote imaging systems.

4.3.2 Common Problems

Sedimentation. Sedimentation and accumulation of debris within components of the cistern and rain barrel system is the most common maintenance concern. In higher loading situations, installation of pretreatment devices can be used to capture larger debris and coarse sediment. These pretreatment devices are typically more accessible and easier to clean than the primary storage area. If high rates of loading are consistently observed, SCMs should be evaluated to identify the source and potential control strategies for reducing long-term loading rates. These may include street sweeping of paved contributing areas, remediation of erosion issues, installation and maintenance of erosion and sediment controls during construction activities, cleaning of roof surfaces, and tree trimming over contributing roof surfaces.

Water Quality. Proper maintenance of cistern and rain barrel systems is essential for maintaining appropriate water quality, particularly for interior uses. Influent water quality requirements for cisterns and rain barrels vary significantly depending on the intended end use. For in-building nonpotable uses such as toilet flushing, some level of treatment and disinfection is commonly required, where as nonpotable use for landscape irrigation wash down, or other exterior nonpotable uses may require little if any treatment beyond settling. Water quality for industrial uses vary widely and are highly dependent on the specific application. For industrial process use, particularly for close loop systems, biofouling of industrial process infrastructure can occur with the use of stormwater containing higher quantities of particulate and dissolved organic matter and nutrients. While treatment and disinfection systems can be used to treat raw water to a variety of finished water standards, proper maintenance and inspections can help to reduce debris and solute loading and buildup, helping to improve the quality of raw water. In particular, testing of raw water quality may help to identify potential water quality issues. Surface foaming or significant odors may also indicate water quality issues and may point to the need for flushing and tank cleaning. If high levels of nutrients, biochemical oxygen demand, and/or organic matter are measured, this may indicate the need for more frequent flushing. Collection of vertical thermal or dissolved oxygen profiles can also identify hypoxic or anoxic conditions that could lead to development of anaerobic bacteria. If these conditions are observed, a bubbler or aeration system may be needed.

Structural Deterioration. Rates of structural deterioration will vary widely based on tank material, whether the tank is exposed to surface elements, enclosed in a building or external façade, or buried. Generally, enclosures are recommended for plastic tanks to reduce exposure to UV light, which can accelerate rates of degradation. Freeze/thaw processes can also place stress on surface tanks or subsurface tanks. To minimize these conditions, tanks should be buried below the frost line. For surface tanks that are not in heated or finished spaces, use of heat tracing elements can provide sufficient heat to prevent freezing.

4.4 Landscaped Roofs (Green Roofs)

Landscaped roofs, also called green roofs, are vegetated roof practices designed to reduce the volume and flowrate of stormwater runoff by absorbing water into a vegetated substrate and drainage media and promoting evapotranspiration. Landscaped roofs are characterized primarily as either extensive or intensive along a continuum of increasing planting media depth. Extensive landscaped roofs typically have less than 150 mm (6 in.) of planting media depth, and intensive landscaped roofs have approximately 150 mm or greater of planting media depth. Planting media depth determines, in part, the species and characteristics of selected vegetation, which guides maintenance needs. Routine maintenance activities and maintenance frequencies are summarized in Table 4.4.

TABLE 4.4 Summary of Routine Maintenance for Landscaped Roofs (Reprinted with permission from AKRF, Inc.)

Maintenance Activity	Maintenance Timing and Frequency	Notes
Sediment, trash, and debris removal	Three times per year; April, July, and October	
Watering	Herbaceous vegetation and shrubs—every 4 days; April through late-October	If site has been planted in the past 24 months, and 4 days have passed without rain
	Sedums and succulents—every 7 days; April through late-October	If site has been planted in the past 12 months, and 7 days have passed without rain
Weeding and Pest Management	Three times per year; April, July, and October	
Plant Care	Removal of dead/damaged vegetation—3 times per year; April, July, and October	
	Pruning and trimming—annually in winter	
Winterization	Annually in October	

4.4.1 Routine Maintenance

Landscaped roof routine maintenance addresses many of the functional, aesthetic, and safety needs typical to vegetated SCMs at ground level as well as considerations specific to rooftop environments. Routine maintenance consists of baseline general care (removal of trash, sediment, and debris from the SCM surface and overflow drains) as well as watering during periods of low precipitation, weeding/pest management, and plant care. The frequency and intensity of such activities may depend on characteristics of the surrounding area, depth of planting media, plant species, and regional climate. The first year of growth for landscaped roof vegetation is the period in which maintenance is particularly critical to long-term effectiveness and resilience of the SCM. In general, extensive landscaped roofs require less routine maintenance than intensive roofs.

Sediment, Trash, and Debris Removal. Sediment, trash, and debris should be removed from SCM surfaces (e.g., roof, planted beds, surface drains) in spring, summer, and fall. Interpretative or safety signage should also be cleaned as needed three times per year.

Watering. While landscaped roofs typically include hardy, drought-tolerant plant species, watering may be necessary to sustain plant health during periods of extensive hot, dry weather. Landscaped roof watering regimes depend on site maturity, species composition, and weather history. Sites with large herbaceous and woody plant species planted in the previous 24 months may require watering if there are 4 or more days without rain or watering. Grasses and sedum, a perennial succulent commonly planted in extensive landscaped roofs, should be watered if there are 7 or more days without rain or watering and the site has been planted in the last 12 months. Landscaped roofs with high temperatures and/or high winds may need to be watered more frequently.

Weeding and Pest Management. Landscaped roofs often have lower pest and weed burdens than ground-level vegetated SCMs. Nevertheless, landscaped roofs should be inspected and weeded at least three times per growing season in the spring, summer, and fall. Weeds should be removed using manual methods (e.g., hand-pulling) unless use of herbicide is approved. Herbicides and preemergent weed controls should generally be avoided unless deemed necessary. More frequent site visits may be required if weeds are present in especially high numbers. To reduce the chances of this happening, weeding activities should be timed to remove nontarget plant species before they flower and set seed, thereby mitigating seed spread. If pests or powdery mildew are present, horticultural spray oils such as neem oil are recommended. Oils should not be applied to plants in temperatures lower than 32 °F or higher than 90 °F.

Plant Care. Landscaped roof plant care consists of routine inspection, trimming, and soil amendments. Routine inspection should occur at least three times per growing season in the spring, summer, and fall. Vegetation should be trimmed at least once per year. Dead or damaged vegetation should be removed from the SCM site three times per year in the spring, summer, and fall. Soil amendments (e.g., organic fertilizer) may be applied on an as-needed basis following annual nutrient test performed by the site manager.

Winterization. If permanent irrigation systems used to water landscaped roofs in regions in which temperatures drops below 32 °F, irrigation systems must be properly winterized in midfall.

4.4.2 Common Problems

Root Penetration. Root intrusion and damage to the impermeable liner may occasionally occur. As plant roots search for water, particularly during dry periods, the roots of vigorous, aggressive plant species may puncture some materials. Prevention is the easiest and most cost-effective solution. For this reason, liners and barriers with high puncture resistance should be used. Watering may also help reduce the likelihood of root invasion.

Foot Traffic. Landscaped roofs can create aesthetically pleasing and inviting environments, potentially leading to high foot traffic and vegetation damage. Managers should first consider whether they want the landscaped roof to be accessible. Many extensive landscaped roofs, which often have shallow-rooted and drought-tolerant species that may grow slowly, are not regularly accessible. In other instances, designated walking paths and interpretive signage may help protect vegetation.

Wind. Wind can cause erosion and pose threats to vegetation through physical damage and, particularly during dry periods, by exacerbating water stress. Frequent watering during hot, windy periods is recommended. Mats or other geotextile fabric can also be used to reduce erosion and limit evaporation because of high wind. In addition, if windy conditions are typical to the site, a plant palette consisting primarily of low-lying, drought-tolerant plants is recommended. If plant damage does occur as a result of wind, large dead or damaged vegetation should be removed for safety and aesthetic reasons.

4.5 Permeable Pavement

Permeable pavement includes a variety of paving technologies that allow stormwater to infiltrate through the paving surface into a storage layer below. The techniques include permeable pavers, porous concrete, and porous asphalt. Routine maintenance activities and maintenance frequencies are summarized in Table 4.5.

4.5.1 Routine Maintenance

Maintenance of permeable pavement most often consists of regularly cleaning the porous surface using a regenerative air sweeper to prevent clogging of the porous surface. While typically used for porous concrete or asphalt, the use of regenerative air equipment on permeable pavers can be effective. However, the sweeper will commonly remove the aggregate in-fill, requiring this material to be replaced following cleaning. Routine cleaning is most commonly performed multiple times per year, typically ranging from quarterly to monthly. Generally, permeable pavement systems installed in higher sediment and debris loading environments, such as right-of-way installations, or installations in the vicinity of mature trees, will require more frequent cleaning.

In addition to regenerative air sweeping, leaves and debris should be routinely removed from permeable pavement before they can decompose and infiltrate into porous voids. This is especially critical during leaf fall and during other periods that produce organic debris (e.g., seeds, pollen). During these times, weekly removal is recommended.

TABLE 4.5 Summary of Routine Maintenance for Permeable Pavement (Reprinted with permission from AKRF, Inc.)

Maintenance Activity	Maintenance Timing and Frequency	Notes
Regenerative air sweeping	Monthly to annually depending on surface loading rates	
Pressure washing and/or air knifing immediately followed by vacuum removal	As needed to deep clean embedded sediment in the surface	Infiltration testing per ASTM C1701 or C1781 should be performed after cleaning to assess efficacy
Replenishment of joint material	As needed following cleaning for permeable pavers	Joint material may be swept or washed in
Surface leaf and debris removal	As needed during leaf fall and pollen season	Use a mechanical blower for most applications
Spot repairs	As needed, but generally at least once annually	Small repairs of porous asphalt and concrete can be made using conventional (nonporous) mixes

Routine maintenance may also include routine flushing and cleaning of underdrain or distribution pipes, structures, and cleanouts associated with the subsurface stone bed or storage chambers beneath permeable pavement systems. These components are addressed in Section 4.2 Subsurface Practices.

4.5.2 Common Problems

Sedimentation. Sedimentation is a typical performance issue that can clog permeable pavement systems and reduce infiltration rates. Routine surface infiltration tests or observation following rain events can help to identify clogging issues. If the porous surface becomes clogged as a result of high rates of sediment loading or deferred maintenance needs, regenerative air sweeping may not be sufficient to restore function and alternative "restorative" cleaning methods using a pressure washer or air knife immediately followed by vacuuming may be required. If permeable segmental pavement systems are used, for extremely clogged surfaces unresponsive to restorative cleaning, individual paving units can be removed for more intensive cleaning and/or replaced with new units. This is particularly helpful along the upstream boundary of a permeable pavement installation, especially if the installation receives significant run-on from upslope drainage areas.

In addition to routine maintenance and restorative cleaning, protection of porous surfaces from sediment loading as a result of adjacent or upstream construction activity is critical to maintaining permeable pavement function. Identifying potential sediment loading hot spots in the drainage area or adjacent areas is a key aspect of preventing sedimentation. It is important to realize that these activities may be small in scale and may not require erosion and sediment control approvals or controls from local jurisdictions. Thus, permeable pavement asset owners may need to work with building permit issuing agencies and local utilities to make sure that permeable protection specifications are included in third-party construction contracts and or as special conditions associated with building permit issuance. This may also require cross-agency geographic information systems collaboration, so that any building permits for sites within a given distance of a permeable pavement can be automatically identified. Specifications may require contractors to line the upstream and adjacent edges of the permeable pavement installation with coir logs or similar products and/or placing plastic sheeting over the installation during construction activities.

Finally, piling of dirt, salt, snow, or other materials that could generate fine particulates should be avoided both on and near permeable pavement surfaces. Additionally, the use of chemical deicers should also be avoided on pervious concrete surfaces, particularly within the first year. If deicing products are needed, they should be used sparingly, and the areas of use should be inspected for signs of wear. Deicers containing magnesium chloride should not be used on any concrete materials. These requirements should be communicated to snow plowing and other public works crews on a routine basis, and incorporated into standardized training.

Surface Wear. If wear is observed on the pervious concrete or porous asphalt surface, small areas, generally less than 4.6 m^2 (50 sq ft), can be replaced using "cold patch" patching compound. Extensive areas of wear, particularly soon after installation, may indicate problems with the installation and/or activities that may be contributing to accelerated surface wear. These activities may include improper use of snow removal equipment on the permeable pavement surface. When removing snow from permeable pavements, the plow blade should be slightly raised up from the permeable surface to prevent direct contact, or a specialty blade with a rubber or polyurethane edge should be used. Extensive areas of wear should be replaced in-kind according to the original design, taking care to avoid any installation or use issues that may have contributed to accelerated wear in the original installation.

Settling and Subsidence. Observation of significant settling or subsidence may indicate subsurface conditions, such as voids or sinkholes that are beyond the scope of this manual. If settling is observed, monitoring of elevation changes over time can help to determine if the settling issue is accelerating or slowing.

5.0 REFERENCES

Adekalu, K. O., Olorunfemi, I. A., & Osunbitan, J. A. (2007). Grass mulching effect on infiltration, surface runoff and soil loss of three agricultural soils in Nigeria. *Bioresource Technology, 98*(4), 912–917.

Angers, D., & Caron, J. (1998). Plant-induced changes in soil structure: Processes and feedbacks. *Biogeochemistry, 42*(1–2), 55–72. https://doi.org/10.1023/A:1005944025343.

Bergman, M., Hedegaard, M. R., Fjendbo, M., Binning, P., Mark, O., & Mikkelsen, P. S. (2010). Evaluation of two stormwater infiltration trenches in central Copenhagen after 15 years of operation. *NOVATECH*, (January), 1–10.

Boyle, M., Frankenberger, W. T., Jr., & Stolzy, L. H. (1989). The influence of organic matter on soil aggregation and water infiltration. *Journal of Production Agriculture, 2*(4), 290. https://doi.org/10.2134/jpa1989.0290

Castellano, M. J., & Valone, T. J. (2007). Livestock, soil compaction and water infiltration rate: Evaluating a potential desertification recovery mechanism. *Journal of Arid Environments, 71*(1), 97–108. https://doi.org/10.1016/j.jaridenv.2007.03.009

Dietz, M. E., & Clausen, J. C. (2006). Saturation to improve pollutant retention in a rain garden. *Environmental Science & Technology, 40*(4), 1335–1340.

Ekwue, E. I. (1990). Organic-matter effects on soil strength properties. *Soil and Tillage Research, 16*(3), 289–297. https://doi.org/10.1016/0167-1987(90)90102-J

Ghestem, M., Veylon, G., Bernard, A., Vanel, Q., & Stokes, A. (2014). Influence of plant root system morphology and architectural traits on soil shear resistance. *Plant Soil, 377*, 43–61. https://doi.org/10.1007/s11104-012-1572-1

Gregory, J. H., Dukes, M. D., Jones, P. H., & Miller, G. L. (2006). Effect of urban soil compaction on infiltration rate. *Journal of Soil and Water Conservation, 61*(3), 117–124.

Gyssels, G., Poesen, J., Bochet, E., & Li, Y. (2005). Impact of plant roots on the resistance of soils to erosion by water: A review. *Progress in Physical Geography, 29*(2), 189–217. https://doi.org/10.1191/0309133305pp443ra

Hatfield, J. L., & Prueger, J. H. (2015). Temperature extremes: Effect on plant growth and development. *Weather and Climate Extremes, 10*(A), 4–10. https://doi.org/10.1016/j.wace.2015.08.001

Horton, R. E. (1933). The role of infiltration in the hydrologic cycle. *Transactions, American Geophysical Union,* 446–460.

Horton, R. E. (1941). An approach toward a physical interpretation of infiltration-capacity. *Soil Science Society of America Journal, 5*(C), 399–418.

Hunt, W. F., & Lord, B. (2006). *Maintenance of stormwater wetlands and wet ponds.* North Carolina Cooperative Extension Service. https://brunswick.ces.ncsu.edu/wp-content/uploads/2013/04/Wetland-and-Pond-Maintenance-2006.pdf?fwd=no

Jenkins, J. K. G., Wadzuk, B. M., & Welker, A. L. (2010). Fines accumulation and distribution in a storm-water rain garden nine years postconstruction. *Journal of Irrigation and Drainage Engineering, 136*(12), 862–869. https://doi.org/10.1061/(asce)ir.1943-4774.0000264

Kay, B. D. (1997). Soil structure and organic carbon: A review. In *Soil processes and the carbon cycle* (pp. 169–197). CRC Press.

Lado, M., Paz, A., & Ben-Hur, M. (2004). Organic matter and aggregate size interactions in infiltration, seal formation, and soil loss. *Soil Science Society of America Journal, 68*(3), 935. https://doi.org/10.2136/sssaj2004.9350

Marin/Sonoma Mosquito and Vector Control District. (2015). *Mosquito, vector and disease control assessment (Assessment No. 3): Engineers's report fiscal year 2015–2016.* http://www.cityofbelvedere.org/DocumentCenter/View/2179/Mosquito-Engineers-Report?bidId=

Minnesota Pollution Control Agency. (2016). *Operation and maintenance of stormwater wetlands.* https://stormwater.pca.state.mn.us/index.php/Operation_and_maintenance_of_stormwater_wetlands

Morin, J., & Benyamini, Y. (1977). Rainfall infiltration into bare soils. *Water Resources Research, 13*(5), 813–817.

National Research Council. (2008). *Urban stormwater management in the United States* (Prepublication Copy). The National Academies Press. https://www3.epa.gov/npdes/pubs/nrc_stormwaterreport.pdf

New York City Department of Environmental Conservation. (2018). *NYC green infrastructure annual report 2018.* https://www1.nyc.gov/assets/dep/downloads/pdf/water/stormwater/green-infrastructure/gi-annual-report-2018.pdf

NJ Pinelands Commission. (2001). *The Mullica River Basin.* https://www1.nyc.gov/html/dep/pdf/green_infrastructure/gi_annual_report_2018.pdfhttps://www.nj.gov/pinelands/infor/reports/Mullica%20River%20Basin%20Report.pdf

Parr, J. F., & Bertrand, A. R. (1960). Water infiltration into soils. *Advances in Agronomy, 12*(C), 311–363. https://doi.org/10.1016/S0065-2113(08)60086-3

Philip, J. R. (1957). The theory of infiltration. Chapter 4: Sorptivity and algebraic infiltration equations. *Soil Science.*

Pimentel, D., Harvey, C., Resosudarmo, P., Sinclair, K., Kurz, D., McNair, M., Crist, S., Shpritz, L., Fitton, L., Saffouri, R., & Blair, R. (1995). Environmental and economic costs of soil erosion and conservation benefits. *Science, 267*(5201), 1117–1123. https://doi.org/10.1126/science.267.5201.1117

Pimentel, D., & Kounang, N. (1998). Ecology of soil erosion in ecosystems. *Ecosystems, 1*(5), 416–426. https://doi.org/10.1007/s100219900035

Reiskind, M. H., & Wund, M. A. (2009). Experimental assessment of the impacts of northern long-eared bats on ovipositing Culex (Diptera: Culicidae) mosquitoes. *Journal of Medical Entomology, 46*(5), 1037–1044.

Schmidt, M. W. I., Torn, M. S., Abiven, S., Dittmar, T., Guggenberger, G., Janssens, I. A., & Trumbore, S. E. (2011). Persistence of soil organic matter as an ecosystem property. *Nature, 478*(7367), 49–56. https://doi.org/10.1038/nature10386

Shammaa, Y., & Zhu, D. Z. (2001). Techniques for controlling total suspended solids in stormwater runoff. *Canadian Water Resource Journal, 26*(3), 359–375.

U.S. Environmental Protection Agency. (2005). Stormwater structures and mosquitoes. https://www3.epa.gov/npdes/pubs/sw_wnv.pdf

Zhu, J.-K. (2002). Salt and drought stress signal transduction in plants. *Annual Review of Plant Biology, 53*(1), 247–273. https://doi.org/10.1146/annurev.arplant.53.091401.14332

5

Inspection and Maintenance During and After Construction (Protocols)

1.0 OVERVIEW OF INSPECTION AND MAINTENANCE PROTOCOLS 121

2.0 TYPES OF STORMWATER CONTROL MEASURES AND COMPONENTS 124

2.1 STORMWATER CONTROL MEASURE TYPES 124

2.1.1 Basins 125

2.1.2 Swales and Strips 125

2.1.3 Filters 126

2.1.4 Infiltrators 127

2.1.5 Gross Pollutant Traps and Mechanical Operations 128

2.2 Stormwater Control Measure Components 129

3.0 INSPECTION AND MAINTENANCE PREPARATION 129

3.1 Health and Safety 129

3.2 Site Location and Access 131

3.3 Permits and Approvals 131

3.4 Personnel Education and Training 132

4.0 DURING CONSTRUCTION PROTOCOLS 133

4.1 Inspections 134

4.1.1 Verification of Proper Stormwater Control Measures 134

4.1.2 Verification of Location and Contributing Drainage Area 135

4.1.3 Verification of Size and Configuration 135

4.1.4 Verification of Elevations, Grades, and Dimensions 135

4.1.5 Verification of Conformance With Plans and Specifications 135

4.1.6 Verification of Structure Safety 136

4.1.7 Verification of Maintainability 136

4.1.7.1 Verification of Accessibility 137

4.1.7.2 Verification of Durability 137

4.1.8 Verification of Noncompaction 138

4.1.9 Verification of Structural Integrity 138

4.1.10 Verification of Soil/Filter Media 138

4.1.11 *Verification of Hydraulic Performance* 139
4.1.12 *Verification of Plant Establishment* 139
4.1.13 *As-Built Drawings, Inspection Documentation, and Records Management* 140
5.0 POSTCONSTRUCTION PROTOCOLS 140
5.1 Inspections 141
5.1.1 *Inspect for Debris and Litter* 142
5.1.2 *Inspect for Sediment Accumulation* 142
5.1.3 *Inspect Vegetation* 143
5.1.4 *Inspect for Erosion* 144
5.1.5 *Inspect for Settling* 144
5.1.6 *Inspect Structural Features* 145
5.1.7 *Inspect Permanent Pool* 146
5.1.8 *Inspect for Damage/Malfunction of Mechanical, Electrical, Pneumatic, and Hydraulic Components* 146
5.1.9 *Inspect Porous Pavement* 148
5.1.10 *Inspect Media* 148
5.1.11 *Inspect for Evidence/Presence of Nuisance Conditions and Animals* 149
5.1.11.1 *Inspect for Undesirable Plant Communities* 149
5.1.11.2 *Inspect for Water Quality Degradation* 150
5.1.11.3 *Inspect for Water Bird Damage* 150
5.1.12 *Inspect for Vectors* 150
5.1.13 *Inspect for Snow and Ice* 151
5.1.14 *Inspect for Miscellaneous Site Damage* 152
5.2 Routine Maintenance Protocols 152
5.2.1 *Debris and Litter Removal Control* 152
5.2.2 *Sediment Removal and Disposal* 153
5.2.3 *Vegetation Maintenance* 153
5.2.3.1 *Weed Control* 154
5.2.3.2 *Mowing* 154
5.2.3.3 *Dead and Damaged Vegetation Removal* 155
5.2.3.4 *Pruning and Trimming* 155
5.2.3.5 *Soil Management* 155
5.2.3.6 *Reseeding and Replanting* 156
5.2.3.7 *Mulching* 158
5.2.3.8 *Watering* 158
5.2.4 *Minor Erosion* 158
5.2.5 *Settling Repair* 159
5.2.6 *Structure Maintenance* 160
5.2.6.1 *Pretreatment Device, Inlets, Outlet Structures, Chambers, and Subsurface Structures* 160
5.2.6.2 *Screens and Trash Racks* 161
5.2.6.3 *Pipes* 161
5.2.6.4 *Standing Water* 162
5.2.6.5 *Permanent Pool* 162
5.2.7 *Mechanical, Electrical, Pneumatic, and Hydraulic Maintenance* 162
5.2.7.1 *Valves, Orifices, and Aerators* 162
5.2.7.2 *Pumps and Switches* 164

5.2.8 Porous Pavement Cleaning and Winter Maintenance 164
5.2.9 Media Maintenance 166
5.2.10 Nuisance Control 168
5.2.10.1 Animals 168
5.2.10.2 Water Birds 168
5.2.10.3 Undesirable Plant Communities 169
5.2.10.4 Water Quality Degradation 169
5.2.11 Vector Management 170
5.2.12 Snow and Ice Removal 171
5.2.13 Miscellaneous Site Damage 171
5.3 Nonroutine/Emergency Maintenance Protocols 171
5.3.1 Structural Repairs 172
5.3.2 Mechanical Equipment Repairs 172
5.3.3 Dam, Embankment, and Slope Repairs 172
5.3.4 Dewatering 172
5.3.5 Pond Maintenance 173
5.3.6 Fence Repair 173
5.3.7 Elimination of Woody Vegetation 173
5.3.8 Spills 173
5.4 Aesthetic Maintenance 176
5.4.1 Graffiti Removal 176
5.4.2 Vegetation Maintenance 176
5.4.3 Overall Site Maintenance 176
6.0 PRIORITIZING CORRECTIVE MAINTENANCE 177
7.0 MAINTENANCE THRESHOLD INDICATORS 177
8.0 CHECKLISTS 177
9.0 REFERENCES 210
10.0 SUGGESTED READINGS 211

1.0 OVERVIEW OF INSPECTION AND MAINTENANCE PROTOCOLS

The purpose of this chapter is to provide general protocols for inspection and maintenance procedures and practices of stormwater control measures (SCMs). All stormwater systems require proper design, construction, and maintenance to perform successfully. Thorough and consistent maintenance is particularly crucial to the successful performance of stormwater treatment practices for the following reasons:

- Some SCMs are large and complex, not only in their function or operation, but also in the number and types of materials used to construct them. This may even include natural materials such as aquatic vegetation and microorganisms. This increased complexity and variety demands a greater level of maintenance and management to ensure safe and effective operation. Many SCMs achieve their performance goals through impoundment or storage of runoff instead of conveyance. This is accomplished through the use of dams, berms, tanks, or chambers. To successfully impound water, either temporarily (for example, in a dry detention or infiltration basin) or permanently (in a wet detention pond or constructed wetland), requires a greater degree of structural integrity. Safely impounding stormwater requires more safeguards to avoid the possibly catastrophic downstream damage caused by structural failure and sudden release of the impounded water. These increased levels of structural integrity and safety, which must be provided continually throughout the life of the SCM, demand a similarly higher level of maintenance. Also, SCMs are intended to treat runoff and reduce pollutants from smaller, more frequent rainfall/runoff events. As a result, they experience maximum design conditions several times each year. This more frequent and repetitive operation at their design limit creates more stress, which again demands greater attention and commitment to proper maintenance and management.

- Failure to perform adequate maintenance of stormwater management systems not only leads to reductions in expected or desired performance levels but may even create conditions that are worse than if the facility had not been constructed. Implementation of SCMs has become an important part of our efforts to achieve clean water and a safe environment. Neglect of an SCM not only poses a threat to those living downstream, but it can also undermine the entire stormwater management program that led to their creation. The importance of regular inspection and thorough SCM maintenance cannot be overstated.
- Lack of routine maintenance can lead to long-term expense. Proactive or preventive maintenance addresses smaller issues before they become larger. For example, removing woody vegetation on the embankment of an SCM can easily prevent structural damage to the slope, which would be more costly to repair.

Maintenance of SCMs includes regular inspections and maintenance. In general, the frequency of SCM maintenance depends on the pollutant loading rate and the ability of the SCM to remove and retain these pollutants. Most factors that influence pollutant loading rates are site-specific, such as erodibility of native soils and landscaping materials, land use activities, and flow dynamics. Storage capacity is also a significant factor affecting maintenance frequency. Also, there may be occasions where emergencies, such as accidents, spills, or other incidents arise, when critical response is needed and nonroutine or emergency maintenance is required.

It is critical to plan for long-term maintenance. Plans must be put in place to identify sufficient resources to ensure, to the extent practical, inspection and maintenance can be carried out for the life of the SCM so that its design performance will be maintained. In addition, clear and concise inspection and maintenance requirements and specifications need to be provided to prevent sustainable performance degradation resulting from the failure to follow specified operations or maintenance procedures required to maintain the SCM's performance. This type of regression is also known as "backsliding." Without clear guidance on what is required to maintain sustainable performance, future owners and operators may rely on old approaches, processes, and replacement parts simply out of ignorance or convenience.

Three main drivers affect the degree and frequency of maintenance:

- Maintaining SCM functionality;
- Protecting of human health and safety; and
- Maintaining SCM aesthetics.

SCMs require a minimal level of maintenance that must be undertaken to achieve their expected performance. For example, trash and debris need to be removed to prevent components of the SCM measure from being blocked or impeded. The maintenance activity and frequency of the SCM is dependent on the type of SCM and from location to location. Although it may not be possible to accurately predict the maintenance frequency during the planning and design phase, it is still important to determine the minimum thresholds that trigger the maintenance activity. This trigger coupled with routine inspection of the SCM will enable the maintenance team to forecast the timing and frequency of maintenance.

Proper maintenance is also needed to protect health and safety. For example, removing standing water or implementing a vector control plan to manage a permanent pool of water may be required in some locations to prevent mosquitoes from spreading disease.

Some activities have less to do with proper SCM function than with appearance. Many citizens do not understand how the SCM functions but certainly care about its aesthetics. A significant amount of maintenance may be required for publicly visible or privately maintained sites compared to maintaining the SCM for performance to address the citizens' desire for an aesthetically pleasing SCM.

This chapter is organized as follows:

Section 2.0—Types of SCMs and Components: Describes the types of SCMs and their components that require inspection and maintenance.

Section 3.0—Inspection and Maintenance Preparation: Provides guidance on activities to be considered before inspection and maintenance commences.

Section 4.0—During Construction Protocols: Identifies the different aspects of the SCM that need to be verified against design plans and specification.

Section 5.0—Postconstruction Protocols: Describes the protocols that should be implemented when inspecting and maintaining SCMs once they've been constructed or installed. Maintenance activities are organized around routine maintenance, nonroutine and emergency maintenance, and aesthetic maintenance.

Section 6.0—Prioritizing Corrective Maintenance: This section provides guidance on prioritizing corrective actions based on potential failure and consequence.

Section 7.0—Maintenance Threshold Indicators: This section provides detailed guidance on specific thresholds that trigger maintenance for each SCM.

Section 8.0—Checklists: This section describes the different types of checklists that may be needed when inspecting and maintaining SCMs.

2.0 TYPES OF STORMWATER CONTROL MEASURES AND COMPONENTS

The types of SCMs presented in this chapter are consistent with those found in *Design of Urban Stormwater Controls* (WEF et al., 2012). Each SCM has different treatment mechanisms and associated components that require maintenance. Details are presented below.

2.1 STORMWATER CONTROL MEASURE TYPES

SCMs are organized around the following categories:

- Basins
- Swales and Strips
- Filters
- Infiltrators
- Gross Pollutant Traps and Mechanical Operations

A description of each SCM category is presented below.

2.1.1 Basins

The term "basin," as used in *Design of Urban Stormwater Controls* (WEF et al., 2012), refers to controls that primarily store stormwater, reduce magnitude of peak flows, provide water quality treatment primarily by sedimentation, and discharge stormwater to another SCM or surface waterbody.

The duration of detention varies from a few hours to several days, depending on the basin type, stormwater control objectives, and unit processes used. A portion of the stormwater may be evaporated, transpired, or infiltrated. The basin may also receive base flow during dry weather.

Detention basins are dry basins designed to discharge all of the stored stormwater to a surface waterbody within a given time. Retention basins (e.g., wet basins) have a permanent pool, where all or some of the stormwater captured remains until the next storm. This manual provides inspection and maintenance protocols for the following types of basins:

- Cisterns and rain barrels—function as water conservation systems by harvesting stormwater to supplement nonpotable water use.
- Forebays—a small basin designed to remove course sediment and is typically used for pretreatment.
- Vaults and swirl concentrators—used as primary or pretreatment controls, depending on their size. Vaults typically have radial baffles, and internal chambers. Swirl concentrators are cylindrical vaults, which move stormwater in a circular fashion before exiting.
- Oil and water separators—specialized vault designed to maximize the removal of oil, grease, sand, and grit. Two types exist: (1) American Petroleum Institute separators, and (2) coalescing plate separators.
- Dry basins—temporarily detain all or a portion of stormwater from each storm event by placing a restricted outlet at the bottom of the basin.
- Wet basins—an artificial lake or pond designed to promote sedimentation.
- Wetlands—a basin that includes shallow pools that store stormwater between events and promote growth of rooted vegetation.

2.1.2 Swales and Strips

Swales are shallow channels with mild longitudinal slopes and flow depths below the height of vegetation that grows within them or rocks that line them. Strips are vegetated surfaces over which stormwater flows in a thin sheet. Swales convey concentrated flow (i.e., water starts to accumulate and does not flow as a thin sheet of water flow), whereas strips convey overland flow (i.e., water flows over the plane surface as a more or less uniformly thick film or sheet of water). Both swales and strips are designed to slow down and strain suspended pollutants from stormwater.

2.1.3 Filters

A filter is a unit operation with the following design characteristics: a bed of specified filter porous media, storage to temporarily hold runoff until it is processed through the filter media, an underdrain system, and a bypass or secondary spillway. Discharge from filters may enter waterbodies, shallow aquifers, other SCMs, or storm drains. Filters are divided into two groups: slow- and rapid-rate. This manual provides inspection and maintenance protocols for the following types of filters:

- Surface sand filter—uses clean sand or gravel for the filter media. Influent stormwater flows into a forebay to a surface filter cell where it flows vertically through the sand media. Filtrate can infiltrate into the ground or be discharged to a waterbody of storm drain.
- Subsurface sand filter—both forebay and sand filter cells are located below ground in a vault. Stormwater moves through the sand media similarly to a surface sand filter.
- Bioretention filter—a class of filters that supports plants to mimic the original site hydrology more closely through evapotranspiration. Bioretention facilities are landscaped shallow depressions that capture and filter stormwater runoff. As stormwater passes down through the planting soil, pollutants are filtered, adsorbed, and biodegraded by the soil and plants. Regardless of the form the bioretention may take, there are several basic design components that are present to ensure the practice's ability to reduce runoff and remove pollutants. These may include a ponding area, filter bed (or soil media), stone layer (with or without underdrain), an inlet, overflow device or outlet, and vegetative cover. The runoff's velocity is reduced by passing over or through a buffer strip and subsequently distributed evenly along a ponding area. Stored water in the bioretention area planting soil exfiltrates into the underlying soils.
- Landscaped roofs—also known as green roofs, vegetated roofs, and eco roofs that collect, store, and evapotranspirate precipitation on building rooftops, thereby reducing the amount of runoff compared to impervious roofs. Roofs can be vegetated or nonvegetated.

Components of a landscaped roof include plants, soil media, root barrier, drainage layer, and an impermeable membrane.

- Drain inlet inserts—filters located in drains or catch basins and are typically manufactured proprietary devices that consist of inert filter material, and a support structure or housing.
- Manufactured filters—composed of a variety of shapes, functions, and sizes owing to the various manufacturers and their products in the marketplace. Most use courser media than sand filters.
- Subsurface gravel wetland—consists of a belowground stone or gravel media bed in which stormwater flows are directed horizontally through the media. A wetland and associated soil media are placed on top of the stone or gravel media bed. Stormwater enters a forebay, travels to the first of two subsurface gravel wetland cells, and flows into a slotted distributor pipe where stormwater is distributed across the stone. Stormwater then flows to the downstream end of the second cell where it is discharged to a waterbody or storm drain.

2.1.4 Infiltrators

Infiltrators are unit operations in which the entire design capture volume infiltrates to the soil and percolates to shallow aquifers. Captured stormwater is also evapotranspired. There are two types of infiltrators: surface infiltrators and underground infiltrators. Surface infiltrators capture stormwater in an aboveground, engineered impoundment and then infiltrate the stormwater to the underlying soil. Underground infiltrators are composed of belowground reservoirs that are either empty or filled with rock or other material providing support, and infiltrate through the bottom and sides of the reservoir. This manual provides inspection and maintenance protocols for the following types of infiltrators:

- Infiltration basins—a dry basin with the soil-air interface as the outlet rather than orifices or weirs.
- Infiltration trenches and vaults—small-scale infiltration systems designed to collect runoff and infiltrate it to the soil. The length of infiltration trenches is greater than its width and depth. Trenches are filled with rock to support the earthen walls. Plastic lattice structure is also used in lieu of rock to increase the pore space.
- Dry wells—underground structures typically designed to infiltrate small volumes of stormwater. Dry wells are typically configured as

excavated pits or boreholes filled with aggregate to prevent collapse of the side walls.

- Permeable pavement—consists of load bearing, durable but permeable paving surface course that rapidly passes rainwater falling on it and runoff flowing to it into an underlying layered structure where it is temporarily stored until it infiltrates to the underlying soil or is released to an underdrain.

2.1.5 Gross Pollutant Traps and Mechanical Operations

A gross pollutant trap (GPT) is a unit operation designed to remove trash, litter, debris, course sediment, vegetation, and other large pollutants from stormwater. This group of SCMs primarily use screening or skimming to remove pollutants. Screening devices include screens, nets, baskets, and racks; hoods or skimmers remove pollutants by skimming. This manual provides inspection and maintenance protocols for the following types of GPTs and mechanical operations:

- Screens—a sieve or mesh-like device used to separate gross pollutants from stormwater. Screens may be mounted on flat or curved frames, or on a drum that rotates. Screen features such as percent open area, smoothness, materials, aperture geometry can affect clogging rates.
- Nets—composed of mesh-like material, somewhat less rigid than screens that trap gross pollutants as stormwater flows through them. They may be placed within the drainage system, outfall, or within a waterbody.
- Baskets—are manufactured filter or fabric placed in a storm drain inlet to remove sediment and debris. Baskets also include inserts of various shapes and configurations and fall into one of the following groups: socks, boxes, and trays. Socks are meant to be placed in inlets and consist of fabric, typically polypropylene attached to the frame or grate of the inlet. Boxes are constructed of plastic or wire mesh. Trays hold different types of media such as polypropylene, porous polymer, treated cellulose, activated carbon, peat, and zeolite.
- Racks—consist of a series of circular or rectangular bars on a frame, spaced to trap gross solids. They are traditionally designed to protect drain inlets and for use as headworks to treatment plants.
- Hoods—devices that cover the entrance to a pipe, which leaves a basin. The hood is placed in a structure such that the bottom extends below the invert of the discharge pipe.

2.2 Stormwater Control Measure Components

Each SCM has one or more components that serve to facilitate the SCM's treatment mechanism(s). Understanding the treatment mechanism and associated SCM component is necessary to establish the specific inspection and maintenance needs of the SCM. Tables 5.4 through 5.8 summarize the five different SCM categories and their associated treatment mechanisms and components.

3.0 INSPECTION AND MAINTENANCE PREPARATION

Before the commissioning of an SCM, an operation and maintenance (O&M) plan must be prepared that defines the procedures to operate and maintain the SCM. The O&M plan typically includes:

- Health and Safety Plan (H&SP);
- Site location and access;
- Features that are provided to facilitate inspection (e.g., observation ports, cleanouts, silt posts, or other features that allow the inspector to view necessary components of the SCM and compare to maintenance thresholds);
- Description of SCM features and components, including manufacturer and part number for proprietary parts;
- Vector management (if appropriate);
- O&M;
  - Inspection protocols
  - Routine maintenance protocols
  - Nonroutine/emergency maintenance protocols
  - Aesthetic maintenance protocols
  - Maintenance threshold indicators
- Required permits; and
- Required personnel training and experience.

3.1 Health and Safety

As part of the O&M plan, the health and safety of personnel involved in the inspection and maintenance program must be considered a high priority. Maintenance activities and equipment operation are to be performed in accordance with all applicable laws and regulations including, but not limited to, those of:

- Occupational Safety and Health Administration (OSHA);
- State and local requirements; and
- The owner/operator's H&SP.

In the event of a conflict between health and safety regulations, maintenance personnel shall follow the most stringent/protective requirements. Personnel shall utilize personal protective equipment such as head, eye, and ear protection, as well as protective gloves, footwear, high-visibility clothing, and all other applicable protective equipment consistent with all OSHA standards. Personnel are responsible for maintaining safe and healthy working conditions as part of their daily activities.

Persons accessing the site for operation, inspection, and maintenance must adhere to the requirements of the H&SP. Stormwater control measures may be placed in challenging locations, and planning for human health and safety is a top priority. Some potential considerations include

- Traffic hazards;
- Wet conditions;
- Hot conditions;
- Cold and icy conditions;
- Biological concerns;
- Transients;
- Physical obstructions that complicate access to the site (e.g., steep slopes, vegetation overgrowth);
- Confined spaces (e.g., manholes that might contain toxic, explosive, or otherwise unsafe conditions);
- Flooding and fast-moving water;
- Dim lighting;
- Slippery conditions;
- Contact with water that could be harmful (e.g., caustic, pathogenic);
- Lifting and carrying heavy and bulky pieces of equipment; and
- Electrical hazards.

Based on the hazard assessment, the appropriate equipment and procedures to protect field personnel from the potential hazards must be included in the O&M plan. The H&SP shall be an appendix of the O&M plan.

Before maintenance events, maintenance personnel must assess sites for safety issues. If safety issues are identified, maintenance personnel must report them to the owner/operator immediately. Personnel are responsible for temporarily securing the safety hazard using cones and safety tape.

Storm drain structures and SCM vaults pose potential health hazards. No personnel shall for any reason enter a confined subsurface structure (such as a manhole or access port) without valid confined space entry certification. Maintenance personnel are to follow OSHA confined space entry protocols and utilize air quality monitors whenever entering a confined subsurface structure.

If any hazardous materials or wastes are encountered, work must be stopped, and the owner/operator notified. Hazardous materials shall be handled only by trained personnel.

3.2 Site Location and Access

The location and access to an SCM must be provided so that field personnel can easily and safely access the site. Photographs of the site and site plans/location maps should be included in the O&M plan. Site-specific information that is important for field personnel to know about includes:

- Coordination with appropriate landowner personnel;
- Location (address, GPS coordinates, Post Mile) with site map;
- Driving directions from the agency office/yard;
- City or county jurisdiction;
- Regulatory agency jurisdiction;
- Parking location;
- Traffic control requirements;
- Gates, locks, keys, combinations;
- Sensitive habitat or species;
- Safety considerations;
- Other features of the site, including distance from roadway(s), slopes, ground cover, overhead concerns, and so on (include photographs of the site); and
- Notification requirements.

3.3 Permits and Approvals

In some cases, it may be necessary to obtain permits and approvals to access, inspect, and maintain the SCM. Permits fall within two major categories:

those issued by landowner or agency to allow access to the SCM; and those issued by other environmental regulatory agencies. The owner/operator and/or maintenance personnel must obtain all required permits and approval before commencement of work and have hard copies of documents on site during inspection and maintenance events.

Maintenance personnel should immediately notify the owner/operator if access to inflow inlets is obstructed by vehicles parked in the right-of-way during a maintenance event. For sites where vehicle obstructions are commonplace, the owner/operator may choose to redirect parking using restrictive signage before a maintenance event. Blocking of public streets should be avoided unless prior arrangements have been made with the local agency and coordination with appropriate departments has been established. Traffic control is the responsibility of maintenance personnel and must be in compliance with state, country, and local highway construction codes.

Regulatory agencies, such as the U.S. Army Corps of Engineers, the U.S. Fish and Wildlife Service, and the Bureau of Indian Affairs, may become involved depending on the project's location or other circumstances. It is essential that all possible permits and approvals be evaluated and obtained before inspecting and maintaining the SCM, as the respective agency can halt the activity, or impose fines, for failure to secure the necessary permit, certification, and/or agreement.

3.4 Personnel Education and Training

Education and training are an essential part of O&M of SCMs. Many SCMs are often implemented by local governments, private landowners, and nonprofit organizations, and may rely on private residents or volunteers to conduct project maintenance. In these cases, many of the individuals may not have experience performing the maintenance activities required for the project to function optimally. To prevent this from causing problems, successful implementation involves not only having an O&M plan in place, but having also conducted public education efforts, outreach campaigns, and training programs.

The maintenance of SCMs is typically labor-intensive and needs to be performed by trained and knowledgeable staff. Maintenance personnel should possess the appropriate training and experience. Personnel operating equipment should possess the appropriate and applicable certifications and licenses. Personnel handling regulated materials must possess the appropriate and applicable certifications and licenses. Personnel performing work on public sites should also be clearly identified by clothing, equipment, and information.

Effective O&M training should be provided in an easy-to-understand format, occur at regular intervals, and target the activities employees, residents, or volunteers are expected to perform. Education and training can also provide information on the water quality and environmental benefits that green infrastructure can yield when properly maintained.

Maintenance activities are accessible to entry-level personnel, provided they receive appropriate training and can demonstrate a base level of applicable knowledge and skill. The entry-level, accessible nature of SCM maintenance jobs offers an opportunity to support job creation and long-term employment opportunities in communities where the SCMs are being implemented. SCM maintenance requires investments in the physical and material aspects of the infrastructure and investments in training responsible staff. Ultimately, the skills and knowledge acquired through training and professional development should be captured in a certification reflecting professional expertise. Similar to other professional credentials that separate training and testing/certification, it is recommended that O&M staff are competently trained and certified while providing livable wages, professional growth, and job portability. Additionally, it would raise the level of professionalism in the sector for those who inspect and maintain SCMs. The National Green Infrastructure Certification Program (NGICP) is one such program that provides the base-level skill set needed for entry-level workers to properly construct, inspect, and maintain green stormwater infrastructure; following is the weblink to NGICP: https://ngicp.org/. In 2019, Congress enacted the Water Infrastructure Improvement Act, which defines green infrastructure as "the range of measures that use plant or soil systems, permeable pavement, or other permeable surfaces or substrates, stormwater harvest and reuse, or landscaping to store, infiltrate, or evapotranspirate stormwater and reduce flows to sewer systems or to surface waters" (DC Water & Water Environment Federation, 2015).

4.0 DURING CONSTRUCTION PROTOCOLS

Construction of most SCMs includes excavation, grading, placement and compaction of fill material, pipe laying, construction of reinforced concrete structures, and installation of appurtenant components. Construction must be performed by qualified and experienced contractors. Implementation of proper construction techniques and use of quality materials are necessary to ensure the durability and maintainability of the SCM. Construction-related maintenance problems cannot be simply avoided by entrusting a qualified contractor to build the SCM from a set of plans and specifications.

Unforeseen situations can arise during the construction phase, which require either deviation from the original plans or modified construction techniques. As a result, a direct link between the contractor and SCM designer is needed to ensure that the best possible SCM is constructed. This link is provided by the construction inspector. The value of thorough construction inspection procedures cannot be overemphasized. Poor SCM construction can lead to many serious maintenance and safety problems, including standing water, wet bottoms, slope erosion, channel scour, mosquito breeding, and even structural failure. It can also lead to poor treatment. It is much easier and less expensive to construct an SCM correctly the first time than it is to repair, reconstruct, or deal with construction defects and the facility maintenance problems they create. This section describes the common inspections that should be conducted to verify the SCM has been properly constructed.

4.1 Inspections

Before construction of the SCM, the construction inspector should become familiar with the SCM plans and specifications and note especially complex components, difficult site conditions, and other potential problem areas that may require special attention. Soon after the award of the construction contract, a preconstruction meeting should be held between the SCM owner, contractor, project engineer, and inspector. These individuals play key roles in the construction of the SCM. Many problems and misunderstandings can be avoided by engaging the same group of people throughout the entire construction period. During the construction phase, the inspector has the ability to alert the contractor to potential problems that lie ahead and to work with the contractor to develop alternate methods or techniques that can avoid the problems without affecting the progress of the work. Presented below are common inspections that should be conducted to avoid construction-related defects or flaws, which can cause additional SCM maintenance and/or premature facility deterioration.

4.1.1 Verification of Proper Stormwater Control Measures

The selection and design of SCMs is done intentionally to comply with regulatory requirements and to meet specified performance objectives, such as capture efficiency, volume reduction, and concentration reduction. Deviation in the type of SCM can lead to noncompliance. To avoid noncompliance, the inspector should verify that the SCM is consistent with the plans and specifications. This is especially important for proprietary SCMs. In some cases, regulatory or permitting agencies require SCMs to meet certain performance standards as certified through third-party, field scale evaluation from organizations such as Washington State Technology Acceptance

Protocol-Ecology Program, Technology Acceptance Reciprocity Partnership, or New Jersey Corporation for Advance Testing.

4.1.2 Verification of Location and Contributing Drainage Area

The location of the SCM, site layout, and drainage patterns based on actual site grading need to be verified by the inspector. This is necessary to confirm that the SCM has been properly placed to receive stormwater runoff from the contributing drainage area originally planned for during the design phase. The overall site layout allocates space for the SCMs and promotes drainage patterns that are effective for hydrologic control and pollutant source control. Changes to the location of the SCM and drainage patterns can result in more or less flow volume and/or flowrate than was originally intended to be treated by the SCM; deviation can lead to noncompliance.

4.1.3 Verification of Size and Configuration

Stormwater control measures are designed to a specific size and configuration to detain, infiltrate, reuse, or filter pollutants from a specified flowrate or flow volume. The inspector should verify that the size and configuration of the SCMs are consistent with the plans and specifications. Verification of size should be done through direct field measurements. Changes to the size of the SCM can result in more or less flow volume and/or flowrate than was originally intended to be treated by the SCM. Furthermore, configuration of SCM features such as inlet and outlet locations can have an effect on pollutant removal. Deviation can lead to noncompliance.

4.1.4 Verification of Elevations, Grades, and Dimensions

The accuracy of the placement and size of pipes, orifices, and low flow channel inverts, weir crests, bottom slopes, outlet structure dimensions, and other SCM components should be verified by the inspector. While some of the specified values are not critical to the performance of the SCM and, therefore, some variation is acceptable, the tolerance on critical components such as orifice inverts, low flow channel grades, and bottom slopes can have serious adverse effects on the performance of the SCM and its required maintenance.

4.1.5 Verification of Conformance With Plans and Specifications

Although relatively small in size, such components as orifice plates, hinges, anchor bolts, and hasps are vital to the correct functioning and low maintenance of an SCM. Careless installation of these components can complicate maintenance efforts and require otherwise avoidable repairs. Also, not all SCM components are visible once the facility has been completed.

The omission or incorrect installation of items such as compacted fill, concrete quality, geotextile fabrics, reinforcing steel, pipe jointing, gabion lacing and diaphragms, quality of other materials, and stone bedding can only be detected through close inspection of each construction step. The effects of these omissions or errors may not show up for several years. The maintenance problems and expenses they cause may continue for many more. As a result, the inspector should be diligent in verifying the SCM has been constructed in conformance with the plans and specification.

4.1.6 Verification of Structure Safety

Because of the inherent dangers of storing runoff and the exceptionally large quantities of runoff that can be produced by these extreme events, SCMs are designed with the goal of safety by ensuring that the facility will also function properly under such extreme conditions. Extreme conditions may be defined as either extreme weather or storm conditions where rainfall exceeds normal design values or where equipment or components fail structurally or operationally. Addressing extreme conditions at an SCM will typically include the provision of an emergency spillway or other auxiliary outflow device that will safely convey the extreme event runoff that exceeds the capacity of the facility's normal outflow structure. It will also include protection of critical portions of any embankment, dam, or discharge points that may be subject to scour or erosion from the high flow velocities generated by this storm event. Protection of such critical areas from damage will not only increase safety but reduce and even eliminate the need for poststorm maintenance and repairs.

Consideration of extreme conditions is also important when reviewing the accessibility of system components to maintenance personnel. For example, if a trash rack is blocked or damaged during a storm event and is causing dangerous water levels in a facility, will maintenance personnel be able to reach it safely? Will inspectors be able to reach the system itself during an extreme storm event to evaluate the potential for overtopping and failure? These questions can only be answered satisfactorily if the facility's performance under such extreme conditions is thoroughly analyzed by the designer. However, it is the inspector's responsibility to ensure the SCM components have been constructed as intended so that it can be safely operated.

4.1.7 Verification of Maintainability

Maintainability can be expressed in three ways:

- Every effort should be made to minimize the amount and frequency of regular maintenance at a stormwater management system.

- Performance of the remaining maintenance tasks should be as easy to perform as possible.
- All efforts should be made to eliminate the need for emergency or extraordinary maintenance at the facility.

The inspector should verify the maintainability of the SCM by inspecting the following:

4.1.7.1 Verification of Accessibility

The biggest problem maintenance staff encounter is not the amount or frequency of maintenance they must perform, but the difficulties they have in simply reaching the location of the required maintenance work. To facilitate maintenance the various components of the SCM and, indeed, the facility itself, must be accessible to both maintenance personnel and their equipment and materials. Physical barriers such as fences, curbs, steep slopes, and lack of adequate and stable walking, standing, climbing, and staging areas can seriously hinder maintenance efforts and drastically increase maintenance difficulty, cost, time, and safety hazards. If potential access issues are noted up front, the maintenance personnel can be warned and can plan accordingly. Risers and manhole access can be particularly challenging and dangerous, particularly when access steps are missing, or no manhole access has been provided. Features such as depressed curbs, hand and safety rails, gates, access roads, hatches, and manholes will expedite both inspection and maintenance efforts. Many access issues should be addressed during design. The inspector should verify that the SCM is accessible so that proper inspection and maintenance can be performed. The inspector should also look for opportunities to improve accessibility during construction that may not have been considered by the designer.

4.1.7.2 Verification of Durability

The use of strong, durable, and noncorroding materials, components, and fasteners can greatly expedite facility maintenance efforts. These include strong, lightweight metals such as aluminum for trash racks, orifice and weir plates, and access hatches; reinforced concrete for outlet structures and inlet head walls; hardy, disease-resistant vegetation for bottoms, side slopes, and perimeters; and durable rock for gabions and riprap linings. In most instances, the extra investment normally required for more durable materials will pay off over time.

4.1.8 Verification of Noncompaction

To help preserve the natural infiltration rate of the subgrade soils before excavation, the infiltration area should not be excessively traveled by heavy construction equipment that causes excessive compaction of soil pores. The area should be marked off and traffic kept off it to the greatest extent possible. Excavation should be done by lightweight equipment to minimize the potential of soil compaction. Tracked, cleated equipment does less soil compaction than tired equipment. The inspector should ensure the contractor follows these practices.

4.1.9 Verification of Structural Integrity

Ground settlement following construction can be the result of many factors, including but not limited to, incomplete compaction, unsuitable backfill materials, poor subsurface conditions unknown at the time of design, and unnecessary disturbance during construction of subsurface soils, which must act as foundations for SCM. Settlement of the facility bottom can create localized ponding areas, which can create a situation whereby the ponded water cannot be drained to the facility's outlet structure or low flow channel. This can unnecessarily complicate, delay, or even prevent required grass mowing. It can also create mosquito breeding habitats, which will require expensive treatment by trained specialists. Settlement of side slopes can create opportunities for rills and gullies to form. Settlement of dams, embankments, and outlet structure foundation soils can result in serious structural damage and total facility failure. In any case, ground settlement can require additional expense in the form of extra maintenance and/or repair efforts. The inspector should verify proper techniques are being employed by the contractor to ensure the integrity of the SCM.

Concrete is a versatile and durable building material. However, proper handling, placing, and curing are vital to achieving that durability and longevity. Premature failure of a concrete structure can result in the need for expensive repairs. Many defects in a concrete structure are not readily discernible immediately after the structure is completed, and it may take several years for the defect to become apparent. Close inspection of each step of the actual construction, therefore, is vital to ensure the longevity and reliability of the concrete structure.

4.1.10 Verification of Soil/Filter Media

Many different types of soil/filter media are available. Bioretention soil media (BSM) is one example, which is a formulated soil mixture intended to filter stormwater and support plant growth while minimizing the leaching of chemicals found in the BSM itself. BSM consists of 70% to 85% by volume washed sand and 15% to 30% by volume compost or alternative organic amendment. Alternative proportions may be justified under certain conditions. The inspector should verify that soil/filter is mixed thoroughly using a mechanical mixing system at the plant site before delivery. To reduce the potential for leaching of nutrients, the proportion of compost or alternative organic amendment must be held to a minimum level that will support the proposed vegetation in the system.

Soil/filter media should be provided from an approved vendor and stored on an adjacent impervious area or plastic sheeting. Soil/filter media should be applied in 305-mm (12-inch) lifts until the desired top elevation of the bioretention area is achieved. If heavy machinery is used, the inspector should make sure the machinery works from the edges to avoid compacting any soils or side slopes.

The inspector should verify filter media is hydraulically compacted to avoid future settling. This process involves flooding the filter media after the initial installation to facilitate settling under natural operation conditions. Additional media should be added a few days later, as needed, to achieve the design elevation.

Other types of pretreatment and membrane filtration are also available and are commonly an integral component of proprietary SCMs. These filtration membranes should be checked for damage before use.

4.1.11 Verification of Hydraulic Performance

The hydraulic performance of the SCM should be verified during the commissioning phase and before accepting the contractor's work. Verification should include checking to see that stormwater runoff enters the facility and does not short-circuit, there is no unintentional bypass or overflow, detention times are met, drain down times are met, there is no scouring of filter media, pumps are functional, and equipment does not leak.

Additionally, the American Society for Testing and Materials (ASTM) developed ASTM C1814/C1814M-20, Standard Test Method for Measurement of Hydraulic Characteristics of Stormwater Filtration Elements. This test determines the hydraulic capacity of stormwater filtration systems. Test results are not an indicator of the filtration performance with respect to the capture of solids or other materials.

4.1.12 Verification of Plant Establishment

Normally, the SCM contractor is responsible for establishing and maintaining suitable grass and other vegetative covers for a specified period of time after construction has been completed. However, inadequate or unsuitable topsoil, lack of fertilizer, and insufficient watering may result in weak plant covers that are unable to withstand more than one seasonal cycle. Once the contractor's responsibility for the vegetation establishment has ended, the cost of any required repair or replacement must come from the facility's maintenance budget. It is therefore critical that the inspector verify that the required plant survival and coverage is achieved during the plant establishment period.

4.1.13 As-Built Drawings, Inspection Documentation, and Records Management

A log of all pertinent construction activities should be kept by the inspector. When the construction of an SCM is substantially complete, but before final cleanup has begun, a complete and thorough inspection of the site should be undertaken by the inspector, who should then prepare a list (commonly called a punch list) of items that require additional work or attention. The punch list is an effective tool that the inspector can use to help ensure that all facility construction is complete and correct even before the contractor demobilizes and leaves the project site. After the punch list items have been completed and final payment made to the contractor (except for any retained percentage), the contractor should be contractually obligated to correct or repair the new SCM as warranted for a period of at least 1 year. During this time, the inspector should perform periodic inspections of the facility and immediately bring any problems to the contractor's attention. Having done so, the inspector should then regularly encourage the contractor to perform the warranted repairs in a timely manner.

As-built plans should be completed promptly following construction of a facility. These plans should show all actual as-built dimensions, elevations, and locations of all facility components. Generally, the as-built plans are produced by making appropriate revisions to the construction plans. The as-built plans should be made available to the owner, municipality, maintenance staff, and all agencies that have any jurisdiction over the facility. Aside from providing a permanent record of the actual facility constructed, these plans are important for establishing maintenance procedures, and will also facilitate any future rehabilitation or modifications of the facility. Finally, the construction documents should be filed by the inspector.

5.0 POSTCONSTRUCTION PROTOCOLS

Once construction is satisfactorily completed, the long-term assurance of adequate facility performance begins. Stormwater control measures are expected to perform their stormwater quality and quantity control functions for their useful life. Failure to maintain these systems can create the following adverse effects:

- Increased discharge of pollutants;
- Increased risk of flooding;
- Increased downstream channel instability, which increases sediment loadings and affects habitat for aquatic organisms;
- Potential loss of life and property, resulting from catastrophic failure of the facility; and
- Aesthetic or nuisance problems, such as mosquitoes.

These adverse effects can be avoided through proper and timely maintenance of the SCM. The most common cause of SCM failure is the lack of adequate and proper operation, maintenance, and management.

Routine or preventive maintenance refers to procedures that are performed on a regular basis to keep the SCM in proper working order and aesthetically pleasing. Routine maintenance may include removing debris, removing silt and sediment, and clearing control devices to prevent clogging. Routine maintenance also includes maintaining healthy vegetation. Dead or unhealthy vegetation needs to be replaced or restored. Connections, fittings, valves, joints, screws, and other mechanical parts may need to be adjusted, repaired, or replaced. SCMs with chemical additives may require removal of spent materials and/or addition of new chemicals

5.1 Inspections

Inspections help the stormwater manager monitor the safety, longevity, and effectiveness of an SCM over time. Inspection requirements vary from jurisdiction to jurisdiction, depending on the specific SCM. For example, some sand filtration systems require monthly inspections while other SCMs can be inspected on a yearly basis. Some agencies provide inspections of all facilities within their jurisdiction while others require that the responsible party arrange for an inspection and send the results for confirmation. The local agency should be contacted to determine specific requirements including qualified inspectors.

Inspectors should identify the extent and location of problems identified during inspection. They should also aid maintenance staff to locate repairs both at the site and on design plans. While all maintenance and inspection items are important, some maintenance concerns actually pose an immediate safety concern. Many of these are caused by missing or damaged components that would normally prevent access by the public. Examples include missing manhole covers or trash racks, missing or damaged fencing that prevents access to the SCM, or a missing or damaged grate at an inlet or outlet. Another immediate concern is addressing basin-type SCMs that pose dam safety or flooding hazards. If an SCM shows signs of embankment failure, then it should be immediately repaired. Similarly, cracks in a riser that drains a large area may pose a dam safety threat.

The inspector should bring a copy of the as-built plan to mark areas of needed maintenance. The inspector should also take photographs of the SCM being inspected. During the inspection, the inspector should highlight key areas of concern with spray paint or other markers. This is particularly helpful for problems that may otherwise be difficult to find by others. Marking should be used as discreetly as possible so not to distract from the facility's aesthetics. The following sections provide detailed descriptions of the different types of inspections.

5.1.1 Inspect for Debris and Litter

Trash and debris removal should occur during the regularly scheduled maintenance to reduce the chance of outlet structures, trash racks, and other components becoming clogged and inoperable during storm events. Proper preventive maintenance includes removal of debris from pond bottoms, embankments and side slopes, perimeter areas, and access areas that can lead to clogging, as well as debris jams at outlet structures and trash racks.

Clogging can be identified through routine visual inspection. Clogging within low-flow pipes and underdrains can be more difficult to find. The openings of a trash rack should be clear of debris. Trash racks should show little or no corrosion and should be completely visible. A weir or orifice is intended to set the permanent pool. The water surface elevations should be inspected to determine if the permanent pool levels are staying higher than designed for longer periods than expected following a rainfall event. If pool levels are higher than expected for long durations, then a clogged low flow pipe or orifice, or internal clogging of a low flow drain may be the problem.

5.1.2 Inspect for Sediment Accumulation

Inspection for sediment accumulation should be done to assess if it needs to be removed before it threatens the operation or storage volume of the SCM in its ability to reduce suspended solids. The inspector should determine when sediment cleanout is needed and should specify where the removed sediments are to be placed.

Certain types of basins, such as wet ponds and constructed wetlands, may need to be dredged. This may be indicated by sediment plumes or deltas at storm drain inlets that feed the SCM. Accumulated sediment can also be measured through use of a staff gauge. The best way to determine if a pond or wetland needs dredging is to perform a bathymetric study, which involves taking field measurements to calculate the volume of water within a pond or lake. The survey is similar to a topographic measurement of the contours below the permanent pool surface of a pond. The survey will result in a two-dimensional map indicating depth contours at locations within the permanent pool. Bathymetric surveys indicate the amount of silt or muck that has accumulated within a pond or wetland, and the amount of material that needs to be dredged.

5.1.3 Inspect Vegetation

Vegetation management is often the most frequent type of maintenance conducted on SCM. The inspector should look for the following to determine if vegetation maintenance is needed:

- Standing water and emergent plant growth where none should be present;
- Monoculture vegetation;
- Poor or spotty grass growth or completely bare areas;
- Soggy surfaces;
- Excessive sedimentation at inlets or outfalls with corresponding emergent plant growth;
- Limited visibility or access to the principal spillway or embankment areas because of vegetation;
- Deep-rooted woody vegetation (trees and shrubs) on any areas of embankments or slopes;
- Woody vegetation growing in riprap on slope areas meant for erosion protection;
- Signs of seepage around any tree stumps or decaying root systems on embankment areas;
- Changes in vegetative color, species, or height because of possible groundwater or seepage problems;
- Pond embankments with newly planted ornamental trees or shrubs not originally included in the design;
- Damaged or torn erosion control blanket;

- Ruts or erosion channels in vegetated swales or level spillways;
- Tree or shrub growth in or around permanent pools appurtenances such as the principal spillway; and
- Damaged irrigation systems.

5.1.4 Inspect for Erosion

Erosion problems can occur within an SCM. For the most part they start as small rills, and if uncorrected, can grow into large gullies that threaten the integrity of the SCM. Inspections to locate erosion problems should be done at least annually or after major storms. A stable embankment is important to ensure that erosion does not contribute to water quality problems and that embankments are not breached, resulting in downstream flooding. Maintaining a healthy vegetative cover and preventing the growth of deep-rooted (woody) vegetation on embankment areas is an important component of stabilization. Outlet structures are particularly prone to undercutting and erosion. Unchecked, a small problem can easily result in the need to replace the entire structure. Evidence of significant foot or bike traffic in areas where vegetation has died indicates potential erosion areas in the future. Specific areas that should be checked include

- Inlet;
- Side slope;
- Bed or invert; and
- Outlet.

5.1.5 Inspect for Settling

SCMs have several structural components that can settle. Settlement in the structure is defined as the failure or the dislocation of the portion as a result of an unequal compression happening in the foundation or displacement of soil underneath the structure because of filling a cavity and a new void space being created. Generally, the settlement of the structure occurs because of the settlement of the foundation. In the uniform settlement of foundation, the whole structure moves vertically downward at a uniform rate. There will be no cracks in the structure with uniform settlement. In the tipping and differential settlement of the foundation, there may be cracks in the structure. The inspector should inspect the following SCM features that may encounter settlement:

- Head walls;
- Pipes;

- Outlet structures; and
- Embankments.

5.1.6 Inspect Structural Features

Structural features including inlets, outlets, pipes, vaults, chambers, weirs, screens, riser structures, and trash racks are the backbone of SCMs. These features should be inspected to verify their structural integrity, that they are not clogged, and that they are not damaged. Pipes and other belowground features should be inspected for the following:

- Joint tightness—The types of joints and their tightness depend on their application (i.e., culverts, underground detention/retention systems, and storm sewers) and the pipe material (e.g., corrugated metal pipe, concrete pipe, and plastic pipe). *Standard Practice for Pipe Joint Selection for Highway Culvert and Storm Drains* (AASHTO, 2017) is an excellent resource. This practice provides definitions of joint performance terms, methodology to determine appropriate joint performance requirements, and uniform criteria for manufacturers' joint qualification and contactors' postinstallation pipe joint testing.
- Misalignment—Pipe segments can be misaligned because of differential settlement, freeze–thaw cycles, and dynamic loads, which are more likely to occur shortly after construction.
- Pitting and corrosion—Pitting is the localized corrosion of a metal surface confined to a point or small area that takes the form of cavities. Pitting is one of the most damaging forms of corrosion. Erosion is the combined effect that occurs as a result of corrosion and erosion and is caused by the rapid flow of any turbulent fluid on a metal surface (Corrosionpedia, 2019). Pitting and corrosion can be addressed by streamlining the pipe to reduce turbulence, controlling stormwater velocity, using more resistant materials, and using correction inhibitors or cathodic protection.
- Staining and calcification—Rust stains on concrete structures often indicate that moisture has reached the steel rebar and is corroding it. Repairs should be made to stop the moisture from infiltrating through the concrete to the rebar. Calcification or spalling occurs when moisture, salt, and magnesium chloride cause concrete to break down and crumble. Application of sealers and coatings can prevent surface water from penetrating concrete and help reduce the permeability of concrete.
- Root intrusion—Roots initially find their way into storm drain lines through small cracks, holes, pipe joints, or gaps. Once the roots are

inside, they began to reach out and spread within the pipe. Root intrusion can be addressed using trenchless repair (cured-in-place piping and hydrojetting) (AASHTO, 2017; Contech Engineering Solutions, 2020).

By inspecting structures for the indicators listed previously, the inspector can better understand the types of problems likely to affect the structural integrity of SCMs and determine the course of corrective action.

5.1.7 Inspect Permanent Pool

Maintaining the permanent pool of a wet pond or constructed wetland is critical because it is the primary treatment mechanism (i.e., promotes settling). The elevation and fluctuations of water level elevation should be inspected.

The following observations indicate clogging of orifices and outlet structures:

- The water level is higher than its base water level (i.e., water level during dry periods) for several days following a storm event and
- Side slopes and plants normally visible are submerged.

The following observations indicate that the permanent pool is too low:

- Water level is below stains or water marks caused by the base water level (i.e., water level during dry periods) on the outlet/flow control structure;
- The pond bottom is exposed; and
- Plant density has increased.

Maintaining a record of permanent pool elevation measurements can aid in assessing whether the wet pond or constructed wetland is clogged or seeping (U.S. EPA, 2009). Other environmental factors such as burrowing animals and the preponderance of trash in the watershed should be considered when establishing the inspection frequency.

5.1.8 Inspect for Damage/Malfunction of Mechanical, Electrical, Pneumatic, and Hydraulic Components

To ensure the useful life of mechanical components, careful inspection is needed. Signs of common mechanical failures include

- Loose components;
- Rusted, pitted, and corroded parts;

- Degradation or damage to protective coatings;
- Loose or corroded bolts;
- Leaking valves and connections;
- Valves and actuators in a stuck position;
- Loose or exposed wires; and
- Standing water.

Pumps and other electrical, pneumatic, and hydraulic components should be inspected for the following:

- Unusual noise;
- Unusual vibration;
- Unusual temperature;
- Leaks in pump or piping;
- Pressure gauge readings;
- Visual inspection of equipment general condition;
- Anytime a pump is opened, inspect the running clearances;
- Anytime a pump is opened, inspect the impeller for corrosion or excessive wear;
- Packing box—verify slight leakage;
- Mechanical seal (should be no leakage);
- Drain lines are working properly;
- Coupling integrity;
- Drive shaft integrity;
- Verify proper operation of oil drip lubricator (vertical wet pit pumps so equipped);
- Verify proper operation of automatic grease lubricator (vertical wet pit pumps so equipped);
- Operate the pump (note—for vertical wet pit pumps first verify proper lubrication);
- Tightness of foundation and hold-down bolts;
- Check coupling alignment and integrity;
- Verify free movement of packing glands (packed pumps);
- Universal joint shafting and steady bearings wear check;
- Check and flush seal water and drain piping;
- Perform a comparative field test (flow, pressures, and power) with calibrated instruments;

- Perform a comparative vibration test;
- Remove packing and inspect sleeve(s);
- Remove pump handhole covers and inspect impeller for corrosion and excessive wear;
- Remove handhole covers to inspect the wear ring clearances;
- Examine running clearance between propeller and propeller housing;
- Inspect the impeller running clearance and impeller housing for excessive wear;
- Inspect batteries and battery charger for proper charge;
- Observe operation of fans and dampers such that the fans and dampers operate at set temperature, and damper opens upon operation of the diesel engine;
- Inspect operation of all valves in the system;
- Check system air pressure is above minimum actuator operating pressure;
- Check that the valve is aligned with the flanges and not binding.
- Check that power is applied;
- Check that voltages are correct for supply; and
- Check coil is not an open circuit using a multimeter (Patterson Pump Company, 2020).

5.1.9 Inspect Porous Pavement

Regular inspection and maintenance are critical to the effective operation of porous pavement. Individual systems may have more, or less, frequent maintenance needs, depending on a variety of factors including the occurrence of large storm events, seasonal changes, and traffic conditions. Pavement should be monitored to ensure water drainage, debris accumulation, and surface deterioration. The inspector should check the following:

- Standing water on the surface of the pavement after a precipitation event;
- Debris accumulating on pavement; and
- Damage to porous pavements from nondesign loads.

5.1.10 Inspect Media

Regular inspections are critical to schedule sediment removal operations, replace filter media, and relieve any surface clogging. Frequent inspections are especially needed for underground and perimeter filters because an organic mat can quickly clog the filter surface. Depending on the level of traffic or the particular land use, a filter system may become clogged within a few months of normal rainfall. Frequent maintenance can quickly establish a routine frequency acclimated to the land use. Maintenance inspections should be conducted within 24 hours following a storm that exceeds 13 mm (½ in.) of rainfall to evaluate the condition and performance of the filtering practice, including checking for the following:

- Trash and debris accumulation on the filter bed;
- Sediment accumulation in the sedimentation chamber;
- Check for a hardened or brittle media surface in the absence of solids accumulation;
- Evidence of standing water on filter bed for more than 48 hours after a storm;
- Dig a small test pit in the sand filter bed to determine whether the first 76 mm (3 inches) of sand are visibly discolored and need replacement;
- Inspect whether the contributing drainage area to the filter is stable and not a source of sediment; and
- Ensure that the filter bed is level.

5.1.11 Inspect for Evidence/Presence of Nuisance Conditions and Animals

Burrowing animals can compromise the integrity of the SCM because their burrows or dens can collapse and create large holes in the bank of the slope. Burrowing animals also consume shoreline vegetation, causing bank erosion, especially when large numbers are confined to small ponds. Burrows and dams found during inspection should immediately trigger corrective action to include removal of the animals and repair of the SCM (U.S. EPA, 2009).

5.1.11.1 Inspect for Undesirable Plant Communities

Native plants are encouraged in SCMs because these species have evolved over time to survive in the region's condition and require less maintenance and replacement than exotic species that have adapted to other climates. Many municipalities and states have adopted policies and strategies to manage and eliminate species that are classified as invasive or noxious. Undesirable plant communities (e.g., cattails) in a wet pond or constructed wetland are typical monocultures, which can result in mosquito breeding. Unacceptable plant species in SCMs should be removed as they are identified during inspection and maintenance.

5.1.11.2 Inspect for Water Quality Degradation

Fertilizing lawns, pet waste, washing cars, painting, pressure washing, construction, automotive maintenance, pesticides, and feeding wildlife are some activities that contribute to the degradation of water quality in wet ponds and constructed wetlands. Nutrients from fertilizers and animal wastes produce visual cues such as algae growth, changes in water color and clarity, or as floating mats of algae. Another visual indicator of poor water quality is the formation of suds or films on the water surface. Evidence of algal growth, odor, or other visual clues mentioned previously should trigger actions to improve water circulation within the SCM as well as investigate and address upstream sources.

5.1.11.3 Inspect for Water Bird Damage

Wet ponds and constructed wetlands are suitable habitats for waterfowl. Concentrations of ducks, geese, or other waterfowl can destabilize banks of wet ponds and constructed wetlands because they eat shoreline vegetation and trample the bank. They also churn sediments near the bank as they sift for insects in the mud and can increase bacteria because of their droppings.

The inspector should look for signs of damage caused by waterfowl. Educating residents to stop feeding ducks and geese can cause the birds to eventually move on. If waterfowl are persistent, even if the community curtails all feeding, then it may be necessary for the inspector to implement bird exclusionary and deterrent devices.

5.1.12 Inspect for Vectors

Mosquito problems are typically brought to the attention of the maintenance authority by adjacent homeowners, or where there is a mosquito control or abatement district. Stormwater control measures can cause mosquito infestation. Stormwater control measures should be periodically checked to determine if there are excessive amounts of mosquitoes.

Stormwater ponds typically will not have mosquito production problems in a central pool deeper than 1.8 meters (6 feet), as long as it does not dry out or become depleted. A relatively large, deep pool helps promote and maintain aquatic predators of mosquito larvae (e.g., larvivorous fishes, dragonfly naiads, predacious diving beetles, water boatmen, backswimmers, salamander larvae). However, in some locations, even an abundance of natural predators may not be enough to control mosquito populations. A deep central pool also inhibits vegetation colonization within the pool, allowing wind to agitate the surface water, which discourages mosquito egg-laying. The primary areas of mosquito production are in the shallow aquatic bench areas that form the pond's periphery and margins. Fluctuation in the pond's water levels can cause isolated areas or pockets within the aquatic bench to cycle in a wet-dry-wet manner, creating conditions under which peripheral low spots, swales, or potholes may become mosquito-rearing habitats. Sites like these that have fluctuating water levels for extended periods of time can favor the production of mosquitos.

Maintaining relatively high and stable water levels over the aquatic bench helps reduce mosquito populations. In many locations, however, it may not be possible to achieve or maintain such high-water level. In some cases, thick mats of vegetation that cover aquatic and safety benches, emergent plants, submerged aquatic vegetation, or floating algae, can also promote mosquito production. Thick vegetation can inhibit access of mosquito predators to mosquito rearing sites, creating a refuge within the aquatic or safety benches where either permanent ("standing") water mosquitoes or more ephemeral floodwater mosquitoes can develop and emerge. As such, without unduly sacrificing water quality goals, the aquatic and safety benches should not be allowed to develop excessively thick screens or layers of aquatic vegetation. In some situations, mosquito production may still be high despite these precautions.

Like stormwater ponds, wetlands have similar concerns and remedies with mosquito production. Of particular concern is a stormwater wetland's smaller and possibly shallower central pool, and an expanded high marsh pond periphery containing less than 152 mm (6 in.) of water. Even the wetland's low marsh zone, being only 152 to 457 mm (6 to 18 in.) deep, could form problematic breeding spots during times of drought and subsequent rewetting. In some instances, limited amounts of larvicides may need to be used.

When the inspector encounters the situations described above, the inspector should contact the Vector Control agency to abate the pond, as necessary.

5.1.13 Inspect for Snow and Ice

Accumulations of snow and ice can threaten the functioning of an SCM, particularly at inlets, outlets, and emergency spillways. The inspector should monitor and call on maintenance crews to remove snow and ice from these critical areas to ensure the continued functioning of the facility during the winter months.

5.1.14 Inspect for Miscellaneous Site Damage

The inspector should inspect the overall SCM and ancillary facility damage. Features to inspect for damage include, but are not limited to, the following:

- Fences;
- Access roads;
- Trails;
- Lighting;
- Signage (e.g., no trespassing, emergency notification contact information, etc.);
- Nest boxes; and
- Platforms.

5.2 Routine Maintenance Protocols

Routine maintenance (i.e., preventive maintenance) includes activities associated with preventive maintenance (i.e., functional maintenance) that should be conducted at regular intervals. Routine maintenance is important for performance and safety reasons. To be effective, routine maintenance should be performed on a regularly scheduled basis and includes routine procedures such as vegetation management, silt and debris removal, and upkeep of moving parts. Because it is performed on a regular basis, routine maintenance is simpler to schedule and budget for and, ultimately, is easier and less expensive to perform than corrective maintenance. Routine maintenance items vary according to each SCM and are not required to be performed on the same schedule.

5.2.1 Debris and Litter Removal Control

A regularly scheduled program of debris and litter removal from SCMs will reduce the chance of outlet structures, trash racks, and other components becoming clogged and inoperable during storm events. Debris and litter should be removed from pretreatment devices, inlets, forebays, SCM surfaces, trash racks, and outlet structures. Additionally, removal of litter and debris will prevent possible damage to vegetated areas and eliminate potential mosquito breeding habitats. The technique for removing a clog depends on the accessibility and severity of the clog. These include

- Manual removal of debris by hand or by machine; and
- Jetting, back flushing, or routing a clogged pipe using high velocity spray and hydraulic head pressure devices.

Disposal of debris and litter must comply with all local, county, state, and federal waste flow control regulations. Only suitable disposal and recycling sites should be used.

5.2.2 Sediment Removal and Disposal

Sediment should be removed before it threatens the operation or storage volume of an SCM. Sediment should be removed from pretreatment devices, inlets, outlets, forebays, from inverts of SCMs, and from the top of filters. Sediment removal from infiltrators must also include provisions for monitoring the porosity of the subbase, and replacement or cleansing of the pervious materials as necessary.

Sediment removal from wet ponds and wetlands will require dewatering via pumping, or other means may be necessary to reveal the source of clogging and allow access. Necessary permits should be obtained before conducting dewatering activities. Once dewatered, sediment can begin to dry in place. After the material is dried, heavy equipment can remove the sediment from the bottom of the wet pond or wetland. This process is known as mechanical dredging. Mechanical dredging may be accomplished with a standard or long reach backhoe, front end loader, dipper, bucket dredge, drag line, or clamshell dredge. Care should be taken to minimize soil compaction around the wet pond or wetland that can be caused by the heavy machinery. Where dredging cannot be accomplished mechanically from the shore, it may be necessary to remove sediment using hydraulic dredging methods. Larger ponds that cannot be drained can be dredged using a hydraulic suction or with the use of draglines operated from barges.

Disposal of sediment must comply with all local, county, state, and federal regulations. Only suitable disposal sites should be utilized. Sediment should be tested to determine how it should be disposed. Uncontaminated sediment can be incorporated on site or disposed of in a land fill. It is typical to spread this material out on a site for use as a soil amendment. On-site disposal typically entails digging a pit, wasting the muck material, covering the pit with previously removed topsoil, and planting the appropriate native plantings. Wet sediment is typically not accepted at many disposal sites; therefore, the material must be dewatered before disposal.

5.2.3 Vegetation Maintenance

Many SCMs rely on vegetation to filter sediment and to prevent erosion of the banks and the bottom of the facility. Vegetation management is one of the most laborious and costly maintenance activities to be undertaken at an SCM. Maintenance includes many tasks including weed control, mowing, removal of dead and damaged vegetation, pruning and trimming, soil management, reseeding and replanting, mulching, and watering. Vegetation maintenance includes both routine maintenance and aesthetic maintenance. Protocols for each of these activities are discussed below (Philadelphia Water, 2016).

5.2.3.1 Weed Control

Weed control is necessary to stop weeds, especially noxious weeds, from competing with desired flora and fauna. There are several methods for weed control, including:

- Hand pulling of mature annual and tap-rooted herbaceous plants and tree seedlings;
- Hand pulling of aquatic weeds;
- Application of herbicides in accordance with manufacturer's instructions and recommended safety procedures;
- Cut stem treatments by cutting stems at or near ground level and then immediately applying an appropriate herbicide;
- Foliar treatments by applying herbicide to leaves and stems of target plants;
- Basal bark treatments by applying herbicide to a basal stem diameter of less than 76 mm (3 in.); and
- Preemergent treatments by applying preemergent herbicide early spring, late summer, or early fall; or immediately following cultivation.

The maintenance staff should consult with a landscape architect or botanist to determine the most appropriate approach to managing weeds.

5.2.3.2 Mowing

Most grass is hardiest if it is maintained to a height of 152 to 203 mm (6 to 8 in.). If a more manicured look is desired, special attention to the health of the turf is needed. Grass should not be cut below 102 mm (4 in.). There are several methods for weed control, including:

- Mowing warm season grasses to a height of 152 to 203 mm (6 to 8 in.) to discourage the establishment of woody species and to encourage the new growth of target grasses and forbs;
- Mowing cool season grasses to a height of 102 mm (4 in.) to discourage the growth of woody species and maintain height/aesthetic conditions as preferred by the owner/operator; and

- String trimming herbaceous vegetation to approximately 102 to 152 mm (4 to 6 in.) above the ground surface.

5.2.3.3 Dead and Damaged Vegetation Removal

Dead or damaged vegetation, especially woody vegetation, present problems for dams or embankments. The root system of woody vegetation can undermine dam or embankment strength. If the vegetation dies and the root system decomposes, voids can be created in the dam or embankment, which weaken the structure. Routine maintenance to avoid this issue should include the following:

- Large shrub removal;
- Tree removal; and
- Herbaceous vegetation and small shrub removal.

5.2.3.4 Pruning and Trimming

Pruning and trimming is necessary to remove dead, damaged, diseased, or dying branches, and to maintain proper clearances between the plant or tree and the SCM. Pruning and trimming include the following:

- Nonstructural pruning of shrubs and trees to remove all dead, damaged, diseased, or dying branches;
- Structural pruning of shrubs and trees to promote proper growth habit and to train the growth of young trees to achieve target clearances; and
- Cutting back of herbaceous species, as needed, to maintain safe lines of sight for pedestrians.

5.2.3.5 Soil Management

Good soil management ensures that mineral elements do not become deficient or toxic to plants. There are a number of techniques that can be used to maintain healthy soils, including:

- Application of soil amendments by spreading them evenly over the target area, and avoiding clumping or piling of material, and taking care not to injure target vegetation;
- Tilling amendments into existing soil where vegetation will be seeded or planted;

- Decompaction of tree pit soil; and
- Remediation of accumulated salt in soils.

The maintenance team should consult a landscape architect or botanist to determine the best method to maintain soil health.

5.2.3.6 Reseeding and Replanting

Reseeding and replanting are necessary to replace dead or dying vegetation and to fill in bare spots. The following protocols should be used:

Reseeding

- Prepare seedbed
  - Avoid seeding on frozen ground or when the temperature is 32 °F/ 0 °C or lower;
  - If herbicide is necessary, apply well in advance (several days to weeks) of site preparation;
  - Well-grade areas and remove weeds, trash, debris, brush, clods, loose stones, construction debris, and other foreign materials that would interfere with seeding; and
  - Scarify seedbed before seeding; take care to avoid damage to existing tree trunks and roots.
- Seeding
  - Seed only after all other work in an area is complete;
  - Do not apply fertilizer or lime in seeded areas, unless explicitly specified by the landscape architect or botanist;
  - Hand broadcast seeding:
    - Uniformly distribute seed throughout the target area by applying seed in two different directions;
    - Harrow or rake site following seeding to maximize the seed/soil contact; do not cover seed with more than 6 mm (¼ in.) of soil;
    - Immediately after initial seeding, water seeded areas evenly and thoroughly; and
    - Mulch seeded areas within 12 hours in a uniformly, continuous 19 mm (¾ in.) blanket; use tackifier if necessary.
  - Hydroseeding:
    - Calibrate seeding equipment before application so that the materials are applied accurately and evenly to avoid misses and overlaps;

  - Apply seed uniformly and evenly across the entire disturbed area;
  - Apply seed-water mixture within the hydroseeder tank no later than 1 hour after the seed is added to the tank; comply with equipment manufacturer's installation instructions and recommendations;
  - Use approved spraying equipment with fan-type nozzle; and
  - Apply hydroseed using a two-step process to ensure good seed to soil contact:

    Step 1: Apply the first coat evenly and uniformly from opposing directions to the soil surface to cover the entire area;

    Step 2: Apply the second coat evenly and uniformly on top of the first coat, covering the entire seeded area with an erosion resistant coating of mulch.
- Protect newly seeded areas—do not allow seeded areas to be trafficked. Install a temporary fence if necessary.

Replanting Trees and Shrubs:

- Dig the planting pits so the walls are vertical or angled outward from the bottom up;
- Scarify the walls of the pit after digging;
- Excavate the planting pit to at least 1½ times the width of the root mass of the plant to be installed and deep enough to allow the bottom of the root flare to be flush with the final grade;
- Remove debris from the pit and lightly tamp loose soil in the bottom of the pit by foot;
- Remove plant from container and place straight in the center of the planting pit, carrying the plant by the root mass. Avoid handling the plant by the branches, leaves, or stem (or trunk);
- If a tree or shrub is balled and burlapped, carefully remove root ball packing (13 mm [½ in.] of cage and as much burlap as possible) while disturbing the tree as little as possible after tree is set in pit. Cut and remove ropes around the burlapped ball. Remove as much burlap from the ball as possible. Remove all nails. Remove staking adjacent to root ball and trunk before planting, if present;
- Backfill planting pit with soil and tamp firmly to fill all voids and air pockets. Do not overcompact soil. Make sure the plant remains straight during backfilling/tamping procedure. The top of the root mass of the trees/shrubs should be flush with, or slightly elevated (no

more than 6 mm [¼ in.] in height) above the final grade. Root flare must be visible. Do not cover woody stem with soil;
- Water plants thoroughly immediately after planting to saturate backfill;
- Place mulch around the plant; and
- Install stakes and guying material to support the tree.

Replanting Herbaceous Containers and Plugs:

- Dig the planting pit to at least 1½ times the width of the root ball;
- Remove the plants and soil from the pots or plug trays and position in the holes so that the soil level of each plant is flush with the surrounding finished grade soil surface;
- After planting, fill soil in around the plant completely, firming the soil and ensuring there are no air pockets as plants are installed; and
- Water plants thoroughly immediately after planting to saturate backfill.

5.2.3.7 Mulching

Mulching is necessary to conserve soil moisture, improve fertility and health of the soil, reduce weed growth, and enhance the visual appeal of the area. Mulch should be applied over the soil in a 76-mm (3-in.) thick layer. Mulch should be raked away from trunks and woody stems of shrubs to a distance of 76 mm (3 in.).

5.2.3.8 Watering

Watering plants may be necessary during plant establishment and during periods of drought. Watering can be accomplished by using a nearby water source such as a fire hydrant, establishing a temporary irrigation system, and/or tanking water to the SCM. Water should be directed toward the base of plants, allowed to soak into the ground within each area of vegetation by moving slowly through each section. A landscape architect or botanist should be consulted to determine the amount and frequency of watering.

5.2.4 Minor Erosion

Vegetative cover or other protective measures are necessary to prevent erosion. Erosion control is accomplished by a variety of materials and methods, including riprap, gabion lining, sod, seeding, erosion control blankets, concrete lining, and regrading. The specific erosion control technique that should be employed is dependent on the type of erosion. Table 5.1 presents

TABLE 5.1 Erosion Control Methods and Mechanisms

Erosion Type	Erosion Control Technique	Erosion Control Mechanism
Concentrated Flow Erosion	Run-on diversions	Protect bare areas from run-on flows
	Water bars	
	Ditch and channel protection	Protect channel from erosive flows
	Check dams	Prevent downcutting, settle sediment
	Slope drains	Protect slope from erosive flows
	Outlet controls	Protect outlet area from scour erosion
Raindrop and Sheet Erosion	Surface roughening	Increase infiltration, prevent soil transport
	Soil binders	Prevent soil detachment and transport
	Topsoil application	Increase infiltration, support vegetation
	Soil fertility amendments	Promote vegetative growth
	Permanent Seeding	Prevent soil detachment and transport
	Mulches	
	Landscape mulches	
	Hydraulic mulches and tackifiers	
	Erosion control blankets	
	Turf reinforcement mats	
	Sodding	
	Slope protection	

the different types of erosion, control techniques, and mechanisms that maintenance staff should consider when addressing erosion issues.

5.2.5 Settling Repair

Settlement following construction should be immediately addressed so that there is no localized ponding, erosion of side slopes, and serious structural damage and total facility failure. If settling has created a visible depression or a sinkhole in SCM, then the following maintenance actions should take place:

- Remove material over the settled area to access any subsurface voids;
- Remove plants, shrubs, and small trees less than 7.5 cm (3 in.) diameter and retain for replanting;
- Clear around settled area and excavate to the bottom of the depression/void space;

- Fill excavated area with suitable fill material and compact;
- Replant or reseed bare soil areas; and
- For hardscaped areas, replace hardscape subbase and surface over repaired area to match existing grade.

5.2.6 Structure Maintenance

The type and nature of structure maintenance varies significantly depending on the issue. Following is guidance on repairing broken, loose, or compromised concrete or masonry structures.

- Place a tarp over adjacent areas to protect surfaces, soil, and vegetation from area being worked;
- Remove loose debris or material from the repair area;
- To repair hairline/cosmetic cracks in concrete, apply a concrete crack repair product to the surface per the manufacturer's recommendations;
- To repair a large/structural crack in concrete, clean out loose debris, and fill the cracked area; and
- If the damage is too large to support mortar, saw cut concrete and install concrete forms, as needed, and fill repair area with mortar.

5.2.6.1 Pretreatment Device, Inlets, Outlet Structures, Chambers, and Subsurface Structures

Pretreatment devices, inlets, outlet structures, and chambers should be checked to ensure they are not filled and clogged with litter, debris, and sediment. Protocols for litter, debris, and sediment removal are discussed in Sections 5.2.1 and 5.2.2, respectively. These SCM features should also be maintained to ensure their structural integrity and are undamaged. Maintenance of subsurface components may include distribution and underdrain piping, inlets, control structures, weirs, sumps, and similar components. If their integrity is compromised or they are damaged, then the following guidance should be considered:

- Open maintenance port or manhole and inspect structure for damage. If the structure is damaged, then replace the components that are damaged.
- Maintenance staff should consult with the as-built plans and specifications to purchase the correct replacement parts. If the component to be replaced is part of a proprietary SCM, then the maintenance staff should consult with the vendor.

- The new components should be replaced as soon as possible. If there is a long lead time to order and replace the parts, the maintenance staff should assess if the SCM should be taken offline in the interim.

5.2.6.2 Screens and Trash Racks

Screens and trash racks should be checked to ensure they are not clogged with litter, debris, and sediment. Protocols for litter, debris, and sediment removal are discussed in Sections 5.2.1 and 5.2.2, respectively. These SCM features should also be maintained to ensure their structural integrity and that they are undamaged. Screens and trash racks can be damaged by the powerful force of water and the debris that it carries. Metal screens and bar typically have a relatively long design life but are susceptible to erosive scour, pitting, and corrosion on its flow side. These parts should be replaced if pitting and corrosion are so excessive that it compromises the integrity of the part. Any damage to the trash rack, orifice plates, or gratings must be repaired immediately. Screens and racks should also be repositioned and fastened if they have been dislodged.

5.2.6.3 Pipes

There are different methods to rehabilitate and replace pipes. Trenchless technology is a form of underground construction that requires the use of few or no trenches at the surface or street level. Trenchless technology uses new techniques and equipment to install or replace underground infra structure without causing disturbance to the ground above. Its goal is to avoid interfering with surface-level activities, including traffic, businesses, residential areas, or people. An engineer specializing in trenchless technologies should be consulted to determine the most appropriate technique. The chosen technique will depend on the type and severity of failure observed during inspections. Listed below are some pipe repair methods:

- Joint sealing,
- Invert protection,
- Chemical stabilization,
- Folded liners,
- Cured-in-place pipe,
- Ferro-cement,
- Pipe bursting,
- Pipe eating,
- Pipe pulling,

- Slip-lining,
- Modified slip-lining, and
- Spray lining (AASHTO, 2017; Contech Engineering Solutions, 2020).

For additional information please consult the North American Society for Trenchless Technology.

5.2.6.4 Standing Water

Standing water is problematic because it can be a place for vectors to breed. Standing water can be caused by a number of issues such as trash and debris, sedimentation, settling of structures, or excessive vegetation. To address chronic standing water, it is important that a root cause analysis be performed. Once the cause has been determined then the appropriate course of action can take place. This may include simple maintenance activities, such as the removal of vegetation, to more complex actions, such as removal and replacement of a structure following proper soil compaction.

5.2.6.5 Permanent Pool

The depth or elevation of the permanent pool during dry weather should be maintained at the design elevation and not fluctuate. Inspections that find an increase or decrease in water level above the design elevation should trigger corrective actions. These actions will range from simple to complex, depending on the root cause. Properly trained and qualified personnel should perform the inspection and maintenance. Table 5.2 presents different types of problems and potential solutions to address permanent pool fluctuations.

5.2.7 Mechanical, Electrical, Pneumatic, and Hydraulic Maintenance

Stormwater control measure components, such as mechanical valves, bladder valves, compressors, sluice gates, pumps, real time controls, programmable logic controllers, fence gates, locks, ladders, and access hatches, should remain functional at all times. Routine maintenance should be performed in accordance with manufacturers' recommendations. Mechanical components should be operated (exercised) at least once every 3 months to ensure their continued performance. Components and parts should be replaced when found damaged or before the end of their useful life (U.S. EPA, 2009).

5.2.7.1 Valves, Orifices, and Aerators

Exercise and lubrication—Components with moving parts, especially valves, should be exercised (operated) and lubricated according to the manufacturer's recommendation or at least annually. After the valve is operated, it

TABLE 5.2 Permanent Pool Fluctuation Diagnosis and Solution (modified from U.S. EPA, 2009)

Issue	Solution	Degree of Maintenance
Clogged low flow	Clear low flow, install trash rack if not present or inadequate	Minor maintenance
Low flow or pond drain valve opened	Shut valve and lock shut with chain and lock	Minor maintenance
Rodent activity (dams, lodges, burrows)	Fill burrows	Minor to major repair
Leak in riser	Seal leak	Major repair
Leak in barrel	Seal leak	Major repair
Leak in upstream dam face or pond bottom	Drain remainder of permanent pool and install waterproof liner; dye test recommended	Major repair
Leak or seepage in downstream dam face	Dye test recommended; seal leak source if found; liner may need to be installed and dam or principal spillway repair or replacement may be required depending on leak severity	Major repair
Vortexing	Consider a call to civil authorities immediately as dam failure may be imminent and downstream evacuation may be necessary; do not attempt to repair without professional help	Usually, major repair

should be slowly closed, making sure that the gate properly reseats to a watertight closed position or to the appropriate opening position. If a valve gate does not move, it will need to be serviced or replaced.

Rustproofing—Parts that are metal are subject to corrosion, especially when located in wet environments such as wet ponds and constructed wetlands. Rust protection or proofing by removing rust, cleaning the part, and applying galvanizing paint or a coating with bituminous tar or rubber should be applied to metal parts. Where possible, stainless steel parts should be used. Any product applied should be allowed to cure before coming into contact with stormwater.

Tightening bolts and hardware—Loose bolts and hardware need to be tightened. Special care should be used when tightening rusted bolts and in locations where concrete may be spalling. Damaged bolts and hardware should be replaced as soon as possible. Stainless steel bolts and hardware should be used.

Aerators—Electrical and air lines for aerators require careful inspection and maintenance. Electrical components should be checked for exposed wire, proper grounding, and lack of damage. Air lines should be inspected and fixed or replaced when kinks, holes, dry rot, or leaks are discovered. Bubblers, aerators, fountains, or diffusers should be checked for clogging and fouling. The manufacturer should be consulted and and/or used to repair or replace the equipment as appropriate.

5.2.7.2 Pumps and Switches

Pump and switch maintenance will vary depending on the root cause. The inspection should identify the maintenance activities that are needed. These may include

- Adding grease to pump antifriction bearings;
- Adding grease to universal joint shafting u-joint bearings, antifriction steady bearings;
- Adding grease to coupling;
- Changing antifriction bearing oil;
- Replacing packing (all packing; not just the outermost ring);
- Cleaning and oiling gland bolts (packed pumps);
- Replacing bearings;
- Cleaning packing box;
- Adjusting ring clearances to original specifications if so supplied or installing new wear rings;
- Repairing or replacing the housing, housing liner, or propeller as appropriate; and
- Performing impeller adjustment. If the wear is excessive, repairing or replacing the impeller housing.

5.2.8 Porous Pavement Cleaning and Winter Maintenance

Porous pavement requires routine maintenance, restorative maintenance, and winter maintenance. The activities associated with each type of maintenance is described below.

Routine maintenance:

- Manually remove large trash/sediment/organic debris;
- Clean pervious pavement using approved regenerative air sweeper;
- Sweep the entire surface of the pervious pavement moving at a controlled speed of 5 to 11 km/h (3 to 7 mph). Use water as needed for dust control;

- Resweep the surface until all visible material is removed from the surface of the pervious pavement; and
- Use a vacuum attachment as needed for any corners or difficult to access sections.

Restorative maintenance:

- Manually remove large trash/sediment/organic debris;
- Divide the site into 457-mm (18-in.) sections, which is based on the width of the vacuum attachment. Mark the divisions on a map of the site;
- Identify areas with low infiltration rates by spraying water using a hose gun over the entire SCM area until the surface is saturated. If water ponds for more than a few seconds, mark these areas for more intensive maintenance;
- Follow a standard cleaning procedure to maintain the entire pervious pavement area using an approved pressure washer with a vacuum attachment;
- Set up equipment at the upstream end of the SCM; maintain the entire site with a steady pace with two passes for each 457-mm (18-in.) wide sections;
- Follow an intensive cleaning procedure to maintain the pervious pavement identified as having low infiltration rates using an approved pressure washer with vacuum attachments;
- Set up equipment at the identified areas with low infiltration rates; maintain the identified areas at a steady pace with at least two passes in at most 305-mm (12-in.) wide sections; and
- Spray water over the entire SCM area until the surface is saturated to confirm maintenance was performed to an adequate level. If water ponds, repeat the process.

Winter maintenance:

- Apply deicer as pre- and posttreatment for every snow event greater than 6 mm (0.25 in.), for sleet and freezing rain events, and after every plowing event; deicer should be applied at the following rates:
  - Sodium formate applied at a rate of 0.05 kg/m^2 (10 lb/1000 sq ft);
  - Permeable interlocking concrete pavements can be treated with a lower application rate of road salt 0.024 kg/m^2 (5 lb/1000 sq ft);

  - Calcium chloride in flake form applied at a rate of 0.1 kg/m^2 (21 lb/1000 sq ft);
- Repeat as requested by owner/operator for the duration of the storm;
- Plow pervious pavement for snow events with snow accumulation of more than 51 mm (2 in.) as directed by the owner/operator;
- Raise rubber plow blade to 13 mm (0.5 in.) above the surface; and
- Repeat as requested by owner/operator for the duration of the storm (Philadelphia Water, 2016).

5.2.9 Media Maintenance

Maintaining the filter media is an essential step in achieving optimal results. In most cases, the media can be maintained either by cleaning and leveling the surface or replacing specific layers of media. The type of maintenance required is based upon the flowrate through the filter and/or the type of pollutants entering the system. Media maintenance is done to provide uniform flow downward through the media, preventing preferential flow and utilizing the entire surface area of the media bed. By providing uniform flow, treatment is maximized. Some filters have multiple media layers, each of which provide treatment for specific pollutants.

Routine surface maintenance should be conducted when the water level within filter begins to pond. Routine surface maintenance may need to be done as frequently as every 3 to 4 weeks depending on the amount of loading to the filter. Following are the routine surface maintenance steps:

1. Clean the entire surface of the media by shoveling off the accumulated solids and the top 6 to 13 mm (¼ to ½ in.) of media (approximate). The newly exposed media should look cleaner than the removed media. Remove more depth if necessary.
2. Dispose of the removed media and accumulated debris.
3. Level the surface of the media.
4. Measure the depth of the remaining inert media layer by inserting a shovel or a probe directly down into the media until it reaches the lower lying fabric layer. This will indicate the depth of the inert media layer. Other methods specific to the SCM may also be used to measure the depth of the media layer.
5. Replenish the removed media with new media if less than 178 mm (7 in.) of the inert layer remains (more than 51 mm [2 in.] of the inert layer has been removed over the course of several surface maintenances).

If the filter is equipped with inert media below the top sand filter layer, then it will require seasonal maintenance. The inert media is replaced to restore the proper flowrate through the filter. Typically, dirt and debris are trapped within the top layer of media, which eventually causes the media to plug. Maintenance is recommended when stormwater sampling shows consistent pollutant reductions and solids loading is not appreciable. Following are the steps to conduct a seasonal maintenance:

1. Set up safety equipment if the system is near vehicle and pedestrian traffic.
2. Sparingly pressure-wash or hand-wipe the side walls of the filter before removing any media. Cleaning the inside walls of the filter will allow the operator to observe the system's most recent operating water level based upon the scum line left behind inside of the filter. No detergent or hot water should be used when cleaning the insides of the filter.
3. Excavate the spent filter media (top layer) down to the first layer of geotextile fabric. A shovel or vactor truck may be used to remove the filter media.
4. Remove the filter fabric separating the top layer from the inert layer and inspect the underlying filter media.
5. Rake the top 152 mm (6 in.) of media to regenerate inert media. Level and smooth the filter media.
6. Reinstall the filter fabric on top of the inert media.
7. Place new inert filter media (top layer). Media should be added in uniform, level layers using the level indicators on the side walls of the filter as a guide. Each media layer should be leveled before adding the next media layer.

A full maintenance replaces all of the filtration media (top layer and inert media) not including the underdrain gravel. The filtering capacity of the media can be exhausted because of a combination of heavy loading, inadequate maintenance of the filter, and extended filter run-times. Full maintenance is recommended when a decline in treatment is observed in the water quality sampling, and routine surface maintenance is no longer capable of restoring the proper flow. Significant loading in the lower lying media layers will often accompany a decline in treatment. Following are the steps to conduct a full maintenance:

1. Set up safety equipment if the system is near vehicle and pedestrian traffic.

2. Sparingly pressure-wash or hand-wipe the side walls of the filter before removing any media. Do not use any detergents. Cleaning the inside walls of the filter will allow the operator to observe the system's most recent operating water level based upon the scum line left behind inside of the filter. No detergent or hot water should be used when cleaning the insides of the filter.
3. Use a vacuum truck or shovel to remove all spent media (top and bottom media). Stop at the filter fabric above the underdrain gravel. The underdrain gravel should not be removed.
4. Pressure-wash the insides of the underdrain to flush its insides.
5. Install new filter fabric on top of underdrain gravel.
6. Install the new media layers and filter fabric layers. Media should be added in uniform, level layers using the level indicators on the side walls of the filter as a guide. Each media layer should be leveled before adding the next media layer.

5.2.10 Nuisance Control

Nuisance control depends on the type of animal, bird, plant, or water quality issue encountered. Once the extent of infestation and damage is understood, maintenance staff should select the most specific control for the pest to avoid harming beneficial organisms. The least toxic measure should be implemented first. Actions to control these types of nuisances are described below (U.S. EPA, 2009).

5.2.10.1 Animals

Rodent management is a contentious issue with strong feelings both for and against the presence of these animals in a suburban setting. There are many types of measures that can be used to ensure that the animals will not continue to negatively affect the SCM. Existing burrows should be plugged by filling with material similar to the existing material. If plugging of burrows does not discourage the animals from returning, further measures should be taken to either remove the animal population or make critical areas of the facility unattractive to them.

5.2.10.2 Water Birds

Waterfowl can damage vegetation by overgrazing and can degrade water quality because of their droppings, which cause high fecal coliform counts. The following actions can control waterfowl effects:

Modify landscaping. Geese and ducks, in particular, are grazers and need short, green grass for food. Allow grass to grow longer so it is unattractive to birds. Along water edges, plant less-attractive vegetation, such as pachysandra, periwinkle, and euonymus.

Discontinue feeding. Wild birds can find their own food and will survive without handouts. Once people stop feeding them, waterfowl will revert to better quality natural foods. In many cases, the birds will leave.

Install barriers. Waterfowl prefer to land on water and walk onto adjacent grassy areas to feed and rest. The most effective tools for controlling waterfowl movement are fences, hedgerows, and other physical barriers.

Use scaring devices. Scarecrows with movable parts, bird-scaring reflecting tape, mylar flags, screamer sirens, whistle bombs, shell crackers, and automatic exploders will help keep geese and other waterfowl from feeding and resting on property. Move these items periodically. Before using noisemakers or pyrotechnics, check local and state regulations for permit requirements and any other limits on using firearms and pyrotechnics.

Prevent nesting. It can help control local populations of waterfowl if property owners keep them from nesting. Nest treatment typically involves manipulating eggs so they do not develop. Methods include addling (shaking), oiling with corn oil, puncturing, chilling, or replacing eggs. Waterfowl are protected by state and federal laws, so SCM owners should first consult with resource agencies.

5.2.10.3 Undesirable Plant Communities

Special care should be taken to remove invasive plants during the establishment of the SCM. This should be in conjunction with replanting with other appropriate native species. A botanist should be consulted before planting new species.

Other techniques include regular application of algaecides and herbicides to eradicate existing weed species. A licensed applicator should be hired, and the chemical should be applied according to the manufacturer's recommendations.

Another vegetation management technique is through the establishment of buffer strips or "no mow areas" around the perimeter of wet ponds and constructed wetlands. These zones help filter nutrients in stormwater runoff and stabilize wet pond and constructed wetland banks.

5.2.10.4 Water Quality Degradation

To address water quality degradation in wet ponds and constructed wetlands, it is first important to determine the source of the problem and the constituent causing the degradation. This should be done while inspecting the SCM. Following are some solutions to address water quality degradation:

Diffusers and surface aerators—Can restore wet pond and constructed wetland water quality by restoring aerobic conditions to the entire water column, including the bottom layer, which interacts with sediment. A pond aerator system consists of three components: (1) a cabinet with an air compressor, (2) weighted tubing, and (3) a diffuser head. Air is pumped by the compressor, through the tubing, and then released from the diffuser head, which is located at the bottom of the pond. As the air rises from the diffuser head, water is lifted by bubbles, and the movement of the rising water creates circulating currents within the pond.

Flocculants—Chemicals applied to a wet pond or constructed wetland that cause phosphorus and other materials suspended in the water column to settle. Removing phosphorus from the water column will prevent algal growth. The application of flocculants may require a permit and should be applied with caution. Accordingly, check with local authorities before application.

5.2.11 Vector Management

The most effective mosquito control program is one that eliminates potential breeding habitats. Most stagnant pools of water can be attractive to mosquitoes and the source of a large mosquito population. Ponded water such as open cans and bottles, debris and sediment accumulations, and areas of ground settlement provide ideal locations for mosquito breeding. A maintenance program dedicated to eliminating potential breeding areas is preferable to controlling flying mosquitoes. Whenever excessive mosquito production is encountered in a stormwater structure, a state, county, or local mosquito control or abatement district should be contacted to request appropriate control actions. In areas where such organized mosquito control programs do not exist, contract with a private company for control actions. Organized mosquito control or abatement districts typically provide comprehensive, integrated pest management remedies for addressing excessive mosquito production, involving source reduction, application of larvicide and adulticide techniques. Adulticides that are applied to more widespread areas by aircraft or truck-mounted sprayers include organophosphates and synthetic pyrethroids and should be used only when source reduction or larvicide application efforts are not working. Application of any pesticides must be in accordance with the requirements specified on the pesticide's label.

Seasonal stocking of predatory fish that eat mosquito larvae is also undertaken in many areas by mosquito control or abatement districts, relying upon mosquitofish (*Gambusia spp.*) in warmer climates, and on the black-striped topminnow (*Notrophus fundulus*), in colder climates.

5.2.12 Snow and Ice Removal

Accumulations of snow and ice can threaten the functioning of an SCM, particularly at inlets, outlets, and emergency spillways. Providing the equipment, materials, and personnel to monitor and remove snow and ice from these critical areas is necessary to ensure the continued functioning of the facility during the winter months. There are also a series of other maintenance activities that should take place including the following:

- Clean and lubricate bolts and moving parts;
- Drain, clean, and seal any surface cisterns, tanks, and rain barrels or any subsurface storage systems that are located above the frost line in the fall;
- Install bollard or markers to protect stormwater bump-outs (e.g., bioretention basins) from snowplows; and
- Drain and seal any irrigation systems that are located above the frost line.

5.2.13 Miscellaneous Site Damage

General housekeeping and miscellaneous site maintenance are necessary to maintain the SCM. These activities include

- Painting;
- Cleaning and lubricating of nuts and bolts;
- Cleaning and lubricating of locks;
- Replacing broken or seized bolts;
- Replacing missing or damaged appurtenances, such as rods, washers, bolts, caps, and gaskets;
- Replacing missing or damaged safety bars; and
- Installing hinged metal grate over headwall and end wall openings.

5.3 Nonroutine/Emergency Maintenance Protocols

Nonroutine maintenance (i.e., corrective maintenance) activities can be defined as the activities that are performed as a reaction to correct a problem or malfunction at an SCM and to restore the facility's intended operation and safe condition. Based upon the severity of the problem, nonroutine maintenance must be performed on an as needed or emergency basis and includes such procedures as structural repairs, mosquito control, restoration of vegetated and nonvegetated linings, replacing a sign or traffic delineator that has been damaged, or irrigating an SCM during a drought.

5.3.1 Structural Repairs

Structural damage to outlet and inlet structures, trash racks, and head walls from vandalism, flood events, or other causes must be repaired promptly. Equipment, materials, and personnel must be available to perform these repairs on short notice. The immediacy of the repairs will depend upon the nature of the damage and its effects on the safety and operation of the facility. The analysis of structural damage and the design and performance of structural repairs should only be undertaken by qualified personnel.

5.3.2 Mechanical Equipment Repairs

Similar to structural repairs, mechanical equipment must be repaired as soon as possible to maintain the safety and operation of the facility. Maintenance staff should consult as-built drawings and manufacturer's literature when making repairs to mechanical equipment.

5.3.3 Dam, Embankment, and Slope Repairs

Damage to dams, embankments, and side slopes must be repaired promptly. This damage can be the result of rain or flood events, vandalism, animals, vehicles, or neglect. Typical problems include settlement, scouring, cracking, sloughing, seepage, and rutting. Equipment, materials, and personnel must be available to perform these repairs on short notice. The immediacy of the repairs will depend upon the nature of the damage and its effects on the safety and operation of the facility. The analysis of damage and the design and performance of geotechnical repairs should only be undertaken by qualified personnel.

5.3.4 Dewatering

It may be necessary to remove ponded water from within a malfunctioning SCM. This ponding may be the result of a blocked principal outlet (detention facility), inoperable low-level outlet (retention facility), loss of infiltration capacity (infiltration facility), or poor bottom drainage. Portable pumps may be necessary to remove the ponded water temporarily until a permanent solution can be implemented. Dewatering activities should be done in accordance with local and state regulatory requirements.

5.3.5 Pond Maintenance

Problems such as algae growth, excessive siltation, and mosquito breeding should be addressed and corrected in a timely manner. The sooner the problem is corrected, the easier it will be to restore a balanced environment in the pond. Section 5.2.6.5 provides maintenance protocols. As a result of the complex environment in a pond, it is also recommended that agencies such as the U.S. Fish and Wildlife Service be consulted for corrective maintenance procedures.

5.3.6 Fence Repair

Fences are damaged by many factors, including vandalism and storm events. Timely repair is necessary to maintain the security of the SCM.

5.3.7 Elimination of Woody Vegetation

The stability of dams, embankments, and side slopes can be impaired by large roots and animal burrows. Additionally, burrows can present a safety hazard for maintenance personnel. Trees and brush with extensive, woody root systems should be promptly removed to prevent sumps and potential failure of the SCM.

5.3.8 Spills

A spill should be contained to minimize the discharge of pollutants to SCM, drainage systems, or waterbody by stopping them at the source, containing and cleaning up the spill, and properly disposing of spill materials. To the extent that the work can be accomplished safely, spills of oil, petroleum products, substances listed under 40 CFR parts 110, 117, and 302, and sanitary and septic wastes should be contained and cleaned up immediately. Following are spill response protocols that should be implemented.

Cleanup

- Clean up leaks and spills immediately.
- Use a rag for small spills on paved surfaces, a damp mop for general cleanup, and absorbent material for larger spills. If the spilled material is hazardous, then the used cleanup materials are also hazardous and must be sent to either a certified laundry (rags) or disposed of as hazardous waste.
- Use the appropriate type of absorbent pad for the type of spill that occurred. Absorbent pads come in three basic types—to deal with

(1) oil, (2) chemicals, and (3) water or general tasks. There's a color-coding system to explain which one does what job:

  - Oil absorbent pads are white.
  - Chemical absorbent pads are yellow.
  - General purpose and water absorbent pads are black or gray; these are also known as "maintenance" absorbent pads.

- Never hose down or bury dry material spills. Clean up as much of the material as possible and dispose of it properly.
- Properly dispose of spilled material, absorbent pads, and other equipment that are contaminated. This may include properly containerizing, labeling, transporting, and disposing of the material as a hazardous waste.

Minor spills: Minor spills typically involve small quantities of oil, gasoline, paint, and so on, which can be controlled by the first responder at the discovery of the spill.

- Use absorbent materials on small spills rather than hosing down or burying the spill.
- Absorbent materials should be promptly removed and disposed of properly.
- Follow the practice below for a minor spill:
  - Contain the spread of the spill.
  - Recover spilled materials.
  - Clean the contaminated area and properly dispose of contaminated materials.

Semisignificant spills: Semisignificant spills still can be controlled by the first responder along with the aid of other personnel such as laborers and the supervisor. This response may require the cessation of all other activities.

- Spills should be cleaned up immediately:
  - Contain spread of the spill.
  - Notify the project foreman immediately.
  - If the spill occurs on paved or impermeable surfaces, clean up using "dry" methods (absorbent materials, cat litter, and/or rags). Contain the spill by encircling with absorbent materials and do not let the spill spread widely.

  - If the spill occurs in dirt areas, immediately contain the spill by constructing an earthen dike. Dig up and properly dispose of contaminated soil.
  - If the spill occurs during rain, cover spill with tarps or other material to prevent contaminating runoff.

Significant/hazardous spills: For significant or hazardous spills that cannot be controlled by personnel in the immediate vicinity, the following steps should be taken:

- Notify the local U.S. emergency response by dialing 911. In addition to 911, the contractor will notify the proper county officials. It is the contractor's responsibility to have all emergency phone numbers at the construction site.
- For spills of federal reportable quantities, in conformance with the requirements in 40 CFR parts 110, 119, and 302, the person who discovered the spill should notify the U.S. National Response Center at (800) 424-8802.
- Notification should first be made by telephone and followed up with a written report.
- The services of a spill contractor or a hazmat team should be obtained immediately. Maintenance personnel should not attempt to clean up until the appropriate and qualified staffs have arrived at the job site.
- Other agencies that may need to be consulted include, but are not limited to, the Fire Department, the Public Works Department, the Coast Guard, the Highway Patrol, the City/County Police Department, Department of Toxic Substances, California Division of Oil and Gas, Cal/OSHA, and so on.

Reporting

- Report significant spills to local agencies, such as the Fire Department; they can assist in cleanup.
- Federal regulations require that any significant oil spill into a water body or onto an adjoining shoreline be reported to the U.S. National Response Center at (800) 424-8802 (24 hours).

Before the SCM is placed in operational mode, it must be cleaned so that there is no spill residual.

5.4 Aesthetic Maintenance

Aesthetic maintenance, although not required to keep an SCM operational, will maintain the visual appeal of a facility and will benefit everyone within the local community. This is particularly true for those SCMs that are also used by members of the community for athletic and recreational purposes. Aesthetic maintenance can also reduce the amount of required preventive and corrective maintenance.

5.4.1 Graffiti Removal

The timely removal of this obvious eyesore will restore the aesthetic quality of an SCM. Removal can be accomplished by painting or otherwise covering it, or removing it with scrapers, solvents, or cleansers. Timely removal is important to discourage further graffiti and other acts of vandalism.

5.4.2 Vegetation Maintenance

Although time consuming, trimming of grass edges around structures and fences will provide for a neat and attractive appearance of the facility. Regular grass maintenance program will keep weed intrusion to a minimum; however, some weeds will invariably appear. Periodic weeding, either chemically or mechanically, will not only help to maintain a healthy turf, but will also keep grassed areas looking attractive.

5.4.3 Overall Site Maintenance

Overall site maintenance, beyond that of maintaining the SCM, is important for a number of reasons. One of the most important ones is safety. An SCM and surrounding area that is damaged or run down gives off the appearance that it's not cared for properly, which can lead to a lack of use by community members and further deterioration and disrepair. It can also lead to the citizens questioning the value of their tax investment to maintain the SCM.

Items such as proper lighting surveillance and graffiti-resistant materials are crucial to making the SCM and surrounding area feel safe to visitors. These measures help park guests feel safer and at ease while also helping to prevent vandalism. In cases where SCMs do experience vandalism or damage, it is important to fix the problems quickly, lest they end up as hot spots for inappropriate or illegal activity.

6.0 PRIORITIZING CORRECTIVE MAINTENANCE

Corrective maintenance is the highest priority over routine and aesthetic maintenance. Each of these forms of maintenance are needed, but prioritizing is necessary, especially when there is a safety or potential safety concern, or when there are limited resources. Table 5.3 is an example prioritization system.

7.0 MAINTENANCE THRESHOLD INDICATORS

Tables 5.4 through 5.9 summarize the five different SCM categories and their associated treatment mechanisms and components. Tables 5.10 through 5.14 summarize thresholds for specified and implied criteria, which "trigger" maintenance activities for specific SCMs. The maintenance activity shown is for those times when the field measurement exceeds the maintenance indicator. These thresholds do not preclude taking other actions needed to mitigate the given thresholds or taking actions needed to correct unanticipated problems.

8.0 CHECKLISTS

Checklists are important to ensure that system components are functioning as originally constructed. They are important not only during facility inspection, but they also provide a historical record of facility function. Inspection checklists help to ensure a degree of consistency. It can be expected that different individuals will inspect a facility over the years. By providing common

TABLE 5.3 Maintenance Prioritization System (Watershed Management Institute, Inc., 1997)

Priority	Criteria
A	Hazard to life or health—a situation presenting substantial likelihood of injury
B	Hazard to structures—a situation presenting a reasonable likelihood of damage to structures
C	Hazard to property—a situation presenting a reasonable likelihood of property damage
D	Nuisance

TABLE 5.4 Basin Components (WEF et al., 2012)

SCM Type	Treatment Mechanism																						SCM Components
	Quantity Control					Pollutant Control									Biological				Other				
	Peak Flow Attenuation	Runoff Volume Reduction	Infiltration	Dispersion	Evapotranspiration	Runoff Collection and Usage	Sedimentation	Flotation	Laminar Separation	Swirl Concentration	Sorption	Precipitation	Coagulation	Filtration	Plant Metabolism	Nitrification/Denitrification	Sulfate Reduction	Organic Compound Degradation	Pathogen Die-off	Temperature Reduction	Disinfection	Screening	
Cisterns and Rain Barrels		X					X																• Inlet Screen • Vessel • Outlet • Valve • Pump
Forebays							X	X															• Pretreatment Unit • Inlet • Outlet (Riser/Principle Spillway, Emergency Spillway, and Low-Flow Orifices) • Embankment and Abutments • Vegetation
Vaults and Swirl Concentrators	X						X	X		X													• Inlet • Outlet • Vault • Baffles • Screens

Oil and Water Separators						X	X	X								• Inlet • Outlet • Vault • Coalescing Plates • Baffles
Dry Basins	X	X	X			X										• Energy Dissipator • Forebay • Inlet • Outlet (Riser/Principle Spillway, Emergency Spillway, and Low-Flow Orifices) • Skimmer • Screen • Embankment and Abutments • Vegetation
Wet Basins	X	X		X	X	X	X		X	X	X	X	X	X	X	• Energy Dissipator • Forebay • Inlet • Outlet (Riser/Principle Spillway, Emergency Spillway, and Low-Flow Orifices) • Skimmer • Screen • Embankment and Abutments • Vegetation
Wetlands	X	X		X	X	X	X		X	X	X	X	X	X	X	• Energy Dissipator • Forebay • Wetland Cells and Pools • Inlet • Outlet (Riser/Principle Spillway, Emergency Spillway, and Low-Flow Orifices) • Skimmer • Screen • Embankment and Abutments • Vegetation

TABLE 5.5 Swale and Strip Components (WEF et al., 2012)

SCM Type	Treatment Mechanism																						SCM Components
	Quantity Control					Pollutant Control									Biological				Other				
	Peak Flow Attenuation	Runoff Volume Reduction	Infiltration	Dispersion	Evapotranspiration	Runoff Collection and Usage	Sedimentation	Flotation	Laminar Separation	Swirl Concentration	Sorption	Precipitation	Coagulation	Filtration	Plant Metabolism	Nitrification/Denitrification	Sulfate Reduction	Organic Compound Degradation	Pathogen Die-off	Temperature Reduction	Disinfection	Screening	
Swales			X	X			X								X					X			• Energy Dissipator • Inlet • Outlet • Side Slopes and Invert • Vegetation
Strips			X	X			X								X					X			• Level Spreader • Inlet • Outlet • Side Slopes and Invert • Vegetation

TABLE 5.6 Filter Components (WEF et al., 2012)

	Treatment Mechanism																						
	Quantity Control					Pollutant Control									Biological				Other				
SCM Type	Peak Flow Attenuation	Runoff Volume Reduction	Infiltration	Dispersion	Evapotranspiration	Runoff Collection and Usage	Sedimentation	Flotation	Laminar Separation	Swirl Concentration	Sorption	Precipitation	Coagulation	Filtration	Plant Metabolism	Nitrification/Denitrification	Sulfate Reduction	Organic Compound Degradation	Pathogen Die-off	Temperature Reduction	Disinfection	Screening	SCM Components
Surface Sand Filter	X						X	X						X		X					X		• Energy Dissipator • Forebay • Inlet • Outlet (Riser/Principle Spillway, Emergency Spillway, and Low-Flow Orifices) • Filter Media • Underdrain • Embankment and Abutments • Vault/Structure • Pumps/Controls
Subsurface Sand Filter	X						X	X						X		X					X		• Forebay • Inlet • Outlet • Overflow Weir • Filter Media • Baffles • Underdrain • Vault/Structure • Pumps/Controls • Inspection and Access Grating and Manholes

(*continued*)

TABLE 5.6 Filter Components (WEF et al., 2012) (*continued*)

SCM Type	Treatment Mechanism																						SCM Components
	Quantity Control					Pollutant Control									Biological				Other				
	Peak Flow Attenuation	Runoff Volume Reduction	Infiltration	Dispersion	Evapotranspiration	Runoff Collection and Usage	Sedimentation	Flotation	Laminar Separation	Swirl Concentration	Sorption	Precipitation	Coagulation	Filtration	Plant Metabolism	Nitrification/Denitrification	Sulfate Reduction	Organic Compound Degradation	Pathogen Die-off	Temperature Reduction	Disinfection	Screening	
Bioretention Filter	X	X	X		X	X	X	X			X	X	X	X	X	X		X		X	X		• Energy Dissipator • Forebay • Inlet • Outlet (Riser/Principle Spillway, Emergency Spillway, and Low-Flow Orifices) • Embankment and Abutments • Media Mix • Vegetation • Underdrain
Landscaped Roofs	X			X	X						X				X					X			• Flashing • Waterproof Membrane • Drainage Layer • Soil • Vegetation • Roof Drain

Drain Inlet Inserts					X			X							• Insert Frame/Structure • Fabric/Media
Manufactured Filters					X			X							• Forebay • Inlet • Flow Distributor • Outlet • Filter Media • Baffles • Underdrain • Vault/Structure • Pumps/Controls
Subsurface Gravel Wetland	X	X	X	X	X	X	X		X	X	X	X	X	X	• Energy Dissipator • Forebay • Wetland Cells • Inlet • Outlet (Riser/Principle Spillway, Emergency Spillway, and Low-Flow Orifices) • Embankment and Abutments • Media Mix • Vegetation • Underdrain

TABLE 5.7 Infiltrator Components (WEF et al., 2012)

	Treatment Mechanism																						
	Quantity Control					Pollutant Control									Biological				Other				
SCM Type	Peak Flow Attenuation	Runoff Volume Reduction	Infiltration	Dispersion	Evapotranspiration	Runoff Collection and Usage	Sedimentation	Flotation	Laminar Separation	Swirl Concentration	Sorption	Precipitation	Coagulation	Filtration	Plant Metabolism	Nitrification/Denitrification	Sulfate Reduction	Organic Compound Degradation	Pathogen Die-off	Temperature Reduction	Disinfection	Screening	SCM Components
Infiltration Basins	X	X	X				X	X			X	X	X			X		X	X	X	X		• Pretreatment Unit • Energy Dissipator • Forebay • Inlet • Bypass/Overflow Structure • Embankment and Abutments • Vegetation

Infiltration Trenches and Vaults	X	X	X	X	X	X	X	X	X	X	X	X	X	• Pretreatment Unit • Inlet • Bypass/Overflow Structure • Trench/Vault Structure
Dry Wells	X	X	X	X	X	X	X	X	X	X	X	X		• Pretreatment Unit • Inlet • Bypass/Overflow Structure • Drywell Structure
Permeable Pavement	X	X	X		X	X	X		X	X	X	X		• Pervious material ◦ Pervious Asphalt Pavement (PAP) ◦ Pervious Concrete Pavement (PCP) ◦ Permeable Interlocking Concrete Pavement (PICP) ◦ Concrete Grid Pavement (CGP) ◦ Reinforced Grass Pavement (RGP)

TABLE 5.8 Gross Pollutant Traps and Mechanical Operations Components (WEF et al., 2012)

	Treatment Mechanism																						
	Quantity Control					Pollutant Control									Biological				Other				
SCM Type	Peak Flow Attenuation	Runoff Volume Reduction	Infiltration	Dispersion	Evapotranspiration	Runoff Collection and Usage	Sedimentation	Flotation	Laminar Separation	Swirl Concentration	Sorption	Precipitation	Coagulation	Filtration	Plant Metabolism	Nitrification/Denitrification	Sulfate Reduction	Organic Compound Degradation	Pathogen Die-off	Temperature Reduction	Disinfection	Screening	SCM Components
Screens																						X	• Inlet • Bypass/Overflow Structure • Outlet • Screen/Mesh • Screen Structure
Nets																						X	• Inlet • Bypass/Overflow Structure • Outlet • Net • Net Structure

Baskets		X	• Inlet • Bypass/Overflow Structure • Outlet • Screen/Mesh • Basket Structure
Racks		X	• Inlet • Bypass/Overflow Structure • Outlet • Rack • Rack Structure
Hoods	X		• Hood • Outlet

TABLE 5.9 SCM Inspection Requirements

Inspection and Corrective Action	Basins							Swales and Strips		Filters							Infiltrators					GPTs and MOs			
	Cisterns and Rain Barrels	Forebays	Vaults and Swirl Concentrators	Oil and Water Separators	Dry Basins	Wet Basins	Wetlands	Swales	Strips	Surface Sand Filter	Subsurface Sand Filter	Bioretention Filter	Landscaped Roofs	Drain Inlet Inserts	Manufactured Filters	Subsurface Gravel Wetland	Infiltration Basins	Infiltration Trenches and Vaults	Dry Wells	Permeable Pavement	Screens	Nets	Baskets	Racks	Hoods
Inspect for Sediment Accumulation	X	X	X	X	X	X	X	X	X	X	X	X		X	X	X	X	X	X	X	X	X	X	X	X
Inspect for Dead/Dying Vegetation and Bare Spots						X	X	X	X			X	X			X	X								
Inspect for Vegetation Damage due to Pests						X	X	X	X			X	X			X	X								
Inspect for Irrigation System Malfunction/Damage						X	X	X	X			X	X			X	X								
Inspect for Erosion		X			X	X	X	X	X			X	X			X	X								

Inspect for Settling		X			X	X	X	X	X	X	X	X			X	X	X		X						
Inspect Inflow, Outflow, and Overflow Infrastructure for Damage	X	X	X	X	X	X	X	X		X	X	X		X	X	X	X	X	X		X	X	X	X	
Inspect Chamber Structure for Damage	X	X	X	X			-			X	X				X										
Inspect Screens and Trash Racks for Damage																					X	X	X	X	
Inspect Pipes for Damage		X	X	X	X	X	X			X	X	X			X	X			X						
Inspect for Standing Water		X	X		X			X	X			X	X		X		X	X	X						
Inspect for Evidence/Presence of Nuisance Animals and Vectors	X	X	X	X	X	X	X	X	X	X			X		X		X	X	X						
Inspect for Presence of Algal Blooms						X	X																		
Inspect for Damage of Bird Exclusionary/Deterrent Devices						X	X																		
Inspect for Loss of Permanent Pool						X	X																		
Inspect for Damage/Malfunction of Mechanical, Electrical, Pneumatic, & Hydraulic Components			X	X											X										
Inspect for Miscellaneous Site Damage	X	X	X	X	X	X	X	X	X	X	X	X	X	X	X	X	X	X	X	X	X	X	X	X	X

TABLE 5.10 Inspections and Maintenance Indicators for Basins

Inspection Type	Maintenance Indicator Type	Qualitative/Quantitative Measure: Cisterns/ Rain Barrels	Forebays	Vaults and Swirl Concentrators	OWS	Dry Basins	Wet Basins	Wetlands	Measurement Type	Frequency	Corrective Maintenance
Inspect for proper drainage/ infiltration	Inspect for debris/ litter accumulation in screens, basin interior, inlet/outlet/ overflow/bypass structures	Evidence of debris and litter clogging gutters, screen, diverter, etc.	Evidence of debris and litter clogging structure components	Evidence of debris and litter clogging structure components	Evidence of debris and litter clogging structure components	Evidence of debris and litter clogging structure components	Evidence of debris and litter clogging structure components	Evidence of debris and litter clogging structure components	• Visual observation	• Quarterly	• Remove debris and dispose of properly
	Sediment accumulation in screens, downspouts, basin/ structure interior, inlet/outlet/ overflow/bypass structures	NA	Remove accumulated sediment when 50% of the original volume has been reduced	Remove accumulated sediment when 50% of the original volume has been reduced or as specified by the manufacturer	Remove accumulated sediment when 50% of the original volume has been reduced or as specified by the manufacturer	Remove accumulated sediment when 50% of the original volume has been reduced	Remove accumulated sediment when 50% of the original volume has been reduced	Remove accumulated sediment when 50% of the original volume has been reduced	• Visual observation • Ruler/indicator measurement	• Semiannually	• Remove accumulated sediment • Analyze material to identify proper disposal procedures • Dispose of sediment according to analysis results and disposal protocols
	Standing water in basin/structure interior that exceeds design drainage times	NA	Standing water for more than 72 hours	Standing water for more than 72 hours	Standing water for more than 72 hours	Standing water for more than 72 hours	NA	NA	• Visual observation	• Semiannually	• Drain/remove clogging • Add mosquito fish if unable to drain immediately
	Settling of screens, basin interior, basin exterior structure, inlet/outlet/ overflow/bypass structures	Evidence of cracks, low areas, ponding, sediment accumulation	Evidence of cracks, low areas, ponding, sediment accumulation	Evidence of cracks, low areas, ponding, sediment accumulation	Evidence of cracks, low areas, ponding, sediment accumulation	Evidence of cracks, low areas, ponding, sediment accumulation	Evidence of cracks, low areas, ponding, sediment accumulation	Evidence of cracks, low areas, ponding, sediment accumulation	• Visual observation	• Annually	• Fill and compact low areas • Repair cracks and other damage • Contact engineer for more extensive settlement and damage that may require redesign or reconstruction
	Overgrown vegetation blocking drainage/ conveyance	NA	Vegetation height exceeds 305 mm (12 in.), emergence of trees or woody vegetation	NA	NA	Vegetation height exceeds 305 mm (12 in.), emergence of trees or woody vegetation	50% reduction in the original open water surface area occurs	50% reduction in the original open water surface area occurs	• Visual observation	• Quarterly	• Trim as appropriate • Harvest vegetation from wet basin or wetland

	Snow or ice accumulation	Prior to freezing temperatures	Snow or ice impedes functionality of SCM	Snow or ice impedes functionality of SCM	Snow or ice impedes functionality of SCM	Snow or ice impedes functionality of SCM	Snow or ice impedes functionality of SCM	Snow or ice impedes functionality of SCM	• Visual observation	• Monthly during freezing conditions or recent snow	• Drain cisterns/rain barrels and prevent new water from entering system • Disinfect cistern/rain barrel storage tank • Remove snows/ice as needed
Inspect for proper erosion/ sediment control	Presence of rills, gullies, or sediment accumulation within basin interior	NA	Evidence of erosion	NA	NA	Evidence of erosion	Evidence of erosion	Evidence of erosion	• Visual observation	• Semi-annually	• Remove sediment • Fill/compact/regrade areas • Address any upstream causes
	Presence of rills, gullies, or sediment accumulation within inflow/ outflow/overflow/ bypass conveyance or inlet/outlet/ overflow/bypass structures	NA	Evidence of erosion	NA	NA	Evidence of erosion	Evidence of erosion	Evidence of erosion	• Visual observation	• Semi-annually	• Remove sediment • Fill/compact/regrade areas • Address any upstream causes
	Loss of vegetation or presence/ evidence of burrowing animals within basin interior, along embankments	NA	Evidence of bare spots, burrows, holes, mounds	NA	NA	Evidence of bare spots, burrows, holes, mounds	Evidence of bare spots, burrows, holes, mounds	Evidence of bare spots, burrows, holes, mounds	• Visual observation • Test irrigation system turns on/ off according to programming	• Semi-annually	• Remove dead/dying vegetation • Replant/reseed as appropriate • Inspect for irrigation system malfunction/damage • Fill or compact mounds or burrows • Coordinate with fish and wildlife agencies if needed • Repair/replace any malfunctioning/damaged irrigation component
	Loss of vegetation or presence/ evidence of burrowing animals within vegetated pretreatment	NA	Evidence of bare spots, burrows, holes, mounds	NA	NA	Evidence of bare spots, burrows, holes, mounds	Evidence of bare spots, burrows, holes, mounds	Evidence of bare spots, burrows, holes, mounds	• Visual observation • Test irrigation system turns on/ off according to programming	• Semi-annually	• Remove dead/dying vegetation • Replant/reseed as appropriate • Fill or compact mounds or burrows • Inspect for irrigation system • Repair/replace any malfunctioning/damaged irrigation component

(continued)

TABLE 5.10 Inspections and Maintenance Indicators for Basins (*continued*)

Inspection Type	Maintenance Indicator Type	Qualitative/Quantitative Measure							Measurement Type	Frequency	Corrective Maintenance
		Cisterns/ Rain Barrels	Forebays	Vaults and Swirl Concentrators	OWS	Dry Basins	Wet Basins	Wetlands			
Inspect for structural integrity	Damage to structure, screens, mesh, nets, racks, inlets, outlets, overflow/bypass	Structural failure or damage (e.g., broken or open pipes, vessels, etc.)	Structural failure or damage (e.g., broken or open structures, exposed subsurface elements, or failure of walls, walkways, or roadways)	Structural failure or damage (e.g., broken or open structures, exposed subsurface elements)	Structural failure or damage (e.g., broken or open structures, exposed subsurface elements)	Structural failure or damage (e.g., broken or open structures, exposed subsurface elements, or failure of slopes, walkways, or roadways)	Structural failure or damage (e.g., broken or open structures, exposed subsurface elements, or failure of slopes, walkways, or roadways)	Structural failure or damage (e.g., broken or open structures, exposed subsurface elements, or failure of slopes, walkways, or roadways)	• Visual observation	• Quarterly	• Repair or replace
Inspect for proper pollutant control	Presence of algae within permanent pool	N/A	N/A	N/A	N/A	N/A	Evidence of algae blooms	Evidence of algae blooms	• Visual observation	• Semi-annually	• Reduce/eliminate upstream fertilizer applications • Remove algal to extent possible • Weed, trim, or prune vegetation to allow more sunlight access • Plant emergent vegetation • Introduce air using diffusers or surface aerators
	Loss of permanent pool design depth	NA	NA	NA	NA	NA	Stain marks on the riser or flow control structure. Exposure of a non-vegetated pond bottom around the pool perimeter.	Stain marks on the riser or flow control structure. Exposure of a non-vegetated pond bottom around the pool perimeter	• Visual observation • Depth/height measurement	• Semi-annually	• Shut and lock low flow drain valve if open • Fill burrows • Repair leak in riser • Repair leak in barrel • Drain permanent pool and install liner • Consult with design engineer

							Swirling action of water caused by submerged orifice flow, usually in the vicinity of the dam, riser, or principal spillway.	Swirling action of water caused by submerged orifice flow, usually in the vicinity of the dam, riser, or principal spillway.			
	Dead/dying vegetation	NA	Damaged, diseased, and/or dead vegetation	NA	NA	Damaged, diseased, and/or dead vegetation	Damaged, diseased, and/or dead vegetation	Damaged, diseased, and/or dead vegetation	• Visual observation	• Semi-annually	• Remove dead/dying vegetation • Replant/reseed as appropriate • Inspect for irrigation system malfunction/ damage
	Bare spots within vegetation	NA	Evidence of bare spots, burrows, holes, mounds	NA	NA	Evidence of bare spots, burrows, holes, mounds	Evidence of bare spots, burrows, holes, mounds	Evidence of bare spots, burrows, holes, mounds	• Visual observation	• Semi-annually	• Replant/reseed as appropriate • Inspect for irrigation system malfunction/ damage
	Undesired vegetation	NA	Evidence of weeds and woody vegetation	NA	NA	Evidence of weeds and woody vegetation	Evidence of weeds and woody vegetation	Evidence of weeds and woody vegetation	• Visual observation	• Semi-annually	• Remove undesired vegetation • Replant/reseed as appropriate
Inspect for proper mechanical, electrical, pneumatic, hydraulic function	Per manufacturer recommendations (baffles, skimmers, pumps, valves, coalescing plates, etc.)	NA	NA	Damage or clogging of baffles and hydraulic structures	Damage or clogging of coalescing plates	Damage or clogging of skimmers and valves	Damage or clogging of valves	Damage or clogging of valves	• Per manufacturer recommendations	• Per manufacturer recommendations	• Per manufacturer recommendations
Inspect absorbent pads	Saturated absorbent pad	N/A	N/A	Saturated or spent pad					• Replace when saturated with oil, every 6 months or more frequently as needed		

(*continued*)

TABLE 5.10 Inspections and Maintenance Indicators for Basins (*continued*)

		Qualitative/Quantitative Measure									
Inspection Type	Maintenance Indicator Type	Cisterns/ Rain Barrels	Forebays	Vaults and Swirl Concentrators	OWS	Dry Basins	Wet Basins	Wetlands	Measurement Type	Frequency	Corrective Maintenance
Inspect for proper vector & nuisance controls	Standing water within basin interior that exceeds local vector control agency thresholds	N/A	Standing water for more than 72 hours	Standing water for more than 72 hours	Standing water for more than 72 hours	Standing water for more than 72 hours	NA	NA	• Visual inspections	• Within threshold established by local vector agency	• Drain SCM or otherwise remove standing water • Check for clogging of outlet structure or other downstream conveyance • Check with design engineer • Use mosquito fish for temporary solution if needed
	Damage to bird exclusionary devices	NA	NA	NA	NA	NA	Evidence of birds or damage to exclusionary devices	Evidence of birds or damage to exclusionary devices	• Visual observation	• Semi-annually	• Repair/replace devices or components as appropriate
	Loss of mosquito fish	NA	NA	NA	NA	NA	Evidence of mosquitos or lack of mosquito fish	Evidence of mosquitos or lack of mosquito fish	• Visual observation	• Quarterly	• Replace fish
	Presence or indication of nuisance animals (rats, moles, gophers, rabbits, birds, etc.)	NA	Presence of nuisance animals	NA	NA	Presence of nuisance animals	Presence of nuisance animals	Presence of nuisance animals	• Visual observation	• Semi-annually	• Fill and compact burrows and holes as appropriate • Remove nests • Coordinate with local fish and wildlife agencies if necessary • Fill gaps/holes allowing access within enclosures • Conduct standing water inspections and correction maintenance
Inspect for proper site aesthetics and safety	Fence damage	Damaged fence	Damaged fence	Damaged fence	Damaged fence	Damaged fence	Damaged fence	Damaged fence	• Visual observation	• Semi-annually	• Repair/replace materials/ components/equipment as appropriate
	Access road damage	Asphalt or concrete is severely degraded or shows significant dents or scars	Asphalt or concrete is severely degraded or shows significant dents or scars	Asphalt or concrete is severely degraded or shows significant dents or scars	Asphalt or concrete is severely degraded or shows significant dents or scars	Asphalt or concrete is severely degraded or shows significant dents or scars	Asphalt or concrete is severely degraded or shows significant dents or scars	Asphalt or concrete is severely degraded or shows significant dents or scars	• Visual observation	• Semi-annually	• Repair/replace materials/ components/equipment as appropriate

Trail damage	Trail is eroded	Trail is eroded	Trail is eroded	Trail is eroded	Trail is eroded	Trail is eroded	Trail is eroded	• Visual observation	• Semi-annually	• Remove sediment • Fill/compact/regrade areas • Address any upstream causes
Light damage	Light does not work	Light does not work	Light does not work	Light does not work	Light does not work	Light does not work	Light does not work	• Visual observation	• Semi-annually	• Repair/replace materials/components/equipment as appropriate
Sign damage	Dust, grime, or other residue is present on signage	Dust, grime, or other residue is present on signage	Dust, grime, or other residue is present on signage	Dust, grime, or other residue is present on signage	Dust, grime, or other residue is present on signage	Dust, grime, or other residue is present on signage	Dust, grime, or other residue is present on signage	• Visual observation	• Semi-annually	• Wipe down signage • Repair/replace materials/components/equipment as appropriate
Graffiti	Evidence of graffiti	Evidence of graffiti	Evidence of graffiti	Evidence of graffiti	Evidence of graffiti	Evidence of graffiti	Evidence of graffiti	• Visual observation	• Semi-annually	• Remove graffiti from SMP signage, structures, or surfaces
Nest box damage	Damaged net box	Damaged net box	Damaged net box	Damaged net box	Damaged net box	Damaged net box	Damaged net box	• Visual observation	• Semi-annually	• Repair/replace materials/components/equipment as appropriate
Platform damage	Damaged platform	Damaged platform	Damaged platform	Damaged platform	Damaged platform	Damaged platform	Damaged platform	• Visual observation	• Semi-annually	• Repair/replace materials/components/equipment as appropriate
Overgrown vegetation	N/A	Vegetation height exceeds 305 mm (12 inches), emergence of trees or woody vegetation	NA	NA	Vegetation height exceeds 305 mm (12 inches), emergence of trees or woody vegetation	50% reduction in the original open water surface area occurs	50% reduction in the original open water surface area occurs	• Visual observation	• Quarterly	• Trim as appropriate • Harvest vegetation from wet basin or wetland
Undesired vegetation	NA	Evidence of weeds and woody vegetation	NA	NA	Evidence of weeds and woody vegetation	Evidence of weeds and woody vegetation	Evidence of weeds and woody vegetation	• Visual observation	• Semi-annually	• Remove undesired vegetation • Replant/reseed as appropriate
Evidence of pest damage to vegetation	NA	Evidence of bare spots, burrows, holes, mounds	NA	NA	Evidence of bare spots, burrows, holes mounds	Evidence of bare spots, burrows, holes, mounds	Evidence of bare spots, burrows, holes, mounds	• Visual observation	• Semi-annually	• Replant/reseed as appropriate • Inspect for irrigation system malfunction/damage

TABLE 5.11 Inspections and Maintenance Indicators for Swales and Strips

Inspection Type	Maintenance Indicator Type	Qualitative/Quantitative Measure		Measurement Type	Frequency	Corrective Maintenance
		Swales	Strips			
Inspect for proper drainage/infiltration	Inspect for debris/litter accumulation inlet/outlet/overflow/bypass structures	Evidence of debris and litter clogging structure components	Evidence of debris and litter clogging structure components	• Visual observation	• Quarterly	• Remove debris/litter and dispose of properly
	Sediment accumulation in inlet/outlet/overflow/bypass structures	Sediment at or near vegetation height, channeling of flow, inhibited flow due to change in slope	Sediment at or near vegetation height, channeling of flow, inhibited flow due to change in slope	• Visual observation • Ruler/indicator measurement	• Semi-annually	• Remove accumulated sediment • Analyze material to identify proper disposal procedures • Dispose of sediment according to analysis results and disposal protocols
	Standing water in swale or strip	Standing water for more than 72 hours	Standing water for more than 72 hours	• Visual observation	• Semi-annually	• Drain and regrade to prevent standing water
	Settling of swales and strip inverts and swale slopes	Evidence of low areas, ponding, sediment accumulation	Evidence of low areas, ponding, sediment accumulation	• Visual observation	• Annually	• Fill and compact low areas • Contact engineer for more extensive settlement and damage that may require redesign or reconstruction
	Overgrown vegetation blocking drainage/conveyance	Vegetation height exceeds 305 mm (12 inches), emergence of trees or woody vegetation	Vegetation height exceeds 305 mm (12 inches), emergence of trees or woody vegetation	• Visual observation	• Quarterly	• Trim as appropriate
	Snow or ice accumulation	Snow or ice impedes functionality of SCM	Snow or ice impedes functionality of SCM	• Visual observation	• Monthly during freezing conditions or recent snow	• Remove snows/ice as needed
Inspect for proper erosion/sediment control	Presence of rills, gullies, or sediment accumulation within the swale or strip	Evidence of erosion	Evidence of erosion	• Visual observation	• Semi-annually	• Fill/compact/regrade areas • Address any upstream causes
	Presence of rills, gullies, or sediment accumulation within inflow/outflow/overflow/bypass conveyance	Evidence of erosion	Evidence of erosion	• Visual observation	• Semi-annually	• Remove sediment • Address any upstream causes
	Loss of vegetation or presence/evidence of burrowing animals within swale or strip	Evidence of bare spots, burrows, holes, mounds	Evidence of bare spots, burrows, holes, mounds	• Visual observation • Test irrigation system turns on/off according to programming	• Semi-annually	• Remove dead/dying vegetation • Replant/reseed as appropriate • Fill or compact mounds or burrows • Inspect for irrigation system • Repair/replace any malfunctioning/damaged irrigation component

Inspect for structural integrity	Damage to swale slopes, inlets, outlets, overflow/bypass	Structural failure or damage to swale side slopes	NA	• Visual observation	• Quarterly	• Repair
	Dead/dying vegetation	Damaged, diseased, and/or dead vegetation	Damaged, diseased, and/or dead vegetation	• Visual observation	• Semi-annually	• Remove dead/dying vegetation • Replant/reseed as appropriate • Inspect for irrigation system malfunction/damage
	Bare spots within vegetation	Evidence of bare spots, burrows, holes, mounds	Evidence of bare spots, burrows, holes, mounds	• Visual observation	• Semi-annually	• Replant/reseed as appropriate • Inspect for irrigation system malfunction/damage
	Undesired vegetation	Evidence of weeds and woody vegetation	Evidence of weeds and woody vegetation	• Visual observation	• Semi-annually	• Remove undesired vegetation • Replant/reseed as appropriate
	Presence or indication of nuisance animals (rats, moles, gophers, rabbits, birds, etc.)	Presence of nuisance animals	Presence of nuisance animals	• Visual observation	• Semi-annually	• Fill and compact burrows and holes as appropriate • Remove nests • Coordinate with local fish and wildlife agencies if necessary • Fill gaps/holes allowing access within enclosures • Conduct standing water inspections and correction maintenance
Inspect for proper site aesthetics and safety	Fence damage	Damaged fence	Damaged fence	• Visual observation	• Semi-annually	• Repair/replace materials/components/equipment as appropriate
	Access road damage	Asphalt or concrete is severely degraded or shows significant dents or scars	Asphalt or concrete is severely degraded or shows significant dents or scars	• Visual observation	• Semi-annually	• Repair/replace materials/components/equipment as appropriate
	Trail damage	Trail is eroded	Trail is eroded	• Visual observation	• Semi-annually	• Remove sediment • Fill/compact/regrade areas • Address any upstream causes
	Light damage	Light does not work	Light does not work	• Visual observation	• Semi-annually	• Repair/replace materials/components/equipment as appropriate
	Sign damage	Dust, grime, or other residue is present on signage	Dust, grime, or other residue is present on signage	• Visual observation	• Semi-annually	• Wipe down signage • Repair/replace materials/components/equipment as appropriate
	Graffiti	Evidence of graffiti	Evidence of graffiti	• Visual observation	• Semi-annually	• Remove graffiti from SMP signage, structures, or surfaces
	Overgrown vegetation	Vegetation height exceeds 305 mm (12 inches), emergence of trees or woody vegetation	Vegetation height exceeds 305 mm (12 inches), emergence of trees or woody vegetation	• Visual observation	• Quarterly	• Trim as appropriate
	Undesired vegetation	Evidence of weeds and woody vegetation	Evidence of weeds and woody vegetation	• Visual observation	• Semi-annually	• Remove undesired vegetation • Replant/reseed as appropriate
	Evidence of pest damage to vegetation	Evidence of bare spots, burrows, holes, mounds	Evidence of bare spots, burrows, holes, mounds	• Visual observation	• Semi-annually	• Replant/reseed as appropriate • Inspect for irrigation system malfunction/damage

TABLE 5.12 Inspections and Maintenance Indicators for Filters

		Qualitative/Quantitative Measure									
Inspection Type	Maintenance Indicator Type	Surface Sand Filters	Subsurface Sand Filters	Bioretention Filters	Landscaped Roofs	Drain Inlet Inserts	Manufactured Filters	Subsurface Gravel Wetlands	Measurement Type	Frequency	Corrective Maintenance
Inspect for proper drainage/ infiltration	Inspect for debris/ litter accumulation in screens, inlet/ outlet/overflow/ bypass structures, and chambers	Evidence of debris and litter clogging structure components	Evidence of debris and litter clogging structure components	Evidence of debris and litter clogging structure components	Evidence of debris and litter clogging SCM	Evidence of debris and litter clogging structure components	Evidence of debris and litter clogging structure components	Evidence of debris and litter clogging structure components	• Visual observation	• Quarterly	• Remove debris and dispose of properly
	Sediment accumulation in screens, inlet/ outlet/overflow/ bypass structures, and chambers	Sediment caking on media surface	Sediment caking on media surface	Sediment caking on media surface	NA	Sediment blinds insert	Sediment caking on media surface	Sediment filling voids of gravel	• Visual observation • Ruler/indicator measurement	• Semi-annually	• Remove accumulated sediment • Analyze material to identify proper disposal procedures • Dispose of sediment according to analysis results and disposal protocols
	Standing water in structure, basin, or chambers	Standing water for more than 72 hours	Standing water for more than 72 hours	Standing water for more than 72 hours	Standing water for more than 72 hours	Standing water for more than 72 hours	Standing water for more than 72 hours	Standing water for more than 72 hours	• Visual observation	• Semi-annually	• Drain/remove clogging • Rehabilitate media • Remove and dispose of media following proper testing and handling procedures • Replace media
	Ponding volume and depth	NA	NA	Ponding volume, depth, and surface area less than 25% of design	NA	NA	NA	NA	• Ruler/indicator measurement	• Annually	• Adjust grade by removal or addition of mulch and/or media • Regrade the facility to meet design areas and volumes
	Settling of structure, basin, chamber, inlet/ outlet/overflow/ bypass structures	Evidence of low areas, ponding, sediment accumulation	Evidence of low areas, ponding, sediment accumulation	Evidence of low areas, ponding, sediment accumulation	Evidence of low areas, ponding	NA	Evidence of low areas, ponding, sediment accumulation	Evidence of low areas, ponding, sediment accumulation	• Visual observation	• Annually	• Fill and compact low areas • Repair cracks and other damage • Contact engineer for more extensive settlement and damage that may require redesign or reconstruction • Spot mulch and repair media

	Overgrown vegetation blocking drainage/ conveyance	NA	NA	Vegetation height exceeds 305 mm (12 inches), emergence of trees or woody vegetation	Vegetation height exceeds 305 mm (12 inches), emergence of trees or woody vegetation	NA	NA	NA	• Visual observation	• Quarterly	• Trim as appropriate
	Snow or ice accumulation	Snow or ice impedes functionality of SCM	Snow or ice impedes functionality of SCM	Snow or ice impedes functionality of SCM	Snow or ice impedes functionality of SCM	Snow or ice impedes functionality of SCM	Snow or ice impedes functionality of SCM	Snow or ice impedes functionality of SCM	• Visual observation	• Monthly during freezing conditions or recent snow	• Remove snow/ice as needed
Inspect for proper erosion/ sediment control	Presence of rills, gullies, or sediment accumulation	Channelization of media or sediment accumulation	Sediment accumulation	Sediment accumulation	Channelization of SCM	Sediment accumulation	Sediment accumulation	Sediment accumulation	• Visual observation	• Semi-annually	• Fill/compact/regrade areas • Address any upstream causes
	Loss of vegetation or presence/ evidence of burrowing animals	NA	NA	Evidence of bare spots, burrows, holes, mounds	Evidence of bare spots, burrows, holes, mounds	NA	NA	NA	• Visual observation • Test irrigation system turns on/ off according to programming	• Semi-annually	• Remove dead/dying vegetation • Replant/reseed as appropriate • Inspect for irrigation system malfunction/ damage • Fill or compact mounds or burrows • Repair/replace any malfunctioning/ damaged irrigation component
Inspect for structural integrity	Damage to structure, basin, or chambers	Structural failure or damage (e.g., broken or open structures, chambers, etc.)	Structural failure or damage (e.g., broken or open structures, chambers, etc.)	Structural failure or damage to basin	Structural failure or damage to green roof structure	Damage to drain inlet insert	Structural failure or damage (e.g., broken or open structures, chambers, etc.)	Structural failure or damage (e.g., broken or open structures, chambers, etc.)	• Visual observation	• Quarterly	• Repair or replace
	Damage to inlets, outlets, overflow/bypass, conveyance channels/pipes, and underdrains	Structural failure or damage (e.g., broken or open inlets, outlets, overflow/ bypass, conveyance channels/ pipes, and underdrains)	Structural failure or damage (e.g., broken or open inlets, outlets, overflow/ bypass, conveyance channels/ pipes, and underdrains)	Structural failure or damage (e.g., broken or open inlets, outlets, overflow/ bypass, conveyance channels/ pipes, and underdrains)	Structural failure or damage (e.g., broken or open outlets and underdrains)	Damage to drain inlet insert	Structural failure or damage (e.g., broken or open inlets, outlets, overflow/ bypass, conveyance channels/ pipes, and underdrains)	Structural failure or damage (e.g., broken or open inlets, outlets, overflow/ bypass, conveyance channels/ pipes, and underdrains)	• Visual observation	• Quarterly	• Repair or replace

(continued)

TABLE 5.12 Inspections and Maintenance Indicators for Filters (*continued*)

		Qualitative/Quantitative Measure									
Inspection Type	Maintenance Indicator Type	Surface Sand Filters	Subsurface Sand Filters	Bioretention Filters	Landscaped Roofs	Drain Inlet Inserts	Manufactured Filters	Subsurface Gravel Wetlands	Measurement Type	Frequency	Corrective Maintenance
Inspect for proper pollutant control	Dead/dying vegetation	NA	NA	Damaged, diseased, and/or dead vegetation	Damaged, diseased, and/or dead vegetation	NA	NA	NA	• Visual observation	• Semi-annually	• Remove dead/dying vegetation • Replant/reseed as appropriate • Inspect for irrigation system malfunction/ damage
	Bare spots within vegetation	NA	NA	Evidence of bare spots, burrows, holes, mounds	Evidence of bare spots, burrows, holes, mounds	NA	NA	NA	• Visual observation	• Semi-annually	• Replant/reseed as appropriate • Inspect for irrigation system malfunction/ damage
	Undesired vegetation	NA	NA	Evidence of weeds and woody vegetation	Evidence of weeds and woody vegetation	NA	NA	NA	• Visual observation	• Semi-annually	• Remove undesired vegetation • Replant/reseed as appropriate
	Evidence of pest damage to vegetation (including presence of pests)	NA	NA	Evidence of bare spots, burrows, holes, mounds	Evidence of bare spots, burrows, holes, mounds	NA	NA	NA	• Visual observation	• Quarterly	• Replant/reseed as appropriate • Inspect for irrigation system malfunction/ damage
Inspect for proper mechanical, electrical, pneumatic, hydraulic function	Per manufacturer recommendations (baffles, pumps, valves, etc.)	Damage or clogging of baffles and hydraulic structures	Damage or clogging of baffles and hydraulic structures	NA	NA	NA	Damage or clogging of baffles and hydraulic structures	NA	• Per manufacturer recommendations	• Per manufacturer recommendations	• Per manufacturer recommendations
Inspect for proper vector and nuisance controls	Standing water within structure, basin or chamber that exceeds local vector control agency thresholds	Standing water for more than 72 hours	Standing water for more than 72 hours	Standing water for more than 72 hours	Standing water for more than 72 hours	Standing water for more than 72 hours	Standing water for more than 72 hours	Standing water for more than 72 hours	• Visual inspections	• Within threshold established by local vector agency	• Drain SCM or otherwise remove standing water • Check for clogging of outlet structure or other downstream conveyance • Check with design engineer

	Presence or indication of nuisance animals (rats, moles, gophers, rabbits, birds, etc.)	Presence of nuisance animals	Presence of nuisance animals	Presence of nuisance animals	Presence of nuisance animals	Presence of nuisance animals	Presence of nuisance animals	Presence of nuisance animals	• Visual observation	• Semi-annually	• Fill and compact burrows and holes as appropriate • Remove nests • Coordinate with local fish and wildlife agencies if necessary • Fill gaps/holes allowing access within enclosures • Conduct standing water inspections and correction maintenance
Inspect for proper site aesthetics and safety	Fence damage	Damaged fence	Damaged fence	Damaged fence	Damaged fence	Damaged fence	Damaged fence	Damaged fence	• Visual observation	• Semi-annually	• Repair/replace materials/components/equipment as appropriate
	Access road damage	Asphalt or concrete is severely degraded or shows significant dents or scars	Asphalt or concrete is severely degraded or shows significant dents or scars	Asphalt or concrete is severely degraded or shows significant dents or scars	NA	NA	Asphalt or concrete is severely degraded or shows significant dents or scars	Asphalt or concrete is severely degraded or shows significant dents or scars	• Visual observation	• Semi-annually	• Repair/replace materials/components/equipment as appropriate
	Trail damage	Trail is eroded	Trail is eroded	Trail is eroded	NA	NA	Trail is eroded	Trail is eroded	• Visual observation	• Semi-annually	• Remove sediment • Fill/compact/regrade areas • Address any upstream causes
	Light damage	Light does not work	Light does not work	Light does not work	NA	NA	Light does not work	Light does not work	• Visual observation	• Semi-annually	• Repair/replace materials/components/equipment as appropriate
	Sign damage	Dust, grime, or other residue is present on signage	Dust, grime, or other residue is present on signage	Dust, grime, or other residue is present on signage	NA	NA	Dust, grime, or other residue is present on signage	Dust, grime, or other residue is present on signage	• Visual observation	• Semi-annually	• Wipe down signage • Repair/replace materials/components/equipment as appropriate
	Graffiti	Evidence of graffiti	Evidence of graffiti	Evidence of graffiti	NA	Evidence of graffiti	Evidence of graffiti	Evidence of graffiti	• Visual observation	• Semi-annually	• Remove graffiti from SMP signage, structures, or surfaces

(*continued*)

TABLE 5.12 Inspections and Maintenance Indicators for Filters (*continued*)

Inspection Type	Maintenance Indicator Type	Qualitative/Quantitative Measure: Surface Sand Filters	Subsurface Sand Filters	Bioretention Filters	Landscaped Roofs	Drain Inlet Inserts	Manufactured Filters	Subsurface Gravel Wetlands	Measurement Type	Frequency	Corrective Maintenance
Inspect for proper site aesthetics and safety (*continued*)	Overgrown vegetation	NA	NA	Vegetation height exceeds 305 mm (12 inches), emergence of trees or woody vegetation	Vegetation height exceeds 305 mm (12 inches), emergence of trees or woody vegetation	NA	NA	NA	• Visual observation	• Quarterly	• Trim as appropriate
	Undesired vegetation	NA	NA	Evidence of weeds and woody vegetation	Evidence of weeds and woody vegetation	NA	NA	NA	• Visual observation	• Semi-annually	• Remove undesired vegetation • Replant/reseed as appropriate
	Evidence of pest damage to vegetation	NA	NA	Evidence of bare spots, burrows, holes, mounds	Evidence of bare spots, burrows, holes, mounds	NA	NA	NA	• Visual observation	• Quarterly	• Replant/reseed as appropriate • Inspect for irrigation system malfunction/damage

TABLE 5.13 Inspections and Maintenance Indicators for Infiltrators

Inspection Type	Maintenance Indicator Type	Qualitative/Quantitative Measure: Infiltration Basins	Qualitative/Quantitative Measure: Infiltration Trenches and Vaults	Qualitative/Quantitative Measure: Dry Wells	Qualitative/Quantitative Measure: Pervious Pavement	Measurement Type	Frequency	Corrective Maintenance
Inspect for proper drainage/infiltration	Inspect for debris/litter accumulation in screens, basin interior, inlet/outlet/overflow/bypass structures	Evidence of debris and litter clogging SCM	Evidence of debris and litter clogging SCM	Evidence of debris and litter clogging SCM	Evidence of debris and litter clogging SCM	• Visual observation	• Quarterly	• Remove debris and dispose of properly
	Sediment accumulation in screens, downspouts, basin/structure interior, inlet/outlet/overflow/bypass structures	Sediment caking on surface	Sediment caking on surface	Sediment caking on surface	Sediment entrained in pervious pavement	• Visual observation • Ruler/indicator measurement	• Semi-annually	• Remove accumulated sediment • Analyze material to identify proper disposal procedures • Dispose of sediment according to analysis results and disposal protocols • Vacuum pervious pavement surface • Perform restorative vacuum cleaning of pervious pavement
	Standing water in basin/structure interior that exceeds design drainage times	Standing water for more than 72 hours	Standing water for more than 72 hours	Standing water for more than 72 hours	Standing water for more than 72 hours	• Visual inspections	• Within threshold established by local vector agency	• Drain SCM or otherwise remove standing water • Check for clogging of outlet structure or other downstream conveyance • Check with design engineer
	Settling of basin interior, basin exterior structure, vaults, inlet/outlet/overflow/bypass structures	Evidence of low areas, ponding	Evidence of low areas, ponding	Evidence of low areas, ponding, sediment accumulation	Evidence of low areas, ponding, sediment accumulation	• Visual observation	• Annually	• Fill low areas • Repair cracks and other damage • Contact engineer for more extensive settlement and damage that may require redesign or reconstruction
	Overgrown vegetation blocking drainage/conveyance	Vegetation height exceeds 305 mm (12 inches), emergence of trees or woody vegetation	Vegetation height exceeds 305 mm (12 inches), emergence of trees or woody vegetation	Vegetation height exceeds 305 mm (12 inches), emergence of trees or woody vegetation	NA	• Visual observation	• Quarterly	• Trim as appropriate

(continued)

TABLE 5.13 Inspections and Maintenance Indicators for Infiltrators (*continued*)

Inspection Type	Maintenance Indicator Type	Qualitative/Quantitative Measure				Measurement Type	Frequency	Corrective Maintenance
		Infiltration Basins	Infiltration Trenches and Vaults	Dry Wells	Pervious Pavement			
Inspect for proper drainage/infiltration (*continued*)	Snow or ice accumulation	Snow or ice impedes functionality of SCM	Snow or ice impedes functionality of SCM	Snow or ice impedes functionality of SCM	Snow events > 0.64 cm (0.25 in.), sleet and freezing rain events, and after any plowing event 5 cm (2 in.)	• Visual observation	• Monthly during freezing conditions or recent snow	• Remove snows/ice as needed • Apply deicer to pervious pavement surface • Plow snow from surface
Inspect for proper erosion/sediment control	Presence of rills, gullies, or sediment accumulation within basin interior	Evidence of erosion	NA	NA	NA	• Visual observation	• Semi-annually	• Fill/compact/regrade areas • Address any upstream causes
	Presence of rills, gullies, or sediment accumulation within inflow/outflow/overflow/bypass conveyance or inlet/outlet/overflow/bypass structures	Evidence of erosion	Evidence of erosion	Evidence of erosion	Evidence of erosion	• Visual observation	• Semi-annually	• Remove sediment • Address any upstream causes
	Loss of vegetation or presence/evidence of burrowing animals within basin interior, along embankments	Evidence of bare spots, burrows, holes, mounds	NA	NA	NA	• Visual observation • Test irrigation system turns on/off according to programming	• Semi-annually	• Remove dead/dying vegetation • Replant/reseed as appropriate • Inspect for irrigation system malfunction/damage • Fill or compact mounds or burrows • Coordinate with fish and wildlife agencies if needed • Repair/replace any malfunctioning/damaged irrigation component

Inspect for structural integrity	Damage to basin including embankments	Structural failure or damage to basin	NA	NA	NA	• Visual observation	• Quarterly	• Repair or replace
	Damage to inlets, outlets, overflow/bypass, conveyance channels/pipes	Structural failure or damage (e.g., broken or open inlets, outlets, overflow/bypass, conveyance channels/pipes)	Structural failure or damage (e.g., broken or open inlets, outlets, overflow/bypass, conveyance channels/pipes)	Structural failure or damage (e.g., broken or open inlets, outlets, overflow/bypass, conveyance channels/pipes)	NA	• Visual observation	• Quarterly	• Repair or replace
	Damage to Porous pavement (raveling)	NA	NA	NA	Pervious asphalt or concrete is severely degraded or shows significant dents or scars	• Visual observation	• Quarterly	• Replace the degraded area of pavement • Consult an engineer for possible system redesign, and a construction contractor to perform repairs
Inspect for proper pollutant control	Dead/dying vegetation	Damaged, diseased, and/or dead vegetation	NA	NA	NA	• Visual observation	• Semi-annually	• Remove dead/dying vegetation • Replant/reseed as appropriate • Inspect for irrigation system malfunction/damage
	Bare spots within vegetation	Evidence of bare spots, burrows, holes, mounds	NA	NA	NA	• Visual observation	• Semi-annually	• Replant/reseed as appropriate • Inspect for irrigation system malfunction/damage
	Undesired vegetation	Evidence of weeds and woody vegetation	NA	NA	NA	• Visual observation	• Semi-annually	• Remove undesired vegetation • Replant/reseed as appropriate
	Evidence of pest damage to vegetation (including presence of pests)	Evidence of bare spots, burrows, holes, mounds	NA	NA	NA	• Visual observation	• Quarterly	• Replant/reseed as appropriate • Inspect for irrigation system malfunction/damage

(continued)

TABLE 5.13 Inspections and Maintenance Indicators for Infiltrators (*continued*)

		Qualitative/Quantitative Measure						
Inspection Type	Maintenance Indicator Type	Infiltration Basins	Infiltration Trenches and Vaults	Dry Wells	Pervious Pavement	Measurement Type	Frequency	Corrective Maintenance
Inspect for proper vector and nuisance controls	Standing water within basin, trench or drywell that exceeds local vector control agency thresholds	Standing water for more than 72 hours	Standing water for more than 72 hours	Standing water for more than 72 hours	Standing water for more than 72 hours	• Visual inspections	• Within threshold established by local vector agency	• Drain SCM or otherwise remove standing water • Check for clogging of outlet structure or other downstream conveyance • Check with design engineer
	Presence or indication of nuisance animals (rats, moles, gophers, rabbits, birds, etc.)	Presence of nuisance animals	Presence of nuisance animals	Presence of nuisance animals	Presence of nuisance animals	• Visual observation	• Semi-annually	• Fill and compact burrows and holes as appropriate • Remove nests • Coordinate with local fish and wildlife agencies if necessary • Fill gaps/holes allowing access within enclosures • Conduct standing water inspections and correction maintenance
Inspect for proper site aesthetics and safety	Fence damage	Damaged fence	Damaged fence	Damaged fence	Damaged fence	• Visual observation	• Semi-annually	• Repair/replace materials/components/equipment as appropriate
	Access road damage	Asphalt or concrete is severely degraded or shows significant dents or scars	Asphalt or concrete is severely degraded or shows significant dents or scars	Asphalt or concrete is severely degraded or shows significant dents or scars	Asphalt or concrete is severely degraded or shows significant dents or scars	• Visual observation	• Semi-annually	• Repair/replace materials/components/equipment as appropriate

Trail damage	Trail is eroded	Trail is eroded	Trail is eroded	Trail is eroded	• Visual observation	• Semi-annually	• Remove sediment • Fill/compact/regrade areas • Address any upstream causes
Light damage	Light does not work	Light does not work	Light does not work	Light does not work	• Visual observation	• Semi-annually	• Repair/replace materials/components/equipment as appropriate
Sign damage	Dust, grime, or other residue is present on signage	Dust, grime, or other residue is present on signage	Dust, grime, or other residue is present on signage	Dust, grime, or other residue is present on signage	• Visual observation	• Semi-annually	• Wipe down signage • Repair/replace materials/components/equipment as appropriate
Graffiti	Evidence of graffiti	Evidence of graffiti	Evidence of graffiti	Evidence of graffiti	• Visual observation	• Semi-annually	• Remove graffiti from SMP signage, structures, or surfaces
Overgrown vegetation	Vegetation height exceeds 305 mm (12 inches), emergence of trees or woody vegetation	NA	NA	NA	• Visual observation	• Quarterly	• Trim or mow as appropriate
Undesired vegetation	Evidence of weeds and woody vegetation	NA	NA	NA	• Visual observation	• Semi-annually	• Remove undesired vegetation • Replant/reseed as appropriate
Evidence of pest damage to vegetation	Evidence of bare spots, burrows, holes, mounds	NA	NA	NA	• Visual observation	• Quarterly	• Replant/reseed as appropriate • Inspect for irrigation system malfunction/damage

TABLE 5.14 Inspections and Maintenance Indicators for Gross Pollutant Devices and Mechanical Operations

Inspection Type	Maintenance Indicator Type	Qualitative/Quantitative Measure					Measurement Type	Frequency	Corrective Maintenance
		Screens	Nets	Baskets	Racks	Hoods			
Inspect for proper drainage/ infiltration	Inspect for debris/ litter accumulation in screens, nets, baskets, racks, inlet/ outlet/overflow/ bypass structures	Evidence of debris and litter clogging SCM	Evidence of debris and litter clogging SCM	Evidence of debris and litter clogging SCM	Evidence of debris and litter clogging SCM	Evidence of debris and litter clogging SCM	• Visual observation	• Quarterly	• Remove debris and dispose of properly
	Inspect for sediment accumulation in screens, nets, baskets, racks, inlet/ outlet/overflow/ bypass structures	Evidence of sediment clogging SCM	Evidence of sediment clogging SCM	Evidence of sediment clogging SCM	Evidence of sediment clogging SCM	Evidence of sediment clogging SCM	• Visual observation • Ruler/indicator measurement	• Semi-annually	• Remove accumulated sediment • Analyze material to identify proper disposal procedures • Dispose of sediment according to analysis results and disposal protocols
	Settling of screens, nets, baskets, racks, inlet/outlet/ overflow/bypass structures	Evidence of cracking or distortion of SCM	Evidence of cracking or distortion of SCM	Evidence of cracking or distortion of SCM	Evidence of cracking or distortion of SCM	Evidence of cracking or distortion of SCM	• Visual observation	• Annually	• Contact engineer and manufacturer for more extensive settlement and damage that may require redesign or reconstruction
	Snow or ice accumulation	Snow or ice impedes functionality of SCM	Snow or ice impedes functionality of SCM	Snow or ice impedes functionality of SCM	Snow or ice impedes functionality of SCM	Snow or ice impedes functionality of SCM	• Visual observation	• Monthly during freezing conditions or recent snow	• Remove snows/ice as needed
Inspect for structural integrity	Damage to screens, nets, baskets, racks,	Structural failure or damage to SCM	Structural failure or damage to SCM	Structural failure or damage to SCM	Structural failure or damage to SCM	Structural failure or damage to SCM	• Visual observation	• Quarterly	• Repair or replace
	Damage to inlets, outlets, overflow/ bypass	Structural failure or damage (e.g., broken or open inlets, outlets, overflow/bypass, conveyance channels/pipes)	Structural failure or damage (e.g., broken or open inlets, outlets, overflow/bypass, conveyance channels/pipes)	Structural failure or damage (e.g., broken or open inlets, outlets, overflow/bypass, conveyance channels/pipes)	Structural failure or damage (e.g., broken or open inlets, outlets, overflow/bypass, conveyance channels/pipes)	Structural failure or damage (e.g., broken or open inlets, outlets, overflow/bypass, conveyance channels/pipes)	• Visual observation	• Quarterly	• Repair or replace

Inspect for proper mechanical, electrical, pneumatic, hydraulic function	Per manufacturer recommendations (baffles, mechanical components, etc.)	Damage or clogging of SCM	Damage or clogging of SCM	Damage or clogging of SCM	Damage or clogging of SCM	Damage or clogging of SCM	• Per manufacturer recommendations	• Per manufacturer recommendations	• Per manufacturer recommendations
Inspect for proper vector and nuisance controls	Presence or indication of nuisance animals (spiders, rats, moles, gophers, rabbits, birds, etc.)	Presence of nuisance animals	Presence of nuisance animals	Presence of nuisance animals	Presence of nuisance animals	Presence of nuisance animals	• Visual observation	• Semi-annually	• Remove nests • Coordinate with local fish and wildlife agencies if necessary • Fill gaps/holes allowing access within enclosures
Inspect for proper site aesthetics and safety	Fence damage	Damaged fence	Damaged fence	Damaged fence	Damaged fence	Damaged fence	• Visual observation	• Semi-annually	• Repair/replace materials/ components/equipment as appropriate
	Access road damage	Asphalt or concrete is severely degraded or shows significant dents or scars	Asphalt or concrete is severely degraded or shows significant dents or scars	Asphalt or concrete is severely degraded or shows significant dents or scars	Asphalt or concrete is severely degraded or shows significant dents or scars	Asphalt or concrete is severely degraded or shows significant dents or scars	• Visual observation	• Semi-annually	• Repair/replace materials/ components/equipment as appropriate
	Trail damage	Trail is eroded	Trail is eroded	Trail is eroded	Trail is eroded	Trail is eroded	• Visual observation	• Semi-annually	• Remove sediment • Fill/compact/regrade areas • Address any upstream causes
	Light damage	Light does not work	Light does not work	Light does not work	Light does not work	Light does not work	• Visual observation	• Semi-annually	• Repair/Replace materials/ components/equipment as appropriate
	Sign damage	Dust, grime, or other residue is present on signage	Dust, grime, or other residue is present on signage	Dust, grime, or other residue is present on signage	Dust, grime, or other residue is present on signage	Dust, grime, or other residue is present on signage	• Visual observation	• Semi-annually	• Wipe down signage • Repair/replace materials/ components/equipment as appropriate
	Graffiti	Evidence of graffiti	Evidence of graffiti	Evidence of graffiti	Evidence of graffiti	Evidence of graffiti	• Visual observation	• Semi-annually	• Remove graffiti from SMP signage, structures, or surfaces

important items in an inspection report, continuity is more easily provided. Inspection reports should always be provided to the individual responsible for facility maintenance so that they are aware of the status of their SCM. Refer to Chapter 9 detailed checklists, forms, and logs.

SCMs will function only as well as its component parts. Each component must be inspected to ensure effective overall operation and facility performance. Checklists, when completed and filed, provide proof that an inspection was done on a routine basis. This documentation is important in case an outside party requests to review the information, or for liability reduction to demonstrate responsible care. The inspection report also identifies needed maintenance activities and establishes a schedule for their completion. Finally, the inspection report forms the basis for reinspection following maintenance activities to ensure satisfactory completion of the activities.

When inspections are regularly conducted, checklists can provide information on the nature of the contaminants being addressed by the SCM, an assessment of facility performance, and they can help to determine maintenance scheduling and needs. Rates of sedimentation can be determined by comparing data from previous inspection reports. This can assist in scheduling periodic sediment removal. In a stabilized watershed, the rates of accretion should be fairly consistent. If there is a subsequent increase in the rate of sedimentation, then areas contributing stormwater to the facility should be inspected for erosion problems or sediment sources and corrective steps taken.

9.0 REFERENCES

American Association of State Highway and Transportation Officials. (2017). *Standard practice for pipe joint selection for highway culvert and storm drains* (AASHTO R 82).

Corrosionpedia. (2019, October 16). *Erosion corrosion.* https://www.corrosionpedia.com/definition/469/erosion-corrosion

DC Water & Water Environment Federation. (2015, July 14). *White paper: The need for national green infrastructure training and certification.*

Contech Engineering Solutions. *Pipe joints and critical performance requirements.* Retrieved June 2020 from conteches.com

Patterson Pump Company. *General pump inspection and maintenance schedule.* Retrieved September 2020 from pattersonpumps.com

Philadelphia Water. (2016). *Green stormwater infrastructure maintenance manual. Version 2.0.*

U.S. Environmental Protection Agency. (2009, February). *Stormwater wet pond and wetland management guidebook* (EPA 833-B-09-001).

Water Environment Federation, American Society of Civil Engineers Environmental, & Water Resources Institute. (2012). *Design of urban stormwater controls* (WEF Manual of Practice No. 23, ASCE/EWRI Manuals and Reports on Engineering Practice No. 87). Water Environment Federation.

Watershed Management Institute, Inc. (1997, August). *Operation, maintenance, and management of stormwater management systems.*

10.0 SUGGESTED READINGS

American Water Works Association. (2016). *Urban stormwater management* (2nd ed.).

California Department of Transportation. (2002). *BMP retrofit pilot program maintenance indicator document* (Version: Threshold17.Doc).

California Department of Transportation. (2009). *BMP pilot study guidance manual* (CTSW-RT-06-171.02.1).

Charlotte-Mecklenburg Stormwater Services. (2010). *Post construction controls: Best management practices maintenance handbook.*

City of Charlotte/Mecklenburg County. (2014). *Post construction controls best management practices maintenance handbook.*

City of Long Beach Development Services. (2013). *Low impact development (LID) best management practices (BMP) design manual* (2nd ed.).

Feehan, C., P.E., LEED AP. (2013). *A survey of green infrastructure maintenance programs in the United States. Hixon Fellowship final report.*

National Cooperative Highway Research Program. (2014). *Report 792, Long-term performance and life-cycle costs of stormwater best management practices.*

Northern Virginia Planning District Commission, Division of Environmental Services. (2000). *Maintaining your BMP: A guidebook for private owners and operators in Northern Virginia.*

Northern Virginia Regional Commission. (2000). *Maintaining BMPs: A guidebook for private owners and operators in Northern Virginia.*

Ocean County Planning and Engineering Department. (1989). *Stormwater management facilities maintenance manual.*

Office of Water Programs at California State University, Sacramento. (2018). *Guidance for stormwater capture (California practices to use runoff effectively) at schools.*

Port of San Diego Environment. (2018). *BMP design manual for permanent site design. Stormwater treatment and hydromodification management.*

Seattle Public Utilities. (2009). *Green stormwater operations and maintenance manual.*

Seattle Public Utilities and Department of Planning and Development. (2011). *Green stormwater restoration and repair manual.*

State of New Jersey, Department of Environmental Protection Division of Water Resources. (1989). *Ocean County demonstration study. Stormwater management facilities maintenance—Manual.*

Stormwater Maintenance and Consulting & Chesapeake Stormwater Network. (2013). *CSN Technical Bulletin No. 10. Bioretention illustrated: A visual guide for constructing, inspecting, maintaining and verifying the bioretention practice* (Version 2.0).

U.S. Environmental Protection Agency & Green Infrastructure Technical Assistance Program, Milwaukee Metropolitan Sewerage District. (2015). *Elements of a green infrastructure maintenance business plan: A stakeholder-driven process to determine the preferred approach to green infrastructure maintenance in southeast Wisconsin* (EPA 832-R-15-005).

U.S. Environmental Protection Agency, Office of Water Office of Wastewater Management Water Permits Division. (2016). *Summary of state post construction stormwater standards.*

University of New Hampshire Stormwater Center. (2011). *Regular inspection and maintenance guidance for porous pavements.*

University of New Hampshire Stormwater Center. *Winter maintenance guidelines for porous pavements.* http://www.unh.edu/unhsc/sites/unh.edu.unhsc/files/pubs_specs_info/winter_maintenance_fact_sheet.pdf

6

Asset Management and Tools

1.0 OVERVIEW OF ASSET MANAGEMENT 213
1.1 Needs 213
1.2 Definitions 214
1.3 Benefits 215
1.4 History 215
1.5 United States Environmental Protection Agency 10-Step Asset Management Process 217
2.0 EVALUATE CURRENT STATE OF ASSETS 219
2.1 Types of Assets 219
2.2 Asset Characteristics 219
2.3 Asset Organization 221
2.4 Gathering Asset Information 222
3.0 IDENTIFY THE APPROPRIATE LEVEL OF SERVICE 225
4.0 EVALUATE CRITICAL ASSETS 226
5.0 EVALUATE INVESTMENT STRATEGIES 231
5.1 Categorizing Assets for Operations and Maintenance or Capital Programs 232
5.2 Identifying Other Program Costs 233
5.3 Gathering Cost Data 233
5.4 Optimizing Operations and Maintenance Investments 235
5.5 Optimizing Capital Investments 236
6.0 EVALUATE LONG-TERM FUNDING OPTIONS 241
6.1 Funding Strategies 241
6.2 Documenting the Asset Management Plan 243
7.0 ADAPTIVE MANAGEMENT 244
7.1 Strategies 244
7.2 Tracking Performance Over Time 245
7.3 Feedback 245
7.4 Update of Asset Management Program 246
8.0 REFERENCES 247

1.0 OVERVIEW OF ASSET MANAGEMENT

1.1 Needs

Communities throughout the United States are facing growing demands in managing stormwater. Municipalities must manage and build systems to provide flood protection and comply with municipal separate storm sewer system (MS4) permits, and even develop watershed management plans to protect and restore habitat, develop green infrastructure, and supplement water supply through capture and use and/or recharge to groundwater. In addition to managing and paying for new features, municipalities must plan to replace many components of existing systems that are now failing. Within all these responsibilities, many MS4 programs struggle to find adequate funding, especially for planning and tracking long-term expenditures and revenues. There is a need for improving long-term planning to optimize the dollars spent with the goals achieved. Asset management, as a process that identifies and prioritizes community goals and tracks associated costs, is a key tool that can be used to meet the various needs of MS4s, specifically:

- Regulatory compliance;
- System data needs;
- Stormwater program cost efficiency from planning through construction and operations and maintenance (O&M);
- Health and safety of residents;
- Flood management and resiliency; and
- Improved long-term technical, managerial, and financial planning.

1.2 Definitions

Asset management is a practice that is broadly used by municipalities, utilities, industries, commercial enterprises, and other organizations to manage the operation, maintenance, and replacement of physical infrastructure assets. It has been recognized by many federal, state, and local agencies and organizations as having particular value for managing long-term planning for drinking water, wastewater, and stormwater programs. Dr. Richard Harvey of the University of Guelph provided perhaps the simplest definitions in the context of drinking water, wastewater, and stormwater systems (Harvey, 2015):

- *Asset: something that has potential or actual value to an organization.*
- *Asset management: coordinated activity to realize asset value.*

U.S. Environmental Protection Agency (2020b) clarifies this definition, describing asset management as a process "utilities can use to make sure that planned maintenance can be conducted and capital assets (pumps, motors, pipes, etc.) can be repaired, replaced, or upgraded on time, and that there is enough money to pay for it." It is important to note that asset management does not just involve tracking assets and their maintenance but evaluates various options and selects between them to identify a long-term plan for maintaining and replacing assets so that the utility can continue to function at a level of service that satisfies customers, optimizes costs, and maximizes benefits.

1.3 Benefits

In addition to meeting the needs as listed above, stormwater asset management can help communities better inform asset investment decisions, improve management of risk, provide improved services and outputs, improve program efficiency and effectiveness, enable better long-term planning, and communicate intentions and needs. The latter—communicate intentions and needs—is a key benefit in that it provides justification for funding and fundraising decisions, including the need for a change to existing revenue sources or identification of new revenue sources.

To achieve these benefits, communities can use sophisticated software or programs to track extensive asset and system information, but simpler asset management approaches and tools can also be used with similar results. The latter approach can often be the most practical, especially for small communities, as it can start with a shorter list of priority assets and use some basic assumptions. The asset management program can then be expanded over time if desired, as the investments and benefits of asset management are better understood by those implementing it.

1.4 History

In 2002, the U.S. EPA and Water Environment Research Foundation (WERF), now part of the Water Research Foundation (WRF), held a workshop that set the national asset management research agenda (WERF & U.S. EPA, 2002). The initial focus of these asset management proceedings was on water and wastewater systems, primarily in relation to physical condition assessments and maintenance considerations. Over time, asset management has expanded to consider and incorporate business risk, service levels, business cases, and other program management functions. In 2006, WRF launched the Strategic Asset Management (SAM) Program, whose intent is to provide useful products to support planning, acquiring, operating, maintaining, rehabilitating, and building water infrastructure while maximizing performance and minimizing the life-cycle cost at an acceptable level of risk (WERF, 2008). Two key asset management products WRF has developed under the SAM program are described in Figure 6.1

KEY STRATEGIC ASSET MANAGEMENT PRODUCTS

SIMPLE: Sustainable Infrastructure Management Program Learning Environment (03CTS14):
An online knowledge base with more than 16,000 pages of best practices and processes from around the world, offering state-of-the-art asset management strategies, tactics, tools, and resources that correspond with each of the 10 steps of asset management.

Practitioners Guide to Economic Decision Making in Asset Management (SAM1R06b1, b2):
A two-volume guide containing approaches to economic decision making related to asset management and guidance on the use of core economic principles at each stage of asset management development.

FIGURE 6.1 Key WRF Asset Management Products (WRF, 2020) (Reprinted with permission. © The Water Research Foundation)

and include the Sustainable Infrastructure Management Program Learning Environment (SIMPLE) and Practitioners Guide to Economic Decision Making in Asset Management. While these resources were developed with a focus on drinking water and wastewater systems, the information can be applied to stormwater systems as well.

Various elements associated with asset management have been included in the stormwater regulatory processes to date. For example, MS4 permits require developing maps of permittee outfalls, as well as creating inventories of MS4 collection system assets. As another example, in 2014, the Water Resources Reform and Development Act made development and implementation of an asset management plan a requirement for receiving Clean Water State Revolving Fund loans desired to fund capital improvements (WERF, 2014). More recently, MS4 permits issued to the City of Salinas, CA, and Guam have required development and implementation of asset management programs. The California Central Coast Regional Water Quality Control Board (2019), the agency that issued the Salinas MS4 permit, summarized the benefits and justification for using asset management by citing the definition from the Association of Metropolitan Sewerage Agencies as a process of "managing infrastructure assets to minimize the total cost of owning and operating them, while continuously delivering the service levels customers desire, at an acceptable level of risk" (Association of Metropolitan Sewerage Agencies, 2002). The California Central Coast Regional Water Quality Control Board also justified inclusion of the asset management requirements in the Salinas permit by referencing relevant sections established in the Federal Code of Regulations.

The U.S. EPA has been a recent advocate of using asset management for complying with various provisions of MS4 permits, as mandated by the Clean Water Act. Such requirements include developing and implementing financial planning and O&M protocols that support long-term operation of stormwater systems, particularly priority components.

Many municipal stormwater programs have decided to pursue asset management based on its own merits (i.e., even though asset management is not required by their MS4 permits). In 2013, the City of Grand Rapids, MI, developed a 20-year asset management plan (updated in 2016) for its public stormwater infrastructure system, covering both gray and green infrastructure. "The plan demonstrates how the city's goal of establishing and delivering certain levels of service may be achieved through effective and sustainable management of the stormwater system. By developing a proactive long-term plan for stormwater asset management, the city will have a sustainable system ensuring the well-being of the community, environment and future generations" (City of Grand Rapids, MI, 2016). Anticipating a need to justify current and future costs and funding needs for federal, state, and location regulations, the City of San Diego also developed an asset management plan for its stormwater program, incorporating both water quality and flood control needs over the next few decades (City of San Diego, CA, 2021). Clearly many entities have found value in developing and implementing asset management programs.

1.5 United States Environmental Protection Agency 10-Step Asset Management Process

The U.S. EPA and WERF (now part of WRF) developed a 10-step integrated planning process, shown in Figure 6.2, that provides a solid framework for municipalities and utilities to manage their assets and optimize their investments. While this approach was initially intended for water and wastewater systems, it is just as well suited for planning various technical, managerial, and financial aspects of stormwater programs. The remainder of this chapter summarizes and supplements this 10-step process. Detailed training courses on each step are available from WERF's (2005b) SIMPLE tool for U.S. EPA Asset Training Management Material and U.S. EPA's (2020a) website.

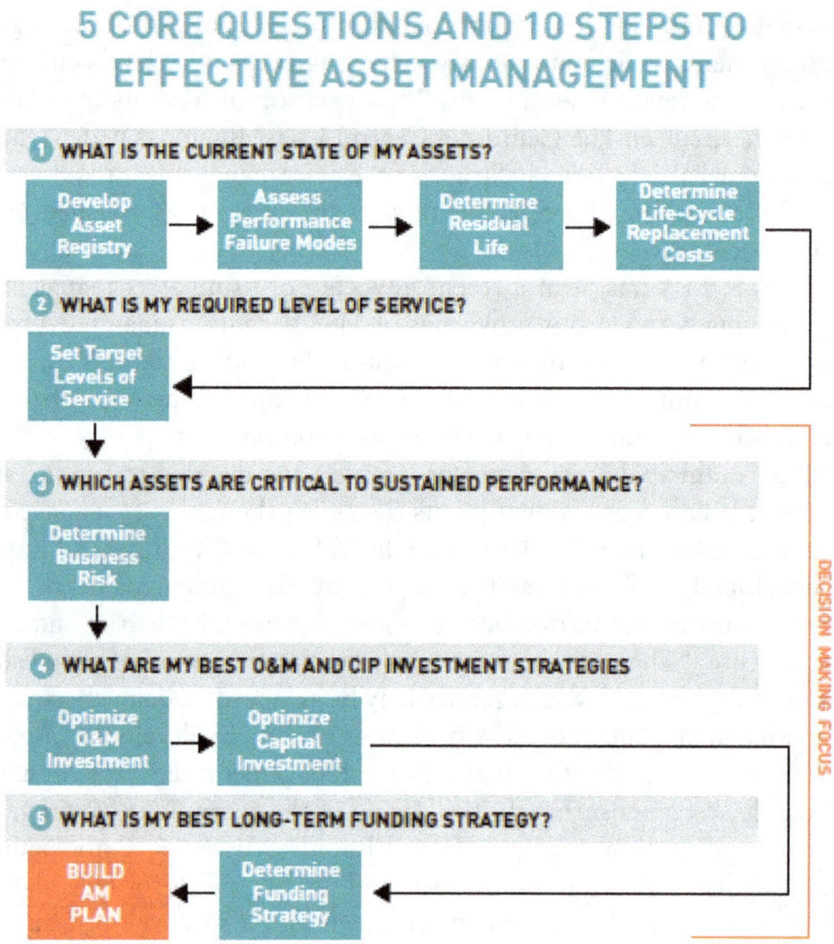

FIGURE 6.2 U.S. EPA/WERF 10-Step Integrated Planning Process (U.S. EPA, 2020b)

The subsections below summarize the various steps and refer to U.S. EPA training materials for specific details. Some of the content covered is fairly advanced, so for smaller systems with presumably fewer resources or those just getting familiar with asset management, WERF's SIMPLE provides simpler instructions that cover just 5 steps:

What Is the Current State of My Assets?

What Is My Required Level of Service?

What Assets Are Critical to Sustained Performance?

What Are My Best O&M and CIP Investment Strategies?

What Is My Best Long-Term Funding Strategy?

2.0 EVALUATE CURRENT STATE OF ASSETS

The first four steps in asset management planning established by WERF (2005a)/U.S. EPA (2020b) are:

- Step 1: Develop Asset Registry
- Step 2: Assess Performance Failure Modes
- Step 3: Determine Residual Life
- Step 4: Determine Life-Cycle Replacement Costs

The result is an asset inventory that documents all assets of interest and relevant information that will be used in later steps to define maintenance and replacements schedules and costs. In developing the inventory, managers must identify the various types of assets that are of interest, decide how to organize the assets, obtain relevant asset characteristics, and finally, establish how the data will be stored.

2.1 Types of Assets

There are a large variety of stormwater assets that extend across the entire drainage system, including buried conveyance infrastructure, surface conveyance, and stormwater control measures (SCMs). Table 6.1 provides examples of asset categories and types. An individual asset that is tracked can be either a unit or device that consists of many components, such as a bioretention filter, or the individual components of a unit, such as the vegetation, forebay, overflow, and underdrains of a bioretention filter. Which types of assets are recorded and how they are categorized is at the discretion of the program manager or owner. If one is just starting an asset management program, a few primary assets or "unit-level assets" may be recorded first, and asset components can be added as the understanding of asset management possibilities and decisions for its application grows.

2.2 Asset Characteristics

Specific characteristics of each asset will need to be gathered to complete other asset management steps. Common characteristics across assets include asset dimensions, condition, material, installation date, estimated effective life, and cost of replacement. A summary of typical asset information for a bioretention facility is provided as Table 6.2.

The information that is recorded includes not only specific asset details such as size, age, and useful life but can also include maintenance items such as frequency, crew size, hours required, and cost. Any information that can

TABLE 6.1 Examples of Typical Stormwater Asset Categories and Types

Conveyance Infrastructure	SCMs*
• Storm sewer pipe	• Bioretention filters
• Manhole	• Filter strips
• Catch basin	• Infiltration basins
• Head wall	• Wet basins
• Flume	• Dry basins
• Junction box	• Constructed wetlands
• Drop inlet	• Permeable pavement
• Pump	• Vaults and swirl concentrators
• Gate	• Manufactured filters
• Valve	
• Concrete ditch/channel	

**A full list of SCMs, as defined by WEF, is provided in Chapter 1.*

TABLE 6.2 Typical Asset Information for Bioretention Facility

Data Field	Data Type	Data Field	Data Type
Asset ID	Text	Hydraulic Loading Rate (gal/sf)	Number
Owner	Text	Soil Media Type	Text
Decimal Latitude	Number	Storage Area (sf)	Number
Decimal Longitude	Number	Storage Depth (ft)	Number
Installation Date	Date	Vegetation Type	Text
Asset Type	Text	Underdrain	Text
Total Tributary Area (ac)	Number	Typical Maintenance Performed	Text
Impervious Tributary Area (ac)	Number	Maintenance Frequency	Text
Pervious Tributary Area (ac)	Number	Maintenance Crew Size	Number
Treatment Volume (cf) or Flowrate (cfs)	Number	Maintenance Crew Rate ($)	Number
SCM Surface Area (sf)	Number	Typical Maintenance Duration (hr)	Number
Storage Volume (cf)	Number	Typical Annual Maintenance Cost ($)	Number
Pretreatment Device	Text	Anticipated Effective Life (yr)	Number
Drawdown Time (hr)	Number		

be effectively used to maintain and increase the longevity and performance of stormwater assets is worth tracking.

2.3 Asset Organization

Assets can be organized into various categories and subcategories as desired by the asset manager or owner. Such asset hierarchy is used to establish relationships of assets, allowing assets with similar characteristics to be grouped for various purposes. For department specific asset management programs, potential hierarchy levels from top to bottom may include municipality/agency, municipal department, area/location, address, group, type, and component, with each component being assigned a unique asset ID, as shown in Table 6.3. Some larger municipalities have integrated asset management across various municipal departments, and Step 1 of U.S. EPA's Asset Training Management Material (WERF, 2005a) provides good examples and further descriptions of this asset management style.

The data collected for asset management can be stored in simple tables or spreadsheets or more complex databases. A digital dataset can be connected with a data dictionary and interface with geographic information systems (GIS) to provide visual perspectives and improve data sharing and communication.

The data may also be integrated with other software, such as computerized maintenance management systems (CMMS), to standardize and

TABLE 6.3 Example Asset Hierarchy

Hierarchy Level	Hierarchy Level Name	Description	Example Values
1	Owner	Roll-up for all assets owned by entity	• Municipality/Department Name
2	Area/District/Neighborhood	Roll-up to separate assets by location	• North side • South Side
3	Address/Intersection	Used to help identify asset location	• Varies depending on location
4	Asset Category	Asset categories as defined by municipality/agency	• Conveyance • SCMs
5	Asset Type/Unit	Individual asset type as defined by municipality/agency	• See Table 6.1 for examples
6	Unit/Component (with unique ID#)	Individual asset units or components of units as defined by municipality/agency	• See Chapter 5 for SCM components

simplify data entry, saving time, improving accuracy and clarity, and simplify reporting. Table 6.4 compares the advantages and disadvantages of CMMS with the simpler asset management checklist and spreadsheet tools.

It is important to note that an expensive asset management system is not mandatory for program success; asset management is about optimizing current and long-term needs with costs. It may be most practical for some systems to start with simple spreadsheets and track only a handful of critical assets (see Table 6.4). However, having more detailed information on your system and using applications that can track, compare, and synergize program elements can be beneficial in an economy of scale sense. Table 6.5 lists several asset management resources from U.S. EPA that are specific to stormwater programs.

2.4 Gathering Asset Information

The data needed to populate asset management systems can come from a number of sources, including

- As-built/design drawings,
- Manufacturers' manuals,
- Bid documents,
- Schedules of quantities,
- Staff—current and previous,

TABLE 6.4 Comparison of Asset Management Tools

Tool Type	Advantages	Disadvantages
Checklists	• Simple to use • Requires little to no training • Inexpensive	• More prone to user error and inconsistent data • Severely limits ability to efficiently compare and use data
Spreadsheets	• Relatively simple to use • Allows for sorting and analyzing of data • Inexpensive	• Limited for reporting, managing, and comparing data
CMMS	• Standardizes and simplifies management of data • Improves accuracy and clarity • Simplifies reporting • Synergizes program elements	• Expensive • Requires training • Requires consistent use to be effective at using software

TABLE 6.5 U.S. EPA Stormwater Asset Management Resources

Resource Name	Summary	Source Link
Asset Management: A Best Practices Guide	This guide explains what asset management means, the benefits of asset management, best practices in asset management, and how to implement an asset management plan. It is for owners, managers, and operators of public water systems, local officials, technical assistance providers, and state personnel.	http://nepis.epa.gov/Exe/ZyPDF.cgi/P1000LP0.PDF?Dockey=P1000LP0.PDF
Building an Asset Management Team	This guide explains how having a team can help your system successfully implement asset management and the components of a successful asset management team. It is for local officials, owners and operators of public water systems, technical assistance providers, and state personnel.	http://nepis.epa.gov/Exe/ZyPDF.cgi/P1000LTZ.PDF?Dockey=P1000LTZ.PDF
Asset Management: A Handbook for Small Public Water Systems—STEP Guide Series	Learn how to inventory system assets and develop a long-term maintenance plan to save money and avoid unexpected problems.	http://nepis.epa.gov/EPA/html/DLwait.htm?url=/Exe/ZyPDF.cgi/2000261D.PDF?Dockey=2000261D.PDF
Asset Management Programs for Stormwater and Wastewater Systems: Overcoming Barriers to Development and Implementation	This paper presents information from case studies and input from utilities at various stages of asset management program implementation.	https://www.epa.gov/sustainable-water-infrastructure/asset-management-programs-stormwater-and-wastewater-systems

- Photographs and videos, and
- Site visits/field inspections.

A number of mobile apps and software are available for assisting with gathering and recording asset characteristics. Table 6.6 lists free and proprietary applications. In selecting appropriate tools, managers should consider the following:

- **Cost.** Many expensive commercial products exist, including software available for direct purchase as well as software licenses available via monthly fee-based subscriptions. Operators or managers of small stormwater systems often have limited resources and may prefer to start with open-source products. Refer to Section 5.0 of this chapter for existing cost resources.

TABLE 6.6 Example Mobile Applications That Support Asset Management Activities for Water Utilities (Environmental Finance Center at Sacramento State, 2019a)

Software	Description	Source
CUPSS Mobile App	Free mobile assistant developed by the Water Innovation Network for Sustainable Small Systems, which allows for field data collection and export (to email) for use on the U.S. EPA's desktop software.	https://www.umass.edu/winsss/research/project-b-non-treatment-technologies/cupss-mobile-app
ESRI Collector	Mobile assistant data collection application developed by the creator of ArcGIS web and desktop mapping software. Includes software for interfacing with ESRI web services software and creating geodatabases for storing data.	http://www.esri.com
Fulcrum and CARTO	CARTO is an online user-friendly mapping platform for visualizing and analyzing spatial data. It provides an application programming interface for third parties to develop additional applications that utilize browser-based maps from CARTO. The Fulcrum company has developed a suite of mobile applications for asset management that are subscription-based services, with clients paying monthly fees based on the number of users.	http://www.fulcrumapp.com/integrations/carto/
Maximo	Enterprise asset management software from IBM for use in a variety of business and utility applications. Maximo's hybrid application model allows for mobile connectivity to support work management and data collection.	https://www.ibm.com/products/maximo
QGIS	QGIS is a free, open-source software that utilities can use for mapping and analysis with GIS.	https://qgis.org/en/site/
Q Ware CMMS eMaint CMMS City Reporter PubWorks CityWorks Trimble	These are commercial municipal asset management software packages with robust desktop and mobile applications for use by cities and companies to schedule and organize long-term asset management and field crew work tasks.	Various

- **Adaptability.** The ability to use data collected in the field and translate it to other platforms, such as GIS or spreadsheet software, is important for use.
- **Platform Integration.** For existing mobile apps or platforms that could support mobile apps, current software and modules that facilitate data transfers among platforms are important.
- **Robustness.** Factors such as the level of detail available for inputting data, the ability to upload attachments such as photographs, or the ability to use the program in the field when offline are important capabilities.

3.0 IDENTIFY THE APPROPRIATE LEVEL OF SERVICE

The WRF's fifth asset management step seeks to define a series of goals the program will strive to achieve. These goals will help in making future decisions on prioritizing assets and optimizing costs. The fifth step is:

- Step 5: Define Target Level of Service

Level of service (LOS) is a measure of the quality or expected reliability that must be provided by an agency to meet a community's basic needs and expectations (City of Grand Rapids, MI, 2016). It describes the extent of capital improvement and O&M activities performed for assets and can have varying degrees of scope and scale. An LOS can be reactive and meet maintenance and repair needs as they arise or can proactively undertake system maintenance and renewal activities before failures. Whatever LOS is selected, it must meet administrative and community expectations for performance and equity.

To determine LOS, O&M activities should be categorized to help distinguish and define multiple levels for possible selection (Environmental Finance Center at Sacramento State, 2019a). Defining multiple levels allows municipalities to compare options and solicit stakeholder input in determining how to best serve the community and make proper investments. The categories of O&M activities are:

- Inspections,
- Preventive maintenance,
- Corrective maintenance, and
- System renewal.

The LOS process should include at minimum the development of a baseline LOS. This represents the minimum service effort needed based on a limited O&M budget and typically without an asset management plan. There are no scheduled preventive maintenance operations or system renewals planned. Instead, assets are replaced or repaired as they fail.

It is also beneficial to determine a "high end" approach—one that is proactive and addresses most if not all of the desired O&M and capital improvement plan (CIP) activities to provide the upper limit of what is possible with an asset management program. While this is often unattainable because of cost, it provides a target with which to frame the range of LOS possible.

Most communities will move forward with an LOS that is somewhere between the baseline and high-end LOS. As the LOS increases above the baseline, the type and frequency of inspections and maintenance is increased and the process of replacing assets is accelerated. A more proactive (higher) LOS would repair/replace assets before their end-of-life and reduce the risk of failures and outages. A proactive LOS plan may have larger upfront costs for maintenance but be more cost effective when considering total life-cycle costs that preserve assets for a longer period. A comparison of three levels of service for a community is shown in Table 6.7.

For a community that is just starting out with an asset management program, they may want to consider establishing the baseline LOS as their current O&M activities. However, having more a proactive O&M and CIP program provides system efficiencies and leads to a more cost-effective asset management program. For higher LOS plans, a community should establish system renewal schedules, inspection schedules, and preventive maintenance schedules.

4.0 EVALUATE CRITICAL ASSETS

WERF's next asset management step intends to identify the system's critical assets by assessing overall business (program) risk:

- Step 6: Determine Business Risk

TABLE 6.7 Level of Service Comparison

No.	Description	Annual Budget		
		Baseline	Moderate	High End
Capital Improvements				
1	Minor Drainage Improvements	$200,000	$300,000	$500,000
2	Major Stormwater System Repair/Replacement	$0	$100,000	$500,000
3	Culvert Repair/Replacement	$0	$50,000	$250,000
4	Green Infrastructure (GI)/Stormwater Control Measures (SCMs)	$50,000	$100,000	$250,000
5	Regional Water Quality Projects	$0	$0	$500,000
	Subtotal	**$250,000**	**$550,000**	**$2,000,000**
Operations and Maintenance				
1	Stormwater Collection System Minor Repairs	$100,000	$150,000	$400,000
2	Stormwater Collection System Cleaning	$0	$50,000	$100,000
3	Stormwater Collection System CCTV	$0	$50,000	$100,000
4	Routine Maintenance of GI/SCMs	$20,000	$50,000	$150,000
5	Routine Maintenance of Surface Conveyance (ditches, culverts, etc.)	$0	$50,000	$250,000
	Subtotal	**$120,000**	**$350,000**	**$1,000,000**
	Total	**$370,000**	**$900,000**	**$3,000,000**

Critical assets are those whose damage or failure would greatly disable a system and make a program unable to meet some or all of its targeted LOS. Comparing overall risk of failure for each asset can be used to prioritize assets for repair and replacement scheduling. Various approaches can be used to assign a numeric value of risk for each asset.

Simple approaches assume that risk is equivalent to an asset's likelihood, or probability of failure (POF). A value of POF can be determined by using estimated remaining life of each asset, which is the difference between the expected life of the asset and its current age. Older assets would be prioritized for replacement. Growing in complexity, other approaches consider the condition of each asset, with or without consideration of an asset's estimated remaining life. The condition may be given a numeric value based on a qualitative scale of "poor," "fair," "good," or "excellent" (e.g., poor = 1; fair = 2; good = 3; excellent = 4). More sophisticated numeric assignments can be developed based on physical measurements such as depth of sediment accumulation, amount of erosion, health of vegetation, and so on. If multiple factors are used in calculating a POF value, each factor can be assigned a weighted value if desired.

More complex approaches to evaluating risk of failure will consider, in addition to POF, the consequence of failure (COF) for the asset and whether or not the overall system has redundancy (R) for the asset. Like POF, numeric values can be assigned to COF and R, and the three variables are multiplied to obtain and overall score for risk. The equation is:

$$\text{Risk} = \text{POF} \times \text{COF} \times R$$

The COF estimates the effects of a component outage, based on knowledge of the difficulty and cost for replacement, as well as effect on other community assets, services, and resources. The overall risk, then, helps prioritize assets for repair and replacement.

Figure 6.3 demonstrates how POF and COF influence risk. Those assets that are in good physical condition (low POF) and are not critical to the overall performance of the stormwater system (low COF) are at the bottom left of the graph. Like a traffic light, assets in good shape are shown in green (move forward: no concern), and as the POF and COF rises, the assets move into the yellow zone (use caution: may require preventive maintenance) and finally into the red zone (warning: requires repair/replacement).

The COF of an asset can include a triple bottom line (TBL) analysis that considers environmental and social considerations as well as an asset's repair/replacement cost. Table 6.8 provide examples of environmental, social, and economic attributes that can be evaluated, including criteria and scoring for each. While scoring can be modified or weighted to favor attributes that are most important to a municipality or agency, for a true TBL analysis, no

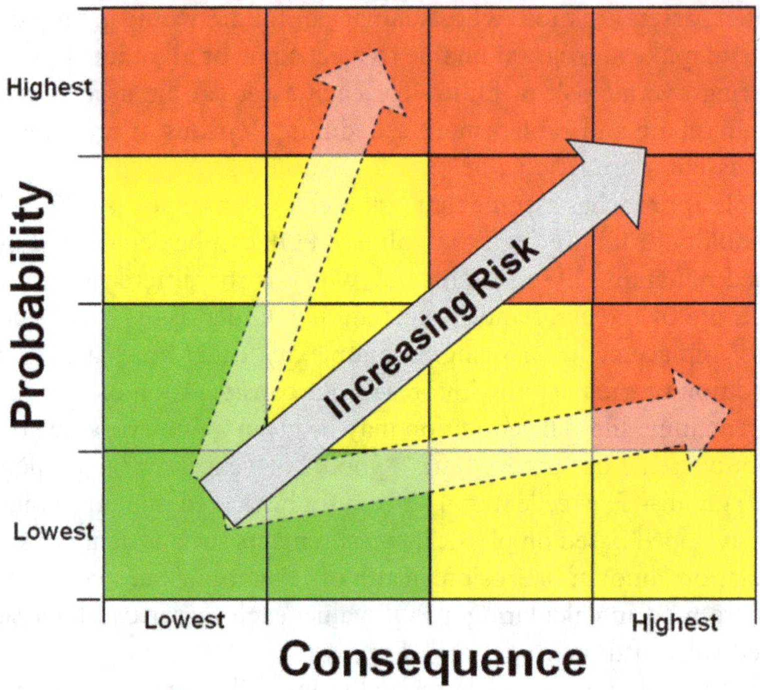

FIGURE 6.3 Effect of Probability and Consequence of Failure on Risk

individual criteria (cost, social, environment) should be more than half of the total score. Scores and weighting of POF and COF should properly reflect the overall program goals as well as the target LOS proposed.

Failure mode is defined as "a systematic series of sequential and interrelated causal steps that can lead to the failure of an asset" (U.S. EPA, 2017b). Failure of stormwater pipes, pumps, and other traditional gray assets is generally easy to identify: a pipe collapses, a pump breaks down, and so on. Degraded and poorly maintained streams and channels are more challenging to assess, although many municipalities have been evaluating them for decades so there is experience there, especially for relatively simple tasks like identifying blockages of culverts and erosion of streams along roadways. However, what constitutes failure of an SCM is harder to gauge. Plugging of permeable pavement with fine sediment will cause a sharp reduction in drainage and decrease in filtration performance, but inspection crews will need specific criteria or conditions to assess for to determine this reduction has occurred. Plugging of risers in wet ponds as a result of debris and sediment may not be visible, and crews will need to know the design intention of the SCM to know to look for that problem as part of routine maintenance. See Chapter 5 for a range of maintenance indicators that should be considered.

TABLE 6.8 Common Triple Bottom Line Elements

ENVIRONMENTAL		
Effect on Impaired Stream	**Criteria**	**Score**
Flows to an impaired stream with a pollutant of concern	> 230 m (750 ft)	1
	> 150 m (500 ft) and ≤ 230 m (750 ft) to impaired stream	3
	≤ 150 m (500 ft) feet to impaired stream	5
Distance to NWI	**Criteria**	**Score**
System is a potential source of impairment	> 230 m (750 ft)	1
	> 150 m (500 ft) and ≤ 230 m (750 ft) to stream	3
	≤ 150 m (500 ft) to stream	5
Distance to Outfall/Discharge Point	**Criteria**	**Score**
System is at or near an outfall/discharge point	> 15 m (50 ft)	1
	≤ 15 m (50 ft) from discharge point	2
	> 7.5 m (25 ft) and ≤ 15 m (50 ft) from outfall	3
	< 7.5 m (25 ft) from outfall	5
SOCIAL		
Degree of Flooding	**Criteria**	**Score**
Design storm frequency where flooding typically occurs within the project area	1% (100-year) Storm	1
	2% (50-year) Storm	2
	4% (25-year) Storm	3
	10% (10-year) Storm	4
	50% (2-year) Storm	5
Disruption of Service	**Criteria**	**Score**
Effect of flooding on traffic in the project area	No potential effect	1
	Minor/isolated flooding	3
	Impassable road(s)	5
Effect to Public	**Criteria**	**Score**
Number of properties affected by flooding in project area	None	1
	1 to 5	2
	6 to 10	3
	10 to 20	4
	> 20	5

(*continued*)

TABLE 6.8 Common Triple Bottom Line Elements (*continued*)

Critical Facility Effect	Criteria	Score
Number of critical facilities (i.e., hospitals, schools, fire stations, etc.) within a 2.4-km (1.5 mile) radius	0 Facilities	1
	≤ 3 Facilities	2
	≤ 6 Facilities	3
	≤ 9 Facilities	4
	> 9 Facilities	5
Population Density	**Criteria**	**Score**
Population density of Census Block Group where asset is located. Measured in population per hectare (acre) of land, as calculated from 2010 U.S. Census Block Groups.	≤ 1.043 906	1
	≤ 3.103 96	2
	≤ 5.013 605	3
	≤ 9.289 872	4
	> 9.289 872	5
	ECONOMIC	
Pipe Location	**Criteria**	**Score**
Does the system run under the road?	Not under road	1
	Under road	5
Conveyance Replacement Cost	**Criteria**	**Score**
Estimate of cost of labor and materials to replace the asset	< $10,000	1
	$10,000 to < $25,000	2
	$25,000 to < $50,000	3
	$50,000 to < $100,000	4
	> $100,000	5
Economic Effect	**Criteria**	**Score**
Economic effect if the project does not move forward	Low	1
	Medium	3
	High	5

The redundancy factor (R) in the overall risk equation is much simpler to quantify than COF. Assets that have backups online or readily at hand can be assigned a value based on the number of backups. For assets with one backup, R can be assigned 0.5. For assets with two backups, R can be assigned 0.33. For assets with no backups, R will default to a value of 1.0.

Example: A community is evaluating six different assets across a range of stormwater groups and types to determine the highest risk assets in a problem watershed (Watershed 1). These include two pipes, an outfall, a ditch, a filter strip, and a wet pond. The scoring in each category goes from 1—best condition to 5—worst condition, with the maximum value from the range of criteria examined selected for each item. The highest risk item, shown in the first line of Table 6.9, is a 0.9-m (36-in.) culvert that is in average condition (physical score), severely undersized as a result of significant upstream development (performance score), and located along a primary evaluation route (Consequence of Failure score). The risk score for the asset is provided below:

$$\text{Risk} = \text{POF} \times \text{COF} \times R$$
$$\text{Risk} = 5 \times 4 \times 1 = 20$$

By understanding potential failure modes for each asset type and identifying those that are likely to drive a given asset to fail, communities and agencies can focus assessment on those attributes of the asset that provide the most telltale signs of failure and time the assessment as cost effectively as possible. Please reference Section 5.0 or WRF's SIMPLE for methods/modes that can be used for failure analysis.

5.0 EVALUATE INVESTMENT STRATEGIES

The next WRF/U.S. EPA steps are intended to consider what types of maintenance, repair, or replacement, or augmentation are needed for the various assets, when they should be done, and whether it's appropriate to have the work done as part of an O&M program or capital improvements program.

- Step 7: Optimize O&M Investment
- Step 8: Optimize Capital Investment

TABLE 6.9 Sample Community Asset Risk Scoring Comparison

Location	Asset Group	Asset Type	Physical Score	Performance Score	POF Score	COF Score	R	Risk Score
Watershed 1	Pipe	Pipe	3	5	5	4	1	20
Watershed 1	Pipe	Outfall	1	5	5	3	1	15
Watershed 1	Pipe	Pipe	2	2	2	2	1	4
Watershed 1	Open Channel	Ditch	4	5	5	3	1	15
Watershed 1	SCM/GI	Filter Strip	2	3	3	2	1	6
Watershed 1	SCM/GI	Wet Pond	4	2	4	3	0.5	6

Note. The POF score is the higher of the physical and performance scores. This is done to prevent having too many scores clumped together in the middle and not moving forward with true problem assets.

5.1 Categorizing Assets for Operations and Maintenance or Capital Programs

Asset management supports both O&M of stormwater infrastructure as well as development of a capital improvements program. The risk-based analysis incorporated into asset management provides comparison between the many assets of a municipal program and helps determine those assets that should be repaired/replaced (as capital improvement projects) versus those that should fall under a preventive or predictive maintenance program. The practices not only include storm sewers, culverts, and pump stations but stream segments, biofiltration systems, and permeable pavement. Figure 6.4 demonstrates how stormwater asset assessment results support both O&M and CIP programs. Those assets with low risk (low POF and COF values) fall under a routine O&M program, those with high risk (high POF and COF values) should be part of a stormwater CIP program, and those in between with increasing risk will need to be monitored more closely to see if/when they need to move from a routine O&M program to a CIP program.

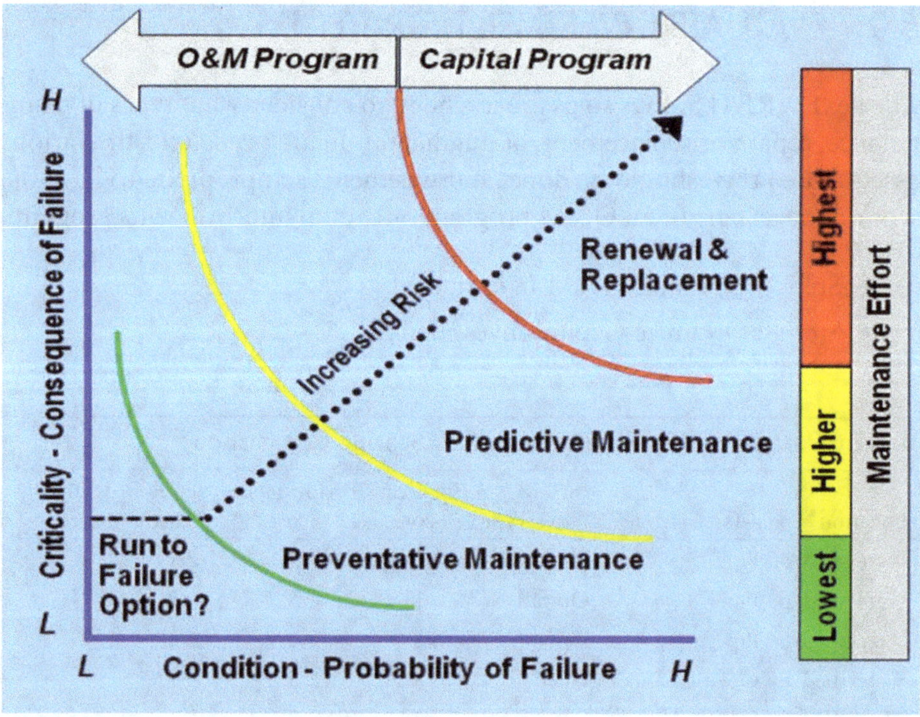

FIGURE 6.4 Asset Management Program Support of Operations and Maintenance and Capital Improvement Plan

5.2 Identifying Other Program Costs

Most stormwater programs provide services that do not fall into the traditional capital or O&M investment categories. For example, most programs must comply with National Pollutant Discharge Elimination System (NPDES) permit requirements outlined by state or federal regulators. Specific activities include construction site runoff control, illicit discharge detection, pollution prevention, public education, and water quality monitoring, as well as associated materials and equipment. Permit compliance activities should also include labor costs for program administration and staff. Additional program costs that may not fall into the CIP or O&M investment strategies might include power and water services. The following section summarizes resources for gathering cost data of all types.

5.3 Gathering Cost Data

It is important to have good cost data when developing O&M and CIP budgets for a stormwater program, and using historical data is imperative to an effective use of stormwater funds. Recording costs by asset type, maintenance type, maintenance crew, and so on creates dynamic spending information for future use. If possible, costs should be as detailed as possible and include crew size, crew hourly rates, maintenance duration, material costs, labor costs, and a detailed description of work performed. Those costs can be rolled up into an overall cost tracking program that looks at total annual maintenance cost and average maintenance cost per asset type and work performed. Data can also be used from U.S. EPA and other national and regional sources to provide a range of expected O&M and capital costs, especially for recent technologies like green infrastructure and other features/facilities that may be new to a community/agency.

There are several sources of cost data or tools to determine capital, O&M, and other life-cycle costs for stormwater projects and programs. Table 6.10 describes several that were compiled in *Estimating Benefits and Costs of Stormwater Management Part I: Methods and Challenges* (Environmental Finance Center at Sacramento State, 2019b). Additional resources include cost books and online data centers that provide line-item cost estimates. Examples include RSMeans and Sierra West Group. Such materials are updated annually or every few years (Office of Water Programs at California State University, Sacramento, 2018). Finally, California practitioners are beginning to establish summaries of full stormwater program costs that include capital projects, O&M, as well as other MS4 permit-required activities like reporting, bookkeeping, monitoring, public outreach, and participation (Environmental Finance Center at Sacramento State, 2020). Although

TABLE 6.10 Stormwater Capital, Operations and Maintenance, and Life-Cycle Costs (Adapted from Environmental Finance Center at Sacramento State, 2019b)

Source	Description
ASCE EWRI Survey of BMP O&M Costs	A 2017 book that reports results of a survey on maintenance costs of green infrastructure and compiles many existing resources.
WRF CLASIC Community-Enabled Lifecycle Analysis of Stormwater Infrastructure Costs Tool	A user-informed screening tool that utilizes a life-cycle cost framework to support implementation of stormwater infrastructure, including green, hybrid green-gray, and gray infrastructure practices.
WERF-AWWA-UKWIR Whole-Life Cost Model	A joint product from U.S. and UK industry organizations to estimate the life-cycle costs of several types of SCMs, including retention ponds, detention basins, vegetated swales, bioretention, porous pavement, and others.
U.S. EPA National Stormwater Calculator	A software tool for calculating stormwater runoff that uses the stormwater management model for planning and includes tools to estimate construction costs, maintenance costs, and averted costs.
University of Minnesota/Weiss BMP Cost Estimation Algorithm	A tool for estimating the construction and annual O&M costs of stormwater capture measures, including total present costs.
University of New Hampshire Maintenance Expenditure Study	A 2013 study that characterized and quantified maintenance costs of several types of low-impact development (LID) over a multiyear period.
The National Cooperative Highway Research Program Whole-Life Cost Models	A spreadsheet-based model covering 50 state departments of transportation to estimate life-cycle costs of stormwater capture measures.
Denver Urban Drainage and Flood Control District's BMP-REALCOST Tool	An Excel-based life-cycle costing model to support life-cycle cost analysis of structural stormwater management facilities in cities.
Wossink and Hunt Empirical Cost Evaluation of SCMs in North Carolina	A 2003 study that collected empirical cost equations for O&M activities across 40 stormwater capture facilities in North Carolina.
U.S. EPA Water Financing Clearinghouse LID and GI Case Study Inventory	A comprehensive list of LID and green infrastructure studies to provide communities with a central repository for verified studies and data.
NPDES Stormwater Cost Survey	A 2005 study in California that reports survey findings for municipal stormwater management costs to comply with NPDES requirements.
Green Values National Stormwater Management Calculator	A 2009 free tool for use in calculating and comparing costs of conventional stormwater management practices with green infrastructure and new types of stormwater control measures. Includes an expansive list of construction, maintenance, and component unit costs.

the data collected to date is not comprehensive and was based on publicly available information (easily accessible data, which represents only a fraction of the spending within California), the California stormwater program costs that were synthesized provide a good glimpse at how costs can be categorized and evaluated for future decision making, including serving as a resource for projecting future costs. The California State Water Resources Control Board is planning to continue the effort in gathering and assessing stormwater program costs through their Strategy to Optimize Resource Management of Stormwater program, Phase II Project 4c: Identify Stormwater Municipal Permit Compliance Costs (California State Water Board, 2020b). The outcomes of this project may serve as useful resources of cost data and collection/assessment methodology for programs throughout the United States.

While larger scale cost estimate tools and resources continue to be developed, it would behoove MS4 program managers to begin tracking costs from within their own program, and perhaps even other departments on which the stormwater program depends (e.g., waste management/street sweeping). This can be done simply in a spreadsheet or within CMMS.

5.4 Optimizing Operations and Maintenance Investments

Many stormwater programs throughout the United States use a reactive approach to O&M, fixing or replacing assets when damage or failure has been identified. Asset management can be used to alter such practices into planned O&M practices to prevent and even predict asset failure, optimizing its life span, and ultimately the long-term costs of the overall program. In fact, in Step 7 of its asset management training, U.S. EPA (2020a) reports that "roughly speaking, planned maintenance costs one third less than unplanned maintenance for the same task."

Step 7 of U.S. EPA's (2020a) training provides detailed information on strategies that can be used for managing O&M programs and optimizing investments. The strategies include identifying and defining program goals and metrics and establishing targets for each. Figure 6.5 shows examples.

Once the goals, metrics, and targets have been defined, data will of course need to be collected to gauge actual performance against desired targets. This can require a certain level of sophistication in determining data type, sources, collection and reporting methods, and an overall data management system. Many communities use CMMS to help guide this step.

Upon establishing the baseline level for each goal/metric, potential for improvements can be done by identifying and assessing causes of failure for various assets, and then identifying opportunities to conduct preventive maintenance. This will include developing schedules using insight from both manufacturer or vendor specifications or recommendations, as well

Metric	*Definition*	*Target*
Availability	The portion of time that a plant or major system is available for producing output of the required quality and quantity	95 – 99%
% Failure analysis	The portion of equipment downtime events that undergo a thorough analysis of failure modes, effects, and root causes	85 – 100%
% Planned work	The portion of corrective maintenance work hours that are planned and scheduled in advance (not unplanned breakdowns)	85 – 95%
% Overtime	The portion of maintenance work hours that are performed at an overtime rate	5 – 8%
Relative maintenance cost	Annual maintenance spending as a percentage of asset replacement value of the plant being maintained	1.5 – 2.5%
Technician productivity	The percent of work hours spent on productive activities versus nonproductive (rework, waiting for parts, etc)	70 – 85%
% Rework	The portion of maintenance work that has to be redone due to poor installation, shoddy workmanship or incorrect diagnosis	2 - 5%

FIGURE 6.5 Examples of Metrics, Definitions, and Targets to Use in Optimizing O&M Investments (U.S. EPA, 2020a)

as a program's specific experiences. Developing a preventive maintenance schedule should consider location of assets relative to others in their proximity. The manager should look at balancing required timing for maintenance with proximity of assets.

Overall, optimizing O&M investments is an iterative process of identifying goals, collecting data, identifying areas for improvement, developing preventive maintenance schedules, and then continually refining the program based on new data and/or needs. The reader is directed to Step 7 of EPA's training for detailed information (U.S. EPA, 2020a).

5.5 Optimizing Capital Investments

Traditional capital improvement projects often come about by various stakeholders identifying needs and championing solutions. The result is a "wish list" of projects that may not have been thoroughly validated or considered against other solutions such as improved O&M practices or other nonasset possibilities, which could have resulted in reduced long-term costs to the overall stormwater program. Opportunities that seek multiple benefits for projects or identify projects that can be combined to optimize benefits can also be missed.

A simple approach for optimizing capital investment can include using the typical championed wish list of projects and incorporating validation and prioritization practices that focus on life-cycle costs and/or benefit-cost analyses (BCA). *Estimating Benefits and Costs of Stormwater Management Part I: Methods and Challenges* (Environmental Finance Center at Sacramento State, 2019b) provides detailed instructions on conducting BCA for stormwater projects and looking for ways to achieve multiple benefits.

Step 8 of EPA's asset management training (U.S. EPA, 2020a) provides an advanced level for optimizing investments in capital projects, which can result in a more cost-effective CIP program. The approach instructs asset development plan coordinators to think of capital investments as having two purposes:

1. Renew assets through repair, refurbishment, restoration, or replacement.
2. Augment an asset's functionality (to improve LOS and/or efficiency) or increase/improve its capacity.

The data, findings, and decisions collected and gathered through asset management can support a structured and methodical approach for identifying renewal and augmentation projects. These can be combined with the less methodical but still valuable "wish list" (i.e., desired) of projects proposed by various community stakeholders. Figure 6.6 shows how the champion and structured models can lead to optimal project development.

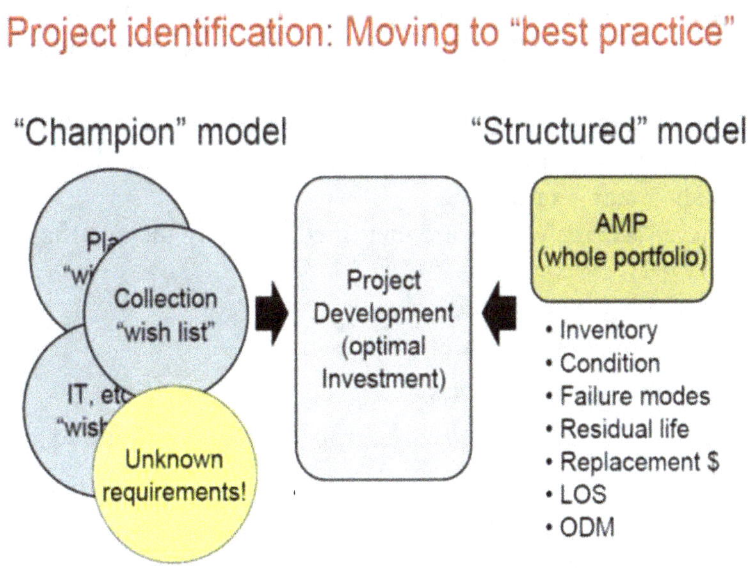

FIGURE 6.6 Asset Management Components That Support a Methodical Approach for Project Identification (U.S. EPA, 2020a)

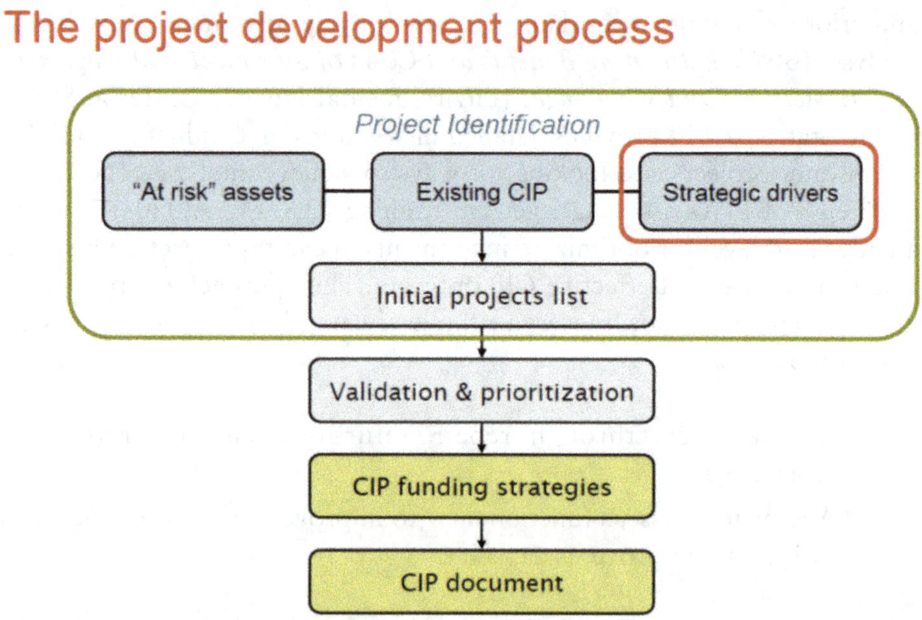

FIGURE 6.7 Identifying Capital Improvement Projects Using Asset Management Information (U.S. EPA, 2020a)

Figure 6.7 shows the project identification process recommended by U.S. EPA (2020a). The process begins with using asset management information and practices to identify strategic drivers and "at risk" assets that will inform an initial project list. Projects from the initial list are then validated and prioritized, followed by consideration and selection of funding sources and documentation of the CIP.

First, asset data are used to define possible modes of failure and align each mode to a management strategy (e.g., redesign, renewal, replacement). Figure 6.8 shows an example.

From here, "at risk" assets are identified and may include the following traits:

- High business risk exposure scores
- Low remaining useful lives
- Poor conditions scores/scores approaching designated minimum acceptable limits
- Poor performance scores
- No redundancy
- Imminent major failure mode of capacity or LOS

The "primary failure mode" gives insight into "strategic drivers" at work

Failure Mode	*Definition*	*Tactical Aspects*	*Management Strategy*
Capacity	Volume of demand exceeds design capacity	Growth, system expansion	(Re)design
LOS	Functional requirements exceed design capacity	Codes & permits: NPDES, CSOs, OSHA, noise, odor, life safety; service, etc.	(Re)design
Mortality	Consumption of asset reduces performance below acceptable level	Physical deterioration due to age, usage (including operator error), acts of nature	O&M optimization, renewal
Efficiency	Operations costs exceed that of feasible alternatives	Pay-back period	Replace

NPDES is National Pollutant Discharge Elimination System, CSOs are combined sewer overflows, and OSHA is Occupational Safety and Health Administration

FIGURE 6.8 Defining Failure Modes and Management Strategies to Inform Project Identification (U.S. EPA, 2020a)

For each "at risk" asset identified, the management strategy can then be applied to develop a conceptual project. The conceptual project information to gather and identify should include the project scope, location, background and context, rationalization, fiscal requirements, design issues, and permit requirements.

Next, projects are validated by considering life-cycle costs; conducting a TBL analysis of the economic, social, and environmental benefits and costs; and evaluating business risk of exposure (BRE) and acceptable levels of confidence. The ultimate goal of project validation is to reduce the CIP costs by eliminating projects, deferring projects by instead changing O&M practices, or finding nonasset (CIP) solutions. Step 8 of EPA's asset management training (U.S. EPA, 2020) provides detailed information on how to do these. The results are BRE and confidence level rating (CLR) scores that can be used to make final project determinations based on scoring and cost, as shown in Figure 6.9.

Validated projects are then prioritized by either using factors and weights (Figure 6.10) or project risk (as determined by each project's CLR and BRE) and CIP budget (Figure 6.11).

Moving forward: Project validation decision matrix

	High BRE (>1M)	*Medium BRE*	*Low BRE (<50K)*
High CLR (>84)	Proceed with project, no changes	Consider proceeding with project if financial criteria are met and funding is available	Consider • Deferral or delay • Project breakup • Cancellation • Increase CLR
Medium CLR (56-84)	Consider • Proceed with project • Deferral or delay • Increase CLR	Consider • Deferral or delay • Breakup project and proceed with parts • Increase CLR	Consider • Deferral or delay • Project breakup • Cancellation • Increase CLR
Low CLR (<56)	Consider • Deferral or delay • Project breakup • Proceed with project using design consultant • Increase CLR	Consider • Deferral or delay • Project breakup • Increase CLR	Consider • Mothball • Deferral or delay • Cancellation • Increase CLR

FIGURE 6.9 Using BRE and CLR Scores to Validate Projects (U.S. EPA, 2020a)

Example: Possible prioritization factors & weights

Factor	Weight
Public Health/Safety	15
Federal or State Mandated Program	15
Local Irrevocable Commitment	15
Business Risk Exposure	10
Service Delivery Impact	10
Fiscal Impact	10
Conformance with Plan / Policies; Phase Completion/	8
Efficiency Improvement	7
Leverage	6
Project Interdependence	4
Total Maximum Score	**100**

FIGURE 6.10 Prioritizing Projects Using Factors and Weights (U.S. EPA, 2020a)

Alternative to prioritization factor weighting

"Risk"

No	Project description	Cost $M	B/C ratio	PBP yrs	CLR	BRE
256	South trunk renewal	4.2	2.42	2.5	83	610
102	Expand plant automation	6.5	2.35	3.5	63	411
16	Renew digester heaters	2.8	2.10	4.0	74	219
205	New CMMS	8.5	1.95	5.0	69	712
167	Office accommodation	4.7	1.35	6.2	72	813
150	Siphon renewals	2.6	1.30	7.2	73	471

Assume agency CIP limit of $25M

FIGURE 6.11 Prioritizing Projects Using Project Risk and CIP Budget (U.S. EPA, 2020a)

Upon having validated and prioritized projects, the funding and financing sources for each project need to be determined. The following section presents relevant strategies.

6.0 EVALUATE LONG-TERM FUNDING OPTIONS

The final WERF/U.S. EPA asset management steps seek to finalize and document the asset management plan so it may be implemented and refined in the future. The plan will include comprehensive costs and funding sources for each expenditure type. The steps are:

- Step 9: Determine Funding Strategy
- Step 10: Build AM Plan

6.1 Funding Strategies

A number of documents and tools have been developed for understanding and implementing various funding strategies specific to stormwater programs. U.S. EPA's (2006) *Guidance for Municipal Stormwater Funding* as well as Chapter 4, Financing Strategies, of WEF's (2014) *Green Infrastructure Implementation* are comprehensive resources for understanding strategies for stormwater funding, and the reader is highly encouraged to refer to these documents for specific information. These guides provide detailed considerations and recommendations regarding funding strategies, funding methods and mechanisms, trends, and legal considerations. Particular funding strategies described include

- Projecting needs and costs over a multiyear time period,
- Using a variety of funding methods and mechanisms,
- Basing services fees on actual costs,
- Identifying links and dependencies for program components to inform scheduling,
- Incorporate community expectations,
- Selecting stable and dedicated funding, and
- Adaptively managing funding plans.

The U.S. EPA guidance also lists and describes the following funding methods and mechanisms:

- General revenue appropriations
- Stormwater user (service) fees
- Plan review, development inspection, and special user fees
- Special assessments
- Bonding for capital improvements
- In-lieu of construction fees
- Capitalization recovery fees
- Impact fees
- Developer extension/latecomer fees
- Federal and state funding opportunities such as grants, loans, and cooperative programs

Trends and topics discussed in the guidance include the increasing complexity of stormwater program responsibilities and expectations; opportunities to blend funding; use multijurisdictional funding; cost sharing with other public programs; incorporation of broader private sector participation; and increased influence of technology and data. Legal considerations cover topics such as who is subject to fees/taxes (and who is not), special tax payer approvals, legal precedents (and case studies), and how funds can be used.

The California Stormwater Quality Association (CASQA, 2020) Funding Resources webpage provides a thorough summary of funding sources and strategies for various investment types. CASQA's sustainable funding sources for O&M and regulatory compliance and administrative needs include general funds, stormwater utility fees, realignment of services, local development fees, and special taxes. Capital investments can be covered by these sources as well as grants and loans.

The Environmental Finance Center (EFC) at California State University, Sacramento's (Sacramento State's) Office of Water Programs (OWP) is one of 10 centers throughout the United States that is partially funded by U.S. EPA to support utilities, municipalities, counties, and states in long-term sustainability of services. The OWP EFC webpage includes material intended to get those just started in stormwater asset management and funding familiar with these topics and provide free tools to make the concepts and implementation more accessible. Tools and resources include a stormwater asset management toolkit, which includes a stormwater rate development spreadsheet; a stormwater funding story board; and listings of various stormwater funding opportunities. The EFC at the University of Maryland (2020) webpage provides several examples and case studies of financial feasibility studies conducted for municipal stormwater programs throughout Maryland. The Northeast EFC at the University of Southern Maine (2020) provides resources for education and outreach, stakeholder engagement, technical assistance, and education on green infrastructure and financing options to achieve water quality goals.

California State Water Board's (2020a) Stormwater Program—Urban Runoff Program Funding webpage provides links to many other webpages that provide additional stormwater funding resources.

U.S. EPA (2017a) tabulates several state and federal programs that provide funding for stormwater and green infrastructure projects, and in 2018, U.S. EPA Region 9 hosted two stormwater funding forums in California that presented in detail various funding options (U.S. EPA, 2018).

Finally, the National Association of Clean Water Agencies (2016) discusses some funding trends, methods, and mechanisms as well as many case studies in *Legal Considerations for Enacting, Implementing, and Funding Stormwater Programs*.

6.2 Documenting the Asset Management Plan

Recall that the goal of asset management is to provide a specified LOS at the lowest life-cycle cost. Documenting the Asset Management Plan (AMP) allows program managers to communicate the planning conducted, data gathered, and process and strategies to be implemented to achieve this goal. Particular topics to highlight include the program goals, services, and requirements; asset inventory; baseline and desired LOS; long-term needs and costs; funding strategy; and adaptive management approach.

The AMP document can be as simple or complex as appropriate for the program's size, capacity, and expectations. Step 10 of U.S. EPA's (2020a) asset management training provides details on more complex AMPs, but a simple outline may include

- Program Description: Goals, services, and drivers for the program
- AMP Intent and Content: Goals and measurable objectives of the AMP and presentation of document elements
- Program Activities and Assets: Descriptions and tabulations of the asset inventory, O&M activities, CIP projects, permit compliance, and administrative duties
- LOS: Descriptions of the baseline and target LOS
- Operational Strategies and Scheduling: Approach for coordinating all services and schedule for services
- Program Costs: Estimates for all services according to the strategies and schedule to be implemented
- Funding Strategies: Explanation of types of funding sources to be used for various services
- Adaptive Management: Description of how data will be tracked, evaluated, and compared with target objectives and how and when the AMP will be updated to reflect new needs or optimize strategies

Suggestions for adaptively managing the AMP are provided in Section 7.0.

7.0 ADAPTIVE MANAGEMENT

7.1 Strategies

The majority of municipalities across the country, especially small communities with nondedicated stormwater funding, address stormwater issues on a reactionary basis, where O&M is performed sporadically, typically in reaction to customer complaints. Adaptive management in contrast is a proactive approach where communities/agencies use system data to continually update their program. Adaptive management is defined as a structured process of learning by doing and adapting based on what's learned (Walters & Holling, 1990) and is a flexible decision-making process that can be adjusted as outcomes from management actions, system monitoring, and other events become better understood. It allows modification of O&M protocols based on an iterative decision-making process with a goal of optimizing functional outcomes and resource expenditures (City of Lancaster, PA, 2019). Adaptive management is based on system data collected by O&M crews, which yields inspection-driven decisions, and observations of management staff, which are typically systematic or large-scale adaptations. It differs from interval-based management where reviews and modifications are driven exclusively by the time elapsed between maintenance events. Interval-based management strategy is most effective when there is little variability between assets and when maintenance strategies are simple and well-established. This is generally not the case with the wide range of surface and subsurface assets present within a stormwater management program, which is why adaptive management is preferred.

7.2 Tracking Performance Over Time

An important element of adaptive management is tracking the performance of stormwater assets over time. Collecting data at the individual group and type level allows for comparison across assets at different resolutions. This type of data collection process provides valuable information on which type of sites, assets, and components may require more frequent (or proactive) maintenance and when or over what time period this maintenance is required. Ultimately, asset data can be used to determine appropriate maintenance frequencies and plan for the future of the program.

For pipe systems, field inspections typically look at condition of the structure/surface and evidence of erosion, blockage, odor, algae, and other similar problems. For the structures themselves, material type, location within the system, and function can be as telling as evidence of degradation, cracking, excessive deposition, root intrusion, and other factors.

For conveyance systems, location and function play a large part in expected maintenance requirements over time. Streams and channels downstream from current or recent development are more likely to be affected than natural systems in upstream or more mature areas. Consistent visual observations are important across the entire conveyance system to prevent blockages, erosion, and other issues that can cause localized flooding.

Monitoring the maturation of individual surface SCMs from year to year provides valuable insight on expected performance of similar asset types and asset locations. Newly constructed or modified SCM sites are likely to require more attention, especially those with vegetative practices. Mature sites that have been maintained for an extended period may self-maintain, require less maintenance, and perform more effectively.

7.3 Feedback

The gain in understanding from monitoring and assessment can be used to inform the selection of management actions to improve performance and reduce costs. As understanding evolves, so too does the decision making that is influenced by improved understanding. In this way, the iterative cycle of decision making, monitoring, and assessment leads gradually to improved management as a consequence of improved understanding.

Whether done in-house or contracted out, performing routine inspections of all stormwater assets by trained inspection professionals is critical to this process. This includes routine inspection of assets and collection of data following individual storm events to further inform system performance and O&M procedures. Use of a CMMS can simplify this process by digitally generating work orders that request inspections, obtaining detailed information, and addressing asset issues. However, visual inspections of known problem areas by stormwater staff and a robust public education/involvement program that promotes active reporting of drainage problems by citizens can help build the case for problem assets that need more detailed inspection and prioritize limited funds to address the most problematic areas.

An inspector's responsibility is not only to determine what issues are currently affecting an asset, but also to look for signs of future issues. By identifying these issues early and providing feedback through a CMMS or even handwritten field notes, the inspector can recommend measures that prevent functional issues and reduce the cost to remedy them.

Upholding proper aesthetic of assets, especially surface stormwater facilities, is also important. By maintaining the proper aesthetic, the community will be more likely to have a positive perception of the stormwater system. Unruly plantings, defaced surfaces, and damaged components should be encouraged to be reported by field staff as well as the general public and incorporated into the O&M program.

7.4 Update of Asset Management Program

To properly update a stormwater asset management program, inspection-driven decisions and systematic adaptations should be initiated and implemented on a regular basis. Program updates should promote both short- and long-term goals.

For example, inspection results may indicate that the crew size, material cost, and/or duration of maintenance for cleaning of catch basins in a downtown area is inadequate to prevent routine flooding. A change in inspection frequency may be enough to identify the problem earlier using the same cleaning process. However, field results may indicate that a change in equipment type, crew size, or maintenance method is required to more cost effectively address the issue.

An example of a systematic adaptation could be the decision to provide photo documentation of all assets during inspection and before/after maintenance or repairs to better track the condition of assets over time, document the improvement level required for properly maintained assets, and improve maintenance performance to reduce costs.

Adaptive management has been framed, often implicitly, on the assumption that the structural or managerial features of the system and the effects on them are stable over time. However, complications can arise on a number of fronts involving economic, social, and environmental issues. An obvious example is a change in administration or budget where resources toward a stormwater management system are dramatically reduced. Another is climate change, where increases in volumes and intensities of major climatic events affect assets in ways beyond their original design. System managers should adapt to these situations as necessary and, as stated above, incorporate program updates that address both short- and long-term goals.

8.0 REFERENCES

Association of Metropolitan Sewerage Agencies. (2002). *Managing public infrastructure assets to minimize cost and maximize performance.* https://books.google.com/books/about/Managing_Public_Infrastructure_Assets_to.html?id=VLktGwAACAAJ

California Central Coast Regional Water Quality Control Board. (2019). *National Pollutant Discharge Elimination System permit and waste discharge requirements for City of Salinas municipal stormwater discharges* (NPDES No. CA0049981. Order No. R3-2019-0073). https://www.waterboards.ca.gov/centralcoast/water_issues/programs/stormwater/docs/salinas/r3-2019-0073_final_order.pdf

California State Water Board. (2020a). CA State Water Board stormwater program—Urban runoff program funding webpage. https://www.waterboards.ca.gov/water_issues/programs/stormwater/funding_stormwater.html

California State Water Board. (2020b). *Strategy to optimize resource management of stormwater.* https://www.waterboards.ca.gov/water_issues/programs/stormwater/storms/

California Stormwater Quality Association. (2020). California Stormwater Quality Association funding resources webpage. https://www.casqa.org/resources/funding-resources

City of Grand Rapids, MI. (2016). *Stormwater asset management and capital improvement plan.* https://www.google.com/url?sa=t&rct=j&q=&esrc=s&source=web&cd=&cad=rja&uact=8&ved=2ahUKEwjK1oiuj9_rAhWMsJ4KHSSiCh8QFjAAegQIARAB&url=https%3A%2F%2Fwww.grandrapidsmi.gov%2Ffiles%2Fassets%2Fpublic%2Fdepartments%2

Fenvironmental-services%2Ffiles%2Fstormwater%2Fenvironmental-services-resources%2Fstormwater-misc%2Fstormwater-and-asset-management-and-capital-plan-2016.pdf&usg=AOvVaw0s62qkq_ONiC4bVygFNK5a

City of Lancaster, PA. (2019). *City of Lancaster green infrastructure O&M plan.*

City of San Diego, CA. (2021). *Watershed asset management plan 2.0. Transportation and Stormwater Management Department.* https://www.sandiego.gov/sites/default/files/watershed_asset_mgmt_plan_01262021.pdf

Environmental Finance Center at Sacramento State. (2019a). *A toolkit for stormwater asset management and funding.*

Environmental Finance Center at Sacramento State. (2019b). *Estimating benefits and costs of stormwater management part I: Methods and challenges.* https://www.efc.csus.edu/reports/efc-cost-project-part-1.pdf

Environmental Finance Center at Sacramento State. (2020). *Estimating benefits and costs of stormwater management part II: Evaluating municipal spending in California.* https://www.efc.csus.edu/reports/efc-cost-project-part-2.pdf

Environmental Finance Center at the University of Maryland. (2020). Environmental Finance Center at the University of Maryland webpage. https://arch.umd.edu/research-creative-practice/centers/environmental-finance-center/programs/stormwater-financing-and-outreach

Harvey, R. (2015). *An introduction to asset management tools municipal water. Wastewater and stormwater systems.*

National Association of Clean Water Agencies. (2016). *Legal considerations for enacting, implementing, and funding stormwater programs.* https://www.google.com/url?sa=t&rct=j&q=&esrc=s&source=web&cd=&ved=2ahUKEwix4OaPwunrAhVLL6wKHXXQDwgQFjADegQIAxAB&url=https%3A%2F%2Fwww.nacwa.org%2Fdocs%2Fdefault-source%2Fdefault-document-library%2F2016-12-08stormwaterwhitepaper.pdf%3Fsfvrsn%3D0&usg=AOvVaw2TIJpijOlmTb1jcmbnJhBl

Northeast Environmental Finance Center at the University of Southern Maine. (2020). Northeast Environmental Finance Center at University of Southern Main webpage. https://neefc.org/stormwater-nutrients-management/

Office of Water Programs at California State University, Sacramento. (2018). *Guidance for stormwater and dry weather runoff capture.* https://www.google.com/url?sa=t&rct=j&q=&esrc=s&source=web&cd=&cad=rja&uact=8&ved=2ahUKEwiMkNqpvN_rAhUBqJ4KHYgnDugQFjAAeg

QIARAB&url=https%3A%2F%2Fwww.waterboards.ca.gov%2Fpublications_forms%2Fpublications%2Flegislative%2Fdocs%2F2018%2Fstormwater_capture_at_schools_with_appendices.pdf&usg=AOvVaw2o7YHkhwu-YCBx55WeaJa7

U.S. Environmental Protection Agency. (2006). *Guidance for municipal stormwater funding.* https://www.google.com/url?sa=t&rct=j&q=&esrc=s&source=web&cd=&ved=2ahUKEwjc-pa3xuHrAhXUvJ4KHfuGB50QFjABegQIBRAB&url=https%3A%2F%2Fwww.epa.gov%2Fsites%2Fproduction%2Ffiles%2F2015-10%2Fdocuments%2Fguidance-manual-version-2x-2.pdf&usg=AOvVaw2qU684wKi20lrjn_cCWz6P

U.S. Environmental Protection Agency. (2017a). *Federal and state funding programs—Stormwater & green infrastructure projects.* https://www.google.com/url?sa=t&rct=j&q=&esrc=s&source=web&cd=&ved=2ahUKEwiJ4uSwlunrAhWEJDQIHedxDHUQFjAGegQICBAB&url=https%3A%2F%2Fwww.epa.gov%2Fsites%2Fproduction%2Ffiles%2F2017-05%2Fdocuments%2Ffederal-and-california-sw-funding-programs.pdf&usg=AOvVaw1sbI2RFXij5X9RmIiU_mS0

U.S. Environmental Protection Agency. (2017b). *Fundamentals of asset management session 2—Assess condition, failure modes.* https://19january2017snapshot.epa.gov/sites/production/files/2016-01/documents/assess-performance-failure-modes.pdf

U.S. Environmental Protection Agency. (2018). Stormwater finance forum presentations. https://www.efc.csus.edu/finance-forums/

U.S. Environmental Protection Agency. (2020a). *Sustainable infrastructure management program learning environment. EPA asset management training material.* https://www.epa.gov/sustainable-water-infrastructure/asset-management-workshops-training-slides

U.S. Environmental Protection Agency. (2020b). *Sustainable water infrastructure: Asset management for water and wastewater utilities.* https://www.epa.gov/sustainable-water-infrastructure/asset-management-programs-stormwater-and-wastewater-systems

Walters, C. J., & Holling, C. S. (1990). *Large-scale management experiments and learning by doing.*

Water Environment Federation. (2014). *Green infrastructure implementation.*

Water Environment Research Foundation. (2005a). *A step-by-step approach to discovering and applying asset management in a utility environment.* https://simple.waterrf.org/simple/media/EPAAsset/Storyline%20Text.pdf

Water Environment Research Foundation. (2005b). *EPA asset training management material.* https://simple.waterrf.org/Books/Contents/Interactive-Training/EPA-Asset-Management-Training-Material

Water Environment Research Foundation. (2008). *Sustainable infrastructure management program learning environment* (SIMPLE). *Version 1.1.* https://www.waterrf.org/research/projects/sustainable-infrastructure-management-program-learning-environment-simple-version

Water Environment Research Foundation. (2014). *Practitioner's guide to economic decision making in asset management: Part I background.* https://www.waterrf.org/research/projects/practitioners-guide-economic-decision-making-asset-management-part-i-background

Water Research Foundation. (2020). *Asset management.* https://www.waterrf.org/system/files/resource/2020-07/4949-AssetManagement_0.pdf

Water Environment Research Foundation & U.S. Environmental Protection Agency. (2002, March 21–22). Asset management workshop, Crystal City, VA, United States.

7

Personnel, Equipment, and Cost Considerations

1.0 PERSONNEL AND EQUIPMENT REQUIREMENTS 251
- 1.1 Surface Inspection and Maintenance 252
  - *1.1.1 Crew Requirements* 252
  - *1.1.2 Equipment* 253
  - *1.1.3 Materials* 254
- 1.2 Subsurface Inspection and Maintenance 254
  - *1.2.1 Crew Requirements* 254
  - *1.2.2 Equipment and Materials* 255
- 1.3 Porous Pavement Inspection and Maintenance 256
  - *1.3.1 Crew Requirements* 256
  - *1.3.2 Equipment* 256
  - *1.3.3 Materials* 256
- 1.4 Nonroutine and Specialty Maintenance 257
  - *1.4.1 Crew Requirements* 257
  - *1.4.2 Equipment* 257
  - *1.4.3 Materials* 258

2.0 BUDGETING CONSIDERATIONS FOR OPERATIONS AND MAINTENANCE PROGRAMS 258
- 2.1 Budget Components 258
- 2.2 Estimating/Budgeting Program Costs 260
  - *2.2.1 Factors Affecting Budget Estimates* 260
  - *2.2.2 Estimating Life-Cycle Costs* 265

3.0 MAINTENANCE CAPITAL IMPROVEMENT PROGRAM 266

4.0 REFERENCES 268

5.0 SUGGESTED READING 269

1.0 PERSONNEL AND EQUIPMENT REQUIREMENTS

The type of personnel and their skill sets, as well as the equipment requirements to conduct maintenance of stormwater control measures (SCMs), are evolving. This evolution is a result of the changes in the design of SCMs from simple passive systems with concrete trickle ditches to convey stormwater from the inlet to the outlet structures and little or no vegetation to more complex systems that include forebays and different types of vegetation to enhance pollutant removal and control stormwater volume, while making them more resilient to extreme precipitation events and climate change. The typical public works maintenance crews are also evolving from "pipe and ditch" crews to crews that understand the function of SCMs and are familiar with vegetation maintenance requirements.

The types of personnel and equipment required for the execution of maintenance activities are typically organized into four categories:

1. *Surface inspection and maintenance,* which focus on surface elements of vegetated systems like rain gardens or ponds.
2. *Subsurface inspection and maintenance,* which focus on maintenance of subsurface features such as distribution pipes, inlets, underdrains, and subsurface storage chambers.
3. *Porous pavement inspection and maintenance*, which focus on maintenance of porous pavement systems such as porous concrete and porous pavement.
4. *Specialty maintenance*, which focuses on a broad range of repair activities that fall outside of the scope of routine maintenance.

Maintenance of structural elements of SCMs is addressed in Chapter 5, Sections 4.1.6, Verification of Structure Safety; 4.1.9, Verification of Structural Integrity; and 5.2.6, Structure Maintenance. Forms for inspections and maintenance are presented in Chapter 9.

1.1 Surface Inspection and Maintenance

Surface maintenance inspection and maintenance is composed of tasks related to maintenance of surface features associated with SCMs, most typically vegetated areas, swales, curb cuts, fencing, signage, inlet grates, and so on. A large portion of surface maintenance is typically focused on vegetative care and general site cleanup, including removal of trash, sediment, and debris from surface features.

1.1.1 Crew Requirements

Surface maintenance crews are typically composed of a crew chief, or foreman, and one or more surface maintenance technicians/laborers or crew members. The crew foreman is a critically important position within the surface maintenance team. Crew foremen are responsible for both executing and directing surface maintenance. Foremen are also commonly responsible for performing site inspections to identify critical work items, escalating issues that cannot be handled using available resources, and implementing emergency safety protocols, as well as enforcing standard operating procedures and safety protocols. Crew foremen are also typically responsible for vehicle operation, communication with scheduling and administrative staff, and interaction with the public. Crew foremen should have prior familiarity/facility with the operation and maintenance of landscaping hand and power tools such as string trimmers, leaf blowers, as well as experience with managing field crews and strong communication skills. Foremen will also typically be required to have a valid driver's license and the ability to safely operate a pickup truck or landscaping stake body truck. Foremen will also need a strong working understanding of common surface maintenance issues and solutions, a strong understanding of stormwater management system function, some level of horticultural training including the identification common weeds and pests and basics of vegetation care, and familiarity with surface maintenance protocols for sediment and debris removal, vegetative care, and minor structural repairs.

Crew members/laborers within surface maintenance teams are responsible for execution of surface maintenance under the direction of a crew foreman. A typical surface maintenance crew will be composed of one to three crew members in addition to the crew foreman, although larger crews are sometimes deployed to maintain larger vegetated sites.

In addition to a standard surface maintenance crew, additional specialty positions may be required to implement certain aspects of surface maintenance. These include a certified arborist, which is typically required to oversee pruning operations, a licensed civil/environmental engineer to perform periodic performance inspections and evaluations including infiltration testing or simulated runoff testing, and a horticulturalist, botanist, landscape architect, or ecologist to perform periodic detailed vegetation health assessments.

1.1.2 Equipment

Most routine surface maintenance visits focus on the removal of sediment and debris and weeding or removal of undesirable plants. As such, the most used equipment for surface maintenance includes landscaping tools such as shovels, rakes, push brooms, garden shears/loppers, tampers, digging bars, leaf blowers, and string trimmers. Brush hogs and/or riding mowers may be needed to maintain turf areas and/or to remove vegetation from overgrown sites, although mowing of large areas is relatively uncommon.

Surface maintenance crews and equipment are commonly transported from site to site via heavy duty crew cab pickup truck or landscape stake body trucks. Trucks with articulated or dump beds and or lift gates are commonly used to support routine surface maintenance work.

During the spring and/or fall, surface maintenance crews may be also replanting areas of poor vegetation establishment and mulching new beds. Common winter tasks include vegetation cutbacks and structural pruning, while watering of newly established plants is a common additional task in the summer months. More specialized equipment is sometimes needed for these focused activities. In the case of watering, for example, if water is sourced from hydrants, a hydrant key, flow meter, and backflow preventor are commonly needed. Alternatively, portable water totes, commonly in the 757 to 1136 L (200 to 300 gal) range, can be filled and transported via small truck to watering sites. The use of small excavators and/or skid steers may be useful in loading trucks for spring mulching. Additional information about surface maintenance is included in Chapter 5, Inspection and Maintenance During and After Construction (Protocols).

1.1.3 Materials

Surface maintenance crews commonly focus efforts on vegetative care and sediment and debris removal. As such, materials required for surface maintenance are typically minimal and include trash bags or other receptacles to collect trash and debris. Other common materials include erosion fabric and small quantities of soil, stone for small erosion control repairs, hardwood mulch, concrete/mortar filler/sealant for minor concrete repairs, and graffiti removal products. Preemergent herbicides are sometimes used by surface maintenance crews to prevent weed growth and development. Insecticides and fungicides are also sometimes used to address vegetative pests but are rare in practice.

1.2 Subsurface Inspection and Maintenance

Subsurface inspection and maintenance most commonly consist of inspection of pipes and surface hydraulic control and storage structures using closed circuit television (CCTV) camera equipment followed by removal of accumulated sediment and debris using hydraulic jetting and vectoring using a combination jet/vac sewer cleaning truck. Subsurface inspections, which are also facilitated with cleanouts, are provided to monitor performance of SCMs, where applicable.

1.2.1 Crew Requirements

Although there are many potential crew arrangements for subsurface work, subsurface maintenance crews typically consist of a combination truck operator, and one or more laborers. The operator also typically serves in a crew chief/foreman role and is responsible for directing work on the site, communication with the public, managing and directing crew members, communicating unresolved issues with program managers, coordinating ancillary work such as vehicle towing, and documenting the completion of work. The crew chief/operator should have a commercial driver's license, prior experience, or focused training in the operation of heavy equipment and specific experience with driving and operating combination jet/vac trucks or similar equipment. Supporting crew members may assist with setup for vacuum cleaning and hydraulic jetting operations, setup and teardown of safety and/or maintenance of traffic measures, removal and cleaning of pretreatment devices, assisting with decanting, and general cleanup. In some cases, separate crews may be setup for vacuum cleaning of inlets, while other crews may be dedicated to hydraulic jetting of pipes and storage structures. In other cases, a single crew may implement both vacuum cleaning and hydraulic jetting work.

Inspection crews typically consist of a CCTV foreman/operator and one CCTV technician. The crew foreman and members are typically National Association of Sewer Service Companies (NASSCO) certified in video pipe inspection. The CCTV foreman/operator is responsible for operation of the CCTV unit, typically either a push camera or crawler camera, including field defect coding. Alternatively, defect coding may be performed by a NASSCO-certified video inspection technician in an office setting. The crew technician commonly assists with camera unit setup and teardown, removal of pretreatment services, grate tops, manhole lids, or cleanout caps required to access and implement safety and/or traffic control measures.

Surface maintenance and inspection activities may occur simultaneously, with CCTV immediately preceding cleaning, or CCTV crews sometimes perform inspections on an independent schedule with combination truck cleaning crews scheduling field visits based on CCTV inspection results.

1.2.2 Equipment and Materials

Equipment for surface maintenance commonly includes a combination sewer cleaning truck. There are a wide variety of truck sizes, models, and features available for combination trucks. Common specifications include maximum water pressure, hose length, debris holding tank size, telescoping boom length, and water tank capacity. In some cases, vacuum-only trucks are used to clean catch basins, which can permit a faster workflow for this type of work, while pipe cleaning is performed separately using a combination sewer cleaning truck or stand-alone hydraulic jetting truck. In some cases, tow behind and non-commercial driver's license (CDL) models can be used for smaller maintenance portfolios or hard to reach sites. CCTV equipment commonly consists of either a robotic crawler camera or push camera unit and laptop or tablet with video-inspection software. Additional information about subsurface general maintenance is included in Chapter 5.

1.3 Porous Pavement Inspection and Maintenance

1.3.1 Crew Requirements

Porous pavement maintenance typically involves periodic cleaning of porous pavements using a regenerative air sweeper or vacuum sweeper. Typical crew make up includes an equipment operator and one crew assistant/laborer. The operator also typically serves in a crew chief/foreman role and is responsible for directing work on the site, communication with the public, managing and directing crew members, communicating unresolved issues with program managers/office staff, coordinating ancillary work such as vehicle towing, and documenting the completion of work. The crew chief/operator should have a CDL, prior experience or focused training in the operation of heavy equipment, and specific experience with driving and operating regenerative air trucks, street sweepers, or vacuum cleaning trucks. Supporting crew members may assist with preparation of the porous surface for cleaning, which may include manual cleanup of larger debris, setup/teardown of maintenance or traffic and safety perimeters, as well as small-scale patching of areas of cracking or wear, replacement of broken pavers, and sweeping in replacement joint material.

1.3.2 Equipment

Typical equipment associated with porous pavement inspection and maintenance includes a regenerative air sweeper truck, mixing and spreading tools for small asphalt and concrete patching, and push broom for sweeping joint material. Additional information about pervious pavement general maintenance is included in Chapter 5.

1.3.3 Materials

Materials for porous pavement maintenance include patching materials for small repairs (e.g., cold patch), replacement precast panels or pavers, and replacement joint material.

1.4 Nonroutine and Specialty Maintenance

Nonroutine and specialty maintenance includes maintenance that exceeds the typical scope of routine maintenance. Nonroutine and specialty maintenance is often associated with failing or poorly performing systems and can include

- Major replanting and reseeding of vegetated areas;
- Replacement or refurbishment of filtration or storage media;
- Structural repairs and replacement or major repair of hydraulic control structures, piping, buried storage vaults or chambers, perimeter fencing, or other structural elements;
- Filling or otherwise mitigating sinkholes or areas of settlement;
- Major erosion control repairs;
- Pond and forebay dredging and sediment removal;
- Aeration system repairs; and
- Bank stabilization.

Nonroutine or specialty maintenance may include specialized investigations, analysis, engineering, and permitting that are beyond the scope of this manual. These may include underground utility exploration, geotechnical testing, dye testing, hydrologic and hydraulic modeling, structural engineering design, geotechnical engineering design, and civil engineering design.

1.4.1 Crew Requirements

Crew requirements for nonroutine or specialty maintenance are highly variable but typically include experienced heavy equipment and truck operators and various types of construction laborers. The crew foreman may or may not be the same individual as one of the equipment operators. Additional specialty maintenance crew members may include masons, carpenters, electricians, and plumbers.

1.4.2 Equipment

Equipment associated with nonroutine or specialty maintenance is highly variable based on the type of work, but can commonly include excavation, site work, and hauling equipment such as excavators, front end loaders, skid steers, back hoes, dump trucks, cement mixers, sheeting and shoring equipment, and concrete forms.

1.4.3 Materials

Materials associated with specialty maintenance are highly variable based on the type of work but may include

- Engineered media (see Chapter 5 or design manuals for media information),
- Soil fill,
- Sand,
- Flowable fill,
- Aggregate,
- Riprap,
- Plantings,
- Seed,
- Soil amendments,
- Mulch,
- Erosion fabric,
- Geotextile fabric,
- Concrete,
- Concrete reinforcing steel,
- Replacement piping, and
- Replacement structures (e.g., precast inlets, fencing, etc.).

2.0 BUDGETING CONSIDERATIONS FOR OPERATIONS AND MAINTENANCE PROGRAMS

2.1 Budget Components

Budgeting for operations and maintenance (O&M) programs is critical for understanding and planning for expected program resources, particularly as programs are developing and expanding. Depending on the jurisdiction, budgeting is commonly performed for 1- and 5-year time periods and includes several additive components that reflect overall program costs. These include

- **Program Development**—upfront and ongoing investments in the development of program resources such as standard operating procedures, workflows, guidance materials, asset management systems, and so on. Some of these costs may be reflected in staffing costs, but any outside consulting support, as an example, would be added as an additional program development cost.

- **Staffing**—Costs related to onboarding, training, recruiting, salaries, and benefits for field staff and office administration and management staff. Staffing costs are typically expressed in full-time equivalent (FTE) terms and can be either in-house or contracted labor costs. Differences in costs between full-time and part-time labor must be included in staff estimates, as well as any anticipated staff level changes to reflect seasonal changes in workflows. Shared staff should be represented as fractions of an FTE.
- **Field Equipment**—Costs related to purchase or renting of equipment including landscaping trucks, pickups, regenerative air sweepers, excavation equipment, landscaping tools, watering storage containers, hose, field computers, and personal protective equipment. Program managers may want to budget for truck and equipment rentals in lieu of capital purchases early in program implementation. As more sites come online, vehicle purchasing or long-term leasing is typically the preferred option. Shared vehicle or field equipment resources should be prorated as appropriate.
- **Office Equipment**—Costs related to purchase and rental of office equipment such as desktop computers, printers, internet, software, and so on.
- **Materials**—Costs related to purchase of materials including mulch, erosion fabric, plants, replacement pavers, concrete and asphalt patching materials, graffiti remover, trash bags, herbicide, as well as office-related materials.
- **Equipment and Facilities Maintenance**—Costs related to maintenance and upkeep of the vehicle fleet, equipment, and yard. Costs should be prorated as needed for shared resources.
- **Disposal**—Costs related to disposal of materials.
- **Facilities**—Costs related to purchase or rental of yard space and associated office space, including rental of storage bins, office trailers, and utilities. Costs should be prorated as needed for shared resources.
- **Other**—Insurance, public relations, debt service, depreciation, contingency, etc. Costs should be prorated as needed for shared resources.

For long range forecasts, budgets should reflect expected rates of escalation in labor and material costs, inflation, as well as a discount rate for future cash flows, and depreciation of capital purchases. The effect of natural disasters can also affect future maintenance costs and should be considered, if appropriate. Contingency for major repairs of at least 10% is recommended on an annual basis. Capital and operating costs are typically provided in separate worksheets/tables.

2.2 Estimating/Budgeting Program Costs

Accurately projecting O&M program costs is critical to program success. Under-budgeting for O&M can lead to system failures, disgruntled residents, and an overall lack of support for the program. Over-budgeting can lead to unnecessary spending that could be used to support other functions.

Methods. There are a wide variety of methods used to estimate O&M costs ranging from using unit costs available in literature, estimating annual costs as a percentage of construction costs, benchmarking using pilot studies, or building "bottom-up estimates" using detailed line item estimating methods. In the case of the last method, productivity estimates for common tasks like planting and watering can be sourced from cost estimating guides such as RS Means, or from local contractors. When working with contractors, program managers should be sure that costs reflect portal-to-portal costs including travel and mobilization. There are also tools developed by the Water Research Foundation to estimate life-cycle cost estimates as described below, in Section 2.2.2.

Operation and maintenance program costs typically scale with the increase in program assets as program implementation proceeds. So, interfacing with design and construction teams to estimate the projected pace and rate of project delivery is integral to forecasting O&M costs. Depending on the estimating methods used, detailed information on project asset characteristics (e.g., pipe lengths and sizes, etc.) may also be needed from design and construction program managers.

Regardless of the method used, managers must understand that the composition, size, and nature of their program can result in widely different costs than other seemingly similar programs. O&M program costs are highly dependent on a few major factors, which can lead to large differences in total expenditures over time.

2.2.1 Factors Affecting Budget Estimates

The following factors should be understood and evaluated when developing program level budgetary estimates:

- **Portfolio size.** Larger O&M portfolios may allow for investment in specialized crews, more sophisticated training, and onboarding programs, as well as the purchase of capital equipment (versus rental).

Economies of scale associated with larger programs will tend to drive down unit costs relative to smaller programs. However, increasing complexity of asset management and reporting systems associated with large programs can result in increasing costs that somewhat offset anticipated economies of scale.

For small programs, maintenance work can sometimes be incorporated into existing workload for existing parks, schools, roadway maintenance, or facilities staff, reducing the need to hire additional staff.

- **Stormwater control measures (practice) size and distribution.** Small, highly decentralized SCMs or practices tend to have much higher unit maintenance costs than larger, centralized SCMs. This is because of the relative exposure of small SCMs to external factors such as windblown trash, vandalism, weed, sediment loading, and so on and the relative high visibility of many smaller SCMs to pedestrians and residents (which drives aesthetic expectations). Diseconomies of scale associated with relatively high mobilization and travel costs, and the need for smaller, less efficient equipment can also drive high unit costs for small SCMs. As a result of these factors, estimating unit costs by asset size class is often needed to develop an accurate predictive understanding of cost.
- **Visibility and aesthetic expectations.** Stormwater control measures located in highly visible areas with high levels of aesthetic expectations, particularly in rights-of-way (ROWs) adjacent to residential areas, tend to have higher unit costs than SCMs in less visible areas such as off ROW areas. Residents may be highly sensitive to relatively small amounts of trash and debris within installations located within ROW environments close to their homes, whereas similar amounts of trash and debris within a large regional SCM in a less visible setting, for instance, would not drive similar reactions. The frequency of trash removal needed to maintain public acceptance in residential settings in particular can drive maintenance frequency, significantly driving up overall program costs.
- **Urban density.** Stormwater control measures located in highly dense urban centers tend to have higher unit costs than those in more suburban environments. In dense urban areas, SCM sizes are typically smaller and located in higher traffic areas that receive more sediment and litter loading. Also, installations are often exposed to vandalism and accidental damage. There are also often higher costs associated with permitting, logistics, and travel in dense urban areas, in addition to higher labor costs.

- **Pretreatment.** Extensive implementation of pretreatment devices such as forebays or inlet filter bags can substantially drive up maintenance costs, particularly if these devices need to be maintained manually and the frequency of maintenance is high (i.e., because of high rates of sediment loading). However, pretreatment may result in a longer service life, particularly for large ponds or systems within underground storage beds that require full replacement if they become clogged with sediment. The trade-offs between pretreatment costs and increased service life are complex but can have significant effects on total program implementation costs.
- **Vegetated versus subsurface stormwater control measures.** Subsurface practices tend to have lower unit maintenance costs than similarly sized vegetated, surface SCMs. This may be due in part to the aesthetic expectations associated with vegetated SCMs that require frequent maintenance visits during the growing season.
- **Program specific policy decisions.** Considerable discretion associated with individual programs' policies can lead to significant differences in cost. For instance, programs may differ with respect to mulching depth preferences, watering triggers, use of preemergent herbicides to reduce weeding, planting preferences (e.g., plugs versus container plantings), and many other discretionary program policies. Careful review of these policies may help to identify opportunities for cost savings.
- **Sediment loading.** Stormwater control measures with higher rates of sediment loading tend to have higher unit maintenance costs. Some of these costs can be avoided by locating SCMs in areas with lower sediment loading, particularly in combined sewer areas, where sediment removal is not always a goal. Sediment removal in combined sewer areas can be a priority as human waste with sediments may develop sludge that must be removed. In these areas, managing rooftop impervious areas can be a good way of limiting sediment loading and reducing maintenance costs. Limiting hydraulic loading ratios, which lessen the unit area loading of sediment within the SCM, limiting the use of subsurface gravel beds (which cannot be cleaned without full replacement), and implementing street sweeping can all be good ways to lessen the effect of sediment on maintenance costs.
- **Prevailing wages.** Labor and equipment costs differences among regions and metropolitan areas can drive differences in maintenance costs. Differences prevailing wages can result in large differences in base labor rates of twofold or greater, as can the specific labor category chosen. In many cases, jurisdictions do not have labor categories that correspond directly to stormwater maintenance work,

so the choice of labor category can be an important determinant of labor costs. Differences between prevailing wage rates for landscaping labor associated with construction are typically much higher than those associated with maintenance. So, if a maintenance-related labor rate is not available, communities may need to use a much costlier construction-related labor rate.

- **Regulatory drivers.** Local or state regulations may in some cases dictate maintenance frequency. For example, local ordinances may have specific maintenance requirements and agreements that dictate the frequency of maintenance activities and reporting requirements. In addition, state or U.S. EPA issued municipal separate storm sewer system (MS4) permits also have maintenance requirements for stormwater infrastructure, as discussed in Chapter 2. It is important to evaluate all maintenance requirements and align them to the overall program goals to ensure efficient implementation of the maintenance activities.
- **Contracted labor versus in-house labor.** Programs that rely on third-party contractors may have differing costs versus in-house labor. When comparing contracted labor costs with in-house costs, it is important to consider the full cost of in-house labor, including the costs of administration, benefits, and so on.

The factors listed above can combine to produce vast differences (i.e., one or more orders of magnitude) in maintenance frequency and level of effort, which may in turn result in profound differences in unit and total program costs. Even within programs, costs may vary substantially among installations. For instance, a 2016 analysis of maintenance data for green infrastructure systems in Philadelphia showed that annual base maintenance costs varied from less than $2,000 per impervious 0.4 ha (1 ac) managed per year to more than $20,000 per directly connected impervious 0.4 (1 ac) managed per year (Philadelphia Water Department, 2016). Around the same time, Houle et al. (2013) tracked annualized maintenance costs associated with seven types of low-impact development practices within a controlled field experiment setting and found annualized maintenance costs ranging from $923 to $3,170 per 0.4 ha (1 ac), substantially below the reported range of costs in the Philadelphia study. These cost comparisons serve to illustrate the difficulties in comparing costs across programs and applying these costs to estimating costs for other programs. Following from this example, caution should be used in applying O&M cost ranges found in literature sources, as these costs may reflect partial costs (i.e., only the field component of maintenance), may be dated, and most importantly may not reflect the program characteristics that drive costs listed above. At minimum, adjustments should be made to account for differences in consumer price index across localities as well as escalation to account for inflation. Also, practitioners should review the maintenance frequencies associated with any published maintenance cost data before using it to estimate costs.

If cost data from literature sources is used for estimating program costs, raw data is typically first converted into unit cost data so it can be scaled and used for cost estimating. Caution must be used in developing or applying unit cost data, particularly with respect to the units of measure. Typically, unit costs are provided in units per drainage area managed or per square meter (square foot) of SCM area, but, less frequently, some organizations may report data in terms of costs per unit pollutant load reduction or volume reduction. For instance, a study by Minnesota Pollution Control Agency (2011) provided cost estimates in terms of cubic meters (cubic feet) of water quality volume. In both typical cases (drainage area or size of the SCM), these units may not be consistent from program to program. In the case of drainage area managed units, differences in the precipitation depth managed per unit drainage area or other sizing factors may influence the difference between unit cost and SCM sizes among programs. Details such as whether SCMs are sized for static storage, for which the SCM storage is equal to the size of the design storm event volume, or dynamic storage, for which the sizing of SCMs reflects a routing analysis of a design storm, can produce significant differences in the relationship between SCM sizing and drainage area.

The use of unit costs that reflect costs per unit of SCM constructed can be used as a more straightforward measure of costs that does not depend on drainage area. Here again, however, caution must be used in applying unit costs, particularly if there is uncertainty as to whether the unit cost was accurately measured (e.g., based on as-built data versus design data), or it is unclear what physical quantity the unit cost represents. For instance, it is sometimes unclear whether an area unit chosen to represent the size of an SCM includes the surface area, subsurface area, or vegetated footprint, and whether this measure includes the area of conveyance systems into and out of the facility.

Caution should also be used when assuming that maintenance costs will reliably be a fixed percentage of construction costs per year. For instance, Minnesota Pollution Control Agency (2011) did a cost comparison study of three cost estimation studies and reported that annual maintenance costs range from 0.02% to 20% of construction costs depending on the data source and type of SCM.

As a result of the methodological problems associated with applying unit costs from literature or estimating maintenance as a percentage of construction costs, benchmarking and tracking maintenance costs is recommended early in program development. Benchmarking unit costs for typical SCMs can help inform long range budgeting, but also can be effective in identifying SCMs with excessive maintenance costs, which in turn can be useful in identifying design and siting improvements to drive future implementation. Cost tracking should continue during the expansion of program assets to quantify efficiency gains as the maintenance program expands and workflows and protocols are standardized.

Tracking O&M costs. The Environmental & Water Resources Institute (EWRI) of the American Society of Civil Engineers (ASCE) and the Water Research Foundation (WRF) published a guidance tool with recommended O&M parameters to track for SCMs, including both activities and cost data. These parameters form the basis of data entry spreadsheets and a companion database that can be used to store collected data. The report titled *Recommended Operation and Maintenance Activity and Cost Reporting Parameters for Stormwater Best Management Practices Database* (WRF, 2018) provides an overview of the database structure including tables and fields for storing maintenance records and a narrative description of the reporting parameters. The use of this type of tool will improve the basis for recommended SCM maintenance activities and frequencies, as well as whole life-cycle cost estimation. Through development of a standardized set of parameters forming a reporting protocol, practitioners will have a common basis for cost estimation and maintenance activity planning (WRF, 2018).

2.2.2 Estimating Life-Cycle Costs

The Water Research Foundation has conducted several projects to support the development of life-cycle costs of stormwater infrastructure, including SCM maintenance. The Water Research Foundation, though its researchers, found that the annual maintenance costs of SCMs varied considerably between agencies, for different SCM types, sizes, and by party responsible. One of the reasons for this variation were the wide range of maintenance practices and preferences that were noted over the many agencies and organizations in the United States and the United Kingdom that participated in the WRF study. As expected, differences in geography (climate, topography, soils, etc.), culture (aesthetics, materials, program goals, etc.), and economics (availability and willingness to use financial resources) necessarily prompted a wide variety of choices in selecting and maintaining SCMs. Maintenance budgets were found to be established largely by market-driven factors rather than based on technical or functional inputs. Essentially no agency or council interviewed by WRF researchers had the resources to fully maintain the best management practice (BMP)/sustainable urban drainage system in their jurisdiction to the level expected or hoped for in their maintenance guidelines (WRF, 2005).

The Environmental and Water Resource Institute and WRF have worked for several years to implement enhancements to the International BMP Database and to develop life-cycle cost tools. The following reports are good references that can be used to develop life-cycle costs:

- *Performance and Whole Life Costs of Best Management Practices and Sustainable Urban Drainage Systems* (WRF, 2005). This report includes information on basins, swales, and permeable pavements.
- *User's Guide to the BMP and LID Whole Life Cycle Cost Models, Version 2.0* (WRF, 2009). This report expands the original suite of models and includes additional SCMs (e.g., cisterns, residential rain gardens, curb-contained bioretention, and in-curb planter vaults).
- *Recommended Operation and Maintenance Activity and Cost Reporting Parameters for Stormwater Best Management Practices Database* (WRF, 2018).
- *Community-enabled Lifecycle Analysis of Stormwater Infrastructure Costs (CLASIC).* CLASIC was developed by the WRF and Colorado State University and is a user-informed screening tool that utilizes a life-cycle cost framework to provide feasibility analysis of stormwater infrastructure (Colorado State University, 2021).

3.0 MAINTENANCE CAPITAL IMPROVEMENT PROGRAM

Stormwater management requirements have been in place for many years throughout the nation, resulting in the construction of stormwater infrastructure (system and SCMs). To operate safely and effectively, SCMs require thorough maintenance performed on a regular basis as described in previous chapters. As both the number of SCMs and the reliance upon them to comply with regulatory requirements and build community resilience grows, the importance of SCM maintenance grows accordingly. However, for several reasons, SCM maintenance is often neglected or, at best, performed only sporadically. This maintenance deficiency poses a serious threat to the safe and effective operation of SCMs and to the health and safety of the people and environment they protect. The primary cause of maintenance neglect is a lack of adequate maintenance funds.

> Reliable funding, including funding for SCM maintenance, is the foundation of a successful stormwater program. Inadequate funding is the primary reason we have inadequate stormwater infrastructure and ineffective stormwater programs.

The problem of inadequate funding manifests itself in several ways, including insufficient manpower, inadequate equipment, limited inspections, and reactive and ineffective maintenance activities. There are also several reasons for the problem, including shortage of funds, poor stormwater program planning, and legal and regulatory constraints, even though most MS4 permits require that the permittee submit a copy of each fiscal year's budget including its proposed capital and O&M expenditures necessary to accomplish the activities required by the state's permit. One remedy to address this problem is to think of SCMs and the overall stormwater infrastructure as true assets that require proper planning, maintenance, and funding (New Jersey Department of Environmental Protection, 1989).

To develop sound SCM maintenance budgets and determine adequate funding levels, the use of a detailed breakdown of costs and a comprehensive database to track those costs, described above, as well as the use of an asset management system (see Chapter 6), will facilitate the development of a maintenance capital improvement program (CIP). The cost of maintaining SCMs depend on several variables such as:

- SCM type, size, and the number of SCMs;
- SCM location within the watershed (i.e., area served or loading ratio);
- Annual precipitation;
- Age of the SCM;
- Design and construction standards used that influence the materials selected; and
- Frequency of maintenance.

A maintenance CIP can be used by a utility or municipality to prioritize which SCM or system maintenance projects should be funded each year within the planning horizon (e.g., 5 to 10 years). Typical maintenance CIPs include (adapted from a Freese and Nichols blog post in 2020):

- A list of proposed CIP projects prioritized based on an established criteria developed in coordination with management and with the support of elected officials. The criteria can be equally weighted or include weights to reflect community priorities. Examples of criteria used to rank projects include life and structure safety, potential infrastructure damage, project cost, frequency of flooding, and maintenance needs.
- Descriptions of the CIP proposed projects focusing on the benefits to the citizens of the stormwater program and the maintenance projects and describing how these projects address specific community problems.

- Estimated costs for each project (planning, design, permitting, construction) and maintenance project (using the budget components described earlier in this chapter).

It is important to align the maintenance CIP to the requirements and priorities of the utility or municipality CIP and budget development process. The tracking of maintenance cost data and the use of a criteria that has internal and external buy-in will facilitate acceptance of the projects and approval of the maintenance CIP.

Maintenance CIP projects are focused on SCMs that are publicly maintained. However, some communities are assuming the maintenance of some or all of the privately constructed and maintained SCMs. For example, Prince William County, VA, and Montgomery County, MD, developed programs to take over maintenance of different types of privately maintained facilities as part of the adoption of stormwater utilities. A principal reason for this trend appears to be a desire for better maintenance programs. There also seems to be a generally held perception among stormwater professionals that it is impractical to hold private property owners responsible for the full range of maintenance functions required to keep SCMs operating as designed over their useful life, particularly when major corrective or nonroutine maintenance and repairs are needed (Metropolitan Washington Council of Governments, 1983). In these cases, the need for a maintenance CIP becomes even more important to ensure that appropriate funding is available to take the additional maintenance responsibilities.

4.0 REFERENCES

Colorado State University. (2021). *Community-enabled lifecycle analysis of stormwater infrastructure costs* (CLASIC).

Houle, J. J., Roseen, R., Ballestero, T., & Puls, T. (2013). Comparison of maintenance cost, labor demands, and system performance for LID and conventional stormwater systems. *Journal of Environmental Engineering, 139*(7), 932–938.

Metropolitan Washington Council of Governments. (1983). *An evaluation of the costs of stormwater management pond construction and maintenance.*

Minnesota Pollution Control Agency. (2011). *Best management practices construction costs, maintenance costs, and land requirements.*

New Jersey Department of Environmental Protection. (1989, June). *Ocean county demonstration study: Stormwater management facilities maintenance manual.*

Philadelphia Water Department. (2016). *Green city, clean waters evaluation and adaptation plan.*

Water Research Foundation. (2005). *Performance and whole life costs of best management practices and sustainable urban drainage systems* (Final report for phase 2 of project 01-CTS-21T).

Water Research Foundation. (2009). *User's guide to the BMP and LID whole life cycle cost models, version 2.0* (Project SW2R08).

Water Research Foundation. (2018). *Recommended operation and maintenance activity and cost reporting parameters for stormwater best management practices database* (Project Number: SIWM22T17/4851).

5.0 SUGGESTED READING

Clary, J., & Piza, H., eds. (2017). *Cost of maintaining green infrastructure.* American Society of Civil Engineers.

8

Maintenance Scheduling

1.0 INTRODUCTION 271
1.1 Maintenance Scheduling Scenarios 272
1.1.1 Regularly Scheduled or Routine Maintenance 272
1.1.2 Postinspection Ad-Hoc Maintenance 272
1.1.3 Maintenance During Inspection 272
1.1.4 Emergency or Nonroutine Maintenance 273
1.1.5 Inspection During Maintenance 273
2.0 CONSIDERATIONS, PRIORITIES, AND TOOLS FOR SCHEDULING MAINTENANCE 273
2.1 Considerations for Setting Schedules for Activities, Crews, Equipment, and Routes 273
2.1.1 Predictability of Maintenance Activity 274
2.1.2 Availability of Workforce and Equipment 274
2.1.3 Availability of Maintenance Products and Materials 275
2.1.4 Seasonal Workload 275
2.1.5 Seasonal Species Conflicts 276
2.1.6 Seasonal Access 276
2.1.7 Logistics and Work Schedules 276
2.1.8 Regional Factors 277
2.2 Prioritization 277
2.3 Scheduling Tools 278
3.0 ADAPTIVE MANAGEMENT PROCESS TO OPTIMIZE SCHEDULING 278
4.0 REFERRAL TO THE DESIGN PROFESSIONAL 280
5.0 REFERENCES 281

1.0 INTRODUCTION

Strategic and informed inspection and maintenance scheduling of stormwater control measures (SCMs) is critical to minimizing cost while maintaining an adequate level of service. Cost inefficiencies are the result of unnecessary inspections and maintenance, suboptimal logistics, or scheduling more staff and equipment than necessary to complete a job. The goal of scheduled maintenance is to minimize these inefficiencies and needless inspections while avoiding substantial loss of service. However, where service life is unknown or unpredictable, reactive maintenance may save costs until a schedule can be predicted. For example, in one study, scheduling the scraping of a sand filter annually would result in maintenance being performed two to three times more frequently than needed, which was determined by letting the system operate to failure (Caltrans, 2004). The same study also demonstrated that with frequent inspections, the desired annual maintenance frequency for certain drain inlet inserts was not frequent enough to maintain the desired level of service. In that case, drain inlet inserts required cleaning after most storm events, but cleaning also varied by location rather than by inlet insert type. This suggests that scheduled maintenance is difficult to predict without a fairly frequent inspection program that can then be later relaxed once regular maintenance intervals are established. This chapter therefore presents an adaptive management process for determining the optimal inspection and maintenance cycle for SCMs, as well as scenarios where unexpected maintenance may necessitate consultation with a design professional for a problematic SCM location.

1.1 Maintenance Scheduling Scenarios

Four maintenance scheduling scenarios are described to support the discussion in this chapter: regularly scheduled, postinspection, during inspection, and emergency maintenance.

1.1.1 Regularly Scheduled or Routine Maintenance

Regularly scheduled or routine maintenance is not predicated by an inspection; instead, it is predictable (e.g., seasonal mowing). Regularly scheduled or routine maintenance is also known as preventive maintenance because the associated activities reduce the development of larger, more expensive maintenance issues. For example, regular litter and debris removal from detention basins may reduce the fouling of screens that protect the discharge orifice.

1.1.2 Postinspection Ad-Hoc Maintenance

Ad-hoc maintenance is scheduled after a need is identified during an inspection. It is challenging to develop an optimal daily schedule for ad-hoc maintenance activities that might occur across several locations. Section 2 presents logistical strategies.

1.1.3 Maintenance During Inspection

Performing minor maintenance during a routine inspection can greatly improve the overall efficiency of maintaining SCMs by eliminating a stop by maintenance crews. Candidate maintenance activities for an inspector can be performed quickly and safely with hand tools and basic personal protective equipment. For example, sometimes a detention basin orifice will clog when small material like pine needles passes through the protective screen and bridges the opening. In this case, major maintenance is not needed and simply poking through the orifice with a slender rod will restore the function of the basin. A thoughtful equipment list for inspectors can enhance their capability to perform minor maintenance during an inspection (see Chapter 9).

1.1.4 Emergency or Nonroutine Maintenance

Emergency or nonroutine maintenance requires the immediate diversion of maintenance crews to address a condition that threatens life or property. Emergency or nonroutine maintenance needs can be identified during an SCM inspection, by first responders to accidents or other hazardous situations, by citizen complaints, or by personnel from other departments (e.g., flood control). Embankment repairs are an example of emergency or nonroutine maintenance.

1.1.5 Inspection During Maintenance

Inspections can also occur during maintenance visits. At least one of the maintenance crew must be cross-trained to perform the inspections needed at that time. Regularly scheduled maintenance visits may be better candidates to include an inspection than ad-hoc maintenance visits because they can be more easily aligned with the required inspection frequency.

2.0 CONSIDERATIONS, PRIORITIES, AND TOOLS FOR SCHEDULING MAINTENANCE

Determining an initial schedule for inspection and maintenance is challenging without direct experience. When developing an initial SCM inspection and maintenance schedule, consider local factors, regional experience, and priorities. Then, scheduling tools can be used to develop specific crew and equipment assignments.

2.1 Considerations for Setting Schedules for Activities, Crews, Equipment, and Routes

Some considerations for setting a maintenance schedule include predictability, availability, seasonal workload, seasonal species, logistics, and regional factors.

2.1.1 Predictability of Maintenance Activity

The more predictable a maintenance activity, the easier it is to include that activity in a regular schedule and reduce ad-hoc and emergency maintenance activities. Seasonal vegetation management is one example. Other items may be predictable with experience. For example, it is common to scrape off the top 50 mm (2 in.) of sand filters, but only experience will determine which locations need scraping every other year or longer. Over time, the cost difference becomes substantial, even if the frequency is extended by just a year for some of the filters. So, honing in on the optimal maintenance frequency will maximize service while minimizing cost.

2.1.2 Availability of Workforce and Equipment

Crews and equipment should be scheduled based on capability and availability. By considering the operations and maintenance (O&M) needs of all SCMs, strategically equipping vehicles (see Chapter 7) can allow crew and equipment combinations to serve multiple needs and improve overall efficiency. This must be balanced against the increased cost of assigning a higher value crew and equipment combination to a lower value activity.

A key factor in scheduling crews and equipment is travel time and length of activity. For example, if a two-person crew and a service truck has completed a half-day job an hour away from the corporation yard, it may be more efficient for them to cycle through inspections and minor repairs in the vicinity of that job rather than to deploy a single person in an inspection vehicle. To illustrate these trade-offs, Table 8.1 details potential crew and equipment assignments for activity types. Assigning a high-cost crew and equipment combination to a lower cost activity may be advantageous in cases where the higher cost crew is already deployed near the target location. The total cost of maintenance by that crew at that location is compared

TABLE 8.1 Matrix of Activity Types and Potential Crew and Equipment Assignments

			Equipment-Related Cost		
Activity Type	Relative Frequency	Relative Cost	Inspection Vehicle $	Service Truck $$	Service Truck + Heavy Equipment $$$
Inspections	High	$	X	X	
Minor repairs	High	$	X	X	
Major repairs	Medium	$$		X	X
Reconstruction or rehabilitation	Low	$$$		X	X

to the cost of a lower cost crew that may have a longer travel time. Other issues affecting logistics are discussed in Section 2.1.7.

Another factor to consider is the capability and training of personnel to perform a variety of tasks because many tasks require specialized training. A cross-trained workforce can enable both maintenance during inspection and inspection during maintenance. Specialized inspector training is of particular importance because of the need to understand the maintenance threshold, the operation of the SCM, and assigning the appropriate level of maintenance. Safety training can also be a limiting factor. Confined-space entry, materials handling, and equipment operation each require specific training that may limit the ability of staff to cover a multitude of activities. The cost of cross-training staff should be weighed against the cost of separate trips for specialized staff.

Rent or own decisions are also important, especially for optimizing maintenance programs for smaller municipalities that may not be able to consistently use equipment. Renting becomes more economically attractive when equipment is not used regularly. For smaller municipalities, sharing equipment across departments may be another solution. In this case, increased coordination will be required to schedule shared equipment.

2.1.3 Availability of Maintenance Products and Materials

Maintenance should also be scheduled around the availability of the product required for the activity. If the product is seasonally available, then consider the storage requirements or schedule the maintenance around the availability of the product. Mulch, woodchips, and certain plantings are examples of products that have variable availability in some communities. For both scheduled and emergency maintenance, consider the products that are needed and order them in advance.

2.1.4 Seasonal Workload

Seasonal activities are difficult to defer because some of them can have an immediate effect on proper drainage and public safety. The most common example is leaf fall. Also consider tourism and the effect of large gatherings and scheduled events on trash and debris. Scheduling seasonal workloads can be challenging when using municipal staff because of other ongoing maintenance requirements, limitations on available work hours, and increased cost of overtime work. Consequently, consider scheduling annual maintenance items throughout other parts of the year and reserve time for seasonal workload activities. Where nonseasonal maintenance activities cannot be adequately scheduled throughout the year to accommodate a high seasonal workload, contracted services may prove cost effective.

2.1.5 Seasonal Species Conflicts

Species conflicts are common throughout the United States. In the Caltrans BMP Retrofit Pilot Study, nesting seasons (least tern) and larval development (salt marsh skipper) affected maintenance schedules for several SCMs (Caltrans, 2004). Consultation with resource agencies or a professional biologist may be helpful in identifying potential conflicts. In some cases, those conflicts are site-specific and may require field surveys.

2.1.6 Seasonal Access

Seasonal access must also be considered when scheduling. In some cases, SCMs are integrated into existing flood control features, which may be inundated for prolonged periods during the wet season.

2.1.7 Logistics and Work Schedules

Logistics should be optimized to minimize cost rather than merely considering travel times. Route scheduling, work sequencing, and crew and equipment assignments can be optimized by commercially available computer software, such as MS Excel add-ins Solver, Evolver, What'sBest, CPLEX, or LINDO. More information on optimization and routing can be found in references by Toth and Vigo (2002) and Rardin (1998). The length of the maintenance activity affects logistics and scheduling of appropriate crew and equipment combinations. For example, an activity that requires a two-person crew for a day and half requires four-person trips. If the activity can be accomplished in a single day by a three-person crew, only three-person trips would be required. The primary cost savings, in this case, is the roundtrip travel time of one person to the job site. Logistics could also inform whether an alternative work schedule might be beneficial. For example, cost could be minimized if a 10-hour workday would reduce the number of days spent on typical maintenance projects.

The type of maintenance activity also affects logistics. It may be more efficient to assign crews and equipment for a specific type of maintenance activity for cases where more than one site can be serviced in a single day. Take, for example, three different routine maintenance activities: vegetation management, mulching, and sediment removal. A single crew and equipment combination may not have the capacity to perform more than one of these activities. Vegetation management will require equipment for trimming and removal, as well as the ability to transport material off site. A mulching operation may require spreading equipment and the ability to transport material to the site. Sediment removal operations may require heavier equipment to remove and transport sediment. Creating separate routes for each activity increases efficiency when more than one location can be serviced in a day. The resulting routes may not be for a specific SCM because maintenance activities can be common across SCM types. For example, vegetation management commonly occurs for SCM types with earthen components such as strips, swales, detention basins, bioretention, and infiltration basins.

The logistics for ad hoc maintenance can be difficult to optimize for smaller maintenance activities. If possible, consider planning a lag between inspections and maintenance scheduling. The lag will create a small but manageable backlog of ad-hoc maintenance work items. Then, the logistics of scheduling from that backlog of maintenance items can be optimized by assigning items to more efficient routes.

2.1.8 Regional Factors

Climate and landcover will cause different inspection and maintenance needs within a particular SCM. For example, vegetation management and mulching vary substantially with climate. Typical frequencies are presented in Table 8.2. Neighboring jurisdictions may have more experience with some SCMs and may also share common factors, such as climate and landcover. Chapter 5 presents maintenance indicators and a typical inspection schedule, which provides a good starting point that can be adjusted based on climate and then revised with experience.

2.2 Prioritization

Prioritization only works when maintenance crews are adequately staffed, and the asset condition information is available. If not, an unsustainable

TABLE 8.2 Typical Inspection and Maintenance Schedule for Vegetation Management and Mulching by Generalized Climate Conditions

Maintenance Category	Arid/Desert/ Mediterranean (Limited Wet Season and Extended Dry Season)[a]	Rainforest or Year-Round Growth/Rain	Harsh Winter, Humid/Wet Summer[c]
Vegetation trimming or mowing	Annually to biannually	Quarterly	Monthly, except winter
Mulching	2–3 years	Annually[b]	Biannually

[a]California Stormwater Quality Association, 2003
[b]Herrera Environmental Consultants & Washington Stormwater Center, 2013
[c]Prince George's County, Environmental Services Division, 2007

backlog of lower priority maintenance items will be left untouched until neglect eventually raises maintenance to a higher priority (at higher cost and lower level of service). A ranking system can be developed for prioritization, but it should also factor in delays so that service requests rise in priority over time. This will help keep small problems from becoming big ones. Asset management (Chapter 6) tools often provide prioritization function because the risk calculation within those tools considers service, consequences of failure, and probability of failure. Potential prioritization considerations include

- Safety of people and property,
- Cost of deferred maintenance,
- Hydraulic level of service,
- Water quality level of service,
- Multibenefit level of service (ecology, community, etc.),
- Aesthetics, and
- Customer complaints.

2.3 Scheduling Tools

Scheduling tools communicate what needs to be done, where, and when by generating work orders or service tags. Many asset management tools (e.g., Maximo) can accomplish this by generating work orders that get picked up by maintenance supervisors and assigned to staff (see Chapter 6). Simpler tools like Gantt charts and electronic calendar tools can be used to schedule, assign, and track maintenance.

3.0 ADAPTIVE MANAGEMENT PROCESS TO OPTIMIZE SCHEDULING

Adaptive management of an SCM maintenance program offers greater efficiency because optimal maintenance is often determined by regional or even location-specific experience. Maintenance activities will vary by SCM type, and these activities are fairly well known (Chapter 5). However, the frequency of maintenance activities for a single SCM type can vary substantially by location. Consequently, the same SCM type may have different frequencies of maintenance activities based on location-specific factors. Location-specific factors (e.g., vegetation type and density within the drainage area) have an effect on maintenance frequency that is difficult to quantify, so maintenance frequency must be determined by experience.

An adaptive management process, which complements or is served by the asset management functions of a stormwater O&M program (see Chapter 6), is illustrated in Figure 8.1. The first step is SCM commissioning (SWC for stormwater control in Figure 8.1), including a maintenance plan with minimum inspection frequencies and expected maintenance intervals.

In Step 2, a break-in period is suggested following the commissioning of the SCM to allow a period of intense inspection and maintenance that is sometimes needed in the early life of an SCM. Break-in operations (typically 1 to 3 years) include a period for vegetation establishment and seasoning of filtration media, if used in the SCM.

In Step 3, trends are evaluated toward the end of the break-in operations. If maintenance needs become less or more frequent, inspection frequency and maintenance plans should be updated. If regular maintenance needs increase with time, this may indicate a design flaw and consultation with a design professional may help identify potential structural improvements (see Section 4.0).

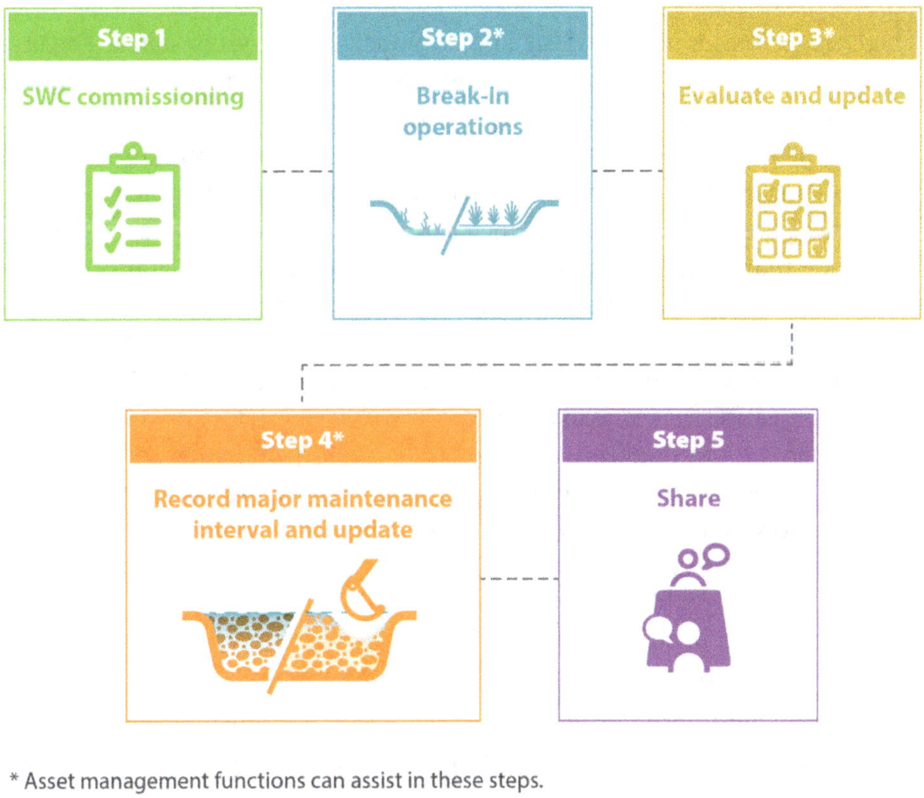

FIGURE 8.1 Adaptive Management Process to Determine Optimal Maintenance Scheduling

The revised maintenance plan is implemented in Step 4 until a major maintenance interval has occurred, such as reconditioning of media or reconstruction of subsurface storage. Compare this interval to the expected interval and adjust the maintenance plan as needed. If the major maintenance interval is substantially less than expected, consider consulting with a design professional.

Finally, in Step 5, findings are shared. Potential target audiences include staff and consultant teams that perform asset management planning, community involvement, procurement, personnel, staff supervision, and maintenance activities. Also, consider publishing your results so that other municipalities can benefit from your experience.

Chapter 9 suggests recordkeeping and data management protocols that will assist in the refinement of O&M scheduling. Maintenance staff will provide critical feedback throughout this process, so consider how that feedback can be captured in your recordkeeping.

4.0 REFERRAL TO THE DESIGN PROFESSIONAL

There are two cases where a design professional should be consulted. The first is for major SCM rehabilitation that involves the reconstruction of drainage features. This is a good opportunity for the design professional to consider advancements in the design of that particular SCM and integrate them into the reconstruction of the SCM. The other is an excessive maintenance burden, where the required maintenance activity is occurring at a much higher frequency than anticipated in the maintenance plan. This scenario is more likely where no SCM commissioning standards are in place. In these cases, the SCM may need to be redesigned, reconstructed, or even decommissioned in favor of an SCM at an alternative location. Inadequate O&M access is a common cause for excessive maintenance because of increased labor or requirements for specialized access training and equipment.

Just a few examples of potential structural improvements that could mitigate inordinately frequent maintenance include

- Improving scour protection for influent and effluent;
- Improving drainage or infiltration to reduce emergent vegetation and vector control activities;
- Reducing internal SCM erosion by engineered options such as curbing, reinforced matting, benching, contour grading, or retaining walls; and
- Adding sediment or litter pretreatment areas to focus maintenance activity location.

5.0 REFERENCES

California Stormwater Quality Association. (2003). *Stormwater best management practice handbook: New development and redevelopment.*

Caltrans. (2004). *BMP retrofit pilot program: Final report.* California Department of Transportation.

Herrera Environmental Consultants & Washington Stormwater Center. (2013). *Western Washington low impact development (LID) operation and maintenance (O&M).* Washington State Department of Ecology.

Prince George's County, Environmental Services Division. (2007). *Bioretention manual.*

Rardin, R. L. (1998). *Optimization in operations research.* Prentice Hall.

Toth, P., & Vigo, D. (2002). *The vehicle routing problem.* Society for Industrial and Applied Mathematics.

9

Operations and Maintenance Forms, Logs, and Reporting

1.0 IMPORTANCE OF TRACKING AND REPORTING INSPECTIONS AND MAINTENANCE 284
- 1.1 Importance of Inspections and Maintenance During Construction 284
- 1.2 Importance of Inspections and Maintenance During Operation 287

2.0 COMPONENTS OF STANDARD OPERATING PROCEDURES FOR THE SUCCESSFUL OPERATIONS AND MAINTENANCE OF STORMWATER CONTROL MEASURES 292
- 2.1 Coordination, Responsibilities, and Communication Protocols 292
- 2.2 Health and Safety Plans and Incident/Near-Miss Reporting 293
- 2.3 Data Collection, Processing, Reporting, and Recordkeeping 294
  - *2.3.1 Data Collection* 294
  - *2.3.2 Reporting and Processing* 294
  - *2.3.3 Recordkeeping* 295
- 2.4 Public Outreach 295
- 2.5 Enforcement 296

3.0 CONSIDERATIONS FOR THE DEVELOPMENT OF INSPECTION FORMS 297
- 3.1 Stormwater Control Measure Inventory and Relevant Information 298
- 3.2 Importance of Rainfall Data 300
- 3.3 Tools, Databases, and Systems Utilized for Inventory and Data Management 301
- 3.4 Typical Stormwater Control Measure Concerns During Construction 301
  - *3.4.1 Vegetated Swales and Strips* 301
  - *3.4.2 Basins* 302
    - *3.4.2.1 Dry Basins* 302
    - *3.4.2.2 Wet Basins* 302
    - *3.4.2.3 Swirl Concentrators and Vaults* 302
  - *3.4.3 Filters* 303
    - *3.4.3.1 Media Filters* 303
    - *3.4.3.2 Bioretention Filters* 303
    - *3.4.3.3 Inlet Basket* 304
    - *3.4.3.4 Landscaped Roofs* 304
  - *3.4.4 Infiltration* 304
    - *3.4.4.1 Infiltration Trench* 304
    - *3.4.4.2 Infiltration Basin* 305
    - *3.4.4.3 Pervious Pavement* 305
  - *3.4.5 Catch Basins* 306
  - *3.4.6 Gross Pollutant Controls* 306
- 3.5 Typical Stormwater Control Measure Concerns During Operation 307

3.5.1 *Vegetated Swales and Strips* 307
3.5.2 *Basins* 308
3.5.2.1 *Dry Basins* 308
3.5.2.2 *Wet Basins* 309
3.5.2.3 *Swirl Concentrators and Vaults* 309
3.5.3 *Filters* 310
3.5.3.1 *Media Filters* 310
3.5.3.2 *Bioretention Filters* 310
3.5.3.3 *Inlet Basket* 310
3.5.3.4 *Landscaped Roofs* 311
3.5.4 *Infiltration* 311
3.5.4.1 *Infiltration Trench* 311
3.5.4.2 *Infiltration Basin* 311
3.5.4.3 *Pervious Pavement* 312
3.5.5 *Catch Basins* 312
3.5.6 *Gross Pollutant Controls* 312
4.0 SAMPLE INSPECTION AND MAINTENANCE REPORTING FORMS 313
4.1 Inspection Forms During Construction 313
4.2 Inspection Forms During Operations and Maintenance 314
5.0 SUMMARY 316
6.0 REFERENCES 344

1.0 IMPORTANCE OF TRACKING AND REPORTING INSPECTIONS AND MAINTENANCE

Section 1.0 introduces the importance of tracking, recordkeeping, and reporting inspections and maintenance activities to achieve an effective operations and maintenance (O&M) program for stormwater control measures (SCMs) and streamline the implementation of the inspection forms. The discussion includes the difference between preventive and corrective maintenance and presents typical activities encountered during both construction and operation.

1.1 Importance of Inspections and Maintenance During Construction

During construction, it is important to ensure the SCMs have been manufactured, installed, and/or constructed according to plans and specifications. SCM failure is not always related to design, operation, or maintenance; at times, failure is attributed to inadequate construction.

Going from the obvious need of appropriate grading to ensure stormwater flows in the right direction for the SCM to operate correctly, to others that are less obvious, such as appropriate layering of different components in a media, all are important construction factors to ensure the long-term operation for the SCM.

Examples of the different parameters that are critical during construction have been discussed in Chapters 4 and 5 and typically include basic specifications such as location, dimensions, grading of the site (flow lines or elevation of different components), type and density of plantings, establishment of vegetation (including irrigation needs), soil media amendments, rock gradation, and so on.

There are other, less intuitive, and yet important specifications typically required during construction that the stormwater professional would need to verify to ensure the proper functioning of the SCM. Some examples are provided below.

For some SCMs, there may be instruments and controls specified during construction that are a critical component for its O&M. Those instruments and controls may be as simple as a catch basin or vault paint markings or as sophisticated as electrical or solar panel real-time controllers that may transmit real-time information related to flood stage, pressure, velocity, total suspended solids, or other parameters. Instructions for the installations would typically be provided as part of the specification and bid documents for the SCM project.

Additionally, there would be other temporary controls during construction necessary to protect water quality and potentially to comply with other regulatory requirements. For example, there may be necessary temporary erosion and sediment control practices, buffer zones to protect sensitive areas, and other permit requirements that should be considered. These elements are not directly related to the long-term O&M of the SCM; however, they are important additional measures that should be in place during construction, so there are no additional concerns.

Finally, besides the prescribed planting plans associated with some vegetated SCMs, there will typically be some final stabilization plans associated with many SCMs (unless the SCM occurs in asphalt or concrete covered areas) where the disturbed areas are revegetated to prevent long-term erosion issues. Inspections would verify that both planting plans and stabilization measures have been completed and that the vegetation has been established. In general, ground stabilization is typically considered completed when a minimum of a 70% coverage has been achieved. It is not unusual to have a multiyear maintenance contract with the installation contractors to ensure that vegetation and stabilization are established for an SCM. Inspections must ensure that progress is being made toward achieving a stable and healthy, vegetative plant coverage.

Figure 9.1 may be utilized to illustrate critical design features to verify during construction or installation for a snout and a rain garden. For a swirl concentrator (for trash and sediment removal), major inspection items during construction would include verifying the vault and pipes sizes, appropriate flow lines to ensure positive flow, and access points for inspection. For the rain garden, critical factors will include ensuring the grading is correctly placed so runoff flows according to plans and specifications, type and distribution

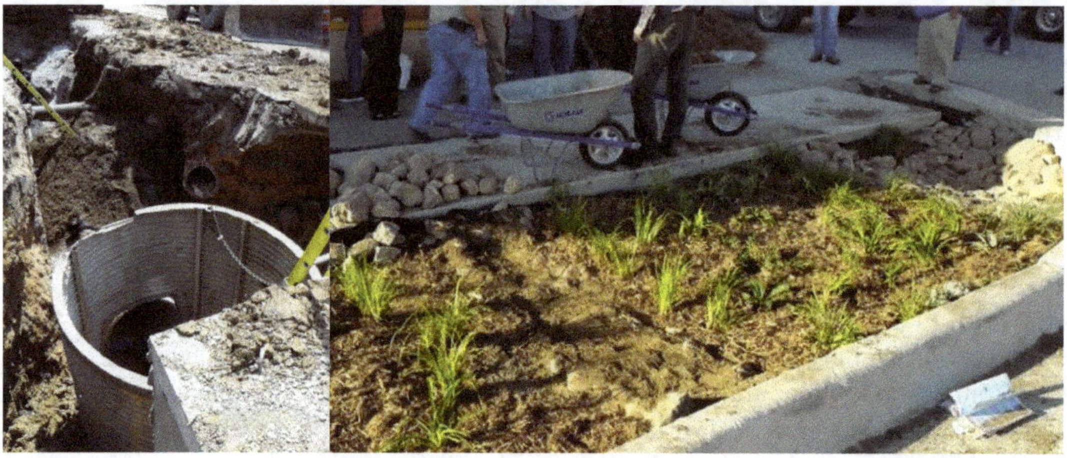

FIGURE 9.1 Swirl Concentrator and Rain Garden During Construction Installation

of plants, soil amendments (topsoil, mulch, engineering soil, etc.), size and distribution of rocks, verifying underdrain and overflow structures, filter placement and media condition, and use of geotextiles or other materials.

It is understood the SCMs will not be in operation until construction is finalized. Therefore, maintenance activities during construction would be limited to the maintenance practices necessary to keep up the temporary erosion and sedimentation control practices as well as any other good housekeeping practices typically practiced during construction. Therefore, only inspection forms and not maintenance forms would be needed during construction phases, as the maintenance activities for erosion control and plantings will typically be performed by those constructing/installing the SCM.

The inspection forms during construction would generally collect the following information:

- Conformance with plans and specifications (SCM location, configuration, measurements, grading, anchoring, configuration, type of materials employed, equipment, construction of access areas needed for O&M, verification of compliance with planting plan).
- Necessary testing: Operation of moving parts, testing of hydraulic performance and structural integrity, and noncompaction of soils.
- Verification of conformance with temporary erosion and sedimentation controls and any other temporary measures. Verification of removal of those temporary measures upon completion of construction.
- Completion of permanent final stabilization.
- Postconstruction: If an as-built survey is prepared, an inspection may be conducted to ensure the as-built conforms to the original plans and

specifications. If there is a variance from them, verify that the variance will not affect the performance of the SCM.

1.2 Importance of Inspections and Maintenance During Operation

To ensure proper design performance and achievement of intended water quality objectives, SCM require inspection, operation, and maintenance in perpetuity. However, the nature of the need for maintenance activities is dynamic in nature, as they are highly influenced by a variety of factors affecting both runoff discharges and the nature and loading of pollutants present in such discharges.

For any given SCM, and assuming no changes in the drainage area contributing to such an SCM, runoff discharges change not only according to seasons but also according to climatologic patterns and trends. While an area may have months within a given year that are wetter than others, some years are wetter than others. Unless the SCMs are properly maintained, some SCM will accumulate pollutants transported by runoff (e.g., sediment, nutrients, trash, leaves, and other floatable debris), decreasing its removal efficiency over time. In many instances, this accumulation could also result in a reduction in the efficiency to convey flow, as many of these pollutants could also plug or block the SCM. The more runoff received by the SCM, the more frequently maintenance will be needed to sustain optimal operation.

For a runoff contributing area that does not change through time, given the runoff remains constant, the nature of pollutants loading to an SCM may vary based on different factors related to the activities taking place within the drainage area. For example, changes in land use or zoning would produce a different composition of the pollutants received by the SCM. Construction activities within an SCM drainage area would typically increase the loading of sediment or total suspended solids expected at that control. Even a special event, such as a city parade, may generate a higher load of floatables and other trash as compared to the loadings occurring during routine days in the city.

Inspection activities would ensure the SCMs are working satisfactorily and safely—or otherwise would determine the needs of maintenance. Conducting inspections over time would determine trends that would help optimize frequencies for maintenance. However, it is important to keep in mind that a large portion of the cost associated with an O&M program is the mobilization of the crew and equipment to conduct such operations. Therefore, the efficiency of an O&M program would be in great part determined by the frequency with which these inspections and O&M activities would be conducted. Optimal frequency will be dependent on the factors discussed above (e.g., contributing drainage area, expected runoff, activities taking place within the watershed, etc.). Frequency of maintenance for each SCM is discussed in detail in Chapter 5.

Tracking, reviewing, and analyzing historical records of inspection and O&M activities would allow the stormwater professional to identify trends and determine site-specific and condition-specific frequencies with which to conduct inspection and O&M activities. This is comparable to having a lifelong experienced employee conducting this activity who has developed a "feel" of when the SCMs need to be inspected and maintained. However, keeping these records and analyzing them more systematically allows for independence from this institutional knowledge, which might be accumulated in just a few individuals and could be lost if those individuals leave without passing that knowledge to others in the institution, thus making the process more systematic and controlled so it can become programmatic and adaptive. Adaptive management can be adopted once the user from these records can determine trigger events that may lead to increased or decreased O&M. It also allows an O&M program to be proactive in providing preventive maintenance, as opposed to allowing the SCM to become overloaded. An overload condition can either produce an overflow, which can lead to a violation of a water quality requirement; or even result in a more complicated maintenance issue and subsequently a more intense need for corrective measures, which could have been prevented had action been taken sooner.

In the absence of historical maintenance data, or conjunction with the analysis of this data, an ArcGIS data analysis is a useful tool to help the stormwater professional determine an adequate site-specific frequency for inspection and O&M activities. Predictions could be determined from the analysis of key watershed factors including the type of soils and their relative degree of erodibility, canopy cover, percent of impervious area, proximity to riparian protected areas, and impaired streams. What this means is that, in the absence of historical inspection information, the stormwater professional could use tools such as ArcGIS data analysis to develop a maintenance predictive analytics tool to help better forecast routine and nonroutine maintenance scheduling (Caldwell, 2020).

The inspection forms will collect the type of maintenance the SCM will require at a given point in time. Maintenance needs could be either preventive (or routine), or corrective (nonroutine or major). For additional information regarding the different types and frequencies of maintenance, please refer to Chapters 4 and 5 of this manual. Preventive maintenance activities are routine and needed on a relatively frequent basis to promote the continuous proper operation of the SCM. Corrective maintenance activities are more involved and occur when something has broken or requires a more intense and time-consuming operation to bring the SCM back to the appropriate level of service. Although corrective maintenance generally can be minimized with good preventive maintenance practices, every SCM during its life cycle will require corrective maintenance at some point. Corrective maintenance may simply be a long-term need for the SCM to conserve its proper function. For example, a wet pond, irrespective of how well it is designed and preventively maintained, will accumulate sediment through time. Eventually, the accumulation may be such that the dredging of the material may be warranted. Dredging represents corrective maintenance, but the need for it is not necessarily associated with a poor preventive maintenance program.

The inspection forms will capture the information necessary to assess the overall condition of the SCM. At times, whether maintenance will be routine or corrective will depend on the degree of malfunctioning of the issue observed during the inspection. A good form will provide mechanisms to capture those details. The forms provided in this chapter will guide the user to ensure those strategies are carefully captured in the forms. During the operation of an inspection, the inspector would generally collect the following information:

- The general appearance of the SCM (evidence of tampering, vandalism, broken or missing pieces, failures, securing confined spaces, missing locks or gates, etc.).
- Evidence of erosion.
- Evidence of flooding/overtopping.
- Evidence of excessive vegetation overgrowth or invasive weed growth.
- Presence of trash or any other debris or waste.
- Evidence of blockage, fouling, or other obstructions in any of the components of the SCM.
- Presence of any odors.
- Presence of any unusual soil discoloration.
- Presence of unusual sheen or other unusual discoloration in the water.
- Accumulation of sediment or dirt.
- Distressed vegetation.

The type of preventive or routine maintenance expected are SCM-specific, but generally would collect information regarding the following activities:

- Minor debris and litter removal.
- Sediment and dirt removal and disposal.
- Vegetation maintenance and control.

- Erosion control.
- Minor structural maintenance (inlets, pretreatment devices, inflow and outflow structures, chambers, screens and trash racks, and pipes).
- Minor mechanical maintenance (valves, orifices, aerators, pumps, and switches).
- Porous pavement cleaning and winter maintenance.
- Media maintenance.
- Nuisance control.
- Vector management.

Figure 9.2 illustrates an example of a couple of gross pollutant removal screen devices. The first one illustrates a screen located at a stormwater outfall in which sediment and debris have accumulated—triggering the need for preventive maintenance. During an inspection, the operator would verify the level of debris in the gross pollutant removal device to determine whether preventive maintenance, in this case, debris removal, is necessary. For trash devices, preventive maintenance would occur typically between 50% and 60% trash level with respect to the screen height. Stenciled markings are typically placed next to the devices to determine the need for maintenance.

Corrective or major maintenance include the following:

- Major removal of sediment and debris.
- Major structural repairs.

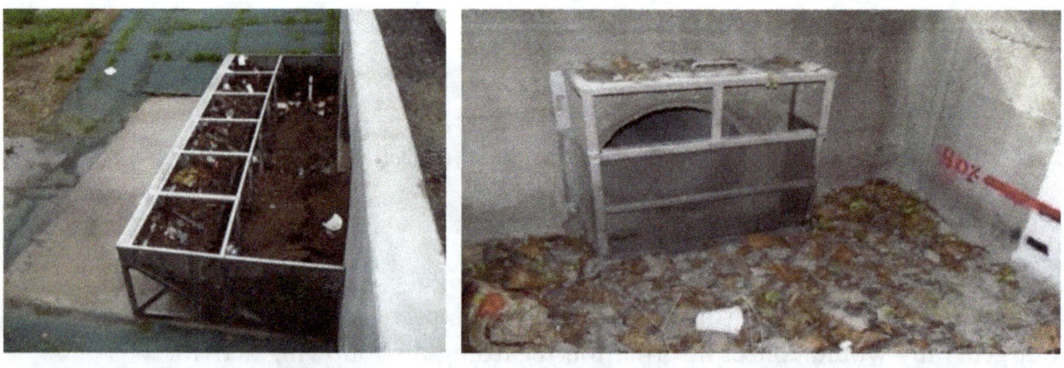

FIGURE 9.2 Gross Pollutants Screens at Outfall. Heavy Debris Accumulation Show Need of Routine or Preventive Maintenance (left); Gross Pollutant Screen Shows Stenciling Marking; the 60% Stenciling Mark Shows the Debris Level at Which the Catch Basin Will Need Routine or Preventive Maintenance (right)

- Major mechanical equipment repairs.
- Dam, embankment, and slope repairs.
- Dewatering.
- Pond maintenance.
- Vector abatement.
- Erosion/scour repair.
- Fence repair.
- Elimination of woody vegetation.
- Removal of burrowing animals.
- Snow and ice removal.
- Spills.

Figure 9.3 illustrates a form of corrective maintenance caused by scouring at an outlet flume and erosion at the inlet from two different wet detention basins.

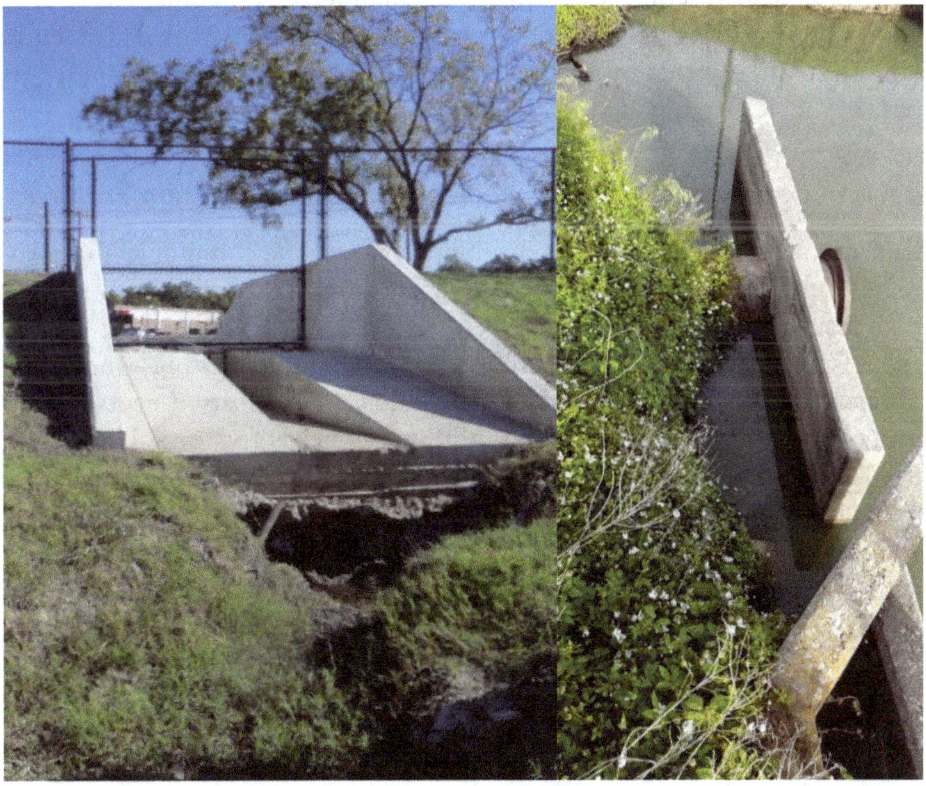

FIGURE 9.3 Scouring and Erosion at Outlet Flume and Inflow Lines from Two Wet Ponds Requiring Corrective Maintenance

As described above, the forms developed in this chapter will allow the user to determine whether the maintenance needed is simply routine or major corrective maintenance is necessary.

2.0 COMPONENTS OF STANDARD OPERATING PROCEDURES FOR THE SUCCESSFUL OPERATIONS AND MAINTENANCE OF STORMWATER CONTROL MEASURES

Section 2.0 covers the overall communication framework necessary for the implementation of an SCM O&M program and the effective use of the inspection forms. Coordination, communication, and awareness are key to the implementation of an effective and efficient O&M protocol. In many places, notifications along the forms and protocols developed for inspection and maintenance are all organized and managed as a single document in the form of standard operating procedures (SOPs) or the form of a stormwater management inspection, operation, and maintenance manual—generally defined here as SCM O&M SOP or manual (Pazwash, 2016). This section will discuss the different notifications that will need to be considered as part of the SOP manual.

2.1 Coordination, Responsibilities, and Communication Protocols

It is important to establish responsibilities, determine communication protocols, and set coordination times to ensure that necessary activities will take place and any difficulties are resolved timely.

Responsibilities must be established clearly and in writing—indicating events triggering the need for reporting and communication protocols. In writing, also, the standard should indicate the needs for formal coordination in the form of reporting (email reporting may be enough) and meetings (regularity determined on an as-needed basis). These should occur regularly so team members can ensure they are up-to-date on the status of the O&M activities—everyone at the level that should be informed.

Typical members of the O&M team may include

- O&M manager or stormwater manager,
- Field operations inspector and maintenance leader,
- Field operations inspector and maintenance crew member,
- Data manager/data analyst,

- Public outreach coordinator, and
- Code enforcement personnel.

The roles of some of these members are discussed in the next sections.

2.2 Health and Safety Plans and Incident/Near-Miss Reporting

Health and Safety Plans (H&S Plans), introduced in Chapter 4, and Incident/Near-Miss Reporting are important when conducting inspection and maintenance activities as individuals conducting these activities may be prone to incidents in the field. The entity may already have in place an H&S Plan and Incident Report system for these activities. If so, it may just be integrated as part of the SOP for the O&M activities. If one is not available, one must be developed.

Contents of the H&S Plans and Incident Reports are out of the scope of this manual, but in general, H&S Plans and Incident Reports should include the following assessment and information:

- Conduct an overall Task Hazard Assessment identifying the potential hazard for each work activity, the mitigation actions, protective measures, and stop-work criteria. An example follows:
  - For the work activity "pedestrian walking/hiking":
    - The hazards may be "exposure to traffic, exposure to heat, exposure to cold, falls/slips, confrontation with hostile residents or inhabitants, exposure to aggressive dogs or animals, exposure to natural landscape hazards—branches, debris, dust, ultraviolet exposure, exposure to venomous snakes/insect bites poisonous plants."
    - The mitigation actions may be "wear traffic personal protective equipment (PPE), long sleeves/long pants, wear layered clothing, schedule work appropriately to minimize exposure, take smaller steps, notify landowners ahead of time, keep a cell phone charged, do not react in a heated or threatening manner, use three-point contact when climbing, plan your path, use insect repellent, use PPE, tuck pants in boots and duct tape."
    - The stop-work criteria may be "escalating altercation, an aggressive animal within your immediate area, eye injury, heat stress, severe burn, injury, bites/infection, reaction to plant oil."
- Summarize all hazards identified for the project. Besides the typical hazards identified for any project such as those outlined above,

hazards associated with SCMs include exposure to vehicular traffic, confined-space entry, fall hazards, operation of heavy equipment, hearing protection around vacuum motors, and contact with contaminants, biological waste, and sharp objects.

- Summarize other safety equipment or other additional considerations (e.g., fire extinguisher, first-aid kit, portable eyewash, traffic control measures, sunscreen, bleach, disinfectant soap, and hand sanitizer).
- Indicate whether the job requires any specific training or certifications (e.g., confined-space entry, HAZWOPER, OSHA 10-hour Construction Safety, Excavation Safety Competent person, Heavy Equipment Safety).
- Emergency References: Identify ambulance, fire, and police phone numbers and the address and directions to the nearest hospital or neighborhood emergency center.
- Identify and provide contact information for personnel to report an incident or a near-miss incident.

All people who are subject to the H&S Plan and Incident Report should read and sign it.

2.3 Data Collection, Processing, Reporting, and Recordkeeping

2.3.1 Data Collection

Data collection and analysis is extremely important as it would allow the entity to learn from the process of inspection and maintenance to make it more efficient and streamline the efforts. As discussed in Section 1.2, inspection and maintenance frequencies may be recommended for an SCM, but they are only a guideline. Data collection, processing, analyzing would allow for the identification of trends and streamlining of processes.

Responsibilities were identified as part of Section 2.1. Generally, the field operations inspector and maintenance crew member or inspector would collect the information in the inspection and maintenance forms. The form may be either in paper form or electronic, depending on the level of sophistication for data collection of the entity (whether they use paper forms or tablets).

2.3.2 Reporting and Processing

If data collection is manual or semiautomatic, it would typically require some level of reporting and processing. Entities that have tablets and geodatabases or an asset management system may collect the data in the field and may be automatically uploaded into their geodatabase system and even automatically processed. More traditionally, some may collect the information in a paper or spreadsheet format. Generally, the field operations inspector and maintenance crew member or inspector and may need to report this data to someone else, typically the data manager/data analyst, who then captures and processes the data. Processing may take some form of organization and analysis, where needs may be identified. For example, a report of inspection or routine maintenance may indicate that corrective maintenance activities are needed. These may be identified by the data manager/data analyst, who in turn may need to report to someone else per the communication protocol defined as these activities are costly and may need additional approval. The data manager/data analyst would inform either the O&M manager/stormwater manager or field operations inspector and maintenance leader (as determined in 2.1) of the needed corrective issue. In turn, also as determined in 2.1 and in the timelines established, the O&M manager/stormwater manager or field operations inspector and maintenance leader would then schedule and coordinate with the field operations inspector and maintenance crew member the development of the corrective maintenance activity.

2.3.3 *Recordkeeping*

Inspection, preventive, and corrective processed data should be kept in a system so trends can be analyzed and studied. It is best to code information with numbers and to avoid text to better support easy processing of information. Instead of using traditional paper forms, users can opt to develop applications that can be used for data collection utilizing tablets or smart phones. Technology and the use of these applications would maximize the efficiency of data processing and data analytics and help the user make predictive and adaptive management. This would allow for predicting more appropriate inspection and maintenance frequencies and variations to streamline the O&M program. Recordkeeping can also help plan for expenditures and long-term plans for capital improvement projects.

2.4 Public Outreach

Public outreach has gained more importance as the community and the public are more informed and involved than ever. Public outreach has also obtained different dimensions, as it has changed from the traditional position of letting people know what is happening, to integrating the community to the new projects to make them their own. This makes more successful projects overall.

From the O&M perspective, it is important to educate the public on what the SCM is and why it needs to be operated and maintained. When they understand that, it needs act accordingly—avoiding activities that are detrimental to the proper operation of such an SCM. Also, they would understand actions that otherwise they may be traditionally against such as no mowing zones, or wildflower or wild prairie areas. This may be essential for the development of an efficient O&M program. As much as 80% of the total staff hours spent in the field in many jurisdictions are associated with grass mowing, as opposed to sediment, debris, and trash removal, or structural repair (WEF et al., 2012). While much of this effort has little effect on control performance, it is driven by the expectations of residents living near the SCM.

The public would also be more cooperative when routine and corrective maintenance may need to be conducted, and these activities may affect temporarily traffic or other areas of the community.

The best way to engage neighbors and community is through education and community outreach events. City projects such as adopt-a-stream, trash bash events, and storm inlet signage are excellent methods to actively involve the community in stormwater projects. Signage of SCMs is also recommended; it is not only needed for safety reasons, but it also helps educate the community directly on the purpose of the SCM and the way it operates—promoting good stormwater practices in the neighborhood. Signage for SCMs is helpful. For example, in "Complete Street" or "Green Infrastructure Street" projects, where the public may be educated about the different types of SCM, its goal and education about the role of the different SCMs are used in the project (Figure 9.4).

Other ideas for public outreach include engaging institutions and nonprofit organizations in different activities. For example, SCMs are abundant in schools, which are highly visible and hold a strong community identity promoting stewardship of such community. Institutions successfully involved in the past include independent school districts that participate directly in activities with stormwater in their communities (Sanchez, 2012). Nonprofits may provide resources for outreach events that also promote community stewardship to help bring awareness and promote outreach to others.

2.5 Enforcement

Code enforcement personnel may need to be involved as part of the O&M effort—specifically when there is something related to an illicit discharge or illegal dumping in connection to the SCM or the stream or stormwater network directly associated with the SCM. At instances during inspections or maintenance activities, it may be evident that some of these issues may

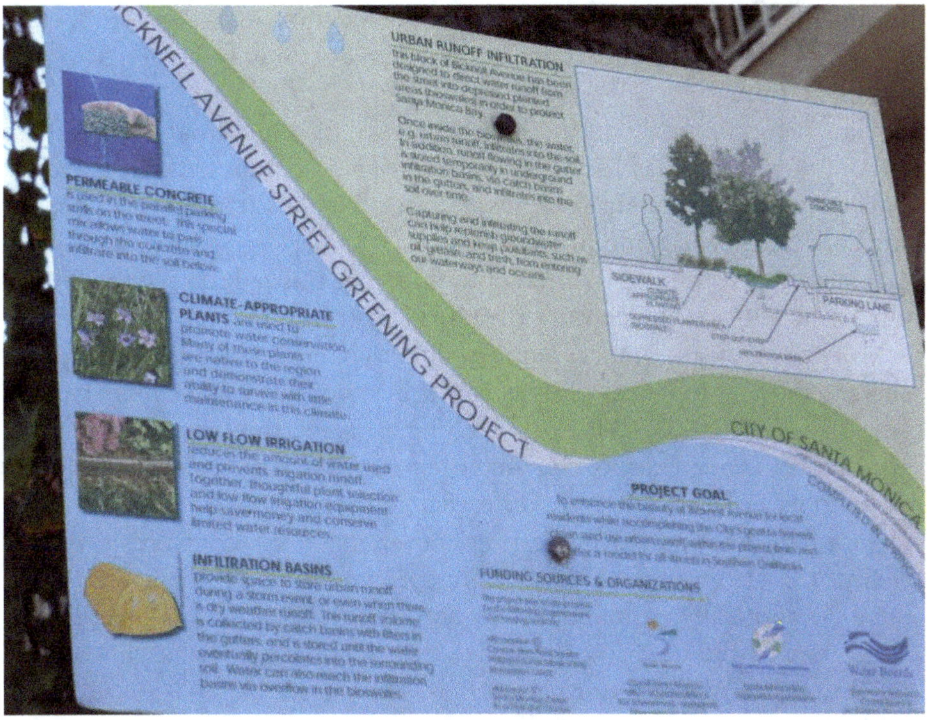

FIGURE 9.4 Signage Utilized to Provide Outreach for a "Complete Street" or "Green Infrastructure Street" Project—Each Element of Green Infrastructure Is Explained for the General Public at the "Complete Street" Project Site

be occurring at the site as indicated by unusual discharges, discoloration, odors, or even objects observed during the O&M activities.

The O&M protocols should identify what activities should take place when illicit discharges or dumping occur in the field. For example, the field operations inspector and maintenance crew member may inform the field operations inspector and maintenance leader who, depending on the severity, may indicate or take corrective action or may inform the O&M manager/stormwater manager, who may have to inform code enforcement personnel.

3.0 CONSIDERATIONS FOR THE DEVELOPMENT OF INSPECTION FORMS

Section 3.0 discusses the general considerations when developing the forms needed for the efficient O&M of SCMs. Discussion includes the inventory information of SCMs that needs to be available for the inspection and maintenance (information about their location, characteristics, etc.), data to be collected, and other supporting documentation (e.g., photo documentation).

This section also discusses the importance of rainfall data and the use of technology to display the SCM inventory (asset database/tablets) and for data collection (asset management software/tablets) that may streamline the data collection/processing process.

In terms of technology, different tools can be utilized to keep the inspection forms and for the capture of information on an O&M program for SCM. The most traditional can utilize simple spreadsheets and paper forms, whereas more sophisticated ones can utilize complex asset management tools such as those described in Chapter 6. Nevertheless, the forms and information needed to develop such templates are the same irrespective of the tools utilized. The only difference is that sophisticated tools allow for more automatic data processing and analysis, which makes for more efficient use of resources. However, irrespective of whether the data is collected electronically or manually, the information that is produced is only as effective as the quality of the data that is collected. Thus, this section emphasizes the type of information that is collected.

Although Section 4.0 provides forms for each of the SCMs discussed in this manual, it is important to note these are comprehensive and detailed forms, covering as many components for the SCM as possible. The user may use the forms as presented or may customize the forms to better conform to their needs. This section may help further refine the user's need to formulate a better suited form as it presents a section of SCM-specific concerns encountered both during construction and O&M.

3.1 Stormwater Control Measure Inventory and Relevant Information

The first step in the planning of an O&M program consists of having an adequate inventory of the SCM. Inventory of an asset first identifies ownership and ensuing responsibility for inspection and maintenance but also includes other pieces necessary to complete an efficient and effective O&M program.

- Type of SCM: What control is being inspected/maintained. Vegetated swale/strip, wet or dry basin, biofilter, inlet basket, landscaped roofs, infiltration trench, infiltration basin, pervious pavement, and catch basin.
- Location: Exact location of the SCM (could be addressed but may also provide geographic coordinates and any identifier if available).

Typically, we would have a graphic display of its location, preferably on a map that indicates not only the location of the SCM but also the drainage area contributing to the SCM and other immediate stormwater infrastructure associated with the control such as immediate pipes, inlets, manholes, and so on. This information is helpful as it would help us identify the source of a problem if one is encountered during the inspection.

- Configuration: Dimensions, orientation, and specific type (dry versus wet). Typically, as-builts are a great piece of information for inspectors, and these can be available electronically. King County, Washington, makes as-built drawings available for their inspector personnel. The New York City Department of Environmental Protection has developed maintenance cards for each control that include as-built drawings with inspection and clean-out procedures (WEF et al., 2012).
- Components: The type of components would be specific for each kind and each SCM. Components could include forebay, inlet, outlet, swale, embankment, spillway, outfall, channel, basin, catch basin, trash rack, filter, vegetation, filter media, gates, valves, pumps, and so on.
- Baseline photo documentation for each of the components of the SCM showing the preferred orientation of the photograph (e.g., looking northwest). This allows continuity during each inspection and maintenance visit to obtain new photographs showing the same orientation and same zoom for each of the components, preventing any guesswork by the personnel or contractor.
- Access, Right-of-Way, Limits, and Traffic Control: All components of the SCM must be readily accessible for inspection and maintenance. Therefore, trees, shrubs, underbrush pruning, and trimming must be included as part of the maintenance plan as necessary to maintain access to the SCM. Roadways, paths, ramps, and easements must be available and indicated in the graphic display used during maintenance activities. Additionally, the exact limits of inspection and maintenance easements and rights-of-way should be specified. Needs for traffic control measures should be clearly indicated for each SCM and maintenance activity.
- Historical Data or Stormwater Management Master Tracking Database: Typically, O&M programs combine inspection data for all SCMs into a master database that serves as the control tracking document for the stormwater program. This contains historical O&M for the SCM and may also contain reporting data from the public

(e.g., 311 hotline system to report SCM issues) that may give the inspector a snapshot of the typical issues associated with the control, assess whether there is any particular follow-up compliance issue that needs to be verified, etc. In this master database, key facility functionality issues are tracked. These can include sedimentation, pipe separation, erosion, and debris accumulation. When considered with previous years databases through the use of software such as Excel and Dashboard, trends are easily identified. This information informs routine maintenance scheduling and predictions of facility functionality "life," allowing nonroutine work to be done before a facility's functionality fails.

3.2 Importance of Rainfall Data

Rainfall data is an indicator of the runoff that will be received by an SCM. The easiest way of keeping up with rainfall data is to find the nearest source of rain gauge data to the different SCM. Many jurisdictions have their own rain gauge data that can be utilized for this purpose. Additionally, there are different rain data sources publicly available that can be helpful to provide information. The most widely used sources for rain data in the United States corresponds to the National Oceanic and Atmospheric Administration National Weather Service (https://hdsc.nws.noaa.gov/hdsc/pfds) and United States Geological Survey (https://waterdata.usgs.gov/nwis). If rain patterns are unknown by the one developing the O&M protocols, it is good practice to investigate historical climate data and/or keep a precipitation log as an indicator and predictor of the relative frequency of inspection and maintenance. On that note, it is important to document that rainfall varies not only temporally, but variations can also be apparent spatially and relatively within a small vicinity. Therefore, care should be exercised when making decisions based on information related to rainfall data considering the proximity to the location of the SCM. In any event, rainfall prevalence will directly affect the need for more frequent inspection and maintenance needs.

Rainfall data analysis and logs are simple and typically include information related to the source of rainfall recording (gauge station location or ID), date, and precipitation depth (in). Depending on the instruments used, precipitation depth is measured with different frequencies. For O&M, daily precipitation records (24-hour increments) are adequate. In the inspection forms, it is typical to record the date since the last rainfall and depth of such rainfall. The forms presented in this manual have a section to record this information. The information may be helpful to also form an idea of the relative frequency of rainfall, its relative depth, and its associated effects on the SCM maintenance needs. An area to record information on the date and depth of the last rainfall event is included in the forms presented in this manual.

3.3 Tools, Databases, and Systems Utilized for Inventory and Data Management

As described earlier in this chapter, inspection forms and data management, in general, may be collected, processed, analyzed, and kept utilizing different tools or systems, from the simplest paper and cabinet files to the most robust asset management system. Each user has different resources and will utilize those as efficiently as possible. Chapter 6 of this book provides an extensive overview of asset management and tools that can help the user of this manual better understand the advantages of such systems. However, as previously described, the information presented herein would be useful for any user irrespective of the type of tool, database, or system utilized for inventory and management of their SCM.

3.4 Typical Stormwater Control Measure Concerns During Construction

Ensuring the SCMs are adequately constructed or installed is the first step of an overall successful O&M program. Issues that are encountered later during the operation of an SCM can sometimes be associated with poor construction or installation of the SCM. For example, failure of stabilization areas may be associated with the inadequate anchoring of temporary erosion control mats that would have otherwise allowed an opportunity for vegetation to grow in a particular area. For additional information related to general verification protocols during construction phases for any SCM, refer to Chapter 5 in this manual. Below are SCM-specific items that must be verified during construction.

3.4.1 Vegetated Swales and Strips

Major concerns during construction include

- Proper utilization of topsoil to promote vegetation growth;
- Seeding mix according to plans and specifications;
- Vegetation establishment (ensuring the proper source of water during establishment, including temporary irrigation as needed);
- Grading according to plans and specifications; and

- Adequate anchoring of temporary erosion controls including erosion control mats, etc.

3.4.2 Basins

3.4.2.1 Dry Basins

Major concerns during construction include

- Verifying adequate grading and sizing of components (inflow line, outfall/spillway, forebay, berm, trickle, or low-flow channel);
- Verifying side slopes (typically 3:1 or less);
- Verifying embankments according to plans and specifications;
- Verifying establishment of vegetation on slopes and basins, stabilization and anchoring of inflow and outfall structures, the lining of the trickle or low-flow channel (vegetation/riprap, preferable; or concrete);
- Anchoring of berm to protect forebay;
- Protection of erosion at the outfall riser with concrete wing walls and apron; and
- Verifying enough access provided to monitor components.

3.4.2.2 Wet Basins

Major concerns during construction include

- Verifying adequate grading and sizing of components (inflow line, outfall/spillway, forebay, permanent pool, and berm),
- Verifying side slopes,
- Embankments according to plans and specifications,
- Establishment of vegetation on slopes,
- Stabilization and anchoring of inflow and outfall structures,
- Anchoring of berm to protect forebay,
- Protecting fencing installed (if applicable), and
- Verifying enough access provided to monitor components.

3.4.2.3 Swirl Concentrators and Vaults

Swirl concentrators are typically premanufactured SCM. Preoperational control is related to the installation of these devices. They are installed in a concrete vault and are installed either in-line or off-line. Therefore, the typical construction issues are associated with the construction of the vault itself, and the connection of the stormwater lines. Major concerns during construction include

- Following the flow lines as directed by the plans and specifications to ensure the vault and manhole are constructed correctly;
- If there are markings associated with the operation of the swirl, ensuring they are displayed adequately on a position that is visible to the operator once the maintenance is being conducted; and
- Verifying enough access provided to monitor components.

3.4.3 Filters

3.4.3.1 Media Filters

Major concerns during construction include

- Ensuring adequate sizing of the basin,
- Placing and layering components according to plans and specifications,
- Vegetation established around the filter as specified,
- Ensuring stabilization of the surrounding area is achieved to prevent major sediment reaching media filters, and
- Verify enough access provided to monitor components.

3.4.3.2 Bioretention Filters

Major concerns during construction include

- Adequate grading and sizing of components (inlet area, erosion control, planting area, slopes, overflow system, and outfall),
- Placing and layering of components (mulch, soil mix, sand or finer mix, gravel, and underdrain),
- Ensuring vegetation establishment (ensure the proper source of water during establishment, including temporary irrigation as needed),
- Ensuring stabilization of area around the bioretention area is achieved to prevent major sediment from reaching the area, and
- Verifying enough access provided to monitor components.

3.4.3.3 Inlet Basket

Inlet baskets come in the form of inserts to be placed inside the catch basin inlets. They are typically premanufactured, and preoperational care is more related to installation than construction.

- Verifying the baskets are properly anchored to the inlet according to specifications and in a way that they capture all stormwater flow coming into the inlet (this is the most critical aspect to verify).
- Ensuring stabilization of the surrounding area is achieved to prevent major sediment reaching the basket and overloading it quickly.

3.4.3.4 Landscaped Roofs

Major concerns during construction include

- Verifying placement and layering of components (impermeable membrane, root membrane, drainage, soil, vegetation, mulch, roof drains, and other) according to plans and specifications,
- Considering the use of galvanized steel as a material to greatly increase the life of the structure,
- Using a hinge attachment to increase access,
- Ensuring vegetation establishment, and
- Verifying enough access provided to monitor components.

3.4.4 Infiltration

3.4.4.1 Infiltration Trench

Major concerns during construction include

- Using topsoil to promote vegetation growth;
- Seeding mix according to plans and specifications;
- Establishing vegetation;
- Grading according to plans and specifications;
- Placing and layering sand media (if applicable) according to plans and specifications;
- Placing outlet pipe according to specifications, if applicable; and
- Verifying enough access provided to monitor components.

3.4.4.2 Infiltration Basin

Major concerns during construction of an infiltration basin (Figure 9.5) include

- Adequate grading and sizing of components (inflow line, spillway, forebay, berm, side slopes, and embankments) according to plans and specifications,
- Establishing vegetation on slopes and basin,
- Stabilizing anchoring structures,
- Anchoring of berm to protect forebay, and
- Verifying enough access provided to monitor components.

3.4.4.3 Pervious Pavement

Major concerns during construction include

- Ensure an appropriate mix of paving, aggregates, subgrades, and bases are placed according to specifications;

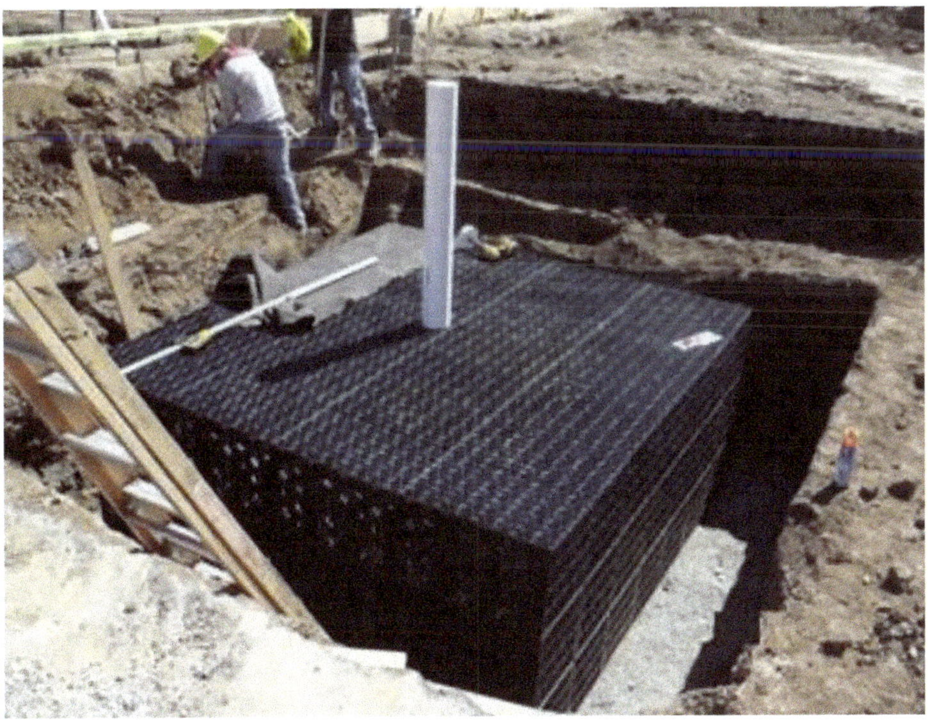

FIGURE 9.5 Installation of an Infiltration Basin

- If a pretreatment area has been specified (e.g., stabilized strip), ensure this is constructed according to specifications;
- During installation, pavement should be inspected and approved to be free of damage and any visual abnormalities;
- Ensure there are no edges that present a tripping hazard; and
- More than any other type of SCM, proper construction and installation is critical to facility functionality. Permeable pavements should be installed by a qualified, experienced contractor. Installer certifications for pervious concrete pavements are held by the National Ready Mixed Concrete Association. A current list of certified vendors can be obtained at https://www.nrmca.org/certifications/pervious-certification-search/. Installer certifications with designations as a specialist in the construction of permeable interlocking concrete pavements is held by the Interlocking Concrete Pavement Institute. A current list can be obtained at https://ams.icpi.org/icpissa/icpicenssa installerlkup.query_page. Concrete paving blocks should meet or exceed the latest standard published by the American Society for Testing and Materials of ASTM C936 Standard Specification for Solid Concrete Interlocking Paving Units to minimize the risk of abrasion and damage (WEF et al., 2012).

3.4.5 Catch Basins

Typical issues associated with catch basins during construction are associated with the construction of the vault itself, and the connection of the stormwater lines, inlet throats, and manholes. Major concerns during construction include

- Ensuring flow lines and grading are constructed as directed by the plans and specifications;
- Ensuring the vault, manhole, and inlet throat are constructed correctly; and
- Verifying enough access provided to monitor components.

3.4.6 Gross Pollutant Controls

Major concerns during construction include the following.

- The most important aspect of installing gross pollutant controls is proper anchoring.

- Irrespective of how much customization took place, the controls must be adjusted in the field to properly fit and anchor properly to the walls of the containing structure. Appropriate tools must be available to ensure fitting is adequate so the gaps between the controls and structure are below an acceptable threshold.
- Because gross pollutant controls maintenance will be typically associated with reaching some debris level on the control (e.g., 50% to 75% capacity), markings will also typically be part of the construction activities. Therefore, ensuring that markings are displayed adequately on a position that is visible to the operator once the maintenance is being conducted would also be a maintenance activity conducted during this phase.
- Verify enough access provided to monitor components.

3.5 Typical Stormwater Control Measure Concerns During Operation

The following are the most commonly reported concerns or most repetitive maintenance activities associated with each SCM that allows the user of this manual to predict those activities that may be predominant during the operation of SCMs and that may constitute the main components in the inspection forms. The user may also understand the differences or variations between the needs of maintenance for a given component between different SCMs. This information will help the user further understand their needs and customize the maintenance forms in a way that best suits those needs. For additional information related to general verification protocols during operation for any SCM, refer to Chapter 5 in this manual. Below are SCM-specific items that must be verified during operation.

3.5.1 Vegetated Swales and Strips

The most common maintenance activities during operation include

- Removal of sediment, litter, or debris;
- Ensuring proper vegetation establishment;
- Removing overgrown vegetation;
- Ensuring no standing water; and
- Addressing erosion concerns (more for swales as they are typically deeper than strips) obstruction or damage to inlet/outlets, weirs, or berms.

3.5.2 Basins

3.5.2.1 Dry Basins

The most common maintenance concerns during operation include

- Damaged embankment and/or outlet and need for stabilization outlet;
- Excess sediment buildup;
- Outlet/inlet blockages (with removal made easier by implementation of a concrete apron and wing wall);
- Broken or clogged low-flow channels;
- Standing water or wet soils and associated mosquito breeding, floatables, or debris;
- Weeds or woody vegetation;
- Excessive mowing and landscaping costs;
- Aesthetics or safety issues;
- Sediment buildup on the forebay area; and
- Blockage of trash rack if one is provided.

Figure 9.6 illustrates excess vegetation growth at the outfall of a dry basin, which can lead to obstruction. This example is also applicable to a vegetated swale.

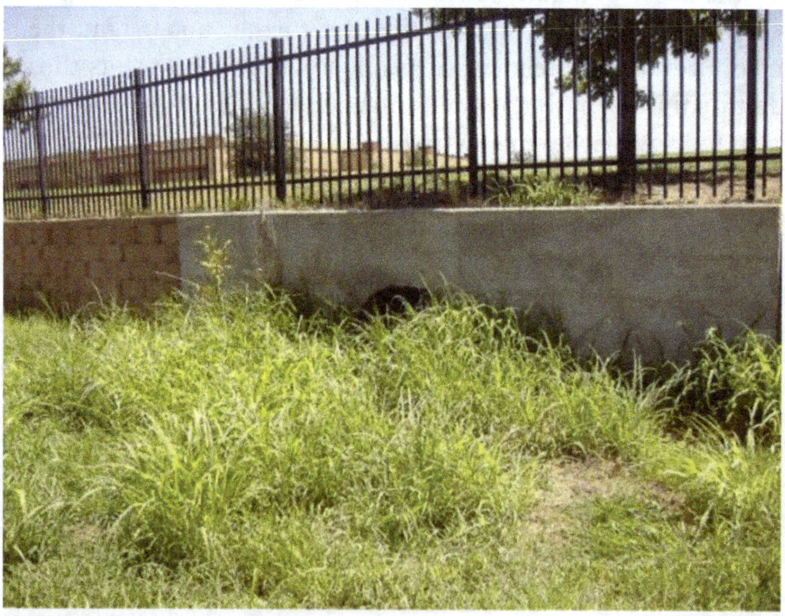

FIGURE 9.6 Excessive Vegetation Dry Basin

3.5.2.2 Wet Basins

The most common maintenance concerns during operation include

- Eroded embankment and inlets and outlets (need for stabilization);
- Excess sediment buildup, outlet/inlet blockages;
- Excess algae growth;
- Floatables or debris;
- Vegetation growth inside the permanent pool area. Invasive plant control is increasingly important in routine maintenance;
- Sediment buildup on the forebay area;
- Blockage of trash rack if one is provided; and
- Damage to weirs, flume, spillway, or outfall structure.

Figure 9.7 provides an example of a wet pond where the riprap originally placed for erosion protection is starting to show signs of erosion.

3.5.2.3 Swirl Concentrators and Vaults

The most common maintenance concerns during operation include

- Resuspension of sediments because of excess loading,
- Accumulation of floatables (trash, plastics, and leaves),

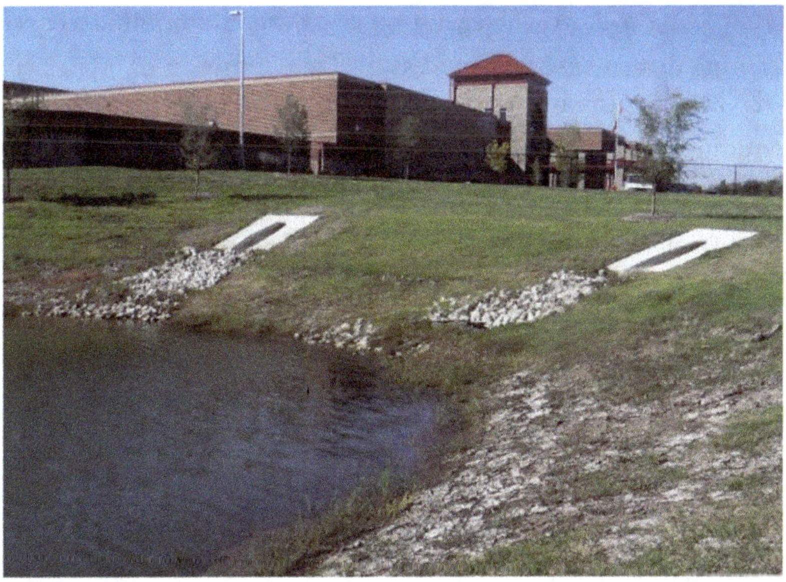

FIGURE 9.7 Riprap Failure and Beginning of Erosion at Inlets of a Wet Pond

- Mosquito breeding in standing water, and
- Fouling odors because of organic matter (leaves and grass).

3.5.3 Filters

3.5.3.1 Media Filters

The most common maintenance activities during operation include

- Maintenance of obstructed media (typically by removing the top of thickening media forming on the top),
- Maintenance of obstructed inlet or outlet structure,
- Removal of floatables (litter or debris),
- Replacement/regeneration of media (e.g., backflushing) and other components (e.g., geotextiles, geomembranes, etc.), and
- Checking if plant root systems may be interfering with the filter system.

3.5.3.2 Bioretention Filters

The most common maintenance activities during operation include

- Removing litter or debris;
- Ensuring proper vegetation establishment (watering/replanting as needed);
- Removing overgrown vegetation (mowing and pruning as needing);
- Tilting dirt to ensure no excess of fine deposition on upper layers of the bioretention media;
- Adding mulch;
- Addressing erosion concerns (if the filter has embankment);
- Addressing obstruction or damage to inlet/outlets, weirs, berms, or overflow system;
- Cleaning outlets; and
- Cleaning out accumulated sediment when over 38 mm (1.5 in.) or when no longer draws down within a specified period.

3.5.3.3 Inlet Basket

The most common maintenance activities during operation include

- Removal of floatables (litter or debris), replacing/regenerating filter media, or insert material and

- Removal of other obstructions at the street level that may be blocking the inlet, damage to components of the filter basket.

3.5.3.4 Landscaped Roofs

The most common maintenance activities during operation include

- Removing floatables (litter or debris), sediment, and other waste material;
- Trimming of vegetation;
- Addressing any erosion or scour;
- Removing any unwanted vegetation; and
- Repairing any cracking, subsidence, or spalling of any of the layers in the roofing system.

3.5.4 Infiltration

3.5.4.1 Infiltration Trench

The most common maintenance activities during operation include

- Mowing and maintaining upland vegetation areas (if applicable),
- Removing grass clippings and floatables (litter or debris),
- Maintaining swale or vegetated strip installed on top of infiltration trench,
- Removing accumulated sediment,
- Removing obstruction of inlet and outlet pipe (if one is provided),
- Cleaning of overflow or spillway structure (if one is provided),
- Replacing stone aggregate,
- Maintaining porosity of the substrate, and
- Removing accumulated sediment from forebays and sediment storage areas when 50% of the original volume has been lost.

3.5.4.2 Infiltration Basin

The most common maintenance activities during operation include

- Mowing and maintaining upland vegetation areas (if applicable);
- Removing accumulated sediments to rejuvenate infiltration capacity;
- Removing accumulated sediment from forebays and sediment storage areas when 50% of the original volume has been lost;

- Removing sediments from vaults, strips, or swales used as pretreatment unit (if applicable);
- Clearing of obstruction of inlet and outlet (if one is provided for peak conditions);
- Replacing stone aggregate; and
- Maintaining porosity of the substrate.

3.5.4.3 Pervious Pavement

The most common maintenance activities during operation include

- Periodic vacuuming (dry and/or wet) to restore infiltration capacity;
- Street sweeping;
- For pavers where there are spaces between pavers filled with gravel for infiltration, if this material is displaced because of runoff and plugged with debris or fine material, it should be replaced with fresh material that may provide infiltration capacity;
- Trash, sediment, and debris removal; and
- Replacement of damaged pavement because of traffic.

3.5.5 Catch Basins

The most common maintenance activities during operation include the following.

- Routine maintenance includes vacuuming the stormwater (if any) and solid (floatables—debris, levees, grass clippings, trash, plant materials, sediment, dirt, etc.) captured in the catch basins typically utilizing vactor trucks (vacuum trucks), which are trucks equipped with water and a vacuum system.
- Corrective maintenance may include correcting major inlet or outlet structural issues like a collapsed pipe or a broken inlet.

3.5.6 Gross Pollutant Controls

The most common maintenance activities during operation include

- Removal of floatables (litter or debris);
- Removal of accumulated sediment/clay mixed with grass clippings attaching to the traps (screens, bars, racks, or baskets);
- Removal of other major obstructions (tree branch/limb, vehicle tires, shopping carts, etc.); and

- Corrective maintenance, which may include fixing a screen, bar, rack, or basket damaged because of a major obstruction.

4.0 SAMPLE INSPECTION AND MAINTENANCE REPORTING FORMS

Section 4.0 provides sample forms for each of the different SCMs presented in this manual. Both forms to be utilized during construction and operation are presented.

There are many ways to configure an appropriate inspection and maintenance form. The best configuration is dictated by several different variables related particularly to the degree of experience and variability of the inspection crew conducting the inspections. The benefit of a complex form is that it minimizes any degree of subjectivity, and it also allows for easier automation if that is what is envisioned for the O&M program. In general, the forms are developed to recognize:

- SCM component.
- A comprehensive inspection of items for issues found either during construction or operation.
- Level of experience of inspection/maintenance crew.
- Variability of the inspection/maintenance crew to ensure a consistent degree of automation (asset management).

Forms may be adapted to asset management systems.

4.1 Inspection Forms During Construction

This manual presents a generic and comprehensive form containing the general inspection elements discussed for each SCM under Section 3.4 for the development of SCM-specific inspection forms to use during construction. The SCM Construction Inspection Form (Figure 9.8) may be used as is, or customized for any specific SCM. To do so, the user may choose to eliminate from the form those components that may not be applicable. Additionally, the user can also make the form more specific by adding detailed elements as described under Section 3.4.

The forms are generally organized into three basic parts. The top part covers general information about the SCM, including facility identification and description, information on the inspector, date of inspection, a summary on the condition of the SCM and its score, and general notes. Scorings for the condition of the SCM during an inspection are given utilizing the following ranking: a value of 1 is assigned for high priority, major noncompliance; 2 for moderate compliance; and 3 for minimal noncompliance. There are also a couple of indicators for compliant conditions, and not applicable. Along with the name of the inspector, the user may identify whether the inspector is certified and the type of certification.

The middle part represents general information about the site, including the condition of the signage, weather conditions, and accessibility. This part ensures the SCM is fully identified and that general site conditions, including information about the last rainfall and the current meteorological conditions, are noted.

The bottom part contains information about the condition of each component of the SCM during construction, documenting the SCM condition, implementation, vegetation establishment, construction items, and final inspection items.

4.2 Inspection Forms During Operations and Maintenance

The forms to be used during O&M presented in this manual are SCM-specific and intended to be detailed and comprehensive. The thought of presenting detailed forms is that it would be easier to develop a more general form if desired by the user. Parting from the forms presented in this manual, the user may select those details they wish to exclude for their use. Similarly, the forms are comprehensive in the sense that they cover all the anticipated components of an SCM, some of which may or may need to be present. Therefore, the user will need to customize, to a certain extent, these forms for ease of application—deleting those components/sections that may not apply for the SCM to be inspected. More generic forms and checklists are encountered in many different green infrastructure guidelines publicly available, including but not limited to several of the references noted in this chapter (City of Frisco, 2019; City of New Jersey, 2018; City of Poway, 2016; City of San Diego, 2012; San Antonio River Authority, 2019; Tarrant Regional Water District, 2018). The forms presented in this manual were developed based on professional experience with substantial collaboration from Fairfax County, Virginia Stormwater Management Branch.

The O&M forms presented in this manual are generally organized in three basic parts. The top part covers general information about the SCM including facility identification and description, information on the inspector, date of inspection, a summary on the condition of the SCM and its score, and overall notes. Scorings for the condition of the SCM are given utilizing the following ranking: a value of 1 is assigned for high priority, nonfunctional SCM; 2 for those approaching nonfunctionality; and 3 to those for low priority, with the SCM being functional. There are also a couple of indicators for no priority/continue routine maintenance, and not applicable. Along with the name of the inspector, the user may identify whether the inspector is certified and the type of certification.

The middle part represents general information about the site including the condition of the signage, weather conditions, and accessibility. This part ensures that the SCM is fully identified and that general site conditions, including information about the last rainfall and the current meteorological conditions, are noted. The middle part also includes a section to record the last rainfall recorded before an inspection and the general meteorological conditions during the inspection.

The bottom part contains information about the condition and operability of each component of the SCM. The order of such components is generally organized starting with the most upstream component of the SCM, followed by components found as the stormwater moves downstream or infiltrates and typically finalizing with the outfall and/or bypass. This order is suggested to provide an intuitive progression through the SCM. And, although the form may be filled in any the order that the inspector may choose, the order in the structure of the form is also proposed for the ease of finding each component in it. Note that for each component, there is a cell to note the number of photographs associated with that SCM with observations. Consider highlighting certain components because of their importance for facility safety and protection of property. Using a dry pond as an example, a blockage will create a water pool that may be a drowning hazard. A primary spillway pipe separation may lead to dam failure. Each facility type will uniquely have important components that should be readily recognized in an inspection form.

Inspection forms are included for each of the following SCMs:

- Vegetated Swales and Strips (Figure 9.9)
- Basins
    - Dry Basins (Figure 9.10)
    - Wet Basins (Figure 9.11)
- Filters
    - Media Filters (Figure 9.12)
    - Bioretention Filters (Figure 9.13)
    - Inlet Baskets (Figure 9.14)
    - Landscaped Roofs (Figure 9.15)

- Infiltration
  - Infiltration Trenches and Infiltration Basins (Figure 9.16)
  - Pervious Pavement (Figure 9.17)
- Catch Basins (Figure 9.18)
- Gross Pollutant Controls
  - Swirl Separators and Vaults (Figure 9.19)
  - Gross Pollutant Screens (Figure 9.20)

5.0 SUMMARY

The overall purpose of this chapter is to provide an overview of the importance of maintaining an effective O&M program for SCM—with the main focus of presenting recommended forms to conduct those activities during construction and operation of the SCM. For the adequate development of effective inspection programs and streamlining the use and implementation of the forms, this chapter outlines consideration of:

- External factors that may affect O&M practices including, for example, the dynamic nature of construction activities within the watershed and weather fluctuations. These factors may affect the frequency of inspection and may allow for an adaptive O&M program.
- Baseline information needed to develop the O&M program, including an inventory of SCMs (along with information about their location, characteristics, as-builts, maps, etc.). This critical information is needed for the user of the forms to conduct effective inspections.
- Assess accessibility to technology to record and manage the SCM inventory (asset database/tablets) and for data collection (asset management software/tablets) that may streamline the data collection/processing process. Advanced technology is not needed for an effective O&M program. However, an assessment of the technology resources available could help streamline the O&M program. Nevertheless, the forms and information needed for an effective O&M program are the same irrespective of the technology tools available.
- The overall communication framework necessary for the implementation of an effective SCM O&M program through the development of SOPs, or in the form of a stormwater management inspection, operation, and maintenance manual.

SWC Construction Inspection Form

Inspector: ______________________ Cert

Inspector: ______________________ Cert

Name of Entity ______________________

Date: ______________________

Site ID: ________ Facility ID: ________ Facility Name: ______________________

Address: ______________________ Coordinates / ParlD : ______________________

Watershed: County/District:

Compliant? ☐ Yes ☐ No

Score Totals: | 1 | 2 | 3 |

Scoring Key	
①	High Priority / Major Non-Compliances
②	Moderate Priority / Moderate Non-Compliances
③	Low Priority / Minor Non-Compliances
⊙	No Priority / Compliant
⊗	Not Applicable

Notes / Specifications: | Facility Specific Info:

Facility Type / Addl Facility Info:

Signs

SCORE	PHOTO	DESCRIPTION
③⊙⊗		Facility Sign
③⊙⊗		Facility Labeling

Weather Conditions

Last Rainfall	Date:	Amount:
Current weather conditions?		

Accessibility

Access Comments:

ACCESS PROBLEMS (Circle)	NEXT STEP (Circle One)
Locked Gate / Fence	Coordinate with Owner
Heavy Vegetation	Return for Re-inspection
Stuck / Broken Cover	Request Photos from Owner
Equipment Needed: ________	Request Maintenance
Other:__________	Other:__________

SCORE	PHOTO	DESCRIPTION
① ⊙⊗		Overall Facility Access
①②③⊙⊗		Component Access: ______________

SWC Condition

SCORE	PHOTO	DESCRIPTION	COMMENTS / SPECIFY INFLOW NUMBER OR ID
①②③⊙⊗		Inlet and Outlet Clear of Debris and Trash	
①②③⊙⊗		Sediment / trash or debris accumulation	
①②③⊙⊗		Condition of SWC Media	
①②③⊙⊗		Condition of Basin Structure (erosion, damange)	
①②③⊙⊗		Mulch Applied and Verify Condition (if applicable)	
①②③⊙⊗		Other:	

SWC Implementation

SCORE	PHOTO	DESCRIPTION	COMMENTS / SPECIFY INFLOW NUMBER OR ID
①②③⊙⊗		Postive Grade from inlet to Outlet	
①②③⊙⊗		Verify Slopes and grading	
①②③⊙⊗		Consistent with Design and Specs	
①②③⊙⊗		Correct component sizing	
①②③⊙⊗		Proper anchoring	
①②③⊙⊗		Concrete structures built appropiately	
①②③⊙⊗		Manholes or Inspection Ports Installed	
①②③⊙⊗		Other:	

Vegetation Establishment

SCORE	PHOTO	DESCRIPTION	COMMENTS / SPECIFY INFLOW NUMBER OR ID
①②③⊙⊗		Sufficient Water	
①②③⊙⊗		Application of top soil or other soil amendments	
①②③⊙⊗		Seeding mix and Plant as Specified	
①②③⊙⊗		Plant Condition/ Survival	
①②③⊙⊗		Inspection by certified arborists performed	
①②③⊙⊗		Other:	

SWC Construction

SCORE	PHOTO	DESCRIPTION	COMMENTS / SPECIFY INFLOW NUMBER OR ID
①②③⊙⊗		Prevent Vehicle Travel across Bioretention Area	
①②③⊙⊗		Excess Material Stocked in Approved Areas	
①②③⊙⊗		Material Storage Areas Protected	
①②③⊙⊗		Protection for Excacation Areas	
		Protect Active SWC Areas from Compaction (Trucks)	
①②③⊙⊗		Protection From Construction	
①②③⊙⊗		Other:	

FIGURE 9.8 SCM Construction Inspection Form

SWC Construction Inspection Form **Page 2**

Site ID:_______ Facility ID:_________ Facility Name:_______________________

Final Inspection Items			
SCORE	PHOTO	DESCRIPTION	COMMENTS / SPECIFY INFLOW NUMBER OR ID
①②③⊙⊗		Underdrain Operational and Clear	
①②③⊙⊗		Observation Wells Operational and Clear	
①②③⊙⊗		Clean-outs Operation and Clear	
①②③⊙⊗		Stockpiled Materials Removed	
①②③⊙⊗		Bioretention Soils Covered (Mulch or Vegetation)	
①②③⊙⊗		Other:	

Other			
SCORE	PHOTO	DESCRIPTION	LOCATION
①②③⊙⊗		Encroachments	
①②③⊙⊗		Modifications	
①②③⊙⊗		Mosquito Habitat	
①②③⊙⊗		Evidence Possible Illicit Discharge, Call to Report	

INSPECTOR COMMENTS

FIGURE 9.8 SCM Construction Inspection Form (*continued*)

Vegetated Swale and Vegetated Strip Inspection Form

Inspector: ________ Cert
Inspector: ________ Cert
Date: ________

Name of Entity: ________

Site ID: ________ Facility ID: ________ Facility Name: ________

Coordinates / ParID: ________

Address ________

Watershed: ________ County/District: ________

Functional? ☐ Yes ☐ No

Score Totals: ☐ 1 ☐ 2 ☐ 3

Scoring Key	
①	High Priority / Non-functional
②	Moderate Priority / Approaching Non-functional
③	Low Priority / Functional
⊙	No Priority / Continue Routine Maintenance
⊗	Not Applicable

Notes / Specifications:

Facility Specific Info:

Facility Type / Addl Facility Info:

Signs			Weather Conditions		
SCORE	PHOTO	DESCRIPTION	Last Rainfall	Date:	Amount:
③⊙⊗		Facility Sign	Current weather conditions?		
③⊙⊗		Facility Labeling			

Accessibility

Access Comments			ACCESS PROBLEMS (Circle)	NEXT STEP (Circle One)
			Locked Gate / Fence	Coordinate with Owner
			Heavy Vegetation	Return for Re-inspection
SCORE	PHOTO	DESCRIPTION	Equipment Needed: ________	Request Photos from Owner
① ⊙⊗		Overall Facility Access	Other: ________	Contact MSMD
①②③⊙⊗		Component Access ________		Other: ________

Upstream Inflow(s)

SCORE	PHOTO	DESCRIPTION	COMMENTS / DIMENSIONS
①②③⊙⊗		Trash / Debris / Sediment Removal	
①②③⊙⊗		Erosion/undercutting	
①②③⊙⊗		Displacement/sedimentation of fabric or rip-rap	
①②③⊙⊗		Pipe Condition	
①②③⊙⊗		Other: *Description:*	

Pre-Treatment / Energy Dissipators

Type(s): Check dams / Flow spreader / Forebay / Gravel diaphragm / Grass filter strip / Grass channel / Leaf screen / Level spreader / Other: ________

SCORE	PHOTO	DESCRIPTION	COMMENTS / DIMENSIONS
① ⊙⊗		Missing / Non-Functional *Description:*	
① ⊙⊗		Inconsistent with Plans *(Area / Vertical Drop / etc.)*	Observed: Specified:
①②③⊙⊗		Damage / Deterioration *Description:*	
①②③⊙⊗		Trash / Debris / Sediment *Description / Amount:*	
①②③⊙⊗		Other:	

Vegetated Swale or Strip

SCORE	PHOTO	DESCRIPTION	COMMENTS / DIMENSIONS
①②③⊙⊗		Trash / Debris / Sediment	
①②③⊙⊗		Bare spots/erosive gullies	
①②③⊙⊗		Sediment accumulation	
①②③⊙⊗		Vegetation length: (too short/too long)	
①②③⊙⊗		Invasive vegetation	
①②③⊙⊗		Erosion/Damage to outlet	
①②③⊙⊗		Other: *Description:*	

Outfall Structure

Material: ________ Size: ________ End Type: ________

SCORE	PHOTO	DESCRIPTION	COMMENTS / DIMENSIONS
①②③⊙⊗		Blockage	
①②③⊙⊗		Trash / Debris / Sediment	
①②③⊙⊗		Erosion / Undermining	
①②③⊙⊗		Spalling / Deterioration	
①②③⊙⊗		Separation / Misalignment	
①②③⊙⊗		Overgrown Vegetation / Tree Removal	
①②③⊙⊗		Manhole Condition	
①②③⊙⊗		Ladder / Steps Condition	
①②③⊙⊗		Downstream Channel Condition	
①②③⊙⊗		Other:	

FIGURE 9.9 Vegetated Swale and Vegetated Strip Inspection Form

Vegetated Swale Inspection Form **Page 2**

Site ID: ______ Facility ID: _______ Facility Name: ____________________

Underdrain(s)			
SCORE	PHOTO	DESCRIPTION	COMMENTS / DIMENSIONS
		Specified on Approved Plans?	
① ⊙⊗		Missing	
①②③⊙⊗		Blockage (③ < 25% < ② < 75% < ①)	
①②③⊙⊗		Spalling / Deterioration	
①②③⊙⊗		Separation / Misaligned Joints	
①②③⊙⊗		Other:	

Other			
SCORE	PHOTO	DESCRIPTION	LOCATION
①②③⊙⊗		Encroachments	
①②③⊙⊗		Modifications	
①②③⊙⊗		Mosquito Habitat	
①②③⊙⊗		Evidence of Possible Illicit Discharge, Call to Report	

INSPECTOR COMMENTS

FIGURE 9.9 Vegetated Swale and Vegetated Strip Inspection Form (*continued*)

Dry Basin Inspection Form

Name of Entity: ______________________

Inspector: ______________ Cert

Inspector: ______________ Cert

Date: ______________

Site ID: ________ Facility ID: ________ Facility Name: ______________

Coordinates / ParID : ______________

Address: ______________ Watershed: ______________ County/District: ______________

Functional? ☐ Yes ☐ No

Score Totals: ☐ 1 ☐ 2 ☐ 3

Scoring Key	
①	High Priority / Non-functional
②	Moderate Priority / Approaching Non-functional
③	Low Priority / Functional
⊙	No Priority / Continue Routine Maintenance
⊗	Not Applicable

Notes / Specifications: | Facility Specific Info:

Facility Type / Addl Facility Info:

Signs

SCORE	PHOTO	DESCRIPTION
③⊙⊗		Facility Sign
③⊙⊗		Facility Labeling

Weather Conditions

Last Rainfall	Date:	Amount:
Current weather conditions?		

Accessibility

Access Comments:

SCORE	PHOTO	DESCRIPTION	ACCESS PROBLEMS (Circle)	NEXT STEP (Circle One)
			Locked Gate / Fence	Coordinate with Owner
			Heavy Vegetation	Return for Re-inspection
			Stuck / Broken Cover	Request Photos from Owner
① ⊙⊗		Overall Facility Access	Equipment Needed: ________	Request Maintenance
①②③⊙⊗		Component Access: ______________	Other: ____________	Other: ____________

Inflow Points

Type (Circle all that apply): Pipe/Flume/Swale/Other: __________ Size(s):

SCORE	PHOTO	DESCRIPTION	COMMENTS / SPECIFY INFLOW NUMBER OR ID
①②③⊙⊗		Obsturctions: vegetation, debris, sediment	
①②③⊙⊗		Erosion/undercutting	
①②③⊙⊗		Structural condition	
①②③⊙⊗		Displacement /sedimentation of fabric/rip rap	
①②③⊙⊗		Pipe condition	
①②③⊙⊗		Other:	

Forebay (as applicable)

SCORE	PHOTO	DESCRIPTION	COMMENTS / SPECIFY TYPE AND IFLOW POINT
①②③⊙⊗		Sediment / trash or debris accumulation	
①②③⊙⊗		Bare soil/erosion (displacement of turf or rip rap)	
①②③⊙⊗		Woody vegetation	
①②③⊙⊗		Invasive / Overgrown Vegetation	
①②③⊙⊗		Turfgrass maintained as mowed	
①②③⊙⊗		Weir Condition	
①②③⊙⊗		Other:	

Main Detention Area

SCORE	PHOTO	DESCRIPTION	COMMENTS / DIMENSIONS
① ⊙⊗		Standing water (>5-days after storm)	
①②③⊙⊗		Trash / Debris / Sediment *Description / Amount:*	
①②③⊙⊗		Overgrown / Invasive Vegetation *Description:*	
①②③⊙⊗		Tree Removal *Number / Size:*	
①②③⊙⊗		Erosion / Bare Spots *Area:*	
①②③⊙⊗		Vegetative shelf thriving?	
①②③⊙⊗		Other: *Description:*	

	Trickle Ditch / Low Flow Channel (if applicable)	Shown on Plans: 'es / No	Ditch Material:	Ditch Total:
① ⊙⊗	Not Found / Completely Covered			
①②③⊙⊗	Trash / Debris / Sediment *Description / Amount:*			
①②③⊙⊗	Blockage *(③ < 25% < ② < 75% < ①)*			
①②③⊙⊗	Erosion / Trenching / Roots *Description:*			
①②③⊙⊗	Detoured Flow Line *Description:*			
①②③⊙⊗	Damage / Deterioration *Description:*			
①②③⊙⊗	Other: *Description:*			

FIGURE 9.10 Dry Basin Inspection Form

Dry Basin Inspection Form

Page 2

Site ID: ______ Facility ID: ______ Facility Name: ______

Perimeter/Side Slopes/Embankment			
Type (Circle all that apply):		Perimeter/Side Slopes	Location:
SCORE	PHOTO	DESCRIPTION	COMMENTS / LOCATION/SURFACE AREA/ VOLUME IMPACTED
①②③⊙⊗		Sediment/debris accumulation	
①②③⊙⊗		Bare soil/erosion/loss dam material	
①②③⊙⊗		Shrubs/trees present (>3'tall)	
①②③⊙⊗		Grass cover eroding/unhealthy	
①②③⊙⊗		Animal burrows	
①②③⊙⊗		Signs of seepage on downstream face	
①②③⊙⊗		Signs of structural failure: i.e., horizontal/vertical	
①②③⊙⊗		cracks	
①②③⊙⊗		Upslope, top, and downslope maintained/mowed	
①②③⊙⊗		Other:	

Dam / Berm and Emergency Spillway										
								Sep Auxillary Spillway:		
SCORE	PHOTO	DESCRIPTION	FACE SLOPE		TOP OF DAM		BACK SLOPE		EMERG. SPILLWAY	
			Score	*Comments*	*Score*	*Comments*	*Score*	*Comments*	Material:	
①②③⊙⊗		Toe Soft Spots							*Score*	*Comments*
①②③⊙⊗		Cave-In								
①②③⊙⊗		Slope Erosion *Area:*								
①②③⊙⊗		Bare Spots *Area:*								
①②③⊙⊗		Animal Holes								
①②③⊙⊗		Tree Removal *Num/Size:*								
①②③⊙⊗		Loss of dam material								
①②③⊙⊗		Woody Vegetation								
①②③⊙⊗		Overgrown Non-woody Veg.								
①②③⊙⊗		Signs of seepage on downstream								
①②③⊙⊗		Trash / Debris / Sediment								
①②③⊙⊗		Alterations: *Description:*								
①②③⊙⊗		Other: *Description:*								
①②③⊙⊗		Blockage at Emergency Spillway *(③ < 25% < ② < 75% < ①)*								
①②③⊙⊗		Damage / Deterioration at Emergency Spillway *Description:*								

Outfall Structure / PSP Downstream End			
Material:		Size: End Type:	
SCORE	PHOTO	DESCRIPTION	COMMENTS / LOCATION/SURFACE AREA/ VOLUME IMPACTED
①②③⊙⊗		Blockage *(③ < 25% < ② < 75% < ①)*	
①②③⊙⊗		Trash / Debris / Sediment *Description / Amount:*	
①②③⊙⊗		Erosion / Undercutting *Area:*	
①②③⊙⊗		Structural Condition: Spalling / Deterioration	
①②③⊙⊗		Separation / Misalignment	
①②③⊙⊗		Overgrown Vegetation / Tree Removal	
①②③⊙⊗		Handrail Status	
①②③⊙⊗		Manhole Condition	
①②③⊙⊗		Ladder / Steps Condition	
①②③⊙⊗		Joint failure/loss of joint material, soil piping	
①②③⊙⊗		Leaking devices	
①②③⊙⊗		Downstream Condition (displacement of fabric/rip	
①②③⊙⊗		rap or other)	
①②③⊙⊗		Other:	

Other			
SCORE	PHOTO	DESCRIPTION	LOCATION
①②③⊙⊗		Encroachments	
①②③⊙⊗		Modifications	
①②③⊙⊗		Evidence of routine maintenace being performed?	
①②③⊙⊗		Fence condition (if applicable)	
①②③⊙⊗		Evidence Possible Illicit Discharge, Call to Report	

INSPECTOR COMMENTS

FIGURE 9.10 Dry Basin Inspection Form (*continued*)

Wet Basin Inspection Form

Inspector: ____________ Cert

Inspector: ____________ Cert

Date: ____________

Name of Entity: ____________

Site ID: ______ Facility ID: ______ Facility Name: ____________

Address: ____________ Coordinates / ParID : ____________

Watershed: ____________ County/District: ____________

Functional? ☐ Yes ☐ No

Score Totals: ☐ 1 ☐ 2 ☐ 3

Scoring Key	
①	High Priority / Non-functional
②	Moderate Priority / Approaching Non-functional
③	Low Priority / Functional
⊙	No Priority / Continue Routine Maintenance
⊗	Not Applicable

Notes / Specifications:

Facility Specific Info:

Facility Type / Addl Facility Info:

Signs

SCORE	PHOTO	DESCRIPTION
③⊙⊗		Facility Sign
③⊙⊗		Facility Labeling

Weather Conditions

Last Rainfall	Date:	Amount:
Current weather conditions?		

Accessibility

Access Comments:

SCORE	PHOTO	DESCRIPTION
① ⊙⊗		Overall Facility Access
①②③⊙⊗		Component Access: ____________

ACCESS PROBLEMS (Circle)	NEXT STEP (Circle One)
Locked Gate / Fence	Coordinate with Owner
Heavy Vegetation	Return for Re-inspection
Stuck / Broken Cover	Request Photos from Owner
Equipment Needed: ________	Request Maintenance
Other:____________	Other:____________

Inflow Points

Type (Circle all that apply): Pipe/Flume/Swale/Other: __________ Size(s):

SCORE	PHOTO	DESCRIPTION	COMMENTS / SPECIFY INFLOW NUMBER OR ID
①②③⊙⊗		Obsturctions: vegetation, debris, sediment	
①②③⊙⊗		Erosion/undercutting	
①②③⊙⊗		Structural condition	
①②③⊙⊗		Displacement /sedimentation of fabric/rip rap	
①②③⊙⊗		Other:	

Forebay (as applicable)

Function: Orifice Size: Type (Circle): Pipe/Flume/Swale/ / Other: ______

SCORE	PHOTO	DESCRIPTION	COMMENTS / SPECIFY TYPE AND IFLOW POINT
①②③⊙⊗		Sediment / trash or debris accumulation	
①②③⊙⊗		Bare soil/erosion (displacement of turf or rip rap)	
①②③⊙⊗		Woody vegetation	
①②③⊙⊗		Invasive / Overgrown Vegetation	
①②③⊙⊗		Turfgrass maintained as mowed	
①②③⊙⊗		Weir Condition	
①②③⊙⊗		Other:	

Pond Floor / Pool

SCORE	PHOTO	DESCRIPTION	COMMENTS / DIMENSIONS
① ⊙⊗		Water Level Inconsistent with Plans (returns to norm pool elevation after 5 days rain event)	
①②③⊙⊗		Trash / Debris / Sediment *Description / Amount:*	
①②③⊙⊗		Overgrown / Invasive Vegetation *Description:*	
①②③⊙⊗		Tree Removal *Number / Size:*	
①②③⊙⊗		Erosion / Bare Spots *Area:*	
①②③⊙⊗		Visible pollution/muddines (Water quality)	
①②③⊙⊗		Vegetative shelf thriving?	
①②③⊙⊗		Alge cover (%)	
①②③⊙⊗		Other: *Description:*	

Perimeter/Side Slopes/Embankment

Trickle Ditch / Low Flow Channel (if applicable) Shown on Plans: Yes / No Ditch Material: Ditch Total:

SCORE	PHOTO	DESCRIPTION	
① ⊙⊗		Not Found / Completely Covered	
①②③⊙⊗		Trash / Debris / Sediment *Description / Amount:*	
①②③⊙⊗		Blockage *(③ < 25% < ② < 75% < ①)*	
①②③⊙⊗		Erosion / Trenching / Roots *Description:*	
①②③⊙⊗		Detoured Flow Line *Description:*	
①②③⊙⊗		Damage / Deterioration *Description:*	
①②③⊙⊗		Other: *Description:*	

Wetland Habitat Signs Posted: Yes / No Plants in Inventory:

SCORE	PHOTO	DESCRIPTION	
		Type of Wetland (Emergent/Forested)	
①②③⊙⊗		Unhealthy / Damaged	
①②③⊙⊗		Overgrown Vegetation / Tree Removal	

FIGURE 9.11 Wet Basin Inspection Form

Wet Basin Inspection Form

Page 2

Site ID: ______ Facility ID: ______ Facility Name: ______

Perimeter/Side Slopes/Embankment

Type (Circle all that apply): Perimeter/Side Slopes Location:

SCORE	PHOTO	DESCRIPTION	COMMENTS / LOCATION/SURFACE AREA/ VOLUME IMPACTED
①②③⊙⊗		Sediment/debris accumulation	
①②③⊙⊗		Bare soil/erosion/loss dam material	
①②③⊙⊗		Shrubs/trees present (>3'tall)	
①②③⊙⊗		Grass cover eroding/unhealthy	
①②③⊙⊗		Animal burrows	
①②③⊙⊗		Signs of seepage on downstream face	
①②③⊙⊗		Signs of structural failure: i.e., horizontal/vertical	
①②③⊙⊗		cracks	
①②③⊙⊗		Upslope, top, and downslope maintained/mowed	
①②③⊙⊗		Other:	

Dam / Berm and Emergency Spillway

Sep Auxillary Spillway:

SCORE	PHOTO	DESCRIPTION	FACE SLOPE		TOP OF DAM		BACK SLOPE		EMERG. SPILLWAY	
			Score	*Comments*	*Score*	*Comments*	*Score*	*Comments*	Material:	
①②③⊙⊗		Toe Soft Spots							*Score*	*Comments*
①②③⊙⊗		Cave-In								
①②③⊙⊗		Slope Erosion *Area:*								
①②③⊙⊗		Bare Spots *Area:*								
①②③⊙⊗		Animal Holes								
①②③⊙⊗		Tree Removal *Num/Size:*								
①②③⊙⊗		Loss of dam material								
①②③⊙⊗		Woody Vegetation								
①②③⊙⊗		Overgrown Non-woody Veg.								
①②③⊙⊗		Signs of seepage on downstream								
①②③⊙⊗		Trash / Debris / Sediment								
①②③⊙⊗		Alterations: *Description:*								
①②③⊙⊗		Other: *Description:*								
①②③⊙⊗		Blockage at Emergency Spillway *(③ < 25% < ② < 75% < ①)*								
①②③⊙⊗		Damage / Deterioration at Emergency Spillway *Description:*								

Outfall Structure

Material: Size: End Type:

SCORE	PHOTO	DESCRIPTION	COMMENTS / LOCATION/SURFACE AREA/ VOLUME IMPACTED
①②③⊙⊗		Blockage *(③ < 25% < ② < 75% < ①)*	
①②③⊙⊗		Trash / Debris / Sediment *Description / Amount:*	
①②③⊙⊗		Erosion / Undercutting *Area:*	
①②③⊙⊗		Structural Condition: Spalling / Deterioration	
①②③⊙⊗		Separation / Misalignment	
①②③⊙⊗		Overgrown Vegetation / Tree Removal	
①②③⊙⊗		Handrail Status	
①②③⊙⊗		Manhole Condition	
①②③⊙⊗		Ladder / Steps Condition	
①②③⊙⊗		Joint failure/loss of joint material, soil piping	
①②③⊙⊗		Leaking devices	
①②③⊙⊗		Downstream Condition (displacement of fabric/rip	
①②③⊙⊗		rap or other)	
①②③⊙⊗		Other:	

Other

SCORE	PHOTO	DESCRIPTION	LOCATION
①②③⊙⊗		Encroachments	
①②③⊙⊗		Modifications	
①②③⊙⊗		Mosquito Habitat	
①②③⊙⊗		Evidence Possible Illicit Discharge, Call to Report	

INSPECTOR COMMENTS

FIGURE 9.11 Wet Basin Inspection Form (*continued*)

Media Filter Inspection Form

Inspector: Cert

Inspector: Cert

Name of Entity

Date:

Site ID: Facility ID: Facility Name:

Address: Coordinates / ParID :

Watershed: County/District:

Functional? Yes No

Score Totals: 1 2 3

Scoring Key

①	High Priority / Non-functional
②	Moderate Priority / Approaching Non-functional
③	Low Priority / Functional
⊙	No Priority / Continue Routine Maintenance
⊗	Not Applicable

Notes / Specifications:

Facility Specific Info:

Facility Type / Addl Facility Info:

Signs

SCORE	PHOTO	DESCRIPTION
③⊙⊗		Facility Sign
③⊙⊗		Facility Labeling

Weather Conditions

Last Rainfall	Date:	Amount:
Current weather conditions?		

Accessibility

			ACCESS PROBLEMS (Circle)	NEXT STEP (Circle One)
Access Comments:				
New Access Comments for EAM:			Locked Gate / Fence	Coordinate with Owner
			Parked Cars	Return for Re-inspection
SCORE	PHOTO	DESCRIPTION	Stuck / Broken Cover	Request Photos from Owner
① ⊙⊗		Overall Facility Access	Equipment Needed: ________	Contact MSMD
①②③⊙⊗		Component Access: ____________	Other:__________	Other:__________

Inflow(s)

SCORE	PHOTO	DESCRIPTION	COMMENTS / SPECIFY INFLOW NUMBER OR ID
①②③⊙⊗		Obstructions: vegetation, debris, sediment	
①②③⊙⊗		Structural condition of grate & covers	
①②③⊙⊗		Trash/debris covering	
①②③⊙⊗		Other: *Description:*	

Sediment Chamber

SCORE	PHOTO	DESCRIPTION	COMMENTS
① ⊙⊗		Sediment exceeds O&M manual tolerance	
①②③⊙⊗		Access hatch condition	
①②③⊙⊗		Vault/pipe structural condition	
①②③⊙⊗		Baffles and/or weir condition	
①②③⊙⊗		Access ladder/steps condition	
①②③⊙⊗		Oil accumulation	
①②③⊙⊗		Leaking Device	
①②③⊙⊗		Proper Drainage	
①②③⊙⊗		Trash/Debris	
①②③⊙⊗		Other: *Description:*	

Filter Chamber

SCORE	PHOTO	DESCRIPTION	COMMENTS
① ⊙⊗		Holding water >24 hours after rain event?	
①②③⊙⊗		Spalling / Deterioration	
①②③⊙⊗		Cleanout(s) Condition	
①②③⊙⊗		Cleanout(s) Condition	
①②③⊙⊗		Emergency Overflow	
①②③⊙⊗		Manhole / Bilco Door Condition	
①②③⊙⊗		Ladder / Steps Condition	
①②③⊙⊗		Other:	
	Filter Bed		
①②③⊙⊗		Filter Media is Silt-in and Needs Replacement	
①②③⊙⊗		Filter Media Color Profile (if discolored >3" deep, remove and replace with clean sand)	
①②③⊙⊗		Filter Media Eroded or Displaced (rake to level) OR Exposed Filter Fabric	
①②③⊙⊗		Filter Media Level	
①②③⊙⊗		Trash / Debris / Sediment *Description / Amount:*	

FIGURE 9.12 Media Filter Inspection Form

Media Filter Inspection Form — Page 2

Site ID: ________ Facility ID: ________ Facility Name: ________________

Filter Chamber			
	Observation Well / Clanout(s)		
① ⊙⊗		Missing / Not Found	
①②③⊙⊗		Damage / Deterioration	
①②③⊙⊗		Access hatch condition	
①②③⊙⊗		Vault/pipe structural condition	
①②③⊙⊗		Access ladder/steps condition	
①②③⊙⊗		Trash/Debris	
①②③⊙⊗		Other: *Description:*	

Outfall Structure / Other

Outfall Structure			
Material:		Size: End Type:	
SCORE	PHOTO	DESCRIPTION	COMMENTS / DIMENSIONS
①②③⊙⊗		Obstruction: vegetation/debris/sediment	
①②③⊙⊗		Erosion/undercutting	
①②③⊙⊗		Joint failure/loss of joint material	
①②③⊙⊗		Leaking device	
①②③⊙⊗		Control valve operation	
①②③⊙⊗		Emergency by-pass condition	
①②③⊙⊗		Displacement	
①②③⊙⊗		Other: *Description:*	

Control Structure			
SCORE	PHOTO	DESCRIPTION	COMMENTS / DIMENSIONS
①②③⊙⊗		Damage / Deterioration *Description:*	
①②③⊙⊗		Vegetation / External Obstructions	
①②③⊙⊗		Other: *Description:*	
	Low-Flow Orifice and Trash Rack		Orifice Size:
① ⊙⊗		Orifice Plate Missing / Non-Functional	
① ⊙⊗		Trash Rack Missing / Non-Functional	
①②③⊙⊗		Blockage *(③ < 25% < ② < 75% < ①)*	
①②③⊙⊗		Damage / Deterioration *Description:*	
	Top Trash Rack and Anti-Vortex Plate		
① ⊙⊗		Pad Lock Missing	
①②③⊙⊗		Blockage *(③ < 25% < ② < 75% < ①)*	
①②③⊙⊗		Damage / Deterioration *Description:*	
	Riser Interior		
①②③⊙⊗		Trash / Debris / Sediment *Description / Amount:*	
①②③⊙⊗		Ladder / Steps Condition	
	Principal Spillway Pipe, Upstream End		
①②③⊙⊗		Blockage *(③ < 25% < ② < 75% < ①)*	
①②③⊙⊗		Spalling / Deterioration	
①②③⊙⊗		Separation / Misaligned Joints	

Dam / Berm and Emergency Spillway

Sep Auxillary Spillway:

SCORE	PHOTO	DESCRIPTION	FACE SLOPE		P OF DAM		BACK SLOPE		EMERG. SPILLWAY	
			Score	*Comments*	*Score*	*Comments*	*Score*	*Comments*	Material:	
①②③⊙⊗		Toe Soft Spots / Cave-In							*Score*	*Comments*
①②③⊙⊗		Slope Erosion / Bare Spots								
①②③⊙⊗		Animal Holes								
①②③⊙⊗		Tree Removal *Num/Size:*								
①②③⊙⊗		Overgrown Vegetation								
①②③⊙⊗		Other: *Description:*								
①②③⊙⊗		Blockage at Emergency Spillway *(③ < 25% < ② < 75% < ①)*								
①②③⊙⊗		Damage / Deterioration at Emergency Spillway *Description:*								

FIGURE 9.12 Media Filter Inspection Form (*continued*)

Media Filter Inspection Form Page 3

Site ID: ______ Facility ID: ______ Facility Name: ______

Ponding Area			
SCORE	PHOTO	DESCRIPTION	COMMENTS / DIMENSIONS
①②③⊙⊗		Erosion / Bare Spots *Area:*	
①②③⊙⊗		Trash / Debris / Sediment *Description / Amount:*	
①②③⊙⊗		Overgrown Vegetation	
①②③⊙⊗		Tree Removal *Number / Size:*	
①②③⊙⊗		Gabion Wall Condition	
①②③⊙⊗		Other: *Description:*	

Other			
SCORE	PHOTO	DESCRIPTION	LOCATION
①②③⊙⊗		Hazardous fumes or odors present	
①②③⊙⊗		Other: *Description:*	
①②③⊙⊗		Evidence of Possible Illicit Discharge, Call to Report	

INSPECTOR COMMENTS

FIGURE 9.12 Media Filter Inspection Form (*continued*)

Bioretention Filters Inspection Form

Inspector: ____________ Cert

Inspector: ____________ Cert

Date: ____________

Name of Entity ____________

Site ID: ______ Facility ID: ______ Facility Name: ____________

Address: ____________ Coordinates / ParID : ____________

Watershed: ____________ County/District: ____________

Functional? ☐ Yes ☐ No

Score Totals: ☐ 1 ☐ 2 ☐ 3

Scoring Key	
①	High Priority / Non-functional
②	Moderate Priority / Approaching Non-functional
③	Low Priority / Functional
⊙	No Priority / Continue Routine Maintenance
⊗	Not Applicable

Notes / Specifications: | Facility Specific Info:

Facility Type / Addl Facility Info:

Signs

SCORE	PHOTO	DESCRIPTION
③⊙⊗		Facility Sign
③⊙⊗		Facility Labeling

Weather Conditions

Last Rainfall	Date:	Amount:
Current weather conditions?		

Accessibility

Access Comments:			ACCESS PROBLEMS (Circle)	NEXT STEP (Circle One)
			Locked Gate / Fence	Coordinate with Owner
			Heavy Vegetation	Return for Re-inspection
SCORE	PHOTO	DESCRIPTION	Stuck / Broken Cover	Request Photos from Owner
① ⊙⊗		Overall Facility Access	Equipment Needed: ______	Request Maintenance
①②③⊙⊗		Component Access: ____________	Other: ______	Other: ______

Inflow Points

Type (Circle all that apply): Pipe/Flume/Swale/Other: ______ Size(s): ☐ ☐ ☐ ☐

SCORE	PHOTO	DESCRIPTION	COMMENTS / SPECIFY INFLOW NUMBER OR ID
①②③⊙⊗		Obstructions: vegetation, debris, sediment	
①②③⊙⊗		Erosion/undercutting	
①②③⊙⊗		Structural condition	
①②③⊙⊗		Displacement /sedimentation of fabric/rip rap	
①②③⊙⊗		Other: *Description:*	

Perimeter/Side Slopes/Embankment

Type (Circle all that apply): Perimeter/Side Slopes

SCORE	PHOTO	DESCRIPTION	Perimeter	Side Slopes
			LOCATION / SURFACE AREA and/or VOLUME IMPACTED	
①②③⊙⊗		Sediment/debris accumulation		
①②③⊙⊗		Bare soil/erosion		
①②③⊙⊗		Woody vegetation		
①②③⊙⊗		Turfgrass maintained as mowed		
①②③⊙⊗		Other: *Description:*		

Pre-Treatment Area (Forebay, gravel diaphragm, grass filter strip, grass channel, leaf screen, level spreader, others)

Type (Circle all that apply): Flow spreader / Forebay / Gravel diaphragm / Grass filter strip / Grass channel / Leaf screen / Level spreader / Other

SCORE	PHOTO	DESCRIPTION	TYPE / LOCATION / SURFACE AREA and/or VOLUME IMPACTED
① ⊙⊗		Sediment/debris accumulation	
①②③⊙⊗		Erosion/gullies present	
①②③⊙⊗		Invasive vegetation	
①②③⊙⊗		Flow is by-passing pretreatment	
①②③⊙⊗		Other: *Description:*	

Bioretention Cell

SCORE	PHOTO	DESCRIPTION	LOCATION / SURFACE AREA IMPACTED
①②③⊙⊗		Overgrown vegetation (requires pruning)	
①②③⊙⊗		Plants dead/diseased/distressed (replace per specs)	
①②③⊙⊗		Mulch decomposed/displaced	
①②③⊙⊗		Lack proper drainage (e.g. dead plants, water marks)	
①②③⊙⊗		Bare or eroded areas	
①②③⊙⊗		Other:	

FIGURE 9.13 Bioretention Filter Inspection Form

Bioretention Filter Inspection Form

Page 2

Site ID: ________ Facility ID: ________ Facility Name: ________

Control Structure (as applicable)

		Orifice Size:	Type (Circle): Riser Structure / Pipe End / Weir / Other:________
SCORE	PHOTO	DESCRIPTION	TYPE / COMMENTS / SURFCE AERA IMPACTED
①②③⊙⊗		Damage / Deterioration *Description:*	
①②③⊙⊗		Vegetation / External Obstructions	
①②③⊙⊗		Other: *Description:*	
	Low-Flow Orifice and Trash Rack		
① ⊙⊗		Orifice Plate Missing / Non-Functional	
① ⊙⊗		Trash Rack Missing / Non-Functional	
①②③⊙⊗		Blockage *(③ < 25% < ② < 75% < ①)*	
①②③⊙⊗		Damage / Deterioration *Description:*	
	Top Trash Rack and Anti-Vortex Plate		
① ⊙⊗		Pad Lock Missing	
①②③⊙⊗		Blockage *(③ < 25% < ② < 75% < ①)*	
①②③⊙⊗		Damage / Deterioration *Description:*	
	Riser Interior		
①②③⊙⊗		Trash / Debris / Sediment *Description / Amount:*	
①②③⊙⊗		Ladder / Steps Condition	
①②③⊙⊗		Manhole Condition	

Dam / Berm and Overflow Spillway (as applicable)

SCORE	PHOTO	DESCRIPTION	COMMENTS / DIMENSIONS	
① ⊙⊗		Missing	Observed:	Specified:
①②③⊙⊗		Slope Erosion *Area:*		
①②③⊙⊗		Bare Spots *Area:*		
①②③⊙⊗		Animal Holes		
①②③⊙⊗		Overgrown Vegetation / Tree Removal		
①②③⊙⊗		Trash / Debris / Sediment *Description / Amount:*		
①②③⊙⊗		Other: *Description:*		

Underdrain(s) and Principal Spillway Pipe

SCORE	PHOTO	DESCRIPTION	UNDERDRAIN(S)	PRINCIPAL SPILLWAY PIPE
		Specified on Approved Plans?		
① ⊙⊗		Missing		
①②③⊙⊗		Blockage *(③ < 25% < ② < 75% < ①)*		
①②③⊙⊗		Spalling / Deterioration		
①②③⊙⊗		Separation / Misaligned Joints		
①②③⊙⊗		Other: *Description:*		

Outfall Structure

Material:		Size: End Type:	
SCORE	PHOTO	DESCRIPTION	COMMENTS / DIMENSIONS
①②③⊙⊗		Blockage *(③ < 25% < ② < 75% < ①)*	
①②③⊙⊗		Trash / Debris / Sediment	
①②③⊙⊗		Erosion / Undercutting *Area:*	
①②③⊙⊗		Structural Condition: Spalling / Deterioration	
①②③⊙⊗		Separation / Misalignment / Joint Failure	
①②③⊙⊗		Overgrown Vegetation / Tree Removal	
①②③⊙⊗		Manhole and/or Pipe Condition	
①②③⊙⊗		Ladder / Steps Condition	
①②③⊙⊗		Downstream Condition (Displacement fabric or rip rap, sediment build up)	
①②③⊙⊗		Other: *Description:*	

Other

SCORE	PHOTO	DESCRIPTION	LOCATION
①②③⊙⊗		Encroachments	
①②③⊙⊗		Modifications	
①②③⊙⊗		Mosquito Habitat	
①②③⊙⊗		Evidence of Possible Illicit Discharge, Call to Report	

INSPECTOR COMMENTS

FIGURE 9.13 Bioretention Filter Inspection Form (*continued*)

Inlet Basket Inspection Form

Name of Entity	Inspector:	Cert
	Inspector:	Cert
	Date:	

Site ID:	Facility ID:	Facility Name:	
Address:		Coordinates / ParID :	
		Watershed:	County/District:

Functional? ☐ Yes ☐ No

Score Totals: ☐ 1 ☐ 2 ☐ 3

Scoring Key	
①	High Priority / Non-functional
②	Moderate Priority / Approaching Non-functional
③	Low Priority / Functional
⊙	No Priority / Continue Routine Maintenance
⊗	Not Applicable

Notes / Specifications:	Facility Specific Info:

Facility Type / Addl Facility Info:

Signs			Weather Conditions		
SCORE	PHOTO	DESCRIPTION	Last Rainfall	Date:	Amount:
③⊙⊗		Inlet ID Mark	Current weather conditions?		
③⊙⊗		No Dumping Site			

Accessibility

			ACCESS PROBLEMS (Circle)	NEXT STEP (Circle All Applied)
Access Comments:			Locked Inlet Manhole	Notify Responsible Party
			Physical Obstruction	Return for Re-inspection
SCORE	PHOTO	DESCRIPTION	Stuck / Broken Manhole Cover	Request Photos from Owner
① ⊙⊗		Overall Facility Access	Equipment Needed: ________	Request Maintenance
①②③⊙⊗		Component Access: ____________	Other:____________	Other:____________

Curb and Gutter

Type (Circle all that apply):		Flow Length	Left side of Inlet	ft	Right side of Inlet	ft
SCORE	PHOTO	DESCRIPTION		COMMENTS		
①②③⊙⊗		Street Flooding *Depth*				
①②③⊙⊗		Sediment / trash, debris *Depth/Volume*				
①②③⊙⊗		Other:				

Drain Basket Insert

SCORE	PHOTO	DESCRIPTION	COMMENTS / DEPTH
①②③⊙⊗		Flow into Curb Inlet *Depth*	
①②③⊙⊗		Standing Water *Depth*	
①②③⊙⊗		Basket Overflowing	
①②③⊙⊗		Odor(s)	
①②③⊙⊗		Inlet Clogged	
①②③⊙⊗		Bypass Evident	
①②③⊙⊗		Tears in basket material	
①②③⊙⊗		Structural Condition	
①②③⊙⊗		Sediment / trash, debris *Depth/Volume*	
①②③⊙⊗		Other:	

Outfall Structure / Other

Outfall and Overflow Structures

Material:	Size:	End Type:	
SCORE	PHOTO	DESCRIPTION	COMMENTS / DIMENSIONS
①②③⊙⊗		Blockage *(③ < 25% < ② < 75% < ①)*	
①②③⊙⊗		Trash / Debris / Sediment	
①②③⊙⊗		Damage *Area:*	
①②③⊙⊗		Spalling / Deterioration	
①②③⊙⊗		Separation / Misalignment	
①②③⊙⊗		Manhole Condition	
①②③⊙⊗		Ladder / Steps Condition	
①②③⊙⊗		Downstream Channel Condition	
①②③⊙⊗		Other:	

Other

SCORE	PHOTO	DESCRIPTION	LOCATION
①②③⊙⊗		Modifications/Alteration Basket	
①②③⊙⊗		Mosquito Habitat	
①②③⊙⊗		Evidence Possible Illicit Discharge, Call to Report	

INSPECTOR COMMENTS

FIGURE 9.14 Inlet Basket Inspection Form

Landscaped Roof Inspection Form

Name of Entity		Inspector:	Cert
		Inspector:	Cert
		Date:	
Site ID:	Facility ID:	Facility Name:	
Address:		Coordinates / ParID :	
		Watershed:	County/District:

Functional? ☐ Yes ☐ No

Score Totals: ☐ 1 ☐ 2 ☐ 3

Scoring Key	
①	High Priority / Non-functional
②	Moderate Priority / Approaching Non-functional
③	Low Priority / Functional
⊙	No Priority / Continue Routine Maintenance
⊗	Not Applicable

Notes / Specifications:

Facility Specific Info:

Facility Type / Addl Facility Info:

Signs			Weather Conditions		
SCORE	PHOTO	DESCRIPTION	Last Rainfall	Date:	Amount:
③⊙⊗		Facility Sign	Current weather conditions?		
③⊙⊗		Facility Labeling			

Accessibility

			ACCESS PROBLEMS (Circle)	NEXT STEP (Circle One)
Access Comments:			Locked Access Door	Coordinate with Owner
New Access Comments for EAM:			Broken / Unsafe Ladder	Return for Re-inspection
SCORE	PHOTO	DESCRIPTION	Too Tall for Standard Ladder	Request Photos from Owner
① ⊙⊗		Overall Facility Access	Equipment Needed: ________	Roofing Contractor/Bucket Truck
①②③⊙⊗		Component Access: ________________	Other:____________	

Roof Surface

SCORE	PHOTO	DESCRIPTION		COMMENTS / DIMENSIONS		
①②③⊙⊗		Ponding Water (after dry weather)	Depth			
①②③⊙⊗		Visible Damage to Surface				
①②③⊙⊗		Erosion / Bare Spots	Area:			
①②③⊙⊗		Trash / Debris / Sediment	Volume/Depth			
①②③⊙⊗		Leaking roof				
①②③⊙⊗		Other:	Description:			
	Plant Material			Plants in Inventory:		Total % of Plant Material Coverage:
①②③⊙⊗		Trees Missing		Observed:	Specified:	
①②③⊙⊗		Shrubs Missing		Observed:	Specified:	
①②③⊙⊗		Grass / Groundcover Missing	Area:	Observed:	Specified:	
①②③⊙⊗		Unhealthy / Damaged				
①②③⊙⊗		Overgrown / Invasive Vegetation				
①②③⊙⊗		Other:	Description:			
		For Multi-Level Rooftop Detention Systems, Describe Stormwater Flow:		Notes:		

Roof Drains

SCORE	PHOTO	DESCRIPTION		1	2	3	4	5	6	7	8	9	10	11	12
① ⊙⊗		Debris Cage or Trap Missing													
①②③⊙⊗		Blockage	(③ < 25% < ② < 75% < ①)												
①②③⊙⊗		Damage / Deterioration													
①②③⊙⊗		Vegetation / External Obstructions													
①②③⊙⊗		Other:	Description:												

Scupper Ports / Emergency Overflow

SCORE	PHOTO	DESCRIPTION		1	2	3	4	5	6	7	8	9	10	11	12
①②③⊙⊗		Blockage	(③ < 25% < ② < 75% < ①)												
①②③⊙⊗		Damage / Deterioration													
①②③⊙⊗		Vegetation / External Obstructions													
①②③⊙⊗		Other:	Description:												
① ⊙⊗		Insufficient Emergency Overflow		Observed:						Specified:					

Other

SCORE	PHOTO	DESCRIPTION	LOCATION
①②③⊙⊗		Modifications	
①②③⊙⊗		Mosquito Habitat	
①②③⊙⊗		Other:	

INSPECTOR COMMENTS

FIGURE 9.15 Landscaped Roof Inspection Form

Infiltration Trench and Infiltration Basin Inspection Form

Inspector: ______ Cert

Inspector: ______ Cert

Date: ______

Name of Entity ______

Site ID: ______ Facility ID: ______ Facility Name: ______

Address: ______ Coordinates / ParID : ______

Watershed: ______ County/District: ______

Functional? [ ] Yes [ ] No

Score Totals: [ ] 1 [ ] 2 [ ] 3

Scoring Key	
①	High Priority / Non-functional
②	Moderate Priority / Approaching Non-functional
③	Low Priority / Functional
⊙	No Priority / Continue Routine Maintenance
⊗	Not Applicable

Notes / Specifications: ______ Facility Specific Info: ______

Facility Type / Addl Facility Info: ______

Signs			Weather Conditions		
SCORE	PHOTO	DESCRIPTION	Last Rainfall	Date:	Amount:
③⊙⊗		Facility Sign	Current weather conditions?		
③⊙⊗		Facility Labeling			

Accessibility

Access Comments:			ACCESS PROBLEMS (Circle)	NEXT STEP (Circle One)
			Locked Gate / Fence	Coordinate with Owner
			Parked Cars	Return for Re-inspection
SCORE	PHOTO	DESCRIPTION	Stuck / Broken Cover	Request Photos from Owner
① ⊙⊗		Overall Facility Access	Equipment Needed: ______	
①②③⊙⊗		Component Access: ______	Other: ______	Other: ______

Surface Trench Components

Pre-Treatment for Energy Dissipators & Gross Pollutant Traps

Type(s): Gravel diaphragm / Grass filter strip or channel / Leaf screen / Level spreader / Plunge pool / Sediment trap or Forbay / Rip Rap/ Gross Pollutant Trap/Sump pit / Other: ____

SCORE	PHOTO	DESCRIPTION		COMMENTS / DIMENSIONS	
① ⊙⊗		Missing / Non-Functional	*Description:*		
① ⊙⊗		Inconsistent with Plans	*(Area / Vertical Drop / etc.)*	Observed:	Specified:
①②③⊙⊗		Erosion/ Rip rap displaced	*Area*		
①②③⊙⊗		Damage / Deterioration	*Description:*		
①②③⊙⊗		Trash / Debris / Sediment	*Description/Volume/Depth:*		
①②③⊙⊗		Other:			

Gravel Bed Surface and Sand Layer

SCORE	PHOTO	DESCRIPTION		COMMENTS / DIMENSIONS	
		Surface Cover:	Gravel / Grass / Both / Other: ____		
① ⊙⊗		Slope according to plans			
① ⊙⊗		Trench Eliminated			
① ⊙⊗		Gravel Not Found Under Turf		Depth to Gravel (if applicable):	
① ⊙⊗		Gravel Footprint		Area Observed:	Area Specified:
① ⊙⊗		Bottom Sand Layer filtrating (< 72 hours)			
①②③⊙⊗		Deterioration	*Type: cracking, subsidence, spalling*		
①②③⊙⊗		Trash / Debris / Sediment	*Description / Amount:*		
①②③⊙⊗		Bare Spots / Erosion	*Area:*		
①②③⊙⊗		Condition of Grass or Gravel			
①②③⊙⊗		Repair Filter Fabric			
①②③⊙⊗		Other:	*Description:*		

Vegetated Areas

SCORE	PHOTO	DESCRIPTION		COMMENTS / DIMENSIONS	
① ⊙⊗		Unplanned Vegetation Growth			
①②③⊙⊗		Unauthorized Planting	*Description:*		
①②③⊙⊗		Bare Spots / Erosion/Scour			
①②③⊙⊗		Grass / Groundcover Missing	*Area:*	Observed:	Specified:
①②③⊙⊗		Unhealthy / Damaged			
①②③⊙⊗		Overgrown / Invasive Vegetation			
①②③⊙⊗		Trash / Debris / Sediment	*Description / Amount:*		
①②③⊙⊗		Other:	*Description:*		

FIGURE 9.16 Infiltration Trench and Infiltration Basin Inspection Form

Infiltration Trench/Basin Inspection Form

Page 2

Site ID: ______ Facility ID: ______ Facility Name: ______

Observation Well / Cleanout(s)

SCORE	PHOTO	DESCRIPTION	COMMENTS / DIMENSIONS	
① ⊙⊗		Missing / Not Found	Observed:	Specified:
① ⊙⊗		Cap Missing / Stuck		
①②③⊙⊗		Water / Sediment Observed in Well?		
①②③⊙⊗		Damaged		
①②③⊙⊗		Other: *Description:*		

Dam / Berm and Emergency Spillway

			Required by Plans?	Yes / No
SCORE	PHOTO	DESCRIPTION	COMMENTS / DIMENSIONS	
① ⊙⊗		Missing	Observed:	Specified:
①②③⊙⊗		Erosion / Bare Spots *Area:*		
①②③⊙⊗		Cave-In		
① ⊙⊗		Emergency Spillway or Overflow Obstructed		
①②③⊙⊗		Animal Holes		
①②③⊙⊗		Overgrown Vegetation / Tree Removal		
①②③⊙⊗		Trash / Debris / Sediment *Description/Volume/Depth:*		
①②③⊙⊗		Other: *Description:*		

Surface Inflows and Roof Drains

SCORE	PHOTO	DESCRIPTION	1	2	3	4	5	6
	Inflow Type (Sheet Flow, Curb Cut, Roof Downspout, Pipe, etc.):							
		Pipe Material:						
		Pipe Size:						
① ⊙⊗		Roof Drain Downspout Disconnected						
①②③⊙⊗		Blockage (③ < 25% < ② < 75% < ①)						
①②③⊙⊗		Spalling / Deterioration						
①②③⊙⊗		Erosion / Undermining						
①②③⊙⊗		Trash / Debris / Sediment Removal						
①②③⊙⊗		Overgrown Vegetation / Tree Removal						
①②③⊙⊗		Other:						

	Inflow Summary			
① ⊙⊗		Curb Cuts Missing / Inconsistent with Plans	Observed:	Specified:
① ⊙⊗		Inflow Diverted Away From Trench	Observed:	Specified:
①②③⊙⊗		Other:		

Underground Trench or Basin Components

Control Structure

[illegible]	[illegible]	[illegible]		Structure # on Plans:		Label(s) on Sketch:	

SCORE	PHOTO	DESCRIPTION	COMMENTS / DIMENSIONS	
①②③⊙⊗		Standing Water (after dry weather)		
①②③⊙⊗		Trash / Debris / Sediment *Description / Amount:*		
①②③⊙⊗		Spalling / Deterioration		
①②③⊙⊗		Manhole / Bilco Door Condition		
①②③⊙⊗		Ladder / Steps Condition		
①②③⊙⊗		Other: *Description:*		
	Low-Flow Orifice and Trash Rack			
① ⊙⊗		Orifice Plate Missing / Non-Functional		
① ⊙⊗		Trash Rack Missing / Non-Functional		
①②③⊙⊗		Blockage (③ < 25% < ② < 75% < ①)		
①②③⊙⊗		Damage / Deterioration *Description:*		
	Higher-Flow Orifice / Weir			
① ⊙⊗		Missing / Not Found	Observed:	Specified:
①②③⊙⊗		Blockage (③ < 25% < ② < 75% < ①)		
①②③⊙⊗		Other: *Description:*		
	Outlet Pipe			
①②③⊙⊗		Blockage (③ < 25% < ② < 75% < ①)		
①②③⊙⊗		Spalling / Deterioration		
①②③⊙⊗		Separation / Misalignment		

FIGURE 9.16 Infiltration Trench and Infiltration Basin Inspection Form (*continued*)

Infiltration Trench/Basin Inspection Form **Page 3**

Site ID: ______ Facility ID: ______ Facility Name: ______

Detention Pipe / Vault								
SCORE	PHOTO	DESCRIPTION	1	2	3	4	5	6
		Structure # on Plans:						
		Label on Sketch:						
①②③⊙⊗		Standing Water (after dry weather)						
①②③⊙⊗		Trash / Debris / Sediment *Description / Amount:*						
①②③⊙⊗		Spalling / Deterioration						
①②③⊙⊗		Separation / Misalignment						
①②③⊙⊗		Inflow Pipes, if any *Pipe Direction / Problem:*						
①②③⊙⊗		Manhole / Bilco Door Condition						
①②③⊙⊗		Ladder / Steps Condition						
①②③⊙⊗		Blockage *(③ < 25% < ② < 75% < ①)*						
①②③⊙⊗		Other: *Description:*						

Outfall Structure / Other

Outfall and Overflow Structures			
Material:		Size: End Type:	
SCORE	PHOTO	DESCRIPTION	COMMENTS / DIMENSIONS
①②③⊙⊗		Blockage *(③ < 25% < ② < 75% < ①)*	
①②③⊙⊗		Trash / Debris / Sediment	
①②③⊙⊗		Erosion / Undermining *Area:*	
①②③⊙⊗		Spalling / Deterioration	
①②③⊙⊗		Separation / Misalignment	
①②③⊙⊗		Overgrown Vegetation / Tree Removal	
①②③⊙⊗		Manhole Condition	
①②③⊙⊗		Ladder / Steps Condition	
①②③⊙⊗		Downstream Channel Condition	
①②③⊙⊗		Other:	

Other			
SCORE	PHOTO	DESCRIPTION	LOCATION
①②③⊙⊗		Encroachments	
①②③⊙⊗		Modifications	
①②③⊙⊗		Mosquito Habitat	
①②③⊙⊗		Evidence of Possible Illicit Discharge, Call to Report (703-877-2800: Inspection, Maint., & Enforc. Section)	

INSPECTOR COMMENTS

FIGURE 9.16 Infiltration Trench and Infiltration Basin Inspection Form (*continued*)

Pervious Pavement Inspection Form

Name of Entity ____________________	Inspector: ________	Cert
	Inspector: ________	Cert
	Date: ________	

Site ID: ______ Facility ID: ______ Facility Name: ____________

Address: ____________ Coordinates / ParID : ____________

Watershed: ______ County/District: ______

Functional? ☐ Yes ☐ No

Score Totals: ☐ 1 ☐ 2 ☐ 3

Scoring Key	
①	High Priority / Non-functional
②	Moderate Priority / Approaching Non-functional
③	Low Priority / Functional
⊙	No Priority / Continue Routine Maintenance
⊗	Not Applicable

Notes / Specifications:

Facility Specific Info:

Facility Type / Addl Facility Info: Filterra

Signs			Weather Conditions		
SCORE	PHOTO	DESCRIPTION	Last Rainfall	Date:	Amount:
③⊙⊗		Facility Sign	Current weather conditions?		
③⊙⊗		Facility Labeling			

Accessibility

Access Comments:			ACCESS PROBLEMS (Circle)	NEXT STEP (Circle One)
			Locked Gate / Fence	Coordinate with Owner
			Blocked by Parked Vehicles	Return for Re-inspection
SCORE	PHOTO	DESCRIPTION	Equipment Needed: ________	Request Photos from Owner
① ⊙⊗		Overall Facility Access	Other: ________	Contact MSMD
①②③⊙⊗		Component Access: ________		Other: ________

Parking Lot

SCORE	PHOTO	DESCRIPTION	COMMENTS / DIMENSIONS
①②③⊙⊗		Trash / Debris / Sediment *Description /Volume/Depth*	
①②③⊙⊗		Asphalt / Concrete Condition	
①②③⊙⊗		Other: *Description:*	

Permeable Pavement

SCORE	PHOTO	DESCRIPTION	COMMENTS / DIMENSIONS
	Type (Paver/Concrete/Asphalt):		Infiltration: Underdrain:
① ⊙⊗		Ponding Water (after dry weather)	
①②③⊙⊗		Trash / Debris / Sediment *Description /Volume/Depth*	
①②③⊙⊗		Unwanted Vegetation	
①②③⊙⊗		Pavement Functionality (Infiltration)	*Test infiltration of system with 5-gallon bucket of water*
①②③⊙⊗		Appropriate Grading/Slopes	
①②③⊙⊗		Surface Damage *(Cracking/ Settlement/Spalling)*	
①②③⊙⊗		Broken or Missing Pavers	
①②③⊙⊗		Mud or Sediment Tracked Into Permeable Area	
①②③⊙⊗		Tree Dripline Over Pavement	
①②③⊙⊗		Structural Edge Resttrain or Toe	
①②③⊙⊗		Filter Fabric Condition	
①②③⊙⊗		Evidence of Sand/Salt/De-Icing Materials Applicatio	
①②③⊙⊗		Other:	
	Observation Well / Cleanout (if applicable)		
① ⊙⊗		Missing	
① ⊙⊗		Cap Missing / Stuck	
① ⊙⊗		Water / Sediment Observed in Well	
①②③⊙⊗		Damaged	
①②③⊙⊗		Other:	

Emergency Overflow / Outfall Structure

SCORE	PHOTO	DESCRIPTION	COMMENTS / DIMENSIONS
			Emegency Overflow Provided? Yes / No
①②③⊙⊗		Blockage *(③ < 25% < ② < 75% < ①)*	
①②③⊙⊗		Trash / Debris / Sediment *Description / Amount*	
①②③⊙⊗		Damage / Deterioration	
①②③⊙⊗		Overgrown Vegetation / External Obstruction	
①②③⊙⊗		Manhole Condition	
①②③⊙⊗		Ladder / Steps Condition	
①②③⊙⊗		Downstream Pipe Condition	
①②③⊙⊗		Other: *Description:*	

FIGURE 9.17 Pervious Pavement Inspection Form

Pervious Pavement Inspection Form **Page 2**

Site ID: ________ Facility ID: ________ Facility Name: ________

Emergency Overflow / Outfall Structure			
	Underdrain Pipe/Overflow Grate		Required by Plans? Yes / No
① ⊙⊗		Missing / Not Found	
① ⊙⊗		Flow-Reduction Orifice Missing (if required)	
①②③⊙⊗		Blockage (③ < 25% < ② < 75% < ①)	
①②③⊙⊗		Damage / Deterioration	
①②③⊙⊗		Other: *Description:*	

Other			
SCORE	PHOTO	DESCRIPTION	LOCATION
①②③⊙⊗		Encroachments	
①②③⊙⊗		Modifications	
①②③⊙⊗		Mosquito Habitat	
①②③⊙⊗		Evidence of Possible Illicit Discharge, Call to Report	

INSPECTOR COMMENTS

FIGURE 9.17 Pervious Pavement Inspection Form (*continued*)

Catch Basin Inspection Form

Name of Entity ______________________

Inspector: ______________ Cert

Inspector: ______________ Cert

Date: ______________

Site ID: ________ Facility ID: ________ Facility Name: ______________

Address: 9107 Horner Ct. Coordinates / ParID: ______________

Watershed: ________ County/District: ________

Functional? ☐ Yes ☐ No

Score Totals: ☐ 1 ☐ 2 ☐ 3

Scoring Key

①	High Priority / Non-functional
②	Moderate Priority / Approaching Non-functional
③	Low Priority / Functional
⊙	No Priority / Continue Routine Maintenance
⊗	Not Applicable

Notes / Specifications: | Facility Specific Info:

Facility Type / Addl Facility Info:

Signs

SCORE	PHOTO	DESCRIPTION
③⊙⊗		Facility Sign
③⊙⊗		Facility Labeling

Weather Conditions

Last Rainfall	Date:	Amount:
Current weather conditions?		

Accessibility

Access Comments:

New Access Comments for EAM:

SCORE	PHOTO	DESCRIPTION
① ⊙⊗		Overall Facility Access
①②③⊙⊗		Component Access: ______

ACCESS PROBLEMS (Circle)	NEXT STEP (Circle One)
Locked Gate / Vehicle Parked	Coordinate with Owner
Heavy Vegetation	Return for Re-inspection
Stuck / Broken Cover	Request Photos from Owner
Equipment Needed: ______	
Other: ______	Other: ______

Curb and Gutter

Type (Circle all that apply): ______ Flow Length | Left side of Inlet ______ ft | ht side of In ______ ft

SCORE	PHOTO	DESCRIPTION		COMMENTS
①②③⊙⊗		Street Flooding	*Depth*	
①②③⊙⊗		Sediment / trash, debris	*Depth/Volume*	
①②③⊙⊗		Other:		

Inflow Structures

SCORE	PHOTO	DESCRIPTION		1	2	3	4	5	6
① ⊙⊗		Disconnected							
①②③⊙⊗		Damaged / Leaking							
①②③⊙⊗		Blockage	*(③ < 25% < ② < 75% < ①)*						
①②③⊙⊗		Other:	*Description:*						

Catch Basin

Type: ______ Size: ______ Location: ______

SCORE	PHOTO	DESCRIPTION		COMMENTS / DIMENSIONS
	Pre-Treatment Device		*Type:*	
① ⊙⊗		Missing / Non-Functional		
①②③⊙⊗		Damage / Deterioration		
①②③⊙⊗		Trash / Debris / Sediment	*Description / Amount:*	
①②③⊙⊗		Other:	*Description:*	
	Storage Tank			
①②③⊙⊗		Damage / Deterioration		
①②③⊙⊗		Trash / Debris / Sediment	*Description / Amount:*	
①②③⊙⊗		Other:	*Description:*	

Outfall Structure / Other

Outfall and Overflow Structures

Material: ______ Size: ______ End Type: ______

SCORE	PHOTO	DESCRIPTION		COMMENTS / DIMENSIONS
①②③⊙⊗		Blockage	*(③ < 25% < ② < 75% < ①)*	
①②③⊙⊗		Trash / Debris / Sediment		
①②③⊙⊗		Damage	*Area:*	
①②③⊙⊗		Spalling / Deterioration		
①②③⊙⊗		Separation / Misalignment		
①②③⊙⊗		Manhole Condition		
①②③⊙⊗		Ladder / Steps Condition		
①②③⊙⊗		Downstream Channel Condition		
①②③⊙⊗		Gross Pollutant Trap at Outfall		
①②③⊙⊗		Other:		

FIGURE 9.18 Catch Basin Inspection Form

Catch Basin Inspection Form **Page 2**

Site ID: ______ Facility ID: ______ Facility Name: ______

Other			
SCORE	PHOTO	DESCRIPTION	LOCATION
①②③⊙⊗		Encroachments	
①②③⊙⊗		Modifications	
①②③⊙⊗		Mosquito Habitat	
①②③⊙⊗		Evidence of Possible Illicit Discharge, Call to Report	

INSPECTOR COMMENTS

FIGURE 9.18 Catch Basin Inspection Form (*continued*)

Swirl Separators & Vault Inspection Form

Name of Entity ______

Inspector: ______ Cert

Inspector: ______ Cert

Date: ______

Site ID: ______ Facility ID: ______ Facility Name: ______

Coordinates / ParID: ______

Address: ______

Watershed: ______ County/District: ______

Functional? [ ] Yes [ ] No

Score Totals: [ ] 1 [ ] 2 [ ] 3

Scoring Key	
①	High Priority / Non-functional
②	Moderate Priority / Approaching Non-functional
③	Low Priority / Functional
⊙	No Priority / Continue Routine Maintenance
⊗	Not Applicable

Notes / Specifications:

Facility Specific Info:

Facility Type / Addl Facility Info: Filterra

Signs

SCORE	PHOTO	DESCRIPTION
③⊙⊗		Facility Sign
③⊙⊗		Facility Labeling

Weather Conditions

Last Rainfall	Date:	Amount:
Current weather conditions?		

Accessibility

Access Comments:

SCORE	PHOTO	DESCRIPTION	ACCESS PROBLEMS (Circle)	NEXT STEP (Circle One)
			Locked Gate / Fence	Coordinate with Owner
			Parked Cars	Return for Re-inspection
			Stuck / Broken Cover	Request Photos from Owner
① ⊙⊗		Overall Facility Access	Equipment Needed: ______	Contact MSMD
①②③⊙⊗		Component Access: ______	Other: ______	Other: ______

Manufacturer-Specific Items

Look for these items as you inspect each chamber of the Manufactured BMP facility.

SCORE	PHOTO	DESCRIPTION	COMMENTS / DIMENSIONS
	Vortechs Hydrodynamic Separator (Swirl concentrators)		
①②③⊙⊗		Inspection Port (manholes access and structural condition)	
①②③⊙⊗		Swirl Chamber (depth of sediment)	
①②③⊙⊗		Floatables Chamber (Floatable layer thickness)	
①②③⊙⊗		Orifice Plates for High and Low Flows	
	Stormceptor		
①②③⊙⊗		Inspection Port (Manhole - access and structural condition)	
①②③⊙⊗		Fiberglass Insert (oil and grease removal)	
①②③⊙⊗		Weir (directing water to low chamber)	
①②③⊙⊗		Oil level (inserting a dipstick in the oil inspection/cleanout port	
①②③⊙⊗		Sediment level (insert dipstick tube through the riser pipe)	
①②③⊙⊗		Safety Grate (optional)	
	Downstream Defender		
①②③⊙⊗		Inspection Port (Manhole - access and structural condition)	
①②③⊙⊗		Inspect Vessel (irregularities)	
①②③⊙⊗		Remove floatables and oil and grease from floatable port (use skimmer net)	
①②③⊙⊗		Cylindrical Baffle	
		simple probe such as a Sludge Judge® can be used to determine the level of accumulated solids stored in the sump	

Inflow Points

Inflow Structure

Material: ______ Size: ______ End Type: ______ Structure # on Plans: ______

SCORE	PHOTO	DESCRIPTION	COMMENTS / DIMENSIONS
①②③⊙⊗		Overgrown Vegetation / Tree Removal	
①②③⊙⊗		Structural Condition	
①②③⊙⊗		Filter Condition	
①②③⊙⊗		Other (Describe)	

Inspect Chambers from Upstream to Downstream, Providing Identifying Information for Each

Chamber 1

Structure # on Plans: ______ Chamber Name on Plans: ______ Label on Sketch: ______

SCORE	PHOTO	DESCRIPTION	COMMENTS / DIMENSIONS	
① ⊙⊗		Inconsistent with Plans	Observed:	Specified:
①②③⊙⊗		Trash / Debris / Sediment *Description / Amount:*		
①②③⊙⊗		Blockage *(Full of water after dry weather, no permanent pool on plans.)*		
①②③⊙⊗		Access hatch condition		
①②③⊙⊗		Separator structural condition		
①②③⊙⊗		Central shaft condition		
①②③⊙⊗		Ladder / Steps Condition		
①②③⊙⊗		Oil accumulation		
①②③⊙⊗		Standing water		
①②③⊙⊗		Spalling / Deterioration		
①②③⊙⊗		Connecting Pipes, if any	Pipe Direction:	Problem:
①②③⊙⊗		Manhole / Bilco Door Condition		
①②③⊙⊗		Other:		

FIGURE 9.19 Swirl Separators and Vault Inspection Form

Swirl Separators & Vault Inspection Form **Page 2**

Site ID: ________ Facility ID: ____________ Facility Name: ______________________________

Chamber 2

Structure # on Plans:		Chamber Name on Plans:	Label on Sketch:	
SCORE	PHOTO	DESCRIPTION	COMMENTS / DIMENSIONS	
① ⊙⊗		Inconsistent with Plans	Observed:	Specified:
①②③⊙⊗		Trash / Debris / Sediment *Description / Amount:*		
①②③⊙⊗		Blockage *(Full of water after dry weather, no permanent pool on plans.)*		
①②③⊙⊗		Access hatch condition		
①②③⊙⊗		Separator structural condition		
①②③⊙⊗		Central shaft condition		
①②③⊙⊗		Ladder / Steps Condition		
①②③⊙⊗		Oil accumulation		
①②③⊙⊗		Standing water		
①②③⊙⊗		Spalling / Deterioration		
①②③⊙⊗		Connecting Pipes, if any	Pipe Direction:	Problem:
①②③⊙⊗		Manhole / Bilco Door Condition		
①②③⊙⊗		Other:		

Chamber 3

Structure # on Plans:		Chamber Name on Plans:	Label on Sketch:	
SCORE	PHOTO	DESCRIPTION	COMMENTS / DIMENSIONS	
① ⊙⊗		Inconsistent with Plans	Observed:	Specified:
①②③⊙⊗		Trash / Debris / Sediment *Description / Amount:*		
①②③⊙⊗		Blockage *(Full of water after dry weather, no permanent pool on plans.)*		
①②③⊙⊗		Access hatch condition		
①②③⊙⊗		Separator structural condition		
①②③⊙⊗		Central shaft condition		
①②③⊙⊗		Ladder / Steps Condition		
①②③⊙⊗		Oil accumulation		
①②③⊙⊗		Standing water		
①②③⊙⊗		Spalling / Deterioration		
①②③⊙⊗		Connecting Pipes, if any	Pipe Direction:	Problem:
①②③⊙⊗		Manhole / Bilco Door Condition		
①②③⊙⊗		Other:		

Chamber 4

Structure # on Plans:		Chamber Name on Plans:	Label on Sketch:	
SCORE	PHOTO	DESCRIPTION	COMMENTS / DIMENSIONS	
① ⊙⊗		Inconsistent with Plans	Observed:	Specified:
①②③⊙⊗		Trash / Debris / Sediment *Description / Amount:*		
①②③⊙⊗		Blockage *(Full of water after dry weather, no permanent pool on plans.)*		
①②③⊙⊗		Access hatch condition		
①②③⊙⊗		Separator structural condition		
①②③⊙⊗		Central shaft condition		
①②③⊙⊗		Ladder / Steps Condition		
①②③⊙⊗		Oil accumulation		
①②③⊙⊗		Standing water		
①②③⊙⊗		Spalling / Deterioration		
①②③⊙⊗		Connecting Pipes, if any	Pipe Direction:	Problem:
①②③⊙⊗		Manhole / Bilco Door Condition		
①②③⊙⊗		Other:		

Chamber 5

Structure # on Plans:		Chamber Name on Plans:	Label on Sketch:	
SCORE	PHOTO	DESCRIPTION	COMMENTS / DIMENSIONS	
① ⊙⊗		Inconsistent with Plans	Observed:	Specified:
①②③⊙⊗		Trash / Debris / Sediment *Description / Amount:*		
①②③⊙⊗		Blockage *(Full of water after dry weather, no permanent pool on plans.)*		
①②③⊙⊗		Access hatch condition		
①②③⊙⊗		Separator structural condition		
①②③⊙⊗		Central shaft condition		
①②③⊙⊗		Ladder / Steps Condition		
①②③⊙⊗		Oil accumulation		
①②③⊙⊗		Standing water		
①②③⊙⊗		Spalling / Deterioration		
①②③⊙⊗		Connecting Pipes, if any	Pipe Direction:	Problem:
①②③⊙⊗		Manhole / Bilco Door Condition		
①②③⊙⊗		Other:		

FIGURE 9.19 Swirl Separators and Vault Inspection Form (*continued*)

Swirl Separators & Vault Inspection Form Page 3

Site ID: ________ Facility ID: ________ Facility Name: ________

Outfall Structure / Other

Outfall Structure

Material:		Size:	End Type:	Structure # on Plans:
SCORE	PHOTO	DESCRIPTION		COMMENTS / DIMENSIONS
①②③⊙⊗		Blockage	(③ < 25% < ② < 75% < ①)	
①②③⊙⊗		Overgrown Vegetation / Tree Removal		
①②③⊙⊗		Trash / Debris / Sediment		
①②③⊙⊗		Erosion / Undermining	Area:	
①②③⊙⊗		Joint Failure/Loss of Joint Material		
①②③⊙⊗		Leaking Device		
①②③⊙⊗		Emergency By-pass Condition		
①②③⊙⊗		Filter Fabric Present Under Rip Rap?		
①②③⊙⊗		Displacement and Condition of Fabric		
①②③⊙⊗		Rip-Rap: Size, Quantity, Underlying Fabric?		
①②③⊙⊗		Spalling / Deterioration		
①②③⊙⊗		Separation / Misalignment		
①②③⊙⊗		Manhole Condition		
①②③⊙⊗		Ladder / Steps Condition		
①②③⊙⊗		Downstream Channel Condition		
①②③⊙⊗		Other:		

Other

SCORE	PHOTO	DESCRIPTION	LOCATION
①②③⊙⊗		Encroachments	
①②③⊙⊗		Modifications	
①②③⊙⊗		Mosquito Habitat	
①②③⊙⊗		Hazardous Fumes/Odors Present	
①②③⊙⊗		Evidence of Possible Illicit Discharge, Call to Report	

INSPECTOR COMMENTS

FIGURE 9.19 Swirl Separators and Vault Inspection Form (*continued*)

Gross Pollutant Screens

Name of Entity		Inspector:	Cert
		Inspector:	Cert
		Date:	
Site ID:	Facility ID:	Facility Name:	
Address:		Coordinates / ParID :	
		Watershed:	County/District:

Scoring Key	
①	High Priority / Non-functional
②	Moderate Priority / Approaching Non-functional
③	Low Priority / Functional
⊙	No Priority / Continue Routine Maintenance
⊗	Not Applicable

Functional? [ ] Yes [ ] No

Score Totals: | 1 | 2 | 3 |

Notes / Specifications:

Facility Specific Info:

Facility Type / Addl Facility Info:

Signs			Weather Conditions		
SCORE	PHOTO	DESCRIPTION	Last Rainfall	Date:	Amount:
③⊙⊗		Facility Sign	Current weather conditions?		
③⊙⊗		Facility Labeling			

Accessibility

			ACCESS PROBLEMS (Circle)	NEXT STEP (Circle One)
Access Comments:			Locked Inlet Manhole	Notify Responsible Party
			Physical Obstruction	Return for Re-inspection
SCORE	PHOTO	DESCRIPTION	Stuck / Broken Manhole Cover	Request Photos from Owner
① ⊙⊗		Overall Facility Access	Equipment Needed: ________	Request Maintenance
①②③⊙⊗		Component Access: ________________	Other:____________	Other:____________

Curb and Gutter

Type (Circle all that apply):		Flow Length	Left side of Inlet	ft	Right side of Inlet	ft

SCORE	PHOTO	DESCRIPTION	COMMENTS
①②③⊙⊗		Street Flooding	
①②③⊙⊗		Sediment / trash or debris accumulation	
①②③⊙⊗		Other:	

Automatic Retractable Screen

Type (Circle all that apply): Open or Closed

SCORE	PHOTO	DESCRIPTION	COMMENTS / DEPTH
①②③⊙⊗		Structural Condition	
①②③⊙⊗		Trash / Debris / Sediment *Description/Volume/Depth*	
①②③⊙⊗		ARS Open or Closed *Open/Closed*	
①②③⊙⊗		ARS Obstruction *(③ < 25% < ② < 75% < ①)*	
①②③⊙⊗		ARS Flushed with Street *Yes/No*	
①②③⊙⊗		Bypass Evident	
①②③⊙⊗		Retractable mechanisms Working Appropriately	
①②③⊙⊗		Other:	

Catch Basin

SCORE	PHOTO	DESCRIPTION	COMMENTS / DEPTH
①②③⊙⊗		Standing Water	
①②③⊙⊗		Damage / Deterioration	
①②③⊙⊗		Trash / Debris / Sediment *Description/Volume/Depth*	
①②③⊙⊗		Other:	

Connector Pipe Screen or Outlet Screen

Type (Circle all that apply): Open or Closed

SCORE	PHOTO	DESCRIPTION	COMMENTS / DEPTH
①②③⊙⊗		Screen Clogging *(③ < 25% < ② < 75% < ①)*	
①②③⊙⊗		Bypass evident	
①②③⊙⊗		Blockage/Obstruction *(③ < 25% < ② < 75% < ①)*	
①②③⊙⊗		Trash / Debris / Sediment *Description/Volume/Depth*	
①②③⊙⊗		Structural Damage *Area:*	
①②③⊙⊗		Spalling / Deterioration	
①②③⊙⊗		Separation / Misalignment	
①②③⊙⊗		Manhole Condition	
①②③⊙⊗		Ladder / Steps Condition	
①②③⊙⊗		Condition of Outfall Pipe	
①②③⊙⊗		Downstream Channel Condition	
①②③⊙⊗		Other:	

FIGURE 9.20 Gross Pollutant Screens Inspection Form

Gross Pollutant Screens Inspection Form Page 2

Site ID: ______ Facility ID: ________ Facility Name: ______________________________

Other			
SCORE	PHOTO	DESCRIPTION	LOCATION
①②③⊙⊗		Encroachments	
①②③⊙⊗		Modifications	
①②③⊙⊗		Mosquito Habitat	
①②③⊙⊗		Evidence Possible Illicit Discharge, Call to Report	

INSPECTOR COMMENTS

FIGURE 9.20 Gross Pollutant Screens Inspection Form (*continued*)

Finally, the heart of this chapter presents SCM-specific concerns during construction and O&M (Sections 3.4 and 3.5, respectively), followed by comprehensive and detailed inspection forms (Sections 4.1 and 4.2). The SCM Construction Inspection Form (Figure 9.8) may be used either as presented in this manual for all different SCMs, or further customized by the user to make it SCM-specific. The O&M forms presented in this manual are SCM-specific and are intended to be detailed and comprehensive in nature. They may also be used as presented or customized by the user. Different forms of customization are discussed in Section 4.2.

6.0 REFERENCES

Caldwell, E. (2020). *Transitioning stormwater facility maintenance from reactive to proactive: An experiment in risk assessment and predictive analytics. World Water: Stormwater Management.* Fairfax County Stormwater Management.

City of Frisco. (2019). *Best management practices maintenance guidelines—A guideline for homeowner's associations and land managers in Frisco, Texas.* https://www.friscotexas.gov/DocumentCenter/View/19892/HOA-Guidance?bidId=

City of New Jersey. (2018). *New Jersey stormwater best management practices manual.* New Jersey Department of Environmental Protection, Division of Watershed Management. https://www.njstormwater.org/bmp_manual2.htm

City of Poway, CA. (2016). *BMP design manual for permanent site design, storm water treatment and hydromodification management.* https://poway.org/847/BMP-Design-Manual

City of San Diego. (2012). *San Diego storm drain insert pilot study* (Project ID# CSD-RT-12-URS43-03). https://www.sandiego.gov/sites/default/files/legacy/stormwater/pdf/stormdrainpilotstudy.pdf

Pazwash, H. (2016). *AWWA urban stormwater management* (2nd ed.).

San Antonio River Authority. (2019). *San Antonio river basin low impact development technical design guidance manual* (2nd ed.). https://www.sariverauthority.org/sites/default/files/2019-08/SARB%20LID%20Technical%20Design%20Manual%202nd%20Edition.pdf

Sanchez, A. J. (2012). *Update on stormwater BMPs and green infrastructure retrofit case studies in Fort Worth, Texas.* StormCon 2012 Proceedings, Denver, CO.

Tarrant Regional Water District. (2018). *Water quality guidance manual planning and implementing stormwater quality practices.* https://www.trwd.com/wp-content/uploads/2019/04/TRWD-WQ-Guidance-Manual_June-2018-Updated-Sept.-2018-Compressed.pdf

Water Environment Federation, American Society of Civil Engineers/Environmental & Water Resources Institute. (2012). *Design of urban stormwater controls* (WEF Manual of Practice No. 23; ASCE/EWRI Manuals and Reports on Engineering Practice No. 87). Water Environment Federation.

10

Case Studies

1.0 INTRODUCTION 348

2.0 CASE STUDY 1—KANSAS CITY, MO 349

2.1 Stormwater Management Program Overview 349

2.1.1 General Program 349

2.1.2 Operations and Maintenance Activities 350

2.2 Types of Stormwater Control Measures 350

2.2.1 Public Stormwater Control Measures 351

2.2.2 Private Stormwater Control Measures 351

2.3 Maintenance of Stormwater Control Measures 352

2.3.1 Performance of Inspection and Maintenance Activities 352

2.3.2 Lessons Learned 352

2.3.2.1 Green Solutions 352

2.3.2.2 Green Stewards 353

2.3.2.3 Construction Contractor Maintenance 354

2.4 Inspection and Maintenance Responsibilities and Recordkeeping 354

2.4.1 Public Practices 354

2.4.1.1 Maintenance Frequencies and Reporting 354

2.4.1.2 Responsible Parties 355

2.4.1.3 Recordkeeping 358

2.4.2 Private Practices 360

2.4.2.1 Maintenance Frequencies and Reporting 360

2.4.2.2 Responsible Parties 361

2.4.2.3 Recordkeeping 362

2.5 Funding Inspections and Maintenance 362

2.5.1 Public Practices 362

2.5.1.1 Funding Mechanisms 362

2.5.1.2 Summary of Annual Costs 362

2.5.2 Private Practices 363

2.5.2.1 Funding Mechanisms 363

2.5.2.2 Summary of Annual Costs 363

2.6 Challenges and Future Initiatives 364

2.6.1 Asset Management 364

2.6.2 In-House Maintenance 364

2.6.3 Contracted Assistance 364

2.6.4 Green Stewards 365

2.6.5 Overall Operations and Maintenance Program Planning 365

3.0 CASE STUDY 2—CITY OF LANCASTER, PA 365

3.1 Stormwater Management Program Overview 365

3.2 Types of Stormwater Control Measures 367
3.3 Maintenance of Stormwater Control Measures 367
3.3.1 Inspection and Maintenance Activities 367
3.3.2 Lessons Learned 367
3.4 Inspection and Maintenance Responsibilities and Recordkeeping 368
3.4.1 Maintenance Frequencies and Reporting 368
3.4.2 Recordkeeping 369
3.5 Funding Inspections and Maintenance 369
3.5.1 Public Practices 369
3.5.2 Private Practices 369
3.6 Challenges and Future Initiatives 370
4.0 CASE STUDY 3—PHILADELPHIA WATER DEPARTMENT 370
4.1 Stormwater Management Program Overview 370
4.2 Types of Stormwater Control Measures 371
4.3 Maintenance of Stormwater Control Measures 372
4.3.1 Inspection and Maintenance Activities 372
4.3.2 Lessons Learned 372
4.4 Inspection and Maintenance Responsibilities and Recordkeeping 373
4.4.1 Public Practices 373
4.4.1.1 Maintenance Frequencies and Reporting 373
4.4.1.2 Recordkeeping 373
4.4.2 Asset Management Considerations 374
4.5 Funding Inspections and Maintenance 374
4.6 Challenges and Future Initiatives 374
4.6.1 Inspection and Maintenance Challenges 374
4.6.2 Future Initiatives to Ensure Continued Performance 376
5.0 REFERENCES 377
6.0 SUGGESTED READING 377

1.0 INTRODUCTION

This chapter presents case studies to illustrate different approaches to address operations and maintenance (O&M) activities in large and small cities/utilities. The case studies follow the same outline and provide information on the following topics:

- Stormwater Management Program Overview. An overview of the city/utility and general information on the program.
- Types of Stormwater Control Measures (SCMs). The types of SCMs that are being maintained and, when possible, explanation of different procedures used for private and publicly maintained facilities.

- Maintenance of SCMs. A description of how inspection and maintenance activities are performed and lessons learned.
- Inspection and Maintenance Responsibilities and Recordkeeping. An overview of the responsibilities assigned to different groups to illustrate different organizational arrangements and procedures for recordkeeping. Also, this section illustrates different approaches for private and public SCM maintenance.
- Funding Inspections and Maintenance. A description of the funding sources used to conduct O&M activities.
- Challenges and Future Initiatives. A description of the O&M program challenges and plans to overcome them. In addition, the case studies include an overview of initiatives that are being implemented to move the programs forward. Examples of initiatives include the need for updated manuals, implementation of asset management, implementation of in-house and contracted maintenance, workforce development, and program planning.

2.0 CASE STUDY 1—KANSAS CITY, MO

2.1 Stormwater Management Program Overview

2.1.1 General Program

The City of Kansas City, Missouri, manages its water systems using a "one water" approach through KC Water. KC Water manages drinking water, wastewater, and stormwater systems for approximately 826 km^2 (319 sq mi), serving approximately 170,000 residences and businesses (KC Water, 2021).

The city and its regulatory partners have agreed to meet the objectives outlined in a federal consent decree over a 25-year period from 2010 through 2035. The plan involves a list of improvements that are structured to capture for treatment approximately 88% of total wet weather flow in the combined sewer system and eliminate separate sanitary sewer overflows during a 5-year, 24-hour rainfall event. This implementation is referred to as the Overflow Control Program (OCP). Kansas City's Overflow Control program team (Smart Sewer Program) managed by KC Water implements the OCP to monitor compliance with the United States of America v. City of Kansas City, MO consent decree (2010).

Objectives of the consent decree included the construction of green infrastructure facilities as an SCM. As of January 2021, KC Water has constructed 119 green hectares (295 green acres) (a green hectare or acre is impervious area that drains to a green infrastructure facility) and is responsible for maintaining approximately 120 108 m^2 (1 292 822 sq ft or approximately 30 ac) of green infrastructure facility footprint.

KC Water also is responsible for managing compliance with the city's National Pollutant Discharge Elimination System (NPDES) Missouri State operating permit for discharges from its municipal separate storm sewer system (MS4), which include postconstruction stormwater best management practice (BMP) requirements as the SCM.

2.1.2 Operations and Maintenance Activities

The responsibility for green infrastructure maintenance lies with the city department that constructed the facility. While green infrastructure facilities have been constructed as part of a variety of different city department projects, KC Water has built and maintains the majority of green infrastructure facilities.

KC Water currently utilizes four different mechanisms for maintaining green infrastructure that are applicable at different phases in a project's life cycle:

- Construction Contractor
- Green Solutions Crew
- Green Stewards
- Contracted Maintenance Assistance

An inspection team oversees the maintenance activities, providing a consistent review.

Figure 10.1 depicts the current typical use of these maintenance mechanisms.

2.2 Types of Stormwater Control Measures

The city classifies SCMs by type using the same practice terminology as the regional Mid-America Regional Council (2008) *Manual of Best Management Practices for Stormwater Quality*. This provides consistency in nomenclature across technical disciplines. Figure 10.2 provides the list of SCMs (green stormwater infrastructure [GSI] practices) and associated components for maintenance. KC Water is using a standardized component-based approach to provide flexibility for SCMs to be integrated into a range of land uses. This component-based approach is detailed in City of Kansas City, MO (2018) *Green Stormwater Infrastructure Manual*.

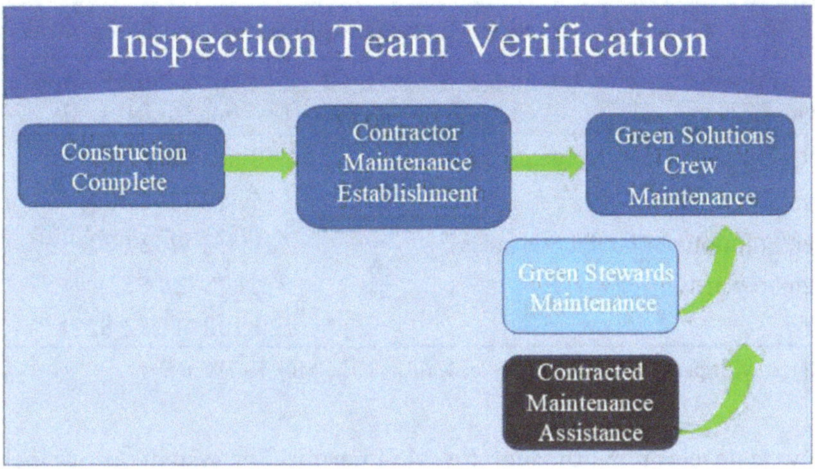

FIGURE 10.1 KC Water Green Infrastructure Maintenance Mechanisms. Reprinted with permission from City of Kansas City, MO, KC Water.

2.2.1 *Public Stormwater Control Measures*

In 2020, KC Water maintained 120 108 m^2 (1 292 822 sq ft or approximately 30 ac) across all maintenance provider types (see Table 10.1).

2.2.2 *Private Stormwater Control Measures*

KIVA was the software application system used by the city to inventory permanent stormwater BMPs and green infrastructure implemented as part

GSI Practice	Inlets	Energy Dissipation & Pretreatment	Above Grade Barriers	Permeable Pavement	Soil & Aggregate Media	Media Liners	Landscaping	Piping	Outlets
Rain Garden	●	●	●		●		●		
Bioretention Basin	●	●	●		●	●	●	●	●
Porous Asphalt		●	●	●	●	●		●	
Pervious Concrete		●	●	●	●	●		●	
Permeable Pavers		●	●	●	●	●		●	
Bioswale/Native Vegetation Swale	●	●	●		●	●	●	●	●
Non-Structural Native Vegetation	●	●	●		●		●		
Infiltration Trench	●	●	●		●	●		●	●
Wetland/Extended Detention Wetland	●	●	●		●	●	●	●	●
Sand Filter	●	●	●		●	●		●	●
Extended Wet Detention Basin	●	●	●		●	●	●	●	●
Extended Dry Detention Basin	●	●	●		●	●	●	●	●
Proprietary Media Filtration	●	●							
Green Roof					●	●	●	●	●

FIGURE 10.2 GSI Practices (City of Kansas City, MO, 2018, p. 7). Reprinted with permission from City of Kansas City, MO, KC Water.

TABLE 10.1 Green Infrastructure Maintenance Providers and Footprint Served.

Green Infrastructure Maintenance Provider Type	Green Infrastructure Footprint (m^2 [sq ft])
Contractor Service Agreement	40 692 (438 000)
Green Solutions	55 184 (594 000)
Green Solutions + Green Stewards	21 554 (232 000)
Green Stewards	2678 (28 822)
Total	120 108 (1 292 822)

Reprinted with permission from City of Kansas City, MO, KC Water.

of private development through the MS4 permit. The system output included site-issued permits from July 2008 through February 2013. Tracking of private green infrastructure since February 2013 has primarily been through permit review processes for private development construction through City Planning and Development in combination with KC Water. Currently, maintenance activities are performed by the property owner at private stormwater BMPs.

2.3 Maintenance of Stormwater Control Measures

2.3.1 Performance of Inspection and Maintenance Activities

Maintenance responsibilities for the KC Water green infrastructure facility footprint are distributed across KC Water's Green Solutions crew, Green Stewards program, and contractor service agreements. In 2020, a portion of the sites in contractor service agreements were nearing the end of the construction contractor maintenance period. Figure 10.3 depicts KC Water's green infrastructure footprint projected growth over the next few years. This growth is determined from known construction and design projects underway.

2.3.2 Lessons Learned

2.3.2.1 Green Solutions

Recruiting and retaining interested team members has been the most significant challenge for the Green Solutions crew. Recruiting for crew job openings is hindered by job classifications and by mismatched interest.

Standard job classifications, specifically the positions titled "Maintenance Worker" and "Equipment Operator," do not set the expectation that the work is primarily landscape-related. These classifications are used for numerous departments within the city, including but not limited to solid

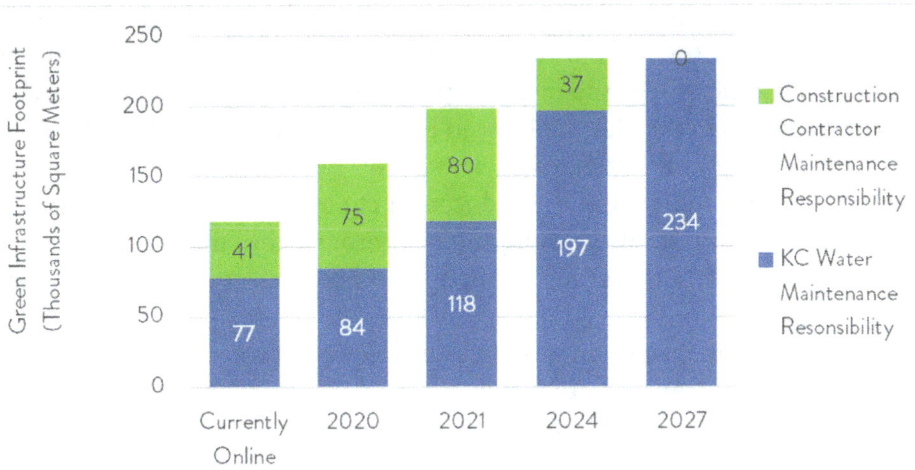

FIGURE 10.3 KC Water Projected Green Infrastructure Asset Growth (2020–2027). Reprinted with permission from City of Kansas City, MO, KC Water.

waste handling, street work, stormwater repair, wastewater preventive maintenance, and stormwater preventive maintenance. The tasks listed for the classifications cover a wide range of job duties, from small machinery repair, operation of backhoes for excavation and trenching, snow plowing and removal, installation and repair of sewer lines, and landscape maintenance for BMPs. There is some ability to add more description within job advertisements, such as to list qualification or skill preferences. However, catching the eye of job applicants with those preferences (such as horticultural, forestry, or landscape-related background) in an advertisement called "Maintenance Worker" or "Equipment Operator" is difficult.

Mismatched interest refers to a situation where a position is found by an applicant who sees "Maintenance Worker" or "Equipment Operator" and envisions pipe work, using heavy equipment, or similar work. Applicants sometimes see the general job descriptions and apply for these positions without realizing that work on the Green Solutions crew is almost entirely related to landscape maintenance and the other tasks listed in the standard descriptions may not regularly be used in these jobs. Experience has shown that some applicants accept employment under these circumstances and end up discontent with the landscape-related work and eager to make lateral transfers to other workgroups in the city.

2.3.2.2 Green Stewards

As a new workforce development program, Green Stewards is continuing to develop and grow based on the lessons learned in the first 3 years of the contract. The city successfully hired one person to the Green Solutions crew. There are hopes for more in the future as skills are honed and positions become available. Over the last few years, several of the Green Stewards have been through the National Green Infrastructure Certification Program training and received certification. There have been other success stories as well, such as pursuing a General Education Diploma or obtaining a driver's license and finding stable housing options through the support of program leadership. Important lessons learned have been related to program size and recruiting.

To stay within the program budget and to offer meaningful positions with health insurance, transportation support, paid vacation, and paid sick leave, the program is small. The number of participants is limited to seven individuals to provide these important benefits while staying within the program budget. Keeping the size limited has also been helpful to avoid having too many people at maintenance sites and disrupting daily life in the project areas.

Recruiting practices have continually refined to reach candidates who are interested in employment, maintaining green infrastructure, and serving the public. It has taken persistence to find candidates who are interested in a job performing physical work in all kinds of weather, answering questions from the public, and learning a new set of skills.

2.3.2.3 Construction Contractor Maintenance

Construction contracts for public green infrastructure through KC Water include a 3-year service agreement in which the construction contractor is required to perform regular maintenance of the green infrastructure sites. The service agreement timeframe was set at 3 years initially to match the 3-year timeframe of the "Correction Period" routinely used for KC Water construction projects.

2.4 Inspection and Maintenance Responsibilities and Recordkeeping

2.4.1 Public Practices

KC Water began continually inspecting, maintaining, and recording green infrastructure assets in 2012. Asset management practices began with paper logs and spreadsheets and have evolved to include an increased reliance on a computerized maintenance management system (CMMS).

2.4.1.1 Maintenance Frequencies and Reporting

General guidance for maintenance frequencies and reporting was compiled for Kansas City's *Green Stormwater Infrastructure Manual (GSI Manual)* in 2018. Before the availability of the *GSI Manual*, green infrastructure project contracts included a green infrastructure service agreement specification, which described required maintenance tasks, frequencies, and reporting requirements for a 3-year period. Reporting consisted of contractor spreadsheet logs that were submitted following a prescribed format when routine invoices were submitted.

After several years of implementing the service agreement specification, KC Water learned there are challenges associated with prescribing maintenance frequencies for some aspects of green infrastructure assets. Weed removal, in particular, could be insufficient if the pace of the weed growth outpaced the contracted weed removal frequency. To address this challenge, a modification was made within the service agreement specification for a small number of tasks that were not effective at the originally specified frequencies. These were weed management, pest/disease management, and watering requirements during drought.

A few years later, an establishment period specification was developed for release with the *GSI Manual*, which expanded on the performance specification idea. The establishment period specification functioned as a performance specification, wherein a contractor prepared a maintenance schedule designed to meet stated performance requirements. The schedule would be updated by the contractor as needed based on the conditions at the particular site. Therefore, for example, maintenance frequencies could become closer together if a particular site is observed to have higher sediment or litter loads. Similar to the original service agreement specification, contractor spreadsheet logs would be submitted with invoices following a prescribed log format.

In addition to the specification included in project contracts, most of KC Water's green infrastructure projects include highly specific, individualized O&M manuals, which are developed by the respective design professional team. The manuals are completed near project closeout to include photographs of the constructed assets. The manuals are reference materials and are not part of service agreement or establishment period contract requirements.

2.4.1.2 Responsible Parties

Maintenance and inspections for green infrastructure facilities built by KC Water are performed through a five-team approach (see Figure 10.1). In-house maintenance, in-house inspection, construction contractor, on-call contractor, and workforce development teams perform maintenance and inspection. This approach to maintenance is designed to be inherently resilient. For example, when one team might be having staff turnover or contract renewal delays, the other teams can temporarily step in to maintain and inspect the assets.

KC Water's in-house maintenance crew, Green Solutions, was formed in 2012 and consists of one utility supervisor, two landscape technicians, and between three and five maintenance workers and equipment operators (depending on staff turnover). Green Solutions crew provides routine maintenance tasks as well as reactive repair tasks, such as repairing damage from vandalism or vehicles. The ability to perform reactive repair tasks is a sometimes overlooked but a critical part of green infrastructure maintenance. Typically, projects transition to this crew when the initial 3-year service agreement or establishment period ends.

Contracted assistance, by the contractor who built the asset (construction contractor), is provided for the first 3 years after an asset is constructed, as described previously. This allows a transition period where the inspection team can become familiar with the asset, has access to the contractor's background knowledge of the project, and can view methods in the field for particular site-specific tasks.

Additionally, KC Water uses an on-call green infrastructure maintenance contract, which includes unit prices for maintenance tasks. This contract is typically implemented in 1-year increments to bridge capacity shortfalls and for unexpected needs, such as repairs beyond the capacity of the Green Solutions crew. One example occurred in 2020, when a number of crew positions became vacant, and the timing unfortunately coincided with a large group of new projects aging out of their 3-year service agreement and handing over to Green Solutions crew. An on-call mowing contract is also used to cover mowing of perimeter lawn at one green infrastructure site.

KC Water started a workforce development program in 2017, called Green Stewards, which is designed to provide on-the-job training to fill a need for skilled maintenance workers who are qualified to apply for contractor or in-house maintenance jobs. Figure 10.4 illustrates the relationship of this team as a source of qualified potential employees. A nonprofit organization, Bridging the Gap, has administered the program on behalf of KC Water since the program inception. The program is advertised for proposals every 3 years. A new contract began with Bridging the Gap in 2021, which will cover 1 year with two optional renewals.

KC Water's plan to promote, maintain, and evaluate green infrastructure includes recommendations for workforce development and job training to support a green collar jobs-related program. The Green Stewards program is designed to help the city meet a portion of those recommendations.

The Green Stewards support the city in day-to-day maintenance and monitoring of a portion of the city's constructed green infrastructure installations (see Table 10.1). The program focuses on the development of the Green Stewards' skills in green infrastructure and landscape maintenance. One program manager, one field manager, and between five and six crew

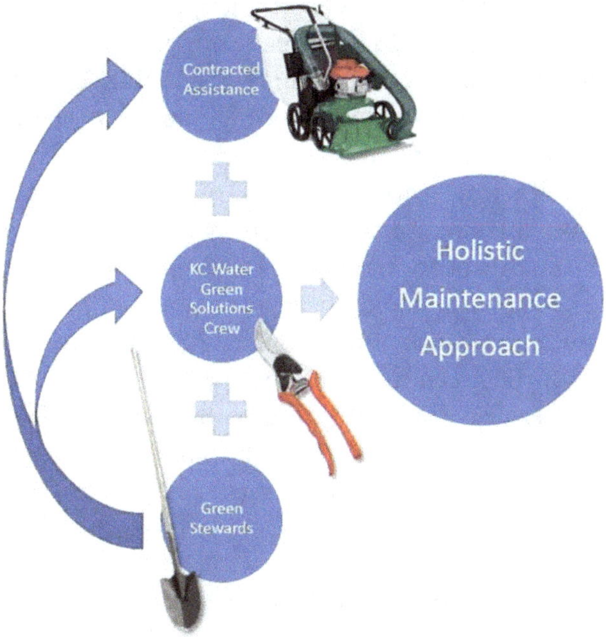

FIGURE 10.4 Green Stewards Program as Source of Qualified Potential Employees (Treese, Brotherton, & Riott, 2019). (Reprinted with permission from City of Kansas City, MO, KC Water.)

members carry out the program year-round in all types of weather. At the same time, the team provides a professional, motivational, and approachable presence in the community that answers questions residents may have about green infrastructure or employment opportunities that might exist to work with green infrastructure.

Inspection is an essential part of green infrastructure maintenance. Self-inspection and third-party inspection are key components to a balanced evaluation of maintenance work.

Self-inspection looks differently for the three categories of maintenance providers. Green Solutions crew inputs inspection information in KC Water's work order management system (or CMMS), Hansen Information Technologies (or Infor Hansen). In 2020, three performance rating indices were added to the inspection form: Functional Index, Litter Index, and Aesthetic Acceptance. These indices allow for an evaluation of function, level of litter, and how aesthetically acceptable each asset appears at each visit. Self-inspections conclude with the crew rating the asset on these three indices. Contractors provide reporting on a spreadsheet log that steps through the tasks and includes prompts to write responses for key inspection items; for example, "Was ponding observed (yes/no)?" Green Stewards input inspection information in a custom-designed form in ArcGIS ArcCollector and Survey123. Since 2018, three rating indices have been included on the Green Stewards inspection form: Functional Index, Litter Index, and Aesthetic Acceptance. Self-inspections conclude with the Green Stewards rating the asset on these three indices.

Figure 10.1 illustrates how the work of an inspection team encompasses the various maintenance mechanisms to monitor and help coordinate the work. The inspections of this third-party inspections team consist of biweekly to monthly field observations by two KC Water personnel from a separate organizational division. The Smart Sewer division builds a large portion of the green infrastructure projects for KC Water and provides inspection services for these projects. Beginning in 2012, one senior landscape architect provided field observations, general logistical support, monthly internal synchronization meetings, contract coordination, invoice processing, troubleshooting, design support, procedural definition, and specialty repair facilitation.

In late 2015, one landscape technician was added to assist with field observation reporting, specialty maintenance tasks, planting coordination assistance, and specialty repair facilitation.

2.4.1.3 Recordkeeping

Three primary asset management systems are used for green infrastructure: Geographic Information System (GIS), PeopleSoft, and Infor Hansen. Each application forms a piece of the asset management whole, and the primary challenge is to keep assets and their attributes consistently named and recorded across the three applications.

GIS software records each asset. The included data consist of asset identification (UNIT ID), location, dimension, responsibility, and as-built drawings. KC Water green infrastructure assets have been recorded in GIS as polygons since 2013, and the data recorded have been relatively consistent for the individual assets. Improvements made in 2018 added point and line components for the assets (such as underdrains, overflow risers, and cleanouts), and an asset grouping layer was added in 2020, which groups assets from individual projects together.

PeopleSoft software records financial information for the green infrastructure assets, primarily related to capital expenditures. Starting in 2012, assets were recorded in PeopleSoft at the project level instead of by individual asset types, which made it difficult to differentiate dollars spent on different asset types. For example, if a project included one (1) rain garden and one (1) bioretention cell, the project's schedule of values includes costs for both of them together as one sum. An average lifespan of 15 years was set for all green infrastructure assets. In 2018, nomenclature and asset categories were defined for use in future project schedules of value to reflect asset costs by asset type. The refined approach meant that a schedule of values would show the costs separately, as could be applied to the example of one rain garden and one bioretention cell. Lifespans were then able to be defined for each asset type, instead of being averaged across different asset types.

Infor Hansen records information related to how assets are being operated and maintained and is the primary CMMS used by KC Water. GIS asset data form the foundation for the assets recorded in Infor Hansen, and the UNIT ID carries over from GIS into this application. Maintenance work orders are created, performed, and closed, and a permanent record is associated with each asset that can be queried to understand asset history. Initially, in 2012, maintenance work was recorded as site-level work orders that did not coordinate with information in GIS. Work order tasks were defined in broad categories based on categories previously defined for levee maintenance activities. In 2016, UNIT IDs were coordinated between GIS and Infor Hansen software applications so that work orders could be recorded at the asset level rather than at the project level. In 2019, after the completion of the *GSI Manual* and the definition of consistent green infrastructure components (see Figure 10.2), refined work order tasks were created to match the tasks defined in the manual. Through a series of coordination efforts, the refined maintenance activities went live in late 2020. Figure 10.5 illustrates the relationship between a green infrastructure asset, its components, and the refined maintenance activities.

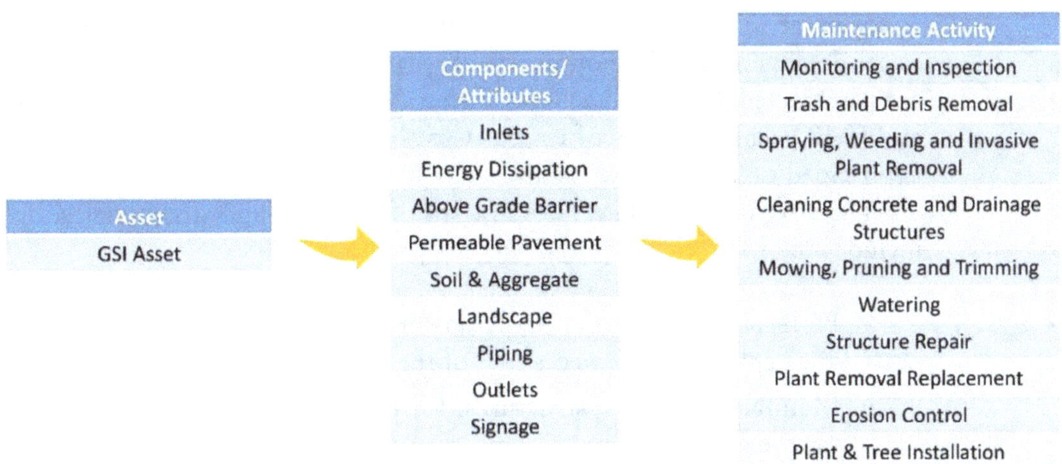

FIGURE 10.5 Green Infrastructure Asset Components and Maintenance Activity Relationship (Iyengar & KC Water, 2019)

2.4.2 Private Practices

The City of Kansas City, Missouri, has ordinances to address postconstruction runoff from new development and redevelopment projects. The ordinances require private developments to mitigate their effects for postconstruction above predevelopment conditions by including permanent postconstruction stormwater BMPs, stream buffers, and maintenance instruments for all sites (KC Water, 2019).

The BMP requirements are enforced by the city's Planning and Development Department during initial planning stages and through construction. "KC Water also provides BMPs guidance during the plan review and approval process" (KC Water, 2019). The city began requiring postconstruction stormwater BMPs to be built as part of private development and redevelopment projects in 2008 (Ordinance #081033) with the integration of the *Manual of Best Management Practices for Stormwater Quality* (*BMP Manual*) (Mid-America Regional Council, 2008) in the city's zoning and development code. Calculations are required for each development and redevelopment project to determine the quantity and type of required stormwater BMPs. Stream Buffer Regulations and Conservation and Open Space Development Regulations were adopted in 2009 with the adoption of a new Zoning and Development code (City of Kansas City, MO, 2019–2020).

Once BMPs have been completed and approved by the city's planning department, the municipal jurisdiction transfers to KC Water for inspection and enforcement.

2.4.2.1 Maintenance Frequencies and Reporting

A covenant is recorded at the respective county office for recording real estate documents for development and redevelopment projects where BMPs are constructed. It is called a "Covenant to Maintain Storm Water Detention and BMP Facilities" (City of Kansas City, MO, 2010). A covenant template is provided on the city's website.

The covenant template does not specify maintenance frequencies, but includes the following requirements for property owners:

a. Be responsible for the perpetual preservation, maintenance, repair and replacement, if necessary, of the facilities.
b. Maintain the pipes, structures, BMPs, grounds, and appurtenances for the facilities.
c. Keep the pipes, structures, BMPs, and appurtenances open and free of silt and nonbeneficial vegetation.

d. Keep the pipes, structures, BMPs, and appurtenances in good working condition or replace same if necessary.

e. Control the growth of the vegetation and grass areas, not identified as beneficial to the BMPs to the limits prescribed by the Kansas City Code of Ordinances.

f. Maintain the grades pursuant to the approved plan on file in the office of the Director of City Planning and Development.

g. Obtain all necessary improvement and repair permits before performing any work on the facilities.

The property owner is not required to report to the city regarding the BMPs. The covenant also states that areas permitted for BMPs shall not be used or built upon in a manner that will interfere with the function of the facilities (City of Kansas City, MO, 2010).

2.4.2.2 Responsible Parties

The covenant requires the property owner to maintain, preserve, and replace BMPs to keep them operational. The covenant stipulates the following related to city inspections and enforcement:

a. City is granted the right but is not obligated to enter upon Tract(s) to inspect, maintain, repair, and/or replace the facilities, including the pipes, structures, grounds, and appurtenances if Owner fails to maintain same. In the event that the city does provide maintenance for the facilities, then the city may:

   1. Charge the costs for such maintenance, repair, or replacement against owner, and/or the owner of specific tract(s) and/or the owners of specific lot(s).
   2. Assess a lien on either the tract(s) or on the lot(s), or both served by the facility.
   3. Maintain suit against owner, and/or the owner of tract(s) and/or the owners of the lot(s) for all costs incurred by the city for such maintenance (City of Kansas City, MO, 2010).

Training provided by the city related to private BMPs is limited. In general, as-needed guidance is provided to property owners who contact the city with questions or for information. Additionally, inspections of private BMP facilities also serve the purpose to educate and give general guidance to property owners related to their covenant obligations.

2.4.2.3 Recordkeeping

Inspection recording practices consist of individual forms and spreadsheets. Terms of the city's MS4 permit require private postconstruction BMPs are inspected for proper function. The goal indicated in the MS4 permit is to inspect all facilities before occupancy and to inspect one-fifth of private BMPs annually. The 2019 MS4 Report states, "During the reporting period, KC Water inspected 20 stormwater detention/retention basins. There are 99 basins on the inspection list" (City of Kansas City, MO, 2019–2020).

2.5 Funding Inspections and Maintenance

Portions of two primary funding sources are used for green infrastructure inspections and maintenance by KC Water. These consist of wastewater funds (for Smart Sewer projects in the combined sewer system area) and stormwater fee funds (primarily for KC Water projects in the MS4 area).

2.5.1 Public Practices

2.5.1.1 Funding Mechanisms

KC Water's wastewater rates are billed to the customer based on rate of water usage, and a small portion of these funds are used for Smart Sewer green infrastructure projects in the combined sewer system area. KC Water's stormwater fee is billed to the customer based on impervious cover at a rate of \$0.50 per 46 m^2 (500 sq ft) of impervious area, and a small portion of these funds is used for green infrastructure projects (primarily in the MS4 area). In 2020, approximately two thirds of green infrastructure inspection and maintenance at KC Water was funded from wastewater rates, and approximately one third was funded from stormwater fee funds.

2.5.1.2 Summary of Annual Costs

Annual costs for green infrastructure maintenance include costs from in-house maintenance (Green Solutions), in-house inspection, construction contractors, on-call contractors, and workforce development contractor (Green Stewards). It is estimated that approximately \$1.2 million were spent in these categories in 2020. This breaks down to approximately \$10/m^2 (\$0.93/sq ft or \$40,600/ac). This estimate includes materials, equipment use, and labor. For purposes of this case study, estimates were made for staff labor hours. Hourly rates were created using the mean pay amount for the appropriate city job classification. Overhead costs for KC Water labor were estimated using a multiplier of 0.42. Figure 10.6 illustrates the approximate proportion of costs associated with each category.

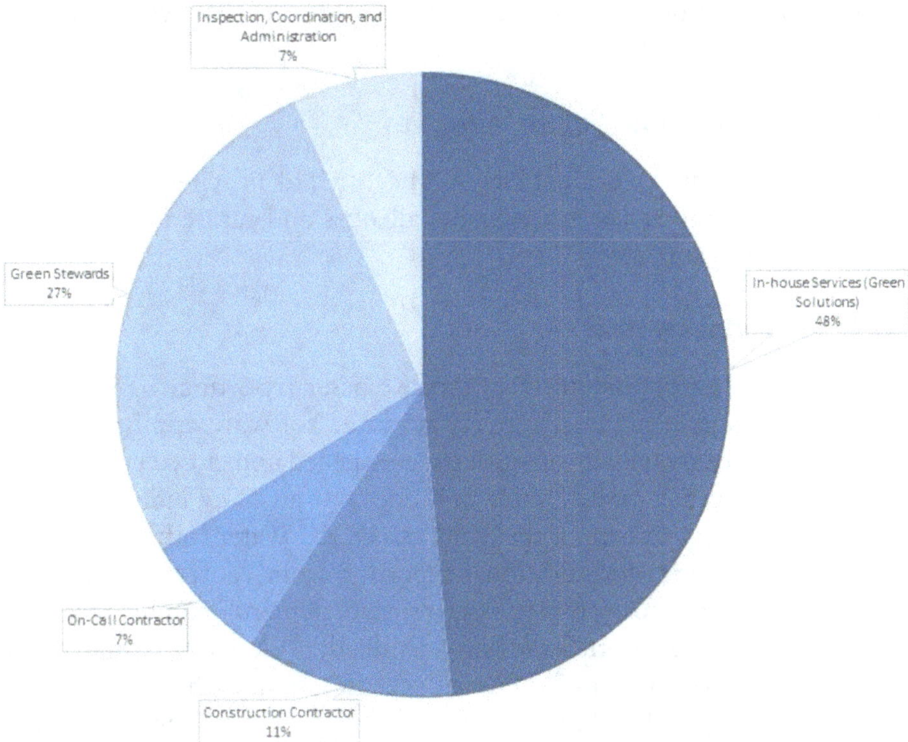

FIGURE 10.6 Proportional Costs by Category for 2020 KC Water Green Infrastructure Maintenance, Inspection, Coordination, and Administration (Reprinted with permission from City of Kansas City, MO, KC Water)

2.5.2 Private Practices

The stormwater fee is the primary funding source used for private BMP inspections by KC Water.

2.5.2.1 Funding Mechanisms

KC Water's stormwater fee is billed based on impervious cover at a rate of \$0.50 per 46 m^2 (500 sq ft) of impervious area and a small portion of these funds is used for private BMP inspections.

2.5.2.2 Summary of Annual Costs

It is estimated that approximately \$23,000 was spent in 2020 for private BMP inspections. This estimate includes materials, equipment use, and labor. For purposes of this case study, estimates were made for staff labor hours. Hourly rates were created using the mean pay amount for the appropriate city job classification. Overhead costs for KC Water labor were estimated using a multiplier of 0.42.

2.6 Challenges and Future Initiatives

KC Water continues to evaluate its SCM O&M, identifying opportunities to improve and grow. The following challenges and future initiatives will drive this improvement.

2.6.1 Asset Management

KC Water sees an opportunity to improve asset reporting to assist both staff and management. Asset reports from the software applications are currently limited to quantity of work orders opened and closed each month. This information has limited value and does not give any indication as to the function or appearance of the SCM assets. KC Water staff continues to identify opportunities for additional reporting from PeopleSoft and Infor Hansen records to inform future asset construction and maintenance decisions. Four desirable reports have been identified: (1) A real-time map that is color-coded to show the length of time since last visit at each asset, indicated by green (1 week), yellow (2 weeks), and red (1 month) with inspection and maintenance visits visually differentiated by shape; (2) A monthly report showing green infrastructure citizen service requests from each project asset group, displayed by month and year totals to show trends; (3) A monthly report ranking all assets by frequency of work orders so that highest input assets can be identified and corrected, also displayed showing month and year totals to show trends; (4) A monthly report showing work order frequency for each green infrastructure asset type (e.g., rain garden, permeable concrete) shown as month and year totals to show trends.

2.6.2 In-House Maintenance

A focus on recruiting processes is needed to improve the ability to recruit interested candidates with compatible skills. The use of different job classifications that could attract applicants with landscape-related background in internet job website searches and the improvement of promotion path definition are options for consideration.

2.6.3 Contracted Assistance

KC Water is evaluating the benefits of having a maintenance transition time that is long enough to get meaningful plant establishment. The establishment of vegetation continues to be a challenge on newly constructed projects. To date, the new establishment period specification has taken effect for KC

Water's two most recent green infrastructure construction contracts. Both projects began their establishment period in late 2020 and will be evaluated over the initial 3-year period for effectiveness at keeping the green infrastructure functional and aesthetically acceptable. During this time, KC Water will evaluate the utilization of this new specification to best establish the function of the vegetative features, and continue to consider other options, such as a separate landscape construction contract or reduced establishment contractual period for the construction contractor. Adjusting the timeframe from 3 years to 1 or 2 years will be considered for the following reasons: (1) the extended time to keep a construction contract open is not preferred, and (2) the ability of the construction contractor to meet the performance specification of maintenance activities requires significant staff enforcement time. Additionally, it is planned that contractor reporting will take place through an application in which contractors can report maintenance activities in real time; however, it is a low priority compared to other planned green infrastructure program efforts.

2.6.4 Green Stewards

The Green Stewards workforce development program has started the first year of its second contract term with the option of two renewals (for a total of 6 years). KC Water will evaluate the workforce development program again in 5 years. Program size is evaluated each year to make sure the number of maintenance sites, funding, and type of work is appropriate to the team's size. Being adaptable and open to learning from employees' feedback and willingness to share will continue to be critical to continually identifying solutions for the best overall success of both the program and the participants.

2.6.5 Overall Operations and Maintenance Program Planning

KC Water plans to formalize its approach to maintenance of green infrastructure as part of a comprehensive O&M Plan for green infrastructure, anticipating the increased management and maintenance needs of SCMs built in the combined sewer system.

3.0 CASE STUDY 2—CITY OF LANCASTER, PA

3.1 Stormwater Management Program Overview

The city of Lancaster is located in south-central Pennsylvania, spanning 19 km^2 (7.4 sq mi) with approximately 60,000 residents. The historic central area of the city, about 45% of the city, is serviced by a combined system, and the remainder of the city is serviced by a separate MS4 system. Combined sewer overflows occur during heavy rainstorms, which is approximately 15% of storms. To address the city's stormwater challenges, the Bureau of Stormwater Management, under the Department of Public Works, oversees the stormwater management and green infrastructure program.

The city's green infrastructure program officially started in 2011 when the first Green Infrastructure Plan was adopted. The development of the Green Infrastructure Plan was driven by regulatory requirements, although the city had already been in communication for several years with the U.S. Environmental Protection Agency (U.S. EPA) to discuss ways to address combined sewer overflows (CSOs). During the planning stages for solutions to comply with regulatory requirements, traditional gray infrastructure was compared with green infrastructure. After a cost analysis was completed, green infrastructure was selected as the approach to address the city's stormwater challenges for the economic and social benefits. The city entered a consent decree with the U.S. EPA in 2017 to prepare an amended Long-Term Control Plan (LTCP), which included green infrastructure program plans and manuals.

When the green infrastructure program started, the city focused on green infrastructure construction throughout the city. In 2015, the city recognized a need to expand its stormwater resources and hired a green infrastructure asset coordinator to prioritize efforts to understand monitoring, maintenance, and performance of green infrastructure systems. The green infrastructure asset coordinator works closely with field maintenance crews to identify common challenges in the field, understand issues from visual inspections, and create protocols for O&M procedures. The city recognized the need for inspections and monitoring to understand how green infrastructure installations were working and how to maintain the systems for continued functionality.

In 2018, the city updated its Green Infrastructure Plan and began developing three manuals, the green infrastructure design manual, green infrastructure operations and maintenance plan, and green infrastructure monitoring plan, to comply with the requirements of the consent decree. The three manuals work together to make sure all goals and requirements within the LTCP are met and serve as references for public and private green infrastructure applications. An adaptive management approach was taken with these green infrastructure documents, as inspection and maintenance procedures are iterative with green infrastructure design.

The city is in the process of implementing the O&M Plan and Monitoring Plan. The city has increased staffing, as recommended in the O&M Plan, to include a green infrastructure maintenance supervisor and two dedicated maintenance workers. Previously, two staff from the Parks Department did the maintenance.

3.2 Types of Stormwater Control Measures

The city has implemented a variety of green infrastructure BMPs, including porous pavement, bioretention systems, green roofs, and subsurface infiltration systems in parking lots, parks, schools, streets, and alleys. In total, the city owns approximately 140 bioretention systems.

3.3 Maintenance of Stormwater Control Measures

3.3.1 Inspection and Maintenance Activities

Inspection and maintenance activities are performed in house. For the city's bioretention systems, three maintenance staff within the Bureau of Stormwater Management predominantly do the work. Operators from the city's Streets Department perform vacuum sweeping of the city's porous surfaces on a monthly basis. Infiltration testing is performed on newly installed projects after construction is completed and then on a 5-year cycle. Plans are in place per the consent decree to televise pipes on a 5-year basis.

3.3.2 Lessons Learned

An adaptive management approach is taken within the city's green infrastructure program for the O&M, monitoring, and design to work collaboratively within a feedback loop to continue improving the program. Lessons learned from the field during O&M and monitoring activities inform changes required in the design strategies for improved system functionalities. One lesson learned from field observations is to more carefully evaluate and avoid proposing porous pavements adjacent to areas with a lot of tree cover because it was noted that decomposing leaves would clog and deteriorate porous surfaces. Bioretention system designs have evolved to include concrete sediment forebays because of field observations of high sedimentation that decrease the functionality of systems.

During the early stages of the city's green infrastructure program, community outreach was prioritized to educate the public of the work being installed throughout the city. This proactive approach with exposure through tours and newspaper articles helped residents understand the projects that were being completed in their areas and valuing the benefits of the work. Through this community outreach, there is more acceptance from the public and less pushback from the community for implementation. The focus on public outreach was highest during the initial phases of the green infrastructure program, but as green infrastructure becomes more of a regular occurrence in the city, there is an identified need to continue to do more public education.

Increasing staffing and allocating dedicated staff to the green infrastructure program has been key to the progress of the city's O&M program. The green infrastructure team has found success with a green infrastructure maintenance supervisor who has specific experience with plant materials for bioretention systems and skilled maintenance crew members. The city is planning to expand the team to a fourth member to have full capacity to meet all maintenance requirements and schedules.

3.4 Inspection and Maintenance Responsibilities and Recordkeeping

3.4.1 Maintenance Frequencies and Reporting

The city has performed a basic level of green infrastructure maintenance since the beginning of the green infrastructure program but formalized the requirements within the green infrastructure O&M Plan in 2018. Standard protocols for individual green infrastructure system maintenance, inspection, data management, reporting, scheduling, equipment, staffing, and budget are included within the O&M Plan. The O&M Plan addresses inspection types and routine maintenance activities and the respective frequencies for each item to ensure each system is maintained properly.

Monthly routine inspections are recommended to visually assess the function, safety, and aesthetic appearance of all surface features. Inspections for vegetation is also recommended to be done monthly during the growing season. Subsurface feature inspections are recommended annually using closed-circuit television (CCTV) to assess pipes and access structures.

Routine maintenance protocols are categorized into monthly, annually, or as needed frequencies. Monthly routine maintenance activities include sediment, debris, and trash removal, mulch and soil amendment, photo documentation, pruning, weeding, vacuum sweeping, and inlet pretreatment clearing. Annual routine maintenance activities include landscaping of green surface features, cleaning of structures and media, and repair of infrastructure. Maintenance activities done as needed include sanitizing of cisterns, watering, porous pavement patching, plowing snow, deicing, concrete repair, mowing, pest management, and erosion and settling repair.

The city provides a semiannual report, which includes the status of any construction, compliance measures, status of permit applications, O&M information, and reports provided to other agencies, to Pennsylvania Department of Environmental Protection per regulations. The data for reporting on O&M tasks is collected through completed data collection forms, which is required to be filled out to close a work order. Data collection forms include sections for work order information, general information, maintenance checklist, equipment and materials list, and associated cost.

3.4.2 Recordkeeping

The Bureau of Stormwater Management is in the process of working with a consultant to develop and implement an asset management tool based in GIS for their stormwater needs. The Bureau of Stormwater Management initially considered using the asset management software Lucity, because other city departments use it. After an assessment of their needs, however, the bureau decided to not move forward with Lucity and switched to a combination of Workforce, Collector, Survey123, ArcGIS, and Excel for asset management.

Green infrastructure installations and assets were already mapped in GIS, and some framework for tracking was already developed for Lucity, so it was an easy transition to the combination of GIS-based tools. Workforce, Collector, and Survey123 provide the framework needed for their field work inspection and work order needs. The long-term goal is to upload plans as attachments to each mapped asset for easy accessibility by staff. This software is only being used within the O&M and monitoring programs, so there are some challenges with integration with other city departments that use Lucity.

3.5 Funding Inspections and Maintenance

3.5.1 Public Practices

The city adopted a stormwater fee in 2015 with the passing of the Stormwater Ordinance. The revenue raised through the stormwater fee funds the city's stormwater management program, which include O&M of existing stormwater systems and capital improvements. The stormwater fee is collected from all property owners based on the amount of impervious surface owned.

3.5.2 Private Practices

Private green infrastructure installations and associated O&M are the responsibility of the owners. The city does, however, provide stormwater credits and rebates for green infrastructure installations, as well as grant funding for qualifying projects. The city continues to do inspections for city-funded or grant-funded projects, and then relays maintenance needs to the private property owners.

In the early stages of the city's green infrastructure program, the city provided vacuum sweeping services on privately owned pervious pavements because of the lack of available local contractors who could perform the task. As the program has grown and capabilities of local contractors expanded, the city has less of a role to fill in performance gaps and has transitioned the responsibility onto the private owners to perform O&M activities.

3.6 Challenges and Future Initiatives

The city faces challenges with funding corrective actions for system issues that are beyond the regular routine maintenance activities, such as redesigning systems that are not functioning, replacing large amounts of soil or plant material, and maintaining systems that have been neglected for several years. For improved cost efficiency, the city prioritizes installing green infrastructure where other capital improvement projects are being completed, such as street repaving or street reconstruction. Although this approach requires additional coordination and oversight to make sure the green infrastructure systems are installed properly, combining efforts streamlines construction activities and increases cost efficiency.

Staffing has also been a challenge for the city to have enough full-time staff dedicated to green infrastructure O&M activities. The staffing analysis completed in the O&M Plan determined four full-time staff are required to complete all the necessary work to stay on schedule for O&M upkeep. The city continues to build the green infrastructure team and currently has three full-time staff. After hiring a green infrastructure maintenance supervisor and two dedicated maintenance workers, the leadership and maintenance crew have been successful in coordinating and completing the required O&M and monitoring work. The city is making progress in staffing to meet the required O&M activities as outlined in the O&M Plan.

4.0 CASE STUDY 3—PHILADELPHIA WATER DEPARTMENT

4.1 Stormwater Management Program Overview

The Philadelphia Water Department (PWD) provides water, stormwater, and wastewater services to the greater Philadelphia region, spanning 337 km^2 (130 sq mi) and approximately 1.6 million individuals. The City of Philadelphia and PWD entered a consent order with the Commonwealth of Pennsylvania in 2011 to address combined sewer overflows. In 2012, the City of Philadelphia and U.S. EPA signed a partnership agreement to formalize the Green City, Clean Waters Plan to use green infrastructure for stormwater management in Philadelphia. Green City, Clean Waters is a 25-year plan with a goal to reduce stormwater pollution entering Philadelphia waterways by 85% and to create environmental, social, and economic benefits for Philadelphia neighborhoods.

Operation of PWD green stormwater infrastructure (GSI) assets began before the consent order with the implementation of several pilot projects in 2008. In response to the new and relatively unknown maintenance needs of these systems, the Green Stormwater Infrastructure Maintenance team (GSIMN) was created to facilitate maintenance operations of the pilot assets while also to develop standard operation procedures for GSI maintenance as well as long-term projections for long-term resource needs (e.g., staff, vehicles, contracts). The pilot projects were initially under the Office of Watersheds, integrated with the Design and Planning Branch, but transitioned to be under the Construction division in 2008. Likewise, GSIMN initially started in the Office of Watersheds before later transitioning into the Operations division. GSIMN started out with four staff members managing 17 to 18 stormwater management practices (SMPs), with activities limited to maintenance of surface features, such as removing trash, weeding, light pruning, and monitoring work. During this time, subsurface inspection and maintenance activities were performed by the Sewer Maintenance unit although the frequency for these activities had yet to be fully established. In 2013, the scope of GSIMN was expanded beyond surface maintenance to subsurface inspection and maintenance as well as retrofit and repair tasks. Each ensuing year, the number of PWD-constructed SMPs increased almost exponentially, while GSIMN worked to also increase the number of staff, develop standard protocols, and increase capacity of staff to specialize in respective roles. As a result of successfully establishing standard protocols and identifying key resource needs for expansion, GSIMN migrated into the Operations division and was reestablished as the Green Stormwater Operations (GSO) unit. This transition enabled GSO to build internal capacity to do maintenance activities and support a grounds maintenance team. As of 2020, GSO serviced 1,041 SMPs.

4.2 Types of Stormwater Control Measures

The focus of the Green City, Clean Waters Plan is the implementation of green infrastructure to intercept and manage stormwater before entering the combined sewer system and local waterways. The SCMs include a variety of green infrastructure practices, such as tree trenches, rain gardens, bumpouts, swales, subsurface storage trenches, porous pavement, and green roofs. The practices are concentrated primarily in the CSO sections of the city. The PWD GSO team maintains PWD's public assets, totaling 1041 SMPs in

2020. The maintenance of other city-owned green infrastructure assets are the responsibility of their respective city agency, with a few exceptions noted by signed memorandums of understanding where PWD maintains on behalf of another agency. Private assets are maintained by their respective owners.

4.3 Maintenance of Stormwater Control Measures

4.3.1 Inspection and Maintenance Activities

The O&M activities are organized into three teams—Surface Operations; Subsurface Operations; and Asset Protection, Retrofit, and Repair. The surface team maintains approximately 5.3 ha (13 ac) of noncontiguous surface area across the service area, including tree trenches, rain gardens, and bump-outs of different sizes. The subsurface team inspects and maintains all underground assets, including inlets, pipes, sewers, and subsurface storage structures. The subsurface team has seven in-house crews for CCTV inspection, inlet cleaning, inlet pretreatment device maintenance, pipe maintenance, and inlet repairs. Approximately half of the total maintenance work is performed by the in-house crews, and the rest of the work is done by external vendors.

The Green Infrastructure Maintenance Manual was developed in 2014 to describe O&M activities for the full range of green stormwater infrastructure projects implemented by the city. A second version of the manual, published in 2016, is more comprehensive, including standard operating procedures, equipment, materials, frequencies, and details for maintenance of surface and subsurface features.

4.3.2 Lessons Learned

Communication with the design branch and GSI implementation unit has been essential to the success and growth of the GSI program. Maintaining a continual feedback loop throughout all stages of projects helps to ensure systems are functioning, issues are not repeated, and specifications are improved upon as needed. GSO has provided input for the Planning & Design Manual so that planners and designers account for O&M considerations throughout the planning and design process. In addition, GSO's surface and subsurface teams review all GSI design projects for O&M factors at the 70% design phase by providing suggestions for design revisions that will improve long-term system functionality while also ensuring proper access and maintainability of key design features. Bringing in GSO earlier on in the design process, during the conceptual stage, is being considered to help guide the process and provide more opportunities to give input on O&M considerations that should be integrated with the design. Through working with the design branch, a lesson learned was that experience should be valued, as systems are able to function the best when there is a consistent feedback loop between the field observations of GSO and the planning and design of the design branch. It is important to incorporate changes to the design based on lessons gathered from GSO and using feedback from operators to inform design decisions.

In addition to working with the design branch, working with the PWD Public Affairs Outreach Team has been important for public acceptance of green infrastructure systems. The Outreach Team communicates to GSO any issues with a constructed system or other complaints from residents or local representatives. The Outreach Team also relays a memorandum of understanding with neighborhoods when systems are built for agreements on maintenance responsibilities. Signage, placards, inlet markers, and access structure covers are standard in branding. Collaboration with the Outreach Team is necessary to problem solve solutions for issues and communicating a standard, consistent message to the public.

4.4 Inspection and Maintenance Responsibilities and Recordkeeping

4.4.1 *Public Practices*

4.4.1.1 Maintenance Frequencies and Reporting

Routine annual maintenance is performed on pipes, inlets, and stormwater structures such as crates, chambers, and infiltrating manholes. Monthly maintenance is done on inlet pretreatment filter bags. Subsurface stormwater crates and chambers are inspected annually, following product maintenance guides.

4.4.1.2 Recordkeeping

The Philadelphia Water Department uses Cityworks as its work order platform. Cityworks is integrated into PWD's ESRI-based asset management platform, which allows integration with GIS data, allowing easy access between PWD and city data. All stormwater management practices are assigned a unique SMP ID, and individual components within the systems are assigned a component ID. The ID numbers are assigned in a standard format across all systems, with the component IDs assigned during the 70% design phase. Work orders are issued through Cityworks, attached to the associated SMP ID and/or component ID to identify to crews what work needs to be completed. All contractors and in-house teams' work orders are standardized through Cityworks. In-house consultants manage the back end data in Cityworks.

4.4.2 Asset Management Considerations

PWD's vision for asset management is to standardize nomenclature for assigning IDs to components of a system and to manage assets within a work order management platform. The Philadelphia Water Department is developing a platform for tracking structural deficiencies that is GIS-based and can tie into Cityworks. This platform will utilize component IDs and store videos in one communal database.

Challenges with asset management include broader decision making regarding integrating with other departments and smaller challenges with work order assignments. Interdepartmental challenges include working with the GIS team on how assets are displayed and working with the records team to decide how to catalog projects, how to document changes to design plans during construction, and how to match work orders in the platform with field conditions. Challenges with work order planning involve prioritization of work orders, delegation of tasks, determination of required equipment, details of field tasks, and delivery and receipt of work orders. Although PWD already used Cityworks for inspection and maintenance assignments for traditional infrastructure, adjustments had to be made to incorporate GSI into the existing workflow.

4.5 Funding Inspections and Maintenance

The transition of bringing the GSO team into the Operations division in 2017 was supported by the PWD commissioner and allowed increased investment from the department into the O&M program. The growth and development of the O&M program is enabled through the support of upper management and the mayor's office, allowing the program to be more proactive in O&M activities. Funding for O&M comes from the Operations budget, which is collected through rate payers. Because the budget is funded by rate payer money, PWD is thoughtful on how the budget is spent, balancing the functionality and aesthetics of systems. Budgets are projected out several years to plan how many in-house staff and how much contracted work is required to ensure the SMPs are serving the people of Philadelphia and managing CSOs as designed.

4.6 Challenges and Future Initiatives

4.6.1 Inspection and Maintenance Challenges

As PWD's GSI program progresses, improvements are made with standardizing components, such as castings and lids for cleanouts, access structures, and observation wells, so inspection and maintenance crews can easily locate and identify the components. When new products or components are introduced, having nonstandard structures and components is a challenge for maintenance activities. For example, stormwater crate systems have not been standardized yet throughout PWD systems, and each manufacturer produces set designs, so it is challenging to procure a standard component that can work with each different manufactured product. These stormwater crate products may also have nonstandard ports that do not conform to PWD guidelines, making it difficult to integrate into standard O&M protocols. The Philadelphia Water Department is working toward having standard lids for all access points to streamline maintenance activities and communicating the need for standardizations with designers.

Prioritizing public safety is an important consideration with PWD's O&M activities. A lot of effort is put into creating physical barriers around systems to protect residents from getting hurt, prevent systems from being damaged, and minimize liabilities associated with these public systems. Fences or shrubs are used as a physical barrier, and maintenance is performed on shrubs to prevent vegetation from growing into the sidewalk. Thought is also put into the design to prevent components, such as rocks and plants, from being taken out of the system by passersby. From these challenges, PWD has been proactive in having crews available to restore systems as needed and having contracts in place to quickly procure plants from a readily available supply.

With systems being in the public right-of-way, PWD also needs to develop remedial plans for potential accidents that could happen, such as if oil is dumped into the system or if a sewer lateral leaks adjacent to a system. Many unknown issues may occur, and so PWD needs to have the proper inspection, repair, and maintenance teams to address any issues that happen. To be able to continue to address maintenance issues, PWD will continue expanding its in-house Grounds Maintenance team over the next 5 to 10 years. As a part of this expansion, PWD understands the need to also purchase additional vehicles and acquire larger space for vehicle parking, equipment storage, and training facilities. By standardizing components and having castings on contract, space is required to store them. Many green infrastructure systems include trees, so there needs to be a way to purchase trees, have a delivery destination for storage, and protocols for how to keep the trees alive before they are planted.

Working with other city departments can be a challenge with coordination. The city's GSI program is a city-wide effort, and PWD works closely with the Streets Department for paving and utility work, with Parks and Recreation for GSI designs in park properties, and Department of Public Property for GSI designs in vacant lots. It has been important to make these relationships early on to discuss and share maintenance responsibilities, especially since typically the focus of interagency coordination is on new capital projects. It is also helpful to create these relationships to get buy-in from other departments for the city-wide issue of cleaning up source water and reducing CSO events. To achieve the goals of the program, the effort must be collective from city agencies.

Another challenge PWD faces is documentation of project history and O&M records. The goal for documentation is to record all the institutional knowledge and project history to pass onto future staff. This documentation would include organizing project-related emails and archiving them into project folders and a document for each project with bullets for the history of each site. Even though PWD's green infrastructure program is a 25-year program, the SMPs will continue to function for the lifetime of the system, so knowledge and the background of each system needs to continue to be accessible.

Integrating subsurface green infrastructure systems into the PA One Call system has been challenging. Stormwater assets are marked with a green color, which is used for sewer. Because sewers are typically 2.5 to 4.5 m (8 to 15 ft) deep and stormwater infrastructure much shallower, using the same color to mark out stormwater and sewer can be confusing. Contractors typically do not expect stormwater plastic pipes, stone media, or shallow utilities with the green mark out, so subsurface green infrastructure assets may be damaged during construction activities. The Philadelphia Water Department is working on figuring out a revised system to mark out stormwater, such as a new color or method of labeling shallow utilities.

Inspection and maintenance protocols are being developed for centralized green infrastructure systems, also known as GSI sewers. Because only one GSI sewer has been in operation for a year and another almost completed construction, PWD is still learning about access issues and maintaining these systems based on the similarities with traditional sewer systems. The GSI program is getting feedback from the Sewer Maintenance team on how to best design and maintain these types of systems.

4.6.2 Future Initiatives to Ensure Continued Performance

A third O&M manual may need to be developed because the green infrastructure systems continue to evolve and grow. Different plant species may be integrated with designs, and maintenance strategies will change as rain gardens and bumpouts mature. Depending on what status is desired for systems, such as keeping systems constantly juvenile or allowing systems to mature, additional O&M activities and protocols may be needed to guide how to maintain systems in a certain status for the system lifespan.

5.0 REFERENCES

City of Kansas City, MO. (2010). *Covenant to maintain storm water detention and BMP facilities.* https://drive.google.com/file/d/1cxmS96w6w_uA9VIurlPfMdrYy8gNJzu-/view

City of Kansas City, MO. (2018, August). *Green stormwater infrastructure manual.* https://www.kcwater.us/wp-content/uploads/2020/01/KCMOGSIManualAugust2018-2.pdf

City of Kansas City, MO. (2019–2020). *NPDES municipal separate storm sewer system (MS4) permit* (MO-0130516). https://www.kcwater.us/wp-content/uploads/2021/05/FY20-Annual-MS4-Report.pdf

Iyengar, P., & KC Water. (2019, October 16). *Green infrastructure leadership exchange asset management workgroup presentation.*

KC Water. (2019). *14th year NPDES annual report permit* (#MO-0130516). https://www.kcwater.us/wp-content/uploads/2020/06/2019-MS4-Report.pdf

KC Water. (2021). About us. https://www.kcwater.us/about-us/

Mid-America Regional Council. (2008, March). *Manual of best management practices for stormwater quality.* https://www.kcwater.us/wp-content/uploads/2020/08/Manual-of-Best-Management-Practices-for-Stormwater-Quality.pdf

Treese, L., Brotherton, R., & Riott, K. (2019, September). *Developing Kansas City's green workforce.* Proceedings of the 92nd Annual Water Environment Federation Technical Exposition and Conference, Chicago, IL. Water Environment Federation.

United States of America v. City of Kansas City, MO. (2010, May 18). *Consent decree.* https://www.epa.gov/sites/production/files/documents/cityofkansascity-cd.pdf

6.0 SUGGESTED READING

City of Kansas City, MO. (2019, August). *Storm water management program plan.* https://www.kcwater.us/wp-content/uploads/2020/07/Stormwater-Management-Program-Plan-20-19-20.pdf

REFERENCES

SUGGESTED READING

Index

A

Adaptive management, 244–247
- feedback, 245–246
- plan, update of, 246–247
- of SCM maintenance program, 278–280
- strategies, 244–245
- tracking performance over time, 245

Adaptive management of SCM maintenance program, 278–280
- break-in period, 279
- revised maintenance plan, 280
- SCM commissioning, 279
- sharing findings, 280
- trends are evaluated, 279

Aesthetic maintenance, 176
- graffiti removal, 176
- overall site maintenance, 176
- vegetation maintenance, 176

Asset maintenance, 213–218
- appropriate level of service, 225–226
- asset characteristics, 219–221
- asset organization, 221–222
- assets, type of, 219
- benefits, 215
- California Stormwater Quality Association Funding Resources, 242–243
- consequence of failure (COF), 227
- critical assets, 226–231
- current state of, 219–224
- definition, 214–215
- EPA 10-step process, 217–218
- failure mode, 228
- funding strategies, 241–243
- gathering asset information, 222–224
- gathering cost data, 233–235
- history, 215–217
- investment strategies, 231–241
- long-term funding options, 241–244
- MS4 permit–required activities, 234–235
- Municipal Separate Storm Sewer System (MS4), 213–214
- O&M investments, 235–236
- O&M or capital programs, 232
- optimizing capital investments, 236–241
- probability of failure (POF), 227
- redundancy factor (R), 230
- stormwater programs, 233
- Triple Bottom Line (TBL) analysis, 227–231

Asset Management Plan (AMP), documenting of, 243–244

B

Basins, 34, 124–125, 302–303, 308–309

Best management practices, 1

Bioretention filter, 90–93, 126
- common problems, 92–93
- routine maintenance, 91–92

Budget components, 258–260
- disposal, 259
- equipment and facilities maintenance, 259
- facilities, 259
- field equipment, 259
- full-time equivalent (FTE), 259
- materials, 259
- office equipment, 259
- O&M programs, budgeting for, 259
- program development, 258–259
- staffing, 259

C

California State Water Board Stormwater Program, 243

Case studies
- City of Lancaster, Pennsylvania, 365–370
- Kansas City, Missouri, 349–365
- Philadelphia Water Department (PWD), 370–376

CASQA's sustainable funding, 242–243

Catch basins, 246, 255, 306, 312

Checklists, 177, 210

Cisterns and rain barrels, 107–110, 125
- common problems, 109–110
- routine maintenance, 108, 109

City of Lancaster, Pennsylvania, 365–370
  challenges and future initiatives, 370
  funding inspections and maintenance, 369–370
  inspection and maintenance responsibilities and recordkeeping, 368–369
  maintenance frequencies and reporting, 368–369
  private practices, 369–370
  public practices, 369
  recordkeeping and SCM, 369
  SCM, maintenance of, 367–368
  SCM, types of, 367
  stormwater management program, 365–367
Combined sewer systems (CSSs), 1
Community-based public private partnerships (CBP3s), 25–26

Construction plans, 48–57
  communication and willingness to adapt, 49
  construction drawings and technical specifications, 54–56
  construction timing and execution constraints, 56–57
  design–bid–build project, 56
  location considerations, 49–50
  preconstruction phase, 49
  stormwater control function and fail points, 50–53
Construction protocols, 133–140
  accessibility, verification of, 137
  as-built plans, 140
  conformance with plans and specifications, verification of, 135–136
  durability, verification of, 137
  elevations, grades, and dimensions, verification of, 135
  hydraulic performance, verification of, 139
  inspections, 135
  location and contributing drainage area, verification of, 134
  maintainability, verification of, 136–137
  noncompaction, verification of, 138
  plant establishment, verification of, 139–140
  proper SCMs, verification of, 134–135
  size and configuration, verification of, 135
  soil/filter media, verification of 138–139
  structural integrity, verification of, 138
  structure safety, verification of, 136
Construction responsibilities, 58–61
  and oversight, 58–59
  quality assurance and quality control (QAQC) parameters, 59
Construction workers, skilled SCM labor, 59–61
  aggregate material, 61
  control and protection, 61
  elevations, 61
  subgrade preparation, 59–61
Corrective maintenance, 177
Cost inefficiencies, 271

D
Design considerations, 35–40
  designer and owner, open communication and collaboration between, 37–38
  designer perspective, 36–39
  function and potential fail points, 39–40
  functional performance with design, 35–36
  infiltration or filtration, 39
  retaining water, 39
  reusing water, 40
  roles and responsibilities of maintenance tasks, 38
  screening/hydromechanics, 40
  thriving vegetation, 39
Design professional, 280
  referral to, 280
Detention basins, 125
Drain inlet inserts, 127
Dry basins, 82–84, 125, 302, 308
  erosion, 84
  routine maintenance, 83
Dry wells, 106–107, 127–128
  common problems, 106–107
  routine maintenance, 106

E
Emergency or nonroutine maintenance, 273
Environmental Finance Center (EFC), 243
Environmental Impact Bonds (EIBs), 25
Erosion and compaction disrupt and disturb vegetation, 69–70

F
Filters, 34, 98, 126–127, 303–304, 310–311
Fine sediments, 72

Forebays, 79–82
erosion and poor vegetation establishment, 82
rapid sedimentation, 82
routine maintenance, 81

G
GI longevity, 71
Grant funding, 26
O&M for SCMs, 26
Grants and assistance programs, 7
Grants and loans, 25
Green infrastructure, 2, 7, 20–21, 24, 27–28, 64, 71–72, 74, 133, 214, 217, 227, 263
city of Lancaster, Pennsylvania, 365–370
guidelines, 314
implementation, 7
Kansas City, Missouri, 349–365
Philadelphia Water Department (PWD), 370–376
"Green Infrastructure Street" projects, 296–297
Green stormwater infrastructure (GI)
practices, 68
high runoff volumes and concentrated sediments, 71
and SCMs, 71
Gross pollutant trap (GPT) and mechanical operations, 128

H
Health and Safety Plan (H&SP), 68, 129–131, 293–294

I
Infiltrating systems, 67, 77–78
Infiltration basins, 64, 82, 93–96, 127
common problems, 95–96
routine maintenance, 94
Infiltration trenches and vaults, 127
Infiltration/Retention Trenches and Vaults, 105–106
pretreatment 105–106
subsurface 105
Infiltrators, 34, 50, 127–128, 153
Inlet basket, 304, 310–311
Inspection and maintenance protocols, 121–124
proper maintenance, 123
stormwater treatment practices, 121–124

J
Job Safety Assessments (JSA), 68
Joint Benefits Authority, 25

K
Kansas City, Missouri, 349–365
asset management, 364
challenges and future initiatives, 364–365
construction contractor maintenance, 354
contracted assistance, 364–365
funding inspections and maintenance, 362–364
green solutions, 352–353
green stewards, 353–354
green stewards workforce development program, 365
in-house maintenance, 364
inspection and maintenance responsibilities and recordkeeping, 354–362
overall O&M program planning, 365
private practices, 363–364
private SCM, 351–352
public practices, 362
public SCM, 351
SCM, maintenance of, 352–354
SCM, types of, 350–352
Stormwater Management Program, 349–350

L
Landscaped roofs (green roofs), 68, 110–113, 126
common problems, 112–113
routine maintenance, 111–112
Leaf litter and plant detritus, 70
Local program maintenance, 18

M
Maintenance goals, 64–68
aesthetics, 66
balancing maintenance level of service, 66–68
BMP (best management practice), 68
level of service, 67
maintenance program managers, 68
sustained function, 64–65
system longevity, 65–66
Manufactured filters, 127
Minnesota Pollution Control Agency, 264

Municipal Separate Storm Sewer System (MS4), 350
collection system assets, 216
communities, 16, 18
needs assessment survey, 2
permit conditions, 3
permits, 214, 216, 217, 263, 267, 352, 362
programs, 214

N
National Association of Clean Water Agencies, 243
National Green Infrastructure Certification Program (NGICP), 9, 27, 133
National Pollution Discharge and Elimination System (NPDES) program, 42
Nonroutine and specialty maintenance, 257–258
crew requirements, 257
equipment, 257
materials, 257
Nonroutine/emergency maintenance protocols, 171–175
cleanup, 173–174
dams, embankments, and side slopes, damage to, 172
dewatering, 172
fence repair, 173
minor spills, 174
pond maintenance, 173
semi-significant spills, 174–175
spills, 173–174
woody vegetation, elimination of, 173

O
O&M activities, 7
O&M, resilience considerations in, 27–28
adaptive strategies, 28
additional strategies, 28
climate change, 27
mitigative efforts, 28
O&M program, tracking and reporting, importance of, 284–292
during construction, 284–287
during operation, 287–292
inspection activities, 287
inspection forms during construction, 286
preventive or routine versus corrective maintenance, 289–291
stabilization plans associated with many SCM, 285
tracking, reviewing, and analyzing historical records, 288
O&M program costs, estimating/budgeting, 258–266
affecting factors, 260–265
bottom-up estimates, 260
contracted labor versus in-house labor, 263
differences in consumer price index (CPI) across localities, 264
estimating life cycle costs, 265–266
EWRI's Municipal Water Infrastructure Council (MWIC), 265
life-cycle costs, 265–266
portfolio size, 260–261
pretreatment, 262
prevailing wages, 262–263
program specific policy decisions, 262
regulatory drivers, 263
SCM (practice) size and distribution, 261
sediment loading, 262
tracking O&M costs, 265
urban density, 261
use of unit costs, 264–265
vegetated versus subsurface SCM, 262
visibility and aesthetic expectations, 261
O&M program funding, 7
O&M training, 26–27
level 1, 27
level 2, 27
level 3, 27
Oil and water separators, 103–105, 125
common problems, 104
routine maintenance, 104
special considerations, 104–105
Operations and maintenance. See O&M
Organic matter content, 70
OWP EFC webpage, 243

P
Performance and longevity, maintenance to optimize, 74–77
erosion and sedimentation processes, 75–76
erosion, scour, and settlement, 76
health vegetation and soils, 74
hydraulics and sediment transport, 75–76

soil and vegetation maintenance, 74
structural components, 76–77
Permeable pavement, 113–115
common problems, 114–115
routine maintenance, 113–114
Personnel and equipment requirements, 251–258
porous pavement inspection and maintenance, 256
specialty maintenance, 257
subsurface inspection and maintenance, 254
surface inspection and maintenance, 252
Philadelphia Water Department (PWD), 370–376
asset management considerations, 374
challenges and future initiatives, 374–376
funding inspections and maintenance, 374
inspection and maintenance responsibilities and recordkeeping, 373–374
O&M activities, 372
public practices, 373
stormwater management program overview, 370–371
SCM, maintenance of, 372–373
SCM, types of, 371–372
Porous pavement inspection and maintenance, 256
crew requirements, 256
equipment, 256
materials, 256
Postconstruction protocols, 140–176
erosion problems, inspection for, 144
inspections, 141
joint tightness, 145
mechanical, electrical, pneumatic, and hydraulic components, damage/malfunction of, 146–148
media, inspection of, 148–149
miscellaneous site damage, inspect for, 152
nuisance conditions and animals, inspect for and evidence/presence of, 149–150
outlet structures, 144
permanent pool, inspection of, 146
porous pavement, 148
routine maintenance protocols, 152–171
routine or preventive maintenance, 141
sediment accumulation, inspect for, 142–143
settling, inspect for, 144
snow and ice, inspection for, 151
structural features, inspection of, 145–146
trash and debris removal, 142
undesirable plant communities, inspection for, 149–150
vectors, inspection for, 150–151
vegetation management, 143–144
water bird damage, inspection for, 150
water quality degradation, inspection for, 150
Postconstruction SCMs, 17
Postinspection ad-hoc maintenance, 272
Potential fail points, designing for, 40
Private and public parties, 18
Private maintenance approach, 18
Program components, 20–23
comprehensive maintenance program, 23
easement and access, 21
local stormwater program, 22
long-term maintenance inspection and reporting, 22
long-term maintenance plan, 21–22
maintenance program, scoping of, 23
maintenance triggers, 20
ordinances, 21
procure equipment, 21
secure funding for maintenance, 20–21
staff resources for inspection and maintenance, 20
standard operating procedures, 20
Program development, 19–27
extent of service (EOS), 19–20
level of service (LOS), 19–20
O&M of SCMs, 19
Program funding, 24–25
Program organization 24
Proper maintenance procedures, 28–29
standard O&M agreement, key elements of, 29
Proper operation and regular maintenance programs, 1–2
Proprietary/manufactured devices, 78–79
replacing parts of, 79
Public and private maintenance, 18
Public and worker safety, 68

R
Regularly scheduled or routine maintenance, 272
Regulatory agencies, roles of, 15–18
  federal, 15
  local, 16
  SCM inspection during construction, 16–18
  state, 15–16
Routine maintenance protocols, 152–171
  debris and litter removal control, 152–153
  fixing pipe problems, 161–162
  folded liners, 161
  general housekeeping and miscellaneous site maintenance, 171
  mechanical equipment repairs, 172
  mechanical, electrical, pneumatic, and hydraulic maintenance, 162
  media maintenance, 166–168
  minor erosion, 158–159
  monolithic plant communities, management of, 169
  nuisance control, 168–170
  permanent pool, 162
  pipe bursting, 161
  pipe eating, 161
  pipe pulling, 161
  porous pavement, 164–166
  pretreatment devices, inlets, outlet structures, and chambers, 160–161
  pump and switch maintenance, 164
  rodent management, 168
  screens and trash racks, 161
  sediment removal and disposal, 153
  settling repair, 159–160
  slip-lining, 162
  snow and ice removal, 171
  spray lining, 162
  standing water, 162
  structural repairs, 172
  structure maintenance, 160–162
  vector management, 170–171
  vegetation maintenance, 153–158
  water quality degradation, 169–170
  waterfowl damage, 168–169

S
Sample maintenance agreements, 28–29
Scheduling maintenance, 273–278
  ad-hoc maintenance, logistics for, 277
  considerations for setting, 273–277
  logistics and work schedules, 276–277
  maintenance activity, predictability of, 274
  maintenance activity, type of, 276
  maintenance products and materials, availability of, 275
  mulching operation, 276–277
  prioritization, 277–278
  regional factors, 277
  scheduling tools, 278
  seasonal access, 276
  seasonal species conflicts, 276
  seasonal workload, 275
  workforce and equipment, availability of, 274–275
Scheduling scenarios, maintenance of, 272–273
  during inspection, 272–273
SCM components, 128
  control and protection measures, 41–48
SCM components, control and protection measures, 41–48
  bypass piping, 45
  enclosed system control, 45–46
  erosion control blankets (ECBs), 48
  erosion control logs, 42
  ground covers, 46
  hydraulic applications, 46
  impermeable liner, 44
  inlet protection, 45
  perimeter controls, 42
  permeable liner, 44
  silt fence, 42
  soil bern, 42–44
  stabilization control, 46–48
  surface controls, 44–48
  turf-reinforcement mats (TRMs), 48
SCM design and maintenance needs, 2
SCM, inspection and maintenance preparation, 129–133
  effective O&M training, 132–133
  H&SP, 129–131
  health and safety, 129–131
  maintenance activities, 132–133
  permits and approvals, 131–132
  personnel education and training, 132–133
  site location and access, 131
SCM installation process, 17–18
SCM loans, 26
SCM maintenance capital improvement program (CIP), 266–268

costs depend on several variables, 267
inadequate funding, 266
projects, 267–268
SCM O&M program, components of SOP, 292–297
coordination, responsibilities, and communication protocols, 292–297
data collection, 294
enforcement, 296–297
health and safety plans (H&S plans) and incident/near-miss reporting, 293–294
public outreach, 295–296
recordkeeping, 295
reporting and processing, 294–295
Task Hazard Assessment (THA), 293
SCM O&M program, considerations for development, 297–313
bioretention filters, 303
catch basins, 306
concerns during operation, 307–313
dry basins, 302
gross pollutant controls, 306–313
infiltration basin, 305
infiltration trench, 304
inlet basket, 304
inspection forms and data management, 301
inventory and relevant information, 298–300
landscaped roofs, 304
media filters, 303
pervious pavement, 305–306
rainfall data, importance of, 300–301
swirl concentrators and vaults, 302–303
typical concerns during development, 301–307
vegetated swales and strips, 301–302
wet basins, 302
SCM O&M program, sample inspection and maintenance reporting forms, 313–316
during construction, 313–314
during O&M, 314–316
SCM rehabilitation, 280
SCMs, designing and constructing, 31–35
five general categories of, 33, 34
functional performance, 32
NOAA precipitation frequency, 33
primary functions, 34–35
Scouring and direct rainfall, 69
Sediment forebays, 72
Slow-release systems, 78
Soil structure, 71
Soil-root matrix, 70
Stormwater control measures (SCMs), 1
and components, 124–129
land development, 13
long-term maintenance, 7, 12
maintenance drivers, 12–15
maintenance of, 2
maintenance of early generations, 12
maintenance requirements, 3
manual overview, 4–6
new generation of, 12
ownership and private and public maintenance, 3
performance, 13
real-time controls, 2
responsibility for operation and maintenance, 12
regulatory drivers, 13
surface practices, 79–100
type, 79–115
Stormwater fees, 26
Stormwater infiltration practices, clogging of, 72
Stormwater MS4, 3
Stormwater Pollution Prevention Plan (SWPPP or SWP3), 16
stormwater projects, innovative financing strategies for, 25
Stormwater runoff, 1
Stormwater utility fee, 26
Stripes, 125
Structural deterioration, 72–74
construction equipment, 73
Structural features, inspect for, 145–146
misalignment, 145
pitting and corrosion, 145
root intrusion, 145–146
staining and calcification, 145
Subsurface gravel wetland, 127
Subsurface inspection and maintenance, 254–256
CCTV camera equipment, 254
CCTV foreman/operator, 255
crew requirements, 254–255
equipment and materials, 255–256
Subsurface practices, 100–102
common problems, 102
drain inlet inserts and filters, 101–102
routine maintenance, 102
Subsurface sand filter, 126

Surface inspection and maintenance, 252–254
  crew requirements, 252–253
  equipment, 253–254
  materials, 254
Surface sand filters, 96–97, 126
  common problems, 97
  routine maintenance, 96–97
Swales and strips, 34, 97–100, 125–126
  common problems, 99–100
  routine maintenance, 98–99

T
Threshold maintenance indicator, 177

U
Undergirds vegetated SCM function, 70
User Fee-Funded Stormwater Programs, 7

V
Vaults and swirl concentrators, 102–103, 125
  subsurface maintenance, 103
Vegetated SCMs, 69
  maintenance, 70
  performance benefits, 70
Vegetation maintenance, 153–158
  dead or damaged vegetation, 155
  mowing, 154–155
  mulching, 158
  pruning and trimming, 155
  reseeding and replanting, 156–158
  soil management, 155
  watering, 158
  weed control, 154
Vegetation–soil interactions, 69

W
Water Environment Federation (WEF) Stormwater Institute, 2
Water quality standards, 1
Watershed Improvement Districts, 25
Watershed Management Department, 24
Wet basins, 84–87, 125, 302, 309
  clogging, 85
  erosion, 85–86
  leaks, 87
  mosquito control, 87
  routine maintenance, 84–85
  safety issues, 87
  sediment, trash, and debris removal, 84
  vegetation maintenance, 84–85
Wetlands (including subsurface gravel wetlands), 88–90, 125
  common problems, 89–90
  routine maintenance, 88–89

www.ingramcontent.com/pod-product-compliance
Lightning Source LLC
LaVergne TN
LVHW060557240526
839643LV00003B/28